Critical Care Medicine

The Essentials

SECOND EDITION

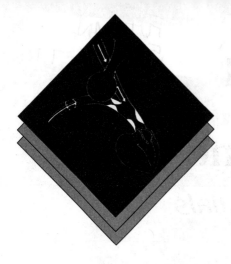

John J. Marini, M.D.

Professor of Medicine
University of Minnesota
Director, Pulmonary and Critical Care Medicine
St. Paul–Ramsey Medical Center
St. Paul, Minnesota

Arthur P. Wheeler, M.D.

Assistant Professor of Medicine
Director, Medical Intensive Care Unit
Vanderbilt University Medical Center
Nashville, Tennessee

Critical Care Medicine

The Essentials

SECOND EDITION

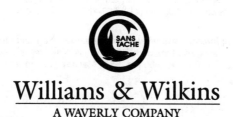

Williams & Wilkins

A WAVERLY COMPANY

BALTIMORE • PHILADELPHIA • LONDON • PARIS • BANGKOK
BUENOS AIRES • HONG KONG • MUNICH • SYDNEY • TOKYO • WROCLAW

Editor: Sharon R. Zinner
Managing Editor: Tanya Lazar
Production Coordinator: Felecia R. Weber
Copy Editor: Denise Wilson
Book Project Editor: Kathleen Gilbert
Designer: Maria Karkucinski
Illustration Planner: Felecia R. Weber
Cover Designer: Maria Karkucinski
Typesetter: Maryland Composition
Printer: Port City Press
Digitized Illustrations: Maryland Composition
Binder: Port City Press

351 West Camden Street
Baltimore, Maryland 21201-2436 USA

Rose Tree Corporate Center
1400 North Providence Road
Building II, Suite 5025
Media, Pennsylvania 19063-2043 USA

Accurate indications, adverse reactions and dosage schedules for drugs are provided in
this book, but it is possible that they may change. The reader is urged to review the package
information data of the manufacturers of the medications mentioned.

Printed in the United States of America

First Edition, 1989

Library of Congress Cataloging-in-Publication Data

Marini, John J.
 Critical care medicine : the essentials / John J. Marini, Arthur
Wheeler. — 2nd ed.
  p.   cm.
 Includes bibliographical references and index.
 ISBN 0-683-05555-0
 1. Critical care medicine—Handbooks, manuals, etc. 2. Surgical
intensive care—Handbooks, manuals, etc. I. Wheeler, Arthur P.
II. Title.
 [DNLM: 1. Critical Care. 2. Emergencies. 3. Life Support Care.
WX 218 M339c 1997]
RC86.8.M386   1997
616'.028—dc21
DNLM/DLC
for Library of Congress   96-46592
                                                          CIP

*The publishers have made every effort to trace the copyright holders for borrowed material.
If they have inadvertently overlooked any, they will be pleased to make the necessary
arrangements at the first opportunity.*

To purchase additional copies of this book, call our customer service department at **(800)
638-0672** or fax orders to **(800) 447-8438.** For other book services, including chapter reprints
and large quantity sales, ask for the Special Sales department.

Canadian customers should call **(800) 268-4178,** or fax **(905) 470-6780.** For all other calls
originating outside of the United States, please call **(410) 528-4223** or fax us at **(410) 528-
8550.**

***Visit Williams & Wilkins on the Internet:* http://www.wwilkins.com** or contact our cus-
tomer service department at **custserv@wwilkins.com.** Williams & Wilkins customer service
representatives are available from 8:30 am to 6:00 pm, EST, Monday through Friday, for
telephone access.

                                                       97 98 99
                                        1 2 3 4 5 6 7 8 9 10

To my sons, a source of wonder, inspiration and great pride, and to my steadfast love, Lisa.

—*A.W.*

To my students, residents, fellows, and younger colleagues, who inspire and educate me on many levels within and outside the discipline of critical care medicine.

—*J.J.M.*

Preface to the Second Edition

Few areas of medicine change as rapidly as the field of critical care. In the years that have elapsed since the first edition of this book, important advances and newly recognized problems have emerged to complicate an already complex field. The expense of providing life support continues to escalate, despite efforts at cost containment. In part, this expenditure is driven by the injudicious use of diagnostic tests and therapeutic options. Never has there been a greater need for thoughtful judgment and timely intervention. Unfortunately, selecting wisely among the extensive and steadily expanding list of alternatives is a difficult assignment.

Knowing that excellent textbooks and manuals already exist in this area, the potential reader may question the uniqueness of ours. This book was written *entirely* by two experienced intensivists who practice, teach, and conduct clinical research in geographically separated academic institutions. The content has been selected for its interest and practical value. Although we tried, whenever possible, to access the definitive literature, many important clinical questions do not lend themselves to formal study. In making our recommendations, we have drawn heavily from our own clinical experience. Every statement has been read aloud and, when appropriate, debated until we reached consensus. Unchanging principles have been emphasized wherever possible.

A similar approach served us well in preparing the first edition. Seven years after its publication, little of the original material required radical modification. On the other hand, we have expanded in many areas to reflect the changes that characterize our discipline. This growth is reflected in a near doubling of the text. Apart from extensive additions to almost every chapter, entirely new chapters have been written in the areas of sepsis, oxygenation and ventilatory failure, mechanical ventilation, cost containment, and general supportive care. Many new tables and figures help clarify key principles and approaches to management. Synopses have been provided for each chapter; selected readings have been updated, and cards are included that succinctly provide the data needed to address selected problems commonly encountered in day-to-day practice.

In writing this book, certain unifying themes and principles spontaneously recurred. Among the more important are these: (1) attempting to quickly restore normal physiology may be a misguided undertaking in the critically ill patient, especially when the efforts to reestablish "normality" incur substantial iatrogenic risk; (2) critical illness is distinguished by rapidly changing physiology and responses, so the clinician must continually question the need for ongoing treatment and reconsider the potential of alternative approaches; (3) because individual responses to an intended treatment can seldom be predicted with absolute certainty, cautious therapeutic challenges are key to scientific management; and, finally, (4) the clinician must be vigilant and thoughtfully proactive. Given a condition that is often tenuous or unstable, therapeutic misadventures are likely, unless management is consistently appropriate and interventions are timely.

We have addressed a broad range of topics but make no pretense to be comprehensive. Ours is not intended as an all-inclusive reference; several excellent multi-authored texts with that primary objective are already available. Moreover, as medical intensivists, we purposely avoided de-scribing details of surgical technique better covered by others. As in the first edition of this text, our aim has been to encourage understanding of the underlying pathophysiology, the most logical diagnostic approaches, and the key principles of management. Whatever the clinical setting, such knowledge forms the core of critical care practice, transports easily across medical/surgical boundaries, and remains current over time.

Acknowledgments

I extend my sincerest thanks to Emily E. Dickman for her expert and enthusiastic help in draft editing and illustrating my contributions to this work.

—J.J.M.

Becoming a physician, practicing critical care, and authoring a text on the topic are difficult and demanding. Far too many people to thank individually have contributed to my education and sanity. Without my parents' dreams, encouragement, and sacrifice, these goals could not have been achieved. I have Scouting to thank for many opportunities and one special leader, George Lee, for his influence on me. I especially thank three dedicated teachers: Frederick Cogswell, for his friendship; Frank Calia, M.D., for his encouragement; and Theodore Woodward, M.D., for his high standards. My gratitude goes to the devoted nurses who have taught me much about caring. I also thank two unique friends, Ernie Glenn and R.E. Duncan, for the gift of flight, my sanctuary. Finally, I thank all of the patients, especially Debbie and Mom, who fight to survive critical illness and, in the process, give us hope and teach us how to do our job better.

—A.W.

Contents

Section 3
SURGICAL CRISES

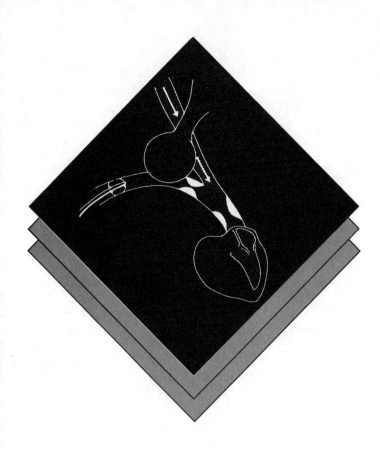

SECTION 1

Techniques and Methods in Critical Care

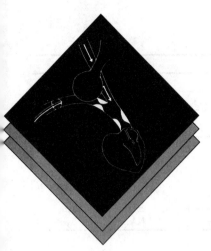

CHAPTER 1

Hemodynamics

CHARACTERISTICS OF THE NORMAL CIRCULATION

ANATOMY

Cardiac Anatomy

The circulatory and respiratory systems are tightly interdependent in their primary function of delivering appropriate quantities of oxygenated blood to metabolizing tissues. The physician's ability to deal with hemodynamic dysfunction requires a well-developed understanding of the anatomy and control of the circulation under normal and abnormal conditions. The blood stream's interface with the environment (the lung) divides the circulatory path into two functionally distinct limbs—right, or pulmonary, and left, or systemic. Except during congestive failure, the atria serve primarily as reservoirs for blood collection rather than as key pumping elements. The right ventricle (RV) is structured differently than its left-sided counterpart (Table 1.1). Because of the low resistance of the pulmonary vascular bed, the normal RV must generate mean pressures only $\frac{1}{7}$ as great as those of the left side in driving the same output. Consequently, the free wall of the RV is normally thin, preload sensitive, and poorly adapted to an acute increase of afterload. The thicker left ventricle (LV) must generate sufficient pressure to drive flow through a much greater and widely fluctuating vascular resistance. The RV and LV share the interventricular septum, circumferential muscle fibers, and the pericardial space; this interdependence has important functional consequences. For example, when the RV swells in response to increased afterload, the LV is made functionally less distensible, and left atrial pressure tends to increase. Ventricular interdependence is enhanced by processes that crowd their shared pericardial fossa: high lung volumes, high heart volumes, and pericardial effusion.

Coronary Circulation

The heart is nourished by the coronary arteries, and its venous outflow drains into the coronary sinus, which opens into the right atrium. The right coronary artery emerges anteriorly from the aorta, distributing to the RV, to the sinus and atrioventricular (AV) nodes, and to the posterior and inferior surfaces of the LV. The left coronary system (circumflex and left anterior descending arteries) nourishes the interventricular septum, the conduction system below the AV node, and the anterior and lateral walls of the LV. If the heart relaxed completely, the difference between mean arterial pressure (MAP) and coronary sinus pressure would drive flow through the coronary circulation. However, because aortic pressure varies continuously and because the wall tension that surrounds the coronary vessels determines the *effective* downstream pressure, perfusion varies with the phases of the cardiac cycle. The LV is perfused most actively in early diastole, when aortic pressure is not at its maximum but myocardial pressures are least. Because the RV generates a much lower compressive force and tissue pressure, right coronary flow tends to be less phasic. The LV myocardial pressure is highest close to

TABLE 1-1

RIGHT VS LEFT HEART PROPERTIES

	Right Heart		Left Heart	
	Normal	Failing	Normal	Failing*
Preload sensitivity	+ + +	+	+ +	+
Afterload sensitivity	+ +	+ + +	+	+ + +
Contractility	+ +	+	+ + +	+ +
Effect on afterload				
Pleural pressure	±	±	+	+ + +
pH	+ +	+ + +	±	±
Hypoxemia	+ + +	+ + + +	±	±
Response to cardiotonic and vasoactive drugs	NA	+ +	NA	+ + + +

* Not including aortic valve disease.

the endocardium and lowest near the epicardium. Hence, under stress, the endocardium is more likely to experience ischemia.

Coronary blood flow normally parallels the metabolic activity of the myocardium. Locally active neural and humoral stimuli cause the coronary circulation to dilate under stress; however, the precise mediators of this linkage are incompletely known. Tachycardia and bradycardia have dual effects on coronary blood flow. Because changes in heart rate are accomplished chiefly by shortening or lengthening diastole, tachycardia reduces the time available for diastolic perfusion while increasing the heart's need for oxygen. This potential reduction in mean coronary flow is normally overridden by vasodilatation. However, coronary disease prevents full expression of this compensation. During bradycardia, longer periods of time are available for diastolic perfusion and metabolic needs are less. However, diastolic myocardial fiber tension rises as the heart expands, and marked bradycardia may lower both mean arterial and coronary perfusion pressures.

Vascular Anatomy

Left Side

Between heartbeats, the continuous flow of blood from the heart to the periphery is maintained by the recoil of elastic vessels distended during systole. Although the aorta is predominately an elastic structure, the peripheral arteries are enveloped by smooth muscle. Arterioles serve as the primary resistive elements, and by adjusting caliber, these small vessels regulate tissue blood flow and aid in the control of arterial pressure.

The capillaries downstream from the arterioles are so numerous that the velocity of flow through them is relatively slow. However, because these vessels are short and narrow, the capillary network accounts for only a minority of the total circulating blood volume—the true capacitance vessels of the circulation are the venules and small veins. At any one time, only a small percentage of the total capacitance bed is distended. The precise distribution of the circulating blood volume among various tissue beds is governed by metabolic or functional requirements and gated by arteriolar vasoconstriction.

Right Side

In the low pressure pulmonary circuit, the central vessels are thinner and the arterioles have little muscle; consequently, few anatomic differences exist between normal arteries and veins. The pulmonary capillary meshwork, however, is even more luxuriant than in the periphery. Flow distribution is influenced by gravity, alveolar pressure, regional pleural pressures, oxygen tension, pH, and other chemical stimuli.

CIRCULATORY CONTROL

Determinants of Cardiac Output

When averaged over time, cardiac output, the product of heart rate and stroke volume, must match metabolic requirements. Output insufficiency results in anaerobic metabolism. In a real sense, metabolic activity regulates the cardiac output of a healthy individual; uncoupling this relationship leads to anaerobiosis that cannot be sus-

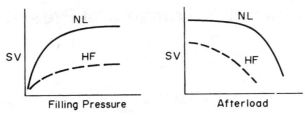

FIG. 1–1. Stroke volume (SV) response of normal (NL) and failing heart (HF) to loading conditions. Impaired hearts are abnormally sensitive to afterload but show blunted responses to preload augmentation.

tained indefinitely. Agitation, anxiety, pain, shivering, fever, and increased breathing workload intensify systemic O_2 demand. In the critical care setting, continued matching of output to demand is often achieved by spontaneous downregulation of tissue oxygen demand or with the help of sedative, analgesic, antipyretic, inotropic, or vasoactive agents. It is important to remember that underlying metabolic activity can change unnoticed, so that increasing or decreasing cardiac output can reflect shifting O_2 demands rather than a change in ventricular loading conditions, pharmacologic action, or response to other therapeutic interventions.

Although the precise mechanism that links output to metabolism remains uncertain, the primary determinants of stroke volume are well defined: precontractile fiber stretch in diastole (preload), the tension developed by the muscle fibers during systolic contraction (afterload), and the forcefulness of muscular contraction under constant loading conditions (contractility) (Fig. 1.1). Factors governing these determinants, as well as their normal values, differ for the two ventricles. For example, because the *average* stroke volume of both ventricles must be equal despite differing end-diastolic volumes, the fraction of end-diastolic blood volume ejected during systole (ejection fraction—an imprecise but widely employed marker of contractility) differs between them. Normally, RV ejection fraction is somewhat less than left ventricular ejection fraction.

Determinants of Stroke Volume—General Concepts

Preload   According to the Frank-Starling principle, muscle fiber length at end-diastole influences the vigor of cardiac contraction. The tendency of ejected volume to increase as transmural filling pressure rises normally constitutes an important adaptive mechanism that enables moment-by-moment adjustments to changing venous return. During heart failure, the Starling curve is flattened and the ventricle is preload insensitive—high filling pressures become necessary to achieve a modest output. Preload changes proportionally to acute changes in end-diastolic ventricular volume. It should be understood, however, that myocardial remodeling can gradually modify the relationship between absolute chamber volume and preload; therefore, muscle fiber stretch within a chronically dilated heart may not differ significantly from normal. End-diastolic volume is determined by ventricular distensibility (compliance) and by the pressure distending the ventricle (the transmural pressure). Transmural pressure is the difference between the intracavitary and juxtacardiac pressures. Viewed alongside the left ventricle, the normal right ventricle operates with a comparatively steep relationship between transmural pressure and ventricular volume. A poorly compliant ventricle, or one surrounded by increased intrathoracic pressure, requires a higher intracavitary pressure to achieve any specified end-diastolic volume and degree of precontractile fiber stretch (Fig. 1.2). The cost of higher filling pressure may be impaired myocardial perfusion or pulmonary edema. Functional ventricular stiffening can result from myocardial disease, pericardial tethering, or extrinsic compression of the heart (Table 1.2). The precise position of the ventricle on the Starling curve is difficult to determine. However, studies of animals and normal human subjects suggest that there is little preload reserve in the supine position and that, once supine, further increases in cardiac output are met primarily by increases in heart rate and/or ejection fraction. Thus, the Starling mechanism may be of most importance during hypovolemia and in the upright position.

Diastolic Dysfunction   Diastole usually is considered a passive process in which transmural pressure distends elastic heart muscle. In normal

Concept of Transmural Pressure

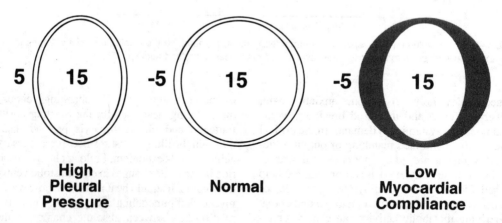

High Pleural Pressure   **Normal**   **Low Myocardial Compliance**

FIG. 1–2. Concept of transmural pressure. The muscle fiber tensions that determine preload and afterload are functions of the pressure difference across the ventricle. In diastole, a measured intracavitary pressure of 15 mm Hg may correspond to a large or small chamber volume and myocardial fiber tension, depending on the compliance of the ventricle and its surrounding pressure.

individuals and many patients with heart disease, this approximation is more or less accurate. However, for some patients, diastole is more properly considered an energy-dependent, active process. Failure of the heart muscle to relax at a normal rate (secondary to ischemia, longstanding hypertension, or hypertrophic myopathy) can cause sufficient functional stiffening to produce pulmonary edema despite preserved systolic function, especially in response to intravascular volume loading, ischemia, or increased metabolic demands. Perhaps one-third or more of adult patients with congestive heart failure develop symptoms on this basis. Diastolic dysfunction often precedes systolic dysfunction and should be considered an early warning sign of deterioration. Although diastolic and systolic impairments often coexist, the

diastolic dysfunction syndrome is an especially likely explanation when congestive symptoms predominate over defects in systolic performance (as gauged by organ perfusion). In all patients with diastolic dysfunction, the early rapid filling phase of ventricular diastole is slowed, and the extent of ventricular filling becomes more heavily influenced by terminal-phase atrial contraction. (Sudden loss of the atrial "kick" often precipitates congestive symptoms.) Diastolic dysfunction should be suspected when congestive symptoms develop despite normal systolic function in patients predisposed by coronary disease, longstanding hypertension, advanced age, or hypertrophic cardiomyopathy. Confirmation, however, requires ancillary testing by echocardiography, Doppler ultrasound, radionuclide angiography, contrast ventriculography, or another imaging method. With all techniques, attention must be focused on diastole, particularly during the phase of rapid filling. In most institutions, echocardiography has become the method of choice for critically ill patients because of its convenience and reliability. Analysis of mitral valve function (deceleration time, early diastolic (E):late diastolic (A) wave velocity ratio, and isovolume relaxation time) is helpful. Reliable signals of the required clarity are often impossible to obtain, however,

TABLE 1–2

REDUCED DIASTOLIC COMPLIANCE

Myocardial Disease	Pericardial Disease	Extrinsic Compression
Ischemia/infarction	Tamponade	PEEP
Hypertrophy	Constriction	Tension pneumothorax
Infiltration		RV dilation

in the critically ill patient. Regarding treatment, calcium channel blockers (e.g., verapamil, diltiazem, nifedipine) have been demonstrated to be useful in animal studies and in humans with hypertrophic cardiomyopathy. Selective β blockers (e.g., metoprolol) can also help certain patients but must be chosen wisely and used with extreme caution when significant systolic dysfunction, conduction system disturbance, or bronchospasm coexist. Predictably, inotropes do not improve diastolic function.

Afterload Although afterload is often equated with altered blood pressure or systemic vascular resistance, it is better defined as the muscular tension that must be developed during systole per unit of blood flow. Moderate changes in afterload usually are countered by increases in contractility, preload, or heart rate, so that the output of the normal heart is usually little affected. Heart size remains small and filling pressures do not rise excessively. However, once preload reserves have been exhausted, raising afterload can profoundly depress cardiac output. Just as the relationship between preload and stroke volume rises more steeply for the right than for the left ventricle, so too is the normal right ventricle more sensitive than the left to changes in its afterload (Fig. 1.3). The dilated chambers of a failing heart—both right and left—are inherently afterload sensitive (Fig. 1.1). Cardiomegaly, pulmonary edema, and mitral regurgitation are clinical findings that help identify potential candidates for afterload reduction. Quantitative assessment of ejection impedance can be made by determining pulmonary vascular resistance (PVR) and systemic vascular resistance (SVR). These indices, the quotients of driving pressure and cardiac output across their respective beds, are calculated as if blood flow fulfilled the assumptions of Poiseuille's law. Because cardiac output must be interpreted relative to body size, both measurements have a wide range of normal values. SVR and PVR indices should be calculated, using cardiac index, rather than cardiac output in the calculation. Although a rising SVR may help support blood pressure when cardiac output falls, elevations in SVR can prove detrimental to a failing heart when the increased impedance itself compromises cardiac output. Judicious reduction of arterial vessel tone may then allow cardiac output to improve, and vital organ perfusion to increase, while maintaining an acceptable blood pressure. Chamber diameter also affects afterload. In a dilated chamber, higher systolic fiber tension must be generated to produce a given intracavitary pressure, especially in fibers on the periphery. Thus, a diuretic or selective venodilator (nitroglycerine) may reduce afterload as well as preload. Apart from vessel length and diameter, blood viscosity is an important determinant of rheology and effective afterload. Blood viscosity rises nonlinearly with hematocrit. With increasing hematocrit,

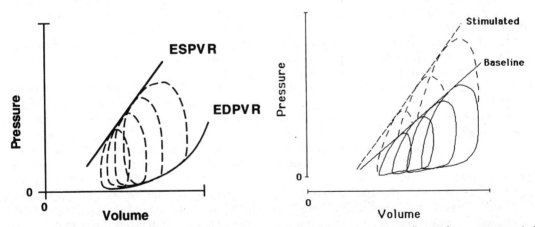

FIG. 1–3. Transmural ventricular pressure volume loops. *Left panel:* four complete cardiac cycles are represented for different states of ventricular filling. The end-diastolic pressure volume relationship (EDPVR) defines the Frank-Starling curve. During each cycle, there are sequential stages of diastolic filling, isovolumic contraction, active systolic ejection, and isovolumic relaxation. The slope of the end-systolic pressure volume relationship (ESPVR) correlates well with contractility. *Right panel:* as the myocardium is stimulated by catecholamines, the slope of the ESPVR increases, resulting in a greater pressure and ejection fraction during systole for any degree of diastolic filling.

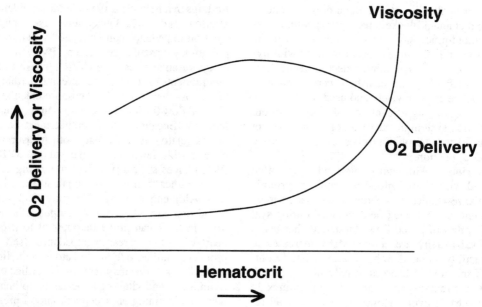

FIG. 1–4. Relationship of O_2 delivery to hematocrit and viscosity. As hematocrit rises, O_2 delivery increases up to the point at which increasing viscosity slows the transit of oxygenated blood through the tissues and impairs cardiac output.

crowded erythrocytes pass more sluggishly through tissues and effective O_2 transport eventually reaches a maximum, the value of which depends on circulating blood volume relative to vascular capacity (Fig. 1.4). Individual tissues have different tolerances to changes in hematocrit and different optimal values for oxygen extraction. Viscosity may also rise dramatically in the setting of hypothermia.

Pleural Pressure and Afterload Systolic pressure is a marker of the intracavitary pressure that must be developed by contracting muscle fibers. The intracavitary pressure is a result of muscular forces and the regional pleural pressure that surrounds the heart. Variations in pleural pressure may significantly alter afterload and, therefore, the function of the compromised left ventricle. Although multifactorial in origin, the paradoxical pulse observed during acute asthma results primarily from inspiratory afterloading of the left ventricle. When the pressure that surrounds the heart declines, greater muscle fiber tension must be developed to generate a given intracavitary and systemic blood pressure during systole. Similarly, vigorous breathing efforts can seriously impair heart function during coronary ischemia. This is a major reason why patients with pulmonary edema

and high breathing workloads respond so well to mechanical ventilation.

Right ventricular afterload tends to rise nonlinearly with increasing lung volume. The pulmonary vascular pressure–flow relationships may differ slightly for positive versus negative pressure breathing. However, the right ventricular afterload corresponding to any given lung volume is not greatly influenced by changes of pleural pressure, because the vessel that accepts its outflow (the pulmonary artery) is subjected to similar variations in pressure.

Contractility Many stimuli compete to influence the contractile state of the myocardium. Sympathetic impulses, circulating catecholamines, acid-base and electrolyte disturbances, ischemia, anoxia, and chemodepressants (drugs, mediators, or toxins) may influence ventricular performance, independent of changes in preload or afterload. Contractility is sometimes impaired transiently after blunt cardiac trauma or when ischemic myocardium is reperfused (e.g., after cardiopulmonary resuscitation, angioplasty, or after lysis of coronary thrombosis). Such "stunned myocardium" may stage a complete recovery after several days of transient dysfunction. In the laboratory setting contractility is best gauged by the slope of the end systolic pressure volume relationship (Fig. 1.3). No physical sign reliably reflects altered contractility. An S_3 gallop, narrow pulse pressure, and poorly audible heart tones suggest impaired contractility but these signs are difficult to quantify and are influenced by myocardial compliance, intravascular volume status, and vascular tone. Radionuclide ventriculograms and echocardiography provide excellent noninvasive means of determining ventricular size and basal contractile properties of the left ventricle but are not well suited to continuous monitoring. The commonly used "ejection fraction" is influenced greatly by the loading conditions of the heart. Moreover, two-dimensional echocardiographic images may misrepresent three-dimensional changes in chamber geometry.

Heart Rate

Changes in the observed heart rate usually result from the interplay between the actions of the two divisions of the autonomic nervous system. Ordinarily, parasympathetic tone predominates. (When both divisions of the autonomic nervous system are blocked, the intrinsic heart rate of young adults rises from approximately 70 to 105 beats/min.) In the supine position, the ability of the heart to respond to an increased demand for cardiac output is determined largely by the ability to raise the heart rate. Furthermore, pathological bradycardias often depress cardiac output and O_2 delivery, especially when a diseased or failing ventricle is unable to call upon a preload reserve. Because two key determinants of oxygen delivery are affected, bradycardia induced by hypoxemia profoundly depresses O_2 delivery and may rapidly precipitate circulatory collapse. Marked increases in heart rate may also lead to circulatory depression when they cause myocardial ischemia or when reduced diastolic filling time or loss of atrial contraction impair ventricular preload. As a rule, sinus heart rates exceeding $(220 - \text{age})$/min reduce cardiac output and myocardial perfusion, even in the absence of ischemic disease or loss of atrial contraction. (For example, heart rate should not exceed 150/min in a 70-year-old patient.)

Peripheral Circulation

Vascular tone and filling are extremely important in controlling the cardiac output—the heart cannot pump what it fails to receive in venous return and may not be able to generate sufficient force to overcome massive elevations in afterload caused by vasoconstriction. In fact, control of cardiac output may be viewed strictly from a vascular perspective (Fig. 1.5), but unlike the indicators of cardiac performance and loading conditions determined by catheter, vascular parameters are less easily measured. Under steady-state conditions, venous return is proportional to the quotient of driving pressure for venous return and venous resistance. Under most circumstances, the downstream pressure for venous return is right atrial pressure. The upstream pressure driving venous return, the mean systemic pressure (P_{MS}), is the volume-weighted average pressure existing in the systemic vascular network. Because a much larger fraction of the total circulating volume is contained on the venous side of the circulation, P_{MS} is much closer to right atrial pressure than to mean arterial pressure (P_{RA}). Were the P_{RA} to rise suddenly to equal the $P_{MS,}$ all blood flow would stop. Indeed, in an experimental setting, P_{MS} can be determined by synchronously clamping the aorta and vena cava to stop flow and opening a wide-bore communication between them. Mean systemic pressure is influenced by intravascular volume and vascular capacitance, which in turn is a function of vascular tone. Thus, P_{MS} rises under conditions of hypervolemia, polycythemia, and right-sided congestive heart failure; it declines during abrupt vasodilation, sepsis, hemorrhage, and diuresis. Up to a certain point, lowering P_{RA} while preserving P_{MS} improves venous return. However, when P_{RA} is reduced below the surrounding tissue pressure, the thin-walled vena cava collapses near the thoracic inlet. Effective downstream pressure for venous return then becomes the pressure just upstream to the point of collapse, rather than the $P_{RA.}$

At any given moment, the cardiac output is determined by the intersection of venous return and Starling curves. In the analysis of a depressed cardiac output, both aspects of circulatory control must be scrutinized. When positive end-expiratory pressure (PEEP) is applied, P_{RA} rises, inhibiting venous return. However, P_{MS} rises simultaneously, and compensatory vascular reflexes are called into action to reduce venous capacitance and expand circulating volume. Therefore, unlike patients with depressed vascular reflexes or hypovolemia, most healthy individuals do not experience a reduction of cardiac output under the influence of moderate PEEP. Although an increase in

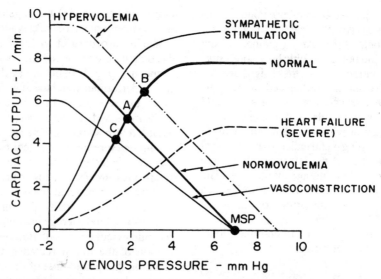

FIG. 1–5. Interaction of Frank-Starling and venous return curves. With normal heart function, observed cardiac output is determined by such vascular factors as filling status (A→B), and vasoconstriction (A→C). Sympathetic stimulation and heart failure have opposing effects on the Starling curve and cardiac output. The mean systemic pressure driving venous return (MSP) is a hypothetical point determined by extrapolating the venous return curve to the venous pressure axis where all cardiac output ceases. Note that venous return improves linearly as central venous pressure falls, up to the point at which central vessels collapse.

venous resistance can also reduce venous return, it is uncommon for venous resistance to increase without an offsetting change in P_{MS}. However, positional compromise of the inferior vena cava by an intraabdominal mass (e.g., during advanced pregnancy) may account for postural changes in cardiac output in such patients.

CHARACTERISTICS OF THE DISEASED CIRCULATION

LEFT VENTRICULAR INSUFFICIENCY

Congestive Heart Failure

Diagnostics

The term heart failure (CHF) is often loosely applied to conditions in which the filling pressures of the left heart are increased sufficiently to cause dyspnea or weakness at rest or mild exertion. However, congestive symptoms can develop when systolic cardiac function is unimpaired (volume overload, diastolic dysfunction, right ventricular encroachment, pericardial effusion) as well as during myocardial failure itself. Unlike the nor-

mal LV, which is relatively sensitive to changes in its preload and insensitive to changes in its afterload, the failing LV has the opposite characteristics (see Fig. 1.1). Changes in afterload can therefore make a major difference in LV systolic performance, whereas preload manipulation usually elicits little benefit, unless it reduces afterload indirectly by shrinking chamber volume and wall tension. Radiographic evidence of acute heart failure includes perivascular cuffing, a widened vascular pedicle, blurring of the hilar vasculature, and diffuse infiltrates that spare the costophrenic angles. These infiltrates tend to lack air bronchograms and are usually unaccompanied by an acute change in heart size. Chronic congestive heart failure is typified by Kerley-B lines, dilated cardiac chambers, and increased cardiac dimensions.

When faced with a patient who seems to have pulmonary venous congestion, a number of key questions should be asked in determining its etiology.

1. **Is forward output adequate to perfuse vital tissues?** When perfusion is severely impaired, consideration should be given to mechanical ventilation and invasive hemodynamic monitoring, especially in the setting of coexisting pulmonary venous congestion. Correction of

disturbances in oxygen content, tissue O_2 demand, serum pH, electrolyte balance, and ventricular loading conditions are of prime importance. Inotropic therapy may be indicated for hypotension, whereas hypertensive patients and those with an elevated SVR may benefit from vasodilators.

2. **Is there evidence of systolic dysfunction?** Adequate perfusion does not necessarily imply intact systolic function—forward output may be maintained at the cost of high preloading pressures and pulmonary vascular congestion. If perfusion is adequate and systolic function of cardiac valves and myocardium remains intact, the patient may simply be volume overloaded or manifesting diastolic dysfunction. Echocardiography helps greatly in this assessment.

3. **What is the LV size and wall thickness?** LV chamber dilation usually indicates a chronic process—most commonly longstanding ischemic heart disease, cardiomyopathy, or LV diastolic overload (aortic or mitral valvular insufficiency). Therapy in such cases should be directed toward optimizing afterload (with systemic vasodilators) or improving myocardial oxygen supply (coronary vasodilators). If there is excessive inspiratory effort, mechanical ventilation can reduce both O_2 demand and left ventricular afterload by raising inspiratory and mean pleural pressures. The clinician should remain alert to the possibility of pericardial effusion as a cause of an enlarged heart shadow. If left ventricular cavity size is normal, mitral stenosis, tamponade, constrictive pericarditis, acute myocardial infarction, or diastolic dysfunction should be suspected. Left ventricular wall hypertrophy, myocardial infiltration, or interdependence with a swollen right ventricle may limit stroke volume and cardiac output, despite normal contractility. A distended left atrium sometimes provides a clue in such cases.

4. **Does the left ventricle show global or regional hypokinesis?** Regional hypokinesis/dyskinesis suggests localized disease (e.g., coronary occlusion). Echocardiography and the precordial electrocardiogram (ECG) are instrumental in this assessment. Generalized hypokinesis of a heart with normal chamber size often reflects the stunned myocardium of trauma, diffuse ischemia, drug overdose, or toxin ingestion.

5. **Is there evidence of valvular dysfunction?** Aortic stenosis may depress cardiac output by causing excessive afterload, myocardial ischemia, or hypertrophic impairment of ventricular filling. Mitral regurgitation impairs forward output and produces congestive symptoms by allowing retrograde venting of the ejected volume. Acute chamber enlargement (regardless of cause) may worsen congestive symptoms by producing transient mitral regurgitation caused by papillary muscle dysfunction or mitral ring dilation.

6. **Is there evidence of increased pulmonary vascular permeability or hypoalbuminemia?** The tendency to form pulmonary edema not only relates to hydrostatic forces (e.g., pulmonary venous pressure) but also to the plasma oncotic pressure and pulmonary capillary permeability. Hence, pulmonary edema may form at a relatively low pulmonary venous pressure if oncotic pressure is reduced or the microvascular endothelium is leaky. Conversely, the lungs may remain dry despite high left heart filling pressures when enlarged lymphatic drainage channels with greater capacity have had time to develop (e.g., mitral stenosis). The radiographic signature of lymphatic dilatation is the presence of Kerley lines.

The physical examination should be directed toward the detection of hypoperfusion (reduced mental status, oliguria) and compensatory vasoconstriction (reduced skin temperature, prolonged capillary filling time, etc.). Rales are often difficult to detect in the bedridden patient who breathes shallowly and in those receiving mechanical ventilatory support. The chest radiograph provides key information regarding heart size, vascular distribution, pulmonary infiltrates, and pleural effusions. Echocardiography and radionuclide ventriculography provide important information regarding chamber size, contractility, diastolic filling, valvular function, P_{RA}, pericardial volume, and filling status of the central pulmonary veins. Although transesophageal echocardiography is not always feasible to perform, the detail it provides is generally superior to its transthoracic counterpart, especially in patients with obstructive lung disease or massive obesity.

Therapeutics

As a general rule, the therapy of congestive heart failure should be geared to documented pathophysiology. Whereas diuretics help in most cases, inotropic agents should be reserved for documented disorders of myocardial function refractory to adjustments of filling pressure, pH, and electrolytes. Angiotensin converting enzyme (ACE) inhibitors (e.g., captopril, enalapril) and/or systemic vasodilators should be used when an elevated systemic vascular resistance is documented in the setting of an adequate preload and blood pressure. Nitrates may aid cardiac ischemia but can precipitate hypotension in patients with borderline or inadequate filling pressures. New-onset atrial or ventricular arrhythmias or conduction disturbances (e.g., atrial fibrillation, atrial flutter, heart block) should be treated aggressively if they reduce forward output.

Although calcium channel blockers can benefit congestive failure by controlling hypertension or reversing coronary spasm, they should only be used in well-selected patients; these agents depress cardiac contractility and may impair conduction or precipitate tachycardia. In similar fashion, β blockers reduce myocardial oxygen consumption by decreasing heart rate and contractility but have the potential to precipitate congestive heart failure, conduction system disturbances, or bronchospasm. β-adrenergic blockade should be reserved primarily for cases of documented ischemia. Without a firm indication, (e.g., thyroid storm, delirium tremens, uncontrolled supraventricular tachycardia) they should *not* be considered first-line measures in other forms of congestive heart failure.

RIGHT VENTRICULAR DYSFUNCTION

Three disease conditions account for most acute problems arising from right ventricular dysfunction: right ventricular infarction; cor pulmonale complicating parenchymal, vascular, or hypoventilatory hypoxemic lung diseases (e.g., sleep apnea); and the acute respiratory distress syndrome (ARDS).

Right Ventricular Infarction

The right ventricle receives most of its blood supply from the right coronary artery. It is not surprising, therefore, that right ventricular infarction complicates as many as 30% of inferior myocardial infarctions, as well as a much smaller percentage of anterior infarctions. The diagnosis should be suspected when there are signs of systemic venous hypertension, an unimpressive or clear chest radiograph, and evidence of ST segment elevation or Q waves over the right precordium (V_4R). A suggestive enzyme profile confirms the diagnosis. Right ventricular infarctions generally require aggressive administration of intravenous fluids. The left ventricle may be required to take up the work of pumping blood through both the systemic circuit (directly) and the pulmonary circuit (indirectly), using ventricular interdependence. Dilatation of the right ventricle and fluid loading tighten these linkages by crowding the two ventricles within the pericardial sac, stretching shared circumferential muscle fibers, and shifting the mobile interventricular septum. Recovery from, accommodation to, or compensation for right ventricular infarction tends to occur over several days. If cardiac output can be supported during this interval, the outlook for patients without other cardiopulmonary disease is generally good. Prognosis depends not only on the size of the infarction but also on the presence or absence of increased pulmonary vascular resistance.

Cor Pulmonale (see Chapter 21)

Pathogenesis

In its purest form, cor pulmonale is defined as hypertrophy, dilatation, or failure of the RV in response to excessive pulmonary vascular resistance. By definition, this term excludes secondary changes in RV function resulting from pulmonary venous hypertension or LV failure. Three reinforcing causes of pulmonary hypertension are a restricted capillary bed, alveolar hypoxia, and acidosis. Although extensive obliteration, constriction, or compression of the capillary bed may be the underlying cause, increased cardiac output and superimposed hypoxemia or acidosis may dramatically elevate pulmonary arterial pressure (P_{PA}). The normal RV cannot sustain adequate forward output at mean pulmonary arterial pressures that exceed ~35 mm Hg. Given sufficient time, however, the right ventricular wall can thicken sufficiently to generate pressures that rival those in the systemic circuit. Arterial smooth muscle also hypertrophies over time, intensifying the response to alveolar hypoxemia and pharmacologic vasoconstrictors. Most diffuse pulmonary insults increase PVR; however, massive pulmonary embolism is the most common cause of acute cor pulmonale in a previously healthy patient.

Chronic cor pulmonale can result from severe lung disease of virtually any etiology (especially disease that obliterates pulmonary capillaries and induces chronic hypoxemia). Acutely decompensated cor pulmonale occurs frequently in patients with chronic obstructive pulmonary disease (COPD). In such patients, P_{PA} can fall dramatically with correction of bronchospasm, hypoxemia, and acidosis. Because ~½ of the normal pulmonary capillary bed can be obstructed without raising resting mean P_{PA} significantly above the normal range, pulmonary hypertension in a normoxemic person at rest usually signifies an important reduction in the number of patent pulmonary capillaries. (This loss is reflected in a reduced diffusing capacity for carbon monoxide.) After the capillary reserve has been exhausted, P_{PA} varies markedly with cardiac output. Thus, elevations of pulmonary artery pressure often signify variations in cardiac output, rather than worsening of lung pathology.

Diagnosis

The measurement of central venous pressure (CVP), pulmonary artery occlusion ("wedge") pressure (P_w), and the computation of PVR help separate right from left heart disease. The physical findings of acute cor pulmonale are those of pulmonary hypertension: hypoperfusion, RV gallop, a loud P_2, pulsatile hepatomegaly, and systemic venous congestion. Deep breathing may accentuate these right heart findings, as inspiratory increases of blood flow returning to the thorax raise P_{PA} and tend to stress the compromised right ventricle. Pulmonic and tricuspid regurgitation, hepatomegaly, a palpable P_2, and a right parasternal lift usually indicate severe subacute or chronic pulmonary hypertension. Unfortunately, many of these signs are difficult to elicit in obese patients and those with hyperinflated or noisy lungs. Clinical suspicion can be confirmed by documenting elevations in P_{RA}, P_{PA}, and PVR and by measuring normal or depressed cardiac output, P_w, SVR, and systemic mixed venous oxygen saturation (SVO_2).

Ancillary Diagnostic Tests Radiographic signs of pulmonary arterial hypertension include dilated central pulmonary arteries with sharp tapering and peripheral vascular "pruning." Although precise measurements are often difficult to make, a right lower lobar artery dimension larger than 18 mm in diameter (on the standard upright PA film) or main pulmonary arteries larger than 25 mm in diameter (judged on lateral) strongly suggest subacute or chronic pulmonary hypertension. Overall heart size may appear normal until disease is advanced, especially in patients with hyperinflation. Encroachment of the RV on the retrosternal airspace in the lateral view is an early but nonspecific sign.

The contrast-enhanced computed tomography (CT) scan of the thorax may confirm right ventricular dilatation. Recent catheter-based techniques allow computation of right ventricular volume and/or RV ejection fraction. Beat-by-beat analysis of the thermodilution temperature profile allows both to be assessed, whereas a double indicator (dye/thermodilution) method permits determination of these indices as well as central blood volume, stroke work, lung water, and others.

ECG criteria for RV hypertrophy are insensitive and nonspecific. In acute cor pulmonale, changes characteristic of hypertrophy are lacking. P pulmonale and a progressive decrease in the R:S ratio across the precordium are sensitive but nonspecific signs. Conversely, the S_1, Q_3, T_3 pattern, right axis deviation $>110°$, R:S ratio in V_5 or V_6 <1.0, and a QR pattern in V_1 are relatively specific but insensitive signs. Radionuclide ventriculography and echocardiography may help document RV chamber size and function noninvasively. In patients with true cor pulmonale, left ventricular systolic function should remain unaffected.

Management of Acute Cor Pulmonale

The key directives in managing cor pulmonale are to maintain adequate RV filling, to reverse hypoxemia and acidosis, to establish a coordinated cardiac rhythm, and to treat the underlying illness. Most patients with decompensated COPD and cor pulmonale have a reversible hypoxemic component. Although oxygen must be administered cautiously, patients with CO_2 retention should not be denied O_2 therapy. Acidosis markedly accentuates the effect of hypoxemia on pulmonary vascular resistance, whereas hypercarbia without acidosis exerts less effect. This should be borne in mind when deciding the need for buffering pH in permissive hypercapnia. Bronchospasm, infection, and retained secretions should be treated. When extreme polycythemia complicates chronic hypoxemia, careful lowering of the hematocrit to ~55% may significantly reduce blood viscosity, decrease RV afterload, and improve myocardial perfusion. To improve viscosity, it may be advisable to rewarm a hypothermic patient.

The effects of digitalis, inotropes, and diuretics

in acute cor pulmonale are variable; these drugs should be employed cautiously. Gentle diuresis helps to relieve symptomatic congestion of the lower extremities, gut, and portal circulation. Diuresis may reduce right ventricular distention and myocardial tension, improving its afterload and perfusion. Any depression of cardiac output resulting from diuresis may also cause a secondary reduction of P_{PA}. In patients requiring extreme right ventricular distention and ventricular interdependence to sustain adequate stroke volume, vigorous diuresis or phlebotomy may have adverse or even disastrous consequences. Central vascular pressures, therefore, should be monitored carefully. The effect of cardiotonic agents in the treatment of acute cor pulmonale is also unpredictable. Digitalis has only a small inotropic effect on the performance of a nonhypertrophied right ventricle but may be valuable in chronic cor pulmonale and for controlling heart rate in atrial fibrillation without depressing myocardial function. Inotropes such as dopamine and dobutamine can improve left ventricular function, boosting the perfusion pressure of the right ventricular myocardium and enhancing the beneficial effects of ventricular interdependence in a dilated ventricle. Furthermore, because the ventricles share the septum and circumferential muscle fibers, it is likely that improved left ventricular contraction benefits the right ventricle through systolic ventricular interdependence. Arrhythmias induced by such agents, however, may disrupt the atrioventricular coordination that maintains effective right ventricular filling and performance.

For a minority of patients, calcium channel blockers (e.g., nifedipine) reduce pulmonary vascular resistance and boost cardiac output by decreasing RV afterload. This effect, however, is highly variable; these drugs may also depress myocardial function or reduce coronary perfusion pressure. For the patient with pulmonary venoocclusive disease, calcium antagonists can prove disastrous because they dilate precapillary arterioles, causing pulmonary edema. For patients with a clearly reversible component to the pulmonary hypertension, inhaled nitric oxide (or aerosolized prostacyclin) may prove to be a useful bridge to definitive therapy or physiologic adaptation. Unfortunately, tolerance to nitric oxide gradually develops and, in itself, does not provide a long-term solution.

Acute Respiratory Failure

Mechanisms of Circulatory Impairment in ARDS   Although cardiac output usually increases in the early stage of acute respiratory distress syndrome (ARDS) in response to the precipitating stress or to compensate for hypoxemia, this is less often true when the illness is far advanced. The performance of one or both ventricles may deteriorate as lung disease worsens, compounding the problem of inadequate tissue O_2 delivery. The cardiac dysfunction that accompanies advanced respiratory failure is incompletely understood. Effective preload may be reduced by PEEP, third spacing, capillary leakage, and myocardial stiffening secondary to ischemia or catecholamine stimulation. Contractility of either ventricle may be impaired by hypotension, ischemia, electrolyte abnormalities, or cardiodepressant factors released during sepsis, injury, or other inflammatory condition. Compression, obliteration, and hypoxic vasoconstriction of the pulmonary vasculature impede ejection of the afterload-sensitive right ventricle, a low pressure–high capacity pump. Increased wall tension also tends to diminish right ventricular perfusion. Severe pulmonary hypertension is an ominous sign in the later stages of ARDS.

Assessing Perfusion Adequacy   The assessment of perfusion adequacy in ARDS is addressed in detail elsewhere (see Oxygenation Failure, Chapter 24). However, a few points deserve emphasis. Individual organs vary widely with regard to O_2 demand, completeness of O_2 extraction, and adaptability to ischemia or hypoxia. Cerebral and cardiac tissues are especially vulnerable to anoxia. In these organs, the O_2 requirement per gram of tissue is high, O_2 stores are minimal, and O_2 extraction is relatively complete—even under normal circumstances. Subtle changes in mental status may be the first indication of hypoxemia, but the multiplicity of potential causes (e.g., early sepsis, dehydration, anxiety, sleep deprivation, drug effects) renders disorientation and lethargy difficult to interpret. Although cool, moist skin often provides a valuable clue to inadequate vital organ perfusion, the use of vasopressors and disorders of vasoregulation common to the critically ill patient reduce the utility of this finding.

The normal kidney provides a window on the adequacy of vital organ perfusion through variation of its urine output, pH, and electrolyte composition. Adequate urine volume and sodium and bicarbonate excretion suggest sufficient renal blood flow when the kidneys are functioning normally. Unfortunately, instead of reflecting adequacy of perfusion, variations in urine volume and alterations of urine composition often result from drug effect, diurnal variations, and or glomerular or tubular dysfunction. As sustained hypoperfusion activates anaerobic metabolic pathways, arterial pH and bicarbonate concentrations decline and lactic acid levels rise, widening the anion gap. Although adequacy of cardiac output can seldom be determined unequivocally by any single calculated index, analysis of the O_2 contents of arterial and mixed venous blood is valuable when addressing questions of tissue O_2 supply and utilization. In recent years, gastric mucosal pH has been investigated as a sensitive marker of insufficient O_2 delivery to vital organs. Despite the value of such indices, inadequacy of systemic O_2 delivery is perhaps best judged from a battery of indicators, including the clinical examination of perfusion-sensitive organ systems (urine output and composition, mental status, ECG, etc.), the cardiac index, systemic vascular resistance, the presence or absence of anion gap acidosis, the mixed venous oxygen saturation (SVO_2), and the calculated O_2 extraction.

Improving perfusion adequacy in ARDS
Apart from efforts to improve cardiac output and arterial O_2 content (e.g., transfusion, inotropic or vasoactive drugs), tissue oxygenation and perfusion may be enhanced by reducing metabolic need and optimizing hemoglobin concentration. Metabolic needs (and perfusion requirements) may be reduced strikingly by controlling sepsis and fever, alleviating anxiety and agitation, and providing assistance (O_2, bronchodilators, ventilatory support) to reduce the work of breathing. Therapy directed at improving cardiac output in the setting of ARDS should be guided by assessing heart rate, contractility, and loading conditions of each ventricle independently. Minor elevations of pulmonary venous pressure may flood the lung, necessitating higher levels of PEEP, mean airway pressure, and supplemental O_2. Every attempt should be made to reduce RV afterload by correcting hypoxemia and acidosis. Although a certain minimum level of PEEP must be maintained in the early phase of ARDS to avoid ventilator-induced lung damage, unnecessary elevations of mean airway pressure may overdistend patent lung units, thereby compressing alveolar capillaries and accentuating the impedance to right ventricular ejection.

PERICARDIAL CONSTRICTION AND TAMPONADE

The pericardium normally supports the heart, shields it from damage or infection, enhances dia-

TABLE 1–3
CAUSES OF PERICARDITIS

Infections	Dissecting	Malignancy
Viral	aneurysm	Trauma
TB	Dressler's	Uremia
Bacterial	syndrome	Radiation
Fungal	Anticoagulation	Drugs
Rheumatologic	Myocardial	
diseases	infarction	

stolic ventricular coupling, and prevents excessive acute dilatation of the heart. In the ICU, three types of pericardial disease are noteworthy: acute pericarditis, pericardial tamponade, and constrictive pericarditis.

Acute Pericarditis

Acute pericardial inflammation can arise from diverse causes (Table 1.3). The characteristic complaint is chest pain, eased by sitting and leaning forward and aggravated by supine positioning, coughing, deep inspiration, or swallowing. Dyspnea, pain referred to the shoulder, and sensations of chest or abdominal pressure are frequent. Unless muffled by effusion, pericarditis usually can be detected on physical examination by a single or multicomponent friction rub. The rub is often evanescent or recurrent, best heard with the patient leaning forward, and easily confused with the mediastinal crunch of pneumomediastinum, a pleural rub, coarse rhonchi, or an artifact of the stethoscope moving against the skin. Early ECG changes include ST segment elevation, which, unlike the pattern in acute myocardial infarction, is concave upward and typically present in all leads except V_1. (The reciprocal depression pattern of regional infarction is absent.) Initially, the T waves are upright in leads with ST segment elevation—another distinction from acute infarction. Depression of the PR segment occurs commonly early in acute pericarditis. The ST segments return to baseline within several days, and the T waves flatten. (Unlike the situation that accompanies acute myocardial infarction, ST segments usually normalize before the T waves invert.) Eventually, T waves normalize, a process that may require weeks or months. Management of uncomplicated pericarditis (without tamponade) includes careful monitoring, treatment of the underlying cause, and judicious use of nonsteroidal anti-inflammatory agents for selected cases. Occasionally, pericarditis is complicated by hydraulic cardiac compression (tamponade) or the development of a constricting pericardial sac.

Pericardial Tamponade

Although pericardial fluid tends to reduce pain and discomfort by buffering the friction between the heart and pericardium, the rapid accumulation of pericardial fluid may compress the heart, resulting in tamponade. At least 250 mL of fluid must collect before an obviously enlarged heart shadow is noted on the chest radiograph; a normal or unchanged chest radiograph does not exclude the presence of a hemodynamically important effusion. Effusions that cause tamponade can be circumferential, asymmetrical, or loculated. In the supine patient, small unloculated effusions pool posteriorly.

As fluid accumulates, nonspecific ECG findings include reduced QRS voltage and T-wave flattening. In this setting, electrical alternans suggests the presence of massive effusion and tamponade. Although echocardiographic quantification of effusion size is imprecise, it is the most rapid and widely used technique. Large pericardial effusions (>350 mL) give rise to anterior echo-free spaces and exaggerated cardiac swinging motions. Diastolic collapse of right heart chambers suggests a critical degree of fluid accu-

mulation and tamponade. Alternative diagnostic techniques include the CT scan with intravenous contrast and the magnetic resonance imaging (MRI) scan (when feasible).

Physiology of Pericardial Tamponade

Pericardial tamponade is a hemodynamic crisis characterized by increased intracardiac pressures, limitation of ventricular diastolic filling, and reduction of stroke volume. Normally, intrapericardial pressure is similar to intrapleural pressure but less than either right or left ventricular diastolic pressures. Rapid accumulation of pericardial fluid causes sufficient pressure within the sac to compress and equalize right and left atrial pressures, reducing maximal diastolic dimensions and stroke volume. Reflex increases in heart rate and adrenergic tone initially maintain cardiac output. In this setting, any process that quickly reduces venous return or causes bradycardia (e.g., hypoxemia, β blockade) can precipitate shock.

Tamponade alters the dynamics of systemic venous return and cardiac filling (Fig. 1.6). As cardiac volume transiently decreases during ejection, pericardial pressure falls, resulting in a prominent X descent on the venous pressure tracing. Tamponade attenuates the normal early diastolic surge of ventricular filling and abolishes the Y descent (its representation on the venous pressure tracing).

Constriction

Tamponade

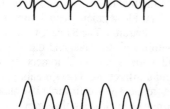

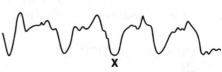

FIG. 1–6. Contrast of pericardial constriction and tamponade in central venous pressure tracings. Unlike the venous pressure tracing of constriction, the "Y descent" is attenuated in tamponade because early diastolic filling is impaired. The systolic "X descent" is well preserved in both conditions.

Pulsus paradoxus, a result of exaggerated normal physiology, may develop simultaneously. Inspiration normally is accompanied by an increase in the diastolic dimensions of the RV and a small decrease in LV volume. These changes reduce LV ejection volume and systolic pressure (<10 mm Hg) during early inspiration. Pericardial tamponade accentuates this normal fluctuation to produce pulsus paradoxus. With an arterial line in place, paradoxical pulse is quantified easily by noting the respiratory variation of systolic pressure during the end-inspiratory and end-expiratory phases of the ventilatory cycle. Paradoxical pulse also can be detected in traditional fashion by lowering the cuff pressure of a sphygmomanometer slowly from a point 20 mm Hg above systolic pressure until the Korotkoff sounds are heard equally well throughout both inspiration and expiration. The "paradox" is the difference between the pressure at which systolic sound is first audible and the point at which the systolic sound is heard consistently throughout the respiratory cycle. Pulsus paradoxus and certain other hemodynamic manifestations of pericardial tamponade depend on inspiratory augmentation of systemic venous return; as the right ventricle swells, it restricts left ventricular chamber volume. Paradox may be absent in pericardial tamponade if underlying heart disease markedly elevates left ventricular diastolic pressure or if the left ventricle fills by a mechanism independent of respiratory variation (e.g., aortic regurgitation).

Clinical Manifestations of Pericardial Tamponade

Reduced systemic arterial pressure and pulse volume, systemic venous congestion, and a small, quiet heart comprise the classic presentation of pericardial tamponade. However, other disorders, including obstructive pulmonary disease, restrictive cardiomyopathy, right ventricular infarction, massive pulmonary embolism, and constrictive pericarditis, may also present with systemic venous distention, pulsus paradoxus, and clear lungs. Hyperactivity of the adrenergic nervous system is evidenced by tachycardia and cold, clammy extremities. The most common physical findings are jugular venous distention and pulsus paradoxus. However, tachypnea may render these signs difficult to elicit.

Laboratory Evaluation

No feature of the chest radiograph is diagnostic of pericardial tamponade. Electrical (QRS) al-

ternans on the ECG in a patient with a known pericardial effusion is suggestive but not definitive evidence. (Electrical alternans also may occur with constrictive pericarditis, tension pneumothorax, severe myocardial dysfunction, and after myocardial infarction.) Adjunctive studies are needed to confirm tamponade physiology. Apart from demonstrating pericardial fluid, the echocardiogram can provide additional clues to pericardial tamponade. These include reduction of the "E to F" slope, brisk posterior motion of the intraventricular septum during inspiration, RV diastolic collapse, and exaggerated inspiratory increases and expiratory decreases in RV size. Yet, however suggestive they may be, the findings of a single echocardiographic study cannot predict the presence or severity of pericardial tamponade. Cardiac catheterization confirms the diagnosis, quantifies the magnitude of hemodynamic compromise, and uncovers coexisting hemodynamic problems. Catheterization typically demonstrates an elevated P_{RA} with a prominent systolic X descent and diminutive or absent Y descent (Fig. 1.6). There is elevation and diastolic equilibration of intrapericardial, right ventricular, and left ventricular pressures. Right ventricular diastolic pressures lack the "dip and plateau" configuration characteristic of constrictive pericarditis. Because the pressure-volume curve of the distended and liquid-filled pericardial sac is very steep, aspirating 50 to 100 mL of fluid usually leads to a striking reduction in intrapericardial pressure and dramatic improvements of systemic arterial pressure and cardiac output. Pericardiocentesis lowers the diastolic pressures in the pericardium, right atrium, right ventricle, and left ventricle and reestablishes normal pressure gradients.

Management

In pericardial tamponade, it is essential to maintain an adequate filling pressure and heart rate. Volume depletion (e.g., excessive diuresis), hypoxemia, β blockade, and other causes of bradycardia can be life threatening. Pericardial fluid can be evacuated by one of three methods: needle pericardiocentesis, pericardiotomy via a subxiphoid window (often under local anesthesia), or pericardiectomy. During pericardiocentesis, the probability of success and the safety of the procedure relate directly to the size of the pericardial effusion. Whereas partial drainage of a massive pericardial effusion may be lifesaving, aspiration of a small pericardial effusion (<200 mL) that is freely mobile within the pericardial sac may be only marginally helpful. A significant hemodynamic effect is also unusual in the absence of a documented anterior effusion or when loculated clot or fibrin inhibits the free withdrawal of fluid. Pericardiocentesis must not be undertaken by inexperienced personnel or in an inappropriate environment. Needle aspiration should be conducted whenever possible in the cardiac catheterization suite by an experienced cardiologist using fluoroscopic and needle electrode ECG guidance. Complications include coronary laceration, pneumothorax, myocardial injury, and life-threatening arrhythmias.

Subxiphoid pericardiotomy can be performed safely under local anesthesia in certain critically ill patients. This procedure often establishes effective continuous drainage of the pericardium as well as enables pericardial biopsy. In many cases, open surgical drainage may be required to definitively relieve pressure. Regardless of drainage method, successful relief of tamponade is documented by the fall of intrapericardial pressure to normal, the reduction of elevated P_{RA}, separation of right from left heart filling pressures, augmentation of cardiac output, and disappearance of pulsus paradoxus. After drainage, most patients should be monitored closely for at least 24 hours in the intensive care unit (ICU) for evidence of recurrent tamponade. Persistent elevation and equilibration of right and left ventricular diastolic pressures after pericardiocentesis or subxiphoid pericardiotomy suggest a component of pericardial constriction. Pericardiectomy may be required for patients with a component of constriction and for those who experience recurrent tamponade despite repeated needle or subxiphoid drainage.

Constrictive Pericarditis

Constrictive pericarditis results from a confining pericardial shell that prevents adequate chamber filling. Although both constriction and tamponade are characterized by elevation and equilibration of right and left ventricular diastolic pressures, they can be differentiated by several key hemodynamic features (see Table 1.4). In chronic constrictive pericarditis, an "M" or "W" contour may be formed by prominent dips in *both* systolic (X descent) and diastolic (Y descent) pressures. (The Y descent is diminutive in tamponade.) Whereas constrictive pericarditis may sometimes demonstrate atrial pressure changes reminiscent of tamponade, the right ventricular pressure contour usually shows a prominent "dip and plateau" ("square root") configuration. Pericardial constriction can be mimicked by restrictive or ischemic cardiomyopathy: in both conditions, right ventricular and left ventricular diastolic pressures are elevated, SV and cardiac output are depressed, left ventricular end-diastolic volume is normal or decreased, and end-diastolic filling is impaired. However, restrictive cardiomyopathy is more likely when marked right ventricular systolic hypertension is present and left ventricular diastolic pressure exceeds right ventricular diastolic pressure by >5 mm Hg. Differentiation between these two entities, however, may require an exploratory thoracotomy. Constrictive pericarditis should be suspected in patients with right-sided congestive symptoms. Supportive (but nondiagnostic) clinical features of constriction include a history of prior cardiothoracic trauma, acute pericarditis, or mediastinal radiation. Physical examination may reveal an early diastolic sound (knock) or mild cardiac enlarge-

TABLE 1–4

TAMPONADE VERSUS CONSTRICTION

Feature	Pericardial Tamponade	Constrictive Pericarditis
Heart size	↑ or ↑↑	↔ to ↑↑
Kussmaul's sign	Usually absent	Usually present
Pulsus paradoxus	Very prominent	May be absent
RV tracing	Prominent X descent	Dip and plateau
RA tracing	Negligible Y descent	M or W Contour
		Prominent Y descent
Pericardial fluid	Always present	May be present
Electrocardiogram	Alternans possible	Low QRS
		T-wave depression

ment. Kussmaul's sign (inspiratory augmentation of the venous pulse wave) is characteristic, but pulsus paradoxus is not. As already mentioned, the right ventricular tracing demonstrates a prominent "dip and plateau" waveform, and the venous or RA waveform shows a prominent Y descent. Common ECG findings include low QRS voltage, generalized T-wave flattening or inversion, and an atrial abnormality suggestive of P mitrale. Because constrictive pericarditis tends to progress inexorably, surgical intervention is eventually required if the patient is an otherwise appropriate candidate. Hemodynamic and symptomatic improvement is evident in some patients immediately after operation; in others, however, improvement may be delayed for weeks or months.

KEY POINTS

1. Because of differences in wall thickness and ejection impedance, the two sides of the heart differ in structure and sensitivity to preload and afterload. The normal right ventricle is relatively sensitive to changes of preload and afterload. By comparison, the normal left ventricle is comparatively insensitive to both. When failing or decompensated, both ventricles are preload insensitive and afterload sensitive.

2. Right ventricular afterload is influenced by hypoxemia and acidosis, especially when the vascular smooth musculature is hypertrophied, as in chronic lung disease. The ejection impedance of the left ventricle is conditioned primarily by vascular tone, except when there is outflow tract narrowing or aortic valve dysfunction.

3. Even when systolic function is well preserved, impaired compliance and failure of the diseased ventricle to relax in diastole can produce pulmonary vascular congestion and "flash pulmonary edema." Diastolic dysfunction often precedes signs of heart failure and commonly develops against the background of systemic hypertension or other diseases that reduce left ventricular compliance.

4. The relationship of cardiac output to cardiac filling pressure can be equally well described by the traditional Frank-Starling relationship or by the venous return curve. The driving pressure for venous return is the difference between mean systemic pressure (the average vascular pressure in the systemic circuit) and right atrial pressure. Venous resistance is conditioned by vascular tone and by anatomic factors influenced by lung expansion. Mean systemic pressure is determined by venous tone and state of vascular filling.

5. Radiographic evidence of acute heart failure includes perivascular cuffing, a widened vascular pedicle, blurring of the hilar vasculature, and diffuse infiltrates that spare the costophrenic angles. These infiltrates tend to lack air bronchograms and usually are unaccompanied by an acute change in heart size. Chronic congestive heart failure is typified by Kerley-B lines, dilated cardiac chambers, and increased cardiac dimensions.

6. The key directives in managing cor pulmonale are to maintain adequate RV filling, to reverse hypoxemia and acidosis, to establish a coordinated cardiac rhythm, and to treat the underlying illness.

7. Pericardial tamponade presents clinically with venous congestion, hypotension, narrow pulse pressure, distant heart sounds, and equalized pressures in the left and right atria. Diastolic pressures in both ventricles are similar to those of the atria.

SUGGESTED READINGS

1. Birnbaum Y, Kloner R. Clinical aspects of myocardial stunning. Coronary Art Dis 1995;6(8):606–612.
2. Bonow R, Udelson J. Left ventricular diastolic dysfunction as a cause of congestive heart failure. Mechanisms and management. Ann Int Med 1992;117(6):502–510.
3. Braunwald E. Regulation of the circulation (parts 1 and 2). N Engl J Med 1974;290:1124–1129, 1420–1425.
4. Clarkson P, Wheeldon N, MacDonald T. Left ventricular diastolic dysfunction. Q J Med 1994;87(3):143–148.
5. Dhainaut J, Brunet F. Right ventricular performance in adult respiratory distress syndrome. Eur Respir J 1990; 11(Suppl):490s-495s.
6. Donovan K, Dobb G, Lee K. Hemodynamic benefit of maintaining atrioventricular synchrony during cardiac pacing in critically ill patients. Crit Care Med 1991;19(3): 320–326.
7. Elkayam U, et al. Calcium channel blockers in heart failure. J Am Coll Cardiol 1993;22(4 Suppl A):139A-144A.
8. Federmann M, Hess O. Differentiation between systolic and diastolic dysfunction. Eur Heart J 1994;15(Suppl D): 2–6.
9. Gaasch W. Diagnosis and treatment of heart failure based on left ventricular systolic or diastolic dysfunction. JAMA 1994;271(16):1276–1280.

10. Gottdiener J. Left ventricular mass, diastolic dysfunction, and hypertension. Adv Int Med 1993;38:31–56.
11. Gropper M, Wiener-Kronish J, Hashimoto S. Acute cardiogenic pulmonary edema. Clin Chest Med 1994;15(3): 501–516.
12. Guyton A. Regulation of cardiac output. N Engl J Med 1967;277:805–812.
13. Howell J. Acute myocardial infarction and congestive heart failure. Emerg Med Clin North Am 1996;14(1): 83–91.
14. Iriarte M, et al. Congestive heart failure due to hypertensive ventricular diastolic dysfunction. Am J Cardiol 1995; 76(13):43D-47D.
15. Johnstone D, et al. Diagnosis and management of heart failure. Can J Cardiol 1994;10(6):613–631.
16. Kinch J, Ryan T. Right ventricular infarction. N Engl J Med 1994;330(17):1211–1217.
17. Klein A, Cohen G. Doppler echocardiographic assessment of constrictive pericarditis, cardiac amyloidosis, and cardiac tamponade. Cleve Clin J Med 1992;59(3):278–290.
18. Lenihan D, et al. Mechanisms, diagnosis, and treatment of diastolic heart failure. Am Heart J 1995;130(1):153–166.
19. Litwin S, Grossman W. Diastolic dysfunction as a cause of heart failure. J Am Coll Cardiol 1993;22(4):49A-55A.
20. Pagel P, et al. Left ventricular diastolic function in the normal and diseased heart. Perspectives for the anesthesiologist. Anesthesiology 1993;79(4):836–854.
21. Parmley W. Pathophysiology of congestive heart failure. Clin Cardiol 1992;15(Suppl 1):15–12.
22. Ross J. Afterload mismatch and preload reserve: a conceptual framework for the analysis of ventricular function. Prog Cardiovasc Dis 1976;18:255–264.
23. Saltissi S, Mushahwar S. The management of acute myocardial infarction. Postgrad Med J 1995;71(839): 534–541.
24. Setaro J, Cabin H. Right ventricular infarction. Cardiol Clin 1992;10(1):69–90.
25. Smith S. Current management of acute myocardial infarction. Dis Mon 1995;41(6):363–433.
26. Tardif J, Rouleau J. Diastolic dysfunction. Can J Cardiol 1996;12(4):389–398.
27. Vasan R, Benjamin E, Levy D. Prevalence, clinical features and prognosis of diastolic heart failure: an epidemiologic perspective. J Am Coll Cardiol 1995;26(7): 1565–1574.
28. Wardrop C, et al. Optimization of the blood for oxygen transport and tissue perfusion in critical care. Postgrad Med J 1992;68(Suppl 2):S2–S6.
29. Yedinak K. Use of calcium channel antagonists for cardiovascular disease. Am Pharm 1993;33(8):49–64.

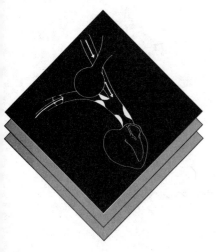

CHAPTER 2

Hemodynamic Monitoring

THE BALLOON FLOTATION (SWAN-GANZ) CATHETER

In one sense, concern for the performance or stability of the cardiorespiratory system helps define the need for intensive care. Reliable data relevant to the heart and vasculature are instrumental in diagnosing problems, in selecting and titrating therapy, and in timing interventions. However, interpreting the complex relationships among vascular pressures and flows is often complicated by spontaneous fluctuations in metabolism and by variations of the respiratory pressures that influence them.

INSERTING THE BALLOON FLOTATION CATHETER

Although detailed descriptions of insertion techniques for the balloon flotation catheter are available elsewhere, a few points are worth emphasizing here. For patients with bleeding disorders, the physician should select a site conducive to applying direct pressure. As opposed to the subclavian and femoral sites, the internal jugular approach tends to be the simplest and least fraught with complications. Several variants of the insertion point can be attempted. The right side provides more direct and reliable access to the superior vena cava than the left, but either approach can be used effectively. For puncture of the internal jugular or subclavian veins, insertion must be accomplished with the patient in the supine position, or preferably in the reverse Trendelenburg position, to ensure vessel distention, and to mini-

mize the risk of air embolism. For a dyspneic patient with orthopnea, this may require prior sedation and endotracheal intubation. If intubation is not an option, the femoral or brachial approach should be considered.

Difficult Insertion and Placement

Problems that occur during placement are generally of two types: (*a*) difficulty entering the central veins of the thorax and (*b*) difficulty directing the catheter tip into the pulmonary artery. Both types of problems can be mastered only by gaining sufficient direct experience. With regard to central vein entry, placement of the introducer/sheath assembly is the crucial step. When difficulty is encountered in locating the internal jugular vein with the probing needle, ultrasonic (Doppler) imaging can be valuable. Sheath insertion must be gentle and never forced. The stab incision made to facilitate the puncture must be sufficiently long and deep to allow easy passage of the easily collapsible and damaged sheath. At several points in the insertion process, luminal positioning of the needle or catheter should be confirmed by the ability to withdraw blood by gentle aspiration. In addition to anatomic aberrations, common reasons for difficulty encountered in floating the catheter tip to proper position include low cardiac output, severe pulmonary hypertension with right ventricular overload and tricuspid regurgitation, and massive right ventricular enlargement. The balloon should always be inflated cautiously and must fill easily, without the need for force.

When the catheter is inserted via the right inter-

RA   **RV**   **PA**   **P_W**

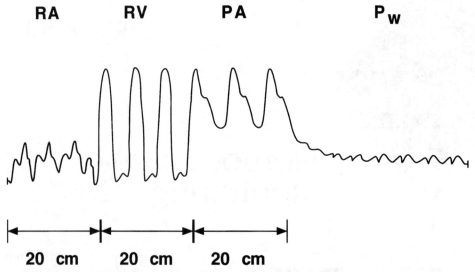

20 cm   **20 cm**   **20 cm**

FIG. 2–1. Sequence of waveforms encountered during placement of the Swan-Ganz catheter. Transitions to the right ventricle and pulmonary artery are marked by sudden changes of systolic and diastolic pressures, respectively. During insertion, the rule of "progressive 20s" applies: the right atrium generally is encountered within 15 to 20 cm of skin entry from the right internal jugular approach (slightly more from the left). The right ventricle generally is entered within 20 cm of the skin, the pulmonary artery (PA) generally is entered within 40 cm, and the wedge is encountered within 60 cm. Failure to achieve these landmarks may indicate misplacement or coiling of the catheter.

nal jugular vein, the balloon is inflated 15 cm from the point of neck entry. The catheter lip should never be advanced more than 20 cm beyond its current position before encountering the next vascular compartment (Fig. 2.1). In other words, a superior vena cava (SVC) tracing should be evident within 20 cm of skin entry and the right ventricle should be entered with far less than 40 cm of catheter. The pulmonary artery should be entered within the first 35 to 50 cm of tip advancement. Coiling within the right ventricle and misdirection of the catheter should be suspected after 45 cm has been advanced without securing an appropriate pulmonary artery (PA) waveform. After the central vein has been entered, the patient can be repositioned (lateral decubitus or Fowler's position) in an attempt to establish favorable balloon orientation and blood streaming. Fluoroscopy can be a helpful adjunct for difficult cases and is especially worthwhile to consider before attempting an insertion from the femoral site, which tends to present more placement problems than brachial, subclavian, or jugular punctures.

INTERPRETING DATA FROM THE SWAN-GANZ CATHETER

The balloon flotation catheter allows acquisition of three types of primary data: central venous, pulmonary arterial, and balloon-occluded ("wedge") pressures; cardiac output (CO) determinations; and sampling of mixed venous or postalveolar capillary blood. This information can be used in its primary form or manipulated to provide useful indices of fluid volume status, right and left ventricular performance and loading conditions, or tissue perfusion (Table 2.1).

Pulmonary Vascular Pressures

Measurement of Pulmonary Vascular Pressures

Used in conjunction with the CO, the pulmonary arterial and wedge pressures yield important

TABLE 2–1

HEMODYNAMIC DATA PROVIDED BY THE PULMONARY ARTERY CATHETER

Direct	Derived*
Cardiac output	Vascular resistance
Mixed venous O_2 saturation	Pulmonary
Vascular pressures	Systemic
Right atrium	Stroke-work index
Right ventricle	Arteriovenous O_2
Pulmonary artery	content difference
Balloon occlusion (wedge)	

* Partial listing.

diagnostic information regarding intravascular filling, the tendency for pulmonary edema formation, the status of the pulmonary vasculature, and the vigor of left ventricular contraction.

System Requirements for Accurate Pressure Measurement

Static Requirements

Zeroing   Accurate recording of intravascular pressure requires error-free measurement of static pressure and faithful tracking of an undulating (dynamic) waveform. Attention must be paid to the technical details of data acquisition to avoid error. For wedge pressure recording, for example, an uninterrupted fluid column must extend from the left atrium (LA) through the catheter lumen to the flexible diaphragm of an electromechanical transducer. The transducer membrane deforms in response to pressure exerted by the fluid column and generates proportional electrical signals for amplification and display. Because this segment of the system is fluid-filled, the vertical distance separating the LA from the transducer dome exerts a hydrostatic pressure against the membrane that adds to or subtracts from the actual (left atrial) pressure (Fig. 2.2). To eliminate bias from transducer positioning, two approaches can be taken that are variants of the same technique. In one

approach, the top of the transducer dome is placed at the LA level. The display is then adjusted to read zero pressure when the dome is closed to the patient and opened to atmosphere. In the second approach, the transducer can be placed at any convenient level. (However, the tubing length necessary to connect the transducer and catheter may impair dynamic response characteristics, setting practical limitations on the actual site of transducer placement.) As before, the fluid line is opened to atmosphere (e.g., by a stopcock held at the LA level). By adjusting the *display* to register zero pressure under those circumstances, any pressure difference developed between the transducer dome and the open stopcock is offset electronically, compensating for the hydrostatic pressure bias with an electrical one. With either method, neither the transducer level relative to the LA nor the zero offset adjustment can be changed without a new "re-zeroing" procedure.

Calibration   After the transducer is balanced ("zeroed") at the LA level, a known pressure is applied to the transducer membrane to complete the calibration. This is accomplished easily by creating an open water column (above the zeroed transducer) of known height, using the connecting tubing that links the transducer and fluid-filled

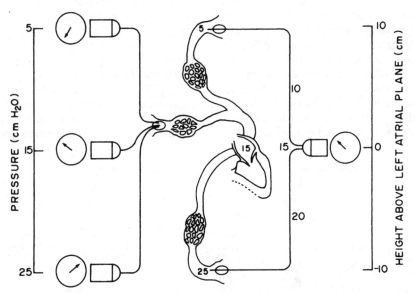

FIG. 2–2. Zeroing the transducer. The transducer must not be moved from its original position after the display has been adjusted to record zero pressure with the liquid-filled system exposed to atmospheric pressure at the left atrial level. After zeroing, a hydrostatic column influences the recorded value when the transducer is lifted or lowered from its original position (*left*). Conversely, when the transducer remains at the "zeroed" position (*right*), movement of the catheter tip makes no difference to the pressure recorded, if a continuous column of fluid extends from the left atrium through the catheter to the transducer dome.

catheter. Because the electronic display expresses pressure in mm Hg, whereas the calibrating pressure is applied in cm H_2O, an appropriate conversion must be made: 1.34 cm H_2O = 1 mm Hg, (or 0.7 mm Hg = 1 cm H_2O). A stopcock is closed to the patient, opened to atmosphere at the LA level, and lifted a known vertical distance. The electronics are then adjusted to display the pressure actually applied by the water column. This calibration can be accomplished quickly before insertion by raising the distal tip of the fluid-filled catheter (on line to the zeroed transducer) a known distance above the mid left atrium. Although automated electronic calibration is integral to many bedside monitors currently in use, the more basic procedures discussed here should be performed whenever utmost accuracy is required or the monitor's output is in doubt.

Dynamic Requirements   Whatever the components and linkages, this newly calibrated system measures static vascular pressure rather accurately, unless the catheter itself becomes kinked or occluded. However, to track dynamic pressures faithfully, the liquid-filled portions of the system must have appropriate frequency-response characteristics. These properties are the natural resonant frequency of the system and its degree of damping. Without an appropriate frequency response, the system may exaggerate or attenuate important subcomponents of complex pressure waveforms. An improperly tuned system often generates erroneous systolic and diastolic pressure values and may not allow differentiation between distorted pulmonary artery and wedge pressure tracings. Moreover, partially occluded catheters connected to "continuous flush" devices can falsely elevate mean pressures as well. Air bubbles, loose or damaged fittings, inefficient

coupling of disposable transducer domes to the sensing membrane, and excessively lengthy or compliant connecting tubing reduce the system's natural resonant frequency, blunting its ability to respond. Damping is produced by air bubbles, defective stopcocks, clot or protein debris within the catheter, impingement of the catheter tip against a vessel wall, and long, narrow, or kinked catheter tubing. Before insertion, vertically whipping the catheter tip can give a simple, qualitative indication of frequency response. After insertion, a simple check for adequate frequency response can be conducted using the rapid flush device of the catheter system (Fig. 2.3). During the rapid flush, a sustained pulse of high pressure is applied temporarily to the transducer membrane. When the flush is terminated suddenly, pressure falls abruptly. Immediately upon release, the tracing from a responsive system should overshoot (plunge below) its normal baseline and briefly (<1 second) oscillate before recovering a crisp, well-defined pulmonary arterial (PA) waveform. A poorly tuned system fails to overshoot or oscillate and recovers to a damped configuration after a noticeable delay.

Accurately calibrated strip-chart records of pulmonary vascular pressure should be examined frequently, particularly when serious diagnostic or therapeutic questions arise. Pressures must be referenced consistently to the same point in the respiratory cycle. For the wedge pressure, this is preferably at end expiration, except during very vigorous breathing when the mean value of the wedge may better reflect average transmural pressure. Influenced by fluctuations of intrathoracic pressure, electronically processed digital displays of "systolic, diastolic, and mean" pressures may be misleading, particularly during forceful or cha-

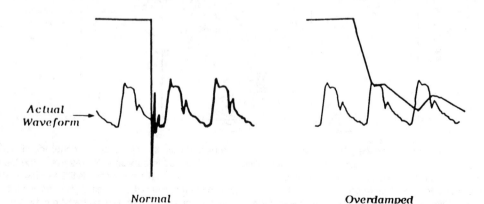

Actual
Waveform →

Normal   Overdamped

FIG. 2–3. The rapid flush test for determining the dynamic response of a catheter transducer system.

otic breathing. The strip-chart record allows the clinician to adjust for the influence of ventilatory effort. The simultaneous recording of pulmonary wedge pressure (P_w), together with airway or (preferably) esophageal pressure, greatly facilitates interpretation.

Types of Pressure Measurement All relevant information provided by the Swan-Ganz catheter should be used. Although there is an understandable tendency to concentrate on the pulmonary arterial and wedge pressures, the experienced clinician recognizes that right ventricular dysfunction often contributes to hemodynamic compromise during critical illness and therefore carefully assesses its loading and performance characteristics as well. Indeed, with current catheter technology, preload, afterload, and contractility can be monitored more directly and completely for the right than for the left ventricle.

Central Venous Pressure Central venous catheters serve a wide variety of clinical purposes. Since the first clinical use of the Swan-Ganz catheter, many physicians have considered these lines primarily as secure and predictable routes for infusing drugs, nutrients, and volume expanders; the "triple lumen" central catheters are invaluable for this purpose. However, by whatever means it is accessed, the central venous pressure (CVP) tracing should not be ignored for the hemodynamic data it provides. In the supine position, the mean CVP is virtually identical to the mean right atrial pressure, which reflects the status of right ventricular (RV) preload. When considered together with RV compliance and pleural pressure, mean CVP serves to index the preload of the right ventricle. A comparison of the central venous and wedge pressures proves helpful in diagnosing right ventricular infarction and cor pulmonale. Furthermore, the contour of the CVP tracing can indicate tricuspid regurgitation caused by right ventricular overload, suggest pericardial restriction and tamponade, or detect the cannon waves of A-V block. Flutter waves evident on the CVP *pressure* tracing sometimes can be detected when the surface electrocardiogram is inconclusive. In the absence of lung or heart disease, CVP serves well to indicate the degree of circulatory filling (e.g., during acute gastrointestinal (GI) hemorrhage). Central venous pressure is a primary component of the systemic vascular resistance calculation.

Interpreted in conjunction with the wedge pressure, CVP can be used to estimate fluctuations in transmural filling pressure. Because the superior vena cava is a flaccid structure embedded in the pleural space, fluctuations in CVP crudely reflect changes in intrapleural and pericardial pressures. It has been suggested that the CVP tracks changes in pleural pressure well enough that the transmission fraction of alveolar pressure to the pleural space can be computed under passive inflation conditions as follows:

Transmission fraction

$$= (CVP_{EI} - CVP_{EE})/(P_{PLAT} - P_{EX})$$

where CVP_{EI} and CVP_{EE} are the end-inspiratory and end-expiratory values of CVP, and P_{PLAT} and P_{EX} are the corresponding static airway pressures recorded during occluded airway (stopped flow) maneuvers. Although the wedge pressure also can be used in this way, respiratory fluctuations in P_w (and estimated transmission fraction) may be exaggerated under non-zone-3 conditions (see below). Sudden and disproportionate elevations of CVP with respect to wedge pressure accompany pulmonary embolism with clot or air, right ventricular infarction, or acute lung disorders (bronchospasm, aspiration, pneumothorax).

Pulmonary Artery Pressure The right ventricle (RV) generates the systolic pulmonary arterial pressure (P_{PA}) in forcing the cardiac output through the pulmonary vascular network against resistance. Because the difference between mean arterial and venous pressures drives flow, P_{PA} can be made to rise by increasing the downstream venous pressure (as in LV failure), the cardiac output, or the flow resistance (as in primary lung diseases). With its large capillary reserve, the normal pulmonary vascular bed offers little resistance to runoff. Consequently, pulmonary artery diastolic pressure (P_{PAD}) seldom exceeds LA pressure by more than a few mm Hg, even when flow is increased. Obliteration of pulmonary vascular channels, however, increases resistance, obligating a larger gradient of pressure. Under these conditions, P_{PAD} may substantially exceed the pressure within pulmonary veins and left atrium. Just as importantly, the lack of recruitable vasculature reduces the compliance reserve that normally buffers P_{PA} against fluctuations in cardiac output. Consequently, major variations in P_{PA} often attend changes in output or vascular tone, making P_{PAD} an unreliable index of LV filling in serious lung disorders. The pulmonary vascular network is designed to accept large (fivefold to 10-fold) variations in CO without building sufficient pressure across the delicate endothelial membrane to cause interstitial fluid accumulation and alveolar flooding. Therefore, the RV normally develops only enough power to pump against modest impedance. As a rule, the normal RV cannot sustain acute loading to mean pressures >35 mm Hg without decompensating. Over long periods, however, as during a protracted course of acute respiratory distress syndrome (ARDS), the RV strengthens and P_{PA} builds. Indeed, the height to which P_{PA} is forced to rise may be a useful prognostic index, correlating inversely with outcome. Given adequate time to adapt to massively increased afterload, systemic levels of arterial pressure can be sustained. After the pulmonary vascular reserve is exhausted, an additional obliteration or narrowing by embolism, hypoxia, acidosis, or infusion of vasoactive drugs may evoke a marked pulmonary pressor response. Such elevations of hydrostatic pressure may cause fluid leakage, even across precapillary and postcapillary vessels. It is certainly possible, therefore, that hydrostatic pulmonary edema can form even when LA and pulmonary venous pressures (reflected by the wedge) remain within the normal range, especially if the serum oncotic pressure is low.

Pulmonary Arterial Occlusion (Wedge) Pressure   Balloon inflation encourages the catheter tip to migrate from a main pulmonary artery into a smaller caliber vessel, where it impacts and wedges. With the distal catheter orifice isolated from P_{PA}, fluid motion stops along the microvascular channels served by the occluded artery (Fig. 2.4). Because no resistive pressure drop occurs along this newly created static column, the pressure at the catheter tip equilibrates with the pressure at the downstream junction ("j" point) of flowing and nonflowing venous blood. It is believed that this junction normally occurs in a vessel of a size similar to that of the occluded artery—that is, in a large vein. Pulmonary wedge pressure, therefore, provides a low-range estimate of the mean hydrostatic pressure within the more proximal fluid-exchanging vessels. (When resistance in the small veins is high, P_w may not accurately reflect the true tendency for edema formation.) Pulmonary capillary pressure is seriously underestimated when mean P_{PA} substantially exceeds P_w. As a crude approximation, the pressure relevant to fluid filtration across the pulmonary vessels generally exceeds P_w by about 40% of the difference between the mean pulmonary arterial and wedge pressures (Fig. 2.5).

The validity of the P_w measurement rests on the assumption that the occlusion of a major vessel by

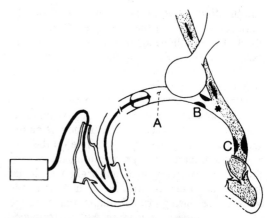

FIG. 2–4. Definition of a wedge pressure (P_w). The P_w, measured at point A, is nearly identical to the pressure at the junction of static and flowing venous blood (*). P_w will not be influenced by partial occlusions of the static column (B) that extends from the catheter tip to the junction. However, obstructions (C) downstream of the junction point dissipate pressure, causing P_w to significantly exceed mean P_{LA}. Although generally in a large pulmonary vein, the junction point may reside in a small pulmonary venule in certain disease states.

the balloon does not reduce the total blood flow through the lungs. This is not always a good assumption when the pulmonary vascular reserve is limited—as after pneumonectomy. In these circumstances, balloon inflation can detrimentally afterload the right ventricle, potentially reducing pulmonary blood flow and P_w during the measurement. Because large pulmonary veins are inherently low-resistance vessels, P_w usually deviates little from P_{LA}. Mean P_{LA}, in turn, closely approximates left ventricular end-diastolic pressure (P_{LVED}) in the absence of mitral valvular obstruction or incompetence or markedly reduced ventricular compliance. Because P_{LVED} is the intravascular pressure component that determines preload, P_w not only provides a low-range estimate of the hydrostatic pressure in the pulmonary venous circuit but, when interpreted in conjunction with an estimate of extramural pleural pressure (e.g., by esophageal balloon), it also gives some indication of presystolic LV fiber stretch.

Obtaining a Valid Wedge Pressure   Unfortunately, a number of technical and physiologic factors encourage errors of data acquisition as well as misinterpretation of recorded values (Table 2.2). The validity of P_w as a measure of pulmonary venous pressure depends on the existence of open vascular channels connecting the LA with the

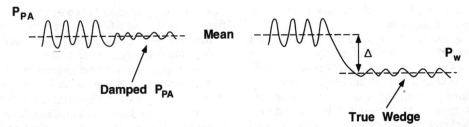

FIG. 2–5. Distinguishing a damped pulmonary artery pressure (P_{PA}) tracing from a true wedge pressure (P_w) during balloon inflation. The mean pressure of a damped P_{PA} tracing should approximate that of the undamped P_{PA} waveform recorded with the balloon deflated (*left*). A true wedge pressure is distinguished by a mean pressure that is substantially lower ($\triangle$) than that of the P_{PA} (*right*).

transducer. However, microvessels exposed to interstitial and alveolar pressures separate the catheter tip from the downstream j point. Because these vessels are collapsible, the interrelation between alveolar gas and fluid pressures governs the patency of the vascular pathway.

Zoning Conceptually, the upright lung can be divided into three zones, viewing the pulmonary vascular network as a variable (Starling) resistor vulnerable to external compression by alveolar pressure (Fig. 2.6). These zones theoretically extend vertically, because regional vascular pressures within the lung are affected by gravity, unlike the uniform gas pressure within the alveoli. In zone 1, near the apex of the upright lung, alveolar pressure exceeds both P_{PA} and pulmonary venous pressure, flattens alveolar capillaries, and stops flow. In zone 2, alveolar pressure is intermediate between P_{PA} and pulmonary venous pressure, so that flow in this region is determined by the arterial-alveolar pressure gradient. In zone 3, near the

lung base, alveolar pressure is less than either vein or artery pressures and does not influence flow. Inflation of the catheter balloon isolates downstream alveoli from P_{PA}. To sense pressure at the j point, the catheter tip must communicate with the pulmonary veins via a channel in which vascular pressure exceeds alveolar pressure. Intuitively, it would seem that only in zone 3 could patent vascular channels remain open to connect the catheter lumen and the LA. Outside zone 3, alveolar pressure would exceed pulmonary venous pressure, collapsing the capillaries in those re-

TABLE 2–2

CHECKLIST FOR VERIFYING POSITION OF PULMONARY ARTERY CATHETER

	Zone 3	Zone 1 or Zone 2
Respiratory variation of P_w	$<\frac{1}{2}\Delta P_{alv}$	$>\frac{1}{2}\Delta P_{alv}$
P_w contour	Cardiac ripple	Unnaturally smooth
Catheter tip location	LA level or below	Above LA level
PEEP trial	$\Delta P_w < \frac{1}{2}\Delta$ PEEP	$\Delta P_w > \frac{1}{2}\Delta$ PEEP
P_{PAD} versus P_w	$P_{PAD} > P_w$	$P_{PAD} < P_w$

LA, left atrium; PEEP, positive end-expiratory pressure.

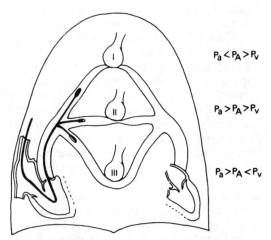

$P_a < P_A > P_v$

$P_a > P_A > P_v$

$P_a > P_A < P_v$

FIG. 2–6. Perfusion zones of the lung and their influence on the recorded wedge pressure. Ascending vertically in the lung, arterial (P_{PA}) and pulmonary venous (P_{PV}) pressures decline relative to alveolar pressure (P_A), which remains uniform throughout the lung. In both zones 1 and 2, P_A exceeds P_{PV} during balloon occlusion, collapsing alveolar vessels. Wedge pressure provides a valid measure of pulmonary venous pressure, only when a continuous fluid column connects the catheter tip with the left atrium (e.g., zone 3).

gions and forcing P_w to track fluctuations in alveolar pressure rather than P_{LA}.

Although conceptually valid, it is now clear that this simple scheme does not always apply. If a portion of the capillary bed in communication with the occluded catheter tip extends below the LA reference level, the hydrostatic column extending down to those vessels will raise their intraluminal pressure sufficiently to maintain a patent channel, even when the tip of the catheter lies at the level of zone 2. Alveolar pressure will not collapse these lowermost vessels until it exceeds P_{LA} plus this hydrostatic pressure (often 5–10 cm H_2O). Moreover, zone 3 conditions tend to be reestablished at end exhalation, even if alveolar distension collapses the capillary bed at the higher lung volumes prevailing during the remainder of the tidal respiratory cycle. Thus, "zoning" is not usually a problem with positive end-expiratory pressure (PEEP) up to 10 cm H_2O, even in patients with nearly normal lungs. This problem seldom occurs so long as the catheter tip lies at or below the level of the LA (its usual position). Furthermore, densely infiltrated or flooded alveoli may protect the patency of vascular channels despite an unfavorable relationship between pulmonary venous pressure and the pressure within gas-filled alveoli. (Shunted blood is not exposed to aerated alveoli.) When a zoning artifact does arise, lateral decubitus positioning can be used to place the catheter tip in a dependent position relative to the left atrium, effectively converting the wedged region from zone 2 to zone 3.

During spontaneous breathing in the supine position, most lung vessels normally remain in zone 3 throughout the respiratory cycle. The extent of zones 1 and 2 will increase when alveolar pressure rises relative to pulmonary venous pressure as during hypovolemia or mechanical ventilation. Because PEEP both augments alveolar pressure and reduces venous return, its application tends to diminish the span of the zone 3 region. Catheter tip positioning in a vertical plane higher than the LA further increases the likelihood of zoning artifacts. A catheter wedged outside zone 3 will show marked respiratory variation and an unnaturally smooth waveform (Table 2.2). In the absence of overt RV overload and failure, the respiratory fluctuation in P_w—influenced by alveolar pressure—will substantially exceed that of the CVP. Although a marked rise in P_w during the respiratory cycle suggests zone 3 positioning, a valid P_w may still be restored at end exhalation as already noted. However, a change in end-expiratory P_w greater than one-half of an applied change in PEEP strongly suggests that end-expiratory P_w reflects alveolar, not left atrial, pressure.

Overwedging Even when the catheter tip is well positioned, asymmetric balloon inflation or transverse orientation of the catheter axis relative to that of the vessel lumen can artifactually elevate P_w ("overwedging") by isolating the catheter tip from the vascular lumen. Often, the catheter is too peripheral. When this occurs, the blind pocket of fluid bounded by the balloon and vascular wall continues to receive inflow from the continuous flushing system, forcing an elevation of the recorded pressure baseline. The overwedged P_w eventually exceeds mean P_{PA}, an event without logical physiologic interpretation. (Such a pressure gradient situation would imply retrograde flow.) Under these circumstances, the balloon should be deflated and the catheter should be gently flushed and repositioned, if necessary.

Wedge Pressure as a Measure of Hydrostatic Filtration Pressure The pressure within the large pulmonary veins, the presumed j point, has long been regarded as a good reflection of the mean pressure within the fluid-filtering vessels. It was believed previously that the small capillaries were the only vessels to conduct significant fluid exchange with the interstitium and that very little pressure drop occurred beyond the capillary level. However, both assumptions now seem doubtful; extra-alveolar vessels clearly participate actively in fluid exchange. Furthermore, as much as 40% of the pulmonary vascular resistance may reside within the capillaries and small veins. It is therefore likely that P_w seriously underestimates the mean filtration pressure under certain conditions. (During permissive hypercapnia, for example, pulmonary vascular resistance rises, with a disproportionate increase occurring in the resistance of the small pulmonary veins. Pulmonary veno-occlusive disease characteristically causes pulmonary edema in the face of a normal P_w.) Such discrepancies may help to account for hydrostatic edema occurring in the face of normal wedge pressure and presumably intact vascular endothelium. Furthermore, the j point may sometimes occur in a small vein (for example, when an underinflated catheter tip wedges within a small pulmonary artery). Under these circumstances, considerable resistance may be interposed between the j point and the LA, leading to a discrepancy between these two pressures. A P_w–P_{LA} discrepancy has been reported to develop in the setting of endotoxemia or sepsis, conditions known to be associated with pulmonary venous constriction.

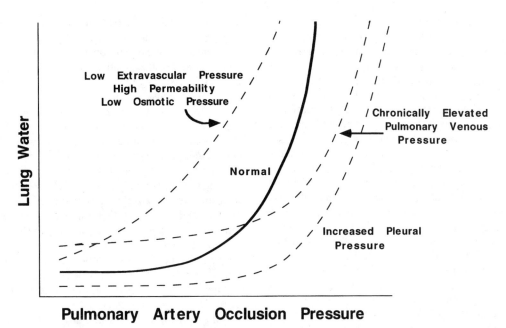

FIG. 2–7. Relationship of lung water to pulmonary artery occlusion pressure for a variety of clinical conditions. Normally, the curve relating lung water to pulmonary artery occlusion pressure (P_w) demonstrates a sharp upward inflexion as P_w exceeds 20 to 25 mm Hg. Leakage is enhanced by high vascular permeability (e.g., ARDS), low serum osmotic pressure, and low extravascular pressure (as during forceful inspiratory effort). Conversely, a high P_w may be well tolerated without excessive lung water accumulation if pleural pressure is increased or if pulmonary venous pressure is elevated chronically.

When P_w is used to estimate the hydrostatic contribution to edema formation, four additional factors should be considered: chronicity of the pathologic process, extravascular pressure, plasma oncotic pressure, and endothelial permeability (Fig. 2.7). Over time, compensatory mechanisms for evacuation of interstitial fluid (e.g., improved lymphatic drainage) may allow high pulmonary venous pressure without frank edema; P_w can be elevated chronically in mitral valvular disease despite a clear chest radiograph. Extramural pressure undoubtedly varies along the length of the filtering segment. For example, recruited capillaries are imbedded within the alveoli, whereas derecruited capillaries and larger filtering vessels may be surrounded by pressures similar to or lower than the mean pleural value. Normal interstitial pressures also vary somewhat across the horizontal plane extending from the hilum to the lateral aspect of the visceral pleura. Moreover, the heterogeneous mechanics of the diseased lung undoubtedly intensify such regional variations, and the magnitude of these variations must fluctuate dramatically in different phases of the tidal ventilatory cycle. Because the hydrostatic gradient across the fluid-exchanging vessels is the difference between intravascular pressure (estimated by P_w) and extravascular pressure, pulmonary edema can form at a normal P_w if the interstitial pressure is reduced sufficiently by markedly negative pleural pressures (for example, during acute reexpansion edema, asthma, or strangulation). Very negative interstitial pressures can be produced locally during the normal ventilation cycle when there is persistent regional microatelectasis adjacent to freely expanding alveoli. Conversely, edema may not form at high pleural pressures (PEEP, auto-PEEP), despite marked elevations of P_w. Therefore, it is wise to interpret P_w in light of possible alterations of intrathoracic and interstitial pressures. One rational but imprecise method is to approximate the change in interstitial pressure to be the change in pleural pressure, measured or estimated at the same point in the respiratory cycle.

An important role for plasma oncotic pressure is predicted by the classic Starling equation that describes transvascular fluid exchange. Capillary oncotic pressure is reduced by the hypoproteinemia of cirrhosis, malnutrition, nephrosis, or the administration of excessive crystalloid. When the ratio of plasma/interstitial protein concentration falls, pulmonary edema forms at a lower transvascular pressure, especially when then the lung is acutely injured. Gross edema formation due to hypoproteinemia alone is unusual when the serum colloid osmotic pressure exceeds P_w by more than 4 mm Hg but is increasingly likely at lower values. Although clearly contributory in many settings, reduced plasma oncotic pressure alone rarely explains edema in the face of normal hydrostatic pressures and an intact capillary membrane.

As already noted, endothelial permeability is a major factor governing the influence of P_w on lung water accumulation. Unlike the curve relating P_w to edema formation when permeability is normal, the steep relationship between these variables exhibits no distinct point of inflection when permeability is increased. Thus, there does not seem to be a "safe range" of rising P_w values over which accelerated edema formation can be avoided completely; when the lung is injured, even small changes in P_w greatly influence the tendency for alveolar flooding.

Wedge Pressure as a Measure of Left Ventricular Preload When afterload and contractility are held constant, end-diastolic muscle fiber length (preload) determines stroke volume. Over brief periods, fiber length parallels ventricular volume, and diastolic ventricular volume is a joint function of myocardial distensibility (compliance) and the net transmural ("inside" minus "outside") pressure stretching the ventricle. Just as extravascular pressure must be considered when judging the hydrostatic tendency for fluid filtration, transmural pressure is the effective force distending the heart. The intracavitary pressure at end-diastole (P_{LVED}) pushes the ventricle outward from within and is helped or hindered by the extramural pressure surrounding the heart (approximated by pleural pressure). Mean left atrial pressure (P_{LA}) closely approximates P_{LVED}, except at high filling pressures ($P_{LVED} > 20$ mm Hg) or in the presence of mitral valve obstruction. In this upper range, atrial systole may boost P_{LVED} significantly above P_{LA}. As a close estimate of P_{LA}, P_w is used clinically to judge the intracavitary filling pressure of the LV and, thereby, to monitor preload.

The other pressure determinant of precontractile fiber stretch, pleural pressure (P_{pl}), varies continuously throughout the respiratory cycle. Pulmonary wedge pressure must be interpreted cautiously, with attention directed toward the fluctuations in P_{pl} that influence its transmural

value. Although P_{pl} is seldom measured directly, changes in P_{pl} can be measured noninvasively with an esophageal balloon catheter. When the signal quality of the esophageal pressure (P_{es}) has been validated (e.g., by recording equivalent pressure deflections during spontaneous efforts against a transiently occluded airway), referencing P_w to esophageal pressure provides an acceptable monitor of changes in LV transmural pressure under most conditions, independent of P_{pl} fluctuation. Under the influence of mediastinal weight, the balloon only senses local pressure and measures neither absolute global pleural pressure nor the mean pressure that surrounds the entire left ventricle. The fiber length achieved by any specific transmural pressure depends on ventricular compliance. Unfortunately, ventricular compliance is rarely known with precision and can change abruptly. The LV and RV are made interdependent by sharing muscle fibers, the septum, and the pericardial sac. Thus, the LV can stiffen when the RV distends in response to changes in pulmonary vascular resistance or volume loading. Ischemia, inotropic drugs, and circulating catecholamines can also produce abrupt but reversible reductions in diastolic compliance. Shrinkage of RV chamber size, relief of ischemia, removal of adrenergic stimulation and the administration of nitroglycerin or nitroprusside produce the opposite (muscle relaxing) effects.

A balloon flotation pulmonary artery catheter is currently available to track right ventricular volume and ejection fraction by thermodilution. Quite recently, a reliable double indicator dilution (thermodilution/dye) system for tracking central blood volume and lung water also has been developed that seems capable of rendering information of potential clinical and research value. The impact on medical practice of either innovation, however, remains to be determined.

Compensating for Elevated Pleural Pressure
Positive End-Expiratory Pressure (PEEP) Regardless of the mode of chest inflation, end exhalation often provides a convenient reference point for P_w interpretation because during quiet breathing, P_{pl} normally returns to its resting baseline. End-expiratory P_{pl} can exceed its normal value when the expiratory musculature actively contracts, tension pneumothorax is present, or when elevated airway pressure at end exhalation increases lung volume (PEEP, auto-PEEP). If PEEP is applied intentionally and exhalation is passive, the relationship between the compliances of the

lung (C_l) and chest wall (C_{cw}) determines the resulting elevation in pleural pressure:

$$P_{pl} = PEEP \times [C_l/(C_l + C_{cw})].$$

For the patient with normal lungs and chest wall, end-expiratory P_{pl} increases by ~$\frac{1}{2}$ of the applied PEEP during passive inflation because C_l and C_{cw} are similar over the tidal volume range. However, under conditions of reduced lung compliance and normal chest wall compliance (e.g., many cases of ARDS), the "transmitted" fraction may be one-quarter of the PEEP value or even less. Thus, if a PEEP of 14 cm H_2O (10 mm Hg) is applied to the airways of a patient with ARDS, P_{pl} and P_w at end exhalation should both increase by ~2.5 mm Hg. (As discussed below, these simple rules cannot be applied during active expiratory efforts.) Some clinicians seek to avoid confusion by discontinuing PEEP transiently and measuring P_w under conditions of ambient end-expiratory pressure. Because venous return usually increases when PEEP is interrupted, a low P_w measured off PEEP should indicate that intravascular filling pressures on PEEP are not excessive. Nonetheless, hemodynamic conditions often change rapidly and unpredictably after PEEP discontinuation, and a P_w in the middle or high range is questionable. When auto-PEEP is present, total PEEP and therefore P_w may not change noticeably after PEEP disconnection unless the next ventilatory breath is also delayed. Lengthy discontinuation of PEEP may also cause oxygenation to deteriorate for some patients with severe lung injury or edema.

The lowest ("nadir") wedge pressure obtained within 1 to 3 seconds of ventilator disconnection has been shown experimentally to reflect the transmural P_w that occurs on PEEP. It is believed that any tendency for increasing venous return during disconnection cannot affect pressures in the pulmonary vasculature for several seconds. This principle is less likely to apply when the lung deflates slowly, as during dynamic hyperinflation in severe airflow obstruction. Although this technique has not been validated adequately in the clinical setting, its simplicity and theoretical rationale are attractive for use in carefully selected patients.

Auto-PEEP (Intrinsic PEEP) When insufficient time is allowed between ventilatory cycles for the chest to deflate to its relaxed volume, airflow continues across critically narrowed airways throughout exhalation, driven by an alveolar pressure higher than airway opening pressure. This results in an occult "auto-PEEP" (intrinsic PEEP) effect at the alveolar level. Auto-PEEP is most likely to occur in patients with airflow obstruction who require high minute volumes, but because the endotracheal tube and exhalation valve are highly resistive elements, it can also develop at any time minute ventilation is significantly elevated—even for normal subjects. Inverse ratio ventilation and high frequency ventilation are other settings in which high levels of auto-PEEP can be encountered. Compliant lungs and stiff chest walls (e.g., obesity, burns, abdominal surgery, ascites) transmit a high percentage of alveolar pressure to the pleural space, producing large fractional increases in P_{pl} and P_w (in the setting of severe airflow obstruction this is often one-half or more of the auto-PEEP value). Unless accounted for, auto-PEEP encourages overestimation of intravascular volume and inappropriate therapy. Although unmeasured during normal ventilator operation, the auto-PEEP level is detectable by the simple bedside maneuver of expiratory port occlusion at the end of passive exhalation (Fig. 2.8).

Active Exhalation Active exhalation and chaotic breathing present other difficult problems in the interpretation of the wedge pressure. For spontaneously breathing patients with airflow obstruction, expiratory effort adds to the recorded "auto-PEEP" value. Vigorous expiratory muscle contraction often elevates end-expiratory P_{pl} during acute respiratory distress of any etiology. Large respiratory fluctuations of P_w (>10 mm Hg) should alert the clinician to this possibility. When the respiratory variation of P_w exceeds 10 mm Hg, the end-expiratory P_w exceeds the postparalysis value in direct (almost 1 for 1) proportion to the respiratory variation observed. During active breathing, the mean wedge pressure averaged over the entire tidal cycle may be a better indicator of the true ventricular filling pressure than the end-expiratory P_w when a reliable estimate of pleural pressure is not available. In theory, the effect of vigorous breathing can be overcome by recording P_{es} simultaneously or by giving short-acting muscle relaxants during the measurement. Silencing respiratory efforts, however, dramatically alters hemodynamic status and may mask any diastolic dysfunction that occurs under the stress (and increased LV afterload) of vigorous breathing. It does, however, give some indication of whether diuresis is indicated. (A high P_w under passive conditions suggests the potential for hydrostatic edema during active breathing.) Even when transmural P_w can be computed with cer-

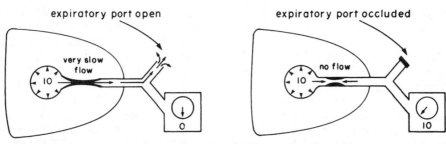

FIG. 2–8. The auto positive end-expiratory pressure (auto-PEEP) affect and its measurement. In the presence of severe airflow obstruction and high ventilation requirements, alveolar pressure at end exhalation remains elevated as flow continues throughout expiration, driven by the recoil pressure of the hyperexpanded lung (*left*). Transiently stopping flow at end exhalation equalizes pressure throughout the lung and ventilator circuit (*right*). Occult alveolar pressure is then detectable by the ventilator.

tainty, effective preload is difficult to estimate without knowledge of the myocardial pressure-volume relationship.

The Fluid Challenge Uncertainty concerning LV compliance is a major reason why absolute P_w values do not track LV volume or preload accurately in the setting of critical illness. Except when the calculated transmural P_w is very high or very low, decisions regarding fluid therapy of a patient in an oxygenation or perfusion crisis are often best made by an empirical trial of rapid volume loading (a fluid challenge). Pulmonary wedge pressure, systemic blood pressure, cardiac output, heart rate, and the physical examination are monitored before and after a rapid infusion of physiologic saline or colloid. A fluid bolus (50–200 mL) is administered over 5 to 20 minutes, depending on the suspected cardiovascular fragility of the patient. If hemodynamic variables improve with little change in the measured P_w, administration of additional volume is prudent. Conversely, marked increases of heart rate or P_w (>5–7 mm Hg), together with marginal improvement in blood pressure and cardiac output, indicates that increasing the rate of volume infusion risks pulmonary edema with little hemodynamic benefit.

Cardiac Output Determination

Measurement

Fick Principle In clinical practice, cardiac output can be estimated by measuring thoracic impedance, or more commonly and reliably, by an indicator–dilution method. In its simplest form, the primary basis for cardiac output determination, the Fick principle, can be explained as follows: The quantity of any marker contained within a static volume is the product of that volume and its concentration. Classically, a dye detectable by spectrophotometry (e.g., indocyanine or "cardio" green) that binds to plasma protein has been used as the indicator. In a dynamic system into which a marker is added continuously and lost, the introduction rate of the marker is the product of flow rate and its concentration difference across the region of loss. In the steady state, no net addition or loss of the marker occurs. For example, if arterial oxygen is being consumed by the body and replenished by the lungs at equal rates, the VO_2 is the product of cardiac output and the O_2 concentration difference between systemic arterial and mixed venous (pulmonary arterial) blood. Therefore, if the O_2 consumption rate is known or estimated readily, determining the O_2 contents in systemic and pulmonary arterial blood samples allows calculation of the flow rate (cardiac output). Under non-steady-state conditions, however, these calculations can be wildly erroneous.

Thermodilution A similar principle applies during determinations of cardiac output by thermodilution, in which the marker that is injected and dissipated is thermal deficit, or "cold," and its rate of disappearance as it is diluted by the warm venous blood is an indication of blood flow. Although all PA catheters can provide a sample of mixed venous blood for use in an oxygen-Fick determination, thermodilution capability allows more convenient, repeatable, and precise measurement of forward blood flow. A sensitive, rapidly responding thermistor bonded to the catheter tip continuously senses temperature, altering its electrical resistance in response to thermal changes within PA blood. As a side benefit, the thermistor provides a highly reliable, continuous readout of core body temperature. When a bolus of cold fluid enters the right atrium (RA), it mixes with warm venous blood returning from the periphery. The churning action of the right ventricle (RV) homogenizes the two fluids, and the thermistor records the dynamic thermal curve generated when the mixture washes past the proximal PA. The relationship linking output to temperature is the Stewart-Hamilton formula:

$$Q = V (T_B - T_I) K_1 K_2 / T_B(t)dt$$

where Q = cardiac output; V = injected volume; T_B = blood temperature; T_I = injectate temperature; $T_B(t)dt$ = change in blood temperature as a function of time; and K_1 and K_2 are computational constants. The components of the numerator are either known constants (V, K_1, K_2) or measured values (T_B, T_I). The denominator is the area beneath the time–temperature curve, derived by computer integration of the thermistor signal. When close attention is paid to the method of data acquisition, thermodilution CO values compare favorably with those obtained by the steady state O_2 Fick method and by dye dilution.

Technical Considerations and Potential Errors

Thermistor Position   Except for a few rather obvious exceptions, most technical errors in cardiac output determination result in overestimates of the true value. To generate a valid estimate of output, the thermistor should sample a well-mixed cold charge of known strength and must lie freely within the lumen of the central pulmonary artery. Impaction against a vessel wall or encapsulation by clot tends to insulate the thermistor from the cool stream, falsely elevating the reported value. A P_{PA} waveform that appears damped or wedged may indicate malpositioning and potential problems. It is good clinical practice to inspect the temperature–time profile periodically, especially when the value conflicts with the rest of the clinical picture, when extreme variability is encountered among serial estimates, or when another question of temperature accuracy exists. A valid curve shows a rapid early descent to a trough value, smoothly returning to baseline within 10 to 15 seconds of injection. Distorted curves should alert the clinician to inadequate blending of injectate with blood, thermistor contact with the wall of the vessel, abnormal respiratory patterns, and arrhythmias or abrupt changes in heart rate. Information from irregular curves should be discarded.

Injectate Volume and Temperature   Icing the injectate accentuates the thermal difference between marker and blood, increasing signal strength. Although icing theoretically enhances output accuracy and reproducibility, the excellent sensitivity of the thermistor/computer systems currently available allows the use of room temperature injectates without appreciable loss of accuracy. Room temperature injectates do not require the 45-minute equilibration period necessary to complete cooling; maintenance of proper injectate temperature is facilitated and errors induced by rewarming during handling are minimized. Furthermore, bradycardia and atrial arrhythmias during injection occur rarely. Although 10-mL injectate volumes are often used with room temperature injectates, 5-mL volumes (with appropriate computer adjustment) can be used with acceptable results when frequent measurements introduce a significant danger of volume overload. Seriously hypothermic patients, however, require the larger volume for an acceptable signal-to-background ratio. Whatever volume is chosen for injection, syringes should be filled carefully; variation in injected volume contributes significantly to measurement error. The crystalloid fluid chosen for injection—saline or dextrose—does not materially influence the output calculation. When completed within 4 seconds, the speed of injection has little influence on outcome; automated, gas-powered injectors offer no convincing advantage over manual technique.

Respiratory Variation   The temperature of PA blood tends to vary throughout the respiratory cycle, particularly during mechanical ventilation. Although it has been suggested that injection be timed to begin consistently at a single point in the ventilatory cycle, the need for this practice is controversial. One logical compromise is to obtain at least three injections spaced equally along the respiratory cycle and to average the results.

Catheter–Computer Mismatch   Coefficients vary widely with the volume and temperature of the injectate and the type of catheter used. Mismatching should be suspected when measured CO does not fit well with the clinical picture, particularly when catheters of varied manufacture are used with the same computer.

Anatomic Variation   Thermodilution values for CO are usually accurate when computational constants are entered correctly, the catheter is well positioned, and appropriate injection technique is used. However, such non-operator-dependent variables as intracardiac shunting, incompetence of the tricuspid valve, or thermistor malfunction due to thermal shielding by wall contact or clot may compromise validity. Errors can also result from inadvertent augmentation of the cold charge by concomitant rapid administration of intravenous fluids near the right atrium.

Clinical Interpretation of Cardiac Output

Important diagnostic information regarding the functional status of the heart and the vasculature often can be obtained by combining measures of CO and ventricular filling pressure. The fluid challenge is particularly helpful for this purpose. However, CO must be interpreted in relation to the mass and the metabolism of the patient. A CO of 3 L/min may suffice for the needs of a hypothermic, cachectic 40-kg patient, but the same CO may be associated with a circulatory crisis in a previously healthy 100-kg burn victim. The cardiac index (CI; cardiac output/surface area) is used to adjust for variations in tissue mass. Body surface area (BSA) can be determined from standard nomograms or can be approximated by this regression equation:

$$BSA = 0.202 \times Wt^{0.425} \times Ht^{0.725}$$

where BSA is expressed in square meters, weight (Wt) is expressed in kilograms, and height (Ht) is expressed in meters. Used alone, however, even the CI is of limited help in assessing perfusion adequacy. Over a broad range, any given value for CI may be associated with luxuriant, barely adequate, or suboptimal tissue O_2 transport, depending on hemoglobin concentration, metabolic requirements, and blood flow distribution. Measures of urine output and metabolic acid production (anion gap, serum lactate) together with indices of tissue O_2 use (e.g. O_2 extraction) provide better guides of perfusion adequacy.

Indices of Vascular Resistance The CO measurement can be used in conjunction with pulmonary and systemic pressure measurements to compute the vascular resistance values needed to gauge ventricular afterload and diagnose the etiology of a hypotensive crisis. These indices of vascular resistance complement mean systemic blood pressure in guiding vasodilator and vasopressor therapy. Pulmonary vascular resistance (PVR) and systemic vascular resistance (SVR) are crude indices, calculated as if blood flow fulfilled the assumptions of Poiseuille's law for laminar flow:

$$PVR = (P_{\overline{PA}} - P_w)/CO \text{ and}$$

$$SVR = (MAP - P_{RA})/CO$$

where CO = cardiac output, MAP = mean systemic arterial pressure, $P_{\overline{PA}}$ = mean pulmonary artery pressure, and P_{RA} = mean right atrial pressure.

Although PVR and SVR are used commonly in the clinical setting, vascular resistance calculations should be referenced, preferably to body surface area, using the cardiac index (instead of cardiac output). The resulting values, the systemic (SVRI) and pulmonary (PVRI) indices, avoid the misleading variations of the raw parameters with body size. Significant elevations of PVRI virtually always indicate underlying lung pathology, reflecting the interplay of constrictive and occlusive forces on a compromised pulmonary capillary bed. Unfortunately, however, the complex relation between PVR and CO often confounds physiologic interpretation. Changes in the PVRI should be evaluated with full awareness that the PVRI is output dependent. In computing PVR, it must be kept in mind that when the pulmonary vascular bed is compromised, resistance may vary as a function of blood flow. In fact, the magnitude of the PVR, as well as its response to an intentional change in cardiac output, may serve as a useful prognostic index in such acute lung diseases as ARDS (Fig. 2.9). Failure of PVR to rise in response to a boost in cardiac output suggests ample reserve; a sharp increase in PVR that parallels cardiac output indicates extensive obliteration of the pulmonary vascular bed. SVR may rise homeostatically to high values in support of suboptimal cardiac output, helping to maintain an appropriate perfusion pressure across vital capillary beds. However, an excessive elevation of SVR can impair the performance of weakened left ventricle.

Oxygen Delivery One of the most useful applications for cardiac output data is the management of hypoxemia. Because tissues attempt to extract the amount of oxygen required to maintain aerobic metabolism, the mixed venous O_2 tension falls when O_2 delivery (the product of CO and arterial O_2 content) becomes insufficient for tissue needs. If the fraction of venous blood shunted past the lung remains unchanged, arterial O_2 tension may fall precipitously as this abnormally desaturated blood is blended with postcapillary blood from better ventilated lung units. Thus, depressed CO values may contribute to hypoxemia, and variations in cardiac output may sometimes explain otherwise puzzling changes in arterial O_2

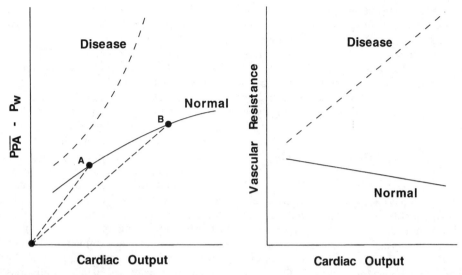

FIG. 2–9. Relationship of cardiac output to the pressure difference driving flow across the pulmonary vasculature ($P\overline{_{PA}} - P_w$) and pulmonary vascular difference. The relationship of $P\overline{_{PA}} - P_w$ to cardiac output does not pass through the origin so that computed values of pulmonary vascular resistance (the slope of this relationship) seem to fall as cardiac output rises in normal subjects. In disease, the relationship of driving pressure to flow is highly curvilinear and, therefore, pulmonary vascular resistance (PVR) may appear unchanged or rising. Calculating pulmonary vascular resistance on the basis of *changes* in ($P\overline{_{PA}} - P_w$) and cardiac output (e.g., slope AB) helps eliminate these interpretive difficulties.

tension. As a primary determinant of O_2 delivery, CO measurements often prove helpful during selection of the appropriate PEEP level for the patient with life-threatening hypoxemia. Depression of venous return coincident with PEEP application may nullify any beneficial effect of improved pulmonary gas exchange on tissue O_2 delivery (see Chapter 9).

Sampling of Mixed Venous Blood

Oxygen Supply and Demand

Analysis of mixed venous blood provides valuable information in evaluating the oxygen supply–demand axis. Blood flow to individual organs (e.g., the kidney) is not governed precisely by metabolic rate, so that venous O_2 content varies widely among sites. Normally, blood from the inferior vena cava is more fully saturated than blood from the superior vena cava. During shock states, however, the converse often occurs. Samples drawn from either of these central vessels or from the incompletely blended pool within the RA are not entirely representative of the true mixed venous value. Blood withdrawn from the proximal pulmonary artery, however, has been blended in the right ventricle and is therefore more appropri-

ate for analysis. Care should be taken to withdraw blood slowly, with the balloon deflated and the catheter tip positioned in the proximal pulmonary artery. Otherwise, contamination from the post-capillary region may artifactually increase the oxygen content.

The value of mixed venous blood analysis is best understood in the framework of tissue O_2 demand–supply dynamics. Briefly, the product of CO and arterial oxygen content defines the overall rate of O_2 delivery. Each organ receives a variable percentage of the total amount, a flow that may be luxuriant, just adequate, or insufficient to satisfy its aerobic metabolic demand. The O_2 tension (PvO_2) and saturation (SvO_2) of the venous effluent reflect the balance between supply and need. When flow does not rise to meet increased tissue demands, more O_2 is extracted from each milliliter of capillary blood, and PvO_2 and SvO_2 fall. Conversely, when the O_2 transport/demand ratio increases, the arteriovenous oxygen difference narrows and PvO_2 and SvO_2 rise. PvO_2 and SvO_2 may not reflect serious perfusion deficits if arterial blood is anatomically or functionally shunted past metabolizing tissue. For example, in cirrhosis, cyanide poisoning, or the early phases of sepsis, non-nutritive flow may cause SvO_2 to be normal or high, despite serious tissue hypoxia.

Because of these distribution and use pitfalls, it is always wise to compute the anion gap and monitor lactate simultaneously. When sustained, low venous O_2 tensions more reliably signal anemia or an impending perfusion crisis. Reduced flow and diminished arterial O_2 concentration (due to reductions in SaO_2 or hemoglobin) depress effective O_2 transport, encouraging lower values for PvO_2 and SvO_2.

Uses and Limits of Mixed Venous O_2 Saturation

The mixed venous oxygen saturation correlates with survival in acute myocardial infarction, acute respiratory failure, and shock. As O_2 delivery is reduced from the normal level without a matching change in O_2 demand, tissues initially compensate by maintaining oxygen consumption (VO_2) at the expense of a falling SvO_2 (i.e., from tissue oxygen extraction ratio: $(SaO_2 - SvO_2)/(SaO_2)$ (Fig. 2.10). However, beyond a certain critical value of O_2 delivery, the O_2 extraction mechanism reaches the limits of compensation, SvO_2 stabilizes, and VO_2 becomes delivery dependent. Once this critical value is reached, SvO_2 becomes an insensitive monitor of changes in perfusion. Such delivery dependence has been demonstrated both in experimental animal models of acute lung injury and in certain clinical settings. Below this critical value of O_2 delivery, anaerobic metabolism must supplement aerobic mechanism. The SvO_2 at which

this limit occurs varies, depending on whether delivery was reduced by anemia, arterial hypoxemia, or falling CO.

Despite the importance of PvO_2 as a global indicator of end-capillary tissue O_2 tension, PvO_2 can vary with alterations in the affinity of hemoglobin for O_2, even when O_2 content remains stable. Therefore, direct assessment of SvO_2 is the preferred index for clinically evaluating the oxygen-perfusion axis; estimation of SvO_2 from PvO_2, pH, and temperature is fraught with error because of the steepness of the O_2 tension–saturation relationship. Traditionally, SvO_2 has been determined on individual blood samples analyzed by laboratory instruments that measure SaO_2 by transmission oximetry (co-oximeter) or O_2 content by fuel cell determination. The application of fiberoptic reflectance oximetry to the balloon flotation catheter has enabled continuous bedside monitoring of SvO_2. O_2 saturation rises when blood is withdrawn past the wedged fiberoptic tip, facilitating the distinction between wedged and damped P_{PA} tracings. (This feature also may help to avoid tissue infarction consequent to inadvertent distal migration of the catheter.) Continuous measurement of SvO_2 also speeds the process of determining the optimal PEEP level, because alterations in net tissue O_2 flux are made apparent quickly.

Changes in SvO_2 have no unique interpretation and must be viewed in light of the variables that determine O_2 transport and demand—the amount and distribution of CO, hemoglobin concentration and function, arterial O_2 tension, and metabolic rate. Although a change in SvO_2 does not indicate which of the multiple factors comprising the Fick equation is responsible, integration of SvO_2 with clinical observations, blood gas information, and cardiac output data often establishes an early, if presumptive, diagnosis (Fig. 2.11). Declining values for SvO_2 and CO, together with unchanging PaO_2, imply hemodynamic deterioration, whereas a rising CO with a falling SvO_2 are consistent with increased metabolic demand or acute loss of circulating blood. Initial experience with the fiberoptic catheter as an on-line monitor has underscored the rapidity with which SvO_2 responds to transient changes in metabolism or altered O_2 delivery. Sensitivity to such changes is undoubtedly enhanced when the heart is unable to raise its output sufficiently in response to stress. Then, SvO_2 must reflect altered arterial oxygenation or increased O_2 demand, undampened by the buffering effect of cardiac compensation. Such wide

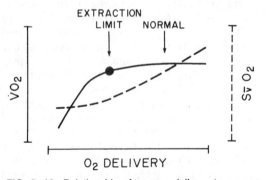

FIG. 2–10. Relationship of oxygen delivery to oxygen consumption ($\dot{V}O_2$) and to the saturation of mixed venous blood ($S\bar{v}O_2$). As oxygen delivery is reduced from the normal value (for example, by reducing cardiac output), metabolic demand remains unchanged. Increased extraction initially can maintain oxygen consumption, at the cost of a falling $S\bar{v}O_2$. At some critical level of oxygen delivery, the limits of extraction are reached, forcing $\dot{V}O_2$ to become delivery dependent.

DETERMINANTS OF S$\bar{v}$O$_2$

$$\dot{V}O_2 \quad = \quad \dot{Q}(C_aO_2 - C_{\bar{v}}O_2)$$

$$\dot{V}O_2 \quad \alpha \quad \dot{Q}\,Hgb\,(SaO_2 - S\bar{v}O_2)$$

$$S\bar{v}O_2 \quad \alpha \quad SaO_2 - \dot{V}O_2/\dot{Q}\,Hgb$$

FIG. 2–11. Determinants of mixed venous oxygen saturation. Oxygen consumption ($\dot{V}O_2$) is a product of cardiac output ($\dot{Q}$) and the oxygen content difference between arterial and mixed venous blood (CaO$_2$ − S$\bar{v}$O$_2$). Hemoglobin concentration (Hgb) and saturation (SaO$_2$, (S$\bar{v}$O$_2$) determine blood oxygen content. Therefore, the saturation of mixed venous blood (S$\bar{v}$O$_2$) is determined by four interacting variables: a decrease in S$\bar{v}$O$_2$ can be caused by reductions in SaO$_2$, $\dot{Q}$, or Hgb or by an increase in $\dot{V}O_2$. Changes in any one of these determinants can be nullified by an offsetting change in another. For example, if metabolism changes, $\dot{V}O_2$ and $\dot{Q}$ can fall or rise in proportion to one another, leaving S$\bar{v}$O$_2$ unchanged.

fluctuations may help to explain why SaO$_2$ often varies markedly in the absence of convincing clinical improvement or deterioration. From initial clinical experience, it seems that SvO$_2$ often falls in advance of detectable changes in the primary hemodynamic variables, and a downward trend may alert the clinician to intervene. A decline in SvO$_2$ may be the first indication of occult bleeding, incipient pump failure, or impending cardiac arrest. Conversely, an increasing SvO$_2$ may signal the onset of sepsis. A growing literature documents rapid and convincing changes in SvO$_2$ accompanying drug therapy (vasopressors, vasodilators, sedatives), intravascular volume manipulation (diuresis, fluid infusion, transfusion), position shifts, and ventilatory changes. Although fiberoptic oximetry has a distinct physiologic rationale and seems to be a useful adjunct to pulmonary artery catheterization, the clinical value of these instruments is still debated.

Gastric Mucosal pH

Measurements of total body oxygen consumption ($\dot{V}O_2$) can now be made with relative ease. Unfortunately, the $\dot{V}O_2$ alone gives little guidance as to its adequacy in meeting tissue oxygen demands, except when the value is extremely low and accompanied by other confirmatory indicators of hypoprofusion. Measurements of mixed venous oxygen saturation and content, interpreted in conjunction with similar data from arterial blood may suggest adequacy or inadequacy of tissue oxygen delivery. Again, however, these data are influenced by blood flow distribution and the ability of the tissues to extract oxygen. In sepsis, for example, nearly normal values of both arterial and mixed venous oxygen saturation may accompany lactic acidosis and shock. No single indicator now in routine clinical use reflects perfusion status in all vital tissues.

Recently there has been enthusiasm for monitoring the pH of the gastric mucosa (gastric tonometry) to provide such essential information. There are two reasons for this enthusiasm. First, the measurement is relatively easy to make using a specialized balloon-tipped catheter (or, according to some reports, by direct analysis of gastric juice obtained via a standard nasogastric tube). Second, unlike skeletal muscle, the intestinal tract tolerates hypoxemia poorly, so the gastric mucosal pH may provide an index of oxygenation in a region of the body that is among the first to initiate anaerobiosis during hypoprofusion and the last to restore normal perfusion after resuscitation.

When conditions are favorable, equilibration seems to be established between luminal and mucosal PCO$_2$. When bicarbonate concentrations are known, intramucosal pH can therefore be calculated from the tonometrically measured PCO$_2$ of the saline within the balloon. These assumptions cannot be made with confidence, however, if acid enters and bicarbonate refluxes from the duodenum, if the patient receives enteral feeding that refluxes into the stomach, or if the stomach is aspirated continuously by a sump tube.

Numerous reports currently in the medical literature suggest the clinical potential of gastric tonometry as an early warning of dysoxic stress and promote its consideration during the management of shock, ARDS, intestinal ischemia, and congestive heart failure. Certain studies suggest that gastric tonometry can provide useful information regarding the prediction of intensive care unit (ICU) mortality and tolerance to attempted weaning from mechanical ventilation. Despite its considerable potential as a sentinal index of dysoxic stress, however, its widespread use cannot yet be recommended. Appropriate interpretation, limitations, and relative advantages of this technique over more standard management practices for assessing perfusion adequacy are still being investigated and debated.

COMPLICATIONS OF THE SWAN-GANZ CATHETER

The Swan-Ganz catheter should never be inserted without a firm indication, and, once inserted, the data must be interpreted skillfully. Misguided decisions resulting from the misinterpretation of data may be the most prevalent serious "complication" of the technique.

In addition to any harm caused by errors in the acquisition or interpretation of data, the complications of pulmonary artery catheterization may arise during insertion, during manipulation of the catheter, and as a result of its residence within the central vascular structures (Table 2.3).

Insertion-Related Complications

Catheter-Related Arrhythmias

Premature atrial and ventricular contractions occur commonly during insertion of the Swan-Ganz catheter, especially when the patient is predisposed to them. Failure to inflate the balloon adequately, slow passage of the catheter through the heart, and insertion of an excessive length of catheter are likely contributors. Special caution should be exercised if the patient is hypoxemic or has an electrolyte disturbance at the time of instrumentation. Complete heart block has been reported to follow insertion of the Swan-Ganz catheter in patients with preexisting conduction system disease because transient right bundle branch block occurs commonly during this procedure. Although the risk is probably not as great as once feared, it is advisable to have a temporary pacemaker available before inserting the catheter in a patient with preexisting left bundle branch block.

Catheter Malpositioning

Experience is the most important determinant of successful catheter placement. Although often difficult and time consuming, vascular access should never require forceful insertion. The clinician must be thoroughly familiar with the pressure tracings that arise from the various cardiovascular structures encountered and should not violate the "rule of progressive 20s" (Fig. 2.1).

Knotting and Fragmentation

Catheter knotting can occur, especially when the catheter is extensively manipulated, an excessive length is inserted, the heart is dilated, or the balloon is not fully inflated during passage. Knotting is most likely to be detected upon attempted catheter withdrawal. The same is true for catheter fragmentation and meteorism. Care to avoid forceful insertion or removal, withdrawal of the catheter through a needle, and cutting of the catheter during wire exchanges generally will prevent this serious complication.

Pulmonary Infarction

Pulmonary infarction is distressingly common. Persistent wedging of the catheter tip or dislodgement of clot formed on the catheter is the most likely explanation. Infarction occurs rarely when the catheter is well positioned (tip within the main pulmonary artery) and the balloon requires its maximum volume (1.25–1.5 mL) for inflation to the wedge position.

Pulmonary Artery Rupture

Pulmonary artery rupture can cause fatal hemoptysis. Several factors predispose pulmonary artery perforation: advanced age, hypothermia, and pulmonary hypertension. Overinflation of a catheter balloon in a small pulmonary artery is the most likely mechanism. Therefore, the balloon should never be inflated abruptly, and inflation should be stopped immediately when there is evidence either of the approach to the wedge position or overwedging. Advancing the catheter tip without balloon inflation should never be undertaken.

Although a variety of therapeutic measures have been suggested (such as the application of PEEP, deliberate balloon inflation, positioning with the catheter with its tip side down), their efficacy is not proven. Maintenance of the airway and support of the circulation are the first priorities, as for any patient with severe hemoptysis.

Complications Related to Long-Term Catheterization

Thrombosis

Although thrombosis around the catheter at its insertion site or at various points along the catheter occurs commonly, serious consequences are seldom encountered. However, thrombosis at or near the insertion site may result in subclavian vein thrombosis, superior vena caval syndrome, or internal jugular vein occlusion. The indwelling

TABLE 2–3

COMPLICATIONS OF THE PULMONARY ARTERY CATHETER

Complication	Cause	Prevention
Arrhythmia	Catheter coiling or excess catheter in RV Catheter tip reentry RV from PA Hypoxemia, coronary ischemia, electrolyte disturbances	ECG monitoring Follow the "rule of 20s" Expedient catheter passage Reverse hypoxemia, electrolyte disturbance Prophylaxis vs. ischemia
Complete heart block	Preexisting left bundle branch block	Temporary pacer on standby
Catheter malpositioning Extracardiac	Forceful insertion	Advance only with caution Consider fluoroscopy
Catheter knotting	Excessive catheter length Extensive manipulation Dilated heart	Follow the "rule of 20s" Do not insert more than 15 cm into the PA Consider fluoroscopy in difficult cases Inflate balloon fully during insertion
Catheter fragmentation and meteorism	Forceful insertion or removal Withdrawal across needle Cutting catheters for wire exchanges	Avoid forceful catheter insertion and withdrawal Follow recommended instructions for insertion Avoid cutting catheter during exchanges
Pulmonary infarction	Persistent wedging of a distally positioned catheter Prolonged balloon occlusion	Wedge with maximal balloon volume (1.25–1.5 mL) Maintain catheter tip in main PA Maintain balloon occlusion for a maximum of 15 seconds Catheter withdrawal if persistent wedge or damped PA tracing Recheck tracings carefully 30–60 minutes after insertion and after patient repositioning Ensure balloon deflation post wedging
Pulmonary artery rupture	Catheter advancement with uninflated balloon Balloon inflation in a distal pulmonary artery Eccentric balloon inflation Balloon inflation with liquid Pulmonary hypertension	Advance catheter only with balloon inflated Slowly inflate to wedge position only with continuous PA monitoring Stop inflation immediately when PA pressure rises or falls significantly during occlusion Limit wedge measurement to 15 seconds Do not flush distal lumen when wedged Maintain catheter in central PA Position catheter to accept >1.25 mL for wedge Inflate balloon only with air Minimize the number of wedge pressures attempted
Thrombosis	Predisposition to clotting	Continuous flush Limited duration of catheter placement
Vascular infection	Prolonged catheterization (>72–96 hours)	Remove catheter when no longer needed Strict attention to sterile technique Frequent inspection of insertion site Remove catheter if persistent fever or bacteremia is detected

ECG, electrocardiogram; PA, pulmonary artery; RV, right ventricle.

catheter also may result in platelet consumption or pulmonary emboli or in right-sided valvular damage. These complications seldom rise to the level of clinical significance in most patients.

Infection

Any indwelling catheter may produce serious infection. The pulmonary artery occlusion catheter is no exception. With strict attention to sterile insertion technique and meticulous care of all catheter lines, stopcocks, transducers, and infusions, most Swan-Ganz catheters can be used for more than 72 hours without serious infectious complications. The incidence of infection tends to rise thereafter. If the local site looks uninflamed and the patient remains afebrile, a catheter can remain in place for 5 days or more without serious risk. Many practitioners, however, change Swan-Ganz catheters over guide wires at approximately 96 hours, but there is no set standard in this regard.

Whenever the patient is febrile or septic, blood cultures should be obtained and the catheter should be removed if it seems to be the most likely source. Assuming that the local site does not appear to be infected, some practitioners insert a fresh Swan-Ganz catheter without changing the site of insertion. This practice, however, is controversial. If the local site seems suspicious, the introducer must be removed, along with the catheter, and a fresh site must be selected (assuming that the catheter is still required).

ECHOCARDIOGRAPHY, RADIONUCLIDE VENTRICULOGRAPHY, AND OTHER IMAGING TECHNIQUES

Neither echocardiography (ECHO) nor radionuclide ventriculography (RVG) provide continuous information and therefore cannot properly be considered true monitoring techniques. However, each has an important place in characterizing the nature of cardiac pathology in the ICU. These methods allow the physician to answer specific diagnostic questions and to categorize the overall structure and performance of the heart as well as to estimate chamber dimensions. In a sense, they can be considered complementary to Swan-Ganz and arterial monitoring.

ECHOCARDIOGRAPHY

General Principles

Echocardiography provides a valuable bedside method for the noninvasive assessment of cardiac function. The ECHO probe both emits a high frequency (1–10 MHz) rapidly pulsed ultrasonic signal and receives its acoustic reflection. These data are then integrated to form an interpretable image. Three different ECHO techniques have been introduced into clinical practice: M-mode, which provides a one-dimensional view of the heart; real time or sector scanning, in which a two-dimensional, dynamic view is produced; and Doppler echocardiography, a technique to quantify blood flow velocity and estimate intravascular pressures. The ejection fraction of the left ventricle can be approximated adequately, but right ventricle performance is assessed less reliably because of its irregular (noncylindrical) geometry. More recently, transesophageal echocardiography has provided high resolution images of regions of the heart that were previously difficult to examine and has given good cardiac images of patients in whom transthoracic (surface) echocardiography is severely limited (obese, hyperinflated). Echocardiography is noninvasive, inexpensive, rapidly performed, and diagnostic in a wide variety of valvular, myocardial, and pericardial disorders. Ambiguity and limited resolution are its most important limitations. Because the ultrasound signal is attenuated by fat and reflected by air–tissue boundaries, ECHO is of limited value for patients with obesity or obstructive lung disease. Chest wall deformities, dressings, and occlusive coverings often prevent optimal transducer positioning. Transesophageal echocardiography may require ventilatory support in patients with cardiorespiratory failure. Skilled technical support and an experienced interpreter are essential for optimal results.

Types of Echocardiogram

M-Mode Echocardiography

M-mode echocardiography provides a one-dimensional "ice pick" view through the heart, forming images from sound reflected along the narrow axis of the beam. M-mode examines the movements of a well-defined tissue core over time. Broad structures lying perpendicular to the ECHO axis reflect the acoustic beam efficiently and are well delineated. The anterior and posterior ventricular walls, intraventricular septum, aortic root, and valve leaflets (particularly the anterior mitral valve) are represented clearly. Conversely, the pulmonic and tricuspid valves are more difficult to visualize; thickening, vegetations, or abnormal motions of the aortic and mitral valve are detected frequently, whereas those of the pulmonic or tricuspid valves are often missed. Although rapidly approaching clinical obsolescence, M-mode echocardiography adequately tracks the selected axis during various phases of the cardiac cycle. Because only a single axis or view can be obtained at any particular instant, M-mode is distinctly inferior to real-time two-dimensional echocardiography for detecting valve or wall motion abnormalities. M-mode usually allows accurate measurement of isolated chamber dimensions, but its narrow sampling window may not accurately reflect the anatomy of the entire atrium or ventricle. Similarly, loculated pericardial effusions, pleural fluid collections contiguous to the pericardial surface, and small intraventricular defects may be missed entirely.

Two-Dimensional Echocardiography

Two-dimensional (real-time) ECHO is the best technique for examining ventricular wall and valve motion. Because two-dimensional ECHO provides a wider field of view than M-mode, any process localized to a segment of the pericardium or myocardium is better seen (e.g., loculated pericardial fluid, small ventricular septal defects, and small left ventricular aneurysms). Diastolic as well as systolic performance of the left heart (and, to a lesser extent, the right heart) can be evaluated. The regional wall motion abnormalities of recent or remote myocardial infarction are well defined. Superior resolution and the ability to delineate valve motion make two-dimensional ECHO superior to M-mode ultrasound for examining right-sided cardiac valves and for detecting mitral prolapse and vegetations. Two-dimensional ECHO is also the preferred technique for calculation of valve area.

Transesophageal Echocardiography

Transesophageal echocardiography (TEE) uses a miniaturized ultrasound transducer inserted into the esophagus via an endoscope to obtain high resolution echocardiographic images. Although TEE is limited by the need to perform endoscopy, frequently it reveals details of valvular motion, diastolic left heart function, chordae abnormalities, and small valvular vegetations missed by surface echocardiography. Transesophageal ECHO imaging is an accurate means of diagnosing aortic dissection, atherosclerosis, and aortic trauma. It is more reliable than transthoracic two-dimensional ECHO for this purpose. Transesophageal echocardiography also offers advantages for patients with

a body habitus that prevents surface echocardiographic imaging, most notably obese patients and those with hyperinflation of the chest.

Doppler Echocardiography

Doppler echocardiography deduces velocity of moving blood by interpreting changes in the frequency of reflected sound waves. Either M-mode or two-dimensional ECHO can be used in conjunction with Doppler technology to estimate cardiac output or flow across a valvular orifice. After valve area is determined and blood velocity is known, flow may be calculated. In many (but certainly not all) patients, pulmonary arterial pressure also can be estimated. Thus, Doppler echocardiography potentially provides a means for estimating cardiac output noninvasively. Pressures in various cardiac chambers may also be inferred from Doppler flow estimates. Finally, Doppler echocardiography helps detect the regurgitant jets of blood characteristic of valvular insufficiency.

Specific Diagnostic Problems

Investigation of Pericardial Effusion and Tamponade

Investigation of pericardial effusion and tamponade is a common use of ECHO in the ICU. Although optimal studies may detect effusions of 25 to 50 mL, delineation of such small pericardial effusions can be difficult, especially when pleural effusions coexist. Normally, the epicardium and pericardium are closely apposed, with only slight separation occasionally seen in systole. Accumulated pericardial fluid separates these two structures throughout both phases of the cardiac cycle. Small amounts of fluid in the pericardial sac pool posteriorly in patients in the supine position and can be missed easily. Two-dimensional is superior to M-mode echocardiography for detecting small amounts of pericardial fluid. In such cases, visualizing the left atrium may be revealing. (Pericardial fluid rarely accumulates behind the left atrium for anatomic reasons.) When larger effusions accumulate, diagnosis becomes much easier because fluid collects anteriorly as well as posteriorly in the pericardial space. When pericardial effusions become very large, the heart may swing to and fro within the sac, producing artifactual wall motion and apparent abnormalities of mitral and tricuspid valve function. The diagnosis of pericardial effusion commonly is missed by ECHO when there is fibroadhesive pericardial disease, simultaneous pleural effusion, or massive left atrial enlargement. The diagnosis of tamponade is a clinical one that cannot be made solely by ECHO criteria. Tamponade physiology may be suspected, however, when a large pericardial effusion is present or when the right atrial or ventricular cavities show intermittent collapse. Evidence of decreased flow through the mitral valve during inspiration and relatively enlarged right ventricular dimensions are also suggestive.

Paradoxical Embolism

Echocardiography also may be used in the ICU to detect intracardiac shunts in patients with refractory hypoxemia or suspected paradoxical embolism. In such cases, the contrast injected is either an echo dense dye or (more commonly) an intravenous fluid containing microbubbles (e.g., agitated saline or sonicated 5% human albumin). In such testing, the acoustic contrast agent is introduced by vein while the ECHO transducer probes the left heart chambers. If a right-to-left cardiac shunt is present, there is prompt appearance of acoustic noise in the left atrium or ventricle shortly after injection. (The legs are used preferentially for such injections because right atrial streaming patterns favor crossing of the contrast material into the left heart.) Although this ''bubble'' technique has relatively high specificity for right-to-left shunt, it lacks the sensitivity of angiographic dye injections. The sensitivity of TEE substantially exceeds that of surface techniques for detection of intracardiac shunts.

NUCLEAR CARDIOLOGY

Nuclear medicine techniques have a very limited place for imaging the heart in critically ill patients. Thallium and technetium scanning detect areas of reversible cardiac ischemia and acute myocardial infarction, respectively. (Both tests are discussed in Angina and Myocardial Infarction, Chapter 21.) Radionuclide ventriculography (RVG) uses radiolabeled red blood cells to define the boundaries of the heart and track changes in its volume. Images may be obtained immediately after injection (single pass scanning) or, more frequently, after a period of equilibration (gated ventriculography). In gated ventriculography, multiple images are acquired at various phases of the cardiac cycle by coupling the detector to an electrocardiography (ECG) trigger. Comparing ven-

tricular volume (count density) during diastole and systole allows calculation of the relative change in ventricular volume resulting from ventricular contraction—the ejection fraction. Ventricular size, contour, and segmental wall motion also may be assessed. Unfortunately, RVG does not visualize the atria or details of valvular anatomy. Radionuclide ventriculography has been proven useful for patients who demonstrate changes in ejection fraction or wall motion during ischemia induced by exercise or provocative pharmacologic agents (e.g., dobutamine); ischemic myocardium becomes dysfunctional and occasionally paradoxic in its motion. ECG-gated RVG studies require a relatively regular ventricular rhythm for computerized data collection. Therefore, patients with atrial fibrillation or frequent premature atrial or ventricular beats are poor candidates for this study. In most instances, RVG also must be performed outside the ICU, necessitating patient transport.

ARTERIAL BLOOD PRESSURE MONITORING

THE ARTERIAL PRESSURE WAVEFORM

Normally, mean arterial pressure (MAP) is similar in all large arterial vessels of a supine subject; there is only a slight pressure gradient between aortic and radial vessels. Posture-related hydrostatic increases of pressure are shared equally between arteries and veins so that perfusion pressure is little affected. Although MAP is largely the same throughout the arterial tree, waveform contours differ with the caliber of the arterial vessel in question. Peak systolic pressure actually rises in the periphery, due to wave reflection. When a vessel is totally occluded by a monitoring catheter, wave reflection may amplify pressure fluctuations to produce sharp spikes of systolic arterial pressure (to over 300 mm Hg in some cases) (Fig. 2.12). Depending on the shape of the arterial pressure waveform, the peak systolic (P_S) and nadir diastolic (P_D) pressures contribute to varying degrees to MAP. At normal heart rates (60–100 beats/min) $MAP \approx P_D + \frac{1}{3}(P_S - P_D)$. (During tachycardia, P_S contributes relatively more, and during bradycardia, it contributes relatively less.) The diastolic pressure, therefore, clearly is the most important contributor to MAP. It is important to remember that pressure imperfectly indexes flow: unlike pressure, flow is largely con-

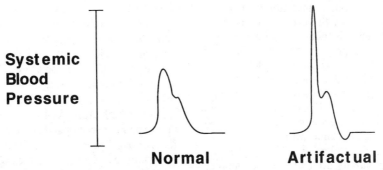

FIG. 2–12. Artifactual elevation of systolic arterial pressure. An underdamped arterial pressure tracing amplified by reflection within an occluded artery may exaggerate the systolic pressure and any mean pressure computed from the raw "systolic" and diastolic pressure values.

tinuous and not pulsatile. More importantly, the ability of any specific gradient between arterial and venous pressures to perfuse tissue depends directly on the resistance of the vascular bed. A MAP of 60 mm Hg may produce luxuriant flow through a widely vasodilated vascular bed, whereas a MAP of 100 mm Hg may be inadequate during accelerated hypertension.

INVASIVE ARTERIAL PRESSURE MONITORING

Indications

The decision to initiate invasive arterial monitoring must be undertaken cautiously. Many critically ill patients can be monitored adequately by intermittent sphygmomanometry (manual or automated). Patients with hemodynamic instability or shock, malignant hypertension, or failure to oxygenate are most likely to benefit from arterial cannulation. A well-adjusted catheter system provides accurate pressure information necessary for hemodynamic monitoring and facilitates blood sampling, often obviating the need for venipuncture.

Although convenient and usually reliable, indwelling arterial catheters occasionally give misleading information—especially when the radial artery has been cannulated for an extended time. Errors are most likely to arise in patients who are elderly, hypotensive, or with underlying vascular disease. An attempt should be made at least once daily to confirm the line pressure by sphygmomanometry. This is especially important for patients receiving vasoactive drugs regulated by radial line pressures. When the cuff-derived value and clinical impression disagree seriously with the

recorded value (generally in the direction of indicating greater pressure than the catheter records), consideration should be given to measuring femoral pressure.

Complications

Serious complications can arise due to local hemorrhage, infection, and thrombosis. (For this reason, the radial artery of the nondominant arm should be used whenever possible.) Although common, regional thrombosis of the radial artery seldom results in tissue-damaging ischemia; digital embolization is the greater hazard. Large catheter size, low cardiac output, preexisting arteriopathy, absence of collateral perfusion, and vasopressors increase the risk. (Artery caliber tends to parallel wrist size.)

The Allen test is performed by raising the wrist well above the heart level and compressing the radial and ulnar arteries simultaneously for 10 seconds, blanching the capillary bed. When the ulnar artery is then released, flushing should occur within a few seconds. Although a positive Allen test (see below) is reassuring, it does not preclude the development of ischemic damage after radial artery thrombosis.

A 20-gauge Teflon catheter is preferred for arterial measurements and sampling because it facilitates insertion, minimizes risk of thrombosis, and tends to exhibit the best dynamic frequency response. (Larger catheters occlude the vessel, creating standing waves; smaller gauge catheters tend to kink or clot off.) Rarely, the arterial catheter may erode the vessel wall to cause aneurysm, localized hematoma, compressive neuropathy, or arteriovenous fistula. Although local colonization is very common, serious soft tissue infections are rare during percutaneous cannulation if the puncture site is kept sterile, the catheter is used for only a few days, and precautions are taken during blood sampling to preserve sterility. Femoral catheters and "cutdowns" are most likely to cause infection. The radial artery is not an appropriate site for injection of any drug. Intra-arterial injections of certain drugs, particularly calcium channel blockers and vasopressors, can cause ischemic necrosis of the hand, which is a functionally devastating injury. Prolonged, high pressure flushing can potentially drive clot or gas bubbles retrograde to produce cerebral embolism.

NONINVASIVE ARTERIAL PRESSURE MONITORING

Sphygmomanometer pressures are notoriously inaccurate when cuff width is less than two-thirds of the arm circumference. Artifactual elevations of blood pressure (BP) occur when measurements are made with an inappropriately narrow cuff and when arteriosclerosis prevents the brachial artery from collapsing under pressure. Conversely, because tight proximal occlusions can artifactually lower the blood pressure, BP should be checked initially in both arms. As noted above, it is always wise to compare readings obtained from an arterial line with a cuff pressure periodically and whenever the monitored number disagrees with the clinical impression. In many hypotensive patients with low cardiac output, the "muffle" and disappearance points of diastolic pressure are poorly audible. In shock, all Korotkoff sounds may be lost. In this setting, Doppler ultrasonography may detect systolic pressures below the audible range.

KEY POINTS

1. Before using hemodynamic information derived from catheter measurements, the transducer system must be zeroed and calibrated. The dynamic pressure response of the catheter–transducer system should be checked by the rapid flush technique.

2. As opposed to a damped PA tracing, a true wedge pressure is significantly less pulsatile and has a value less than the mean PA pressure.

3. All pulmonary artery pressures are influenced, to varying degrees, by fluctuations in pleural pressure. Respiratory fluctuations of pleural pressure are conditioned by the alveolar pressure transmission fraction: $C_L / (C_L + C_w)$. Major respiratory fluctuations in P_w may cause the end-expiratory wedge pressure value to exceed the relaxed value. During active breathing, the mean, nadir, and postparalysis wedge pressures reflect left ventricular filling and pulmonary vascular pressures better than the traditional end-expiratory wedge pressure.

4. The fluid challenge is a key maneuver in determining hemodynamic reserves. During the fluid challenge, the clinician notes symptoms, physical signs, cardiac output, blood pressure, wedge pressures, and PA pressure in response to a fluid bolus. A notable improvement in key target variables (cardiac output, systemic blood pressure) without the development of symp-

toms or excessive cardiac filling pressures encourages the physician to increase the rate of fluid administration.

5. The complete hemodynamic profile should include sampling of mixed venous blood, a comparison of central venous and pulmonary artery wedge pressures, and calculations of systemic vascular resistance and pulmonary vascular resistance. Without such information, adequacy of cardiac output and mechanisms of hemodynamic impairment are often difficult to determine.

6. Echocardiography provides vital data that complement catheterization and physical examination. Wall motion abnormalities, ventricular contractility, chamber dimensions, and valve function are well evaluated by this noninvasive method.

7. Arterial blood pressure monitoring is an invaluable aid to the management of patients with hemodynamic instability. It is always wise to compare readings obtained from an arterial line with a cuff pressure periodically and whenever the monitored number disagrees with the clinical impression. An arterial line is also appropriate for patients with respiratory compromise who are in need of frequent blood pressure or arterial blood gas assessment. Certain modern instruments allow on-line assessment of arterial blood gases and pH as well as provide reliable data for hemodynamic evaluation.

SUGGESTED READINGS

1. Anonymous. European Society of Intensive Care Medicine. Expert panel: the use of the pulmonary artery catheter. Int Care Med 1991;17(3):I–VIII.
2. Astiz M, Rackow E. Assessing perfusion failure during circulatory shock. Crit Care Clin 1993;9(2):299–312.
3. Bossaert L, et al. Hemodynamic monitoring. Problems, pitfalls and practical solutions. Drugs 1991;41(6):857–874.
4. Bridges E, Woods S. Pulmonary artery pressure measurement: state of the art. Heart Lung 1993;22(2):99–111.
5. Carroll G. Blood pressure monitoring. Crit Care Clin 1988;4(3):411–434.
6. Clark C, Gutierrez G. Gastric intramucosal pH: a noninvasive method for the indirect measurement of tissue oxygenation. Am J Crit Care 1992;1(2):53–60.
7. Clark V, Kruse J. Arterial catheterization. Crit Care Clin 1992;8(4):687–697.
8. Cope D, et al. Pulmonary capillary pressure: a review. Crit Care Med 1992;20(7):1043–1056.
9. Dantzker D. Adequacy of tissue oxygenation. Crit Care Med 1993;21(2 Suppl):S40–S43.
10. Ermakov S, Hoyt J. Pulmonary artery catheterization. Crit Care Clin 1992;8(4):773–806.
11. Foster E, Schiller N. Transesophageal echocardiography in the critical care patient. Cardiol Clin 1993;11(3):489–503.
12. Futterman L, Lemberg L. Heart rate variability: prognostic implications. Am J Crit Care 1994;3(6):476–480.
13. Gardner P. Cardiac output: theory, technique, and troubleshooting. Crit Care Nurs Clin North Am 1989;1(3):577–587.
14. Kinefuchi Y, et al. Evaluation of dynamic response of catheter-manometer systems for pulmonary arterial pressure. J Appl Physiol 1994;77(4):2023–2028.
15. Kuecherer H, Foster E. Hemodynamics by transesophageal echocardiography. Cardiol Clin 1993;11(3):475–487.
16. Leatherman JW, Marini JJ. Clinical use of the pulmonary artery catheter. In: Schmidt GA, ed. Principles of critical care medicine. New York: McGraw Hill, 1992;323–342.
17. Leatherman JW, Marini JJ. Pulmonary artery catheter: Pressure monitoring. In: Sprung CL, ed. The pulmonary artery catheter—methodology and clinical applications. Closter: Critical Care Research Associates, Inc., 1993;119–156.
18. Marini J. Acute lung injury. Hemodynamic monitoring with the pulmonary artery catheter. Crit Care Clin 1986;2(3):551–572.
19. Marini JJ. Hemodynamic monitoring using the pulmonary artery catheter. Crit Care Clin 1986;2(3):551–572.
20. Mark J. Central venous pressure monitoring: clinical insights beyond the numbers. J Cardiol Vasc Anesth 1991;5(2):163–173.
21. Matthay M, Chatterjee K. Bedside catheterization of the pulmonary artery: risks compared with benefits. Ann Int Med 1988;109(10):826–834.
22. Mermel L, Maki D. Infectious complications of Swan-Ganz pulmonary artery catheters. Pathogenesis, epidemiology, prevention, and management. Am J Resp Crit Care Med 1994;149(4 Pt 1):1020–1036.
23. O'Quin R, Marini JJ. Pulmonary artery occlusion pressure. Clinical physiology, measurement, and interpretation. Am Rev Respir Dis 1983;128:319–326.
24. Pepe PE, Marini JJ. Occult positive end-expiratory pressure in mechanically ventilated patients with airflow obstruction. Am Rev Respir Dis 1982;126:166–170.
25. Pierce T, Woodcock T. How to insert a pulmonary arterial flotation catheter. Brit J Hosp Med 1989;42(6):484–487.
26. Sharkey S. Beyond the wedge: clinical physiology and the Swan-Ganz catheter. Am J Med 1987;83:111.
27. Shoemaker W. Use and abuse of the balloon tip pulmonary artery (Swan-Ganz) catheter: are patients getting their money's worth? Crit Care Med 1990;18(11):1294–1296.
28. Sladen A. Complications of invasive hemodynamic monitoring in the intensive care unit. Current Prob Surg 1988;25(2):69–145.
29. Smart F, Husserl F. Complications of flow-directed balloon-tipped catheters. Chest 1990;97(1):227–228.
30. Sprung, CL. The pulmonary artery catheter. 1993, Closter: Critical Care Research Associates, Inc.
31. Swan H. The pulmonary artery catheter. Dis Mon 1991;37(8):473–543.
32. Taylor A, Bergin J. Noninvasive assessment of systolic and diastolic function. Important clues to differentiating types of congestive heart failure. Postgrad Med 1993;94(3):55–58.
33. Tuchschmidt J, Mecher C. Predictors of outcome from critical illness. Shock and cardiopulmonary resuscitation. Crit Care Clin 1994;10(1):179–195.
34. Tuman K, Carroll G, Ivankovich A. Pitfalls in interpretation of pulmonary artery catheter. J Cardio Anes 1989;3(5):625–641.
35. Vender J. Clinical utilization of pulmonary artery catheter monitoring. Int Anesthesiol Clin 1993;31(3):57–85.
36. Yelderman M. Continuous cardiac output by thermodilution. Int Anesthesiol Clin 1993;31(3):127–140.

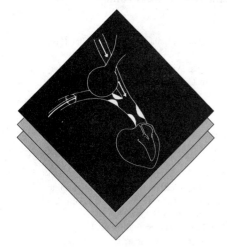

Support of the Failing Circulation

PHYSIOLOGY OF THE FAILING CIRCULATION

CIRCULATORY INSUFFICIENCY

Circulatory insufficiency and shock reflect inadequate perfusion relative to tissue demands. Although certain physical and laboratory parameters may be suggestive, shock is defined by overt dysfunction of vital organ systems—not by such "supply side" parameters as blood pressure (BP) or cardiac output (CO) or by such "demand side" parameters as oxygen consumption (VO_2). What might be considered a normal CO in a healthy patient at rest may inadequately perfuse the tissue beds of a critically ill patient. The prime objective of circulatory support, therefore, is to maintain near optimal vital organ perfusion, as reflected in mental status, urinary output, and systemic pH, at acceptable cardiac filling pressures.

Organ perfusion is governed by driving pressure and vascular resistance. Ordinarily, an adequate pressure gradient is present and vasomotor control regulates individual organ perfusion in proportion to metabolic demand. Under resting conditions, only a small percentage of all vascular channels are fully open. However, when the available pressure fails to maintain adequate flow despite optimal vasodilation (e.g., during a cardiovascular crisis or hypovolemia) or when defective vasoregulation fails to maintain perfusion pressure or flow distribution (e.g., during sepsis), vital tissues are not adequately nourished and the shock syndrome may be initiated. Once under way, vasoactive mediators, some with myocardial depres-

sant properties, may be released into the circulation, perpetuating the circulatory crisis. Even with appropriate treatment, mortality exceeds 50%, both for septic shock and for cardiogenic shock without coronary reperfusion.

DETERMINANTS OF CARDIAC OUTPUT

Although attention usually is focused on the pump that energizes the circulation (the heart), vascular compliance and tone are equally important. Thus, whereas the Frank-Starling relationship offers a restricted perspective on circulatory kinetics, CO can be viewed equally well as a function of the effective pressure driving blood centrally and the resistance to venous return. The upstream force driving venous return, the mean systemic pressure (MSP), is the equilibrium pressure that would exist throughout the vasculature if the heart abruptly stopped pumping. Because of the large capacitance of the venous bed relative to the arterial bed, MSP lies much closer in value to the central venous pressure (CVP) than to mean arterial pressure (normally 7–10 mm Hg). MSP is influenced both by blood volume and by vascular tone. The downstream back pressure to venous return is right atrial pressure (P_{RA}). If MSP fails to rise sufficiently to compensate for an increase in P_{RA}, CO falls. Indeed, the relationship between CO and P_{RA} is linear for any fixed value of MSP, and the slope of this relationship is influenced by the resistance to venous return. The tendency of the vena cava to collapse limits the extent to which effective driving pressure (MSP-P_{RA}) can be increased by reducing P_{RA} (Fig. 3.1). The actual CO observed at any moment is defined by the

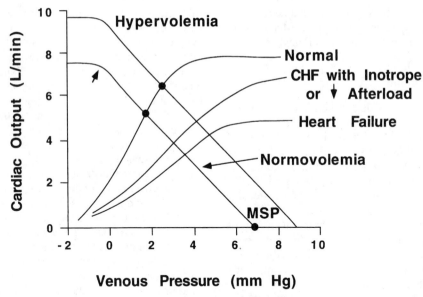

Venous Pressure (mm Hg)

FIG. 3–1. Regulation of cardiac output (CO). Cardiac output is determined by the intersection of the Frank-Starling and venous return curves. Venous return, which is driven by the difference between mean systemic pressure and central venous pressure (CVP), tends to improve as CVP falls, until the point at which venous pressure is insufficient to prevent vessel collapse (arrow). For the same venous return curve, the failing heart reduces its output, despite a higher filling pressure. Cardiac output can be maintained at a nearly normal level by increasing intravascular volume and/or using an inotrope or afterload reducer.

intersection of Starling and VR curves. Thus, both pump factors (heart rate, loading conditions, and contractility) and circuit factors (intravascular volume, vessel tone) affect circulatory performance. Three basic mechanisms may cause or contribute to circulatory failure: (*a*) pump failure; (*b*) failure of vascular tone; and (*c*) hypovolemia.

Pump Failure

Heart Rate

Cardiac output, the product of heart rate (HR) and stroke volume (SV), can be depressed by abnormalities of either factor (see Chapter 1, Hemodynamics). Isolated deficits in either stroke volume or HR are compensated largely by adjustments in the other cofactor over a wide range to meet metabolic demand. Both extremes of HR can cause CO to fall to shock levels. During sinus rhythm, the maximal sustainable physiologic HR can be estimated as ($HR_{max} = 220 - $ age). Heart rates exceeding this value may reduce CO and myocardial perfusion, even in healthy normal people. When the heart is noncompliant or compromised by coronary insufficiency, CO may fall

at much lower heart rates. Furthermore, the loss of atrial contraction that accompanies many tachyarrhythmias (i.e., atrial fibrillation) may cause the circulation to fail on this basis alone.

In the intensive care unit (ICU), hypoxemia, enhanced vagal tone, and high grade conduction block caused by intrinsic disease or pharmacologic agents are three key mechanisms causing marked bradycardia. The normally compliant and contractile heart can adapt to physiologic or pathologic depressions in HR via the Starling mechanism. (For example, young well-conditioned athletes often maintain resting heart rates <40 beats/minute.) However, patients with impaired myocardial contractility or reduced effective compliance (e.g., ischemia, diastolic dysfunction, pericardial disease) may suffer marked depressions in CO and BP when heart rates fall into the low normal range (<60 beats/min). This is especially true when the normally coordinated activation sequence is compromised or metabolic demands are high. It must be remembered that the appropriate physiologic response to hypovolemia is sinus tachycardia; hypotension suspected on the basis of massive gastrointestinal (GI) hemorrhage, therefore, should be accompanied by a compensatory tachycardia. A normal heart rate in this setting implicates an erroneous diagnosis or superimposed vagal, drug, or pathologic explanations.

Stroke Volume

Stroke volume is determined by end-diastolic volume and ejection fraction (see Chapter 1). End-diastolic volume, in turn, is the product of transmural filling pressure and myocardial compliance. Foremost among the primary depressants of contractility and ejection fraction during critical illness are: (*a*) acute ischemia; (*b*) extensive myocardial necrosis; (*c*) tumor necrosis factor and other less well characterized humoral mediators (collectively known as "myocardial depressant factors") released during inflammation and trauma; and (*d*) drugs that impair contractility (e.g., certain β blockers, calcium channel blockers, and antiarrhythmics—most notably of the type Ia class). Cardiogenic shock consequent to acute myocardial infarction implies cumulative tissue losses exceeding 40% of the total myocardial mass.

Structural defects, such as papillary muscle rupture or postinfarction ventriculoseptal defect (VSD), may compromise CO on a mechanical basis, even when there has been subcritical myocardial damage. Because the output of a failing heart is influenced by the impedance to ventricular ejection (afterload), increased vascular tone may improve blood pressure at the expense of tissue perfusion. Patients with "tight" aortic stenosis are especially sensitive to changes in preload and contractility.

To scale for metabolic needs, the CO must be referenced to body surface area. The resulting quotient, the cardiac index (CI), attempts to take the mass of metabolizing tissue into account (normal > 2.5 L/min/m^2). Cardiac output adequacy can be judged only with respect to metabolic demands. Under some circumstances, even a normal CI may be insufficient for vital organ support. Such "high output" cardiac failure can be precipitated by fever, anemia, thiamine deficiency, thyrotoxicosis, and arteriovenous shunting. Patients with extensive burns, septic shock, and cirrhosis also may have vastly higher CO requirements than the average resting patient.

Failure of Vascular Tone

Because organ perfusion depends on the gradient of pressure and the resistance to flow through the tissue bed, failure of vasomotor tone and/or distributive control may produce the shock syndrome, even when the cardiac index is maintained in the normal range. Early sepsis provides a common example of maldistributive shock, characterized by reduced afterload, and normal or elevated CO and VO_2, despite underperfused vital tissue beds. (General and spinal anesthesia, autonomic failure resulting from acute spinal cord injury, and certain drugs may also produce generalized, nonselective vasodilation that leads to underperfusion of critical organs.) Although moderate acidosis is generally well tolerated, severe metabolic acidosis may aggravate the shock state by causing myocardial depression, catecholamine resistance, increased right ventricular afterload, and potentially irreversible precapillary arteriolar dilation. Selective arteriolar dilation produces direct cellular injury and massive transudation of fluid into the extracellular space. Adrenal insufficiency and myxedema are two frequently ignored endocrine problems that may contribute to vasomotor insufficiency and circulatory failure.

Hypovolemia

Although marked inadequacy of circulating blood volume is a primary cause of circulatory failure, relative deficiency of intravascular volume is often a contributing cause in the setting of impaired pump function or reduced vascular tone (e.g., sepsis). Primary hypovolemic shock develops during hemorrhage or when extensive extracellular volume losses result from burns, pancreatitis, vomiting, diarrhea, anaphylaxis, hypoproteinemia, or multiple trauma. Right ventricular infarction and pericardial disease mimic hypovolemia because inadequate fluid primes the left ventricle, despite systemic venous congestion and/or normal wedge pressure.

EFFECT OF SHOCK ON ORGAN SYSTEMS

The closely autoregulated central nervous system of the healthy subject can tolerate marked reductions in mean arterial pressure (to 50–60 mm Hg) without sustaining irreversible tissue damage. However, cerebrocortical functions are among the first to be impaired as shock develops.

As a rule, reductions of mean arterial pressure (MAP) are tolerated poorly by the GI tract. Early in shock, the gut suffers marked reductions in flow, impairing mucosal function and bowel integrity, occasionally to the point of frank ischemic necrosis. A reduction of gastric pH is among the first indications of inadequate perfusion. Translocation of bacteria across the abnormally permeable gut mucosa and into the lymphatic system or bloodstream may be the next step on the path to multisystem organ failure. Hepatic ischemia may elevate liver function tests, alter the metabolism of drugs, and impair removal of toxins and coagulation products. Hypotension and shock may convert uncomplicated pancreatitis into its hemorrhagic variant.

Shock often impairs the clotting system sufficiently to initiate disseminated intravascular coagulation (DIC). The stimulus is multifactorial: vascular endothelial injury, cell death, and impaired hepatic clearance of fibrin degradation products are important contributing factors. In response to hypotension, the kidneys secrete renin to retain sodium and water. Intense vasoconstriction of the afferent arterioles shunts blood from the cortex to the medulla, reducing glomerular filtration to a greater degree than total renal blood flow or cardiac output. If profound or prolonged, underperfusion may culminate in acute tubular necrosis.

During the hyperpnea that accompanies shock, respiratory muscles may consume large amounts of oxygen, outstripping the heart's ability to deliver adequate flow to them. Ventilatory failure and lactic acidosis may result. However, even when the ventilatory pump remains well compensated, intubation and mechanical ventilation during circulatory shock may decrease respiratory muscle O_2 consumption, and increase the blood flow available to other critical organs. Thus, in the vigorously breathing patient, mechanical ventilation often improves circulatory homeostasis.

THERAPY OF THE FAILING CIRCULATION

INDICATIONS FOR MONITORING

Repeated examinations of mental status, urine output, and skin perfusion provide information essential in guiding therapy. Each component of arterial blood pressure (systolic, diastolic and mean) may hold special significance. For example, a widening pulse pressure with a falling diastolic arterial pressure would suggest critical deterioration of aortic valve competence in the setting of acute bacterial endocarditis. Although a specific blood pressure should not be used as the sole endpoint of circulatory support, a MAP of 60 to 70 mm Hg is required for most patients to perfuse the heart and brain adequately; higher pressures are required in those with compromised cerebrovasculature.

Arterial and ventricular filling pressures should be monitored continuously when hypotension produces signs of vital organ dysfunction that are not reversed rapidly. For young patients without underlying heart or lung disease, a CVP catheter may suffice to monitor filling pressures. However, when data are obtained and analyzed carefully, the pulmonary arterial catheter aids in accurate assessment of left ventricular filling pressure, cardiac output, and mixed venous oxygen saturation (see Chapter 2). By enabling calculations of vascular resistance indices, pulmonary artery (PA) catheters can be helpful in diagnosing the etiology of shock and in guiding therapy. Most hypotensive patients requiring vasopressor support should be monitored invasively. Severe peripheral vasoconstriction and the reduced pulse pressure of certain shock states make determination of systemic blood pressure by standard cuff methods difficult and unreliable. Arterial catheterization allows frequent determinations of blood gases, effortless blood drawing, and continuous on-line assessment of BP. A bladder catheter also should be placed in patients with hypotension to monitor urine output as an index of renal perfusion and adequacy of O_2 delivery.

FLUID THERAPY

Water normally comprises 60% of body weight. Of this total, approximately two-thirds are intracellular and approximately one-third is extracellular. Of the extracellular fluid, one-quarter is intravascular and three-quarters are interstitial (Fig. 3.2). Isotonic solutions (e.g., normal saline and Ringer's lactate) initially distribute only into the extracellular space, whereas the distributive space of hypotonic (or potentially hypotonic) fluids approximates that of total body water. Therefore, hypotonic fluids (e.g., one-half normal saline) or fluids subject to rapid metabolism of their osmotic components (e.g., D5W) only affect intravascular volume transiently (i.e., only one-twelfth of the volume of D5W remains intravascular after dextrose metabolism). Because most isotonic crystalloid ultimately migrates to the interstitial space, edema should be expected after massive fluid resuscitation with crystalloid. As a result of normal fluid partitioning, replacing a specific volume of lost plasma requires at least four times as much isotonic crystalloid and even more hypotonic fluid.

When first given, large volumes of fluid initially dilute the packed cell volume (PCV) and serum proteins. As fluid redistributes out of the

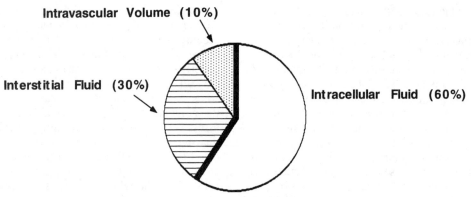

FIG. 3–2. Body fluid distribution.

vascular space, these values tend to return gradually toward their preinfusion baselines. The time required for this equilibration or "circulation dwell time" is brief for crystalloid. Redistribution begins within minutes and is completed within hours.

Hypotension complicating renal insufficiency or anuria presents a difficult challenge, requiring the utmost skill for management. Dialysis often is required for these patients to clear toxins, restore electrolyte balance, allow nutritional support, and offset metabolic acidosis. Continuous hemofiltration (SCUF) can be especially helpful when fluid overloading or acidosis complicate management, because it gently allows the removal of sodium and water—useful characteristics for patients who require frequent saline or bicarbonate infusions.

Use of the Fluid Challenge

Fluid challenge is instrumental for assessing the need for volume replacement in hypotensive patients. In fact, for most newly hypotensive patients without evidence of pulmonary edema, fluid administration is rarely an inappropriate first response. Although some patients respond transiently to simple leg elevation, most require volume infusion to increase cardiac filling pressures. The keys to effective use of the fluid challenge are as follows: (*a*) use crystalloid as the replacement fluid; (*b*) use a relatively large volume (200–500 mL) to maximize chances of detecting a significant hemodynamic effect; (*c*) infuse the fluid rapidly (<20 minutes); and (*d*) closely monitor the patient's response. Because most of an isotonic fluid load diffuses within hours into the interstitial space, crystalloid infusions are a relatively "reversible" method to expand volume. (When it works at all, leg elevation is even more "reversible.") Large volumes of fluid are infused rapidly to maximize the hemodynamic impact before redistribution dissipates the preloading effects. Fluid challenge should not be performed without close monitoring by a clinical caregiver. To safely obtain meaningful information, it is critical that the physical examination, CVP, wedge pressure, CO, and arterial pressure be monitored closely. A marked, sustained increase in filling pressure after fluid infusion signals that the heart is operating on the flat portion of the Starling curve, particularly if CO or MAP fail to rise. In such patients, further administration of intravascular fluid may overload the circulation, causing pulmonary edema. Conversely, if the fluid infusion causes small, transient increases in filling pressure, accompanied by substantial increases in CO and MAP, additional preload augmentation is likely to be beneficial.

Selection of Fluids

Selection of intravenous fluid is controversial; one logical approach is to replace adequate quantities of the missing constituent. For example, blood is the preferred therapy for acute hemorrhage and isotonic crystalloid is appropriate for the dehydrated patient with near-normal electrolytes. The major difference between colloids and crystalloids resides in the tendency for the former to remain within the vascular space. Unlike saline, most infused colloid remains intravascular for many hours; it may require as much as five times more crystalloid than colloid to achieve equivalent intravascular volume expansion. However, colloid is expensive, frequently costing many times more than crystalloid to achieve a similar volume expansion effect. Furthermore, crystalloid is free of allergic risk and is more easily transported and stored.

Crystalloid

Physiologic "normal" saline is the preferred crystalloid for volume expansion, except in patients with hyperchloremic acidosis, a setting in which saline may worsen the problem. Ringer's lactate has a slightly lower Na^+ concentration than normal saline; therefore, less volume remains intravascular. Additionally, it contains 4 mEq/L of K^+ that is undesirable for patients with renal failure, oliguria, or hyperkalemia. Although lactate in Ringer's solution does not potentiate systemic lactic acidosis, its metabolism to bicarbonate occurs slowly in patients with shock or hepatic hypoperfusion. Compared to isotonic solutions, small volumes of hypertonic crystalloid (3% saline) have been used effectively for emergency resuscitations. Although their mechanism of action is not defined clearly, hypertonic crystalloids redistribute total body water into the extracellular compartment. Hypertonic saline risks development of hypernatremia, and its role in resuscitation is debated.

A 5:1 ratio of crystalloid to colloid is sometimes used because it provides more effective volume resuscitation than crystalloid alone at less cost than using colloid exclusively. A crystalloid-containing regimen also helps to replete intracellular fluid losses. Blood is not essential for resuscitation unless there is acute blood loss exceeding 2 units, marked anemia, or ongoing coagulopathy (see Chapter 14, Transfusion and Blood Component Therapy).

Colloid Infusions

Albumin   Albumin is available as a 5% (isotonic) or 25% (hypotonic) solution. Isotonic albumin contains up to 145 mEq/L of sodium. Therefore, the 25% solution contains relatively less salt per unit of colloid effect and therefore may offer an advantage in edematous, volume-depleted patients. The oncotic effect of 1 g of albumin pulls 18 g of H_2O into the vascular compartment. Because albumin leaks gradually from the intravascular space, its circulating half-life in many forms of shock is only about 16 hours. Albumin should not be used as nutritional supplement for hypoalbuminemic patients (e.g., nephrotic syndrome or hepatic failure). Exogenous albumin is catabo-

lized rapidly or excreted in these conditions, negating its nutritional value and blunting its effect on volume expansion. In certain highly unusual circumstances (e.g., anabolism with preexisting hypoalbuminemia), the administration of albumin can raise oncotic pressure for extended periods and should be considered if pulmonary edema is present. Albumin is expensive and carries the risk of allergic reactions. Although once a definite risk for transmitting certain viral infections, albumin is now heat treated, obviating this hazard. It contains no viable coagulation factors.

Fresh Frozen Plasma   Fresh frozen plasma (FFP) provides another source of colloid protein. Because FFP carries a significant risk of allergic reaction and potentially risks infection, it should not be used solely for volume expansion. However, when hypovolemia and coagulopathy coexist, FFP may help reverse both.

Dextran   Dextran is a mixture of heterogenous polysaccharides available as 40,000 or 70,000 molecular weight (MW) solutions. Clearance of small MW fractions occurs rapidly through renal filtration, whereas larger molecules are taken up and metabolized by the reticuloendothelial system. The effect of dextran on circulatory volume is relatively brief, with only 20 to 30% remaining intravascular after 24 hours. Dextran offers several potential advantages: it produces volume expansion greater than the volume infused, promotes "microvascular" flow by coating vessel walls and decreasing red cell–vessel wall interaction, and reduces serum viscosity.

Unfortunately, dextran also has important adverse characteristics. Reductions in platelet adherence and degranulation may incite bleeding most often when doses exceed 1.5 g/kg/day. If urinary flow is sluggish, renal failure may occur secondary to tubular obstruction. Minor allergic reactions are seen in approximately 5% of cases. (Patients with previous streptococcal or salmonella infections are predisposed.) Fatal anaphylactic reactions occur rarely. The osmotic diuresis that follows dextran resuscitation may necessitate ongoing fluid replacement. Finally, dextran interferes with several common laboratory tests, occasionally producing false elevations in the serum glucose, bilirubin, and protein concentrations. Dextran also mimics antibody-induced red cell agglutination, making cross-matching of blood more difficult.

Hydroxyethyl Starch   Hydroxyethyl starch (HES) is a polysaccharide structurally similar to glycogen, supplied as a mixture of MW fractions from 10,000 to 1,000,000. Hydroxyethyl starch expands plasma volume in direct relationship to the amount infused. Small MW fractions of HES are cleared predominantly by the kidney, whereas reticuloendothelial cells metabolize larger MW fractions. Hydroxyethyl starch is also degraded by serum alpha amylase. Trace amounts of HES have been detected more than 4 months after its administration. Prolonged or massive starch infusions may accumulate in phagocytes, resulting in unknown effects on immune function.

Hydroxyethyl starch prolongs the partial thromboplastin time (PTT) modestly for most patients, but the mechanism is uncertain. Hydroxyethyl starch also causes a transient decrease in platelet count and clot tensile strength. Intracerebral hemorrhage has been reported in HES recipients. Clotting abnormalities may be reversed with transfusions of FFP and platelets. Allergic reactions occur in <1% of patients receiving HES; anaphylactic reactions are extremely rare. Hydroxyethyl starch may artifactually increase the sedimentation rate and often doubles the serum amylase. In a minority of patients, indirect bilirubin may be elevated spuriously by up to 1 mg/dL. Hydroxyethyl starch and 5% albumin are similar in cost and both are more expensive than dextran.

VASOPRESSORS

General Principles

The proper goal of vasopressor therapy is to support vital organ perfusion—not to achieve any specific blood pressure. Because vasoactive drugs are relatively ineffective for volume-depleted patients and are partially inhibited in the setting of severe acidosis, an adequate circulating volume and reversal of profound acidosis (pH > 7.0) are needed for maximal pressor effect. Moreover, although poorly studied, it is our impression that vasopressors also may be ineffective when serum concentrations of K^+, Mg^{++}, or Ca^{++} are strikingly abnormal. Making an optimal choice of vasopressor requires a clear understanding of the operative cardiovascular pathophysiology, an understanding of adrenergic receptor distribution and action, and a working knowledge of the pharmacologic alternatives. Alpha effects are vasoconstrictive in the peripheral circulation. $\beta1$ receptor activation is both chronotropic and inotropic. $\beta2$ effects induce vasodilation and

bronchodilation (Table 3.1). Dopaminergic (Δ) receptor activation increases renal blood flow. For any given patient, an optimal choice may involve several vasoactive agents with complementary actions. It is worth considering, however, that certain drugs—notably dopamine—can stimulate both $\beta1$ and α adrenergic receptors, depending on dosage. Moreover, the sensitivity to any specific dosage varies widely among patients. For a volume-repleted hypotensive patient, the problem is either inadequate pump function or insufficient vascular tone. Therefore, dopamine begun in a moderate ($\beta1$ preferential, cardiostimulating) dosage and, if ineffective, rapidly titrated upward to α-stimulating, vasoconstricting dosage, is seldom inappropriate. As a principle, it is desirable to titrate a single well-selected drug to effect (or toxicity) before it is abandoned or supplemented by additional agents. Whatever drug or drug combination is selected, its physiologic impact must be monitored appropriately (see Chapter 2). The need for these potent and potentially hazardous agents, as well as their dosage, must be reassessed frequently. Over time, patients tend to become "dependent" on these agents, so that weaning rather than abrupt termination generally is the most prudent course.

Specific Agents

Drug preparation and dosage ranges for selected vasoactive agents are presented on Therapeutic Card No. 1. Potent vasoconstrictors (e.g., epinephrine, norepinephrine, phenylephrine, and dopamine) are best administered through a central line to avoid tissue necrosis resulting from extravasation.

Epinephrine

Epinephrine has balanced α and β agonist properties and serves as the standard to which all other vasopressors are compared. Epinephrine "coarsens" ventricular fibrillation and augments arterial tone during cardiac arrest. Mean arterial pressure (MAP), systemic vascular resistance (SVR), and CO are boosted in patients with an organized heart rhythm. Potential side effects include palpitations, arrhythmias, and angina caused by increased myocardial oxygen consumption. For patients with hypotension caused by ischemia-induced pump dysfunction, epinephrine may increase myocardial oxygen delivery to a greater degree than it increases myocardial oxygen con-

TABLE 3–1

INOTROPIC DRUGS*

	Adrenergic Receptor Activation	Relative Effects in Midrange of Dosage		
		Inotropic	Chronotropic	Vasoconstrictor
Amrinone	0	+ + +	0	–
Dobutamine	$\alpha\beta1\beta2$	+ + +	+	– to +*
Dopamine	$\alpha\beta1\Delta$	+ + +	+ +	– to + +*
Epinephrine	$\alpha\beta1\beta2$	+ + +	+ + +	+ +
Isoproterenol	$\beta1\beta2$	+ + + +	+ + + +	–
Methoxamine	α	0	0	+ + + +
Norepinephrine	$\alpha\beta1$	+ + +	+ + +	+ + + +
Phenylephrine	$\alpha\beta1$	+	0	+ + + +

* Effect dependent on dosage range.

sumption. Patients taking β-blocking drugs may experience unopposed α effects when given a balanced α and β agonist such as epinephrine.

Norepinephrine

Norepinephrine is primarily an α agonist with mild $\beta1$ activity. Its primary effect, therefore, is to vasoconstrict. Despite increases in SVR and left ventricular afterload, CO usually remains stable because of offsetting augmentation of heart rate and contractility. However, excessive increases in afterload induced by norepinephrine may reduce CO. Side effects include hypertension and increased myocardial oxygen consumption. Norepinephrine is often useful in the early phases of septic shock, a condition in which CO is normal or elevated but SVR is reduced. Norepinephrine frequently is combined with dopamine or other pressor agents in the setting of refractory shock.

Isoproterenol

Isoproterenol has primarily $\beta1$ (chronotropic and inotropic) actions but also possesses the $\beta2$ properties of vasodilation and bronchodilation. It is used most commonly to increase heart rate and CO in the setting of marked bradycardia (e.g., 3° atrioventricular (AV) block). Increases in CO due to isoproterenol result primarily from increases in heart rate. Mean arterial pressure may actually fall, despite rising CO, as a result of peripheral vasodilation. Isoproterenol occasionally is used to increase heart rate and shorten the QT interval in patients with arrhythmias resulting from QT prolongation (e.g., torsades de pointes).

Neosynephrine

Neosynephrine (phenylephrine) is a pure α agonist that lacks cardiac stimulant properties. In high doses, increases in afterload resulting from neosynephrine actually may decrease CO, but such effects are less marked than with norepinephrine. Neosynephrine is useful to increase blood pressure in the treatment of supraventricular tachycardias and has become popular in combination with intravenous nitroglycerin to provide decreased preload and coronary vasodilation while maintaining arterial blood pressure in patients with acute cardiac ischemia.

Dopamine

Dopamine is a naturally occurring precursor of norepinephrine with a spectrum of effects that varies with the infusion rate. At doses of 2 to 5 μgm/kg/min, dopamine has primarily $\beta1$ actions and very mild $\beta2$ effects. At such doses, dopamine independently stimulates renal dopamine receptors, increasing renal blood flow, enhancing glomerular filtration rate (GFR), and promoting Na^+ excretion. Although the dopaminergic effects are not lost, at higher doses, α effects become more prominent. With doses >10 μgm/kg/min, α effects predominate. In still higher doses, dopamine possesses a pharmacologic profile much like that of norepinephrine. Even when using potent α agonists such as norepinephrine, low doses of dopamine may help promote diuresis in some patients, but this point is still debated actively. Dopamine increases the potential for arrhythmias. Dopamine causes intense vasoconstriction and, if extravasated, may induce soft tissue necrosis, an effect antagonized by local infiltration of phentolamine.

Dobutamine

Dobutamine is an isoproterenol analog with primarily $\beta1$ actions. Dobutamine causes much less α stimulation than dopamine and less $\beta2$ activity than isoproterenol. Unlike isoproterenol, dobutamine boosts CO primarily by increasing stroke volume and not heart rate. Dobutamine is best suited to the treatment of low CO states in patients with a near-normal blood pressure. At commonly used doses, dobutamine is less likely than isoproterenol to produce tachycardia, but mild increases in heart rate occur frequently, particularly in hypovolemic patients. In some patients with a very high baseline SVR, dobutamine may cause sufficient peripheral vasodilation to induce hypotension. Rarely, dobutamine increases AV conduction in patients with atrial fibrillation or flutter, leading to accelerated heart rate.

Amrinone and Milrinone

Although the mechanism of action is unclear, amrinone has inotropic properties distinct from the catecholamines or digitalis glycosides. (Its effect may be due to increased cAMP activity.) Amrinone is a positive inotrope and vasodilator that raises CO by increasing stroke volume, not by increasing heart rate. Although renal excretion provides the primary route of clearance, hepatic metabolism is significant. Therefore, the drug may accumulate in patients with either hepatic or renal failure. Increases in inotropic activity may aggravate outflow obstruction in hypertrophic cardiomyopathy. Increased ventricular rates have been reported during atrial fibrillation or flutter, but the chronotropic effect is generally less than with any other currently available inotrope. Thrombocytopenia occurs in a small minority of patients. High doses of amrinone given for long periods of time may elevate liver function tests or cause frank hepatic necrosis.

MECHANICAL INTERVENTIONS AND DEVICES

The output of the failing left ventricle is sensitive to reductions in afterload (the fiber tension developed during systole) and relatively insensitive to reductions in precontractile fiber stretch or preload. Reducing the vigor of respiratory efforts may partially relieve the burden of the failing heart simply by decreasing its output require-

ments. Moreover, conversion to positive-pressure-assisted breathing raises the mean intrathoracic pressure, reducing the afterload to the left ventricle without compromising its effective preload. For similar reasons, the application of positive end-expiratory pressure (PEEP) can be an extremely helpful intervention in this setting.

Pacemakers can boost cardiac output and reduce left atrial falling pressure when used on patients whose heart rate is inappropriately low relative to $\dot{V}O_2$. AV sequential pacemakers are perhaps most physiologic, but require special skills to insert in the ICU setting. Pacemakers are discussed in greater detail in Chapter 4.

Fluid and vasopressors traditionally have been the only options for support of the failing circulation, but recently several mechanical devices have been developed and used on occasion for special indications. Artificial hearts and implanted left ventricular assist devices (LVAD) can provide temporary support options for patients with myocardial failure. Problems of infection, immobility, embolism, and cost have limited use of implantable devices. Much more experience has accumulated with the intra-aortic balloon pump (IABP). This device is inserted in a retrograde fashion through the femoral artery into the descending aorta, above the renal arteries. Cycle-by-cycle diastolic inflation of the large tube-shaped aortic balloon augments both coronary and systemic perfusion pressures. Balloon deflation during systole reduces LV afterload, improving systemic perfusion. Ischemia of renal and peripheral arteries, cholesterol or gas embolism, stroke, coagulopathy, hemolysis, infection, and aortic dissection constitute major hazards. The IABP has been proven to be most useful in temporary support of patients with acute mitral insufficiency, ventricular septal defects, or myocardial ischemia refractory to medical therapy (see Chapter 21, Angina and Myocardial Infarction). Gradual weaning from IABP usually is required and generally accomplished by reducing the ratio of balloon-assisted to unaided cardiac cycles. The intra-aortic balloon pump may be life-sustaining for patients awaiting cardiac transplantation. For patients without appropriate physiology (aortic insufficiency, mitral stenosis) or correctable mechanical defects, IABP and other ventricular assist devices are of unproven benefit and may be harmful.

CONGESTIVE HEART FAILURE

The physiology underlying management of congestive heart failure is detailed in Chapter 1,

Hemodynamics. In essence, the common problem of these conditions relates to an imbalance between the hydrostatic pressure in the fluid-exchanging vessels of the lung (capillaries, small arterioles, and small venules) on one hand and the vascular oncotic forces and lymphatic drainage capacity on the other. Because neither lymphatic drainage nor vascular oncotic pressure can be improved easily or rapidly, clinical attention usually centers on reducing the left atrial pressure that regulates the filtering pressures upstream.

CAUSES

Left atrial pressure can rise for many reasons: reduced compliance of the left heart secondary to hypertrophy, ischemia, catecholamines, or interdependence with a swollen right ventricle; impaired contractility due to intrinsic myocardial disease, circulating depressant factors, or performance-impairing drugs; pathologically slow or rapid heart rates (requiring higher filling pressure to support a higher stroke volume or preventing adequate filling of the left ventricle, respectively); conduction system disease and arrhythmias; or mitral valvular stenosis or insufficiency. Pulmonary congestion may or may not be accompanied by relative insufficiency of forward output, depending on underlying cardiopathology and precipitating cause for the exacerbation.

PRECIPITANTS

For a predisposed patient, decompensation usually is brought on by excessive demands for cardiac output relative to capacity (fever, increased work of breathing, physiologic stress), by medication error or noncompliance, by an adverse change in cardiac preload (renal insufficiency, overly zealous administration of intravascular volume, dietary indiscretion), by a sudden augmentation of cardiac afterload (hypertension, ischemia, forceful inspiratory efforts), or by alterations in myocardial compliance, heart rhythm, or contractility (electrolyte disturbances, ischemia, and sepsis are major offenders in this latter category).

DIAGNOSIS

The key bedside indicators of pulmonary congestion are well known—new crackles, wheezes, and rhonchi; the appearance of an S3 gallop; and, in many instances, distended neck veins, cool extremities, diaphoresis, and tachypnea. Alert patients almost always—but not invariably—express dyspnea. The chest radiograph often exhibits characteristic features: Kerley lines, blurred hilar structures, pleural effusions, a widened vascular pedicle, and diffuse, symmetrical infiltrates with spared costophrenic angles and without prominent air bronchograms. A balloon occlusion wedge pressure confirms an elevated pulmonary venous pressure that rises sharply after volume challenge. The echocardiogram usually provides evidence of a dilated left atrium, distended vena cava, impaired contractility, or diastolic dysfunction (see Chapter 2, Hemodynamic Monitoring).

MANAGEMENT

The sitting position, supplemental oxygen, diuresis, afterload reduction, and relief of an excessive breathing workload by continuous positive airway pressure (CPAP), biphasic airway pressure (Bi-PAP), or mechanical ventilation are fundamental to the care of patients with acute left heart failure. With regard to diuretics, consideration should be given to the use of a furosemide drip to more closely and consistently regulate diuresis (rather than conventional boluses) for patients who are particularly fragile with regard to intravascular volume status. Precipitating causes must be identified and eliminated, if possible. Electrical cardioversion of rapid atrial arrhythmias and slowing of rapid atrial fibrillation with digoxin, verapamil, or even esmolol may sometimes be indicated. Morphine and nitrates have multiple therapeutic effects in carefully selected patients. Morphine relieves anxiety, thereby reducing the $\dot{V}O_2$, and doubles as a venodilator that reduces central vascular volume. Nitrates also increase venous capacitance, simultaneously dilating the coronary vasculature in patients with ischemic disease.

Nitroprusside can be an invaluable agent when congestive heart failure (CHF) is either caused or exacerbated by systemic hypertension. It is also worth considering to offset the augmented preload and afterload that accompany ventilator withdrawal for fragile patients with CHF or coronary ischemia (see Chapter 10, Weaning from Mechanical Ventilation). In less obvious cases, angiotensin-converting enzyme (ACE) inhibitors reduce the ejection impedance of the afterload-sensitive left ventricle and often prove fundamental to successful management. Although calcium channel blocking agents also can be used for this purpose, they also tend to suppress ventricular contractility. (Verapamil is the greatest offender in this regard; nifedipine and nimodepine are better tolerated.)

Digoxin has a definite but limited role in improving the contractility of a dilated heart. In the critical care unit, many practitioners reserve it for control of heart rate in atrial fibrillation. Catecholamine-based inotropes such as dobutamine or dopamine are generally the agents of choice, unless their tendency to increase heart rate overcomes their inotropic benefit by reducing left ventricular filling time or inciting ischemia. Amrinone may be particularly useful in circumstances in which inotropy is desired but concomitant eleva-

tion of heart rate must be minimized. Occasionally, norepinephrine or phenylephrine help maintain coronary perfusion pressure and sustain forward output when hypotension accompanies failure. For patients with florid pulmonary edema, intubation and mechanical ventilation may be a key therapeutic intervention if CPAP and noninvasive ventilation by mask is not feasible or is poorly tolerated, acidosis is progressing, or hypoxemia and the work of breathing are severe.

KEY POINTS

1. Circulatory insufficiency and shock result from inadequate perfusion relative to tissue demands. Although certain physical and laboratory parameters may be suggestive, shock is defined by overt dysfunction of key vital organs—not by parameters that selectively reflect either oxygen supply or demand.

2. Three basic mechanisms may cause or contribute to circulatory insufficiency: pump failure, insufficient vascular tone, and hypovolemia. Heart rate as well as the determinants of stroke volume (preload, contractility, and afterload) should be considered independently for their potential to contribute to cardiovascular dysfunction.

3. The parameters that characterize heart function must be scaled to body size; any specific value of cardiac output, oxygen consumption, or vascular resistance may take on different significance for large and small patients.

4. During shock, the respiratory muscles may outstrip the heart's ability to deliver adequate blood flow to them. Mechanical support may relieve the ventilatory burden, thereby increasing the blood flow available to other marginally perfused organs.

5. Repeated examination of mental status, urine output, and skin perfusion provides information essential in guiding therapy. Invasive monitoring with arterial and pulmonary artery catheters, in conjunction with the fluid challenge, provide the data necessary to wisely select vasoactive agents and regulate the rates of volume and drug infusion.

6. Adequate circulatory volume must be ensured before vasopressors are employed. The type of fluid should be selected by considering the need for blood, the nature of the fluid lost from the vascular space, the acuity of the problem, the urgency of reversal, the financial cost, and the potential risk of the product to the patient.

7. Most (but not all) vasoactive agents used to support the circulation are catecholamine derivatives with α, $\beta 1$, or $\beta 2$ activity, in varying proportions. The relative intensity of each effect may vary with dosage.

8. Mechanical interventions (ventilatory support PEEP, aortic balloon pumping) may be needed to reduce afterload or modify preload. Once initiated, these interventions should be maintained only as long as necessary but should be withdrawn cautiously.

SUGGESTED READINGS

1. Alpert J, Becker R. Mechanisms and management of cardiogenic shock. Crit Care Clin 1993;9(2):205–218.
2. Astiz M, Rackow E. Assessing perfusion failure during circulatory shock. Crit Care Clin 1993;9(2):299–312.
3. Astiz M, Rackow E, Weil M. Pathophysiology and treatment of circulatory shock. Crit Care Clin 1993;9(2):183–203.
4. Blosser S, Stauffer J. Intubation of critically ill patients. Clin Chest Med 1996;17(3):355–378.
5. Camu F, Ivens D, Christiaens F. Human albumin and colloid fluid replacement: their use in general surgery. Acta Anaesthesiol Belg 1995;46(1):3–18.
6. Cone A. The use of colloids in clinical practice. Br J Hosp Med 1995;54(4):155–159.
7. DeGent G, Greenbaum D. Mechanical ventilatory support in circulatory shock. Crit Care Clin 1993;9(2):377–393.
8. DiBona G. Hemodynamic support: volume management and pharmacological cardiovascular support. Semin Nephrol 1994;14(1):33–40.
9. Domanski M, Topol E. Cardiogenic shock: current under-

standings and future research directions. Am J Cardiol 1994;74(7):724–726.

10. Fiddian-Green R. Associations between intramucosal acidosis in the gut and organ failure. Crit Care Med 1993; 21(2 Suppl):S103–S107.

11. Fiddian-Green R, Haglund H, Gutierrez G, et al. Goals for the resuscitation of shock. Crit Care Med 1993;21(2 Suppl):S25–S31.

12. Goldenberg I. Nonpharmacologic management of cardiac arrest and cardiogenic shock. Chest 1992;102(5 Suppl 2): 596S–616S.

13. Gould S, Sehgal LR, Sehgal HL, et al. Hypovolemic shock. Crit Care Clin 1993;9(2):239–259.

14. Grella R, Becker R. Cardiogenic shock complicating coronary artery disease: diagnosis, treatment, and management. Curr Probl Cardiol 1994;19(12):693–742.

15. Haljamae H. The pathophysiology of shock. Acta Anaesthesiol Scand 1993;98:3–6.

16. Haupt M, Kaufman B, Carlson R. Fluid resuscitation in patients with increased vascular permeability. Crit Care Clin 1992;8(2):341–353.

17. Hochman J, et al. Current spectrum of cardiogenic shock and effect of early revascularization on mortality. Circulation 1995;91(3):873–881.

18. Imm A, Carlson R. Fluid resuscitation in circulatory shock. Crit Care Clin 1993;9(2):313–334.

19. Kantrowitz A, Cardona R, Freed P. Percutaneous intra-aortic balloon counterpulsation. Crit Care Clin 1992;8(4): 819–837.

20. Karakusis P. Considerations in the therapy of septic shock. Med Clin North Am 1986;70(4):933–944.

21. Knox J. Oxygen consumption-oxygen delivery dependency in adult respiratory distress syndrome. New Horizons 1993;1(3):381–387.

22. Kulka P, Tryba M. Inotropic support of the critically ill patient. A review of the agents. Drugs 1993;45(5): 654–667.

23. Lee RM, Balk RA, Bone RC. Ventilatory support in the management of septic patients. Crit Care Clin 1989;5(1): 157–175.

24. Lynn W, Cohen J. Management of septic shock. J Infect 1995;30(3):207–212.

25. Mizock B, Falk J. Lactic acidosis in critical illness. Crit Care Med 1992;20(1):80–93.

26. Mueller H. Role of intra-aortic counterpulsation in cardiogenic shock and acute myocardial infarction. Cardiology 1994;84(3):168–174.

27. Mythen M, Salmon J, Webb A. The rational administration of colloids. Blood Rev 1993;7(4):223–228.

28. Pae W. Ventricular assist devices and total artificial hearts: a combined registry experience. Ann Thorac Surg 1993;55(1):295–298.

29. Pinsky M. Beyond global oxygen supply-demand relations: in search of measures of dysoxia. Intensive Care Med 1994;20(1):1–3.

30. Rackow E, Astiz M. Mechanisms and management of septic shock. Crit Care Clin 1993;9(2):219–238.

31. Rodgers K. Cardiovascular shock. Emerg Med Clin North Am 1995;13(4):793–810.

32. Rogers W. Contemporary management of acute myocardial infarction. Am J Med 1995;99(2):195–206.

33. Russell J, Phang P. The oxygen delivery/consumption controversy. Approaches to management of the critically ill. Am J Resp Crit Care Med 1994;149(2 Pt 1):533–537.

34. Shires G, Barber A, Illner H. Current status of resuscitation: solutions including hypertonic saline. Adv Surg 1995;28:133–170.

35. Shoemaker W. Pathophysiology, monitoring, and therapy of acute circulatory problems. Crit Care Nurs Clin North Am 1994;6(2):295–307.

36. Shoemaker WC, Appel PL, Kram HB, et al. Hemodynamic and oxygen transport monitoring to titrate therapy in septic shock. New Horizons 1993;1(1):145–159.

37. Stanford G. Use of inotropic agents in critical illness. Surg Clin North Am 1991;71(4):683–698.

38. Tuchschmidt J, Mecher C. Predictors of outcome from critical illness. Shock and cardiopulmonary resuscitations. Crit Care Clin 1994;10(1):179–195.

39. Vaca K, Lohmann D, Moroney D. Current status and future trends of mechanical circulatory support. Crit Care Nurs Clin North Am 1995;7(2):249–258.

40. Zaloga GP, Prielipp RC, Butterworth JF 4th, et al. Pharmacologic cardiovascular support. Crit Care Clin 1993; 9(2):335–362.

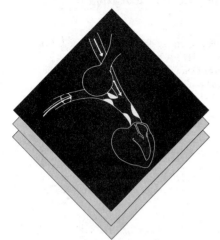

CHAPTER 4

Arrhythmias, Pacing, and Cardioversion

Possibly no field of therapy has changed as much over the last 10 years as that of arrhythmias. Time-honored practices such as administration of prophylactic lidocaine have fallen out of favor. Dramatic and surprising clinical trials proved that antiarrhythmic agents, used for many years, suppress ventricular arrhythmias but paradoxically increase mortality. This decade also saw the development of effective transthoracic pacing, the expanded use of implantable defibrillators and radiofrequency ablation, and the discovery of a genetic cause of at least one arrhythmia (long QT syndrome). A valuable diagnostic and therapeutic drug, adenosine, was also developed for the treatment of several common arrhythmias. Many things have not changed, however: the intensive care unit (ICU) physician must still be able to rapidly interpret an electrocardiogram, separating artifact from reality, while simultaneously weighing clinical findings to decide on an optimal treatment plan; hence, we begin this discussion with the electrocardiogram.

COMPONENTS OF THE ELECTROCARDIOGRAM

The first step in evaluation of the electrocardiogram (ECG) is to identify atrial activity (P waves). P waves are best seen in the inferior leads (II, III, and aVF). P wave shape and pattern should be examined specifically for evidence of atrial flutter or atrial fibrillation. P wave inversion in limb lead II signifies retrograde depolarization. The atrial rate should be examined for regularity.

Once the atrial rhythm has been characterized, ventricular activity (QRS complex) should be examined. If the QRS is narrow, ventricular depolarization most likely occurs in response to normal sequential atrioventricular (AV) conduction. A wide QRS complex (>0.12 second) suggests (*a*) ectopic ventricular origin or (*b*) aberrant supraventricular conduction. The QRS should be examined for regularity and rate. The pattern of grouped beats may suggest a specific arrhythmia. The relationship between the P and QRS components should be determined. If every P wave is not followed by a QRS complex, AV block, ventricular tachycardia, atrial flutter, or atrial fibrillation is likely. Because of the delays associated with AV nodal conduction, a QRS complex occurring <0.1 second after a P wave is unlikely to be related to it.

GENERAL APPROACH TO ARRHYTHMIAS

Cardiac arrhythmias are detrimental when they are symptomatic or when they reduce tissue perfusion or increase myocardial oxygen demand. In making management decisions, the state of perfusion, the risks of treatment versus observation, and a variety of patient factors must be considered. Tachyarrhythmias evoking hypotension, fulminant pulmonary edema, or angina should be terminated immediately with cardioversion or drugs. Symptomatic bradycardia should be corrected with chronotropes or pacing. Each potential therapy and its side effects should be considered carefully. For example, patients with isolated premature ventricular contractions (PVCs) lacking evidence of heart failure or myocardial ischemia have an excellent prognosis without treatment. For such patients, drug suppression of the arrhythmia is unlikely to alter the outcome but is very likely to produce untoward side effects. A history of well-tolerated arrhythmia of a similar type also suggests that acute treatment is not necessary. Conversely, patients with acute myocardial ischemia and those with a history of malignant or degenerative arrhythmias should be treated aggressively. Arrhythmias are often provoked by drugs, electrolyte disturbances, and cardiac ischemia. Thus, hypokalemia, hypomagnesemia, acidosis, alkalosis, anemia, and hypoxemia exacerbate an arrhythmic tendency. Intracardiac catheter irritation, pacemaker dysfunction, digitalis, and theophylline provoke a wide variety of arrhythmias that cease with their removal. It has also become clear that several antiarrhythmic drugs (e.g., quinidine, sotalol, flecanide) can have serious proarrhythmic effects. Electrical stability also may be disturbed by ischemia. For example, hypotension reduces myocardial perfusion, whereas excesses of intravascular volume or ventricular afterload can increase wall tension and oxygen demand.

WHAT TO DO WHEN UNCERTAIN

Asymptomatic narrow complex arrhythmias of supraventricular origin or pulseless ventricular arrhythmias rarely present diagnostic or therapeutic dilemmas. In contrast, being confronted with an unfamiliar arrhythmia in a patient with moderate decreases in blood pressure or symptoms is often anxiety provoking. The first step when confronted with an unfamiliar arrhythmia is to confirm that it is real. Electrical artifacts may occur as a result of poor surface electrode contact or electromechanical devices such as aortic balloon pumps or infusion pumps. Shivering, seizure activity, and tremors of Parkinson's disease can produce ECG artifacts that may be confused with serious arrhythmias. Specialized electrocardiographic techniques may be of particular value in selected patients. These include esophageal, Lewis, and intracavitary recordings to detect occult atrial activity or right-sided chest leads to detect right ventricular (RV) infarction.

The most difficult situation usually is caused by an arrhythmia not clearly of ventricular or supraventricular origin (a wide complex tachycardia [WCT]). In this setting, it is especially important to develop an approach to diagnosis and therapy in advance (Table 4.1). When patients are hemo-

TABLE 4–1

DRUG TREATMENT PLAN FOR WIDE COMPLEX TACHYCARDIA (WCT) OF UNCERTAIN ORIGIN

(Pulseless or symptomatic hypotensive patients should receive immediate synchronized cardioversion.)
Lidocaine (1–1.5 mg/kg × 1, i.v. bolus)
↓
Lidocaine (0.5–0.75 mg/kg i.v. q 5–10 minutes) (maximum dose, 3 mg/kg)
↓
Adenosine (6–12 mg i.v. rapid bolus) (May repeat × 2–3)
↓
Procainamide (20–30 mg/min) (maximum, 17 mg/kg)
↓
Bretylium (5 mg/kg over 10 minutes) (may repeat to total dose of 30 mg/kg/day)
↓
Unresponsive? DC synchronized cardioversion

dynamically compromised, arrhythmias should be treated as if they were life threatening and ventricular in origin. For such patients, however, it is important to exclude the presence of AV block. (Infranodal escape rhythms must not be terminated before treating the underlying heart block.) Most WCTs in ICU patients are ventricular in origin. Hence, patients with WCT in distress initially should receive lidocaine or cardioversion, depending on the urgency of the clinical situation. Failure to respond to lidocaine is one piece of evidence that the arrhythmia is of supraventricular origin with aberrant conduction. Lack of response to lidocaine should prompt a trial of adenosine. (By transiently blocking the AV node, adenosine is very effective at slowing or terminating supraventricular tachycardias.) If neither lidocaine nor adenosine is effective, procainamide is a good therapeutic choice for the patient in distress, because it will control many supraventricular and ventricular arrhythmias. Although procainamide rarely helps clarify the diagnosis, it often controls the rhythm disturbance long enough to get expert advice or perform more sophisticated diagnostic maneuvers. If all of the above measures fail, bretylium or synchronized cardioversion are salvage therapies. In cases of WCT, verapamil or diltiazem are not good choices for empirical therapy, because their cardiodepressant and vasodilating properties often further lower blood pressure in the setting of ventricular arrhythmias and supraventricular arrhythmias using a bypass tract can accelerate. A brief discussion of the most common arrhythmias and their treatment, including an overview of commonly used antiarrhythmic drugs, follows.

TACHYARRHYTHMIAS

SINUS TACHYCARDIA

Sinus tachycardia is the primary means by which cardiac output rises in response to metabolic demands; thus, sinus tachycardia is physiologic in the setting of exercise, fever, or hyperthyroidism. Sinus tachycardia also may be an appropriate physiologic attempt to compensate for hypovolemia, limited stroke volume, or reduced myocardial compliance. Anxiety, pain, circulatory reflexes, and drugs also may be responsible. Unless sinus tachycardia precipitates myocardial ischemia, it should be viewed primarily as a potential indicator of an underlying disorder. Inappropriate sinus tachycardia reduces diastolic perfusion time and increases myocardial oxygen consumption. For patients with symptomatic ischemia, β-blockade may prove helpful. However, β-blockers should be used with extreme caution in the settings of hypotension, acute infarction, or underlying myocardial dysfunction, because sinus tachycardia often reflects incipient heart failure in these settings and is probably a compensatory response.

NONSINUS SUPRAVENTRICULAR TACHYCARDIAS

Reentrant Tachycardias

Diagnosis

The nomenclature surrounding supraventricular tachycardia (SVT) is confusing. SVT usually results from a reentry mechanism and less commonly from the rapid discharge of an ectopic atrial focus. The most common form, by far, is AV nodal reentrant tachycardia in which an atrial reentry circuit involves the AV node. Graphic examples of the most common forms of supraventricular tachycardias are presented in Figure 4.1. Less common forms of SVT include AV reentrant tachycardia, in which the conducting circuit uses a bypass tract circumventing the AV node (e.g., Wolff-Parkinson-White syndrome). This variant may be identified by the short P-R interval and delta waves indicative of ventricular

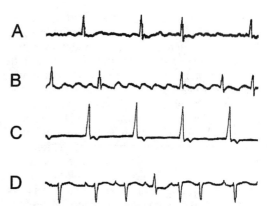

FIG. 4–1. Stylized electrocardiographic tracings illustrating the distinguishing features of the most common supraventricular arrhythmias. (**A**) the irregularly irregular ventricular response and absence of well-defined P waves characteristic of atrial fibrillation. In contrast, (**B**) illustrates the rapid inverted "sawtooth" atrial depolarizations of atrial flutter and the common 2:1 ventricular response resulting in a ventricular rate of 150 beats/minute. (**C**) the most common pattern of AV nodal reentrant tachycardia in which an isolelectric baseline is punctuated by slightly irregular narrow complex ventricular depolarizations. Close examination reveals inverted monomorphic P waves buried in the QRS and T waves. (**D**) the characteristic polymorphic P wave pattern of multifocal atrial tachycardia.

preexcitation occurring via the bypass tract. Moreover, this unusual variant must be recognized because it may respond paradoxically to the approaches that are appropriate for the more common arrhythmias that involve the AV node. Rarely, intrasinoatrial node reentry may occur. Although sometimes confused with atrial flutter with 2:1 conduction, AV nodal reentrant tachycardia usually can be distinguished as a slightly irregular, narrow QRS tachycardia occurring at a rate <200 beats/minute. The inter-QRS baseline is isoelectric. Unlike atrial flutter or fibrillation, in which the ventricular response slows to vagal stimulation or adenosine therapy, AV nodal reentrant tachycardia either remains unaffected or terminates abruptly. QRS complexes frequently exhibit a rate-related, right bundle branch block pattern that may simulate ventricular tachycardia. (P waves are often buried in the QRS complex or T wave.) When visible, P waves frequently are inverted in the inferior leads because atrial depolarization characteristically begins from a focus low in the right atrium and spreads cephalad. The diagnosis of SVT may be confirmed using esophageal or intracavitary electrodes demonstrating atrial activity. Nonsustained SVT is generally well tolerated and requires no treatment.

Treatment

Because AV nodal reentrant tachycardia usually involves the AV node and a refractory atrial pathway, therapy is directed at disrupting the most accessible portion of the reverberating circuit, the AV node. Thus, AV nodal reentrant tachycardia is most commonly terminated by maneuvers or drugs that increase acetylcholine concentration in the AV node, slowing conduction through this region. Conversely, AV reentrant tachycardias are best interrupted by slowing conduction through the bypass tract. An outline of therapy for supraventricular tachycardia is presented in Table 4.2. Massage of the nondominant carotid artery for 10–15 seconds, used alone or in conjunction with the Valsalva maneuver, often interrupts AV nodal reentrant tachycardias. To avoid cerebral ischemia, both carotid arteries should not be compressed simultaneously and vessels with bruits should not be massaged. Other vagal maneuvers (e.g., ocular compression) are potentially dangerous. When vagal maneuvers fail, drug intervention is indicated. Adenosine, an endogenous nucleoside, has now supplanted verapamil as the drug of choice for initial treatment of hemodynamically stable AV nodal reentrant tachycardias. As a potent AV node blocking drug, a 6- to 12-mg i.v. dose terminates nodal reentrant tachycardia with a success rate equal to or greater than that of verapamil. Adenosine will not terminate atrial fibrillation or atrial flutter but, by temporarily blocking the AV node, may reveal unsuspected bypass tracts of AV reentrant tachycardia like Wolff-Parkinson-White syndrome. Verapamil represents second-line therapy but should be avoided when a supraventricular origin is in doubt or for patients with systolic pressures <100 mm Hg. The vasodilating effects of calcium channel blockers may cause hypotension unless rhythm conversion occurs. Doses of verapamil (2.5–5 mg i.v.) usually are adequate. (Appropriate doses of diltiazem may be substituted for verapamil.) Propranolol in doses of 0.5–1.0 mg every 5 minutes (up to a 4-mg total dose) also may be effective. Digoxin has long been used in the treatment of AV nodal reentrant tachycardia but often requires hours for effect, making it most useful for hemodynamically stable patients and for those requiring prophylaxis. By boosting systemic blood pressure, vasoconstrictive drugs may reflexly decrease AV nodal conduction. However, vasopressors may precipitate cardiac or cerebrovascular complications and are therefore usually avoided. Type Ia antiarrhythmics (e.g., quinidine, procainamide, and disopyramide) exert vagolytic effects and may worsen arrhythmias by accelerating AV conduction unless the AV node has been partially blocked. Lidocaine has no effect on SVT. In refractory SVT, temporary overdrive atrial pacing may restore sinus rhythm. Overdrive pacing is particularly convenient when an atrial pacer or pacing Swan-Ganz catheter is already in place, as after cardiac surgery. Hemodynamically unstable SVT should be treated with low-energy synchronized cardioversion.

ECTOPIC SUPRAVENTRICULAR TACHYCARDIAS

Multifocal (Chaotic) Atrial Tachycardia

Diagnosis

Multifocal atrial tachycardia (MAT) occurs most often in association with obstructive lung disease or metabolic crisis, but it also complicates left ventricular failure, coronary artery disease, diabetes, sepsis, and toxicity with digitalis and theophylline. Among patients with lung disease, hypoxemia, hypercapnia, acidosis, right atrial enlargement and β agonist therapy all have been

TABLE 4–2

TREATMENT PLAN FOR PAROXYSMAL SUPRAVENTRICULAR TACHYCARDIA

If unstable, direct current synchronized cardioversion
↓
Vagal maneuvers
↓
Adenosine (6–12 mg rapid i.v. bolus)
(may repeat 2×)

Wide complex?	Narrow complex?
Lidocaine (1–1.5 mg/kg bolus)	Verapamil (2.5–5 mg i.v.)
Procainamide (20–30 mg/ min) (maximum dose, 17 mg/kg)	Verapamil (5–10 mg i.v.) Consider digitalis, β-blockers, diltiazem
Synchronized cardioversion	

identified as risk factors. MAT usually portends a poor prognosis probably more because of its association with underlying illness rather than due to the arrhythmia itself. Because MAT (unlike SVT) is an ectopic tachycardia, measures to increase AV nodal refractoriness are ineffective in control. MAT is recognized by irregular QRS complexes of supraventricular origin, varying P-R intervals, and the presence of at least three morphologically distinct P waveforms on an isoelectric baseline. Comparable heart rates (100–180 beats/minute) and beat-to-beat variation in P-R and R-R intervals often cause MAT to be confused with atrial fibrillation.

Treatment

Although verapamil may temporarily slow or convert MAT, the definitive treatment of MAT is to reverse hypoxemia, acidosis, and other underlying causes. Correction of hypokalemia and supplementing magnesium, even if levels are within the normal range, can be effective. Verapamil therapy can be useful by decreasing the frequency of the atrial impulses, not by blocking their entry to ventricle. Unfortunately, verapamil commonly reduces blood pressure and can adversely affect ventilation perfusion matching in the lung. β-blockade can also abolish or control the rate of MAT but obviously has limitations in a population of patients with lung disease. If β-blockers are used, short-acting agents (esmolol) or cardioselective blockers (metoprolol) make the most sense. Neither cardioversion nor digitalis benefits patients with MAT. Whereas theophylline and β-agonists may occasionally precipitate MAT, their cautious use may improve underlying bronchospasm sufficiently to reverse the arrhythmia. For patients who demonstrate MAT in response to theophylline or β-agonists, corticosteroid or inhaled anticholinergics represent attractive alternative options for treating bronchospasm because they are not cardiostimulatory.

ATRIAL FIBRILLATION

Diagnosis

Atrial fibrillation is a chaotic atrial rhythm in which no single ectopic pacemaker captures the entire atrium. Atrial fibrillation, a rhythm often seen in obstructive lung disease and hyperthyroidism, does not always signify heart disease. Atrial fibrillation classically produces an irregularly irregular ventricular rhythm that may be confused with MAT, frequent premature atrial contractions, sinus tachycardia, or atrial flutter with variable AV block. Because there is no organized atrial depolarization, there is no detectable P wave or effective atrial contraction. By preventing the normal atrial contraction that facilitates left ventricular priming, cardiac output may fall by as much as 30% in patients with impaired ventricular distensibility. Although the atria may depolarize 700 times per minute, the AV node usually fails to conduct impulses at rates higher than 180–200 beats/minute. However, fever, sepsis, vagolytic drugs, and the presence of accessory conduction pathways may increase the ventricular response. On physical examination, atrial fibrillation is suggested by a fluctuating S1 (due to varying mitral valve position at the onset of ventricular systole) and a pulse deficit (due to occasional systoles with low ejection volumes).

Treatment

Treatment is guided by ventricular response rate and hemodynamic status. Acute hemodynamic compromise mandates synchronized cardioversion (200–400 J) to quickly terminate the arrhythmia. Ventricular rates >200 beats/minute suggest accelerated conduction due to vagolytic drugs (e.g., Type Ia antiarrhythmics) or an accelerated conduction pathway. If the ventricular rate is <60 beats/minute, conduction system disease or drug effect (digitalis, β-blockers, calcium channel blockers) should be suspected. There should be no rush to correct chronic, hemodynamically stable atrial fibrillation. Before conversion is attempted, the likelihood of attaining and maintaining sinus rhythm should be assessed. When left atrial diameter exceeds 4–6 cm, conversion to stable sinus rhythm is unlikely. Although many clinicians advocate at least one attempt at restoring sinus rhythm, most patients do well if the resting ventricular response is maintained at <100 beats/minute. The initial therapy of atrial fibrillation is to slow the resting ventricular rate to <100 beats/minute with digoxin alone or in combination with a β-blocker or calcium channel blocker (20% of patients with new onset atrial fibrillation treated with digoxin alone convert to normal sinus rhythm). In chronic atrial fibrillation, anticoagulation should be undertaken for 2–6 weeks before rhythm conversion is attempted to minimize the risk of embolization. For patients with untreated atrial fibrillation and a spontaneous slow ventricular response (<80 beats/minute), electrical cardioversion, digoxin, or verapamil may produce symptomatic bradycardia or even asystole. The risk of bradycardia is sufficiently high that a temporary pacemaker should be inserted before attempting cardioversion in this group. Once the ventricular response is slowed, propofanone, flecanide, quinidine, sotalol, or amiodarone may chemically convert atrial fibrillation to sinus rhythm, but each has specific liabilities. Quinidine should not be used alone, because vagolysis may speed AV conduction and accelerate the ventricular rate to dangerous levels; AV nodal blocking pretreatment should be given first. This combination is effective in ~40% of patients, whereas procainamide is less effective. Added to a stable dose of digoxin, quinidine may increase serum digoxin levels by as much as 50%. Quinidine and sotalol may increase QT intervals, thereby predisposing to Torsades de pointes. Flecanide has been associated with pro-arrhythmic effects, and amiodarone can precipitate pulmonary toxicity, especially when used in high doses or for long periods of time.

Electrocardioversion may change atrial fibrillation to sinus rhythm in patients failing a drug regimen. Atrial fibrillation recurs after cardioversion for most patients, unless pharmacologic suppression is continued; therefore, it makes little sense to cardiovert patients intolerant of the available medications. For patients in whom atrial fibrillation cannot be corrected, long-term anticoagulation with warfarin is indicated to prevent systemic embolism.

ATRIAL FLUTTER

Diagnosis

Atrial flutter, a rhythm that usually implies organic heart disease, arises in a localized region of reentry outside the AV node or, less commonly, in a rapidly firing ectopic focus. Atrial flutter frequently complicates pneumonia, exacerbations of chronic lung disease, and the postoperative course of thoracic surgery patients but seldom occurs after myocardial infarction. Atrial flutter is intrinsically unstable, often converting to atrial fibrillation spontaneously or in response to digitalis. Because the atrial flutter pathway does not involve the AV node, atrial rates usually are rapid (260–340 beats/minute). The ventricular response can be slowed, but the rhythm cannot be terminated by vagal maneuvers. Depolarization usually originates from a focus low in the right atrium, producing inverted P waves in the inferior leads and upright P deflections in lead V1. The frequency of ventricular response depends on the underlying atrial rate and the extent of AV block. Most commonly, a 2:1 AV block leads to a regular ventricular rate of ~150 beats/minute and uncovers the "saw tooth" baseline pattern of atrial depolarization. Examination of the jugular pulse or recording of a right atrial pressure tracing sometimes can reveal the diagnostic flutter "f" waves of atrial contraction.

Treatment

Ventricular rate may be slowed further by conduction system disease or drugs (digitalis, β-blockers). Patients receiving digoxin sometimes show irregular AV conduction or higher degrees of block (3:1 or 4:1). Vagal maneuvers or adenosine administration facilitate the identification of atrial flutter by transiently increasing AV block in stepwise fashion, allowing flutter waves to emerge. Although useful for diagnosis, adenosine rarely terminates atrial flutter. With a success rate higher than 95%, direct current (DC) cardioversion is the most effective method of restoring sinus rhythm, even when low doses of electrical energy are used. Overdrive atrial pacing also effectively terminates this rhythm. Because a high percentage of patients revert to flutter or atrial fibrillation after conversion, prophylaxis with digoxin and quinidine is indicated.

VENTRICULAR EXTRASYSTOLES

Diagnosis

Ventricular extrasystoles are commonly associated with organic heart disease, ischemia, and digitalis toxicity. These autonomous discharges usually occur before the next expected sinus depolarization and are therefore termed premature ventricular contractions (PVCs). A PVC is recognized by an abnormally wide QRS complex accompanied by an ST segment and a T wave, the axes of which are directed opposite to that of the QRS. "Electrically insulated" from the ventricles, the sinoatrial (SA) node continues to discharge independently during the PVC but usually fails to influence the ventricle. Occasionally, when the timing is conducive, a combined supraventricular/ventricular electrical impulse may

TABLE 4-3

TABLE 4-3

FACTORS FAVORING VENTRICULAR ARRHYTHMIAS OVER SUPRAVENTRICULAR ABERRANCY

Monophasic or diaphasic complex in lead V1

Notched QRS complex with R > R'

QS in V6 or an R:S ratio in V6 <1.0

Absent P waves or P-R interval <0.10 seconds

QRS duration >0.14 second

Fully compensatory pause

Fusion beats or capture beats

Extreme left axis deviation (lead I and lead aVF)

Uniform depolarization rate

form a "fusion beat." Because the SA node is not reset by the PVC, the first conducted sinus beat following the PVC appears only after a fully compensatory pause. (A PVC may be interpolated between two sinus beats without a compensatory pause in patients with bradycardia.) It is often difficult to distinguish PVCs from aberrantly conducted supraventricular beats. Factors favoring PVCs are listed in Table 4.3. Aberrantly conducted supraventricular beats (usually in a right bundle branch block configuration) often appear when a short R-R interval follows a long R-R interval in patients with atrial fibrillation or MAT. This "Ashman" phenomenon results from variable, rate-related recovery of the conduction system after depolarization. Occasionally, ventricular extrasystoles are not premature but delayed. These escape beats, usually occurring at a rate of 30–40 beats/minute, function as a safety mechanism to produce ventricular contraction when normal sinus conduction fails. Ventricular extrasystoles that occur in succession at rates <40 beats/minute are referred to as "idioventricular." A rate of 40–100 beats/minute defines an "accelerated" idioventricular rhythm. For obvious reasons, ventricular escape beats should not be suppressed. The primary treatment of idioventricular rhythm is to increase the SA nodal rate with atropine, isoproterenol, or pacing.

The prognosis and treatment of PVCs depends on their cause and frequency. Most PVCs do not require treatment. Indeed, it is clear that pharmacologic suppression of isolated PVCs or minimally symptomatic complex ventricular ectopy in the postmyocardial infarction setting may be associated with a higher likelihood of sudden death.

Although some patterns are clearly more dangerous than others, ventricular tachycardia or ventricular fibrillation often develop without a "warning rhythm." Except in the setting of heart failure or acute myocardial ischemia, there is little evidence that pharmacologic suppression of PVCs improves outcome. Generally accepted indications for acute treatment of PVCs in the critically ill include the following: (a) frequent (>5-minute) or multifocal PVCs in the setting of cardiac ischemia; (b) ventricular tachycardia (three or more closely linked PVCs); (c) ventricular tachycardia or frequent PVCs causing angina or changes in blood pressure; or the once widely accepted but now more controversial (d) "R on T" configuration (PVC interrupts ascending portion of preceding T wave). Common underlying causes of PVCs include ischemia, acidosis, hypoxemia, electrolyte disorders, drugs, and toxins. Surprisingly, "antiarrhythmic" agents have a relatively high frequency (~20%) of worsening existing arrhythmias or causing new rhythm disturbances, the so-called proarrhythmic effect.

Treatment

Intravenous lidocaine is the drug of choice for ventricular extrasystoles requiring acute treatment. Procainamide is an acceptable parenteral alternative. Third-line therapy for ventricular ectopy (usually reserved for refractory ventricular tachycardia) is bretylium. Quinidine should not be used in the acute setting because it is frequently ineffective, has a delayed onset of action, and is available only as an oral preparation. A host of other new antiarrhythmics (flecainide, encainide, mexiletine, amiodarone, etc.) may prove useful in refractory cases but probably should be initiated only with expert consultation.

VENTRICULAR TACHYCARDIA

Diagnosis

Ventricular tachycardia is defined as three or more consecutive ventricular beats occurring at a rate >100/minute (commonly 140–220/minute). Some clinicians prefer the more stringent definition of 10 or more consecutive ventricular beats. The beats of ventricular tachycardia are recognized by wide QRS complexes with T waves of opposite polarity. The ECG hallmark of ventricular tachycardia is AV dissociation (a phenomenon resulting from the independent firing of the SA node and the ventricular focus). Mild beat-to-beat variation in the R-R interval usually is present. Ventricular tachycardia usually is symptomatic and generally occurs in patients with underlying heart disease. "Primary" ventricular tachycardia associated with myocardial infarction or coronary reperfusion carries little prognostic significance; however, late or secondary ventricular tachycardia occurring several days after infarction is associated with a high likelihood of recurrence and a poor prognosis. The mechanism of ventricular tachycardia is the rapid firing of an ectopic ventricular pacemaker or electrical reentry at the level of the His-Purkinje network. Antecedent isolated PVCs are not present consistently. Ventricular tachycardia usually is initiated by a PVC with delayed linkage to the preceding QRS. Occasionally, retrograde atrial depolarization may occur. Differentiating SVT from ventricular tachycardia may be difficult, particularly when supraventricular beats are aberrantly conducted or a bundle branch block is present. Varying S1 or cannon A waves in the jugular venous pulse suggest ventricular tachycardia, as do capture or fusion beats observed on the ECG. The arrhythmia usually is supraventricular if regular, upright P waves occur at an appropriate time before each QRS complex. However, if an inverted P wave follows each QRS, ventricular tachycardia or junctional tachycardia is more likely. In contrast to AV nodal reentrant tachycardia, ventricular tachycardia fails to respond to vagal stimulation. Esophageal or special precordial leads may help to demonstrate atrial activity. The ECG characteristics used to distinguish SVT from ventricular tachycardia are helpful but not infallible (Table 4.3).

Treatment

For the hemodynamically compromised patient, ventricular tachycardia should be treated by synchronized cardioversion, beginning with 100 J of energy, rapidly escalating the energy of the shock. Precordial thump is rarely successful. After cardioversion of ventricular tachycardia to a stable rhythm, lidocaine or procainamide is indicated to prevent recurrence. If the patient is hemodynamically stable, lidocaine, procainamide, or bretylium may be used as primary therapy. For patients with chronic, nonsustained ventricular tachycardia, benefits of drug therapy, electrophysiological testing, and implantable internal defibrillators are unproven. For patients with chronic recurrent sustained ventricular tachycardia or re-

TABLE 4–4
DRUGS ASSOCIATED WITH *TORSADES DE POINTES*
Tricyclic antidepressants
imipramine
doxepin
thioridazine
amitriptyline
Bepridil
Erythromycin
Type Ia antiarrhythmics
quinidine
procainamide
disopyramide
Haloperidol
Sotalol
Pentamidine
Cisapride
Terfenadine
Astemizole

current ventricular fibrillation, either Holter monitoring with empiric drug therapy or electrophysiological testing to demonstrate drug suppression of arrhythmias is an acceptable course of therapy. Unfortunately, an effective drug can be discovered for only 50% of patients. One of the newest antiarrhythmic agents, sotalol, is most likely to provide arrhythmia control in such patients. Internal defibrillator-cardioverters may offer a reduction in mortality for patients with recurrent ventricular fibrillation, but at high financial cost and unpredictable psychological impact.

Torsades de pointes ("the twisting of points") is a specific subset of ventricular tachycardia recognized by its bizarre polymorphism, constantly changing QRS axis, and propensity to begin after the peak of the preceding T wave. Symptomatic Torsades requires immediate treatment. Therapy should include removal of precipitating agents (see Table 4.4) and correction of electrolyte abnormalities (especially hypokalemia and hypomagnesemia). Although lidocaine or cardioversion may be temporarily effective, definitive therapy requires shortening the QT interval, usually by accelerating the normal sinus rate to more than 100 beats/minute. Atropine, isoproterenol, or ventricular pacing can be used as cardioaccelerants.

BRADYARRHYTHMIAS

Except when caused by intrinsic disease of the sinus mechanism or conduction system, bradycardia tends to reflect a noncardiogenic etiology. Such stimuli include vagal reflexes, hypoxemia, hypothyroidism, and drug effects (particularly β-blockers, calcium channel blockers, or digoxin). Bradycardia is usually of little import for patients with normally compliant hearts, adequate preload reserves, and the ability to peripherally vasoconstrict. However, if stroke volume cannot be increased (e.g., dehydration, pericardial disease, noncompliant myocardium, loss of atrial contraction, or depressed contractility), bradycardia may precipitously lower cardiac output and blood pressure.

SINUS BRADYCARDIA

Bradycardia may be physiologic when metabolic demands are reduced (hypothermia, hypothyroidism, starvation). Sinus bradycardia is characterized by normal P wave morphology and 1:1 AV conduction at a rate <60 beats/minute. The association of sinus bradycardia with inferior and posterior myocardial infarctions may be related to ischemia of nodal tissue and increased vagal tone. The vagotonic actions of morphine and β-blockers aggravate bradycardia in such patients. Sinus bradycardia does not require treatment unless it causes hypotension, pulmonary edema, or angina or unless it precipitates ventricular escape beats. However, sinus bradycardia may be a marker of other pathologic processes important to reverse (e.g., hypoxemia, visceral distention, pain, hypothyroidism). Sinus bradycardia may be treated with atropine or catecholamine infusions, but both therapies have the potential to increase myocardial O_2 consumption when used in the setting of myocardial ischemia.

If initial doses of atropine (0.5–1.0 mg i.v. q 3–5 minutes) fail to raise the heart rate to an acceptable level, external pacing or infusion of dopamine (5–20 μg/kg/minute), epinephrine (2–10 μg/minute) or isoproterenol (2–10 μg/minute) dose should be tried. Among patients with sinus bradycardia resulting from β-blocker, calcium channel blocker, or digitalis intoxication, the sequence of treatments offered above is often ineffective. Specific therapy with antidigitalis antibodies in digitalis intoxication, glucagon in β-blocker overdose, or calcium chloride (1–3 gm i.v.) in calcium-channel-blocker overdose usually are effective.

ATRIOVENTRICULAR BLOCK

First-Degree Atrioventricular Block

In itself, first-degree (1°) AV block is physiologically unimportant. However, 1° AV block may signal drug toxicity or progressive disease of the conduction system. In 1° AV block, AV nodal or infranodal conduction is slowed, prolonging the P-R interval (>0.2 second). In the ICU, 1° AV block usually is a temporary phenomenon caused by increased vagal tone or digitalis. Isolated 1° AV block does not require therapy. However, pacing is indicated if 1° AV block accompanies right bundle branch block and left anterior fascicular block in the setting of an acute myocardial infarction (MI). Complete heart block often follows in such patients. Although external transcutaneous pacing may be effective, the more difficult to initiate, transvenous route usually proves more reliable in capturing the ventricle.

Second-Degree AV Block

There are two forms of second-degree (2°) AV block, an arrhythmia in which some atrial impulses are conducted while others are blocked. Mobitz I (Wenkebach) conduction is characterized by sequential and progressive prolongation of the P-R interval, culminating in periodic failure to transmit the atrial impulse. (While the P-R intervals of successive beats progressively lengthen, the R-R intervals shorten.) After QRS depolarization is blocked, the sequence is repeated, resulting in a recurring rhythm. The blockage site almost always resides within the AV node and is most frequently the result of digitalis toxicity or intrinsic heart disease (e.g., infarction, myocarditis, or cardiac surgery). Because the right coronary artery supplies the AV node for almost all patients, Mobitz I block often accompanies inferior MI. In this setting, Mobitz I block usually is benign and self-limited with ventricular escape rates of 40–50 beats per minute. Conversely, Mobitz I block complicating anterior infarction suggests extensive myocardial damage and a guarded prognosis. Although atropine or isoproterenol may be used to improve conduction, no treatment usually is required. Pacemakers are effective but rarely necessary.

Mobitz II AV block originates below the level of the AV node, in the His-Purkinje system, in conduction tissue predominately supplied by branches of the left anterior descending coronary artery. In contrast to Mobitz I block, the P-R interval remains constant. Atrial depolarizations are conducted inconsistently. The QRS complex may be prolonged if the His bundle is the site of blockade. Mobitz II block usually is not transient and, because it often progresses to symptomatic AV block of higher degree, almost always requires treatment. Mobitz II block with 2:1 conduction is difficult or impossible to separate from Mobitz I block in which every other P wave is nonconducted. (One helpful clue may be that QRS prolongation is more common in Mobitz II block.) Atropine fails to influence the infranodal site of blockade, making transvenous pacing necessary in most cases (see below).

Third-Degree AV Block

During complete (third-degree [3°]) AV block, the atria and ventricles fire independently, usually at different but regular rates. Third-degree AV block may result from degenerative myocardial disease or inflammation, myocardial infarction, or infiltration of the conducting system (e.g., sarcoidosis, amyloidosis). Toxic concentrations of digitalis and other drugs may also produce 3° AV block. On physical examination, AV dissociation produces a varying first heart sound and cannon A waves in the jugular venous pulse, the result of occasional simultaneous atrial and ventricular contractions. Blockage of the AV node itself produces a "narrow complex" junctional rhythm at a rate of 40–60 beats/minute and usually results from myocardial infarction. In most cases, it is transient and asymptomatic. On the other hand, infranodal AV block, a pattern associated with a wide QRS (>0.10 second), is almost always symptomatic because it tends to produce slower heart rates (30–45 beats/minute). The inherent instability of pacemakers originating distal to the AV node renders infranodal 3° AV block worthy of treatment, regardless of the rate. Immediate insertion of a transvenous pacemaker is indicated.

ANTIARRHYTHMIC DRUGS

Antiarrhythmic therapy is far from ideal. Antiarrhythmics fail to suppress the rhythm disorder in approximately 50% of cases of serious ventricular arrhythmias and, in many cases, prevention may not improve outcome. Furthermore, antiarrhythmic drugs have a narrow therapeutic window and

TABLE 4–5

CLASSIFICATION OF COMMONLY USED ANTIARRHYTHMICS

Class	Mechanism of Action	Examples
Ia	Depress conduction Accelerate repolarization	Quinidine Procainamide Disopyramide
Ib	Depress conduction Accelerate repolarization	Lidocaine Phenytoin Tocanide Mexilitine
Ic	Marked reduction in conduction	Flecanide Encanide
II	β-receptor blockade	Propranolol Esmolol Metoprolol
III	Repolarization prolonged	Amiodarone Bretylium Sotalol
IV	Block Ca^{++} slow channels, decrease automaticity, and nodal conduction	Verapamil Nicardipine Diltiazem

high incidence of gastrointestinal and central nervous system side effects. Paradoxically, antiarrhythmic drugs exacerbate the underlying problem or cause new arrhythmias in as many as 20% of treated patients ("proarrhythmic" effects). Moreover, preoccupation with the drug management of physiologically insignificant arrhythmias may distract the physician from addressing the primary disorder (e.g., ischemia, electrolyte disturbance, heart failure, thyrotoxicosis, or drug intoxication). Normalizing arterial oxygenation, pH, potassium, and magnesium often improves or abolishes the arrhythmic tendency. For hypotensive or pulseless patients with tachyarrhythmias, electrical cardioversion (not pharmacotherapy) is the initial treatment of choice. Synchronized cardioversion is the preferred method, except for ventricular fibrillation. Amazingly, in the setting of ischemic heart disease, only β-blocking agents have reduced mortality convincingly, and their beneficial effect probably is not related to arrhythmia suppression alone. A simplified version of a standard classification system for antiarrhythmic drugs is presented in Table 4.5, and an overview of drugs used in the treatment of symptomatic arrhythmias is presented in Table 4.6. For patients with sustained ventricular tachycardia or recurrent ventricular fibrillation, automatic implantable

TABLE 4-6

TREATMENT OF SYMPTOMATIC ARRHYTHMIAS

Arrhythmia	Primary Treatment[a]	Alternative or Supplemental Measures	Comment
Atrial fibrillation/flutter	Cardioversion	Rate control with digoxin, propranolol, verapamil	Suppress recurrence with quinidine, procainamide, disopyrimide.
AV nodal reentrant tachycardia	Vagal stimulation adenosine	Verapamil, propranolol, digoxin	Cardioversion useful when drugs fail or reversal is urgent.
Multifocal atrial tachycardia	Correction of metabolic or cardiopulmonary cause	Verapamil	Verapamil slows rate and occasionally reestablishes sinus mechanism. Digoxin or propranolol may slow rate but may prove toxic.
Bradycardia			
Supranodal	Atropine/oxygen	Catecholamine infusion	Hypoxemia and vagal reflexes are common precipitants.
Infranodal	Isoproterenol/pacing		
Ventricular premature contractions	Lidocaine	Procainamide, quinidine, disopyrimide	Many new agents are available.
Ventricular tachycardia	Cardioversion	Lidocaine, procainamide, bretylium	
Ventricular fibrillation	Cardioversion	Lidocaine, bretylium	Success rate correlates inversely with duration of fibrillation.
Digitoxic rhythms	Lidocaine, KCl	Phenytoin, procainamide, propranolol Digibind™	Bretylium is contraindicated.

[a] Correction of hypoxemia, hypotension, disturbances of pH and electrolytes (Ca^{++}, Mg^{++}, K^+) are key elements of therapy for all arrhythmias.

cardiodefibrillators are effective therapy, reducing annual mortality to 1–2%. Unfortunately, an invasive procedure is required for placement; the procedure is costly, and the sporadic, unexpected, painful shocks it delivers can be psychologically disabling.

SPECIFIC ANTIARRHYTHMIC DRUGS

Lidocaine

Lidocaine, a type II antiarrhythmic, effectively suppresses ventricular irritability but has little effect on supraventricular arrhythmias. Because a survival benefit has not been demonstrated and side effects are common, prophylactic therapy in myocardial infarction is no longer recommended for patients in a monitored setting. Lidocaine distributes into multiple compartments; therefore, it requires one or more loading doses to maintain effective serum concentrations. Without loading, constant infusion may require hours to achieve therapeutic serum levels. Loading usually is ac-

complished by giving two to three decremental doses (e.g., 100, 75, and 50 mg) spaced 7–10 minutes apart. For similar reasons, a modified drug bolus should accompany increased infusion rates in the correction of an inadequate serum concentration. Lidocaine doses should be reduced for elderly patients and for patients with heart failure, shock, or liver disease (see Chapter 15). Although no adjustment is needed for renal dysfunction, patients should be monitored closely after institution or withdrawal of drugs interfering with the hepatic metabolism of lidocaine (e.g., cimetidine, propranolol). Neurologic toxicity (confusion, lethargy, and seizures) emerges when lidocaine levels exceed 5 mg/mL. Lidocaine also may exacerbate the neuromuscular blocking effects of paralytic drugs. The hemodynamic effects of lidocaine are usually inconsequential but include mild depression of blood pressure and cardiac contractility. Because of its multicompartment distribution, lidocaine washes out slowly (over 6 hours) after abrupt termination. Therefore, although tapering of the drug is not required, ECG monitoring is indicated for 6–12 hours after discontinuation.

Bretylium

Bretylium is a second- or third-line drug indicated for the treatment of ventricular arrhythmias refractory to lidocaine. Bretylium suppresses PVCs, prevents ventricular tachycardia, increases fibrillation threshold, and may "chemically cardiovert" some patients with ventricular fibrillation. Loading doses of 5–10 mg/kg may be given before initiating a constant infusion of 1–2 mg/minute. Bretylium can produce hypotension if given rapidly. Bradycardia, nausea, vomiting, and orthostatic blood pressure changes are common.

Procainamide

Procainamide is a type Ia antiarrhythmic, in many ways similar to quinidine, useful for both supraventricular and ventricular arrhythmias. It effectively controls PVCs and ventricular tachycardia and may convert supraventricular arrhythmias to sinus rhythm. Like other type Ia drugs (quinidine and disopyramide), procainamide may accelerate the ventricular rate in atrial fibrillation or atrial flutter unless AV conduction is slowed with digitalis or β-blockers. For an average-sized patient, a total loading dose of 1 g is given by injecting sequential boluses of 100 mg every 5 minutes. When continuous intravenous therapy is required, loading may be followed by constant infusion (2–6 mg/minute). Procainamide acts as a vasodilator and negative ionotrope, thereby decreasing blood pressure and contractility. Both the QRS and QT intervals of the ECG often increase modestly. Like quinidine, procainamide may precipitate Torsades de pointes. Procainamide is less likely than quinidine to cause gastrointestinal distress but, over long periods, induces a lupus-like syndrome in as many as one in five patients. A positive antinuclear antibody (ANA) develops in ~50% of all patients using the drug chronically, effects that are reversible with discontinuation of therapy. Rare cases of hemolysis or agranulocytosis have been reported.

Quinidine

Quinidine is a type Ia antiarrhythmic, most effective in restoring sinus rhythm in patients with atrial fibrillation or atrial flutter. Quinidine is not useful for emergent indications; even though it may suppress ventricular ectopy, data suggest a higher mortality rate in quinidine-treated patients with PVCs in the postmyocardial infarction setting. There is little use for quinidine in the ICU because it has limited effectiveness and many side effects and is available only as an oral preparation. Diarrhea is the most common side effect during chronic use. Cardiac toxicity includes (a) AV block; (b) aggravation of ventricular arrhythmias; and (c) negative ionotropy. Quinidine prolongs the QT interval and may precipitate Torsades de pointes in 10–15% of patients treated with the drug. Exacerbation of arrhythmias is more common in patients with deficiencies of potassium or magnesium. (The proarrhythmic effects are idiosyncratic: unrelated to dose or duration of therapy.) When added to a stable regimen, quinidine may double serum levels of digoxin.

Sotalol

Sotalol is an antiarrhythmic that increases the action potential duration and has β-blocking properties. Sotalol is an excellent drug to control AV nodal reentrant tachycardias and is also moderately effective for atrial fibrillation and atrial flutter. In contrast to other β-blockers and AV nodal blocking agents (e.g., digitalis, verapamil), sotalol also can influence AV reentrant tachycardia, which uses an accessory pathway (e.g., Wolff-Parkinson-White syndrome). Sotalol also is one of the few agents demonstrated to decrease the frequency of sustained ventricular tachycardia and ventricular fibrillation and its associated mortality. Because of its QT prolonging effects, use in the setting of hypokalemia or hypomagnesemia or combination with other drugs known to prolong the QT interval is unwise. Sotalol's QT-prolonging and β-blocking actions dictate that it probably should be initiated during ECG monitoring in a hospital. As might be expected because of the QT prolonging effects, sotalol has been associated with Torsades de pointes.

Digitalis

The major use of digitalis in arrhythmia management is to slow AV conduction in atrial fibrillation and atrial flutter. In this role, digoxin usually is given in 0.125- to 0.25-mg doses i.v. every 4–6 hours until the ventricular response rate is <100/minute. (If hemodynamically unstable, cardioversion is indicated.) When used as an antiarrhythmic, digoxin usually is titrated to the desired degree of AV block, with less regard for "standard therapeutic drug levels" than when used as an ionotropic medication. Nonetheless, levels above 3 ng/ml are poorly tolerated and usually not necessary. Heart block, increased myocardial irritability, gastrointestinal distress (nausea and vomiting), and central nervous system (CNS) disturbances (confusion, visual aberrations) are the most common toxic side effects.

Verapamil

Verapamil, a calcium channel blocker, routinely converts AV nodal reentrant tachycardia and slows the ventricular response of atrial fibrillation and atrial flutter. Verapamil often slows or abolishes MAT but rarely converts atrial fibrillation or atrial flutter to sinus rhythm. For hemodynamically compromised patients, cardioversion (not verapamil) is the treatment of choice. Intravenous doses of 2.5–5 mg at 5- to 10-minute intervals are usually promptly effective. Verapamil must be used with extreme caution; even with commonly used doses, high-grade AV block (occasionally asystole) may result. (This effect is more common in ventricular tachycardia than in SVT.) Because of its vasodilating effects, hypotension is common in volume-depleted and elderly patients. The troublesome vasodilation induced by verapamil when used to treat arrhythmias often can be avoided by pretreatment with intravenous calcium preparations.

Phenytoin

Phenytoin is a type II antiarrhythmic most useful in treating digitalis-induced ventricular tachyarrhythmias. Phenytoin shortens the QT and P-R intervals and increases AV block. Phenytoin usually is administered i.v. in loading doses of ~1 g but must be given slowly (<50 mg/minute) as the cardiac rhythm is monitored. The drug and its solvent, propylene glycol, may provoke serious arrhythmias or hypotension during rapid administration. Phenytoin lowers blood pressure by decreasing cardiac output and systemic vascular resistance. Cerebellar ataxia is the major toxicity of phenytoin levels >20 mg/dL. Phenytoin potentiates the effects of other drugs that are highly protein bound (e.g., warfarin, phenylbutazone).

β-Adrenergic Blockers

A wide range of β-adrenergic-blocking drugs is currently available. These differ with respect to speed of onset, receptor selectivity, duration of action, and side effects. The prototype is propranolol, the primary actions of which are shared by most members of the class. Propranolol, a nonspecific β-blocker, is a negative ionotrope and chronotrope. Propranolol decreases the rate of SA node depolarization and conduction velocity. Although useful in states of catecholamine excess (e.g., pheochromocytoma, hyperthyroidism, cocaine toxicity), β-blockade may produce disastrous results in patients who depend on catecholamine stimulation to remain compensated. Such problems are likely to arise in patients with intravascular volume depletion, asthma, impaired cardiac contractility, or stroke volume limited by constriction. Propranolol helps slow the rate in supraventricular tachyarrhythmias such as SVT, atrial fibrillation, atrial flutter, and Wolff-Parkinson-White syndrome. The drug is a poor choice for treating most ventricular arrhythmias, except when these are exacerbated by tachycardia or ischemia. In emergency situations, propranolol may be administered in i.v. doses of 0.5–1.0 mg every 10 minutes. Contraindications include severe bradycardia or high-grade AV block, heart failure, asthma, or digitalis toxicity. β-blocking drugs may aggravate coronary spasm in variant (Prinzmetal's) angina. When selecting a β-blocker, the desired duration of action should be a key consideration. The antiarrhythmic and antihypertensive effects of atenolol may last for 24 hours. Conversely, the ultra-short action of esmolol may help in the acute management of supraventricular tachyarrhythmias (atrial fibrillation, atrial flutter, SVT) without depressing myocardial function for protracted periods.

Amiodarone

Amiodarone is a highly effective antiarrhythmic drug for a wide variety of supraventricular and ventricular rhythm disturbances. At one time, amiodarone was used in high doses only for refractory life-threatening ventricular arrhythmias in large part because of its significant toxicities. Now, lower, less toxic doses, have been shown to be effective for a variety of supraventricular arrhythmias. Paroxysmal supraventricular tachycardia, atrial fibrillation, and atrial flutter are controlled in up to 70% of patients, and ventricular arrhythmias may be controlled almost as frequently. Amiodarone may be the most effective agent for controlling atrial fibrillation, but questions remain about its long-term safety. Up to $\frac{1}{3}$ of all recipients discontinue therapy because of toxicity. The most common side effects are gastrointestinal and neurologic; however, pulmonary toxicity is a well-recognized, potentially fatal complication. On its own, amiodarone may induce SA or AV nodal blockade as well as infranodal conduction system disorders. Unpredictable interactions also can occur with other antiarrhythmics. Amiodarone routinely increases plasma levels of digitalis, quinidine, procainamide, and flecanide and potentiates the anticoagulant effect of warfarin.

ELECTRICAL CARDIOVERSION

Electrical shock terminates reentrant tachycardias and ventricular fibrillation by simultaneously depolarizing the entire myocardium. In pulseless tachyarrhythmias or ventricular fibrillation, unsynchronized shock interrupts the arrhythmia, allowing a more stable pacemaker to emerge (see Chapter 20, Cardiopulmonary Arrest). A stable supraventricular pacemaker is less likely to predominate after cardioversion in patients with slow atrial fibrillation or evidence of infranodal disease. Synchronized cardioversion is preferred whenever an organized rhythm is present. Synchronization times the electrical discharge to occur slightly after the R wave (a "nonvulnerable" point in the cardiac cycle at which shock is unlikely to induce ventricular fibrillation). To trigger the discharge synchronized cardioversion requires monitoring of an ECG lead that demonstrates a tall R wave (usually lead I or II). Rarely, tall, steeply sloping T waves may trigger discharge at inappropriate times. If possible, patients undergoing elective synchronized cardioversion should take nothing by mouth (NPO) for 8 hours before the procedure to minimize the risk of aspiration. An anesthesiologist should be present to monitor airway patency, ventilation, oxygenation, and level of sedation. Benzodiazepines, ultrashort-acting barbiturates, propofol, or short-acting synthetic narcotics can produce sufficient sedation and amnesia for patient comfort. Digitalis preparations should be withheld for 24–48 hours before the procedure to minimize the risk of postcardioversion arrhythmias. Hypokalemia, digitalis toxicity, and unaddressed hyperthyroidism contraindicate elective synchronized cardioversion. Hypoxemia and other electrolyte disorders also should be corrected before the procedure.

It should be emphasized that the appropriate dose of electricity depends on the underlying rhythm. Unsuccessful attempts should be followed by another shock with double electrical energy. Being relatively unstable, atrial flutter may convert with as little as 5 J. Atrial fibrillation may convert with a 50-J shock. Patients with reentrant SVT frequently require >100 J. Ventricular tachycardia often requires 200 J for conversion. For patients with reentrant SVT, electrical "fatigue" of the SA or AV nodes may delay recovery of normal conduction and automaticity. For this reason, the physician should be prepared to initiate transcutaneous pacing and immediately insert a temporary transvenous pacemaker. Adverse effects of cardioversion include skin burns and disorders of conduction and repolarization. The myocardium may be dysfunctional for a variable period afterward. Serum glutamic-oxaloacetic transaminase (SGOT), creatine phosphokinase (CPK), and lactate dehydrogenase (LDH) may rise slightly. The most dreaded complication of cardioversion is systemic embolization, a problem seen most commonly in nonanticoagulated patients with dilated cardiomyopathy, mitral stenosis, or chronic atrial fibrillation.

PACEMAKERS

A thorough discussion of all of the issues surrounding permanent pacemakers is well beyond the limits of this book. Frequently, however, temporary pacemakers are inserted in the ICU; hence, a basic understanding of their use and problems is essential. Temporary pacemakers are indicated for (a) high-grade (especially symptomatic) AV block after myocardial infarction; (b) overdrive suppression of refractory atrial tachyarrhythmias; (c) suppression of Torsades de pointes resulting from bradycardia; (d) sick sinus syndrome; and (e) control of postcardiac surgery arrhythmias.

In emergent situations, noninvasive transthoracic pacing is worth trying but often fails to pace (capture) the ventricle. More likely to be successful is insertion of a transvenous pacing catheter. Effective pacing requires that the catheter electrodes firmly contact the endocardium of the right ventricle. When optimally positioned, the pacer will sense the occurrence of native electrical discharges and achieve ventricular capture (pacing ability) using a very low energy pulse. Although complex pacemakers capable of sequential atrial-ventricular pacing are available, these are rarely necessary in the ICU and often do not function properly when inserted emergently. A simple ventricular pacer will suffice in almost all cases. Three basic kinds of pacing catheters are available: semistiff dedicated pacing "wires," balloon-tipped pacing catheters, and pacing-capable pulmonary artery catheters. (When electively inserting a pulmonary artery catheter in a patient with left bundle branch block, a "pacing capable" catheter should be considered, because insertion can precipitate complete heart block.) The stiff pacing wires may be difficult to place emergently but, once in place, are usually stable. In contrast, the flow-directed balloon catheters usually are easier to place emergently but are less stable. All of these temporary pacing catheters are bipolar (i.e., contain both a distal cathode and proximal anode).

Although the jugular and subclavian sites are the preferred access points, brachial or femoral veins can be used for pacer insertion. Fluoroscopic guidance can be helpful to properly position the catheter but often cannot be arranged emergently. Therefore, in most cases, the pacing catheter is inserted using only electrocardiographic guidance. The ECG can be used in two basic ways to guide pacer placement. For patients with an underlying rhythm, the distal pacer electrode is connected to the V1 lead of the ECG while standard limb leads are attached to the patient. The pacer is then advanced slowly while the ECG signal is monitored continuously. While the catheter is in the superior vena cava, a small negative atrial deflection will be noted. If the catheter "bypasses" the heart, into the inferior vena cava, the atrial deflection will become positive. When the right ventricle is entered, a large ventricular signal will be sensed. Advancing the catheter further results in an "injury" current in the V1 lead when the ventricular wall is encountered. (These findings are most evident if simultaneous recording of one or two limb leads is performed.) The pacer is then disconnected from the ECG machine and an attempt to pace the ventricle is made.

To generate depolarizations, the electrodes are connected to an external pacing generator. The simplest of these devices has three adjustments: discharge rate, output pacing current (in milliamps), and sensitivity (the electrical strength, in millivolts, of the intrinsic cardiac depolarization necessary to inhibit firing of the pacer). For asystolic patients, the pacing catheter can be inserted while pacing in the asynchronous mode is set with a high output (5–10 mA) and a rate of 60–100 beats per minute. Monitoring the surface ECG initially will reveal a pacing "spike" until the catheter encounters the right ventricular wall. When ventricular capture occurs, the ECG will show the typical bundle branch block pattern of depolarizations originating in the ventricle.

After insertion, the generator should be adjusted to achieve three major goals: (a) achieve a heart rate sufficient to meet the patient's cardiac output demands; (b) minimize the pacing threshold (current necessary to achieve capture); and (c) adjust the sensitivity threshold to prevent simultaneous patient and pacer discharge. If spontaneous electrical activity is present, the pacer usually should be operated in the "demand" mode, discharging only when intrinsic activity is deficient. Initially, the sensitivity should be set on the lowest value (usually 1.5 mV) and then increased gradually until the pacer fails to sense the intrinsic beats. The point at which the pacer fails to recognize intrinsic electrical activity is the "sensitivity threshold." To minimize endocardial injury, the minimum current necessary to capture the ventricle should be used. This "pacing threshold" is determined by reducing the output setting from the initial 5–10 mA range until the pacer fails to capture the ventricle. Ideally, capture can be achieved with outputs as low as 0.5 mA. Because a patient's sensitivity to pacing varies with a variety of factors, including catheter position, it is customary to set the output at a value two to three times the pacing threshold. After pacing and sensitivity thresholds have been set, the rate can be adjusted to provide optimal cardiac output.

Several problems may occur with emergent temporary pacemaker placement. Although it is unusual, the pacing catheter can perforate the thin-walled right ventricle. Although perforation can occur at the time of insertion, it more commonly is delayed for hours to days after insertion. Its detection is signalled by an increase in the pacing threshold or failure to capture. Electrical changes may be accompanied by chest or shoulder pain or the development of hiccups as the diaphragm is stimulated by the pacer. Physical examination may reveal a new pericardial friction rub or tamponade; chest radiograph or echocardiogram may confirm puncture by demonstrating a shifted electrode position or accumulated pericardial fluid. The pacer can provoke atrial and ventricular arrhythmias, especially if it is coiled in the ventricle or placed in the right ventricular outflow tract. Again, malposition can be detected by plain chest radiograph. As may occur with any indwelling catheter, infection or thrombosis may develop. Both risks relate predominantly to the duration of the catheterization.

KEY POINTS

1. Correction of hypoxemia and electrolyte disturbances are essential to minimize the risk of arrhythmias and to facilitate conversion to a stable baseline rhythm.

2. Not all arrhythmias require antiarrhythmic drug treatment: those that are asymptomatic, chronic, and stable or related to a temporary physiological disturbance (e.g., transient hypoxemia, electrolyte abnormalities) can be observed while the underlying problems are being corrected.

3. Symptomatic patients with tachyarrhythmias of uncertain origin usually should be treated as if they have ventricular arrhythmias, regardless of QRS complex width, especially if hypotension exists.

4. Narrow complex tachycardias can be diagnosed or terminated in most cases by i.v. adenosine.

5. Many patients treated with antiarrhythmics will develop side effects, which may include new or worsened arrhythmias.

6. Temporary pacemakers are indicated for (*a*) high-grade (especially symptomatic) AV block following myocardial infarction, (*b*) overdrive suppression of refractory atrial tachyarrhythmias, (*c*) suppression of Torsades de pointes resulting from bradycardia, (*d*) sick sinus syndrome, and (*e*) control of postcardiac surgery arrhythmias.

7. Standby pacing capability should be available during high-risk cardioversions and during right heart catheterization in patients with underlying conduction system disease (e.g., left bundle branch block).

SUGGESTED READINGS

1. Ahktar M, Shenasa M, Jazayeri M, et al. Wide QRS complex tachycardia. Ann Intern Med 1988;109:905–912.
2. Echt DS. Mortality and morbidity in patients receiving encanide, flecanide, or placebo—the cardiac arrhythmia suppression trial. N Engl J Med 1991;324:781.
3. Epstein AE. AVID necessity. PACE 1993;16:1773.
4. Levine JH, Michael JR, Guarnieri T. Treatment of multifocal atrial tachycardia with verapamil. N Engl J Med 1985;312:21–25.
5. Mason JW. A comparison of electrophysiologic testing with Holter monitoring to predict anti-arrhythmic drug therapy for ventricular tachycardia. N Engl J Med 1993; 369:445.
6. Mason JW. A comparison of seven antiarrhythmic drugs in patients with ventricular tachycardias. N Engl J Med 1993;329:452.
7. Reiser HJ, Sullivan ME. Antiarrhythmic drug therapy: new drugs and changing concepts. Fed Proc 1986;45: 2206–2212.
8. Roden DM. Risks and benefits of antiarrhythmic therapy. N Engl J Med 1994;331:785.
9. Shaw M, Niemann JT, Haskell RJ, et al. Esophageal electrocardiography in acute cardiac care: efficacy and diagnostic value of a new technique. Am J Med 1987;82: 689–696.
10. Stewart RB, Bardy GH, Greene HL. Wide-complex tachycardia: misdiagnosis and outcome after emergent therapy. Ann Intern Med 1986;104:766–771.
11. Waldo AL. Mechanisms of atrial fibrillation, atrial flutter, and ectopic atrial tachycardias—a brief review. Circulation 1987;75:37–42.
12. Wellens HJJ. The wide QRS tachycardia. Ann Intern Med 1986;104:879.

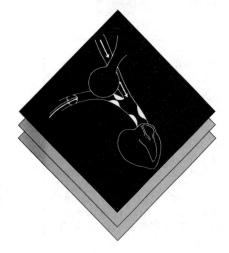

CHAPTER 5

Respiratory Monitoring

Data relevant to the output, efficiency, capacity, and reserve of the respiratory system facilitate appropriate management during cardiorespiratory failure. Monitoring techniques can be classified conveniently into those that characterize pulmonary and systemic exchange of respiratory gases, ventilatory capability, and respiratory impedance (flow, pressures, and breathing workload).

MONITORING GAS EXCHANGE

ARTERIAL BLOOD GAS ANALYSIS

Analysis of arterial blood gases (ABG) provides data that are fundamental to the diagnosis of respiratory and metabolic disturbances and the effect of therapeutic interventions. A typical report includes PaO_2, calculated O_2 saturation, $PaCO_2$, pH, and estimated base excess or deficit. Although certain inferences can be made from the blood gas data alone, a full interpretation and appreciation of the implications for decision making require knowledge of the clinical context, serum electrolyte concentrations, and, in certain settings, the serum albumin and lactate concentrations as well.

Arterial O_2 Tension and Saturation

The relationship of arterial O_2 tension to hemoglobin saturation, blood O_2 content, and tissue O_2 delivery are addressed below. Principles of interpreting the efficiency of transpulmonary O_2 exchange are also discussed. It remains to be empha-

sized that the significance of hypoxemia depends on its chronicity, the integrity of compensatory mechanisms, the hypoxic ventilatory response, and the tolerance of those vital organs most at risk—chiefly the heart and brain. Clearly, a patient with critical coronary stenosis, acute cor pulmonale, or symptomatic cerebrovascular compromise must be kept as fully saturated as feasible, as should patients with dyspnea, circulatory inadequacy, and severe anemia. Conversely, maintaining less than full saturation may be appropriate for patients who depend chronically on moderate hypoxemia to avoid CO_2 retention and for those with intact compensatory mechanisms for whom full O_2 saturation can be achieved only at the expense of very high fractions of inspired oxygen or ventilating pressure.

In the absence of carbon monoxide, methemoglobin, abnormal hemoglobins, etc., arterial O_2 saturation at 37°C (the temperature at which blood is analyzed *ex vivo*) can be calculated with acceptable accuracy from the PaO_2 and pH alone—at least near the upper plateau of the oxyhemoglobin relationship. If the arterial O_2 content is required, if carboxyhemoglobin or methemoglobin concentrations are high, or if the patient is severely hypoxemic, direct analysis by co-oximetry must be requested. (This is particularly important when analyzing mixed venous O_2 saturations, see p. 79.) Whether to "temperature correct" the analyzed specimen is debatable, depending somewhat on the purpose to which such information is put. For example, temperature correction would seem appropriate if the oxygen-exchanging efficiency of the lung were the primary question, whereas the need to correct SaO_2 for temperature is more debatable when tissue O_2 *adequacy* is the concern. Individual hospital laboratories have different practices and reporting policies with regard to these issues.

Acid–Base Status, pH, and $PaCO_2$

Hydrogen ion is a reactive chemical species whose concentration must be regulated carefully to preserve enzyme function. Normally, acids are generated by the hydration of CO_2 ("respiratory" acid) and by other processes of metabolism ("metabolic acids"—primarily phosphate, sulfate, and lactate). In disease states, hydrogen ion concentration can rise secondary to the production of excess lactate (ischemia, hypoxemia), generation of ketoacids (diabetes, starvation), ingestion of certain alcohols, or failure of the body to excrete or metabolize the load of hydrogen ion (ventilatory failure, kidney dysfunction, or liver disease). Occasionally, sufficient hydrogen or bicarbonate ion is lost in the urine or stool or aspirated from the gastrointestinal tract to affect acid–base balance. To address such disorders, the clinician must understand the primary determinants of acid–base homeostasis and deftly interpret the pH, $PaCO_2$, and HCO_3^- components of the blood gas report.

The body defends against radical changes in pH primarily by regulating its two pathways for eliminating acid: respiratory and renal. The Henderson–Hasselbach equation for the bicarbonate buffer system relates pH to the concentrations of bicarbonate and $PaCO_2$:

$$pH = 6.1 + log\{HCO_3^-/(0.03\ PaCO_2)\}$$

In this expression, knowledge of any two variables enables calculation of the third. In practice, $PaCO_2$ (lung excreted) and pH are measured and HCO_3^- (kidney excreted) is estimated. Once formed, hydrogen ions are neutralized partially by combining with bicarbonate ion (producing CO_2) and by reversible oxidation of protein. The bicarbonate buffer system:

$$CO_2 + H_2O \rightleftharpoons H_2CO_3 \rightleftharpoons H^+ + HCO_3^-$$

generates CO_2 when H^+ is added to the extracellular fluid. The rising CO_2 and H^+ concentrations stimulate the respiratory center in an attempt to limit hypercapnea, effectively eliminating H^+ by driving the above equation leftward. Over time (generally, several days are required), the healthy kidney will adapt to hypercapnia or hypocapnia by adjusting the bicarbonate level to help restore the Henderson–Hasselbach-defined $20:1$ normal ratio between bicarbonate concentration and the product of $PaCO_2$ and its solubility coefficient (0.03). Respiratory compensation for metabolic disturbances is generally incomplete and occurs more reliably and vigorously in response to metabolic acidosis than alkalosis.

Despite its functional importance, this bicarbonate buffer system is not the only one available—certain proteins, chiefly hemoglobin, also play a significant role. Thus, a rising $[H]^+$ is partially buffered by hemoglobin, as well as by HCO_3^-, giving rise to a generally small discrepancy between the difference in HCO_3^- relative to normal (24 mEq/dL) and the calculated base excess or deficit, which quantifies the magnitude of the metabolic disturbance or compensation. An acutely rising $PaCO_2$ tends to generate bicarbonate as a portion of the H^+ formed in the hydration of CO_2 is buffered by hemoglobin; the opposite occurs during hyperventilation. Thus, even in the absence of renal activity, the acutely rising $PaCO_2$ of pure hypoventilation is accompanied by a gently rising $[HCO_3^-]$; an acutely falling $PaCO_2$ by a gently falling $[HCO_3^-]$.

Definitions

Acid*osis* and alkal*osis*—the underlying processes that contribute to pH status—may be pathogenic or compensatory. The normal ranges for pH and $PaCO_2$ are 7.38–7.44 and 35–45 mm Hg, respectively. A pH that exceeds 7.45 indicates alkal*emia,* generated either by bicarbonate retention, hyperventilation relative to metabolic need, or both. A pH < 7.35 indicates acid*emia,* caused by metabolic or renal depletion of bicarbonate, hypoventilation relative to metabolic need, or both.

Interpretation

The information available from arterial blood gas analysis allows the clinician to determine pH and the relative contributions of respiratory and metabolic mechanisms. Because compensation is never complete, the dominant underlying mechanism—acidosis or alkalosis—is suggested by the pH. Does a blood gas demonstrating a $PaCO_2$ of 32 mm Hg and a HCO_3^- of 16 mEq/L indicate respiratory alkalosis with renal compensation or metabolic acidosis with respiratory compensation? A major clue is provided by the pH—acidemia would suggest that the fundamental problem is metabolic. Failure of the $PaCO_2$ to fall to the *expected* level would suggest a superimposed problem with ventilatory drive or ventilatory pump.

Chronicity of the process can be judged by comparing the observed values of pH, bicarbonate, and base excess with those *expected* for acute hypercapnia or hypocapnia (see below). To place such information into proper perspective for diagnosis and management decisions, the clinician must take account of the clinical backdrop and examine the serum electrolytes and albumin for evidence of renal insufficiency, renal tubular dysfunction, and an anion gap that indicates the presence of such noncarbonic (metabolic) acids as lactate.

The Anion Gap

The anion gap is the difference between the serum sodium concentration and the sum of chloride and bicarbonate ions. Normally, the gap is 10 mEq or less—a reflection of the sulfates, phosphates, and other unmeasured negatively charged ions that correspond to kidney-excreted "mineral" acids. Because of the anionic nature of serum proteins, the calculated gap should be increased by $\approx$2–2.5 mEq/L for each gram/dL of hypoalbuminemia.

Rules for Compensation

As already noted, primary metabolic disturbances are incompletely compensated by changes in ventilation, and primary respiratory disturbances are partially offset by renal excretion or retention of bicarbonate. Knowledge of these expected compensations allows a judgment to be made regarding the nature and chronicity of the underlying processes.

Respiratory Compensation for Metabolic Disturbances A useful equation for predicting the $PaCO_2$ during a primary metabolic disturbance is as follows:

Metabolic Acidosis : Expected $PaCO_2$
$$= 1.5 \times [HCO_3^-] + 8 \text{ mm Hg}$$

Metabolic Alkalosis : Expected $PaCO_2$
$$= 0.7 \times [HCO_3^-] + 20 \text{ mm Hg}$$

For example, if a measured HCO_3 were 16, the expected compensation would be: $PaCO_2 = 1.5$

$\times [HCO_3^-] + 8 = 24 + 8 = 32$ mm Hg. Note that the pH would be less than 7.40, however, because the HCO_3^- to $(0.03 \times PaCO_2)$ ratio is 16/$(0.03 \times 32) = 16/0.96 = 16.7 < 20$. If measured HCO_3^- were 36 mEq/L, the expected compensation would be $PaCO_2 = 0.7 \times [HCO_3^-] + 20$ mm Hg $= 0.7 \times (36) + 20 = 25.2 + 20$ 45 mm Hg.

Metabolic Adjustments for Primary Respiratory Disturbances The kidney requires time to compensate for a sustained respiratory disturbance and adjusts more successfully to respiratory alkalosis than to respiratory acidosis. The following are simple rules for the HCO_3 expected in the acute and chronic settings.

Acute Rule: $[HCO_3^-]$ rises 1 mEq/L for each 10 mm Hg rise in $PaCO_2$ above 40 mm Hg and falls 2 mEq/L for each 10 mm Hg fall in $PaCO_2$ below 40 mm Hg.

Chronic Rule: $[HCO_3^-]$ rises 4 mEq/L for each 10 mm Hg rise in $PaCO_2$ above 40 mm Hg and falls 3 mEq/L for each 10 mm Hg fall in $PaCO_2$ below 40 mm Hg.

Algorithm for Evaluating Blood Gas Data

A systematic approach to blood gas evaluation incorporates the elements of the forgoing discussion. The first priority is to verify the technical validity of the sample—errors in sampling, sample processing, analysis, and transcription occur commonly. (Is the sample characteristic of a venous rather than the intended arterial specimen? Are the pH, $PaCO_2$, and $[HCO_3^-]$ internally consistent? Does the $[HCO_3^-]$ correlate with the venous blood $[HCO_3^-]$? Is the PaO_2 physically possible given the FiO_2 administered?)

Although there is no best method for interpreting a technically valid report, one logical approach has the following steps:

1. Look at the arterial pH: a pH outside the normal range defines acidemia (<7.35) or alkalemia (>7.45).
2. Look at the $PaCO_2$: if $PaCO_2 < 35$ mm Hg, the patient has primary or compensatory respiratory alkalosis. If $PaCO_2 > 45$ mm Hg, the patient has primary or compensatory respiratory acidosis.
3. Look at the $[HCO_3^-]$ and compute the base excess, knowing that each 10 mm Hg rise in $PaCO_2$ generates 1 mEq/L of bicarbonate via protein buffers and each fall of 10 mm Hg depletes $[HCO_3^-]$ by a similar amount. Compute

the difference between the adjusted [HCO_3^-] and 24 as the base excess or deficit. If the base excess exceeds 2, the patient has a metabolic alkalotic disturbance—primary or secondary. A deficit exceeding 2 indicates a primary or compensatory metabolic acidosis.

4. Look at the serum electrolyte and albumin concentrations. Calculate the albumin-adjusted anion gap for clues to the nature of a metabolic acidosis.
5. Consider the clinical setting and make a judgment regarding the nature of the primary acid–base disturbance. As a general but not infallible rule, pH will be driven in the direction dictated by the primary variable—an alkalemia in conjunction with a low $PaCO_2$ is at least partially driven by a respiratory mechanism; acidemia in conjunction with a low $PaCO_2$ suggests that the respiratory alkalosis is compensatory.
6. Look for evidence of a mixed disorder (as opposed to a simple but compensated disturbance) by calculating the expected value of the variable not involved in the primary disturbance, using the rules given above. Acid–base disorders can be single (e.g., respiratory acidosis, with or without compensation), double (e.g., respiratory acidosis, metabolic alkalosis), or even triple (e.g., respiratory acidosis, metabolic alkalosis, and metabolic acidosis) —as indicated by an anion gap together with CO_2 retention and a disproportionately elevated HCO_3^-. Review the clinical data and electrolytes for clues to the clinical significance of the acid–base data.

MONITORING OXYGENATION

The human eye is not very good at detecting or quantifying arterial hypoxemia. Perhaps the most popular recent innovation in gas exchange monitoring has been the application of oximetry to the on-line assessment of arterial (SaO_2) and mixed venous O_2 saturations (SvO_2). Although intimately linked, O_2 saturation and tension (partial pressure) provide complementary clinical data. PaO_2 reflects the maximal tension driving O_2 to the tissues, whereas saturation reflects O_2 content per gram of hemoglobin. Reflectance oximetry is used when a fiberoptic catheter continuously samples oxygen saturation in the pulmonary or systemic arterial bloodstream. Multichannel fiberoptic chemiluminescent catheter systems for continuously monitoring PaO_2, $PaCO_2$, and arterial pH now have been introduced into clinical practice. These can be quite useful for tracking either rapidly changing clinical events or progress after a clinical intervention (e.g., ventilator adjustment).

Arterial Pulse Oximetry

Transcutaneous photometric oximetry is useful for monitoring patients with marginal or fluctuating oxygen exchange. For patients supported by mechanical ventilation, transcutaneous oximetry continuously measures SaO_2, enabling rapid adjustment of FiO_2, mean airway pressure, and positive end-expiratory pressure (PEEP) and warning of arterial desaturation during weaning, sleeping, or changes of body position. As a general rule, *trends* in oximetry values are of greater significance than the absolute value of saturation, at least over the clinical saturation range usually encountered.

Technical Issues

Lightweight probes direct filtered light of several specific wavelengths onto the surface of the digit, nasal bridge, or earlobe. The relative absorption of these spectrophotometric beams as they pass through the tissue (which differs for O_2 saturated and desaturated blood) is converted into the appropriate saturation value by computer-stored algorithms. Phasic variations separate the incoming arterial component from venous and background absorption. Pulse oximetry probes do not require tissue heating because phasic changes in blood volume and optical density cue the instrument to the arterial component of the blood contained in the vascular bed. Most units also display pulse rate, and many display a simulated arterial waveform or other visual indicator of pulse intensity. The pulse rate should be "correlated" to the ECG measured rate to ensure signal quality. Good correlation does not ensure accuracy, but poor correlation of the heart rate displayed on the ECG and pulse oximeter calls the reported saturation value into question. With a good pulse signal, currently available instruments are quite accurate in their upper range (i.e., saturations > 80%) but become less reliable as the patient desaturates or perfusion deteriorates. Even when accurate, pulse oximetry presents a signal-averaged and therefore delayed report. Probes on the ear tend to respond faster to step changes in arterial O_2 saturation than those placed on the finger (~15 seconds as opposed to ~30 seconds).

Potential Artifacts

Routine arterial blood gas reports of saturation are calculated from the measured PaO_2 and pH. A direct determination of arterial blood saturation (preferably by co-oximetry) is the most definitive check. Motion artifact often is an important problem for patients who are not immobilized. Because separation of the "arterial" segment of the cycle depends on small phasic changes in the tissue volume, large amplitude vibrations of other kinds that are unassociated with arterial pulsation can confuse the sampling algorithm—especially when the frequencies of the rhythmic vibration approximate the patient's own heart rate. When a patient has a rhythmic tremor (Parkinson's disease, anxiety, agitation, seizures, essential tremor, shivering, etc.), tissue volumes can vary phasically in such a way as to invalidate the oximeter's output, which trends toward the default value. In the absence of any detected discrimination between the "baseline" and "arterial" absorption differences, many devices default to a recorded display of 85–88%. Movement of the probe to the ear, nasal bridge, or a nonpulsating site usually improves signal quality.

Anemia and jaundice do not routinely affect the accuracy of pulse oximetry. Pulse oximetry tends to be misleadingly high in some black patients, but by no means all. (The existing literature conflicts on this point.) However, carboxyhemoglobin and methemoglobin can produce falsely high saturation values and specific nail polishes (particularly blue, green, or black) interfere with light transmission and absorbance, as do certain bloodborne dyes, such as indocyanine green and methylene blue. These tend to artifactually reduce the O_2 saturation reported.

Interpretation

Even though used commonly for clinical decision making, many practitioners do not fully understand the oxyhemoglobin dissociation relationship or the value and limitations of transmission oximetry. The relationship of O_2 saturation to O_2 tension and content must be borne carefully in mind (Fig. 5.1). Over the clinically relevant range, the oxyhemoglobin dissociation curve is highly

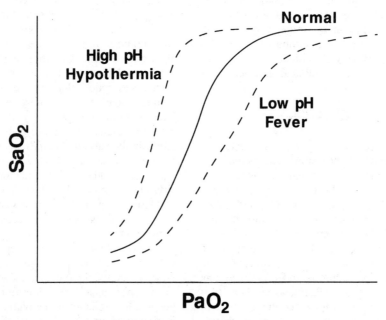

FIG. 5–1. Relationship of blood oxygen saturation (SaO_2) to blood oxygen tension (PaO_2). A normal curve has a sigmoidal shape, with the upper plateau of the relationship (90% saturation) reached at a PaO_2 of approximately 55–60 mm Hg. Alkalemia and hypothermia shift the curve up and to the left; acidemia and fever shift it down and to the right.

alinear, so that a drop of a few percentage points in SaO_2 over the 95–100% interval reflects a much larger change in PaO_2 than does a similar decrement over the 80–85% interval. Pulse oximeters record the relative absorption of light by oxyhemoglobin and deoxyhemoglobin. Therefore, for a fixed value of viable hemoglobin, the saturation parallels its relative O_2 content, but a high saturation guarantees neither its total O_2 content nor the adequacy of tissue O_2 delivery. For example, a patient may have a "full" SaO_2 after inhaling a high concentration of carbon monoxide, and yet, directly measuring arterial oxygen *content* per deciliter of blood (by co-oximetry) may demonstrate profound arterial O_2 depletion. Moreover, a patient in circulatory shock may maintain a perfectly normal SaO_2 despite serious O_2 privation. Cyanide blocks the uptake of oxygen by the tissues, so that O_2 consumption is low even as arterial and mixed venous saturations are normal or increased. Arterial oxygen saturation also bears no direct relationship to the adequacy of ventilation; a patient breathing a high inspired concentration of oxygen will maintain a nearly normal SaO_2 for extended periods in the face of a full respiratory arrest.

Other gas-measuring techniques (e.g., transcutaneous and transconjuctival measurements of O_2 and CO_2) have been used widely in neonatology to monitor tissue gas tensions but are generally less helpful for adults. Transcutaneous techniques require frequent calibration, excellent skin and electrode preparation to ensure transcutaneous gas transfer to the skin surface, and regular site changes to avoid burning the warmed patch of skin they monitor. More importantly, they are profoundly affected by inadequacy of perfusion and therefore track arterial gas tensions unreliably during many critical illnesses. Alert patients tolerate conjunctival probes poorly.

O_2 Consumption

Although a valuable measurement, total body oxygen consumption (VO_2) is often difficult to measure accurately at the bedside of patients receiving mechanical ventilation. Two primary methods are in general use: direct analysis of inspired and expired gases and the Fick method (computation of VO_2 from the product of cardiac output [CO] and the difference in O_2 content between samples of arterial and mixed venous blood). Neither method reflects average oxygen consumption when the patient's metabolic rate fluctuates during data collection.

Methods

Analysis of Inspired and Expired Gases Mechanically ventilated patients often require high inspired fractions (>0.50) of oxygen (FiO_2) and breathe large volumes per minute. Under these conditions, such large quantities of O_2 flush through the lungs each minute that analyses of gas tensions and measurements of V_E must be very accurate to distinguish the small inspiratory-expiratory oxygen deficits that define VO_2. To ensure accuracy, the inspired gas mixture must be blended thoroughly to a uniform and unvarying composition. The ability to determine O_2 consumption on a breath-by-breath basis has improved to such a degree that "metabolic" units with acceptable accuracy and reliability are now available to interface directly with certain mechanical ventilators for ongoing monitoring of VO_2, VCO_2, and other derived variables (e.g., respiratory quotient). Although such technology continues to improve, precise measurement of inspired oxygen tensions and VO_2 in patients requiring high FiO_2 remains a clinical challenge, and variability of metabolism still complicates interpretation, whatever the technical accuracy may be.

Fick Method The Fick method analyzes arterial and mixed venous blood samples for O_2 content (see Chapter 2, Hemodynamic Monitoring). The arteriovenous O_2 content difference is then multiplied by CO to determine VO_2. Unfortunately, this time-honored method is influenced greatly by small changes in either metabolic activity or the CO over the period of the data collection. Furthermore, because of the steepness and interpatient variability of the oxyhemoglobin saturation curve, O_2 content should be measured directly—not calculated. Technical errors in blood analysis and CO determinations are multiplicative, further compromising the accuracy of the method.

Volumetric Analysis Volumetric analysis is a method of estimating VO_2 that uses a closed breathing circuit to absorb CO_2 while metering in sufficient O_2 to keep the total volume of the system constant. This rarely used technique avoids problems of gas tension analysis but imposes significant airway resistance, because all necessary elements must be incorporated into the breathing circuit.

Applications of VO_2

The VO_2 often is useful in determining nutritional requirements and adequacy of O_2 delivery and may occasionally help determine the cause of a high ventilation requirement. Assuming a stable tissue demand for O_2, measurements of VO_2 also may be used to follow the hemodynamic response to therapeutic interventions. (An increasing VO_2 suggests improvement, whereas failure of VO_2 to change implies initial output adequacy or failure of the intervention.) Unfortunately, serial VO_2 measurements are not highly reproducible and are subject to sudden changes in underlying metabolic requirements.

Delivery Dependence of VO_2 Controversy has surrounded the concept of supply dependency of O_2 consumption for patients having sustained trauma, massive surgery, or sepsis. Failure to provide sufficient O_2 delivery may result in anaerobiosis, multisystem organ failure, and an adverse or fatal outcome. Moreover, it generally is agreed that prognosis in these conditions is somewhat better for critically ill patients in whom higher O_2 delivery is manifest. By inference, it has been suggested that in these settings, supranormal O_2 delivery is needed to satisfy the O_2 demands of certain vital organs. Whereas there is little doubt that prompt and vigorous resuscitation must be carried out or that patients who do not spontaneously generate sufficient O_2 delivery or who cannot extract O_2 effectively have a worse prognosis than other patients undergoing the same stress who do, it is highly questionable whether attempts to sustain O_2 delivery at supranormal values are well advised. Some data even suggest potential harm. Specific subgroups of surgical patients could, in fact, benefit; there are no tightly controlled data available to settle this question in either direction. Patients having sustained massive trauma or extensive surgery may represent a fundamentally different physiologic problem and respond more favorably than patients with medical crises. On the strength of a recent well-designed multicenter Italian trial, it now seems clear that maintaining supranormal values for oxygen delivery confers no routine benefit for patients in the latter category. For nonmoribund patients with sepsis and/or acute respiratory distress syndrome (ARDS), supply dependency may not, in fact, exist and, if it did, there are currently no data that convincingly demonstrate that aggressive use of fluids, inotropes, and pressors is helpful. Without better evidence, therefore, maximizing VO_2 can-

not be accepted as the primary target variable for circulatory support in these settings. Nonetheless, it may be worthwhile to follow VO_2 in conjunction with standard measures of perfusion adequacy when assessing the response to therapeutic interventions.

Efficiency of Oxygen Exchange

Computing Alveolar Oxygen Tension

To judge the efficiency of gas exchange, mean alveolar oxygen tension (PAO_2) must first be computed. The ideal PAO_2 is obtained from the modified alveolar gas equation:

$$PAO_2 = PIO_2 - (PaCO_2/R) + [(PaCO_2 \times FiO_2 \times (1 - R)/R)]$$

where R is the respiratory exchange ratio and PIO_2 is the inspired oxygen tension, adjusted for FiO_2 and water vapor pressure at body temperature (47 mm Hg at 37°C).

$$PIO_2 = (\text{barometric pressure} - 47) \times FiO_2$$

Under steady-state conditions, R normally varies from ~0.7 to 1.0, depending on the mix of metabolic fuels. When the same patient is monitored over time, R generally is assumed to be 0.8 or neglected entirely. Under most clinical conditions, the alveolar gas equation can be simplified to:

$$PAO_2 = PIO_2 - (1.25 \times PaCO_2)$$

For example, at sea level with a normally ventilated patient breathing room air:

$$PAO_2 = 0.21 \times (760 - 47) - 1.25 \times (PaCO_2)$$
$$= 150 - (1.25 \times 40)$$
$$\approx 100\text{--}110 \text{ mm Hg}$$

Alveolar-Arterial Oxygen Tension Difference $P(A\text{-}a)O_2$

The difference between alveolar and arterial oxygen tensions, $P(A\text{-}a)O_2$, takes account of alveolar CO_2 tension and therefore eliminates hypoventilation and hypercapnia from consideration as the sole cause of hypoxemia. However, although useful, a single value of $P(A\text{-}a)O_2$ does not characterize the efficiency of gas exchange across all FiO_2s—even in normal subjects. The $P(A\text{-}a)O_2$ normally ranges from ~10 mm Hg (on room air)

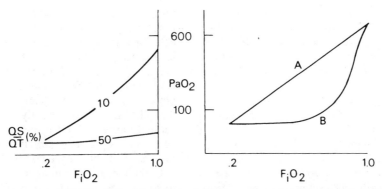

FIG. 5–2. Effect of true shunt (Q_S/Q_T; *left*) and ventilation/perfusion mismatching (*right*) on the relationship between arterial oxygen tension (PaO_2) and inspired oxygen fraction (FiO_2). Hypoxemia caused by true shunt is refractory to supplementary oxygen once the shunt fraction exceeds 30%. Similar reductions in PaO_2 caused by ventilation/perfusion mismatching respond to oxygen; however, the FiO_2 required to boost PaO_2 into an acceptable range depends on whether hypoxemia is caused by an extensive number of units with mildly abnormal ventilation/perfusion mismatching (solid line) or by a smaller number of units with very low ventilation to perfusion ratios (dashed line).

to ~100 mm Hg (on an FiO_2 of 1.0). Moreover, PAO_2 changes alinearly with respect to FiO_2 as the extent of V/Q mismatch increases. Thus, when the V/Q abnormality is severe and inhomogeneously distributed among gas exchanging units, the PAO_2 may vary little with FiO_2 until high fractions of inspired oxygen are given (Fig. 5.2). Finally, the $P(A-a)O_2$ may be influenced by fluctuations in venous oxygen content.

Venous Admixture and Shunt

Under normal circumstances, fluctuations in mixed venous O_2 saturation (SvO_2) do not contribute significantly to hypoxemia. However, as ventilation/perfusion inequality or shunting develop, the O_2 content of mixed venous blood (CvO_2) exerts an increasingly important effect on SaO_2. On-line measurements of SvO_2 with a fiberoptic Swan-Ganz catheter enable venous admixture (Q_s/Q_t) to be computed with relative ease. In the steady state:

$$Q_s/Q_t = (CAO_2 - CaO_2)/(CAO_2 - CvO_2)$$

where the oxygen content of alveolar capillary blood (CAO_2), arterial blood (CaO_2), or mixed venous blood ($CvO2$), expressed in mL of O_2 per 100 mL of blood, equal the sum:

$$[0.003 \times PO_2] + [0.0138 \times (SO_2 \times Hgb)]$$

(In the latter equation, PO_2 (mm Hg) and SO_2(%) refer to the oxygen tension and saturation of blood at the respective sites. Hemoglobin (Hgb) is ex-

pressed in gm/dL.) Like $P(A-a)O_2$, Q_s/Q_t is also influenced by variations in V/Q mismatching and by fluctuations in SvO_2 and FiO_2. If Q_s/Q_t is abnormally high but all alveoli are patent, calculated admixture will diminish toward the normal physiologic value (~5%) as FiO_2 increases. Conversely, if the Q_s/Q_t abnormality results from blood bypassing patent alveoli through intrapulmonary communications or through an intracardiac defect, there will be no change in Q_s/Q_t as FiO_2 increases ("true" shunt).

Simplified Measures of Oxygen Exchange

Several pragmatic approaches have been taken to simplify bedside assessment of O_2 exchange efficiency. The first is to quantitate $P(A-a)O_2$ during the administration of pure O_2. After a suitable wash-in time (5–15 minutes depending on the severity of the disease), pure shunt accounts for the entire $P(A-a)O_2$. Furthermore, if hemoglobin is fully saturated with O_2, dividing the $P(A-a)O_2$ by 20 approximates shunt percentage (at $FiO_2 = 1$). As pure O_2 replaces alveolar nitrogen, some patent but poorly ventilated units may collapse—the process of "absorption atelectasis." Moreover, because shunt percentage is affected by changes in cardiac output and mixed venous O_2 saturation, these simplified measures may give a misleading impression of changes within the lung itself. Whatever its shortcomings, determining shunt fraction is worthwhile because it can alert the clinician to consider nonparenchymal causes of hypoxemia (e.g., arteriovenous malformation, intracardiac right-to-left shunting). Furthermore, because PaO_2 shows little response to variations in FiO_2 at true shunt fractions greater than 25%, the clinician may be encouraged to reduce toxic and marginally effective concentrations of oxygen.

The PaO_2/FiO_2 (or "P/F") ratio is a convenient and widely used bedside index of oxygen exchange that attempts to adjust for fluctuating FiO_2. However, although simple to calculate, this ratio is affected by changes in SvO_2 and does not remain equally sensitive across the entire range of FiO_2–especially when shunt is the major cause for admixture. Another easily calculated index of oxygen exchange properties, the PaO_2/PAO_2 (or "a/A") ratio, offers similar advantages and disadvantages as FiO_2 is varied. Like the P/F ratio, it is a useful bedside index that does not require blood sampling from the central circulation but loses reliability in proportion to the degree of shunting. Furthermore, in common with all measures that calculate an "ideal" PAO_2, even the a/A ratio can be misleading when fluctuations occur in the primary determinants of SvO_2 (hemoglobin and the balance between oxygen consumption and delivery).

None of the indices discussed thus far account for changes in the functional status of the lung that result from alterations in PEEP, auto-PEEP, or other techniques for adjusting average lung volume (e.g., inverse ratio ventilation, lateral or prone positioning). If the objective is to categorize the severity of disease or to track the true O_2 exchanging status of the lung in the face of such interventions, the P/F ratio falls short. The *oxygenation index*,

$$PaO_2/(FiO2 \times \text{mean } P_{aw})$$

which takes the effects of PEEP and inspiratory time fraction into account, has gained widespread popularity in neonatal and pediatric practice but has yet to catch hold in adult critical care. Although preferable, this index, too, is imperfect; mean airway pressure (P_{aw}) and FiO_2 bear complex and alinear relationships to PaO_2 when considered across their entire ranges.

MONITORING CARBON DIOXIDE AND VENTILATION

Kinetics and Estimates of Carbon Dioxide Production

Body stores of carbon dioxide are far greater than those of oxygen. When breathing room air,

only ~1.5 L of O_2 are stored (much of it in the lungs) and some of this stored O_2 remains unavailable for release until life-threatening hypoxemia is under way. Although breathing pure O_2 can fill the alveolar compartment with an additional 2–3 L of oxygen (a safety factor during apnea or asphyxia), these O_2 reserves are still much less than the ≈ 120 L of CO_2 normally stored in body tissues. Because of limited oxygen reserves, PaO_2 and tissue PO_2 change rapidly during apnea, at a rate that is highly dependent on FiO_2.

Carbon dioxide stores are held in several forms (dissolved, bound to protein, fixed as bicarbonate) and distributed in compartments that differ in their volumetric capacity and ability to exchange CO_2 rapidly with the blood. Well-perfused organs constitute a small reservoir for CO_2 capable of quick turnover, skeletal muscle is a larger compartment with sluggish exchange, and bone and fat are high capacity chambers with very slow filling and release. Practically, the existence of large CO_2 reservoirs with different capacities and time constants of filling and emptying means that equilibration to a new steady-state $PaCO_2$ after a step change in ventilation (assuming a constant rate of CO_2 production, VCO_2) takes longer than generally appreciated—especially for step *reductions* in alveolar ventilation (Fig. 5.3). With such a large capacity and only a modest rate of metabolic CO_2 production, the CO_2 reservoir fills rather slowly, so that $PaCO_2$ rises only 6–9 mm Hg during the first minute of apnea and 3–6 mm Hg each minute thereafter. Depletion of this reservoir can occur at a faster rate.

Measurement of CO_2 excretion is valuable for metabolic studies, computations of deadspace ventilation, and evaluation of hyperpnea. Estimates of CO_2 production are representative when the sample is collected carefully in the steady state over adequate time. The rate of CO_2 elimination is a product of minute ventilation (V_E) and the expired fraction of CO_2 in the expelled gas. If gas collection is timed accurately and the sample is adequately mixed and analyzed, an accurate value for excreted CO_2 can be obtained. However, whether this value faithfully represents metabolic CO_2 production depends on the stability of the patient during the period of gas collection—not only with regard to VO_2, but also in terms of acid–base fluctuations, perfusion constancy, and ventilation status with respect to metabolic needs. During acute hyperventilation or rapidly developing metabolic acidosis, for example, the rate of CO_2 excretion overestimates metabolic rate until

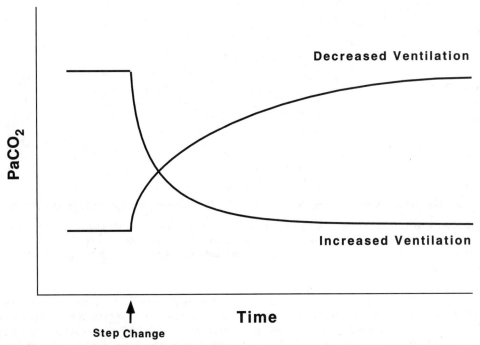

FIG. 5-3. Effect of step changes in ventilation on $PaCO_2$. After an abrupt change in ventilation, $PaCO_2$ either climbs (step decrease in ventilation) or descends (step increase in ventilation) toward a new plateau. Equilibration is reached more slowly after a step decrease in ventilation because the large storage reservoir for CO_2 can be filled only at the rate of CO_2 production. Elimination of CO_2 can occur more rapidly.

surplus body stores of CO_2 are washed out or bicarbonate stores reach equilibrium. The opposite obtains during abrupt hypoventilation or transient reduction in cardiac output.

Efficiency of CO_2 Exchange

The volume of CO_2 produced by the body tissues varies with metabolic rate (fever, pain, agitation, sepsis, etc.). In the mechanically ventilated patient, many vagaries of CO_2 flux can be eliminated by controlling ventilation and quieting muscle activity with deep sedation with or without paralysis. $PaCO_2$ must be interpreted in conjunction with the V_E. For example, the gas exchanging ability of the lung may be unimpaired even though $PaCO_2$ rises when reduced alveolar ventilation is the result of diminished respiratory drive or marked neuromuscular weakness. As already noted, alveolar and arterial CO_2 concentrations respond quasi-exponentially after step changes in ventilation, with a half-time of ~3 minutes during hyperventilation but a slower half-time (16 minutes) during hypoventilation. These differing time

courses should be taken into account when sampling blood gases after making ventilator adjustments.

Deadspace and Deadspace Fraction

Deadspace The physiologic deadspace (V_D) refers to the "wasted" portion of the tidal breath that fails to participate in CO_2 exchange. A breath can fail to accomplish CO_2 elimination either because fresh (CO_2-free) gas is not brought to the alveoli or because fresh gas fails to contact systemic venous blood. Thus, tidal ventilation is wasted whenever CO_2-laden gas is recycled to the alveoli with the next tidal breath. Alternatively, a portion of the tidal volume is wasted if fresh gas distributes to inadequately perfused aveoli, so that CO_2-poor gas is exhausted during exhalation (Fig. 5.4). If this concept is understood, then it becomes clear why V_D cannot be considered accurately as a composite of physical volumes. Nonetheless, wasted ventilation traditionally is characterized as the sum of the "anatomic" (or "series") deadspace, and the "alveolar" deadspace. Because the

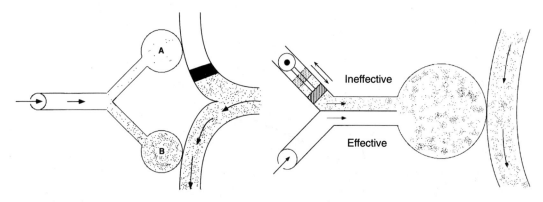

A   **Ventilation Without Perfusion**   B   **Ineffective Ventilation With CO_2 Recycling**

FIG. 5–4. Two definitions of ventilatory deadspace. Tidal ventilation is ineffective in eliminating CO_2 if fresh gas flows to poorly perfused alveoli that cannot deliver CO_2 to the tidal air stream (left). Alternatively, tidal ventilation can be ineffective if the gas flowing to the alveolus during inspiration contains a high concentration of carbon dioxide (right).

airways fill with CO_2-containing alveolar gas at the end of the tidal breath, the physical volume of the airways corresponds rather closely to their contribution to wasted ventilation (the ''anatomic'' deadspace)—provided that mixed alveolar gas is similar in composition to the gas within a well-perfused alveolus. This is almost true for a quietly breathing normal subject, in whom the alveolar deadspace (poorly perfused alveolar volume) is negligible. When the parenchyma is well aerated and well perfused, the anatomic deadspace is relatively fixed at approximately 1 mL per pound of body weight. Quite the opposite is true for patients with most lung diseases, in whom alveolar deadspace predominates. Here, the lung is composed of well and poorly perfused units, so that the *mixed* alveolar gas within the airways at end exhalation has a CO_2 concentration lower than that of pulmonary arterial blood. Although V_D may increase dramatically, the contribution to V_D of stale airway gas is much less important because less airway CO_2 is recycled to the alveoli.

For normal subjects, deadspace increases with advancing age and body size and is reduced modestly by recumbency, extended breath holding, and decelerating inspiratory flow patterns. External apparatus attached to the airway that remains unflushed by fresh gas may add to the series deadspace, whereas tracheostomy reduces it. The supine position reduces deadspace by decreasing the average size of the lung and by increasing the number of well-perfused lung units.

Numerous diseases increase V_D. Destruction of alveolar septae, low output circulatory failure,

pulmonary embolism, pulmonary vasoconstriction or vascular compression, and mechanical ventilation with high tidal volumes or PEEP are common mechanisms that often act in combination.

Deadspace Fraction   In the setting of parenchymal lung disease, deadspace varies in proportion to tidal volume over a remarkably wide range. Series deadspace tends to remain fixed but generally constitutes a small percentage of the total physiologic V_D, overwhelmed by the alveolar deadspace component. Therefore, except at very small tidal volumes, the *fraction* of wasted ventilation (V_D/V_T) tends to remain relatively constant as the depth of the breath varies. The deadspace fraction can be estimated from analyzed specimens of arterial blood and mixed expired ($P\overline{E}CO_2$) gas:

$$(V_D/V_T) = (PaCO_2 - P\overline{E}CO_2)/PaCO_2$$

where $P\overline{E}CO_2$ is the CO_2 concentration in mixed expired gas. (This expression is known as the Enghoff-modified Bohr equation.) As already noted, $P\overline{E}CO_2$ can be determined on a breath-by-breath basis if exhaled volume is measured simultaneously. Alternatively, exhaled gas can be collected over a defined period. The PCO_2 of gas exiting a mixing chamber attached to the expiratory line provides a continuous ''rolling average'' value. In collecting the expired gas sample during pressurized ventilator cycles, an adjustment should be made for the volume of any sampled gas stored in the compressible portions of the ventilator circuit (without gaining exposure to the patient, see p. 125).

In healthy persons, the normal V_D/V_T during spontaneous breathing varies from ≈ 0.35 to 0.15, depending on the factors noted above (position, exercise, age, tidal volume, pulmonary capillary distention, breath holding, etc.). In the setting of critical illness, however, it is not uncommon for V_D/V_T to rise to values that exceed 0.7. Indeed, increased deadspace ventilation usually accounts for most of the increase in the V_E requirement and CO_2 retention that occur in the terminal phase of acute hypoxemic respiratory failure. In addition to pathologic processes that increase deadspace, changes in V_D/V_T occur during periods of hypovolemia or overdistention by high airway pressures. This phenomenon often is apparent when progressive levels of PEEP are applied to support oxygenation. Examination of the airway pressure tracing under conditions of controlled, constant inspiratory flow ventilation may demonstrate concavity or a clear point of upward inflection, indicating overdistention, accelerated deadspace formation, and escalating risk of barotrauma. Small reductions in PEEP or tidal volume may then dramatically reduce peak cycling pressure and V_D/V_T.

Monitoring of Exhaled Gas

Capnography analyzes the CO_2 concentration of the expiratory airstream, plotting CO_2 concentration against time, or more usefully, against exhaled volume. Although most capnometers in clinical use currently display PCO_2 as a function of time, much of the attention here will focus on the CO_2 vs. volume plot because it provides more information of clinical value. After anatomic deadspace has been cleared, the CO_2 tension rises progressively to its maximal value at end-exhalation, a number that reflects the CO_2 tension of mixed alveolar gas. For normal subjects, the transition between phases of the capnogram is sharp, and once achieved, the alveolar plateau rises only gently. Furthermore, when ventilation and perfusion are evenly distributed, as they are in healthy subjects, end-tidal PCO_2 ($PetCO_2$) closely approximates $PaCO_2$. ($PetCO_2$ normally underestimates $PaCO_2$ by 1–3 mm Hg.) This difference widens when ventilation and perfusion are matched suboptimally, so that alveolar deadspace gas admixes with CO_2-rich gas from well-perfused alveoli.

When plotted against a volume axis, as opposed to the more commonly encountered time axis, the capnogram offers data of considerable clinical value. Inspection of such tracings can yield estimates for the "anatomic" (Fowler) deadspace, as well as for the end tidal and mixed expired CO_2 concentrations (Fig. 5.5). Knowing the barometric pressure, the mixed expired value can be expressed as a percentage of the exhaled volume, which is also immediately available from the tracing. If the V_T remains constant, the product of the $P\bar{E}CO_2 : P_B$ ratio and V_E is the VCO_2, and the mixed expired CO_2 concentration can be used in the Enghoff-modified Bohr Equation to estimate the physiologic deadspace fraction.

As with other monitoring techniques, exhaled CO_2 values must be interpreted cautiously. The normal capnogram is composed of an ascending portion, a plateau, a descending portion, and a baseline (Fig. 5.6). In disease, the sharp distinction between phases of the capnogram, as well as the slopes of each segment, are blurred. Moreover, failure of the airway gas to equilibrate with gas from well-perfused alveoli invalidates $PetCO_2$ as a reflection of $PaCO_2$, especially as respiratory frequency fluctuates. (The $PeCO_2$ per cycle, however, remains valid.) End-tidal PCO_2 gives a low range estimate of $PaCO_2$ in virtually all clinical circumstances, so that a high $PetCO_2$ strongly suggests hypoventilation. Abrupt changes in $PetCO_2$ may reflect such acute processes as aspiration or pulmonary embolism, if the V_E and breathing pattern (f, V_T, and I:E ratio) remain unchanged. Although breath-to-breath fluctuations in $PetCO_2$ can be extreme, the trend of $PetCO_2$ over time helps identify underlying changes in CO_2 exchange.

The capnogram also provides an excellent monitor of breathing rhythm. Close examination of the tracing contour and comparison with earlier waveforms may give helpful indications of circuit leaks, patient ventilator dyssynchrony, equipment malfunctions, secretion retention, and changes in underlying pathophysiology. In evaluating the $PetCO_2$, it is essential to record and examine the entire capnographic tracing, not relying on digital readouts alone. Breathing pattern can be as influential as pathology, especially when gas flow is inhomogeneously distributed, as in airflow obstruction. Failure of the tracing to achieve a true plateau can occur because the sampling technique is inappropriate, exhalation is too brief, or ventilation is inhomogeneously distributed. Thus, the $PetCO_2$ may fluctuate for a variety of reasons, not all of which imply changes in lung disease.

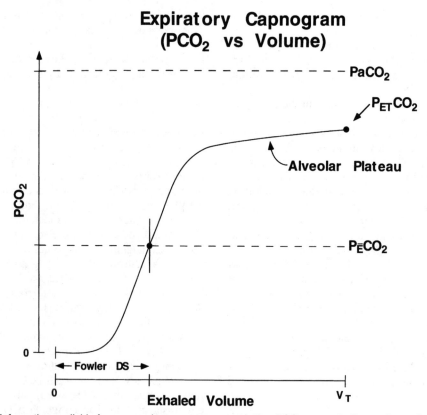

FIG. 5–5. Information available from an expiratory capnogram plotting PCO_2 concentration against exhaled volume. Under steady state conditions, mixed expired CO_2 concentration ($P\bar{E}CO_2$), a key component of the physiologic deadspace fraction and VCO_2, is easily discerned. The slope of the alveolar plateau is a measure of ventilation heterogeneity. The Fowler deadspace (DS) is a close correlate of anatomic deadspace. End-tidal PCO_2 ($P_{ET}CO_2$) reflects the concentration of CO_2 within the alveolar units that are last to empty. Although this value may parallel $PaCO_2$ in normal individuals, it is less reliable in disease.

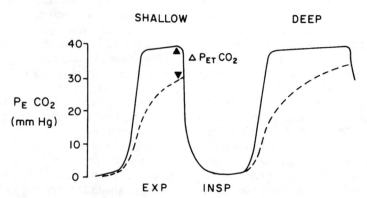

FIG. 5–6. Expired CO_2 (P_ECO_2) as a function of time. Expired CO_2 tension varies markedly during a breathing cycle in four phases. Wide separation of end-expiratory values of end-tidal CO_2 ($\Delta P_{ET}CO_2$) for a normal subject (solid line) and a patient with increased anatomic deadspace (dashed line) narrows during more complete exhalation.

The arterial to end-tidal CO_2 difference is minimized when perfused alveoli are recruited maximally. On this basis, the $(PaCO_2 - P_{ET}CO_2)$ difference has been suggested as helpful in identifying "best PEEP" (Fig. 5.5). This technique may have value for patients in whom a clear inflection point observed on the ascending limb of the airway pressure tracing suggests recruitable volume (see below).

MONITORING LUNG AND CHEST WALL MECHANICS

GENERAL PRINCIPLES

For cooperative ambulatory patients, respiratory mechanics—those properties of the lung and chest wall that determine the ease of chest expansion—are best measured in the pulmonary function laboratory. However, because most patients with critical illness cannot cooperate and are often supported by a mechanical ventilator, the clinician must become the analyst of pulmonary function.

Certain properties (e.g., compliance of the chest wall and respiratory system) can be assessed only under passive conditions; others (e.g., maximal inspiratory pressure) require active breathing effort. The lung's impedance properties can be determined with or without active breathing effort, if an estimate of pleural pressure as well as airway pressure and flow are available. Finally, to separate static (e.g., compliance) from dynamic (e.g., flow resistance) variables, points of zero flow within the tidal cycle must be determined; to accomplish this, the clinician may need to impose a well-timed flow stoppage of appropriate length.

PRESSURE–VOLUME RELATIONSHIPS

A good understanding of static pressure–volume relationships is fundamental to the interpretation of chest mechanics. Although this complex topic cannot be addressed thoroughly here, certain key concepts deserve emphasis. Because the lung is a flexible but passive structure, gas flows to and from the alveoli driven by differences between airway and alveolar pressures—no matter how they may be generated. The total pressure gradient expanding the respiratory system is accounted for in two primary ways: (a) in driving gas between the airway opening and the alveolus and (b) in expanding the alveoli against the recoil forces of

the lung and chest wall. The pressure required for inspiratory flow dissipates against friction; the elastic pressure that expands the respiratory system is stored temporarily in elastic tissues and then dissipated in driving expiratory flow.

Static Properties of the Respiratory System

Increasing the pressure applied across the normal lungs and chest wall increases lung volume, but the relationship between pressure and volume varies markedly over the vital capacity range (Fig. 5.7). Over a small segment, this relationship can be considered approximately linear over most regions of the pressure–volume (PV) curve. Therefore, assuming linearity, the elastic properties of the lung, chest wall, and integrated respiratory system can be described by single values for chord elastance ($\Delta P/\Delta V$) or its inverse, chord compliance ($\Delta V/\Delta P$). (Chord compliance differs from tangential compliance, which is the slope at a single point on the curve.)

The same ΔP will result in a different ΔV for two lungs of identical tissue properties but different sizes. Examination of the pressure volume relationship indicates that chord compliance differs according to the segment over which it is computed. A change in compliance, therefore, could result from a position shift along the pressure–volume relationship (e.g., hyperinflation),

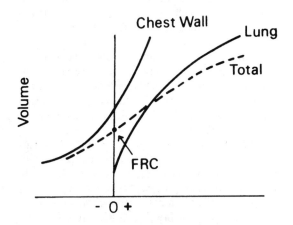

FIG. 5–7. Normal static pressure–volume relationships of the lung, chest wall, and total respiratory system. With no pressure applied to the airway opening, the outward recoil pressure of the chest wall at end-expiration counterbalances the inward collapsing pressure of the lung at functional residual capacity (FRC).

an alteration of tissue elastic properties (e.g., the development of lung fibrosis), or a variation in the aeratable capacity of the lung (e.g., pneumonectomy).

Respiratory System Compliance

The pressure difference (ΔP) required to expand the lung by a certain volume (ΔV) is the corresponding change in transpulmonary pressure: $P = (P_{alv} - P_{pl})$, where P_{alv} = alveolar pressure and P_{pl} = pleural pressure. The lung compliance ($C_L = \Delta V / \Delta P$) is the pressure per unit of inflation volume required to keep the lung expanded under no-flow (static) conditions. The distensibility of the relaxed chest wall is characterized by chest wall compliance ($C_w = \Delta V / \Delta P_{pl}$). The slope of the static pressure-volume relationship for the total respiratory system is C_{RS} ($C_{RS} = \Delta V / \Delta P_{alv}$). In ventilator-derived calculations of compliance, ΔV (normally, the tidal volume) must be measured at the endotracheal tube or expired volume must be adjusted for the volume stored during pressurized inflation in compressible circuit elements. As a useful rule, approximately 3 mL of volume are stored per cm H_2O of peak cycling pressure for a typical adult circuit exposed to a typical pressure range. The physician should be aware, however, that this figure may vary markedly, depending on the peak cycling pressure. The compression factor of the same circuit at 20 cm H_2O of peak cycling pressure may be much less than it is when 60 cm H_2O are required and delivered tidal volume will fluctuate accordingly.

Compliance measurements obtained under passive conditions may have therapeutic and prognostic value for patients with arterial desaturation. When PEEP is applied incrementally, C_L and C_{RS} tend to reach their highest values when lung units are recruited maximally. This point also tends to be that associated with minimal ventilatory deadspace and shunt fraction and often coincides with the point of maximal oxygen delivery. Different tidal volumes may be associated with different "optimal PEEP" values. Although this guideline does not always apply, it is a good rule to avoid using values of end-expiratory pressure or tidal volume that depress thoracic compliance—unless objective evidence of significantly improved oxygen delivery is available. Followed over time, serial changes in the respiratory pressure-volume curve and C_{RS} tend to reflect the nature and course of acute lung injury. Severe disease is implied

when compliance falls to less than 25 mL/cm H_2O. Maximal depression of C_{RS} often requires 1-2 weeks to develop in the setting of acute lung injury. Although C_{RS} provides useful information regarding the difficulty of chest expansion, C_{RS} does not necessarily parallel underlying tissue elastance—both the size of the alveolar compartment and the relative position on the pressure volume curve are important to consider. For example, identical pressures drive greatly different volumes into the chest of a patient before and after pneumonectomy. Ideally, compliance is referenced to a measure of absolute lung volume, such as functional residual capacity (FRC) or total lung capacity (TLC) ("specific" compliance). Furthermore, C_{RS} may differ greatly at the extremes of the vital capacity range, even in the same individual (Fig. 5.8). Thus, most patients with hyperinflated lungs ventilated for acute exacerbations of asthma or chronic obstructive pulmonary disease exhibit depressed C_{RS}, despite normal or "supernormal" tissue distensibility; C_{RS} would be a better indicator of tissue elastic properties if measured in a lower volume range. Because compliances add in parallel, C_{RS} bears a complex relationship to the individual compliances of the lung (C_L) and chest wall (C_w):

$$C_{RS} = (C_L \times C_w)/(C_w + C_L).$$

Chest Wall Compliance

The usual assumption that the pressure-volume characteristic of the chest wall is linear and unchanging throughout its range is often invalid for critically ill patients whose thoracic distensibility may be disturbed by abdominal distention, effusions, ascites, muscular tone, recent surgery, position, binders, braces, and so on. Such changes in C_w are important to consider, in that they influence P_{PL} and hemodynamic data (e.g., pulmonary artery occlusion pressure, P_w) as well as calculations of chest mechanics. Specific values for peak airway pressure and C_{RS} have different prognostic significance, depending on whether the lung or chest wall accounts for the stiffness. Furthermore, the fraction of expiratory airway pressure (PEEP) transmitted to the pleural space depends on the relative compliances of the lungs and chest wall:

$$\Delta P_{pl} = PEEP \times (C_L/(C_L + C_w))$$

Apart from any effect on venous return, the relative stiffness of the lungs and chest wall determines the effect of PEEP on the measured P_w.

Tidal (Chord) Compliance

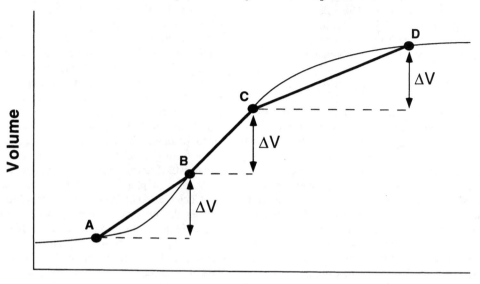

FIG. 5–8. Computation of tidal ("chord") compliance of the respiratory system. An identical tidal volume (ΔV) results in quite different values for compliance (ΔV/Δelastic pressure). In this example, tidal compliance, the inverse of the slope of the chord linking the two volumes over which tidal volume was delivered, is best in the middle third of the curve (BC), worst in the top third of the curve (CD) and intermediate in the bottom third (AB).

Clinical Utility of the Pressure–Volume Curve

In the setting of acute lung injury, virtually all lung units may sustain initial damage, but not all are equally compromised or mechanically equivalent. In severe cases, perhaps only 20–30% of alveoli remain patent; the others are atelectatic or occluded by lung edema, cellular infiltrate, or inflammatory debris. Moreover, the mechanical properties of the lung differ in dependent and nondependent regions. For a supine patient, atelectasis predominates in dorsal sectors, where lung units tend to collapse under the influence of regionally increased pleural pressure and the weight of the overlying lung. This proclivity is greatest at FRC, when transalveolar pressure is least. In this surfactant-deficient lung, there are tendencies for persisting collapse of dependent alveoli and/ or tidal reopening and recollapse of lung units in the middle and dependent zones. The latter process subjects injured tissue to damaging shear forces when high inflation pressures are used. According to current thinking, both persisting collapse of inflamed tissue and the tidal collapse cycle must be avoided. To aid in healing, the objective is to "open the lung and keep it open" without causing overdistention (see Chapter 25, Ventilatory Failure).

Nondependent alveoli remain open and relatively compliant but are subject to overdistention by high peak tidal pressures. These regional differences give rise to a pressure–volume (PV) curve with poor compliance in its initial and terminal segments. Defining the pressure–volume relationship may help guide the ventilator settings needed to avoid the damaging effects of both tidal collapse and alveolar overdistention. Although not everyone agrees, most investigators of barotrauma currently believe that sufficient end-expiratory alveolar pressure (total PEEP, see Chapter 9) should be maintained to surpass the inflection zone ("P_{flex}" region) of the PV curve. Although approximately 10–15 cm H_2O generally suffices to accomplish this in the early stage of ARDS, the requirement will vary with body size, stage and severity of lung injury, as well as chest wall compliance. At the same time, peak tidal alveolar pressure should not encroach on the upper deflection zone that signals widespread alveolar overdistention. (A few sustained inflations to high static pressure may be necessary to open the lung in the initial stages of ARDS, and periodic "recruiting breaths" may be needed when very small tidal volumes are used.) The relevant pressure here may be as low as 25 cm H_2O in some individuals and as high as 50 cm H_2O in others, influenced heavily by chest wall characteristics.

Construction of the PV Curve

No simple rules for choosing optimal PEEP apply to all patients because the compliance characteristics of the lung and chest wall differ so radically. Consequently, there is no completely satisfactory alternative to defining the entire PV curve, even though this is not always feasible or safe to undertake. Disconnection of the ventilator may cause a marked drop in mean and end-expiratory transalveolar pressures that can cause hypoxemia, bradycardia, arrhythmia, and/or flooding of the airway with edema fluid. For this reason, many physicians forgo PV curve measurement entirely in their most severely ill patients or elect to use methods whereby the patient remains connected to the ventilator as PEEP is maintained and varied tidal volumes are administered.

Traditionally, the PV curve is constructed by briefly disconnecting the patient from the ventilator and attaching an oxygen-filled, 2–3 L "super syringe" to the airway opening. After establishing a uniform inflation "history," airway pressure is followed as serial 100-mL volumes are injected until TLC is reached. Static pressures are recorded 2–3 seconds after injection of each increment. The entire process is completed within 60–90 seconds. The P_{flex} and the upper deflection zones used to guide PEEP and applied pressure or tidal volume selections may be defined carefully by using smaller injection steps in the early and late phases.

CALCULATION OF C_{RS} AND R_{AW} DURING MECHANICAL VENTILATION

Inspiratory Resistance and Static Compliance

Although not always elegantly presented or continuously displayed, all ventilators monitor external airway pressure (P_{aw}). When a mechanical ventilator expands the chest of a passive subject, inspiratory P_{aw} furnishes the entire force accomplishing ventilation. Because the pressure–volume relationships of the lung and chest wall are approximately linear over the tidal volume range and because the increment in P_{aw}

necessary to drive gas flow is nearly unchanging under constant flow conditions, the corresponding P_{aw} waveform resembles a trapezoid, a shape composed of a triangle of elastic pressure and a parallelogram of resistive pressure (Fig. 5.9). Although the inspiratory resistance and compliance characteristics of the mechanically ventilated respiratory system can be gauged using esophageal pressure, in clinical practice, these data usually are estimated during volume-cycled constant flow ventilation using P_{aw} alone. It should be emphasized, however, that calculations of C_{RS} and resistance from P_{aw} only can be made when inflation is passive. (During active effort, P_{aw} must be referenced to esophageal pressure to make the relevant calculations.) When gas is prevented from exiting the lung at the end of tidal inspiration, P_{aw} falls quickly to a plateau value. If this end-inspiratory "stop flow," "plateau," or "peak static" (P_S) pressure is referenced to end-expiratory alveolar pressure (total PEEP), the difference determines the component of end-inspiratory pressure necessary to overcome the elastic forces of inflating the chest with the delivered tidal volume. Total PEEP ($PEEP_{TOT}$) is the sum of applied PEEP and auto-PEEP. When tidal volume (adjusted for gas compression) is divided by (P_S − $PEEP_{TOT}$), effective compliance (C_{eff}) can be computed as follows:

$$C_{eff} = [(V_T \times C_{cf}) \\ \times (P_S - PEEP_{TOT})]/(P_S - PEEP_{TOT})$$

where C_{cf} is the circuit compression factor, expressed in mL/cm H_2O.

The maximal pressure achieved just before the end of gas delivery (the peak dynamic pressure, P_D) is the total system pressure required to drive gas to the alveolar level at the selected flow rate and to expand the lungs and chest wall by the full V_T. The difference between P_D and P_S quantifies the gradient driving gas flow ($\dot{V}$) at end-inspiration, a difference that varies with the resistance of the patient and endotracheal tube as well as with the inspiratory gas flow setting. Under these conditions of passive constant inspiratory flow, the ratio of (P_D − P_S)/$\dot{V}_{end\text{-}insp}$ is the airway resistance (R_{AW}). When corrected for the compression volume of the external circuit, the ratio of delivered volume to (P_D − $PEEP_{TOT}$) reflects the overall difficulty of chest expansion, if V_T and inspiratory flow settings do not change and inflation occurs passively. This index had been termed the "dynamic characteristic":

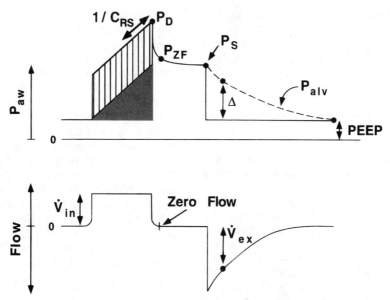

FIG. 5–9. Computation of compliance and resistance of the respiratory system under passive conditions during constant inspiratory flow ($\dot{V}_{IN}$). An end-inspiratory pause is applied to hold the inspired tidal volume before exhalation is begun. Tidal compliance is the quotient of tidal volume and the difference between static plateau pressure (P_S) (equivalent to alveolar pressure, P_{alv}) and total PEEP. In this example, no auto-PEEP is present. The difference between peak dynamic pressure (P_D) and plateau pressures, divided by $\dot{V}_{IN}$, equals maximum inspiratory resistance. The difference between P_D and point at which flow first becomes zero after the pause is applied (P_{ZF}) reflects the least resistance pressure because it excludes stress relaxation, ventilation redistribution ("pendelluft"), and viscoelastic pressures. Expiratory resistance requires measurement or calculation of alveolar pressure (referenced to PEEP, Δ) and the corresponding flow it produces ($\dot{V}_{EX}$). Finally, the slope of the airway pressure tracing at the end of inspiration obtained under constant flow conditions reflects elastance of the respiratory system (1/C_{RS}).

$$DC = V_{Tcorr}/(P_D - PEEP_{TOT}).$$

Because P_D is influenced both by the frictional and elastic properties of the thorax, it serves as a simple yet valuable indicator of bronchodilator response under passive conditions, again provided that flow rate and V_T remain unchanged. During controlled inflation with constant square wave inspiratory flow and stable airway resistance (R_{AW}), the slope of the inspiratory pressure ramp should reflect C_{RS} (see Fig. 5.9). However, estimates of C_{RS} made by this technique (and those by the method described previously) are inappropriately low, unless auto-PEEP is taken into account. When there is occult positive end-expiratory pressure (auto-PEEP) at the onset of inspiration, the relevant pressure for chest expansion is (P_S − $PEEP_{TOT}$), not P_S − PEEP. Whereas P_D and P_S can be measured rather precisely, the flow rate on which the bedside R_{AW} computation depends is not always reflected accurately by the peak flow

setting of the machine. Indeed, flow rates at end-inflation are often lower than set, especially for patients with elevated chest impedance, because many ventilators do not maintain constant flow against increasing back pressure. Of course, a deliberately set decelerating flow profile is subject to a similar misinterpretation.

Expiratory Resistance

For the same average flow rate, expiratory resistance routinely exceeds inspiratory resistance, even in the normal airway. This discrepancy can be much larger in the clinical setting, especially when the patient is connected to a mechanical ventilator. This expiratory resistance arises in the endotracheal tube and exhalation valve as well as in the increased expiratory resistance of the native airway. The resistance across the exhalation valve and external tubing can be monitored easily by recording airway pressure and flow in the external airway. Total expiratory resistance, the quotient of expiratory flow and the difference between alveolar and airway opening pressures (or critical closing pressure if expiration is flow limited), is difficult to measure directly. However, it often can be estimated from knowledge of expiratory flow just before an occlusion of the airway opening and the "stop-flow" pressure (which estimates alveolar pressure). Alternatively, if the time constant of tidal exhalation can be measured under passive conditions, expiratory resistance is the quotient of the time constant and respiratory system compliance.

Expiratory resistance has important consequences, giving rise to auto-PEEP, neuromuscular reflexes, dyspnea, and differences between mean airway and mean alveolar pressures. Average expiratory flow and expiratory resistance increase as V_E rises and the I:E ratio extends, reducing the time available for expiration and boosting average expiratory flow. Except when very mild, the patient must contend with the effects of expiratory resistance by allowing dynamic hyperinflation or by increasing expiratory muscle pressure. For these reasons, certain ventilator manufacturers are now developing techniques to offset the expiratory resistance of the endotracheal tube and circuitry.

Endotracheal Tube Resistance

The endotracheal tube often contributes greatly to R_{AW}. Depending on the nature, length, diameter, patency, and angulation of the endotracheal tube, the resistive properties of the external airway may dominate computed values for R_{AW}. Marked flow dependence of resistance also may be demonstrated in certain patients, a phenomenon usually attributed to turbulence developing in a narrow or partially occluded tube. If endogenous bronchial resistance is the variable of interest, P_{aw} should be sensed at or beyond the carinal tip of the endotracheal tube. This can be accomplished with an intraluminal catheter or by using a tube specially designed for measuring pressures at this site (e.g., tubes designed for jet ventilation or tracheal gas insufflation). Values for C_{RS} (computed under static conditions) remain valid, whatever the resistances of the endotracheal tube or airway may be.

AUTO-PEEP (INTRINSIC PEEP) EFFECT

Definitions of Auto-PEEP, Intrinsic PEEP, and Total PEEP

Considerable confusion has arisen regarding the terms auto-PEEP and intrinsic PEEP. PEEP is the pressure applied to the airway by the clinician. This is also termed extrinsic PEEP by some authors. The pressure measured when all airflow is stopped is equivalent to average alveolar pressure and is termed total PEEP. Auto-PEEP is the difference between total PEEP and PEEP, i.e., that component of total PEEP attributable to dynamic hyperinflation. (The prefix "auto" derives from the Greek term meaning "self.") Different authors use the term intrinsic PEEP as a synonym for total PEEP and others use it as a synonym for auto-PEEP. The latter usage allows specific designation of clinician-set ("extrinsic") PEEP and dynamic hyperinflation-generated ("intrinsic") PEEP without ambiguity. For clarity, we have used the terms PEEP (rather than extrinsic PEEP), auto-PEEP (rather than intrinsic PEEP), and total PEEP throughout this book.

Variants of Auto-PEEP

The need for high levels of ventilation may cause hyperinflation when insufficient time elapses between inflation cycles to reestablish the equilibrium (resting) position of the respiratory system, especially in the presence of increased airway resistance and a lengthy exhalation time constant (Fig. 5.10). Consequently, when a mechanical ventilator powers inflation, alveolar pressure (P_{alv}) remains continuously positive through both phases of the respiratory cycle and airflow does not cease at end exhalation.

Auto-PEEP does not necessarily indicate dynamic hyperinflation, unless expiration occurs passively (Fig. 5.11). Even under passive conditions, the extent of dynamic hyperinflation that results from auto-PEEP is a function of lung compliance. During spontaneous breathing efforts, expiratory muscle activity can raise end-expiratory alveolar pressure, sometimes preventing any hyperinflation at all. Auto-PEEP also is not synonymous with airflow obstruction but, rather, can occur anytime that $\dot{V}_E$ is high enough and/or the combination of frequency and I:E ratio leaves insufficient expiratory time—even for normal subjects. Moreover, auto-PEEP varies markedly from one site to another within the obstructed lung, tending to be greatest in the dependent lung regions. Auto-PEEP can change with variations of body position.

Although deliberate distention of the lungs by dynamic hyperinflation can be used therapeutically for patients with refractory hypoxemia, auto-PEEP usually occurs inadvertently, often with adverse consequences for hemodynamics, respira-

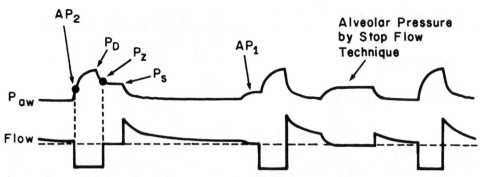

FIG. 5–10. Simultaneous tracings of airway pressure (P_{aw}) and airflow during controlled volume-cycled ventilation with constant inspiratory flow in a patient with airflow obstruction. P_D, P_Z, and P_S represent end-inspiratory airway pressures during dynamic conditions, at the point of flow cessation, and after complete equilibration among all alveolar and airway pressures, respectively. Alveolar pressure can be estimated by the stop-flow technique in mid-expiration or at end-exhalation (AP1). Auto-PEEP also can be estimated under dynamic conditions as the airway pressure above the set PEEP value that is needed to counterbalance elastic recoil and stop expiratory airflow (AP2).

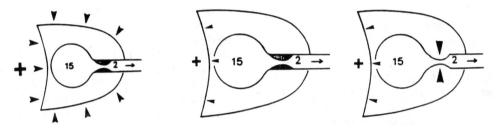

FIG. 5–11. Three forms of auto-PEEP. Auto-PEEP can exist without dynamic hyperinflation (*left*) when vigorous expiratory muscle contraction persists to the end of expiration. Under conditions of passive inflation; however, auto-PEEP *does* imply dynamic hyperinflation—either without (*middle*) or with (*right*) expiratory flow limitation. The response to exogenous PEEP is influenced greatly by the form of auto-PEEP encountered.

tory muscle function, and lung mechanics. Barotrauma is an obvious risk of serious hyperinflation. Unlike restrictive lung disease, obstructive lung disease allows excellent transmission of alveolar pressure to the pleural space. Thus, the hemodynamic consequences of the auto-PEEP effect may be more severe than those incurred by intentionally applied PEEP of a similar level. Immediately after intubation, cardiac output tends to drop as the auto-PEEP impedes venous return during passive inflation. With some exceptions, hypotension occurs routinely after intubating a patient with serious airflow obstruction. This adverse effect of auto-PEEP is particularly important to keep in mind during cardiopulmonary resuscitation, when gas trapping secondary to vigorous ventilation further compromises marginally adequate blood flow.

Auto-PEEP also adds to the work of breathing, presenting an increased threshold load to inspiration, impairing the strength of the inspiratory muscles and depressing the effective triggering sensitivity of the ventilator. For cases in which expiration is flow limited during tidal breathing, the addition of low levels of exogenous PEEP (less than the original auto-PEEP level) effectively replaces auto-PEEP and therefore improves subject comfort and the work of breathing, without increasing lung volume or peak cycling pressure. Substitution of PEEP for auto-PEEP also may improve the distribution of ventilation marginally. At the bedside, total PEEP can be quantified by occluding the expiratory port of the ventilator at the end of the period allowed for exhalation between mechanical breaths. As already noted, the auto-PEEP component is the difference between this measured occlusion pressure and the PEEP value set by the clinician.

Variability of Auto-PEEP

Regional Gas Trapping

Auto-PEEP varies widely throughout a lung composed of individual units with varying time constants. Because pleural pressure follows a gravitational gradient, transpulmonary pressure and alveolar dimensions are least and the tendency for airway closure greatest in the most dependent regions. Therefore, even if the time constants were otherwise perfectly uniform throughout the lung, there would be a tendency for those units in dependent areas to trap more gas than those located above them.

Vulnerability to Changes in Minute Ventilation

Minute ventilation is a powerful determinant of auto-PEEP; in fact, in a uniform lung characterized by a single time constant, variations in frequency or tidal volume that do not change the minute ventilation have little effect on the observed auto-PEEP. On the contrary, relatively small changes in $\dot{V}_E$ can dramatically change the extent of gas trapping in such a single compartment system. In practice, the diseased lung of an asthmatic patient deflates in a pattern that is better typified as bi-exponential or multi-exponential. For these patients, end-expiratory flows from the slowest compartments are so small that increasing the cycling frequency (and increasing the minute ventilation) may have a negligible effect on gas trapping.

Alterations in Resistance and Compliance

For the same minute ventilation, variations in retained secretions, bronchospasm, apparatus resistance, tissue edema, body position, muscle tone, etc. alter the deflation time constant and the extent of gas trapping encountered at an unchanging V_E. Partially for this reason, simple maneuvers such as suctioning the airway or changing the patient from the reclining to the upright position can make a dramatic difference in the level of comfort.

TABLE 5–1
CLINICAL METHODS FOR DETERMINING AUTO-PEEP
End-expiratory port occlusion
Proto-inspiratory counterbalancing
End-inspiratory plateau pressure during volume-cycled ventilation
PEEP substitution
Trapped gas release

Methods for Determining Auto-PEEP (Table 5.1)

The presence of auto-PEEP should be suspected whenever detectable flow persists to the very end of tidal expiration. Such flow often is audible using a stethoscope positioned over the trachea or expiratory valve, and auto-PEEP (if not dynamic hyperinflation) is certain if wheezing persists to the very end of the expiratory cycle. This flow can be transduced and displayed graphically on the bedside monitor. However, the magnitude of end-expiratory flow does not correlate with the magnitude of auto-PEEP, whether comparing patients to one another or when observing the same patient over time. End expiratory flow of a given amount, for example, may result from widespread severe obstruction or from more moderate obstruction confined to a smaller subpopulation of alveoli. Moreover, very high levels of regional hyperinflation and auto-PEEP can lurk behind airways that have been sealed completely by mucus plugs (with collateral ventilation). Others may open during inspiration but seal before end-expiration is reached, preventing all further discharge of their trapped gas.

Because auto-PEEP varies on a breath-by-breath basis during spontaneous breathing, it cannot be quantified precisely unless exhalation is passive and the depth and duration of all breaths are equivalent—conditions that only rarely occur when making spontaneous breathing efforts. Once passive conditions are established, an estimate of auto-PEEP can be determined (or its effects monitored) by a variety of methods. All of these methods are approximations, and all are somewhat lower than the highest values existing within the lung. Two of these methods are based on the principle of counterbalancing auto-PEEP, either by end-expiratory airway occlusion or by a measured dynamic airway pressure (proto-inspiratory counterbalancing, or zero flow method). Alternatively, the auto-PEEP effect can be characterized by directly measuring the change in end-inspiratory plateau (peak alveolar) pressure with a constant tidal volume and inspiratory time. Finally, the excess (trapped) gas volume that exits during an extended deflation interval reflects the corresponding end-expiratory pressure during tidal breaths. Two of the most important effects of auto-PEEP—on hemodynamics and work of breathing—are mediated by pleural pressure, which can be assessed directly by measuring esophageal pressure.

End-Expiratory Port Occlusion Method

For accuracy, occlusion must occur just before the subsequent ventilator-delivered breath and continue for 1.5–2.0 seconds (Fig. 2.8). Such timing of occlusion is easiest to achieve during controlled ventilation at modest breathing rates (<20/minute) and can be approximated manually or, when the patient is totally passive, automated using a three-way inspiratory valve. With the latter technique, a simple (''Braschi'') valve inserted into the inspiratory limb of the circuit can be turned at any time during expiration to block expiratory backflow through the inspiratory path. When the next tidal breath is delivered, the open limb of the valve diverts the ventilator's inflation volume to atmosphere for one breath as automatic tidal closure of the expiratory valve completes the airway occlusion at exactly the appropriate time.

Proto-inspiratory Counterbalancing Method

During passive inflation, inspiratory flow does not begin until the expiratory pressure within the units with the least auto-PEEP is counterbalanced by an offsetting proximal airway pressure. If flow and airway pressure signals are perfectly synchronous, auto-PEEP is the airway pressure at the time of zero flow. This estimate for auto-PEEP is usually less than that given by port occlusion.

End-Inspiratory Plateau Pressure During Volume-Cycled Ventilation

As already noted, auto-PEEP behind occluded airways can be elevated unexpectedly, even if auto-PEEP measured at the airway opening is quite low. End-inspiratory plateau pressure is the sum of PEEP, auto-PEEP, and the quotient of V_T/C_{RS}. Therefore, when tidal volume and PEEP

are accounted for and unchanging, plateau pressure reflects the degree of dynamic hyperinflation of all lung units more faithfully than does direct measurement of auto-PEEP itself, which gives an average of the auto-PEEP values from only those units that remain in communication with the airway opening. For similar reasons, *changes* in plateau pressure that occur after a prolonged expiration or a variation in a machine setting more reliably index changes in hyperinflation than does direct auto-PEEP estimation. Assuming passive inflation with a constant tidal volume and applied PEEP, the easiest clinical method at rapid breathing frequencies is to first measure the plateau pressure at the clinically relevant frequency, and to then resume the clinical pattern (without the measurement pause) for five or more breaths. Next, the frequency is slowed to <5 breaths per minute, waiting 15 seconds before reapplying the end-inspiratory pause. The difference in pause pressures estimates the original auto-PEEP.

PEEP Substitution Method

When PEEP is added downstream from the site of critical flow limitation, end-expiratory alveolar pressure rises only very modestly until the original level of auto-PEEP is surpassed, at which point the alveolar and airway pressures rise together. As PEEP is substituted for auto-PEEP, end-expiratory flow slows or stops completely and audible flow or wheezing ceases before end-expiration. In flow-controlled, volume-cycled ventilation, plateau pressure changes little until the original level of auto-PEEP is approximated. In pressure-controlled ventilation, tidal volume may crest at its maximum as PEEP approaches the critical level and auto-PEEP disappears. Although imprecise and unreliable in (rather unusual) patients with severe airflow obstruction who lack tidal flow limitation, this pragmatic technique lends itself well for both passive and actively breathing patients.

Release of Trapped Gas

A measurement of the *extra* gas released (in excess of the routine tidal volume) in the first exhalation after a sudden and dramatic slowing of ventilatory frequency (to two breaths or less per minute) estimates the amount of the total trapped gas (V_{TR}) that can be expelled. If compliance of the respiratory system (C_{RS}) is known, auto-PEEP can be computed as V_{TR}/C_{RS}.

ESOPHAGEAL PRESSURE MONITORING

Knowledge of intrapleural pressure often facilitates clinical decision making. The thin esophageal catheter (~2-mm diameter) is relatively comfortable, simple to insert, and poses little risk of esophageal perforation. Appropriate placement is achieved by first inflating the 10-cm-long balloon with ~1 mL of air and passing it into the stomach. The catheter is carefully withdrawn 10 cm beyond the position where negative pressure deflections are initially observed during spontaneous inspiratory efforts. The balloon's final position within the lower third of the esophagus is tested by occluding the airway and measuring the simultaneous deflections in P_{aw} and P_{es}. Because no significant change of transpulmonary pressure can occur without a change in lung volume, good balloon position is indicated by nearly identical deflections of esophageal and airway pressures during an occluded spontaneous breath.

As a rule, P_{es} is best measured in an upright position. However, a lateral decubitus position may suffice if the patient must remain recumbent. (The supine position is suboptimal.) Although the absolute value of the average pressure that surrounds the lung cannot be gauged accurately from such a local sampling, fluctuations of average intrathoracic pressure can be estimated acceptably well by an occlusion-tested balloon catheter in any position. Certain systems (e.g., the commercially available BiCore™ and Ventrak™ instruments) are designed to sample esophageal pressure in conjunction with airway pressure and flow, outputting primary and derived mechanics data of clinical interest (e.g., resistance, compliance, and several indices of inspiratory effort during active breathing conditions). Useful graphics of dynamic pressure–volume and flow–volume data are also available. Esophageal pressure enables estimation of force generation during all patient-initiated breaths (spontaneous or machine-assisted) and allows partitioning of transthoracic pressure into its lung and chest wall components during passive inflation. The intrapleural pressure provided by the P_{es} tracing also permits calculation of lung compliance and airway resistance during spontaneous breathing. Furthermore, P_{es} aids in interpreting pulmonary artery and wedge pressures under conditions of vigorous hyperpnea or elevated alveolar pressure (PEEP, auto-PEEP). The P_{es} can be used to compute the work of breathing across the lung and external circuitry or to calculate the product of developed pressure and the duration of inspiratory effort (the pressure–time product). It has been suggested that fluctuations in central venous pressure can serve a similar purpose, but the damped vascular pressure tracing yields a low range estimate of effort. Such underestimation occurs because venous return tends to rise as intrathoracic pressure falls; conversely, venous return declines when intrathoracic pressure rises.

Transdiaphragmatic pressure (P_{di}), the difference between P_{es} and balloon catheter-measured gastric pressure, is generated theoretically by a single inspiratory muscle (the diaphragm) and can be used to quantify its effective contractile force. Clinically, the P_{di} is used occasionally in conjunction with phrenic nerve stimulation or voluntary effort to investigate diaphragmatic paralysis.

VALUE OF CONTINUOUSLY MONITORING P_{aw} AND FLOW

The Flow Tracing

Most modern ventilators offer the option of displaying both airway pressure and airflow. When used in conjunction with a simultaneously recorded airway pressure, the flow tracing is an invaluable aid in determining a number of parameters of clinical interest. A glance at the flow tracing usually is sufficient to determine the inspiratory mode of the ventilator and may be more sensitive than airway pressure in detecting patient–ventilator asynchrony. Flow must be known to compute airway resistance and the work of breathing, as well as to detect (but not quantify) auto-PEEP without airway occlusion. A smoothly linear, biphasic flow profile, rather than a uniexponential one, may give a clear indication of expiratory flow limitation. A rippling inspiratory flow tracing indicates secretion retention within the central airways. The "zero flow" points of the airway and esophageal pressure tracings define the dynamic mechanical limits of the respiratory cycle, which are required in computations of mouth occlusion pressure ($P_{0.1}$, see below), minimum airway resistance and auto-PEEP. The flow tracing also is helpful when adjusting the inspiratory period during time-cycled pressure-preset forms of ventilation (e.g., pressure controlled ventilation), to maximize inspiratory tidal volume while avoiding unintended end-inspiratory pauses and/or excessive auto-PEEP.

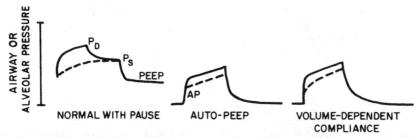

FIG. 5–12. Airway and alveolar pressures during controlled ventilation with constant flow. Airway pressure (solid line) and alveolar pressure (dashed line) are represented. For the passive subject, the airway pressures measured at end inflation and after a brief inspiratory pause provide the data needed to compute airway resistance: $[(P_D - P_S)/\text{inspiratory flow rate}]$. Compliance of the respiratory system: $[V_T/(P_S - \text{Total PEEP})]$ must take auto-PEEP into account to avoid underestimation of actual compliance. Auto-PEEP (AP) and early volume recruitment cause the normally trapezoidal airway pressure contour to "square off."

The Airway Pressure Tracing

A continuous tracing of P_{aw} provides useful information commonly neglected at the bedside (Fig. 5.12). When the ventilator's display does not automatically provide the tracing, airway pressure can be monitored continuously using transducer and display equipment normally used for measuring pressures in the pulmonary vasculature. A dedicated transducer must be used for this purpose, however, to avoid the risk of air embolism.

Apart from enabling estimation of R_{AW} and C_{RS}, the waveform of inspiratory airway pressure traced during a controlled machine cycle provides graphic evidence of the inflation work performed by the ventilator at the particular combination of tidal volume and flow settings in use. When inflation occurs passively during constant flow, the area under the pressure–time curve is proportionate to the work performed by the machine to inflate the chest, and the pressure measured halfway through the cycle ($\overline{P}$) is the work per liter of ventilation under those conditions. When average flow and tidal volume are matched to spontaneous values, $\overline{P}$ is a good estimate of the pressure needed to fully ventilate the patient during a conversion to pressure-supported ventilation.

The shape of the airway pressure tracing also should be examined. Using constant inspiratory flow, concavity of the airway pressure ramp under passive conditions reflects patient effort during triggered cycles. An upward inflection of the terminal portion of the inspiratory airway pressure tracing (concavity) during passive inflation suggests that the combination of end-expiratory pressure and tidal volume chosen generates pressures that risk overdistention and barotrauma. Conversely, marked convexity of the P_{aw} tracing during constant flow indicates that inflation is becoming easier as the breath proceeds. Such a profile can be seen when volume is alternately recruited and derecruited during the breathing cycle, when auto-PEEP is present (requiring a range of counterbalancing pressures before units with different auto-PEEP values are brought "on-line" for inspiration), or when resistance is highly volume dependent (Fig. 5.12). Cycle-to-cycle variations in the peak dynamic pressure of machine-aided breaths suggest that the durations of inspiratory effort and flow delivery are not well matched or synchronous (Fig. 5.13).

MEAN AIRWAY PRESSURE

Under passive conditions, mean alveolar pressure and its only measurable analog, mean airway presssure (mP_{aw}), relate intimately to the forces that drive ventilation and hold the lung distended. When the pressures dissipated in inspiration and expiration are identical, the airway pressure averaged over the entire ventilatory cycle should be the same everywhere—including the alveolus (Fig. 5.14). This mean pressure is the average pressure that distends the alveolus and passive chest wall and therefore correlates with alveolar size and recruitment, as well as with mean intrapleural pressure. Mean alveolar pressure also is the average pressure available to drive expiratory flow, which is indexed by minute ventilation. It follows that mean airway (mean alveolar) pres-

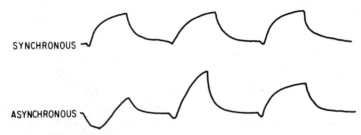

FIG. 5–13. Airway pressure tracings during assist/control ventilation. Variations in contour and peak cycling pressure characterize asynchrony between the respiratory rhythms of the patient and ventilator.

Mean Airway Pressure

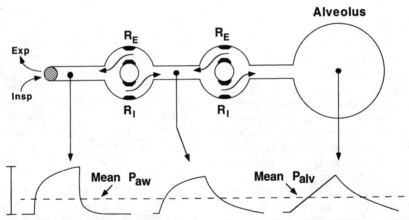

FIG. 5–14. Relationship of mean airway pressure to mean alveolar pressure. In an airway in which inspiratory (R_I) and expiratory (R_E) resistive pressure losses are equivalent, the mean pressure averaged over the entire ventilatory cycle should be equivalent at every point along the path, including airway opening and alveolus. When R_E exceeds R_I, mean alveolar pressure exceeds mean airway opening pressure; when R_I exceeds R_E, mean airway opening pressure exceeds mean alveolar pressure.

sure correlates directly with arterial oxygenation in the setting of pulmonary edema and lung injury, with backpressure to venous return (and consequently with cardiac output and peripheral edema), as well as with minute ventilation.

Mean airway pressure can be raised by increasing $\dot{V}_E$, by raising end-expiratory pressure, or by extending the inspiratory time fraction (see Chapters 9 and 24). To avoid serious and unanticipated problems, mean airway pressure is a crucial variable to monitor when minute ventilation is changed intentionally or when the clinician alters the mode of ventilation, breathing pattern, PEEP, or other ventilator setting.

Although the relationship between mP_{aw} and mP_{alv} is a close one, these pressures are not identical. The actual relationship can be expressed mathematically as:

$$mP_{alv} = mP_{aw} + \dot{V}_E (R_{ex} - R_{in})$$

where $(R_{ex} - R_{in})$ is the calculated difference between expiratory and inspiratory resistances. For reasons already discussed, this pressure difference generally tends to be positive and may be strikingly so in the setting of severe airflow obstruction with high ventilatory requirements or high frequency or inverse ratio ventilation.

OXYGEN CONSUMPTION OF THE RESPIRATORY SYSTEM

The oxygen consumed by the ventilatory pump ($\dot{V}O_2R$) estimates respiratory muscular effort at its most basic level: cellular metabolism. In theory, $\dot{V}O_{2R}$ accounts for all factors that tax the respiratory muscles, i.e., the external workload (W) and the efficiency (e) of the conversion between cellular energy and useful work ($\dot{V}O_{2R}$ = W/e). Two patients with different chest configurations, patterns of muscle activation, or degrees of coordination between the muscles of inspiration and expiration may perform identical external work (W) but consume vastly different amounts of O_2 in the process. Because $\dot{V}O_{2R}$ cannot be measured directly, total body oxygen consumption ($\dot{V}O_2$) is tracked as ventilatory stresses are imposed or relieved, perturbing the respiratory system. Unfortunately, $\dot{V}O_2$ is difficult to measure in unstable patients. Thus, other measures of respiratory muscle effort usually are sought.

DIRECT MEASURES OF EXTERNAL MECHANICAL OUTPUT

External Work of Breathing

Mechanical work is accomplished when a pressure gradient (P) moves the lung or relaxed chest wall (passive structures) through a volume change. At volumes (V_T) above relaxed FRC, pressure dissipates against frictional and elastic forces in the following way:

$$P = R_{AW} \times (V_T/t_i) + V/C_{RS}.$$

Average developed pressure ($\bar{P}$) for the tidal inflation (V_T) can be expressed as follows:

$$\bar{P} = R_{AW} \times (V_T/t_i) + V_T/2C_{RS} + \text{auto-PEEP}$$

and is numerically equivalent to the work per liter of ventilation. (Work per tidal breath [W_b] can be quantified as the product of $\bar{P}$ and V_T.) Thus, if R_{AW}, C_{RS}, t_i, and V_T are known for the spontaneously breathing subject, the external work rate for inspiration can be computed easily. (Exhalation normally proceeds passively, dissipating elastic energy stored during the inspiratory half cycle.) Such computations also serve to conveniently estimate the pressure support level needed to achieve most ventilatory needs. When the ventilator performs the entire workload for a passive patient, total inflation pressure (P) is simply P_{aw}. (When inflation is achieved with a constant flow waveform, it is then approximated by the inflation pressure at midcycle.) However, no exertion must occur during inflation and, to be relevant to unsupported natural breathing, V_T and peak flow rate must approximate the spontaneous values. With pressures and volumes expressed in the customary way, a convenient work unit is the joule (or watt-second) ~10 cm H_2O × 1 L (equivalent to 1 kgm = 10 J). Total inspiratory mechanical work per minute is the product of $\bar{P}$ and minute ventilation or of W_b and f, the breathing frequency.

Influence of Auto-PEEP on Work of Breathing

Auto-PEEP (AP) imposes a threshold load on inspiration in the sense that the patient must supply a pressure sufficient to counterbalance AP before central airway pressure falls low enough to trigger the ventilator or initiate a pressure supported breath. The threshold load imposed by AP effectively reduces the triggering sensitivity of the machine to a value equal to the sum of AP and the set trigger sensitivity value. When expiration is flow limited during tidal breathing, low levels of continuous positive airway pressure (CPAP) or PEEP can help restore triggering sensitivity and reduce the work of breathing (see above). Moreover, during pressure-supported ventilation, PEEP that counterbalances auto-PEEP leaves a greater proportion of the inspiratory pressure available to power inflation, often resulting in an increased tidal volume for the same value of pressure support. Although PEEP also tends to improve the distribution of ventilation, additional PEEP should not be used if it causes the peak dynamic cycling pressure to rise significantly.

Work Measurements

Spontaneous Breathing Cycles An esophageal balloon is required to directly measure work during spontaneous, machine-assisted, or pressure-supported breathing cycles. Fluctuations in P_{es} reflect patient efforts to overcome the impedance of the lung and external circuit. (Clues to the work done against the external apparatus can be gained by examining the P_{aw} tracing). Inspiratory inflections of the P_{aw} waveform quantify the pressure needed to suck gas through the inspiratory cir-

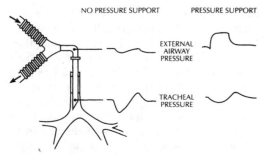

FIG. 5–15. Pressure tracings at the proximal and distal ends of the endotracheal tube during spontaneous breathing. External recordings do not reflect exertion against the endotracheal tube (*left*). The application of pressure support may overcome endotracheal tube resistance during the inspiratory phase but does nothing to offset the expiratory resistance imposed by the endotracheal tube.

cuitry to the point of pressure measurement. To include the resistance of the endotracheal tube, P_{aw} must be sampled between the tube tip and the carina, a site at which much deeper pressure fluctuations may be seen during inspiration (Fig. 5.15). The resistance of standard endotracheal tubes often exceeds 10 cm H_2O/L/sec and is commonly offset during inspiration by pressure support.

Machine-Assisted Breathing Cycles

Volume-Limited Machine Cycles   It is often assumed that patient work becomes negligible during patient-initiated but machine-assisted breathing cycles. Indeed, the ventilator is fully capable of performing the entire work of breathing if the patient were to cease effort immediately after triggering inspiration. However, relaxation does not occur abruptly once the machine cycle begins; instead, patient effort continues in direct proportion to the intensity of respiratory drive. When the ventilation requirement or sense of dyspnea is high (e.g., when the ventilator is poorly adjusted with respect to sensitivity, peak inspiratory flow rate, inspiratory duration, or tidal volume), exertion levels may approach those of unsupported breathing. Interestingly, resistance and compliance do not influence the work of breathing during triggered cycles, provided that the machine fully satisfies the patient's peak inspiratory flow demand ($\approx 4 \times \dot{V}_E$). However, if the patient's flow demand exceeds the delivery rate, the patient works against the resistance of the endotracheal tube and ventilator circuitry, as well as against

the innate impedance characteristics of the chest. Clues to patient exertion during triggered machine cycles are provided by the airway pressure tracing, as already described. When a P_{aw} tracing is not available, the primary indication of excessive patient effort during a triggered cycle may be the stuttering rise of the manometer needle to its peak value. Peak dynamic pressure itself may not be much different from expected, inasmuch as inspiratory effort slackens near the end of inflation.

Pressure-Supported Cycles   During pressure-supported cycles, inspiratory airway pressure is maintained nearly constant by the machine at the preset level. Therefore, patient effort can only be gauged directly from a P_{es} tracing.

Pressure Time Product

Isometric components of muscle tension that consume oxygen without contributing to volume change fail to register as externally measured work, accounting in large part for the lack of agreement between force generation and W_b. A pressure–time product (PTP = $\overline{P} \times t_i$) parallels effort and $\dot{V}O_{2R}$ more closely than W_b because it includes the isometric component of muscle pressure and is less influenced by the afterload to contraction. When average inspiratory pressure ($\overline{P}$, as computed above) is referenced to the maximal isometric pressure that can be generated at FRC (P_{max}) and inspiratory time (t_i) is expressed as a fraction of total cycle length (t_{tot}), a useful effort index is derived:

Pressure–time index (PTI) = $\overline{P}/P_{max} \times t_i/t_{tot}$

Values of PTI that exceed 0.15 identify highly stressful breathing workloads that may not be sustainable.

MONITORING VENTILATORY DRIVE AND BREATHING PATTERN

IMPORTANCE OF ASSESSING VENTILATORY DRIVE

Remarkably little attention has been paid to drive measurement during critical illness. Heightened ventilatory drive increases work expenditure during triggered machine cycles and often signals pain, sepsis, and important perturbations of the cardiopulmonary system. During machine-assisted breathing cycles, ventilatory drive plays a more important role in determining the energy expenditure of the patient than any indicator of ventilatory mechanics—if the flow delivered by the machine exceeds the patient's flow demand. Derangements in ventilatory drive also furnish clues regarding the ability of the patient to wean from ventilator support. Recent clinical studies demonstrate that patients who fail to wean from mechanical ventilation often have elevated drives to breathe and limited abilities of drive to respond to increases in ventilatory loads (e.g., increased $PaCO_2$).

VENTILATORY DRIVE INDICES

Several methods can be used to index drive. When respiratory mechanics and strength reserves are normal, minute ventilation directly parallels the output of the ventilatory control center. Unfortunately, such preconditions are seldom met in the clinical setting. Minute ventilation can be viewed as the product of mean inspiratory flow rate (the quotient of tidal volume and inspiratory time, V_T/t_i) and the inspiratory time fraction or duty cycle (t_i/t_{tot}):

$$V_e = V_T/t_i \times t_i/t_{tot}$$

Both components yield useful and largely ignored clinical information. Mean inspiratory flow (V_T/t_i) provides another potential index of drive but also depends on the mechanical properties of the ventilatory system. The airway pressure generated against a surreptitiously occluded airway 100 msec after the onset of inspiratory effort (the $P_{0.1}$) is measured before the occlusion is recognized consciously, so that the corresponding outflow from the respiratory center is representative of the unimpeded cycles that preceded it. As an isometric measurement, the $P_{0.1}$ is influenced by muscle strength and lung volume but does not depend on respiratory mechanics. The delay imposed by the demand valve systems of certain ventilators in common use provide a quasi-occlusion period long enough to allow close estimation of $P_{0.1}$. However, the measurement of this index requires a sensitive pressure recording system and very rapid recording rates.

BREATHING PATTERN, FREQUENCY, AND DUTY CYCLE

Rapid Shallow Breathing and the f/V_T Ratio

The breathing pattern also offers valuable information. When muscular strength is limited, patients tend to meet $\dot{V}_E$ requirements by increasing frequency (f) without raising V_T. Although smaller breaths require less effort, the cost of rapid, shallow breathing may be increased deadspace ventilation and the need for a higher $\dot{V}_E$ to eliminate CO_2. Thus, although work per breath (W_b) is controlled by limiting tidal volume, total work (the product of f and W_b) per minute tends to increase when f exceeds some optimal value. A very high and continuously rising frequency (to rates >30 breaths/minute) is generally accepted as a sign of ventilatory muscle decompensation and impending fatigue. It should be noted, however, that some patients increase f to a stable value >35 breaths/minute and remain compensated.

In recent years, considerable attention has focused on the f/V_T ratio, a simply computed bedside index that seems to indicate the ability or inability of mechanically ventilated patients to breathe without mechanical assistance. Discontinuation of ventilator support is likely to prove successful if (f/V_T) does *not* exceed ~100 breaths/minute·liters within the first minute of a brief trial of fully spontaneous breathing. Although hardly infallible, this simple guide does seem to have some clinical utility.

As the ventilatory muscles fatigue, the duty cycle (t_i/t_{tot}), the fraction of each breathing cycle spent in inspiration, also changes. When there is a breathing stress, the t_i/t_{tot} of spontaneous breathing normally increases from ~0.35 to a value of 0.40–0.50. ("Inspiratory time" may be fixed by chosen values of inspiratory flow rate and tidal volume during constant flow mechanical ventilation.) At the limits of compensation, the t_i/t_{tot} fails to increase with further stress and may actually decline.

At times of maximal effort, noteworthy alterations may be observed in the pattern of activation and coordination of the ventilatory muscle groups. Although normally passive, expiratory muscles may be called into play whenever the inspiratory muscles face a burden that is stressful in relation to their capability (e.g., during expiratory airflow obstruction, when high levels of PEEP or CPAP are used, when the patient is anxious, when machine-controlled inspiratory duration is excessive, and at high levels of $\dot{V}_E$). Visible use of the accessory muscles, especially the sternocleidomastoid group, may also signal the approach to the limits of ventilatory compensation.

Asynchrony of the Respiratory Muscles

Two indices once believed to always indicate diaphragmatic dysfunction or fatigue—asynchrony between the peak excursions of chest and abdominal compartments and paradoxical inward movement of the abdomen on inspiration—often reflect the normal response of a compensated system to stress. Asynchrony between the excursions of rib cage and abdomen may be a stage in the development of full-blown abdominal paradox. Respiratory alternans, another reported pattern of fatigue in which muscles of the chest cage and diaphragm alternate primary responsibility for achieving ventilation, is observed much less commonly than abdominal paradox.

Inductance or Impedance Plethysmography

Inductance (impedance) plethysmography provides a noninvasive means of monitoring f, V_T, t_i/t_{tot}, and respiratory muscle coordination. With this technique, loose elastic bands encircle the chest and abdomen. Changes in compartmental volume create proportional changes in the cross-sectional areas of electrical inductance loops. Fluctuations of compartmental motion can be summed to estimate overall tidal volume changes. The ratio of maximal compartmental amplitude to tidal volume (the MCA/V_T ratio) correlates with ventilatory distress and provides tangible evidence of mechanical inefficiency. Impedance plethysmography can also be used as an apnea detector in nonintubated patients and may prove helpful in monitoring volume changes during pressure-cycled modes of ventilation (e.g., pressure support, pressure control, and intermittent positive pressure breathing [IPPB]).

MONITORING STRENGTH AND MUSCLE RESERVE (ENDURANCE)

The ability of a patient to sustain independent breathing must not be judged on the basis of any absolute value for workload but rather on workload interpreted against the background of muscular strength and endurance.

STRENGTH MEASURES

The two measures of respiratory muscle strength most commonly used in the clinical setting are the vital capacity (VC) and the maximal inspiratory pressure (MIP) generated against an occluded airway. Maximal activation of the respiratory musculature requires intense voluntary effort. Therefore, without full patient cooperation, it is questionable that any measure of strength can reflect the full capability for pressure development.

Vital Capacity

In cooperative patients, VC tends to be well preserved relative to MIP for two primary reasons. First, the pressure–volume relationship of the thorax is convex to the volume axis, so that small applied pressures achieve relatively large volume changes. Second, whereas many seriously ill patients can generate brief spikes of inspiratory pressure, few can sustain inspiratory effort long enough to achieve the plateau of their volume curve. Vital capacity generally should be mea-

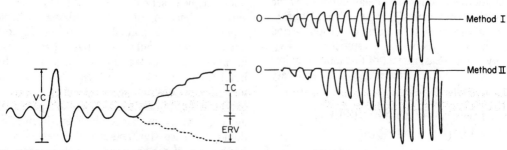

FIG. 5–16. Techniques for testing ventilatory strength in a poorly cooperative patient. *Left,* use of a one-way valve during tidal breathing efforts to measure inspiratory capacity (IC), expiratory reserve volume (ERV), and their sum, vital capacity (VC). *Right,* use of a one-way valve to measure maximum inspiratory pressure. In both instances, the patient's own drive to breathe stimulates forceful effort. From ref. 18 (left) and ref. 19 (right), with permission.

sured upright rather than supine, because certain conditions—diaphragmatic paralysis, for example—may demonstrate a positional reduction of more than 30% (see Chapter 25). Routine measurements of VC involve a single forceful effort from residual volume to total lung capacity (or the converse). However, many weak patients fail to sustain inspiratory effort long enough to achieve their potential maximum. Others simply refuse or cannot fully cooperate with the testing. Thus, for critically ill patients, the VC has proven to be a disappointing measure of strength. A one-way valve can be used to achieve a "stacked vital capacity," even when patients do not cooperate fully with testing (Fig. 5.16).

Maximal Inspiratory Pressure

The maximal inspiratory pressure (MIP, sometimes erroneously referred to as "maximum inspiratory *force*") is an isometric pressure measured in a totally occluded airway after 20 seconds or 10 breathing efforts (Fig. 5.16). A one-way valve directed toward expiration can ensure that inspiratory efforts begin from a lung volume low enough to achieve maximal mechanical advantage. The P_{aw} during the MIP maneuver should be measured continuously, either with a needle gauge or (preferably) by a pressure transducer linked to recording apparatus. Ideally, the MIP is sustained for at least 1 second; a transient isometric pressure may bear little relation to true ventilatory muscle strength and endurance. The MIP is perhaps the only involuntary measure of muscle strength that is even moderately reliable. However, it should be kept in mind that the validity of MIP in uncooperative patients depends on the strength of ventilatory drive, and that the intensity of a voluntary effort in a fully cooperative patient is likely to exceed that elicited by simple airway occlusion. If sufficient ventilatory drive can be elicited (e.g., by the addition of deadspace tubing to the airway), the drive-stimulated involuntary MIP may approximate the voluntary MIP rather closely.

MEASURES OF ENDURANCE

Mechanical Reserve

Two simple indices of ventilatory power reserve—the ratio of Ve requirement to maximal voluntary ventilation (MVV) and the V_T/V_C ratio—have long been used to predict the outcome of machine withdrawal. On empirical grounds, it has been suggested that ratios >50% portend weaning failure. Interestingly, newer laboratory data confirm that only ~50–60% of the MVV can be sustained longer than 15 minutes without ventilatory fatigue.

Electromyography

In the physiology laboratory, an increasing ratio of the integrated diaphragmatic electromyographic (EMG) signal to generated pressure suggests a declining ability of the muscle pump to respond to neural stimulation (i.e., fatigue). Another EMG index of interest characterizes the spectrum of frequencies represented within the diaphragmatic EMG signal. The high frequency to low frequency ratio (H/L) is a good indicator of ventilatory stress and may be a sensitive and specific indicator of developing fatigue. Unfortunately, the diaphragmatic EMG (measured by surface or esophageal electrodes) is not commonly available, and advanced signal conditioning is required to compute the H/L ratio.

Pressure–Time Index

Measured accurately, the MIP can be used in conjunction with to judge endurance and the likelihood of weaning success. In the laboratory setting, a diaphragmatic $\bar{P}/P_{max}$ ratio >40% (with $t_i/t_{tot} = 0.40$) or a pressure–time index (PTI = $\bar{P}/P_{max} \times t_i/t_{tot}$) > 0.15 predicts the inability to indefinitely sustain a target workload. No confirmatory data are available yet for the specific clinical setting of the weaning trial.

Sequential Measurements of Drive

A practical indication of declining power reserve may also be provided by a comparison of drive indices (such as the $P_{0.1}$) measured sequentially during the stress period. Recent work suggests that patients who fail to increase ventilatory drive in response to increasing $PaCO_2$ are prone to alveolar hypoventilation and weaning failure. In the future, monitoring the response of such indices as $P_{0.1}$ to an imposed stress or to CO_2 loading may provide valuable clinical indications of breathing reserve.

KEY POINTS

1. Although pulse oximetry is an invaluable clinical tool, it provides a signal-averaged number, the output of which lags behind the actual physiologic value of interest. Pulse oximetry is influenced by extraneous rhythmic vibration, carbon monoxide, and methemoglobin. Even if the recorded pulse rate correlates exactly with an independently measured value, oximetry loses accuracy when true arterial saturation falls to less than 80%.

2. After a step change in ventilation, a change in arterial carbon dioxide concentration approaches steady-state equilibrium less quickly than does the arterial oxygen tension, because the storage reservoir of the body for CO_2 is far larger than that for O_2.

3. The compliance of the respiratory system is influenced by the number of patent alveolar units as well as by their elasticity. The static and dynamic pressure volume curves of the respiratory system can provide vital information unavailable through computation of simpler indices, such as tidal compliance.

4. The mechanics of breathing (resistance and compliance) are most easily assessed during passive inflation with a known constant flow, using an end-inspiratory pause. During active breathing, the mechanical properties of the lung can be assessed if pleural pressure is recorded using an esophageal balloon.

5. Auto-PEEP, a result of dynamic hyperinflation and/or expiratory muscle contraction, contributes to the work of breathing and can be estimated using a variety of techniques. Because auto-PEEP varies from site to site throughout the lungs of a diseased patient, the externally measured value may not accurately reflect the degree of overdistention. In obstructive diseases (asthma, chronic obstructive pulmonary disease [COPD]), the end-inspiratory plateau pressure indicates the degree of hyperinflation better than does auto-PEEP itself.

6. The flow tracing can be used to detect (but not quantify) auto-PEEP and dysynchrony between the tidal rhythms of patient and ventilator. The zero-flow points of the flow tracing partition the ventilatory cycle into its inspiratory and expiratory phases. The airway pressure tracing complements the flow tracing, helping to detect and quantify the work of breathing.

7. As an index of mean lung and chest wall volumes, mean airway pressure recorded under passive conditions is an important determinant of arterial oxygenation, the back pressure to venous return, and the tendency for gas leakage after barotrauma. Mean airway pressure alone has limited value during active breathing and seriously underestimates mean alveolar pressure when expiratory pressure losses exceed inspiratory pressure losses.

8. The mechanical work of breathing is not synonymous with breathing effort. The pressure–time index better indicates total ventilatory stress, correlating inversely with pump reserve.

9. Respiratory muscle dysynchrony, elevations in the $P_{0.1}$, and an excessive frequency to tidal volume ratio are helpful indicators of respiratory muscle overload and incipient muscle fatigue.

10. The CO_2 challenged $P_{0.1}$, the ratio between spontaneous tidal volume and vital capacity, and the ratio between minute ventilation and maximum voluntary ventilation are helpful indicators of ventilatory reserve.

SUGGESTED READINGS

1. Anonymous. Noninvasive blood gas monitoring: a review for use in the adult critical care unit. Can Med Assoc J 1992;146(5):703–712.
2. Banner MJ, Jaeger MJ, Kirby RR. Components of the work of breathing and implications for monitoring ventilator-dependent patients. Crit Care Med 1994;22:515–523.
3. Benito S, Lemaire F. Pulmonary pressure-volume relationship in acute respiratory distress syndrome in adults: role of positive end expiratory pressure. J Crit Care 1990; 5:27.
4. Branson R. Monitoring ventilator function. Crit Care Clin 1995;11(1):127–143.
5. Broseghini C, Brandolese R, Poggi R. Respiratory mechanics during the first day of mechanical ventilation in patients with pulmonary edema and chronic airway obstruction. Am Rev Respir Dis 1988;138:355–361.
6. Capps JS, Hicks GH. Monitoring non-gas respiratory variables during mechanical ventilation. Respir Care 1987; 32:558–571.
7. Dechman G, Sato J, Bates JH. Factors affecting the accuracy of esophageal balloon measurement of pleural pressure in dogs. J Appl Physiol 1992;72(1):383–388.
8. Gilbert H, Vender J. Arterial blood gas monitoring. Crit Care Clin 1995;11(1):233–248.
9. Harrison RA. Monitoring respiratory mechanics. Crit Care Clin 1995;11(1):151–167.
10. Hendriks J, Ince C, Bruining H. Tonometry to assess the

adequacy of splanchnic oxygenation in the critically ill patient. Intensive Care Med 1994;20(6):452–456.

11. Hubmayr RD, Gay PC, Tayyab M. Respiratory system mechanics in ventilated patients: techniques and indications. Mayo Clin Proc 1987;62:358–368.

12. Jubran A, Tobin MJ. Monitoring during mechanical ventilation. Clin Chest Med 1996;17(3):453–474.

13. Jubran A, Tobin MJ. Use of flow-volume curves in detecting secretions in ventilator dependent patients. Am J Respir Crit Care Med 1994;150:766–769.

14. Marini JJ. Monitoring during mechanical ventilation. Clin Chest Med 1988;9(1):73–100.

15. Marini JJ. Respiratory medicine for the house officer, 2nd ed. Baltimore: Williams & Wilkins, 1987; 1–39.

16. Marini JJ. What derived variables should be monitored during mechanical ventilation? Respir Care 1992;37(9):1097–1107.

17. Marini JJ, Ravenscraft SA. Mean airway pressure: physiologic determinants and clinical importance. Part 2: clinical implications. Crit Care Med 1992;20:1604–1616.

18. Marini JJ, Rodriguez RM, Lamb VJ. Involuntary breath stacking. An alternative method for vital capacity estimation in poorly cooperative subjects. Am Rev Respir Dis 1986;134:694–698.

19. Marini JJ, Smith TC, Lamb VJ. Estimation of inspiratory muscle strength in mechanically ventilated patients: the measurement of maximal inspiratory pressure. J Crit Care 1986;1(1):32–38.

20. Marini JJ, Truwit JD. Monitoring the respiratory system. In: Schmidt GA, ed. Principles of critical care medicine. New York: McGraw Hill, 1991; 197–219.

21. Moxham J, Goldstone J. Assessment of respiratory muscle strength in the intensive care unit. Eur Respir J 1994; 7(11):2057–2061.

22. Pepe PE, Marini JJ. Occult positive end-expiratory pressure in mechanically ventilated patients with airflow obstruction. Am Rev Respir Dis 1982;126:166–170.

23. Roupie E, Dambriosio M, Servillo G, et al. Titration of tidal volume and induced hypercapnia in acute respiratory distress syndrome. Am J Respir Crit Care Med 1995;152:121–128.

24. Stock MC. Capnography for adults. Crit Care Clin 1995; 11(1):219–232.

25. Tobin M. Breathing pattern analysis. Intensive Care Med 1992;18(4):193–201.

26. Truwit J, Rochester D. Monitoring the respiratory system of the mechanically ventilated patient. New Horizons 1994;2(1):94–106.

27. Truwit JD, Marini JJ. Evaluation of thoracic mechanics in the ventilated patient. Part I: primary measurements. J Crit Care 1988;3:133–150.

28. Truwit JD, Marini JJ. Validation of a technique to assess maximal inspiratory pressure in poorly cooperative patients. Chest 1992;102(4):1216–1219.

29. Wahr J, Tremper K. Noninvasive oxygen monitoring techniques. Crit Care Clin 1995;11(1):199–217.

30. Weissman C, Kemper M. Metabolic measurements in the critically ill. Crit Care Clin 1995;11(1):169–197.

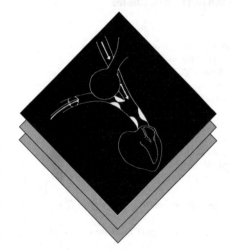

CHAPTER **6**

Airway Intubation

Primary indications for endotracheal intubation include: (*a*) the need for assisted ventilation or the delivery of high levels of inspired oxygen; (*b*) airway protection against aspiration; (*c*) clearance of secretions retained in central airways; (*d*) relief of upper airway obstruction.

NEED FOR ASSISTED VENTILATION AND POSITIVE END-EXPIRATORY PRESSURE (PEEP)

Until quite recently, intubation of the trachea with a cuffed endotracheal tube was the only viable option for both securing the airway and providing effective ventilatory support. Recent advances in noninvasive ventilation, however, suggest that the indications for airway intubation must be defined explicitly (see Chapter 7). Although noninvasive approaches hold promise, tracheal intubation is still required when high levels of airway pressure must be applied to ensure satisfactory oxygen exchange or ventilation. Moreover, noninvasive ventilation may not be appropriate or entirely safe for patients who are obtunded or uncooperative, for those in whom even momentary loss of ventilatory pressure or inspired oxygen might be hazardous, for those requiring high levels of applied pressure, and for those who are hemodynamically unstable. When ventilatory support must be continuous or extended more than a few days, intubation clearly is a better approach.

AIRWAY PROTECTION

Because effective protection of the upper airway cannot be ensured without establishing a tight cuff seal, intubation is required for lethargic or comatose patients at high risk for aspiration. Although an inflated cuff prevents massive airway flooding and luminal occlusion, small quantities of pharyngeal contents are aspirated routinely. Seepage of the infected secretions that pool just above the cuff may help account for the high incidence of pulmonary infections that occur in mechanically ventilated patients. Special tubes that allow continued evacuation of this secretion pool have been reported to reduce the incidence of ventilator-associated pneumonia (see Chapter 26, Severe Infections).

SECRETION CLEARANCE

Retained airway secretions predispose to infection, encourage atelectasis and hypoxemia, and dramatically increase the breathing workload for patients with neuromuscular weakness and/or underlying airflow obstruction. Translaryngeal intubation and tracheostomy facilitate extraction of these secretions.

UPPER AIRWAY OBSTRUCTION

Intubation addresses the immediate physiologic threat of anatomic or functional obstruction of the upper airway and is often the first step taken before attempting definitive treatment (see Chapter 25).

TABLE 6–1

INDICATIONS FOR SUPRAGLOTTIC AIRWAYS

Oral	Nasal
Removal of retropharyngeal secretions	Removal of supraglottic secretions
Maintain patency of oropharyngeal airway	Conscious or unconscious patient
Obtunded without gag	Need for repeated cannulation of trachea
Prevention of biting	Limited value in preventing closure of the oropharynx

TYPES OF AIRWAYS AND ROUTES OF INTUBATION

SUPRAGLOTTIC AIRWAYS

Pharyngeal airways are firm supports placed through the nose or mouth that are intended to bypass the relaxed tongue, thereby splinting open the retropharynx and providing protected access to the hypopharynx (Table 6.1). Well-placed pharyngeal airways allow unimpeded spontaneous or assisted ventilation and facilitate removal of airway or pharyngeal secretions. They are not intended to substitute for endotracheal intubation in patients with firm indications for airway protection or who require uncompromised access to the lower airway.

Oropharyngeal Airways

Oral airways are anatomically contoured plastic devices that displace the tongue from the posterior wall of the pharynx to prevent its closure. Their primary purpose is to wedge open the hypopharynx and to facilitate secretion extraction during spontaneous breathing or bag-mask ventilation. An oral airway can either serve as a ''bite block'' for an orally intubated patient inclined to jaw clenching or as a stabilizer of the artificial airway for an edentulous patient. Because they stimulate the retropharynx and promote gagging, oral airways must not be used in alert patients or in those with intact gag reflexes. (Over time, some accommodation to this foreign object may develop.) Disturbingly, obtunded patients with depressed gag reflexes are just those who are most inclined to aspirate. These oropharyngeal airways must, therefore, be removed as soon as consciousness returns or evidence for an activated gag reflex appears.

Nasopharyngeal Airways

These firm (but compressible), curved, flanged, and hollow tubes are available in a variety of diameters and lengths, but none are designed to extend into the glottis. They are inserted through a lubricated, topically anesthetized, and widely patent nasal passage to facilitate extraction of secretions from the hypopharynx or to guide the passage of tracheal suction catheters. For many patients, they are especially useful in the period immediately after extubation, when swallowing of oropharyngeal secretions and effective coughing are impaired. Because they induce considerably less pharyngeal stimulation than do oral airways, they can be used for conscious patients. Nasopharyngeal airways are best transferred to the alternate nasal passage on a daily basis. Continuous use beyond 48–72 hours is generally inadvisable, due to the escalating risk of infective and erosive complications. Although often effective, they do not reliably maintain airway patency and are not an acceptable alternative to endotracheal intubation for high risk patients.

ENDOTRACHEAL INTUBATION

Orotracheal Tubes

As a rule, orotracheal (OT) tubes are easier to insert than nasotracheal (NT) tubes, making oral placement the method of choice during emergencies. The larger tube that may be passed by the oral route improves both airway resistance and secretion management and allows passage of a standard caliber fiberoptic bronchoscope (FOB) if the need arises. However, oral tubes are less stable and less comfortable than nasal tubes, and they impair swallowing to a greater extent. Most self-extubations occur in patients who are orally intubated. They often require an additional oral appliance or pharyngeal airway for stabilization and to prevent tube occlusion by biting. Insertion of an oral tube incurs a higher incidence of retching, vomiting, aspiration, mainstem bronchial intubation, and self-extubation than the nasal approach, and oral tubes seriously compromise oropharyngeal hygiene. Conventional orotracheal intubation often can not (or should not) be performed for patients with head injury, neck injury, or limited neck mobility (e.g., ankylosing spondylitis, rheumatoid arthritis). Fiberoptic intubating bronchoscopes, illuminated stylets, and a variety of other aids to difficult intubation help make orotracheal intubation feasible for such patients (see below).

Nasotracheal Tubes

Nasotracheal tubes present a comparatively high resistance to airflow because they are relatively long, kink easily, and impose unusually high resistance when lined with thickened secretions. As already noted, the nares do not admit tubes as large as those that the oropharynx will accept. Nasotracheal tubes are often difficult and sometimes painful to insert. In a significant percentage of patients, purulent nasal discharge or sinusitis may develop after several days. Because local trauma tends to disrupt the rich vascular bed of the nasopharynx, bleeding diatheses generally contraindicate nasal intubation. Once in place, however, nasal tubes allow better communication, swallowing, mouth hygiene, and anchoring than their oral counterparts. Nasal intubation offers clear advantages for patients with cervical spine disease and for those with a variety of oral, mandibular, and temporomandibular problems. Many practitioners consider nasal tubes to be the airway of choice for conscious patients when intubation is continued longer than 7–10 days without tracheostomy, particularly if the patient is not comfortable. The relative indications for placing orotracheal tubes and nasotracheal tubes and tracheostomies are summarized in Table 6.2.

PHYSIOLOGIC RESPONSE TO TRACHEAL INTUBATION

During the intubation of a lightly anesthetized normal adult, substantial increases of heart rate and blood pressure are mediated by neural reflexes, catecholamines, and stress hormones. Bradycardia and hypotension are observed less commonly. These cardiovascular effects are blunted by sedatives, analgesics, and systemic or topical anesthetics. Clinically significant laryngospasm and bronchospasm occur infrequently in a well-prepared subject.

By definition, an endotracheal tube cannot exceed the caliber of the larynx, which normally is the site of greatest narrowing within the native airway. Consequently, intubation reduces the deadspace of the upper airway by 20–60 mL but simultaneously increases the resistance to airflow. Moreover, once inserted, the resistance offered by a bent, kinked, and secretion-lined or clot-obstructed endotracheal tube in situ can be considerably greater than its manufacturing specification. Although certain reports suggest that intubation reduces the resting lung volume and alters the breathing pattern, the available evidence is conflicting, and there is no firm consensus on these points.

COMPLICATIONS OF AIRWAY INTUBATION

PHYSIOLOGIC IMPAIRMENT

Endotracheal (ET) tubes bypass the mechanical defenses of the upper airway, contaminate the

TABLE 6–2

INDICATIONS FOR ORAL INTUBATION, NASAL INTUBATION AND TRACHEOSTOMY

Oral	Nasal	Tracheostomy
Emergent intubation (cardiopulmonary resuscitation, unconsciousness, or apnea)	Anticipated long-term translaryngeal tube	Inability to insert translaryngeal tube
	Cervical spine ankylosis, arthritis, or trauma	Need for long-term definitive airway
		Obstruction above cricoid cartilage
	Oral or mandibular trauma, surgery, or deformity	Complications of translaryngeal intubation
Nasal or midfacial trauma		Glottic incompetence
Basilar skull fracture	Temporomandibular joint disease	Inability to clear tracheobronchial secretions
Epiglottitis	Awake intubation	Sleep apnea unresponsive to continuous positive airway pressure
Nasal obstruction	Gagging and vomiting	Facial or laryngeal trauma or structural contraindications to translaryngeal intubation
Paranasal disease	Short (bull) neck	
Bleeding diathesis	Agitation	
Need for bronchoscopy		

lower airways, and severely hamper effective coughing. Despite advances in materials and cuff design, all tubes have the potential of inflicting laryngeal and tracheal injury, and none completely protect the lungs against aspiration of liquids. Furthermore, the bio-film that routinely lines the lumen of the tube serves to repeatedly inoculate the lower airway with potential pathogens.

INSERTION TRAUMA

Inexpert placement of an ET tube may injure delicate laryngeal, nasal, and pharyngeal tissues or cause dental or spinal trauma. Epistaxis occurs in a sizable percentage of patients intubated nasotracheally. Mouth trauma and mandibular dislocation can result from forceful placement of an orotracheal tube. Most laryngeal injuries resulting from intubation with tubes having soft, high volume cuffs are mild and easily healed. The formation of granulation tissue and ulcers by pressure-induced mucosal ischemia, however, can cause major trouble. Tight-fitting (oversized) endotracheal tubes and longer durations of intubation are risk factors for such lesions. Bilateral vocal cord paralysis and arytenoid cartilage dislocation typically present as postextubation hoarseness and upper airway obstruction. Use of a nasogastric tube in conjunction with oral intubation has been associated with a higher incidence of aspiration, erythema, and granuloma formation. Rarely, a tracheoesophageal fistula may form.

HYPOXEMIA AND ISCHEMIA

Patients who require supplemental O_2 often are exposed to room air during intubation, with consequent desaturation of arterial blood. Although this risk is reduced by "preoxygenation," O_2 stored in this way is depleted quickly by deep breathing. Therefore, intubation attempts should not be prolonged beyond 30 seconds before "reoxygenating," especially for patients who continue to breathe actively. Pulse oximetry or, preferably, continuous intra-arterial fiberoptic blood gas analysis, can help warn of developing hypoxemia during the attempt. (Pulse oximetry lags behind the real-time arterial saturation.) Nasal prongs set to deliver 6–10 L of oxygen per minute can provide supplemental O_2 during intubation, as can the use of a laryngoscope adapted for this purpose.

Depletion of the pulmonary oxygen reservoir can be prevented by giving a rapidly acting hypnotic agent (e.g., thiopental, 25–100 mg intravenously or midazolam, 1–5 mg, as required), followed by a muscle relaxant (e.g., succinylcholine, 1 mg/kg) to induce temporary paralysis. (If the patient is at risk for cardiac instability, vecuronium, although somewhat longer acting, is a safer choice) (see also Chapter 17, Analgesia, Sedation, and Paralysis). This apneic intubation technique also facilitates cannulation of the larynx, shortens the time without ventilation, and lessens the hazards of laryngospasm and insertion trauma. Although apneic intubation is often the preferred technique in difficult cases, sedatives and muscle relaxants are not without risk. Relaxed musculature may totally obstruct the upper airway if the intubation attempt is unsuccessful, and barbiturates may depress cardiac contractility; the clinician must be certain that face mask ventilation is effective before committing to muscle relaxation, and expert assistance must be immediately at hand. Tremors, vomiting, and mild hyperkalemia are relatively common; rarely, succinylcholine can induce the syndrome of "malignant hyperthermia."

Ischemia is less well tolerated than hypoxemia alone; therefore, intubation attempts should not interrupt cardiac compression for longer than 10–15 seconds during cardiopulmonary resuscitation, especially if the lungs can be ventilated effectively by mask. In general, the blind nasotracheal approach should not be attempted during emergent intubation because of the uncertain time required to secure the airway. Moreover, blind nasotracheal intubation is exceedingly difficult if the patient is apneic. Fiberoptic bronchoscopy or direct laryngoscopy may facilitate semiemergent placement of either type of ET tube.

GASTRIC ASPIRATION

Stimulation of the oropharynx frequently causes vomiting, especially when the stomach is distended by food or air. Gentle cricothyroid pressure (Sellick maneuver) from the start of mask ventilation helps seal the esophagus against air entry but does not obviate the risk of aspiration. Evacuation of the stomach before intubation can reduce the aspiration risk; however, gastric decompression should not delay emergent intubation.

REFLEX GLOTTIC CLOSURE AND LARYNGOSPASM

Reflex closure of the glottis and true laryngospasm can prevent passage of the ET tube and may severely limit spontaneous ventilation. Prior use of a topical anesthetic (e.g., lidocaine, 4%) minimizes the risk. Rather than attempt forceful intubation (losing valuable time and risking laryngeal trauma), the patient should be ventilated with bag-mask insufflation of oxygen. Spasm usually subsides promptly. However, if adequate ventilation cannot be achieved and the situation becomes urgent, intravenous succinylcholine (1 mg/kg) will relax the contracted muscles during ET placement.

BRONCHOSPASM

Tube placement often stimulates irritant receptors, triggering cough and bronchospasm. Such receptors stop firing shortly after tube placement in most cases, unless the tip of the tube continues to touch the carina. Although coughing is often difficult to arrest, an endotracheal bolus of lidocaine (5 mL of a 2% solution) may be effective. Infused or aerosolized bronchodilators may relieve the bronchospasm but leave the mechanically stimulated coughing reflex unaffected.

RIGHT MAIN BRONCHUS INTUBATION

In emergent situations, there is a natural tendency to advance the ET tube beyond the carina. The right main bronchus is less sharply angulated from the trachea than is the left main bronchus and will be entered in 90% of low placements. Rarely, this tendency may facilitate intentional isolation of the right and left lungs during management of such problems as massive hemoptysis originating distal to the main carina. The underventilated left lung and right upper lobe may collapse rapidly, especially when previously ventilated with oxygen. Although comparative auscultation is helpful, breath sounds often are surprisingly well transmitted to an underventilated lung.

Endotracheal tubes should be advanced a maximum of 2.5–5.0 cm beyond the point at which the tube cuff is seen to pass the cords. Use of a lighted stylet facilitates tip localization to the appropriate level. As a general rule, 22 cm at the second molar, or 24–27 cm at the lips, will approximate the proper position in an adult of average size. A postprocedure chest x-ray is necessary to check position. A generous distance between tube tip and main carina must be allowed for tube movement.

POINTS OF TECHNIQUE

Intubation of a rapidly deteriorating, critically ill patient can be a dramatic clinical event. In these challenging circumstances, success depends on optimal preparation and experience proportional to the anticipated difficulty of successful insertion. Certain important questions should be addressed before the attempt: (*a*) Is intubation of the airway likely to be anatomically challenging? If so, who should attempt the intubation? (*b*) Which is the best approach—oral, nasal, or tracheostomy? (*c*) Should the attempt be made awake, under sedation, or using rapid sequence (apneic) technique? (*d*) Is the patient at unusually high risk for aspiration? (*e*) What is the contingency approach (''backup'' plan)? (*f*) Are all necessary materials and personnel at hand to support both the primary and backup plans?

THE DIFFICULT AIRWAY

In a significant minority of critically ill patients, a practitioner who is well trained in conventional intubation techniques will experience difficulty with mask ventilation or tracheal intubation. Such problems assume particular importance for the critically ill patient who is hypoxemic, acidotic, or hemodynamically unstable. Very obese patients with ''short necks'' often present problems. Certain physical features correlate (imperfectly) with the difficulty of intubation (Fig. 6.1). These include the nonvisibility of key oropharyngeal landmarks: faucial pillars, soft palate, and uvula; poor atlantooccipital joint mobility (<30° excursion of the maxillary teeth, neutral to fully extended); short mentohyoid distance (less than three finger breadths); and restricted temperomandibular joint excursion (maximal oral aperture less than three vertical finger breadths in the saggital midline) (Table 6.3). Helpful techniques are now available for consideration in such circumstances (Table 6.4).

TABLE 6–3

PREDICTORS OF DIFFICULT INTUBATION

Invisibility of facial pillars, soft palate, uvula

Mentohyoid distance less than three finger breadths

Restricted temperomandibular joint excursion

Restricted excursion of atlantooccipital joint

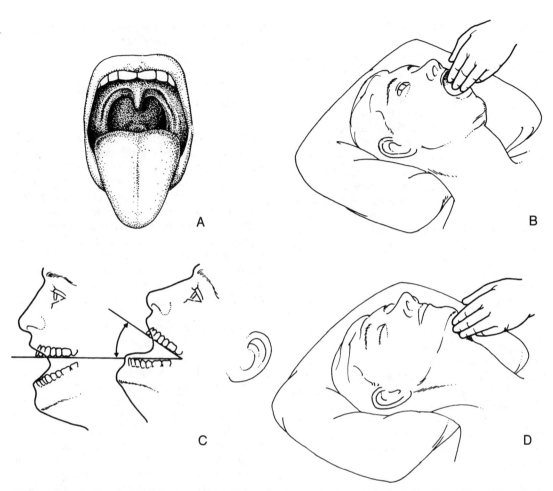

FIG. 6–1. Evaluating the airway for ease of intubation. (A) A patient who can not be intubated easily will have poorly defined oral landmarks (uvula, faucial pillars, and epiglottis) during tongue protrusion. (B) The mouth aperture should be sufficient to allow entry of three finger breadths upon widest opening. (C) Mobility of the atlantooccipital joint is ensured by the ability to incline the occlusal surfaces of the maxillary molars by 30° or more from the neutral position. (D) Finally, the chin should allow separation from the hyoid bone by three finger breadths or more. Failure to meet these criteria indicates a potentially difficult oral (and perhaps nasal) intubation.

TABLE 6–4

TECHNIQUES TO AID DIFFICULT INTUBATION

Forceps guided insertion
Stylet guided insertion
Specialized laryngoscopes
Retrograde intubation

TECHNIQUES TO AID IN DIFFICULT INTUBATION.

Bronchoscope-Guided Airway Management

A fiberoptic bronchoscope may be used to place an oral or nasal tube, position a double lumen or single lumen tube, or assess the feasibility of extubation. Although this procedure may be particularly helpful for patients with difficult airways or poor neck mobility, the field of view is obscured easily by secretions, vomitus, or blood.

Forceps-Guided Intubation

When difficulty is encountered in entering the larynx using a nasal approach (or when exchanging an oral for a nasal tube), McGill forceps can be used to grasp the tip of the nasal tube as it enters the retropharynx, directing it through the vocal cords under direct laryngoscopic observation.

Stylet-Guided Intubation

Various forms of stylet can be used to configure the soft tube to enter the glottic aperture more easily. These deformable metal or plastic rods span a range from the standard aluminum rods and elastic bougies, which allow no alteration *in situ*, to flexible guides with thumb triggers, which give the operator the ability to direct the tube tip at any time during the insertion attempt. A tube changer is a long plastic tube (hollow or solid) that acts as a stent when a fresh endotracheal tube is exchanged for a malfunctioning or less desirable one along the same insertion path. In an emergency, a tube changer can be fashioned by trimming a standard nasogastric tube.

Illuminating Stylets

A battery-operated illuminating stylet ("light wand") has a very bright tip that transilluminates the skin above the thyroid cartilage as it enters the larynx. This "jack-o'-lantern" effect fails to be seen distinctly when the tube enters the esophagus. The light wand accurately guides endotracheal tube passage in a very high percentage of blind endotracheal intubations (reportedly >95%). This device does not require the sniffing position or laryngoscopy and is used commonly to verify the position of a tube recently placed by another method.

Specialized Laryngoscopes

For many years, the primary options for cord visualization were straight and curved blade laryngoscopes, and most clinicians have developed facility with (or preference for) one or the other of them. In response to clinical need, specialized blades that incorporate a variety of desirable features are now available. These range from innovatively shaped blades (V-form, double-angled, tube-shaped, and hinged-tip configurations) to blades that incorporate flexible fiberoscopic bundles to aid visualization or ports for oxygen delivery and suctioning.

Retrograde Intubation

When elective or semielective endotracheal intubation is indicated but the cords defy passage by other methods, a flexible guide wire inserted retrograde through the needle-punctured cricothyroid membrane can be advanced through the mouth to establish the channel. With the current availability of simpler aids to intubation, this method is now seldom used.

DISTINGUISHING TRACHEAL FROM ESOPHAGEAL INTUBATION

Although unquestionably useful, traditional methods for confirming the endotracheal placement of the tube have limited reliability (Table 6.5). These techniques include stethoscopic audibility and symmetry of breath sounds, direct visualization of the cords during insertion, ease of insufflation and recovery of the tidal volume, tidal fogging and clearing of the endotracheal tube, palpation of the endotracheal tube in the larynx, loss of voice, coughing and expulsion of airway secretions, expansion of the upper chest, and failure of the abdomen to progressively distend during gas delivery.

Pulse oximetry, which is useful in ensuring optimal arterial oxygenation during the procedure for patients with adequate cardiac output, may also help in the evaluation of correct placement. To improve reliability and speed of placement, other methods for confirming airway intubation have been developed. These are generally based on the phasic detection of CO_2 during expiration or on the ease or difficulty of gas withdrawal from the airway. One simple device for detecting (but not measuring) CO_2 can be attached quickly to the endotracheal tube and observed for the tidally

---

TABLE 6–5

DISTINGUISHING TRACHEAL FROM ESOPHAGEAL INTUBATION

Conventional
  Symmetrical breath sounds
  Visualization of vocal cords during insertion
  Ease of insufflation and recovery of tidal volume
  Expiratory fogging of ET tube
  Palpation of larynx
  Loss of voice
  Coughing of airway secretions through tube
  Upper chest expansion
  Absence of progressive abdominal distention
Devices and Aids
  CO_2 excretion
    Color detector
    Capnometry
  Tidal gas recovery
    Squeeze bulb
    Syringe

phasic purple to yellow color changes that signal proper placement. Quantitative capnometry is also feasible but less commonly available or portable. Carbon dioxide detection and measurement by these methods occasionally can be misleading—little CO_2 is evolved or expelled during shock or circulatory arrest, and conversely, some CO_2 may be liberated initially after esophageal intubation from gas trapped in the gastric pouch. (However, this concentration falls rapidly as serial tidal volumes are delivered.) Reliability of the detector may be compromised by soiling with gastric secretions.

When compressed, a large capacity squeeze bulb affixed to the endotracheal tube will fail to fill easily if the tube is in the collapsible esophagus. If in good position, however, it recoils effortlessly to its resting volume. Free withdrawal of air via a fitted 50-mL syringe is an equivalent method that is based on this same principle.

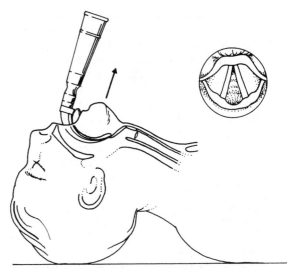

FIG. 6-2. Orotracheal intubation. To align glottis, pharynx, and oral cavity, the neck is flexed and the head is extended. The laryngoscope lifts the tongue and lower jaw away from the posterior pharynx by a motion directed perpendicular to the oroglottic axis.

INTUBATION SEQUENCE

Sedation and Neuromuscular Blockade

Rapidly acting benzodiazepines impart amnesia and induce anesthesia, usually without significantly affecting hemodynamics. Intravenous midazolam, a rapidly acting drug of this class, has a convenient onset (1–3 minutes) and duration (~20 minutes). Fentanyl or similar narcotic agent often provides an effective supplement. When necessary, the effects of both can be reversed rapidly (flumazenil, naloxone). Propofol, given as a bolus of 2 mg/kg, has a near immediate onset of action and a duration of 7–10 minutes. The mild cardiovascular effects of this anesthetic may block any intubation-associated increases of heart rate, systemic vascular resistance and blood pressure. When required, muscle relaxation can be accomplished with depolarizing (succinylcholine) or nondepolarizing (vecuronium, atracurium) agents. Succinylcholine acts quickly, but its depolarizing action may provoke vomiting. In contrast, the more slowly acting nondepolarizers are less likely to stimulate emesis directly but extend the period of vulnerability for aspiration. Etomidate and ketamine are useful drugs preferred by some practitioners.

Oral Intubation

Apart from being well prepared for emergent developments, perhaps the most important thing for the physician to do is to relax and avoid panic. After clearing the airway of secretions and debris, the base of the tongue is dislodged from the retropharynx by lifting at the angles of the jaw. For obtunded or comatose patients, an oropharyngeal airway can be placed to maintain the passage, but such devices may stimulate vomiting in the conscious or agitated subject. Unless contraindicated, the patient should be positioned with the head (not shoulders) resting on a thin pillow or a doubly folded towel. The optimal ''sniffing'' position is with the neck flexed and the head extended (Fig. 6.2). Once positioned, the patient generally can be ventilated by mask without difficulty until the tube is inserted. Bag insufflations should be delivered gently (never forcefully) at a measured rate. During a cardiac arrest in a patient with severe airflow obstruction, special care should be taken to avoid overventilation and iatrogenic ''auto-PEEP.'' If tube placement is not emergent, an alert patient should be lightly sedated, premedicated with atropine (0.4–0.8 mg i.v.) and a topical anesthetic. A cooperative patient can be instructed to pant to concentrate deposition of the drug on the larynx and upper airway. As a rule, agitated or seriously hypoxemic patients should be sedated and paralyzed quickly (apneic intubation technique). However, this method must be used with special caution for patients who are massively obese and for those with upper airway pathology. In such cases, experienced personnel must be available, and the physician should be prepared to undertake cricothyroid puncture in case the airway totally obstructs after paralysis, bag-mask ventilation is unsuccessful, or attempts to intubate repeatedly fail. Even if phasic gas delivery is not undertaken, oxygen insufflated continuously through the needle at 2–4 L/minute can often maintain acceptable arterial oxygenation (and a degree of ventilation) without hyperinflation until a secure airway is established.

A 8.5-mm (internal diameter) tube for an average male and an 8.0-mm tube for an average female are good sizes to try first. The tube selected should generally be the largest that will easily pass through the cords.

Curved laryngoscope blades are directed anterior to the epiglottis (Fig. 6.2). Straight blades are inserted immediately posterior to the epiglottis and allow a better view of the cords. Both instruments should lift the entire jaw upward to expose the larynx. Placement of neither instrument should use the teeth as a fulcrum for leverage. During intubation, firm cricothyroid pressure helps to bring the cords into view and to seal the esophagus.

When flexible stylets are used to direct the tip of the tube into a glottic opening that cannot be visualized clearly and continuously, care must be taken to ensure that the stylet does not project beyond the tip of the tube. After placement, the cuff should be inflated with the minimum volume that seals without leakage under positive pressure. A variety of useful devices is now available to stabilize an orotracheal tube after placement. A standard ET tube can be anchored effectively by a continuous single band of tape wrapped circumferentially around the neck and secured to the tube (and bite block, if used) at both ends. The hands must be restrained if there is any possibility for self-extubation. (This is especially important after orotracheal intubation in a hypoxemic patient requiring high levels of inspired oxygen or airway pressure.) Although a nasogastric or orogastric tube should be used for the orally intubated patient to decompress the stomach when there is gut hypomotility or active air swallowing, its continued use may increase the incidence of aspiration and laryngeal erosion.

Nasotracheal Intubation

Blind nasotracheal intubation is not a technique to be performed by the inexperienced caregiver. It should not be used in emergent situations and is especially inappropriate for establishing the airway during apnea. Because it is usually performed in awake patients, topical anesthesia of the nose, pharynx, and larynx and sedation are mandatory. A topical vasoconstricter (phenylephrine or cocaine) can facilitate tube passage and reduce the risk of mucosal hemorrhage. Selection of a small tube (e.g., size 7.0), generous nasal lubrication, and gentle insertion technique are necessary to prevent nasal, laryngeal, or tracheal injury. The nasotracheal tube should be inserted initially to a level just above the vocal cords. (This tube position can be detected by listening to the intensity of expired air flowing through the tube.) The tube is then rapidly but gently advanced in synchrony with the next inspiratory effort. Entry to the larynx usually is signaled by a vigorous cough and subsequent inability to speak. Vigilance should be maintained against the development of sinusitis, which complicates approximately one-third of placements longer than a few days.

EXTUBATION

Extubation must not be performed casually. Inadvertent extubation can be lethal in acutely ill, agitated patients and must be avoided at all costs. Extubation breaks the seal between the patient's upper and lower airway, potentially allowing purulent secretions pooled above the cuff to enter the lung. Reflex stimulation may also provoke laryngospasm, bronchospasm, or cardiac arrhythmias.

Oxygen should be administered, and the trachea and oropharynx should be cleared of secretions before the cuff is deflated. After a deep inspiration, the tube should be pulled quickly as the patient exhales forcefully from a high lung volume. Postextubation stridor may occur due to laryngospasm or edema. This usually subsides within the first 6–24 hours, but such patients must be observed carefully to assess the need for urgent reintubation. Although not routinely necessary, racemic epinephrine and corticosteroids may be helpful after extubation in selected cases—especially those involving small adults or children.

The ability of the patient to exhale freely around the deflated cuff before extubation gives some assurance that the airway above the cuff is not severely narrowed. (This simple test is useful when upper airway obstruction has been the primary indication for intubation.) A leak around the partially deflated cuff during ventilation is a sensitive predictor of successful extubation for a patient who meets other criteria for ventilator independence, but the absence of a cuff leak does not reliably predict extubation failure secondary to upper airway obstruction. Noninvasive ventilation may provide a useful bridge across the immediate postextubation period. Heliox, a low density helium–oxygen mixture, reduces resistive pressure losses due to turbulence and may prove useful during the period of maximal edema for selected patients.

Women tend to be predisposed to the complications of intubation. Post-extubation stridor may result from vocal cord dysfunction, arytenoid dislocation, laryngospasm, uncleared secretions or blood, or tracheomalacia. If reintubation is needed, a smaller endotracheal tube and a prophylactic epinephrine aerosol directed onto the cords are reasonable measures.

TRACHEOSTOMY

BENEFITS AND INDICATIONS

Tracheostomy improves comfort (potentially allowing the patient to eat, talk, and ambulate), greatly facilitates secretion management, minimizes airway resistance and anatomic deadspace, and reduces the risk of laryngeal injury (Table 6.6). However, tracheostomies have the highest associated risk of serious complications (bleeding, stenosis) and the highest incidence of swallowing difficulty and aspiration postextubation. Unless carried out emergently for acute upper airway obstruction, conventional tracheostomy (but not necessarily *percutaneous* tracheostomy) should be performed over an oral or nasal tube in an operating suite. Except when long-term ventilator dependence or need for ongoing secretion management has been established, most experts defer tracheostomy for at least 10 days after intubation. For selected patients who are comfortable, quiet, and making progress toward extubation, tracheostomy may be deferred for longer than 3–4 weeks.

VARIANTS OF CONVENTIONAL TRACHEOSTOMY

Certain variants of tracheostomy recently introduced to clinical practice may be carried out safely at the bedside.

Needle Cricothyroidotomy

In very rare circumstances, life-threatening upper airway obstruction renders all standard methods of airway control invalid or infeasible: pharyngeal airways, bag-mask ventilation, and translaryngeal intubation. Needle cricothyroidotomy can be performed quickly with a 14-gauge or larger needle to provide a temporary conduit for a high pressure source of oxygen. After the

TABLE 6–6

TRANSLARYNGEAL INTUBATION VERSUS TRACHEOSTOMY

	Translaryngeal Intubation	Tracheostomy
Advantages:	Ease of placement	Comfort
	Inexpensive	Ease of mouth care
	Fewer severe complications	Secretion removal
	No specialized venue needed for insertion	Stability
		Less airway resistance
		Improved communication
		Ease of swallowing and enteral feeding
		Reduced work of breathing
		Improved mobility
		Ease of reinsertion and ventilator reconnection
Disadvantages:	Discomfort	Expense
	Swallowing	Severity of complications
	Secretion clearance	Swallowing impairment
	Greater work of breathing	Reduced cough efficiency postdecannulation
	Impaired speech	
	Upper airway and larynx damage	

cricothyroid membrane is located, prepared antiseptically, anesthetized, and immobilized, a syringe-mounted needle with external cannula punctures the membrane at a 45° angle and air is aspirated to confirm its position. Once inserted, the outer flexible sheath is advanced as the metallic needle is withdrawn. Attachment of a Y-connector and high pressure oxygen source at 40–60 L/minute may then allow manually gated (phasic) insufflations, which usually maintain acceptable gas exchange until a definitive airway can be established.

Percutaneous Dilatational Tracheostomy

An entirely different variant of conventional tracheostomy is gaining considerable popularity as an elective (nonemergent) procedure for establishing long-term airway access, ventilatory support, and secretion clearance for those patients who cannot be transported to the operating room. The tube enters the trachea between the cricoid and first tracheal cartilages or between the first and second tracheal cartilages. After dissecting to the anterior tracheal wall, an introducer, sheath, guide wire, and catheter are used to progressively develop and dilate the stoma for acceptance of a standard tracheostomy tube. Bleeding, subcutaneous emphysema, and paratracheal insertion are reported complications. The incidence of infection is believed to be less than with the open surgical approach.

Mini-Tracheostomy

When secretion retention is the primary concern, a mini-tracheostomy may be performed to allow suctioning through a small-diameter (4.0-mm) cuffless indwelling cannula that can also serve as an O_2 delivery conduit. Although inadequate for ventilation, transtracheal insufflation via the "mini-trach" can be helpful in an emergency, similar to needle cricothyroidotomy, as already described. Candidates for the mini-trach should have an intact gag reflex because the airway is not protected. This device does not seriously impede talking, coughing, or eating.

KEY POINTS

1. Noninvasive ventilation may not be appropriate for patients who are obtunded or uncooperative, for those in whom unexpected loss of pressure or supplemental oxygen might be immediately hazardous, for those who require high levels of applied pressure, or for those who are hemodynamically unstable. In such cases, endotracheal intubation is the indicated intervention.

2. Orotracheal tube placement is the method of choice during emergencies. Nasotracheal tubes are of generally smaller diameter than orotracheal tubes but are more comfortable and stable in the conscious or active patient.

3. Important complications of intubation include a variety of insertion trauma, gastric aspiration, hypoxemia, laryngospasm, esophageal intubation, and right main bronchus intubation.

4. Predictors of difficult intubation include nonvisibility of key oropharyngeal landmarks, poor atlantooccipital joint mobility, short mentohyoid distance, and restricted temporomandibular joint excursion. In such cases, apneic intubation and the need for special expertise should be considered before the attempt.

5. Techniques to aid difficult intubation include bronchoscopy, forceps and stylet guidance, specialized laryngoscopes, and retrograde wire insertion. Traditional methods to confirm tracheal positioning of the endotracheal tube include stethoscopically audible symmetry of breath sounds, ease of manual insufflation, complete recovery of insufflated tidal volume, loss of voice, expansion of the upper chest, and coughing with expulsion of airway secretions. CO_2-sensing indicators and squeeze bulb or syringe recovery of small injected gas volumes effectively complement these techniques.

6. Inadvertent extubation is often a life-threatening event that occurs more commonly in orally intubated, lightly sedated patients (who must be carefully restrained). The ability of the patient to exhale freely around a partially deflated cuff gives some assurance of patency of the larynx above the cuff immediately before a planned extubation.

7. Although its long-term complications can be serious, tracheostomy improves comfort, communication, and secretion management. Certain newer variants of conventional tracheostomy (e.g., needle cricothyroidotomy, percutaneous dilatational tracheostomy, and mini-tracheostomy) do not require an operating room and may, therefore, promise to be safer to perform for well-selected acutely ill patients.

SUGGESTED READINGS

1. Anderson H, Bartlett R. Elective tracheotomy for mechanical ventilation by the percutaneous technique. Clin Chest Med 1991;12(3):555–560.
2. Bach J. Indications for tracheostomy and decannulation of tracheostomized ventilator users. Monaldi Arch Chest Dis 1995;50(3):223–227.
3. Benumof J. Management of the difficult adult airway, with special emphasis on awake tracheal intubation. Anesthesia 1991;75(6):1087–1110.
4. Blosser S, Stauffer J. Intubation of critically ill patients. Clin Chest Med 1996;17(3):355–378.
5. Brimacombe J, Berry A, Verghese C. The laryngeal mask airway in critical care medicine. Intensive Care Med 1995; 21(4):361–364.
6. Chang V. Protocol for prevention of complications of endotracheal intubation. Crit Care Nurse 1995;15(5):19–20.
7. Deem S, Bishop M. Evaluation and management of the difficult airway. Crit Care Clin 1995;11(1):1–27.
8. Einarsson O, Rochester C, Rosenbaum S. Airway management in respiratory emergencies. Clin Chest Med 1994;15(1):13–34.
9. Gallagher T. Endotracheal intubation. Crit Care Clin 1992;8(4):665–676.
10. Godwin J, Heffner J. Special critical care considerations in tracheostomy management. Clin Chest Med 1991;12(3): 573–584.
11. Hansen-Flaschen J. Improving patient tolerance of mechanical ventilation. Challenges ahead. Crit Care Clin 1994;10(4):659–671.
12. Hartley M, Vaughan R. Problems associated with tracheal extubation. Br J Anaesth 1993;71(4):561–568.
13. Heffner J. Airway management in the critically ill patient. Crit Care Clin 1990;6(3):533–550.
14. Heffner JE. Tracheal intubation in mechanically ventilated patients. Clin Chest Med 1988;9(1):23–35.
15. Kaplan J, Schuster D. Physiologic consequences of tracheal intubation. Clin Chest Med 1991;12(3):425–432.
16. Kharasch M, Graff J. Emergency management of the airway. Crit Care Clin 1995;11(1):53–66.
17. Levine S, Niederman M. The impact of tracheal intubation on host defenses and risks for nosocomial pneumonia. Clin Chest Med 1991;12(3):523–543.
18. Lewis R. Tracheostomies. Indications, timing, and complications. Clin Chest Med 1992;13(1):137–149.
19. Mancinelli-Van Atta J, Beck S. Preventing hypoxemia and hemodynamic compromise related to endotracheal suctioning. Am J Crit Care 1992;1(3):62–79.
20. McCulloch T, Bishop M. Complications of translaryngeal intubation. Clin Chest Med 1991;12(3):507–521.
21. Morgan J, Haug R, Holmgreen WC. Awake blind nasoendotracheal intubation: a comprehensive review. J Oral Maxillofac Surg 1994;52(12):1303–1311.
22. Morris I. Fiberoptic intubation. Can J Anaesth 1994; 41(10):996–1007.
23. Morris I. Pharmacologic aids to intubation and the rapid sequence induction. Emerg Med Clin North Am 1988; 6(4):753–768.
24. Pepe P, Zachariah B, Chandra N. Invasive airway techniques in resuscitation. Ann Emerg Med 1993;22(2 Pt 2): 393–403.
25. Plummer A, Gracey D. Consensus conference on artificial airways in patients receiving mechanical ventilation. Chest 1989;96(1):178–180.
26. Rashkin MC, Davis T. Acute complications of endotracheal intubation. Relationship to reintubation, route, urgency and duration. Chest 1986;89:165–167.
27. Sanchez A, Kantor B. New advances in airway management. West J Med 1995;162(1):55.
28. Schwartz D, Wiener-Kronish J. Management of the difficult airway. Clin Chest Med 1991;12(3):483–495.
29. Stauffer J. Medical Management of the Airway. Clin Chest Med 1991;12(3):449.
30. Steitz J, Shapshay S. Airway injury after tracheotomy and endotracheal intubation. Surg Clin North Am 1991;71(6): 1211–1230.
31. Walls R. Airway management. Emerg Med Clin North Am 1993;11(1):53–60.
32. Wenig B, Applebaum E. Indications for and techniques of tracheotomy. Clin Chest Med 1991;12(3):545–554.
33. Weymuller E. Prevention and management of intubation injury of the larynx and trachea. Am J Otolaryngol 1992; 13(3):139–144.

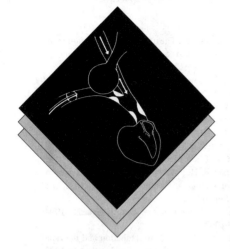

Indications and Options for Mechanical Ventilation

INDICATIONS FOR MECHANICAL VENTILATION

Although often made concurrently, the decisions to institute mechanical support should be made independently of those to perform tracheal intubation or to use positive end-expiratory pressure (PEEP) or continuous posture airway pressure (CPAP). This is especially true considering the recently improved noninvasive (nasal and mask) options for supporting ventilation. As the ventilator assumes the work of breathing, important changes occur in pleural pressure, ventilation distribution, and cardiac output (Fig. 7.1). Mechanical assistance may be needed to achieve the level of ventilation appropriate to the clinical setting, because oxygenation cannot be achieved at an acceptable FiO_2 without manipulating PEEP, mean airway pressure, and pattern of ventilation or because spontaneous ventilation places excessive demands on ventilatory muscles or on a compromised cardiovascular system (Table 7.1).

INADEQUATE ALVEOLAR VENTILATION

Apnea or deteriorating ventilation despite other therapeutic measures are absolute indications for instituting mechanical breathing assistance. In such cases, there usually are signs of respiratory distress or advancing obtundation, and serial blood gas measurements show a falling pH and stable or rising $PaCO_2$. Although few physicians withhold mechanical assistance when the pH trends steadily downward and there are signs of physiologic intolerance, there is less agreement

regarding the absolute values of $PaCO_2$ and pH that warrant such intervention; these clearly vary with the specific clinical setting. In fact, after intubation has been accomplished, pH and $PaCO_2$ may be allowed to drift deliberately far outside the normal range to avoid the high ventilating pressures and tidal volumes that tend to induce lung damage. This strategy—''permissive hypercapnia''—is now considered integral to a lung-protective ventilatory approach to the acute management of severe asthma and adult respiratory distress syndrome (ARDS; see Chapter 24, ''Oxygenation Failure'').

For the nonintubated patient, pH is generally a better indicator than $PaCO_2$ of the need for ventilatory support. Hypercapnia *per se* should not prompt aggressive intervention if pH remains acceptable and the patient remains alert, especially if CO_2 is retained chronically and increases in $PaCO_2$ occur slowly. Many patients require ventilatory assistance despite levels of alveolar ventilation that are appropriate to normal resting metabolism. For example, patients with metabolic acidosis and neuromuscular weakness or airflow obstruction may lower $PaCO_2$ to 40 mm Hg or below but not sufficiently to prevent acidemia. The physiologic consequences of altered pH are still debated and clearly depend on the underlying pathophysiology. However, if not quickly reversible by simpler measures, a sustained pH >7.65 or <7.10 is often considered sufficiently dangerous in itself to require control by mechanical ventilation and sedation (with muscle relaxants, if needed). Inside these extremes, the threshold for initiating support varies with the clinical setting. For example, a lethargic patient with asthma who

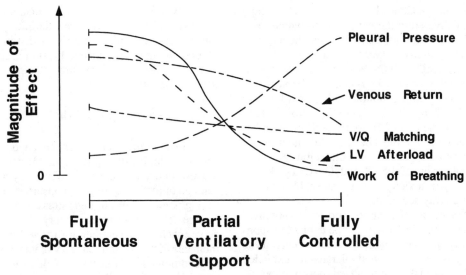

FIG. 7–1. Important physiologic differences between spontaneous and mechanical ventilation. As the proportion of ventilatory support with positive pressure increases, work of breathing falls and pleural pressure rises, influencing venous return, left ventricular (LV) afterload, and ventilation/perfusion (V/Q) matching.

TABLE 7–1

INDICATIONS FOR MECHANICAL VENTILATION

Inadequate ventilation to maintain pH
Inadequate oxygenation
Excessive workload
Congestive failure
Circulatory shock

is struggling to breathe can maintain a normal pH until shortly before suffering a respiratory arrest, whereas an alert cooperative patient with chronically blunted respiratory drive may allow pH to fall to 7.25 or lower before recovering uneventfully in response to aggressive bronchodilation, steroids, and oxygen. In less obvious situations, the decision to ventilate should be guided by trends in pH, arterial blood gases, mental status, dyspnea, hemodynamic stability, and response to therapy.

The ongoing need for ventilatory assistance must be carefully and repeatedly assessed (see Chapter 10, Weaning from Mechanical Ventilation). To cite one specific situation, a comatose patient who is overventilated (backup rate set too high) is frequently mistaken for a pathologically apneic one. The distinction generally can be made during a several-minute trial of unsupported breathing. With the patient well monitored by electrocardiogram (ECG) and oximetry in the as-

sist control mode, the FiO$_2$ is first set to 1.0 for approximately five breaths to avert hypoxemia during the apneic period. The backup rate of the ventilator is then reduced to a very low level for 1 to 3 minutes while the patient is watched carefully for indications of spontaneous effort (e.g., on a pressure or flow tracing), hypoxemia, or arrhythmia. Mean airway pressure also should be monitored before and after such manipulations, because the accompanying fall in $\dot{V}_E$ will tend to reduce it, potentially improving oxygenation while boosting cardiac output.

INADEQUATE OXYGENATION

Arterial oxygenation is the result of complex interactions between systemic oxygen demand, cardiovascular adequacy, and the efficiency of pulmonary oxygen exchange. Improving cardiovascular performance and minimizing O$_2$ consumption (by attending to fever, agitation, pain, etc.) may dramatically improve the balance between delivery and consumption. Transpulmonary oxygen exchange can be aided by supplementing FiO$_2$, by using PEEP, or by changing the pattern of ventilation to increase mean airway (and consequently, mean alveolar) pressure and average lung size (see Chapter 5, Respiratory Monitoring).

Modest fractions of inspired oxygen are administered to nonintubated patients using masks or nasal cannulas. Controlled, low-range O_2 therapy is best delivered to the nonintubated patient by a well-fitting Venturi mask, which can be adjusted for changes in inspiratory flow requirements with minimal change in FiO_2. Without tracheal intubation, delivery of high FiO_2 can only be achieved with a tightly fitting, nonrebreathing mask that is flushed with high flows of pure O_2. Unfortunately, apart from the risk of O_2 toxicity, these often become displaced or must be removed intentionally for eating or expectoration. Intubation facilitates the application of PEEP and CPAP needed to avert oxygen toxicity, as well as enables extraction of airway secretions.

Although positive airway pressure (noninvasive ventilation or CPAP) can be applied to spontaneously breathing, nonintubated patients, these techniques may not be well tolerated for extended periods, especially by confused, poorly cooperative, or hemodynamically unstable patients who require high mask pressures (>15 cm H_2O; see *Noninvasive Ventilation* below). Patients who retain secretions also are poor candidates for these techniques. Moreover, with the airway unprotected, these methods should be used only with extreme caution in patients who are obtunded or comatose. Continuous positive airway pressure is best tolerated at low levels (<7.5 cm H_2O) for less than 48 hours, with sporadic breaks allowed to relieve facial pressure.

EXCESSIVE RESPIRATORY WORKLOAD

A common reason for ventilatory assistance is to amplify ventilatory power. As discussed elsewhere in this volume, the respiratory muscles cannot sustain tidal pressures greater than 40 to 50% of maximal isometric pressure indefinitely. Respiratory pressure requirements rise with minute ventilation and the impedance to breathing; impaired ventilatory drive or muscle strength diminish ventilatory capability and reserve.

CARDIOVASCULAR SUPPORT

Although little work is expended by normal subjects who breathe quietly, the O_2 demands of the respiratory system account for a very high percentage of total body oxygen consumption ($\dot{V}O_2$) during periods of physiologic stress (Fig. 7.2). Experimental animals in circulatory shock that receive mechanical ventilation survive longer than their unassisted counterparts. Moreover, patients with combined cardiorespiratory disease often fail withdrawal of ventilatory support for cardiac rather than respiratory reasons. Such observations demonstrate the importance of minimizing the ventilatory O_2 requirement during cardiac insufficiency or ischemia to rebalance myocardial O_2 supply with requirements and/or allow diaphragmatic blood flow to be redirected to other O_2-deprived vital organs. Moreover, reducing the magnitude of ventilatory effort may improve afterload to the left ventricle (see Chapter 1, Hemodynamics). Therefore, the physician should intervene early to relieve an excessive breathing workload for patients with compromised cardiac output. Most patients who need intubation and positive end-expiratory airway pressure (CPAP or PEEP) for oxygenation also expend considerable energy in meeting ventilatory requirements. Al-

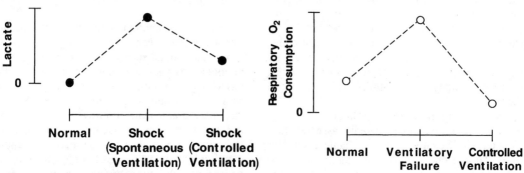

FIG. 7–2. Influence of ventilatory support on perfusion adequacy and oxygen consumed by ventilatory musculature. The work cost of spontaneous breathing and the increased afterload to left ventricular ejection often contribute significantly to anaerobiosis and lactic acid production during circulatory shock (left). A better balance between oxygen delivery and consumption can be achieved when ventilation is controlled, thereby freeing needed oxygen for other organ systems. Conversely, boosting circulatory output in the setting of shock improves oxygen delivery to the fatiguing respiratory musculature, improving their O_2 supply and endurance (right).

though it is possible to use noninvasive ventilation or CPAP alone for mildly to moderately affected patients, fatigue often sets in unless underlying oxygen requirements are reduced substantially, which often requires sedation, paralysis, or higher pressures than can be provided noninvasively. Therefore, most physicians use fully assisted mechanical ventilation in the initial period.

OPTIONS IN MECHANICAL VENTILATION

TYPES OF VENTILATION

Negative Versus Positive Pressure

To accomplish ventilation, a pressure difference must be developed phasically across the lung. This difference can be generated by negative pressure in the pleural space, by positive pressure applied to the airway opening, or by a combination of both. For machine-aided cycles, the physician must determine the machine's minimum cycling rate, the duration of its inspiratory cycle, and either the pressure to be applied or the tidal volume to administer, depending on the "mode" selected.

Although of major historical interest and potential use in isolated instances, conventional negative pressure ventilators (e.g., tanks or body suits) are seldom appropriate for the modern acute care setting. These devices are powerful but inflexible (usually unresponsive to effort) and therefore are difficult to use for patients with dyspnea and severe lung disease. Furthermore, they inhibit nursing access to the patient. They will not be discussed further. In recent years, powerful negative pressure units have become available that, in addition to generating phasic tidal pressure swings, are capable of increasing resting lung volume by sustaining a negative pressure baseline as well as vibrating the chest wall and air column to improve gas exchange and secretion clearance. If perfected, such devices may well see increased use in the ICU setting, either to avoid intubation, to help mobilize secretions, or to provide temporary support post-extubation.

Positive Pressure Ventilation

Positive pressure inflation can be achieved with machines that control *either* of the two determinants of ventilating power—pressure or flow—and terminate inspiration according to pressure, flow, volume, or time limits. (The waveforms of both flow and pressure cannot be controlled *simultaneously,* however, because pressure is developed as a function of flow and the impedance to breathing, which is determined by the uncontrolled parameters of resistance and compliance.) Whereas older ventilators offered only a single control variable and single cycling criterion, positive pressure ventilators of the latest generation enable the physician to select freely among multiple options.

Pressure Cycled Ventilation   Although pressure-cycled ventilators generally have been supplanted by more advanced machines, some are still used, especially in economically depressed regions or developing countries. In their simplest form, pressure cycled (pressure-limited) machines allow gas to flow continuously until a set pressure limit is reached. A pressurized gas source is all that is required to operate many of these machines, making them immune to electrical failure. Small size, portability, and low cost make these machines well suited for applications in transport and respiratory therapy, where they can be used for intermittent delivery of aerosols or for deep breathing (intermittent positive pressure [IPPB]). However, most versions of pressure cycled ventilators have limited power or flow generating capacity, and because they are pressure limited, the delivered tidal volume (V_T) varies with changes in airway resistance, respiratory system compliance, and muscular effort. Therefore, they generally are not adequate to sustain ventilation for hospitalized patients who undergo sudden variations in airway resistance or chest compliance—unless V_T is monitored continuously and the pressure limit is adjusted frequently to maintain exhaled volume approximately constant. A pressure cycled ventilator is a poor choice to support a patient with decompensated asthma or chronic obstructive pulmonary disease (COPD) because changes in body position, airway secretions, bronchospasm, dynamic hyperinflation, or muscular tone can influence V_T. Moreover, many pressure limited ventilators cannot be used for patients with stiff lungs and high ventilatory requirements, because inherent design characteristics of such machines limit the flows of gas that can be moved at the required pressures. For such reasons, hospital use of pressure cycled machines of this type is currently restricted (in adults) to IPPB applications (deep breathing and bronchodilator administration) and, more rarely, to continous support of comatose patients with stable and relatively normal thoracic mechanics. Even in this case, premature pressure limiting (with insufficient delivered volume) occurs very commonly in agitated or hyperventilating patients who attempt to exhale prematurely. For this reason, IPPB cannot be delivered effectively to uncooperative patients.

Pressure Preset (Pressure Targeted) Ventilation Such low capability, pressure cycled ventilators must be distinguished sharply from modern high capacity ventilators that provide pressure preset or pressure targeted ventilatory modes (e.g., pressure control or pressure support) as options for full or partial ventilatory assistance. After the breath is initiated, these modes apply and maintain a targeted amount of pressure at the airway opening until a specified time (pressure control) or flow (pressure support) cycling criterion is met (Fig 7.3). Maximal pressure is controlled, but tidal volume is a complex function of applied pressure and its rate of approach to target pressure, available inspiratory time, and the impedance to breathing (compliance, inspiratory and expiratory resistance, and auto-PEEP). High flow capacity, pressure targeted ventilation compensates well for small air leaks and is therefore quite appropriate for use with leaking or uncuffed

endotracheal (ET) tubes, as in neonatal or pediatric patients. Because of its virtually "unlimited" ability to deliver flow and its decelerating flow profile, pressure-targeted ventilation also is an appropriate choice for spontaneously breathing patients with high inspiratory flow demands, which usually peak early in the ventilatory cycle. Decelerating flow profiles also tend to improve the distribution of ventilation in a lung with heterogeneous mechanical properties (widely varying time constants). Apart from their application in limiting the lung's exposure to high airway pressure and barotrauma, pressure-targeted modes also may prove helpful for adult patients in whom the airway cannot be completely sealed (e.g., bronchopleural fistula).

Flow Controlled, Volume Cycled Ventilation For many years, flow controlled, volume cycled ventilation has been the technique of choice for adult patients. Flow can be controlled by selecting a waveform and setting a peak flow value or by selecting a waveform and setting the combination of tidal volume, and inspiratory time. By controlling the tidal volume, a certain lower limit for minute ventilation can be guaranteed, but the pressure required varies widely with the impedance to breathing (Fig. 7.3). Moreover, once

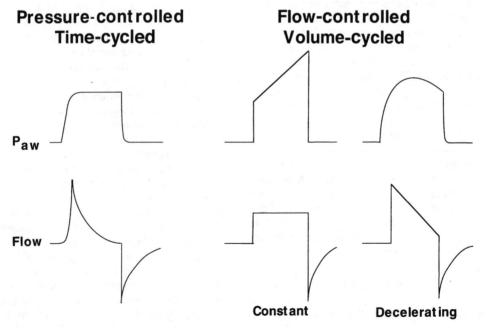

Pressure-controlled Time-cycled   **Flow-controlled Volume-cycled**

P_{aw}

Flow

Constant   Decelerating

FIG. 7–3. Airway pressure (P_{aw}) and flow wave forms during pressure-controlled, time-cycled ventilation and during flow-controlled, volume-cycled ventilation delivered with constant and decelerating flow profiles.

chosen, flow is inflexible to increased (or decreased) inspiratory flow demands.

Differences Between Pressure- and Volume-Targeted Ventilation

After the decision has been made to initiate mechanical ventilation, the physician must decide to use either pressure-controlled ventilation or volume-cycled ventilation. For a well-monitored patient, pressure-targeted and volume-targeted modes can be used with virtually identical effects. With either method, F_iO_2, PEEP, and backup frequency must be selected. If pressure control is used, the targeted inspiratory pressure (above PEEP) and the inspiratory time must be selected (usually with consideration toward the desired tidal volume). If volume-cycled ventilation is used, the physician may select (depending on ventilator) either tidal volume and flow delivery pattern (waveform and peak flow) or flow delivery pattern and minimum minute ventilation (with tidal volume the resulting quotient of $\dot{V}_E$ and backup frequency).

The fundamental difference between pressure- and volume-targeted ventilation is implicit in their names; pressure-targeted modes guarantee pressure at the expense of letting tidal volume vary, and volume-targeted modes guarantee flow—and consequently the volume provided to the circuit in the allowed inspiratory time (tidal volume)—at the expense of letting airway pressure float. This distinction governs how they are used in clinical practice (Table 7.2).

Flow and tidal volumes are important variables to monitor in pressure targeting; pressure is of parallel importance in volume targeting. Gas stored in compressible circuit elements does not contribute to effective alveolar ventilation. For adult patients, such losses (approximately 2–4 mL/cm H_2O of peak pressure) usually constitute a modest fraction of the tidal volume. For infants, however, compressible losses may comprise such a high fraction of the V_T that *effective* ventilation varies markedly with peak cycling pressure. Thus, during volume-cycled ventilation, moment-by-moment changes in chest impedance caused by bronchospasm, secretions, and muscular activity can force peak airway pressure and compressible circuit volume to rise and effective tidal volume to fall. Finally, because airway pressure is controlled, pressure-targeted modes are somewhat less likely to cause barotrauma, which is a life-threatening problem for this age group.

Volume-targeted modes provide a preset volume unless a specified pressure limit is exceeded. Major advantages to volume targeting are the capacity to deliver unvarying tidal volumes (except in the presence of a gas leak), flexibility of flow and volume adjustments, and power to ventilate difficult patients. All ventilators currently used for continuous support in adults offer volume cycling as a primary option. Despite its advantages for acute care, volume cycling also has important disadvantages. Volume-cycled modes cannot ventilate effectively and consistently unless the airway is well sealed. Furthermore, after the flow rate is set, the inflation time of the machine is fixed and remains unresponsive to the patient's native cycling rhythm. Perhaps most importantly, excessive alveolar pressure may be required to deliver the desired tidal volume.

STANDARD MODES OF POSITIVE-PRESSURE VENTILATION

Controlled Mechanical Ventilation

With the sensitivity adjustment turned off during controlled mechanical ventilation (CMV), the machine provides a fixed number of breaths per minute and remains totally uninfluenced by the patient's efforts to alter frequency. This "lockout" mode demands constant vigilance to make appropriate adjustments for changes in ventilatory requirements and is used only for situations in which pH and/or $PaCO_2$ must be controlled tightly. Most patients require sedation to ensure comfort and to ablate breathing efforts. Under these conditions, assist-control ventilation has

TABLE 7–2

PRESSURE CONTROLLED VS. VOLUME CONTROLLED VENTILATION

	Pressure Control	Volume Control
Settings	Pressure target	Tidal volume target
	Inspiratory duration	Flow rate
	Inspiratory rise rate	Flow waveform
Outcome variables	1°—Tidal volume	1°—Airway pressure
	2°—Auto PEEP	2°—Auto PEEP
Common variables	FiO_2	FiO_2
	PEEP	PEEP
	Mode	Mode
	Frequency	Frequency

CONVENTIONAL MODES

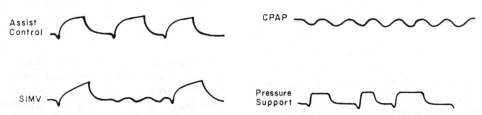

FIG. 7–4. Airway pressure waveforms characteristic of conventional modes of mechanical ventilation.

similar capability and offers additional advantages.

Assist-Control Ventilation

During assist-control ventilation (or assisted mechanical ventilation [AMV]), each inspiration triggered by the patient is powered by the ventilator using either volume-cycled or pressure-targeted breaths (Fig. 7.4). Sensitivity to inspiratory effort can be adjusted to require a small or large negative pressure deflection below the set level of end-expiratory pressure to initiate the machine's inspiratory phase. Alternatively, many of the latest generation machines can be flow triggered, initiating a cycle when a flow deficit is sensed in the expiratory limb of the circuit relative to the inspiratory limb during the exhalation period. Both may be effective. As a safety mechanism, a "backup rate" is set so that if the patient does not initiate a breath within the number of seconds dictated by that frequency, a machine cycle is started automatically. A backup rate set high enough to cause alkalosis blunts respiratory drive and terminates the patient's efforts to breathe at the "apneic threshold" of $PaCO_2$. (For wakeful normal subjects, this threshold usually is achieved when $PaCO_2$ is abruptly lowered to 28–32 mm Hg. It may be higher during sleep.) Note that unlike CMV or synchronized intermittent mandatory ventilation (SIMV; see below), changes in set machine frequency during AMV have no effect on $\dot{V}_E$ unless this "backup" frequency is set high enough to terminate the patient's own respiratory efforts. Hence, AMV is *not* an appropriate mode for weaning.

Synchronized Intermittent Mandatory Ventilation

During intermittent mandatory ventilation (IMV), the intubated patient is connected to a single circuit that allows both spontaneous and mechanical breathing cycles. Ventilator breaths— volume cycled or pressure controlled—are interspersed to supplement spontaneous ventilation. The spontaneous breathing cycles of SIMV can be pressure supported. If breaths from the ventilator are preferentially timed to coincide with spontaneous effort, the mode is termed "synchronized IMV" (SIMV). Because SIMV can provide a wide range of ventilatory support, it can be used either as a full support mode or as a weaning mode, depending on the mandatory frequency selected.

Pressure Support Ventilation

Description

Pressure support ventilation (PSV) is a method in which each breath taken by a spontaneously breathing patient receives a pressure boost. After the breath is initiated, pressure builds rapidly toward an inspiratory pressure target. Inspiratory airway pressure is then maintained constant at the level set by the clinician until flow decays to satisfy the machine's "off switch" criterion. At relatively slow respiratory rates, the resulting airway pressure profile resembles a "square" wave. Because PSV is flow cycled, the patient retains control of cycle length and tidal volume.

Advantages

Pressure support ventilation hybridizes the power of the machine and the patient, providing assistance that ranges from no support at all to fully powered ventilation, depending on the machine's developed pressure relative to patient effort. Because the depth, length, and flow profile of the breath are influenced by the patient, well-adjusted PSV tends to be relatively comfortable. Adaptability to the vagaries of patient cycle length can prove especially helpful for patients with erratic breathing patterns that otherwise would be difficult to adapt to a fixed flow profile or set inspiratory time (e.g., COPD, anxiety). The transition to spontaneous breathing is eased by the gradual removal of machine support (see Chapter 10, Weaning from Mechanical Ventilation). Pressure-support ventilation has its widest application as a weaning mode. Pressure support also is valuable in offsetting the resistive work required to breathe spontaneously through an endotracheal tube, as during CPAP or SIMV. The pressure-support level should be adjusted to maintain an adequate tidal volume at an acceptable frequency (<30 per minute). In theory, PSV would provide sufficient power for the entire work of breathing if set to meet or exceed the average inspiratory pressure required (P_{req}). For a normal subject breathing at a moderate rate, P_{req} is amazingly small, seldom exceeding 5 cm H_2O. For patients who are appropriate for weaning, V_E usually approximates 10 L/minute or less, and P_{req} commonly does not exceed 10 to 15 cm H_2O. This explains why patients seem to be "weaning smoothly" until some rather low threshold value of PSV is reached, at which point further reductions precipitate sudden deterioration. When PSV is greater than P_{req}, the patient performs little work but instead adjusts frequency and tidal volume to minimize effort.

Problems

Pressure-support ventilation requires the ventilatory cycle to be patient initiated and cannot adjust itself to changes in the ease of chest inflation. Therefore, PSV is not an ideal mode for patients with unstable ventilatory drive or highly variable thoracic impedance (e.g., bronchospasm, copious secretions, or changing auto-PEEP). Furthermore, because the ability of most ventilator systems to provide a true square wave of airway pressure tends to deteriorate as ventilatory demands increase, the average inspiratory pressure (and tidal volume) resulting from PSV tends to be frequency sensitive.

VENTILATOR SETUP (TABLE 7.3)

Ventilator "Circuit"

With the upper airway bypassed, pressurized gas must be warmed and humidified before enter-

TABLE 7–3

VENTILATOR SET-UP

Mode

Backup frequency

PEEP

FiO_2

Inspiratory flow rate and wave shape

Target inspiratory pressure (pressure control)

Target tidal volume (volume control)

Alarms
    Apnea
    Low exhaled tidal volume and/or $\dot{V}_E$
    Low inspiratory pressure
    Maximum peak airway pressure

ing the trachea. Disposable low-resistance heat and moisture exchangers ("artificial noses") may be used for patients with modest ventilatory requirements and minimal airway secretions (e.g., in the postoperative setting). By recovering a high percentage of the exhaled water vapor, these units are able to satisfactorily humidify inspired gas for such patients with low ventilation requirements. These devices impose deadspace and increase expiratory resistance, especially when saturated with liquid or contaminated by secretions. Consequently, a given unit performs less well when used for extended periods (>24 hours) or when provided to patients who cough frequently or whose ventilation power is compromised during spontaneous breathing. (Unless purposely designed or used with special attachments, disconnection of the ventilator is necessary to suction the airway.) Therefore, patients requiring high PEEP to maintain arterial oxygenation are also questionable candidates.

Modern "heated wire" circuits maintain a fairly consistent temperature throughout the external circuit, keeping water vapor in its gaseous phase. These are largely successful in keeping condensate from forming before the Y-connector. Because warmed, fully saturated gas cools in unheated connecting tubing, some condensation ("rain-out") should occur in nonheated wire circuits. Using such equipment, a humidifier maladjustment or malfunction should be suspected if fine water droplets are not evident. The inspired temperature of fully saturated gas should be maintained at approximately 34 to 37°C. If airway secretions are thick, temperature should be raised to hydrate them (but not to exceed 37°C). Excessive "rain-out" may result in pooled liquid that can interfere with machine triggering or inadvertently empty into the lung during position changes, thereby injecting a bacterial inoculum or precipitating coughing or bronchospasm.

At the start of inspiration, the exhalation valve closes and pressure builds. PEEP is applied by causing the exhalation valve to close at a preset pressure level. Expiratory valves are often of a diaphragm or scissor type, located on the expiratory side of the Y connection that links the endotracheal (ET) tube to the ventilator. Tubing inserted between the ET tube and the Y connector extends the "anatomic" deadspace with apparatus deadspace.

Ventilator Options and Settings

The ventilator is a device for delivering conditioned gas and assisting ventilation. Therefore, major decisions concern mode, FiO_2, tidal volume, guaranteed ventilator frequency, and baseline airway pressure (PEEP). Although minor adjustments can be made safely on the basis of vital signs, physical examination, subjective response, and pulse oximetry, initial choices and major setting adjustments should be verified by checking arterial blood gases drawn within 20 to 30 minutes of the change.

Mode

The AMV mode generally is the best choice for full support because it allows the patient to control pH and $PaCO_2$ while the machine powers inflation. Trigger sensitivity should be set at the lowest level that avoids autocycling (approximately 0.5 to 1.0 cm H_2O below end-expiratory airway pressure). It should be recognized, however, that effective triggering sensitivity is greatly reduced in the presence of dynamic hyperinflation (auto-PEEP). Although designed primarily as a method to facilitate weaning, SIMV is used for other purposes.

Compared to AMV, SIMV allows lower mean intrathoracic pressure, minimizing inhibition of venous return. Intermittent mandatory ventilation provides an alternative to sedation and control for patients who have difficulty in synchronizing rhythmically with the ventilator or who require some mechanical assistance but who hyperventilate inappropriately when allowed to trigger the machine on every cycle (e.g., central neurogenic

hyperventilation, anxiety). Unless each nonmandated breath is supported with the same pressure used during machine cycles, the ventilatory workload of SIMV increases in proportion to the number of spontaneous breaths taken.

CPAP alone may be appropriate for patients who can comfortably maintain ventilation but require airway protection and/or improved arterial oxygenation (e.g., mild forms of ARDS). Inspiratory flow on CPAP can be regulated by demand valve or by varying continuous flow, a method that tends to be marginally less resistive. All modern ventilators provide the pressure support option that selectively boosts inspiratory airway pressure by an amount set by the physician while allowing the patient to maintain control of cycle timing and depth.

Newer Ventilatory Options   In certain situations, it is desirable either to adjust midinspiratory flow in response to changing patient needs or, alternatively, to restrict maximal cycling pressure but ensure delivery of a specified tidal volume. These needs and microprocessor capability have given rise to such "combination" modes as pressure-regulated volume control, volume support, volume-assured pressure support, and augmented minute volume (Fig. 7.5).

Pressure-Regulated Volume Control   This mode satisfies a tidal volume with the least cycling pressure that accomplishes it within the preset inspiratory time. Pressure is continuously regulated in response to changing inflation impedance to satisfy the tidal volume objective. It should be noted that the patient may receive no help at all from the ventilator if a satisfactory tidal volume can be attained through patient effort alone.

Volume Support   In volume support, flow-cycled pressure support is adjusted up or down, depending on the tidal volume and minute ventilation that result in comparison to the preset minimums. Minute ventilation is the primary target variable and a tidal volume minimum is guaranteed. When breathing frequency falls, tidal volume can increase by as much as 50% over the baseline target in an attempt to satisfy the $\dot{V}_E$ minimum.

Volume-Assured Pressure Support   In volume-assured pressure support (VAPS), a fixed level of pressure support is supplemented by gas from a backup flow generator if the PSV becomes insufficient to meet a minimum tidal volume objective.

Self-Adjusting Modes of Partial Ventilatory Support

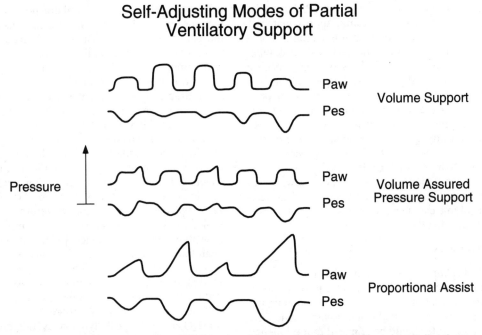

FIG. 7–5. Conceptual representation of recently introduced modes of partial ventilatory support. In volume support, pressure support is automatically regulated to achieve preset targets for minimum tidal volume and minute ventilation. In volume-assured pressure support (also known as pressure augmentation), a fixed pressure-support level may be augmented by constant flow at end inspiration as necessary to achieve a preselected tidal volume target. Proportional assist ventilation increases the pressure output of the ventilator parallel to the vigor of patient effort, thereby acting as an auxiliary set of ventilatory muscles, the strength of which is regulated by the clinician. (P_{aw} = airway pressure; P_{es} = pleural (esophageal) pressure.)

Inspired Oxygen Fraction (FiO$_2$)

Initially, FiO$_2$ should be set to err deliberately on the high side, with later adjustment guided by arterial oximetry or blood gases. Immediately after intubation, for example, it is generally prudent to administer pure oxygen until adequate arterial oxygenation has been confirmed.

Tidal Volume

Inspired tidal volume is either a preset (controlled) parameter or a dependent variable that is taken into account when selecting the controlled pressure during pressure controlled ventilation. For otherwise healthy individuals, large tidal volumes can be given without generating high pressures. Therefore, delivered tidal volumes of 10 to 12 mL/kg of lean body weight usually are appropriate. Of course, obese patients do not have larger lungs, and the tidal volume delivered to a patient with a reduced number of available units must be reduced accordingly (e.g., ARDS, pneumonec-

tomy, interstitial fibrosis). Even higher tidal volumes may be needed to satisfy the demands of a hyperpneic subject with normal ventilatory mechanics. Even in the normal lung, monotonous shallow breaths (<6 mL/kg) encourage microatelectasis, unless interrupted periodically by larger inflations or offset by PEEP. If very small tidal volumes are used, one or more larger breaths (sighs generally 2–3 × V$_T$) may be advisable every 10 to 15 minutes to avert problems, but this is controversial. As pressure builds during inspiration, a fraction of the inspired gas is stored in tubing and other compressible elements of the ventilator circuit (internal reservoirs, filters, humidifiers, etc.). Stored volume is not a major concern when the breath is regulated by pressure rather than flow (volume cycled), but nonetheless, gas storage is sometimes necessary to consider when interpreting delivered tidal volume and $\dot{V}_E$. A typical value for such compressible losses is ≈3 mL/cm H$_2$O of peak system pressure; however, compression volume (CV) varies with ventilator type, peak cycling pressure, and the length, diameter, and composition of the tubing. (Pediatric circuits use less compliant tubing, approximately 1 mL/cm H_2O.) The compression factor is not a fixed number but varies alinearly with peak pressure. Therefore, considerably less of any specific set V_T may actually reach the patient if thoracic compliance falls (requiring an increase in peak airway pressure). Measurements of exhaled volume often include CV because decompression occurs as the airway is exposed to atmospheric pressure. Many modern ventilators compensate for CV on their readout. Under conditions of controlled ventilation, the discrepancy between set or measured inspiratory tidal volume and exhaled tidal volume can quantitate the severity of a bronchopleural fistula.

Frequency

The backup frequency should be chosen in conjunction with V_T or pressure setting to provide a minute ventilation ($\dot{V}_E$) adequate to maintain pH and patient comfort. In the assist mode, the "backup" rate should be adjusted to a frequency sufficient to provide 70 to 80% of usual $\dot{V}_E$, in case of complete failure of the patient to trigger. (In the AMV mode, any adjustments in the set frequency—up or down—have no effect on $\dot{V}_E$ or on the level of machine support, so long as the patient triggers each breath.) To avoid paradoxical motion of a mobile or "flail" chest segment, patients with multiple rib fractures should be supported at a rate that just suppresses spontaneous efforts or at a very sensitive trigger setting.

Other Settings

Volume-cycled ventilators allow the physician to choose the inspiratory flow rate and to define its contour (square or decelerating). Inappropriately rapid inspiratory flow rates may worsen the distribution of ventilation in some patients; however, a decelerating flow waveform helps to compensate for a rapid mean inspiratory flow rate, and the longer exhalation time is a marked advantage for patients with airflow obstruction and those with marginal cardiopulmonary reserve. Although peak pressure rises as flow rate increases, the mean airway pressure averaged over the entire ventilatory cycle may remain unchanged or even fall as flow rate increases. The extent to which the ventilator takes up the inspiratory work of breathing is a function of the margin with which flow delivery exceeds flow demand. It is mandatory that the flow metered by the ventilator always meets or exceeds the patient's inspiratory flow

demand. Otherwise, the ventilator not only fails to reduce the work of breathing but also may force the patient to pull against the resistance of the ventilator circuitry, as well as against his own internal impedance to airflow and chest expansion.

Comfortably rapid inspiratory flow rates also are desirable to ensure that the machine completes inflation before the patient's own ventilatory rhythm cycles into its exhalation phase. Delayed opening of the exhalation valve causes the patient to "fight the ventilator." As a rule, the ventilator's *average* inspiratory flow should be approximately 4.0 times the minute ventilation. Peak flow should be set 20 to 30% higher than this average value when the decelerating waveform is used. Peak airway pressure is influenced by inspiratory flow rate, airway resistance, tidal volume, and total thoracic compliance. The plateau airway pressure reflects the maximum stretching force applied to a typical alveolus. To avoid barotrauma, maximum pressure (alarm and "pop-off" pressure) should be set no more than 15 to 20 cm H_2O above the peak dynamic cycling pressure observed during a typical breath during constant flow. The pop-off alarm should be set more closely than this (5–10 cm H_2O) if a decelerating flow waveform or pressure control is used because end-inspiratory dynamic and static (plateau) pressures are not as widely separated.

Although deleted from most later-generation ventilators, the expiratory retard option is theoretically useful for patients who experience airway collapse during tidal exhalation. The inflation hold setting sustains peak chest volume, raises mean inflation pressure, allows calculation of lung mechanics, and may improve gas distribution for some patients. A typical hold time is 0.1 to 0.5 second. Longer pauses may be tolerated poorly by conscious or nonpassive patients. In theory, an inflation hold helps reverse atelectasis and aids in the distribution of therapeutic aerosols. (A temporary inflation hold also can be used to check for circuit leaks, as circuit pressure will continue to decline during the pause interval rather than "plateau" as gas bleeds off.)

On some pressure-limited, time-cycled machines, the ratio of inspiratory to expiratory time (I : E ratio) can be set directly. However, on volume-cycled ventilators, the I : E ratio usually is set indirectly by specifying inhaled volume, frequency, and mean inspiratory flow rate. In general, shorter I : E ratios allow more time for exhalation and reduce mean intrathoracic pressure. To avoid gas trapping, many ventilators provide a visual warning or auditory alarm when the I : E ratio exceeds 1 : 1 (duty cycle > 0.5). This threshold defines inverse ratio ventilation.

NEWER MODES TO IMPROVE VENTILATION

The primary purposes of mechanical ventilation are to achieve adequate alveolar ventilation and to improve oxygen exchange. Until recently, volume-limited ventilation, used alone (AMV, CMV) or in conjunction with spontaneous breathing (SIMV), has been the only form of machine assistance commonly used for adults. Similarly, enrichment of FiO_2 and the addition of end-expiratory pressure (PEEP, CPAP) have been the primary means of supporting oxygenation. Recently, a number of new techniques have been developed, and a few have been introduced into clinical practice. These innovations take the form of newer modes of ventilation or of adjuncts to ventilatory support. Each has a defensible physiologic rationale but little objective supporting data to document clinical benefit. Because most of these newer modes are pressure cycled, independent flow and volume monitoring is highly desirable.

Variants of Minimum Minute Ventilation

Minimum (or minimal) minute ventilation (MMV) was the forerunner of more modern "servo-adjusted" modes designed to vary machine output to achieve a specific clinical objective (pressure augmentation, volume support [VAPS]). MMV guarantees a certain minute ventilation, whether or not the patient attempts to breathe. Unlike SIMV, MMV does not provide a fixed number of breaths—no machine cycles are delivered if the patient breathes at an adequate pace. MMV was envisioned as a stand-alone "automatic" weaning mode. MMV can be provided by intermittent volume-cycled breaths delivered only as required. Alternatively, a pressure support level for each breath can be adjusted to optimize tidal volume or frequency.

Advantages

In principle, MMV provides a nearly ideal backup mode to PSV. Although ready if needed, MMV does not obligate the patient to receive machine support.

Disadvantages

MMV guarantees $\dot{V}_E$ but may allow fatigue to occur in the attempt to achieve the targeted value.

Indeed, the minute ventilation target can be achieved by increasing frequency, even as exhaustion sets in. (Frequency and tidal volume alarms can be added to warn of deterioration.) The potential for excessive effort also characterizes pressure-regulated volume control and volume support. Modes such as VAPS that adjust or supplement PSV as necessary to accomplish MMV, but limit maximal frequency and/or maintain tidal volume, would seem desirable (but as yet unproven options) for preventing fatigue or in compensating for it.

High-Frequency Ventilation

The collective term "high-frequency ventilation" (HFV) refers to methods of ventilation in which tidal volumes less than or equal to the calculated anatomic deadspace are moved at frequencies ranging from 60 to 3000 cycles per minute. The mechanisms by which these varied forms of HFV establish alveolar ventilation is uncertain and differ among techniques. However, all forms of HFV are characterized by lower peak airway pressures than conventional ventilation. Peripheral airway pressure, however, is generally higher than measured central airway pressure, and mean alveolar pressures may not differ greatly from those observed during conventional ventilation.

Types of High-Frequency Ventilation

High-Frequency Positive-Pressure Ventilation High-frequency positive-pressure ventilation (HFPPV) is identical in concept to conventional ventilation; however, tidal volumes are very small, and cycling frequencies are very fast (60 cycles per minute or greater).

High-Frequency Jet Ventilation High-frequency jet ventilation (HFJV) works differently. A small-diameter injecting catheter positioned in the central airway pulses gas along the luminal axis under high pressure (5–50 psi) at a rapid cycling rate (typically 100–400 cycles per minute). The actual insufflation period, the inspiratory dwell time, is normally set to occupy 20 to 50% of the total cycling period. Conditioned gas is entrained with the pulse, augmenting the effective V_T. Tidal volume is not a set parameter but varies with jet driving pressure, frequency, and dwell time. Exhalation is passive; exhaled gas is expelled more or less continuously through a valveless port. Although HFJV is the most frequently used form of HFV for adults, there is some debate on the mechanism of its action. At the lower set frequencies approved for clinical use (100–150 breaths per minute), most evidence is compatible with modified convective (''bulk'') flow. Efficiency is improved by square-wave delivery, placement of the injector close to the carina, and a jet lumen/exhaust lumen ratio of 1:11 to 1:6. Although external PEEP can be used in conjunction with HFV, additional auto-PEEP often is physiologically important but difficult to quantify safely (unless ventilation can be stopped synchronously with circuit occlusion).

High-Frequency Oscillation High-frequency oscillation (HFO) operates on yet another mechanical principle. Even though used widely for children, the limited power of available machines previously available has severely restricted its applications to adult patients. A very small tidal volume (1–3 mL/kg) is moved to and fro by a piston at extremely high frequencies (500–3000 cycles per minute). Fresh gas is introduced as a continuous flow, and a narrow gauge venting tube (a ''low-pass filter'') provides egress for waste gas. Delivered tidal volume depends on the relative resistances for gas flow through the airway and the bias flow lines. Carbon dioxide elimination is a function of stroke (tidal) volume and, to a lesser degree, vibration frequency. Unlike jet ventilation, both phases of the ventilatory cycle are controlled actively by the oscillator's piston. Consequently, auto-PEEP does not generally present a serious problem. Although fresh gas must be provided through the airway, pulsatility of the air column may originate either in the airway or at the lung surface. In experimental animals, mere vibration of the chest wall has successfully established effective gas exchange. Exactly how HFO accomplishes ventilation continues to be investigated. Although improved gas mixing and facilitated diffusion are undoubtedly important, pulsatility itself does not seem to be a strict requirement for *some* alveolar ventilation to occur. A continuous stream of O_2 introduced just beyond the carina can maintain arterial oxygenation and accomplish significant CO_2 washout in apneic animals, a technique dubbed ''apneic diffusion,'' ''continuous flow apneic ventilation,'' or ''tracheal insufflation of oxygen'' (TRIO). Although not currently advocated for clinical use, apneic ventilation may have some use as a temporizing measure in emergent settings in which standard endotracheal intubation cannot be accomplished.

Applications of High-Frequency Ventilation

High-frequency ventilation can silence the normal respiratory rhythm and phasic variations of chest volume. This feature already has proven advantageous during lithotripsy and certain delicate surgical procedures in which gross thoracic motions must be minimized. Because HFJV does not require a cuffed endotracheal tube, it has been helpful in bronchoscopy and laryngeal surgery. Furthermore, HFJV occasionally is effective in the setting of bronchopleural fistulas that are refractory to closure, in part because of lower peak airway pressures. Fistulas also tend to draw less flow at higher frequencies because the inertance of the fistulous pathway is greater than that of alternative routes. Jet ventilation well synchronized to the heartbeat has been demonstrated to boost the cardiac output of patients with dilated cardiomyopathy, presumably because systolic heart compression decreases left ventricular afterload. Because high airway cycling pressure may be instrumental in causing bronchopulmonary dysplasia, HFV also may have a role in preventing this complication in neonates and perhaps in older children and adults with ARDS as well. ''Recruiting'' maneuvers, in which large peak pressures are applied for 10 to 20 seconds, may be needed to avoid atelectasis and to preserve optimal gas exchange when HFV techniques are used. Although occasionally dramatically effective, HFV generally has proven disappointing in the care of adult patients. With occasional exceptions, HFV seems to offer little advantage with regard to cardiovascular performance, lung water accumulation, or gas exchange at equivalent levels of end-expiratory alveolar pressure. Indeed, many patients with high ventilation requirements or high thoracic impedance cannot be ventilated successfully by HFV. Finally, although initial problems with inadequate humidification, jet-induced mucosal disruption, and mechanical breakdown have been mastered, monitoring alveolar pressure remains a vexing clinical problem during HFV.

NEWER MODES TO IMPROVE OXYGENATION

Pressure-Controlled Inverse Ratio Ventilation

Description and Rationale

To prevent gas trapping, it has long been standard practice to allow at least as much time for exhalation as for inhalation; however, for certain patients, gas exchange may improve markedly when the I:E ratio is extended to values greater than 1:1 (Fig. 7.6). First applied in neonates with

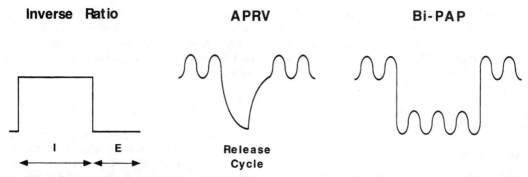

FIG. 7–6. Airway pressure waveforms corresponding to inverse ratio ventilation, airway pressure release ventilation (APRV), and biphasic airway pressure (Bi-Pap). In inverse ratio ventilation, the airway is pressurized for more than one-half of the total cycle length, increasing mean airway pressure. Deep sedation (with or without muscle relaxants) may be necessary to suppress spontaneous breathing efforts. APRV allows the patient to breathe spontaneously around an elevated pressure baseline, which is periodically released and reestablished, thereby aiding spontaneous ventilation. Bi-Pap extends the release cycle, allowing spontaneous ventilation to occur at each of two CPAP levels.

hyaline membrane disease, inverse ratio ventilation (IRV) now has been used for adult patients with refractory ARDS and other forms of hypoxemia. IRV can be applied by slowing the rate of flow delivery during conventional volume-cycled ventilation, by placing an end-inspiratory pause of appropriate length, or more commonly, by maintaining pressure at a controlled level for a fixed time (pressure-controlled ventilation). When using IRV, pressure control has the distinct advantage of safety when compared to flow-controlled, volume-cycled methods that leave alveolar pressure unregulated. All methods sustain the time over which the maximal tidal inflation pressure and stretching force is applied. Because all methods require a passive patient, sedation, overventilation, and/or paralysis usually are necessary. Silencing of spontaneous breathing efforts and carefully set pressure alarms are particularly important during flow-controlled, volume-cycled ventilation, in which pressure is otherwise free to climb to dangerous levels in response to increased impedance of the respiratory system or muscular opposition to the unnatural breathing pattern that IRV imposes.

Mechanism of Action

How IRV improves oxygenation is uncertain. However, raised mean intrathoracic pressure (and increased average lung volume) is almost certainly a primary mechanism. Auto-PEEP is generated in most cases and probably is necessary for optimal oxygenation unless an equivalent level of

PEEP is applied. Sustained tethering forces may recruit lung units that would otherwise remain collapsed, and units with very long time constants may be given sufficient time to ventilate. Despite these theoretical benefits, it remains unclear whether IRV has any important advantage over conventional ventilation applied at an equivalent level of total end-expiratory pressure. IRV is not an appropriate mode of treatment for severely obstructed patients. Although it is commonly used as a technique of last resort in cases of ARDS, IRV has its best rationale and seems to be most effective in the earliest phase, when lung units are most recruitable. At usual frequencies, inverse ratios greater than 2 : 1 are seldom helpful and may be dangerous. IRV should seldom be used for longer than 48 to 72 hours before reassessing its relative advantage over conventional ratio ventilation.

Potential Advantages of IRV

Proposed advantages of IRV are as follows: (*a*) improved oxygenation for the same level of PEEP, FiO_2, and peak alveolar pressure; (*b*) reduced peak cycling pressure when the same tidal volume and mean airway pressures are achieved; (*c*) enhanced gas distribution and ventilation efficiency within the diseased lung; and (*d*) time-dependent recruitment of edematous and atelectatic lung tissues that are refractory to other measures.

Disadvantages of IRV

Sustained maximal tidal pressure and higher mean intrathoracic pressure may impede venous return and contribute to barotrauma, depending on the peak pressure used, the fragility of the lung tissue, and the extent of cardiovascular reserves. Most importantly, IRV usually requires deep sedation or paralysis and close monitoring of gas exchange.

Airway Pressure Release and Biphasic Airway Pressure

Description

Airway pressure release (APRV) and biphasic airway pressure (Bi-PAP) can be thought of as variants of IRV intended for use by spontaneously breathing patients with poor oxygenation (Fig. 7.6). [Biphasic airway pressure should not be confused with the commercial term ''Bi-PAP™,'' which is bi-**level** airway pressure, basically synonymous with pressure support.] The idea here is to provide added ventilatory support for a patient who needs CPAP for oxygenation and can provide most of the ventilatory power requirement without machine assistance. Both APRV and Bi-PAP allow ventilatory efforts around an elevated pressure baseline (CPAP) but also to depressurize the system (partially or completely) for brief periods at a frequency set by the physician. After release, fresh gas enters as CPAP rebuilds to its higher value. Bi-PAP differs from APRV in allowing the option for extended periods of spontaneous breathing at both selected levels of end-expiratory pressure.

Advantages

These techniques can be viewed as methods to aid in ventilation and/or to provide elevated airway pressure to improve oxygenation. Phasic release cycles function in a manner similar to the machine cycles of SIMV, insofar as they augment ventilation. The difference is that high peak cycling pressures are avoided and spontaneous breathing can occur at any time. As with IRV, sustained higher airway pressure may exert traction and improve ventilation in slow time constant units. Unlike IRV, however, maximal alveolar pressures are limited more readily. The patient remains conscious and can adjust alveolar ventilation to the extent that he or she is able to do so. In some configurations of Bi-PAP, pressure support can be added to spontaneous cycles at each pressure baseline. Biphasic airway pressure can therefore provide the entire range of ventilatory support (ranging from completely controlled ven-

tilation to unsupported breathing), depending on the frequency and duration of the release cycles. For this reason, it serves as the primary basis of ventilatory support in at least one modern ventilator system.

Disadvantages

The efficacy of the pressure-release cycle depends on (a) the duration of release, (b) the mechanical properties of the chest, (c) the level to which airway pressure is allowed to fall, and (d) the cycling frequency between the two pressure baselines. As ventilation support increases, mean airway pressure falls, dissipating some of the oxygen-exchange benefit of the higher CPAP level. More importantly, their value is questionable for patients with significant airflow obstruction or severely reduced lung compliance. In the first instance, the brief release cycles of APRV are relatively ineffectual. In the second instance, the work of spontaneous breathing may be too great to sustain. Neither APRV nor Bi-PAP has yet undergone sufficiently rigorous testing to firmly establish its clinical indications.

ADJUNCTS TO MECHANICAL VENTILATION

Techniques to Improve Gas Exchange

Recently, there has been increasing interest in developing techniques capable of maintaining or improving pulmonary gas exchange without the need to elevate alveolar and pleural pressures (Table 7.4). Such methods include the administration of therapeutic gases or aerosols (e.g., nitric oxide and inhaled prostacyclin), alterations of body position (prone repositioning), vibration of the air column (high-frequency ventilation or

TABLE 7–4

ADJUNCTS TO MECHANICAL VENTILATION

Nitric oxide/inhaled prostacyclin

Vibration of airway or chest wall

Tracheal gas insufflation

Partial liquid ventilation

Extracorporeal membrane oxygenation

Extracorporeal CO_2 removal

Intravenacaval gas exchange (IVOX)

Permissive hypercapnia

Prone positioning

chest wall vibration), deadspace bypass or washout (intratracheal pulmonary ventilation, tracheal gas insufflation), alteration of the gas exchange medium (partial liquid ventilation), and extrapulmonary gas exchange (extracorporeal membrane oxygenation, extracorporeal CO_2 removal, and intravenacaval gas exchange via gas-permeable catheter [IVOX]). Most of these techniques are discussed elsewhere in this volume (see Chapters 24 and 25).

Permissive Hypercapnia

One important "adjunct" to ventilation simply relaxes the ventilation target when the system is severely compromised. Permissive hypercapnia is a ventilatory strategy that assigns higher priority to avoiding injurious pressure than to maintaining normal levels of alveolar ventilation. In the setting of acute lung injury and asthma, high alveolar pressures can injure fragile tissues. Allowing $PaCO_2$ to rise above baseline values is perhaps the simplest technique for reducing the ventilatory workload, the pressure cost of breathing, and/or the total number of machine cycles needed per minute. As $PaCO_2$ rises, each exhaled breath of a given volume eliminates more CO_2 than it would during normocapnia, thereby improving CO_2 excretion efficiency (Fig. 7.7). With reduced ventilation requirements, smaller tidal volumes can be delivered, lowering the peak and mean inflation pressures and, consequently, the work of spontaneous breathing. Because ventilatory power varies as the second power of $\dot{V}_E$, small reductions in $\dot{V}_E$ can reduce effort and transpulmonary pressure impressively. If the concomitant fall in mean alveolar pressure causes an unacceptable reduction in arterial oxygenation, raising end-expiratory pressure or extending the inspiratory time fraction may restore it to an appropriate level.

Gradual increases in $PaCO_2$ (extending over a few hours) are accompanied by minimal shifts in *intracellular* pH and are generally well tolerated, even to quite high concentrations of $PaCO_2$ and dramatically low pH values. As a rule, patients without coexisting β blockade, intracranial pathology, hemodynamic instability, severe pulmonary hypertension, or uncorrected hypoxemia function well at pH values greater than or equal to 7.15 (and, at times, even lower). Indeed, elite athletes typically allow acidosis of this magnitude during maximal exercise. Very abrupt reductions in ventilation will cause intracellular pH to fall, however, unless the serum concentration of bicarbonate is augmented by infused buffer. Deep sedation and paralysis are often required during the buildup to the hypercapnic plateau. As clinical status improves, normocapnia is restored gradually. Normalization of pH at a higher level of $PaCO_2$ obligates HCO_3^- retention, which usually blunts ventilatory drive. In single-center retrospective studies, permissive hypercapnia has been reported to be helpful in reducing the mortality of status asthma and ARDS. (At least one single-center prospective, concurrently controlled study of ARDS also indicates impressive benefit.) It seems reasonable to suggest that similar principles should apply to all difficult problems of ventilation. Although still viewed as experimental by some practitioners, an increasing minority consider lower pH to be a natural consequence of a lung-protective ventilation strategy. Consensus may eventually be reached to allow controlled hypercapnia and respiratory acidosis during the acute phase of severe illness or to wean tenuous patients more quickly from mechanical ventilation.

NONINVASIVE VENTILATION

Many patients require only modest pressures to maintain compensated ventilation. With the increasing availability of improved mask interfaces and efficient valving mechanisms, the option of applying ventilatory support noninvasively by occlusive mask has become widely exercised—both for chronic nocturnal support and increasingly for acute in-hospital applications. Noninvasive ventilation may be used as a means by which to offer assistance without reintubating a marginally compensated patient recently weaned from ventilatory support. These methods also are helpful for patients who are not candidates for intubation (e.g., patients with advanced directives for "do not intubate or resuscitate"). For well-selected patients, noninvasive techniques may obviate the need for intubation and help avoid infections and other complications of securing the airway. A few centers report improved mortality rates for patients who are able to accept this treatment. Noninvasive ventilation seems to be particularly helpful when implemented at an early stage for patients with rapidly reversible diseases (e.g., congestive heart failure, moderate asthma) and for patients for whom intubation is not an acceptable option. Despite its clear value for well-selected patients, noninvasive ventilation has important limitations as well (Table 7.5). It helps less consistently in

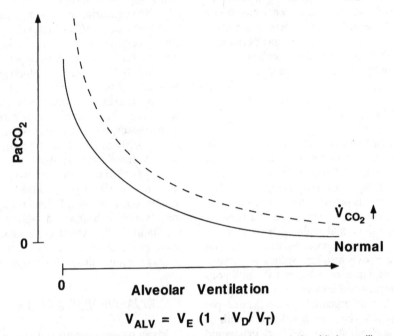

PaCO$_2$ vs Alveolar Ventilation

$$V_{ALV} = V_E (1 - V_D/V_T)$$

FIG. 7–7. Relationship of PaCO$_2$ to alveolar ventilation (V$_{ALV}$). Because this relationship is curvilinear, relatively small changes in V$_{ALV}$ that occur at low levels of ventilation have a dramatic effect on PaCO$_2$. An increase in CO$_2$ production ($\dot{V}_{CO_2}$) results in a higher PaCO$_2$ for any specified level of ventilation.

TABLE 7–5

NONINVASIVE VENTILATION: BENEFITS & LIMITATIONS

Benefits	Limitations
Easy to implement and remove	Psychic distress
	Increased nursing time
Improves comfort	Slow reversal
Reduces need for sedation	Hypoxemia when removed
Preserves speech/swallowing	
Preserves cough	Eye irritation
Avoids tube resistance	Difficult airway hygiene
Avoids tube complications	No airway protection
Upper airway trauma	Facial discomfort
"Mini" aspiration	Gastric distention
Pulmonary infection	Limited ventilatory capability
Dilates upper airway	

acute respiratory failure of other types, particularly when the disease is far advanced. Combative or comatose patients, those who cannot be attended or monitored closely, and those with retained secretions, hemodynamic instability, or massive obesity are decidedly poor candidates. However, noninvasive ventilation often is successful when applied early enough to cooperative patients by vigilant, well-trained personnel.

Noninvasive ventilation allows communication, expectoration, and eating. There is no major penalty for starting and stopping ventilatory support—indeed, brief intervals off the mask every several hours may help improve tolerance. The air stream generally does not require humidification unless high inspired fractions of desiccated O$_2$ are in use. Machines vary in their capability and design purpose; conventional ICU ventilators providing CPAP, pressure control, adequate FiO$_2$ and the entire range of other support modes are often the best choices for the seriously ill patient. (Devices intended for chronic nocturnal prophylaxis against

TABLE 7–6

BEDSIDE EVALUATION OF THE VENTILATED PATIENT

Mental status	pH and gas exchange
Spontaneous breathing rhythm	Breath sounds
	Chest radiograph
Minute ventilation requirement	Mode of cycling
	Cycling pressure (compliance/resistance)
Muscular strength	
Secretion character and volume	Medications
	Complications and practical problems
Breathing effort/ paradox/coordination	

the upper airway obstruction of sleep apnea are not optimal for use in the acute arena. Many machines are limited in the concentrations of inspired oxygen they can provide.) The interface is also important. A nasal mask (or nasal "pillows," e.g., the "Adam circuit") often proves suboptimal in the acute care setting, as the mouth often opens, depressurizing the airway. Although full facial masks usually are more efficient in developing the required pressures, they are generally less comfortable and often impose substantial deadspace.

At high pressures, noninvasive ventilation can cause discomfort, skin necrosis, secretion inspissation, and eye abrasions. For nonagitated patients, gastric distention is unusual at peak mask pressures lower than 20 cm H_2O. The success of noninvasive ventilation varies widely from hospital to hospital, which perhaps is the result of certain key differences in management. In our view, the most important of these are appropriate patient selection, rigorous training of support personnel, early intervention, and vigorous efforts to coax and encourage the patient to accept noninvasive ventilation in the first few hours of its application. As a rule, attempts to make noninvasive ventilation work should not persist longer than 1 to 2 hours without clear evidence for benefit and tolerance.

For marginally compensated patients, noninvasive techniques may prove especially helpful at night, when sleep impairs ventilatory drive or immobilizes the nondiaphragmatic musculature crucial to maintaining adequate ventilation. Indeed, nocturnal nasal ventilation (by nasal mask or other occlusive fitting) seems to be useful over extended periods for selected patients with irreversible neuromuscular disease, sleep apnea, and airflow obstruction. Intermittent rest of fatigued respiratory muscles and, in a minority of cases, improved lung compliance may result. The precise reason for non-

invasive ventilation's benefit during waking hours remains undetermined. From current evidence, however, it seems that the primary benefit of nocturnal support for many patients may be to allow the sleep quality needed to preserve adequate ventilatory drive and muscle strength.

GENERAL APPROACH TO THE VENTILATED PATIENT

The complex interactions of the patient and ventilator must be approached in a systematic fashion to optimize machine performance, establish synchrony, and minimize hazards (Table 7.6). A number of important questions must be asked in the daily assessment of the ventilated patient.

PATIENT STATUS

1. *Are cycling pressures excessive (>50 cm H_2O)?*
   Have they changed? Are changes attributable to alterations in resistance or compliance? (Or, alternatively, are flow, tidal volume, or PEEP different with unchanging mechanics?)
2. *Are there reversible factors impeding airflow (bronchospasm, secretions) or worsening the compliance of the lung (new infiltrate, atelectasis) or the chest wall (agitation, ascites, pleural effusion, abdominal distention)?*
   Do secretion volume and character suggest respiratory infection, pulmonary hemorrhage, or ongoing aspiration of oropharyngeal or gastric contents? Is there any sign of unaddressed congestive heart failure, volume overload, volume depletion, or sepsis?
3. *What is the minute ventilation requirement?*
   To determine whether a high $\dot{V}_E$ is related to drive, metabolic requirement, acidosis, or iatrogenic hyperventilation, $\dot{V}_E$ must be interpreted in conjunction with $PaCO_2$, pH, and the physical examination.
4. *How hard is the patient working to breathe?*
   Is the patient making spontaneous breathing efforts? What is the drive to breathe? Are there signs of fatigue—elevated respiratory rate, abdominal paradox, irregular breathing rhythm? What are the pH and $PaCO_2$? During which mode of ventilation, PEEP level, and position were blood gases assessed? The implications of respiratory acidosis, for example, are much different for CMV (underventilation), AMV (reduced drive), or low-level SIMV (reduced drive, inadequate strength).
5. *Is the patient still ventilator-dependent?*
   What is the ventilatory requirement? Are cy-

cling pressures high or low? Is the patient alert and strong? If the patient is unweanable, is dependency likely to change any time soon? Should a tracheostomy be scheduled? Can noninvasive ventilation be substituted?

6. *What is the patient's comfort level?*
Is there evidence of agitation or distress? Does any discomfort relate to pain, visceral distention, anxiety, fever, or maladjusted ventilator?

VENTILATOR STATUS

1. Are ventilator connections appropriate? Are connectors tight, the ET tube cuff well sealed, and the circuit tubing unkinked and water-free?

2. Is there a need to raise or lower the overall level of machine support for oxygenation or ventilation? Is there an appropriate PAO_2:-PaO_2 ratio? Should PEEP be adjusted? Is a change in ventilation mode or cycling frequency indicated to increase or decrease support?

3. Are machine adjustments in mode, flow rate, corrected tidal volume, or PEEP required? Are airway pressures during ventilator cycles uniform and of expected shape, indicating synchrony of patient and ventilator breathing cycles?

KEY POINTS

1. Prime indications for initiating mechanical ventilation include inadequate alveolar ventilation, inadequate arterial oxygenation, excessive respiratory workload, and acute heart failure with labored breathing.

2. For machine-aided breathing cycles, the physician must determine the ventilator's minimum cycling rate and its response to an appropriate call by the patient for a breath. Other key decisions concern duration of the machine's inspiratory cycle, the pressure or tidal volume to administer, and levels of certain boundary conditions (e.g., end-expiratory pressure and alarm limits).

3. Positive pressure inflation can be achieved with machines that control either of the two determinants of ventilating power—pressure or flow—and terminate inspiration according to pressure, flow, volume, or time criteria. Both pressure and flow cannot be fixed simultaneously because once either is set, the other becomes a dependent variable influenced by the interaction of the inflation impedance with the controlled variable.

4. The fundamental difference between pressure-targeted and volume-targeted ventilation is implicit in their names. Strictly pressure-targeted modes regulate pressure at the expense of letting flow and tidal volume vary; volume-targeted modes guarantee flow and/or tidal volume but let airway pressure float.

5. Standard modes of positive pressure ventilation include controlled mechanical ventilation, assist/control ventilation, synchronized intermittent mandatory ventilation, and pressure support ventilation. The first three can be applied using either flow-controlled or pressure-controlled machine cycles.

6. New ventilatory options include pressure-regulated volume control, volume support, and volume-assured pressure support. Each of these innovations is intended to combine desirable features of pressure preset and flow-controlled, volume-targeted ventilation.

7. High frequency ventilation may be useful for certain patients who have a bronchopleural fistula, refractory hypoxemia and risk for barotrauma, or a specialized need for ventilatory support without conventional intubation and/or conventional ventilation.

8. Despite theoretical advantages, inverse ratio ventilation (a mode usually requiring controlled ventilation) and variants of airway pressure release ventilation (a mode for spontaneously breathing patients) require further testing before their appropriate place in the therapeutic spectrum is ensured.

9. Certain adjuncts to mechanical ventilation, including permissive hypercapnia and prone positioning, are now widely applied in clinical practice. The value of other methods, such as chest wall vibration, tracheal gas insufflation, partial liquid ventilation, and extrapulmonary gas exchange, is yet unproven.

10. Noninvasive ventilation seems to be particularly helpful when initiated early in the course of rapidly reversible diseases that respond to modest airway pressures. It is less often successful for patients whose condition has already deteriorated, for patients who are comatose or noncooperative, and for patients who either cannot be attended closely or who are hemodynamically unstable.

SUGGESTED READINGS

1. Abou-Shala N, Meduri U. Noninvasive mechanical ventilation in patients with acute respiratory failure. Crit Care Med 1996;24(4):705–715.
2. Adoumie R, Shennib H, Brown R, et al. Differential lung ventilation. Applications beyond the operating room. J Thorac Cardiovasc Surg 1993;105:229–233.
3. Blanch PB, Jones M, Layon AJ, et al. Pressure-preset ventilation. Part 1: physiologic and mechanical considerations. Chest 1993;104(2):590–599.
4. Cane RD, Peruzzi WT, Shapiro BA. Airway pressure release ventilation in severe acute respiratory failure. Chest 1991;100:460.
5. Cioffi W, Ogura H. Inhaled nitric oxide in acute lung disease. New Horizons 1995;3:73–85.
6. Downs JB, Stock MC. Airway pressure release ventilation. A new concept in ventilatory support. Crit Care Med 1987;15:459–461.
7. Fuhrman BP. Perfluorocarbon liquids and respiratory support. Crit Care Med 1993;21(7):951.
8. Gammon R, Strickland JH Jr, Kennedy JI Jr, et al. Mechanical ventilation: a review for the internist. Am J Med 1995;99(5):553–562.
9. Gattinoni L, Presenti A, Bombino M, et al. Role of extracorporeal circulation in adult respiratory distress syndrome management. New Horizons 1993;1:603–612.
10. Gattinoni L, Pesenti A, Mascheroni D, et al. Low frequency positive pressure ventilation with extracorporeal CO_2 removal in severe acute respiratory failure. JAMA 1986;256(7):881–886.
11. Hinson JR, Marini JJ. Principles of mechanical ventilator use in respiratory failure. Annu Rev Med 1992;43:341–361.
12. Jobe AH. Pulmonary surfactant therapy. N Engl J Med 1993;328:861–868.
13. Kramer N, Meyer TJ, Meharg J, et al. Randomized, prospective trial of noninvasive positive pressure ventilation in acute respiratory failure. Am J Resp Crit Care Med 1995;151(6):1799–1806.
14. Kreit J, Eschenbacher W. The physiology of spontaneous and mechanical ventilation. Clin Chest Med 1988;9(1):11–22.
15. MacIntyre N. New modes of mechanical ventilation. Clin Chest Med 1996;17(3):411–422.
16. MacIntyre NR, Gropper C, Westfall T. Combining pressure-limiting and volume-cycling features in a patient-interactive mechanical breath. Crit Care Med 1994;22(2):353–357.
17. Marcy TW, Marini JJ. Inverse ratio ventilation in ARDS. Rationale and implementation. Chest 1991;100(2):494–504.
18. Marini JJ. New options for the ventilatory management of acute lung injury. New Horizons 1993;1(4):489–503.
19. Marini JJ. Tracheal gas insufflation: a useful adjunct to ventilation? [editorial]. Thorax 1994;49(8):735–737.
20. Marini JJ, Crooke PS, Truwit JD. Determinants and limits of pressure preset ventilation: a mathematical model of pressure control. J Appl Physiol 1989;67(3):1081–1092.
21. McKibben A, Ravenscraft S. Pressure-controlled and volume-cycled mechanical ventilation. Clin Chest Med 1996;17(3):395–410.
22. Meduri G. Noninvasive positive-pressure ventilation in patients with acute respiratory failure. Clin Chest Med 1996;17(3):555–576.
23. Meduri G, Turner RE, Abou-Shala N, et al. Noninvasive positive pressure ventilation via face mask. First-line intervention in patients with acute hypercapnic and hypoxemic respiratory failure. Chest 1996;109(1):179–193.
24. Meyer T, Hill N. Noninvasive positive pressure ventilation to treat respiratory failure. Ann Intern Med 1994;120(9):760–770.
25. Mira JP, Brunet F, Belghith M, et al. Reduction of ventilator settings allowed by intravenous oxygenator (IVOX) in ARDS patients. Intensive Care Med 1995;21:11–17.
26. Nahum A, Marini JJ. Alternatives to conventional mechanical ventilation in acute respiratory failure. In: Tierney DF, ed. Current pulmonary. Chicago: Mosby-Year Book, 1994; 157–208.
27. Nahum A, Shapiro R. Adjuncts to mechanical ventilation. Clin Chest Med 1996;17(3):491–512.
28. Ost D, Corbridge T. Independent lung ventilation. Clin Chest Med 1996;17(3):591–602.
29. Ravenscraft SA, Burke WC, Marini JJ. Volume-cycled decelerating flow. An alternative form of mechanical ventilation. Chest 1992;101(5):1342–1351.
30. Simbruner G. Lung mechanics and mechanical ventilation. Crit Care Med 1993;21(9 Suppl):S369–S370.
31. Slutsky AS. Mechanical ventilation. American College of Chest Physicians' Consensus Conference. Chest 1993;104(6):1833–1859.
32. Slutsky AS. Nonconventional methods of ventilation. Am Rev Respir Dis 1988;138:175–181.
33. Spessert C, Weilitz P, Goodenberger D. A protocol for initiation of nasal positive pressure ventilation. Am J Crit Care 1993;2(1):54–60.
34. Tobin M. Mechanical ventilation. N Engl J Med 1994;330(15):1056–1061.
35. Younes M, Puddy A, Roberts D, et al. Proportional assist ventilation. Results of an initial clinical trial. Am Rev Respir Dis 1992;145:121–129.
36. Zapol W, Hurford W. Inhaled nitric oxide in adult respiratory distress syndrome and other lung diseases. New Horizons 1993;1:638–650.

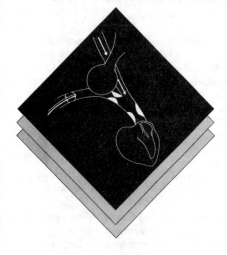

CHAPTER 8

Practical Problems and Complications of Mechanical Ventilation

ACUTE COMPLICATIONS OF MECHANICAL VENTILATION

CARDIOVASCULAR IMPAIRMENT

In general, patients with an uncompromised heart, normal sympathetic reflexes, and normal or increased intravascular volume tolerate mechanical ventilation well. Venous return is driven across the venous resistance by the difference between mean systemic venous pressure (determined by intravascular volume and venous tone) and intrathoracic vena caval pressure. For ventilated patients who make weak inspiratory efforts, mean intrathoracic pressure rises during ventilation with positive pressure, especially when positive end-expiratory pressure (PEEP) is used. This raised intrapleural pressure increases intracavitary right atrial pressure (but reduces the transmural pressure), causing cardiac output to fall unless mean systemic pressure rises sufficiently to compensate (see Chapter 1, Hemodynamics). Moreover, major increases in lung volume could also compress the vena cava and increase resistance in the region of the diaphragm. The mechanisms impairing cardiac output during positive-pressure ventilation are detailed elsewhere in this volume. Forward output is most likely to be compromised in patients who are not making breathing efforts; indeed, relief of the ventilatory burden, in combination with the reduction of left ventricular afterload that positive intrathoracic pressure provides, may dramatically improve forward output and pulmonary vascular congestion for patients with conges-

tive failure. (Conversely, resumption of the ventilatory workload increases O_2 demands and lowers intrathoracic pressure sufficiently to seriously afterload the ischemic or failing heart.) Impairment of cardiac output is particularly likely to occur in patients whose mean intrathoracic pressures rise highest (e.g., those with chest wall restriction and air trapping) and in patients who either are volume depleted or fail to venoconstrict adequately. Most evident shortly after mechanical ventilation or PEEP is instituted, output reduction is minimized by slowly adapting compensatory changes in intravascular volume and vessel tone. Profound deterioration may occur in patients developing auto-PEEP immediately after the institution of positive pressure ventilation.

BAROTRAUMA

Pathogenesis of Alveolar Rupture

The varied forms of pulmonary barotrauma—interstitial emphysema, pneumomediastinum, pneumoperitoneum, subcutaneous emphysema, cyst formation, and pneumothorax (PTX)—are prominent among the iatrogenic causes of critical illness. Although PTX may arise from such diverse medical problems as pulmonary infection or infarction, eosinophilic granuloma (histiocytosis), pneumocystis pneumonia, or spontaneous rupture of a pleural bleb, a confined set of etiologies accounts for most PTX in the intensive care unit: pleural puncture, lung necrosis, and ventilator barotrauma. Missiles, sharp instruments, and displaced rib fractures cause PTX by direct puncture of the visceral pleura. Pneumo-thorax may complicate any medical procedure in which a needle enters the thorax, especially thora-centesis, pleural biopsy, transthoracic aspiration of a pulmonary mass, and central line placement. (Therefore, if a central line must be placed, it is prudent to select the side with an existing chest tube.) Discrete single punctures of the lung are less likely to cause problems than multiple punc-tures or slashing actions of the bevel of the needle. Disruption of the visceral pleura and PTX may follow necrotizing pulmonary infection. Although direct rupture of the visceral pleura undoubtedly occurs in many patients, the barotrauma that com-plicates mechanical ventilation develops fre-quently by a more circuitous path. Rupture of weakened alveolar tissues is particularly likely to occur in "nonpartitional" or "marginal" alveoli, which have bases that abut on relatively immobile structures—vessels, bronchioles, or fibrous sep-tae. During positive-pressure ventilation (or se-vere blunt chest injury that occurs with the glottis closed), alveolar pressures rise more than intersti-tial pressures, allowing pressure gradients to de-velop between marginal alveoli and the contig-uous perivascular connective tissues. If rupture occurs, extra-alveolar gas follows a pressure gra-dient down the path of least resistance, tracking along the perivascular sheaths toward the hilum. The interstitial emphysema produced *en route* may be detected against the radiopaque back-ground of infiltrated lung as lucent streaks and small cysts that do not correspond to the bronchial anatomy. The gas continues to track centrally, forming a pneumomediastinum that may or may not be evident radiographically (see Chapter 11).

In the absence of preexisting mediastinal pa-thology, gas freely dissects along fascial planes, usually decompressing into the soft tissues of the neck (subcutaneous emphysema) or retroperito-neum (pneumoperitoneum). Pneumothorax oc-curs in a minority of such cases (perhaps 20–30%) when soft-tissue gas ruptures into the pleural space via an interrupted or weakened mediastinal pleural membrane. Interstitial emphysema, pneu-momediastinum, and subcutaneous emphysema have little hemodynamic significance and seldom affect gas exchange in adult patients. Because their presence signals alveolar rupture and the po-tential for PTX, these signs are important to detect in the ventilated patient. Pressure gradients usu-ally favor decompression of interstitial gas into the mediastinum. However, when normal bron-chovascular channels are blocked, gas accumu-lates locally or migrates distally to produce sub-pleural air cysts that compress parenchymal vessels, create deadspace, increase the ventilatory requirement, and cause major problems for venti-lation-perfusion matching. The development of cystic barotrauma is a common and ominous find-ing that usually presages tension PTX occurring a short time afterward.

Bronchopulmonary Injury

Until quite recently, the development of bron-chial damage was believed to occur only rarely in adult patients. An important autopsy study of patients ventilated at moderately high pressures for extended periods, however, has demonstrated that small airways unsupported by cartilage can sustain considerable damage at high airway pres-sures. Airway distortion predisposes to cystic pa-renchymal damage, disordered gas exchange, and impaired secretion clearance.

Cystic Barotrauma

Widespread cystic barotrauma is most likely to develop in young patients with necrotizing pneu-monitis, small narrow airways, and retained secre-tions. Alveolar rupture and focal gas trapping are key to its pathogenesis. As predicted by the Law of Laplace ($P = 2T/R$), the pressure (P) required to maintain a fixed tension (T) in the wall of a spherical structure falls as its radius (R) increases. Therefore, it is not uncommon for a cyst created by positive airway pressure to grow quickly to a large dimension (>10 cm in diameter). Once under way, cystic barotrauma tends to be perni-cious and self reinforcing. As cysts develop, they compress normal lung tissue, stiffening the lung and increasing the airway pressure needed for ef-fective ventilation. Furthermore, blood flow di-verts away from areas of cyst expansion, creating deadspace that increases the ventilatory require-ment and mean alveolar pressure. Increased peak and mean ventilatory pressures accentuate the ten-dency for further lung damage, whereas higher requirements for alveolar ventilation tend to keep the patient dependent on the ventilator. Secretion management, treatment of infection, and most im-portantly, reduction of airway pressure are funda-mental to effective management.

Systemic Gas Embolism

For patients with acute respiratory distress syn-drome (ARDS) ventilated with high tidal pressures and maintained with low left ventricular fill-ing pressures ("wedge pressures"), peak and even mean alveolar pressures may exceed pulmo-nary venous pressures in certain lung regions. If alveolar rupture opens a communication pathway to the vascular system, this pressure gradient may drive air into systemic circulation. Irritating mi-crobubbles can then cause neurologic damage or myocardial infarction (MI). Usually, the MI is in-ferior, as the bouyant air percolates into the right coronary artery, which is anterior and superior in the supine position.

Uncomplicated Pneumothorax

Ordinarily, the visceral and parietal pleural sur-faces are approximated closely during both phases of the respiratory cycle. The negative pressure be-tween them is maintained by the joint tendencies of the chest wall to expand and the lung to recoil to their natural resting volumes. At equilibrium, these opposing forces create a moderately nega-tive pleural pressure. Pneumothorax disrupts the normal relationship of the lung to the chest wall. The lung collapses toward its resting volume, which occurs below residual volume at ambient surface pressure. Simultaneously, PTX allows the chest wall to expand toward its unstressed vol-ume, which occurs at approximately 60% of the normal vital capacity. The natural tendency of the chest wall to expand—"the counter-springing ef-fect"—is diminished or lost when thoracic vol-ume increases. Coupling between the lung and chest wall is impaired by the gas buffer separating them. Outward migration of the chest wall puts the bellows at a mechanical disadvantage. Expan-sion of the chest wall shortens the resting length of the inspiratory muscles, placing them on a less advantageous portion of their length-tension rela-tionship. Less obviously, the total force developed by the muscles of the chest wall normally distrib-utes over a larger surface area than that offered by the collapsed lung. Therefore, even if the inspi-ratory muscles generate the same intrapleural pressure, the total force applied to the lung is re-duced, in proportion to the degree of lung col-lapse. As tidal excursions of the unaffected lung increase to maintain ventilation, elastic and flow-resistive work increase. This increase is well toler-ated by healthy patients with adequate ventilatory reserve. However, those with significant airflow obstruction, neuromuscular weakness, or paren-chymal restriction may experience dyspnea, pro-gressive hypoventilation, and respiratory acidosis.

Tension Pneumothorax

The term "tension PTX" implies sustained positivity of pleural pressure. A tension compo-nent can develop when a ball valve mechanism pumps air into the pleural cavity during sponta-neous breathing, but it is much more common when positive pressure provides the ventilatory power. Positive intrapleural pressure expands the ipsilateral chest cage, rendering the muscles less efficient generators of inspiratory pleural pres-sure. Contralateral pleural pressure tends to be maintained near normal levels until rather late in the process. However, a shifting mediastinum may encroach upon and deform the contralateral hemithorax, compromising lung expansion. (Par-enthetically, single lung transplantation per-formed in emphysematous subjects can provoke similar "tension" physiology.) Eventually, rising pleural and central venous pressures impede ve-nous return sufficiently to cause hemodynamic deterioration. Vigorous inspiratory efforts tend to maintain intrapleural pressure (averaged for both lungs over the entire respiratory cycle) at near-normal levels until the patient fatigues, is sedated, or receives increased machine assistance. Then, abrupt hemodynamic deterioration may occur as mean pleural pressure rises sharply. Such consid-erations explain why so many patients who de-velop pneumothoraces while mechanically venti-lated show a tension component and why ventilated patients with PTX who receive sedating or paralytic drugs frequently experience abrupt hemodynamic deterioration. For the nonintubated patient, muscle fatigue and respiratory arrest may precede the cardiovascular collapse described classically with the tension PTX syndrome. It should be emphasized that tension can develop without lung collapse or even major volume loss (e.g., when the lung is heavily infiltrated, air trap-ped, or regionally bound by pleural adhesions).

Risk Factors For Barotrauma

Although the peak airway cycling pressure has been cited frequently as the most important risk factor for ventilator-related barotrauma (VB), it is clearly not the only one (Table 8.1). In fact, height of tidal pressure may be overwhelmed by other cofactors. A necrotizing parenchymal pro-cess, nonhomogeneity of lung pathology, young age, excessive airway secretions, and duration of positive-pressure ventilation are major predispo-

TABLE 8-1

PREDISPOSITIONS TO BAROTRAUMA

Necrotizing lung pathology	High peak cycling pressure
	High mean alveolar pressure
Secretion retention	Minute ventilation requirement
Young age	Nonhomogeneous
Duration of ventilation	parenchymal disease

sitions. The process of alveolar rupture is one that seems to require sustained hyperexpansion of fragile alveoli. Therefore, the mean alveolar pressure, averaged over an entire respiratory cycle, may be an important contributing factor. As major determinants of peak and mean alveolar pressures, minute ventilation requirement and high levels of PEEP contribute to the PTX hazard. (PEEP itself may contribute little to the risk of barotrauma if it is applied within the range in which lung recruitment is its primary action.) Notwithstanding these considerations, peak dynamic (P_D) and static (P_S) airway pressures seem to contribute most to the multivariate risk equation. Peak dynamic airway pressure can be reduced by improving lung compliance, reducing tidal volume (V_T) or PEEP, lowering airflow resistance, or slowing peak inspiratory flow rate. On first consideration, it might seem that P_S (the pressure that, in conjunction with thoracic compliance, determines overall lung volume and alveolar stretch) should correlate even more closely with PTX than P_D. However, although P_S does bear a strong relationship to PTX, airway resistance varies greatly among the bronchial channels of a nonhomogeneously affected lung, so that increasing the dynamic pressure within the central airway may encourage regional overdistention and alveolar rupture in channels with open pathways to weakened alveoli. Therefore, raising the peak flow rate is not risk free. On the other hand, slowing the rate of inspiratory flow prolongs alveolar distention, increasing mean alveolar pressure. This is true especially for patients with critical airflow obstruction. Improving airway resistance or lung compliance and reducing V_T and PEEP are preferable methods for lowering P_D.

As a rule, high peak pressures applied to a stiff lung cause less alveolar stretch than the same pressures applied to a compliant lung. However, the inherent susceptibility of lung tissue to rupture and the degree of regional inhomogeneity play crucial roles. Largely for these reasons, there does not seem to be a sharp threshold value of peak

ventilator cycling pressure below which lung rupture does not occur. Nevertheless, as a rule, PTX becomes much more likely at peak ventilator cycling pressures greater than 40 cm H_2O. A peak static (plateau) pressure greater than 35 cm H_2O usually achieves or exceeds the alveolar volume corresponding to total lung capacity in a patient with a normal chest wall. (Higher pressures, therefore, cause regional overdistention.) Conversely, when the chest wall is stiff, somewhat higher plateau pressures may be well tolerated. Secretion accumulation, blood clots, or foreign objects can increase the degree of nonhomogeneity or create ball-valve phenomena that exacerbate the risk of barotrauma. The crucial role of inhomogeneity of lung injury in producing barotrauma may explain why PTX tends to develop 1 to 3 weeks after diffuse lung injury, a time when some regions are healing while others remain actively inflamed.

Diagnosis of Barotrauma

Clinical Features of Pneumothorax

Early recognition of PTX is of paramount importance for patients ventilated with positive pressure because of their proclivity to develop tension. During episodes of acute clinical deterioration compatible with PTX, the risk of mortality rises when physicians delay intervention, awaiting roentgenographic confirmation. Pleuritic chest pain, dyspnea, and anxiety comprise the most common symptoms of uncomplicated PTX. Symptoms indicative of other forms of extra-alveolar air that may precede PTX include transient precordial chest discomfort, neck pain, dysphagia, and abdominal pain. These nonspecific symptoms often are transient. Tension PTX frequently presents with tachypnea, respiratory distress, tachycardia, diaphoresis, cyanosis, or agitation. For patients receiving volume-cycled ventilation, the airway manometer usually (but not always) shows increased peak inspiratory (and peak static) airway pressures as PTX develops, especially if tension is present, and the calculated compliance of the respiratory system usually falls from previous values. Volume-cycled ventilators may "pressure limit" or "pop off," resulting in ineffective ventilation. During pressure-controlled ventilation, a decreased tidal volume and/or minute ventilation may be the only clue to increasing ventilatory impedance.

Close examination of the affected hemithorax often reveals signs of hyperexpansion with unilateral hyperresonance, diminished ventilatory excursion, and reduced breath sounds on the affected side. The examination must be performed carefully; massive atelectasis can present a similar clinical picture, simulating PTX on the contralateral side. Massive gas trapping and auto-PEEP is another effective mimic of PTX, especially if hyperinflation or infiltration is distributed asymmetrically. Palpation of the pericervical tissues and suprasternal notch is important to detect subcutaneous emphysema or a trachea deviated away from the side of tension. Tension is reflected in elevations of central venous, right atrial, and pulmonary arterial pressures. Such hemodynamic changes generally do not occur during atelectasis.

Radiographic Signs of Barotrauma

Extra-Alveolar Gas   Extra-alveolar air in the lung parenchyma can manifest as interstitial emphysema or as subpleural air cysts. Both are easiest to detect when the parenchyma is densely infiltrated. Sharp black lines that outline the heart, great vessels, trachea, inferior pulmonary ligament, or diaphragm suggest mediastinal emphysema, even when the pleural membrane itself cannot be visualized (see Chapter 4 and Fig. 8.1). The "complete diaphragm" sign indicates that the heart is separated from the diaphragm by a cushion of air. Subcutaneous emphysema, subdiaphragmatic air, and pneumoperitoneum are

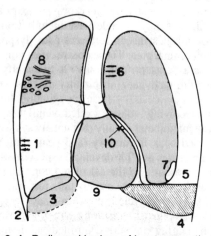

FIG. 8–1. Radiographic signs of barotrauma: 1) visible visceral pleural line; 2) deep sulcus sign; 3) radiolucency localized to the upper abdomen; 4) inverted hemidiaphragm; 5) air–fluid level; 6) mediastinal shift; 7) subpleural air cyst; 8) interstitial emphysema; 9) complete diaphragm sign; 10) pneumomediastinum.

other manifestations of barotrauma that may precede or coexist with PTX. Subpleural air cysts commonly are seen in basilar regions.

Pneumothorax   A number of radiographic signs of PTX deserve emphasis (see Chapter 11). A smooth, two-sided visceral pleural line is roentgenographically diagnostic but must be distinguished from skin folds and other artifacts at the skin surface. A pleural line may be particularly difficult to detect on a standard supine view if pleural air loculates anteriorly or if ribs or mediastinal vessels obscure the pleural margin. Two useful markers of occult PTX visible on supine films are the "deep sulcus" sign and hyperlucency centered over the ipsilateral abdominal upper quadrant. For bedridden patients, a lateral decubitus view allows air to collect along the upper margin of the hemithorax, facilitating visualization. An expiratory chest radiograph also may prove revealing. (Although the volume of intrapleural air remains constant, it occupies a greater percentage of the available space as the volume of the thoracic cage decreases.) Pneumothorax under tension can be suspected strongly from a single film when diaphragmatic inversion or extreme mediastinal shift occurs. A sequence of films demonstrating progressive migration of the mediastinal contents into the contralateral hemithorax indicates that the diagnosis was delayed but confirms its validity. It should be emphasized that life-threatening tension can exist without complete lung collapse or mediastinal displacement if the lung adheres to the pleura, if the lung is densely infiltrated, if the airway is obstructed, or if the mediastinum is immobilized by infection, fibrosis, neoplasm, or previous surgery. The mere presence of a chest tube may not prevent tension from developing if the tube is nonfunctional or inadequate to evacuate a large air leak, if the pocket drained is loculated, if the drainage holes are within the major fissure, or if intraparenchymal tension cysts coexist. In fact, by indicating the *presence* of and tendency for tissue rupture, the presence of a chest tube should reduce the clinician's threshold to suspect pneumothorax on that same side.

Value of the Computed Tomography Scan
The thoracic computed tomography (CT) scan is an invaluable aid in determining whether a lucency represents parenchymal or pleural air. In fact, accurate placement of a chest tube into a loculated pocket of gas or fluid may require insertion under direct CT guidance.

Management of Pneumothorax

General Principles

Pulmonary barotrauma developing in the setting of acute lung injury is a self-perpetuating, auto-amplifying, and highly lethal process that must be prevented. After extra-alveolar air begins to manifest in its cystic form, impaired gas exchange often forces an increase in minute ventilation requirement and, therefore, in mean airway pressure. In turn, higher mean airway pressure may worsen the tendency for alveolar rupture. Key interventions aimed at avoiding barotrauma (Table 8.2) are as follows: (a) treat the underlying disease, especially suppurative processes; (b) maintain excellent bronchial hygiene but minimize unnecessary coughing; (c) reduce the minute ventilation requirement by treating agitation, fever, metabolic acidosis, and bronchospasm (many physicians now advocate deliberate hypoventilation and permissive hypercapnia achieved by sedation or paralysis); (d) reduce peak and mean airway pressures by limiting PEEP and tidal volume and by increasing the percentage of spontaneous versus machine-aided breaths (i.e., reduce the number of ventilator breaths given during synchronized intermittent mandatory ventilation [SIMV]). Ventilator settings for tidal volume should be varied, peak pressures should be measured, and thoracic compliance should be calculated. During volume-cycled ventilation, reducing tidal volume modestly (e.g., 100–300 ml) may greatly reduce P_D and P_S. Peak flow should be set to the lowest value that satisfies inspiratory demand without incurring additional patient work or auto-PEEP, thus lowering peak dynamic (but not peak static or mean alveolar) pressure. Although several modes of ventilation have been advocated to reduce peak airway pressure (high frequency, pressure supported, and pressure controlled ventilation), these forms of positive pressure ventilation do little to alter mean airway pressure, and their therapeutic efficacy in preventing barotrauma is unproven.

Chest Tube Drainage

Indications for Thoracostomy Vigilant observation and conservative management are appropriate options in the spontaneously breathing, uncompromised patient with a small PTX. Simple observation frequently is a useful strategy for well-compensated patients who experience PTX after thoracentesis, aspiration needle biopsy, or central line placement. Many such patients will not require more aggressive management. However, serial radiographs must demonstrate gradual improvement. An air collection that fails to show convincing improvement over several days may indicate an unresolved process, with equilibration between the rates of leakage and absorption. However, spontaneous resolution of PTX is a slow process. After leakage stops, the absorption of intrapleural air occurs at a variable rate (see Chapter 11), averaging approximately (1.5%)/(original %) each day. (For example, a 15% PTX would be expected to reabsorb completely in 15/1.5 = 10 days.) Even a moderate PTX may take weeks to resolve. During this period, the partially collapsed lung clears secretions poorly. Large collections of undrained pleural air predispose to infection of the lung or pleural space, fibrosis, and formation of a restrictive outer shell. Pneumothorax is particularly dangerous for the mechanically ventilated patient. The high risk of tension mandates early decompression. Other patients to consider for early intervention are those with ipsilateral lung infection or secretion retention, ventilatory insufficiency, or high ventilatory requirements.

Tube Options The ideal chest tube system provides a reliable, low-impedance conduit that ensures efficient, unidirectional evacuation of gas and liquid from the chest. It should restore the normal subatmospheric intrapleural pressure and reapproximate the pleural surfaces. To be in best position for drainage of unloculated air, the tube should be directed superiorly and anteriorly. Small tubes can be introduced anteriorly in the second intercostal space. Larger tubes are best introduced laterally in the midaxillary line of the sixth to seventh interspace and directed upward. Starting from a lower interspace, care must be taken to begin far enough posteriorly to avoid sub-

TABLE 8–2

PREVENTING VENTILATOR-RELATED LUNG RUPTURE

Minimize minute ventilation	Normalize lung compliance
Minimize PEEP	
Use lower V_T	Improve chest wall compliance
Decrease I:E ratio	
Decrease bronchial obstruction	Encourage spontaneous breathing
Use newer modes of ventilation (?)	

diaphragmatic placement. When the pneumothorax is distributed evenly (unloculated) and suction is used, the actual position of the tube tip makes little difference. However, if loculations develop, a poorly placed chest tube, especially one not connected to suction, may fail to evacuate the appropriate area. Although large tubes usually are needed to drain substantial collections of fluid, chest tubes placed for simple air drainage are usually 28 French in caliber or smaller. Iatrogenic pneumothoraces without major air leak often can be managed in stable patients with short flexible tubes of very small diameter. Examples of these include the pigtail catheter, the von Sonnenberg catheter, and the McSwain dart. These can be attached to a water-sealed chamber drainage system (with or without suction) or to a lightweight flutter valve (Heimlich valve) to facilitate ambulation. Such small catheters can be introduced with minimal patient discomfort. Larger tubes are selected if liquid drainage is needed. Tube radius is a major determinant of the evacuation capability of the system. However, unless the tube caliber is very small, the leak is very large, or the drainage system is compromised by fibrin or debris, system resistance usually does not limit evacuation. (Tube placement and patency are much more important.)

Drainage Apparatus One-way drainage usually is provided by a water seal (Fig. 8.2). A collection column (or bottle) may be inserted in tandem and proximal to the water seal column, or one "bottle" may serve both functions. In the classical (but now seldom used) "one bottle" sys-

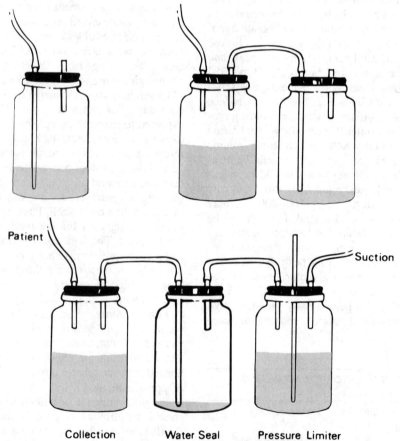

Patient

Suction

Collection   Water Seal   Pressure Limiter

FIG. 8–2. One-, two-, and three-bottle drainage systems. When a single bottle is used to collect fluid and to provide the "water seal," compensation must be made for a rising liquid level. Otherwise, there will be increasing back pressure as the tube submerges, and foaming will occur as air bubbles through the proteinaceous liquid. Separation of collection and water seal functions in a two-bottle system obviate these problems. The addition of a third "pressure-limiting" bottle enables the application of a safe, constant level of suction from any vacuum source.

tem, accumulated liquid drainage makes air leakage difficult to visualize and, more importantly, may create sufficient back-pressure to hinder lung expansion as fluid accumulates. Adjustment of applied suction or periodic liquid removal can obviate this problem. The vertical distance separating the thoracostomy incision and the liquid level must be sufficient to prevent suction of liquid into the pleural space during vigorous inspiratory efforts. Because maximum static inspiratory forces may approach -100 cm H_2O within the pleural space, a one meter vertical separation is appropriate when suction is not applied, as during transport. To avoid back pressure, the end of the water seal tube should be maintained no deeper than 2 cm beneath the fluid surface.

Monitoring Tube Function Fluid movements in the water seal tube reflect tidal variations in regional intrapleural pressure. For the spontaneously breathing patient, fluid rises in inspiration and falls during exhalation. The reverse is true during passive inflation with intermittent positive pressure. The direction of tidal fluctuations during triggered machine cycles varies with the vigor of the respiratory effort. The degree of fluctuation of the water seal without suction applied (''tidaling'') can provide useful clinical information. (Tidal fluctuations generally are smaller during suction.) An abrupt increase in tidaling suggests the development of undrained air surrounding the tube, lobar atelectasis, upper airway obstruction, impaired secretion clearance, or hyperpnea. Decreased fluctuation can reflect resolution of any of these problems, partial outflow obstruction (e.g., by fluid in a dependent loop of tubing), or decreased air leakage through a bronchopleural fistula. Absent fluctuations may be explained by tube obstruction with fibrin, blood clots, or extrinsic compression. Because of the risks of infection, the chest tube should be removed as soon as it no longer fulfills a useful function. Because 25 to 50 mL of liquid will drain each day from the normal pleural space, drainage of this amount is expected through a functioning tube that has full access to the pleural space. (Tubes draining loculated spaces may be patent despite lesser output.) Noticeable fluctuations should occur during respiratory efforts.

A ''dead tube'' (<50 mL per 24 hours of drainage, no gas leak, and no respiratory fluctuation) should be made functional or pulled. A tube that drains fluid can be maintained by periodic stripping. Quite often, a clogged tube can be reopened at least transiently by sterile injection of streptoki-

nase, followed by a brief period of clamping. This maneuver is not entirely without risk, and a tube that clogs repeatedly presents a genuine risk of infection. Another tube should then be placed if the need for drainage is still apparent radiographically. If the water seal level rises (toward the patient) and ceases to fluctuate with respiration after several days of declining drainage, pleural reapposition probably has occurred, and the tube should be removed after radiographic confirmation. The rising level reflects sealing of the air leak and subsequent reabsorption of the air contained within the chest tube. If the liquid column remains patent, fluid will rise until negative pressure within the gas-filled lumen offsets the hydrostatic column.

Persistent bubbling at the water seal signals an air leak within the lung or tubing connections. If the leak is within the lung, its magnitude can be quantified during volume-cycled mechanical ventilation by comparing the set inspiratory volume delivered by the machine cycle to the recovered exhaled tidal volume (corrected for the circuit tubing component). (Some drainage systems also provide crude flow detectors.) If the inspired and expired volumes are equivalent, air leakage is likely to originate external to the lung. Cessation of the air leak when the tube is clamped transiently near the chest wall indicates a bronchopleural fistula or air entry at the incision site. The latter can be excluded by careful approximation of the skin edges and the application of airtight occlusive dressings. If the leak does not stop after clamping near the chest wall, there has been a breach of drainage system integrity. Migratory (transient) clamping of the tubing (moving away from the patient) will then allow more precise localization. All connection sites should be inspected with special care.

Suction

Indications for Suction In certain clinical situations, natural pressure gradients (fluid siphon effects, expiratory contractions) are adequate to empty the pleural space of gas and liquid. However, suction may be needed for large air leaks or for drainage of viscous or clotting fluids. When the lung is surrounded by gas, pressure applied to one portion of the pleural surface distributes equally throughout the hemithorax. However, when normal pleural surfaces are approximated, the negative pressure applied to one area transmits poorly to other regions. The explanation is that lung tissues adjacent to the tube effectively isolate a pocket of negative pressure. In addition, tissue may be drawn into the "eyes" of the tube, preventing general transmission of applied pressure. When this happens, increasing suction only increases the risk for local tissue injury. Adhesions with loculation also may impede pressure transmission. In this instance, multiple tubes in different locations may be required. Unless the draining fluid is unusually viscid, suction usually can be discontinued (but the water seal maintained) when the bubbling stops. The tube itself can be removed safely after 24 to 48 hours of additional observation, provided that no air leakage occurs during coughing and a PTX is not visible radiographically. Some physicians recommend keeping a functioning chest tube in place as long as the patient receives positive-pressure ventilation, but this practice is controversial.

Suction Systems   Two common types of suction systems are used to regulate safe levels of suction pressure (Fig. 8.3). The Emerson suction generator links a servomechanism to a fan. A high-capacity, low-impedance system, it is capable of maintaining essentially constant negative pressure at flow rates up to 40 L/minute. If power is interrupted, air escaping from a bronchopleural fistula can vent between the fan blades, preventing tension. If increased gas leakage develops in the system, the servomechanism increases the evacuation rate in an attempt to maintain constant pressure. It is important to recognize, however, that pressure is sensed within the apparatus itself, and the manometer will continue to register a substantial level of negative pressure, even if the pump becomes completely disconnected from the patient. If set up as recommended by the manufac-

turer, the collection and water seal functions are combined. This efficiently protects the motor against damage but causes problems when there is substantial liquid drainage. If suction must be maintained during transport, special battery-operated pumps should be employed.

Several commercially available units incorporate a pressure-regulated "three bottle" system in a single molded plastic container (Fig. 8.3). A needle valve or a third chamber added in series to fluid collection and water seal columns serves as a pressure governor, modulating excessive wall suction pressures (-80 to -200 cm H_2O) to the desired level (typically <30 cm H_2O). The filling level of the vacuum control column determines and limits the degree of applied suction. Suction is increased until continuous bubbling occurs in the control chamber, indicating that sufficient negative pressure has been applied to the water surface to offset the hydrostatic column. Continuous gentle bubbling in the control chamber must be maintained throughout both phases of the respiratory cycle to ensure the desired level of suction. Increasing the applied vacuum then only serves to increase fluid perturbations in the suction control bottle, leaving the suction applied to the pleural space unaffected. (The magnitude of bronchopleural air leakage must be gauged from the water seal column). As opposed to needle valve controllers, these three bottle units are inherently noisy. If the delivered wall suction increases abruptly, air will rush from the atmosphere through the suction control inlet, preventing undesired transmission of increased suction to the pleural space. A fail-safe mechanism (a positive-

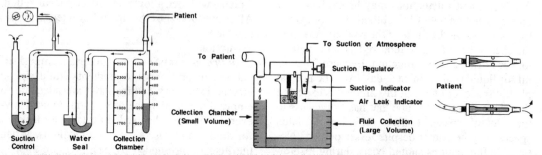

FIG. 8–3. Pleural drainage apparatus. **Left,** the disposable plastic unit is attached to the chest tube and to a high-capacity suction source to form the equivalent of a three-bottle system. Disconnection from the suction source opens the unit to atmosphere, creating a simple water-sealed two-bottle collection system. **Middle,** suction regulation can be achieved by a needle valve, reducing the noise associated with the constant bubbling of a suction control water column and obviating the need to replace evaporative water losses from the suction control column. **Right,** the flutter (Heimlich) valve opens only when sufficient positive pressure builds within the chest tube. Such devices are intended primarily for low-volume pleural air leaks without substantial fluid drainage. They enhance mobility for ambulatory patients.

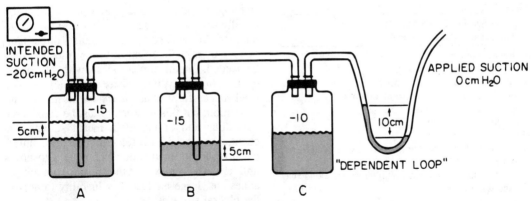

FIG. 8–4. Factors contributing to failure of applied suction. An intended suction pressure of -20 cm H_2O applied in a three-bottle system can be attenuated by evaporation of water from the pressure limiter bottle (A), by submersion of the water seal tube below the appropriate level of 1 to 2 cm below the water surface (B), and by the presence of liquid in a dependent loop of connecting tubing (C).

pressure pop-off valve, 2 cm H_2O) must be provided to open the pressure-control chamber to atmosphere when suction is disconnected. Otherwise, the water column developed within the control tube would impede egress of air from the pleural space. Three easily remediable problems (Fig. 8.4) commonly cause failure to deliver the desired level of negative pressure: fluid accumulation in the water seal chamber (common with Emerson pump), evaporation from the pressure-limiting tube of a three-bottle system, and the development of a fluid-filled dependent loop.

Special Problems of Barotrauma

Extensive Subcutaneous Emphysema A small amount of subcutaneous emphysema frequently is palpable around the chest tube entrance site. However, extensive unilateral emphysema suggests focal accumulation of air under pressure near the thoracostomy wound. Forced exhalation, straining, and coughing tend to drive gas into soft tissues. Extensive subcutaneous emphysema often indicates inadequate evacuation of a large air leak and should prompt careful examination for problems that might decrease system efficiency. In the absence of these, management options include increasing suction pressure, changing to an evacuation system with greater capability (e.g., Emerson suction generator), readjusting tube position, or placing a second chest tube to diminish the impedance to pleural emptying. Another potential cause is migration of the most proximal drainage hole out of the pleural space and into the soft tissues.

Persistent Bronchopleural Fistula Unresolving air leaks occur commonly after rupture of emphysematous blebs, after subtotal pulmonary resection, and during ventilator treatment of ARDS. In the latter setting, the development of a large bronchopleural fistula (BPF) portends a poor prognosis for survival, largely because BPF is a marker of underlying disease severity. Adequate gas exchange usually can be maintained by conventional ventilator adjustments or by one of the techniques outlined below. Interestingly, the effluent from BPF contains considerable CO_2, especially if the lung tissue functions well. Although the ''flow-through'' ventilation provided by the fistula is less efficient than tidal breathing, the gas that exits the fistula has participated in gas exchange and is not entirely ''wasted.'' For this reason, effective tidal volume is somewhat greater than that measured from the exhalation line of the ventilator circuit.

Routine Management of a Bronchopleural Fistula (Table 8.3) To manage a bronchopleural fistula, the underlying pathology must be reversed, the airway secretions must be cleared, $\dot{V}_E$ must be minimized, and good nutrition must be ensured. A large body of clinical data suggests that approximating the visceral and parietal pleura facilitates healing of pleural rents. The initial approach to management may include tube repositioning and/or a trial of increased suction in an attempt to appose the pleural surfaces more tightly. However, in certain situations, excess suction may perpetuate flow through the fistula by increasing the pressure gradient between the air-

TABLE 8–3

TECHNIQUES FOR MANAGING BRONCHOPLEURAL FISTULA

General measures:
  Reverse underlying pathology
  Clear retained airway secretions
  Minimize $\dot{V}_E$ and pressure requirements
  Improve nutritional status
  Change body position
  Reposition chest tubes
  Increase suction force if pneumothorax persists by radiograph
  Trial of decreased suction if high suction is ineffective
  Chest tube PEEP
Specialized measures
  High-frequency ventilation
  Chemical pleurodesis
  Endobronchial occlusion
    Blood clot
    Thrombin/FFP
    Tissue glue
  Pleural "blood patch"
  Operative closure

way and pleural space. If increasing suction fails, lowering or removing the suction may, in rare instances, promote healing by relieving tension on the margins of the tear. Increased lung collapse may compromise gas exchange, however.

Specialized Techniques Management of a life-threatening air leak in the mechanically ventilated patient can prove very difficult. Several techniques have been described for modifying the apparatus, either to prevent flow through the chest tube during inspiration or to maintain a common level of PEEP in the airway and the affected pleural space. None of these has gained widespread support. In some instances, independent lung ventilation has been tried successfully, but this intervention requires heroic supportive efforts. A few studies conducted primarily in children suggest that high-frequency ventilation (HFV) is associated with a lower incidence of barotrauma. Moreover, some reports indicate that HFV can help to close large air leaks by reducing the flow through the low-impedance, high-compliance (leaking) pathway. However, although HFV occasionally is helpful for adults, it is not routinely effective for management of severe lung injury or air leaks that arise. Surgical intervention may be considered, especially for less critically ill patients with cystic or bullous lung disease, after several weeks of observation and manipulation of the drainage system. Primary suturing or

stapling of the injured area and pleural abrasion usually suffice. Thoracoscopic closure can be attempted. In the case of large fistulas, direct tamponade by a pedicle flap or tissue resection may be needed. Chemical pleurodesis with talc, doxycycline, or tetracycline (where available) has been used successfully as an alternative to surgical intervention, but this treatment must be considered hazardous and of uncertain merit. Attempts at chemical sclerosis are seldom successful unless performed with meticulous technique. Closure is unlikely to be achieved in the presence of multiple adhesions, large air leaks, or inability to appose the pleural surfaces.

Occasionally successful, transbronchoscopic techniques that occlude the airway with autologous clot or a mixture of thrombin and fresh frozen plasma may close a persistent BPF and obviate the need for surgery. After identifying a leaking segmental or subsegmental bronchus, occlusion is accomplished by using a balloon-tipped (Fogarty) catheter. Then blood (50 mL) or a similar volume of the thrombin/fresh frozen plasma mixture is instilled. Although seldom effective, results are often immediate. Alternatively, pleural instillation of sterile talc (by insufflation or as a slurry), tetracycline, or autologous blood (a blood patch) using a chest tube may seal a persistent leak, but such pleurodesis is not without risk. Because the procedure requires at least transient clamping of the chest tube, tension physiology may ensue. Both endobronchial occlusion and pleurodesis methods work best; however, when the BPF is small, neither can be accomplished safely in the unstable patient.

VENTILATOR-INDUCED PULMONARY EDEMA, LUNG INJURY, AND VOLUTRAUMA

Pathogenesis

Even when alveolar rupture does not occur, there is little doubt that the application of excessive *regional* volumes are damaging to alveoli—whether produced by positive or negative pressure. Patients with the acute respiratory distress syndrome seem to be at highest risk; the prevalence of barotrauma in this condition may exceed 50%. In experimental animals, the choice of ventilatory pattern influences the morphology of normal and previously injured tissues. Such observations regarding the effects of tidal pressures are of intense interest, especially when it is under-

TABLE 8–4

Risk Factors for Ventilator-Induced Lung Injury

		High Pressure	High Tidal Volume	PEEP	Risk
Normal		No	Yes	No	None
		No	Yes	Yes	Low
		Yes	Yes	Yes	Moderate
ARDS	Early	Yes	Yes	Yes	Moderate
		Yes	Yes	No	High
	Late	Yes	Yes	No	High
		Yes	No	Yes	High
		No	No	No	Moderate

No = Not applied; Yes = applied

stood that an excess of 20,000 tidal cycles are undertaken each day.

Effect of Excessive Peak Pressures

Ventilatory patterns that apply high transalveolar stretching forces cause or extend tissue edema and damage in experimental animals (Table 8.4). Such pressures traditionally have been encountered during conventional management of ARDS. Pressure–volume curves and CT evidence strongly suggest that static airway pressures greater than 30 cm H_2O commonly produce regional overdistention in patients with ARDS and normal chest wall compliance. Peak tidal pressures of this magnitude are known to cause tissue damage in experimental animals when ventilation is sustained for more than 12 to 24 hours. Judging from the substantial delay to peak incidence of pneumothorax, the lung seems to be able to withstand exposure to somewhat higher distending forces in the earliest phase of ARDS without radiographically evident barotrauma (see Chapter 24, Oxygenation Failure). Later in the course of illness, the strong collagen infrastructure of the lung degrades unevenly, so that similar pressures are more likely to result in overt alveolar disruption (pneumothorax, pneumomediastinum, gas cyst formation). Independent of radiographic evidence for extra-alveolar gas, the lung may be susceptible to edematous injury produced by high inflating pressures in both early and late stages.

Importance of End-Expiratory Lung Volume and PEEP

Failure to preserve a certain minimum end-expiratory transalveolar pressure (i.e., total PEEP) in the early phase of ARDS may intensify preexisting alveolar damage, especially when high tidal volumes and high inflation pressures are used. Indeed, the shear forces associated with tidal collapse and reinflation of injured alveolar tissues may be responsible for an important component of ventilator-induced lung damage (Fig. 8.5). The end-expiratory pressure required to avert widespread alveolar collapse varies with the hydrostatic forces applied to the lung; consequently, a higher end-expiratory pressure is required to prevent atelectasis in dependent regions than in the more superior regions. Gravitational factors, therefore, help explain the strikingly dependent distribution of radiographic infiltrates shortly after the onset of lung injury, as well as reversal of these infiltrates and improvement of arterial oxygenation in the prone position. Total PEEP sufficient to place the tidal volume above the initial low compliance region (''P_{flex}'') of the static pressure–volume relationship of the respiratory system seems, in experimental studies, to attenuate the severe hemorrhagic edema otherwise induced by high ventilating pressure.

Experimentally, inflicting severe lung damage requires both the application of high pressure and failure to maintain recruitment with sufficient end-expiratory pressure. What recruits one part of the lung (e.g., dependent regions) is likely to overdistend other parts (e.g., nondependent regions) (Fig. 8.6). Lung recruitment is likely to occur throughout the tidal cycle whenever PEEP or peak alveolar pressure fails to reach a sufficient opening pressure.

Stress failure of the pulmonary capillaries with resulting extravasation of formed blood elements into the lung tissue may occur at transvascular pressures that exceed 40 to 90 mm Hg, depending on animal species. Transcapillary mechanical forces of comparable magnitude may be generated

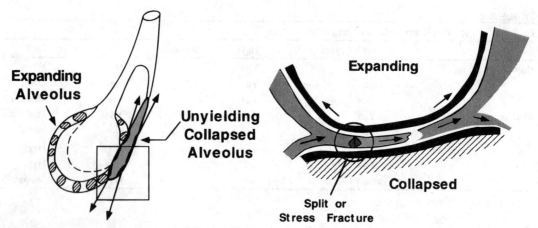

FIG. 8–5. Shearing forces during mechanical ventilation of the heterogeneous lung. **Left,** The targential shearing forces at the junction of expanding and collapsed alveolus may far exceed the tensions experienced in the free walls of expanding units, especially at high inflation pressures. **Right,** When junctional tensions rise high enough, the shearing action may exert sufficient force to cause capillary stress fractures and hemorrhagic edema.

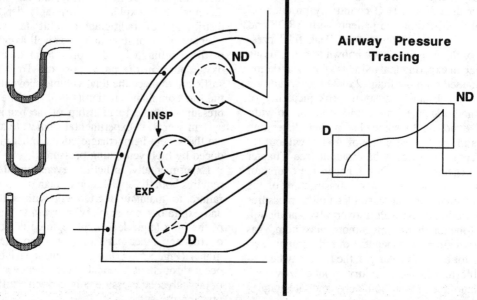

FIG. 8–6. Regional alveolar mechanics during the tidal breath in ARDS. Dependent (D) lung units may be surrounded by sufficiently high pressure to collapse at end-expiration and reexpand at some pressure achieved during the tidal cycle. Nondependent (ND) units that are exposed to low extra alveolar pressures may overdistend at end-inspiration, risking "over-stretch" injury. During controlled ventilation with constant inspiratory flow, the airway pressure tracing may show indirect evidence of these phenomena if it displays segments of rapidly improving and rapidly deteriorating respiratory system compliance.

when high tidal volumes and peak static tidal pressures are used in the setting of heterogeneous lung disease. High vascular pressure and blood flows also may be important determinants of lung injury.

Management

Detailed clinical information is not available for guidance regarding the maximum safe peak and mean alveolar pressures that can be applied for extended periods without inducing alveolar damage or retarding lung healing. Clearly, the answer differs among individual patients (Table 8.4). Alveolar volumes and stresses undoubtedly vary from site to site within the damaged lung (Fig. 8.6). The common airway pressure applied to the endotracheal tube (ET) must account for the distensibility and vulnerability of each type of lung unit. Although failure to preserve a certain minimum end-expiratory transalveolar pressure has been shown experimentally to intensify preexisting alveolar damage, this phenomenon has not yet been demonstrated clearly in humans. Moreover, all are agreed that once recruitment has been completed, additional PEEP is probably ineffectual or damaging. Consequently, expert opinion differs regarding whether applying the least PEEP that accomplishes adequate gas exchange or guaranteeing some minimal value of end-expiratory alveolar pressure is the best course to follow within the first few days of the disease process. Periodic application of sustained high inflating pressures to recruit unstable lung units continues to be advocated by some knowledgeable investigators, especially when small tidal volumes (<4–5 mL/kg) are used or when high-frequency ventilation is employed. PEEP should be withdrawn later in the disease process, especially if no inflection region can be identified on the pressure–volume curve of the respiratory system. Because tidal compliance depends on tidal volume, the appropriate V_T to select undoubtedly varies with the level of PEEP and vice versa. There is no consensus regarding the contribution of vascular pressures, position changes, infection, inspired oxygen concentration, and other clinical variables on the incidence or intensity of ventilator-induced lung injury.

Allowing $PaCO_2$ to rise to supernormal values (permissive hypercapnia) seems to be an effective strategy for limiting the need for ventilatory pressure (see Chapter 24, Oxygenation Failure). The full effects of hypercapnia on such important variables as gas exchange, cardiovascular dynamics, and tissue edema has yet to be determined in the two settings for which it is most commonly applied—asthma and ARDS. Moreover, there are both relative and absolute contraindications for using this technique (Table 8.5). Elevated FiO_2 and high ventilatory pressures often are required to achieve near-complete saturation of arterial blood with oxygen. The conditions (if any) under which arterial O_2 saturation can be allowed to fall to subnormal values without unacceptable clinical consequences have not yet been delineated. There is no clear consensus regarding the most appropriate indicator of regional or global adequacy/inadequacy of O_2 delivery (dysoxia) for routine clinical use. The combinations of O_2 concentration and exposure duration that produce significant lung damage have not been established firmly in the setting of ARDS and may vary with disease severity and individual susceptibility. Similarly, although a considerable body of experimental data has been accumulated, detailed information is not yet available regarding which ventilation pressures and patterns of inflation are safe to apply for extended periods. In the absence of definitive data obtained in a clinical context, some knowledgeable practitioners increase lung volume in an attempt to minimize FiO_2, whereas others prefer to use higher inspired fractions of O_2 rather than increase peak, mean, and end-expiratory airway pressures. At FiO_2 levels less than 0.7, limiting P_{aw} to ''safe'' levels generally takes precedence over limiting FiO_2.

Whether different methods for achieving a similar mean airway pressure (such as PEEP and inverse ratio ventilation) differ with respect to risks and benefits has not been clarified adequately. The extent to which spontaneous (versus controlled) ventilation should be encouraged also has been an area of uncertainty. (Management of ARDS is addressed in detail in Chapter 24, Oxygenation Failure).

TABLE 8–5

CONTRAINDICATIONS TO PERMISSIVE HYPERCAPNIA

Increased intracranial pressure
Severe cardiovascular dysfunction
Severe pulmonary hypertension
Profound metabolic acidosis

FLUID RETENTION AND REDISTRIBUTION

Extravascular fluid retention tends to develop during positive-pressure ventilation for several reasons: (*a*) ventilated patients are relatively immobile; (*b*) as increased intrathoracic pressure limits venous return, stretch receptors located in the atria signal additional antidiuretic hormone (ADH) release to help replenish central vascular volume; (*c*) hypotension induced by positive pressure may curtail renal perfusion, redistribute renal blood flow, reduce glomerular filtration, and promote sodium retention. PEEP may cause a similar redistribution of intrarenal blood flow by reflex mechanisms. The hypoalbuminemia almost routinely present in the ventilated, critically ill patient is also contributory. As positive-pressure ventilation is discontinued, these fluid shifts reverse and may precipitate cardiac decompensation in patients with poor reserve, as fluid translocates from extravascular sites to the central vessels.

The controversy regarding fluid management in ARDS is more than an academic one; data exist to indicate that fluid retention correlates with adverse outcomes in several published studies, either because tissue edema is a marker of disease severity or because it relates integrally to organ dysfunction.

FLUCTUATIONS IN PH

The ventilator can powerfully affect acid–base balance. When support is initiated, special care should be exercised not to reverse acidosis too quickly or to cause marked respiratory alkalosis. Metabolic alkalosis tends to develop in mechanically ventilated patients because of intravascular volume contraction, nasogastric suctioning, use of steroids, etc. If repletion of KCl or intravascular volume fails to correct it, acetazolamide (Diamox) may prove useful in controlling extravascular fluid retention while dumping excess bicarbonate. In the assist/control mode, marked fluctuations in pH and $PaCO_2$ can occur in patients who are alternately agitated and sedated, especially if the ventilator's backup rate is inappropriately low. Mental status and ventilation mode always should be taken into account when interpreting blood gas values.

INFECTIONS

Infections of the lung and upper respiratory tract are exceedingly common during mechanical ventilation. Endotracheal intubation prevents glottic closure, disrupts the laryngeal barrier, slows the mucociliary escalator, impedes secretion clearance, and provides an open pathway for large quantities of aspirated pharyngeal bacteria and fungi to inoculate the lung. Oral and nasal secretions gravitate continuously to the lower tract via the cuff interstices, even though cuff inflation prevents massive gastric aspiration. The oropharynx of critically ill patients quickly recolonizes with hospital-prevalent pathogens, e.g., gram-negative bacteria and staphylococci. Nasogastric tubes commonly used during mechanical ventilation for gastric decompression or feeding serve as a conduit for enteric bacteria to the pharynx and upper respiratory tract. Furthermore, bacterial overgrowth is common when histamine blockers, antacids, or tube feedings buffer the gastric pH to levels greater than 4.0. Some evidence suggests that sucralfate, which requires acid production for optimal action, may be preferable to pH-altering regimens for this reason, but this is controversial (see Chapter 31). Duodenal instillation of liquid feeding reduces the risk of aspiration and largely avoids acid buffering. Condensate within corrugated tubing allows bacteria to multiply. Therefore, great care should be taken to prevent transfer of the condensate into the trachea during manipulations of the ventilator circuit or changes of patient position. Nasotracheal and nasogastric tubes frequently precipitate sinus infection by blocking their ostia, which prevents drainage. In itself, occult sinusitis is a frequent cause for febrile episodes in intubated patients. Furthermore, blocked sinuses also provide a seeding focus for infections of the lung and bloodstream. It should be emphasized that occult sinopulmonary infections often are responsible for the sepsis syndrome in intubated, mechanically ventilated patients, even when organisms cannot be recovered by conventional culturing techniques. Overt pneumonitis, frequently polymicrobial, usually manifests after the first week of hospitalization.

Ventilator-Associated Pneumonia

Although the oropharynx teems with microbes, the upper airway normally is sterile below the vocal cords, swept clean by the mucociliary escalator and protected by an effective cough. Bypass-

TABLE 8–6

PREDISPOSITIONS TO VENTILATOR-ASSOCIATED PNEUMONIA

Sinusitis
Poor dentition
Immobilization
Immune compromise
Supine position
Coexisting nasogastric tube
Lengthy period of ventilation
High gastric pH
Condensate within ventilator tubing
Frequent circuit disconnections

ing the upper airway with an endotracheal tube seriously impairs these defenses while facilitating innoculation of the lower airway and lungs with high concentrations of potential pathogens. The rate of developing a ventilator-associated pneumonia approximates 2 to 3% per day, so that the likelihood of developing a pneumonia is quite high after the first 10 days of ventilatory support, even when appropriate precautions are taken. Poor dentition, impaired nutritional status, age, immobilization, immune compromise, and the supine position predispose pulmonary infection (Table 8.6). Once underway, pneumonia contributes clearly to the mortality resulting from such underlying conditions as decompensated chronic obstructive pulmonary disease (COPD) and ARDS.

Although pneumonia occasionally arises from hematogenous innoculation, most alveolar seeding occurs via the airway. In epidemiologic and experimental studies, the likelihood of developing pneumonia relates to the delivery mechanism as well as to the size of the airway innoculum. Whereas 10^7 aerosolized organisms are needed to initiate a parenchymal infection, liquid aspiration of 10^4 organisms generally is sufficient. The endotracheal tube interferes with the mucociliary escalator and with coughing effectiveness. Given that the colony counts of oral secretions may exceed 10^8/mL, that the interstices of the endotracheal tube cuff may allow continuing seepage of these secretions into the lower airway, and that considerable axial movement of the endotracheal tube may help pump a critical innoculum into the lung, a high incidence of nosocomial pneumonia is hardly surprising. An intriguing body of experi-

mental and clinical data suggests not only that high tidal volume and low PEEP ventilatory patterns predispose the lung damage described earlier but also that lungs injured in this fashion are usually susceptible to pulmonary infections. Moreover, such high shearing stress patterns may cause capillary rupture and allow bacteria, inflammatory products, or mediators to enter the bloodstream.

Sinus drainage is seriously impaired by extended immobility in the supine position. Moreover, nasal tubes of various kinds impede ipsilateral drainage and increase the reservoir of nosocomial pathogens at risk for aspiration. Diagnostic techniques and approaches to management of ventilator-associated pneumonia are detailed in Chapter 26.

DECONDITIONING

Weakening and discoordination of respiratory muscles may occur as the burden, timing, and breathing pattern are machine controlled for prolonged periods. Substantial work is performed in the effort to trigger the ventilator, especially by breathless patients. As a rule, patients receiving assisted mechanical ventilation expend sufficient effort in triggering the ventilator to prevent disuse atrophy, but it is unclear whether original muscle bulk and strength are preserved. The problem of deconditioning seems most serious for those patients who must assume a large workload of breathing when mechanical ventilation is discontinued, for those with preexisting neuromuscular impairment, for those with suppressed ventilatory drive, and for those requiring prolonged sedation or paralysis. Nutritional support, increased spontaneous muscle activity (continuous positive airway pressure [CPAP], intermittent mandatory ventilation [IMV], pressure support), and muscle training may be helpful. Although unproven, periodic ''sprints'' (or 5- to 10-minute CPAP trials) may help preserve bulk and strength, even during the acute stage.

PATIENT-VENTILATOR INTERACTIONS

SPECIFIC "EARLY PHASE" PROBLEMS

Coordination Between Breathing Rhythms of Patient and Ventilator

Initial discomfort may be extreme, due to the ET tube, distended hollow viscera, impaired swallowing, pharyngeal or sinus pain, anxiety, disorientation, inability to speak, or discomfort related to recent invasive procedures. Stimulation of bronchial, laryngeal, and carinal irritant receptors triggers bronchospasm and coughing efforts. Furthermore, mechanical ventilators usually are set to deliver higher (and occasionally lower) tidal volumes than the patient would choose spontaneously, whereas inspiratory pattern, flow rate, and cycling frequency differ from those of the presupport period. Hence, shortly after mechanical ventilation begins, attempts to "fight the ventilator" are the rule in alert, awakening, and mildly obtunded patients. Initial mismatching usually abates spontaneously (within minutes) as the settings are adjusted and the patient becomes accustomed to the machine. Constant attendance by trained medical personnel is necessary throughout this period, however, to calm the patient, adjust the settings to the patient's requirements, and ensure that the agitation neither interferes with gas exchange nor has a more serious origin. It is extremely important to secure all tubing connectors and restrain the arms of an intermittently agitated or rousable patient. Ventilator disconnection or self-extubation is a potentially lethal and distressingly common event, especially when nursing resources are stretched too thin. When the patient is connected initially, sensitivity should be adjusted so that the minimal effort that avoids "autocycling" is required to trigger a ventilator breath. Inspiratory flow rate is adjusted to a level commensurate with the vigor and frequency of the patient's efforts. (A flow setting $\approx 4 \times \dot{V}_E$ usually satisfies flow demands.) Tidal volume may need to be reduced temporarily to achieve an adequate matchup between patient and ventilator frequencies. With the machine properly adjusted, mechanical malfunctioning ruled out, the patient examined, the initial set of blood gases analyzed, and the chest radiograph checked for position of the tube tip and pneumothorax, an opiate, benzodiazepine, or propofol may be given to assist smooth linking of endogenous respiratory and ventilator rhythms. Intratracheal lidocaine (2–4 mL of 2% concentration) can briefly arrest coughing spasms and reduce pain. A nasogastric tube helps to decompress the gastrointestinal tract and is particularly helpful for patients with gastrointestinal motility impaired by opiates or disease who swallow air around orotracheal tubes.

Special Problems of Patients with High Ventilatory Requirements

Patients with high ventilatory requirements may overtax the capacity of the ventilator to deliver gas and, hence, may work against the machine as well as their intrinsic respiratory mechanics. If a more powerful machine is not effective or available, this is one of the few situations that justifies heavy sedation and use of the control mode. Hyperpnea strains the capacity of the machine to coordinate with the patient, forcing major deviations between intended and delivered waveforms. Asynchrony markedly elevates the breathing workload and tachypnea accentuates the importance of resistance within the ET and other circuit elements. Active use of the expiratory musculature may cause hypoxemia by combatting the volume recruitment effect of PEEP, altering ventilation–perfusion relationships and desaturating mixed venous blood. In these circumstances, reducing active effort can improve arterial oxygenation. Although deep sedation and paralysis can be helpful, prolonged immobility encourages regional atelectasis and secretion retention (especially in dependent areas), as well as muscle atrophy. For the paralyzed patient, undetected ventilator disconnections can be rapidly lethal. Under extreme circumstances, adequate ventilation is difficult to achieve, even with paralysis and full machine support. A steady infusion of bicarbonate may allow pH to remain compensated as CO_2 is permitted to stabilize at a higher level. It is not commonly realized that the PEEP valves used with most ventilators offer substantial airflow resistance, which increases with the level of PEEP. In part, this expiratory retard effect is an unavoidable consequence of the fact that such valves are pressure activated and must sense a pressure difference across the valve to block further exhalation at the preset level. If exhalation is passive, this resistance slows airflow but does not influence the amount of ventilatory work performed by the patient. During active exhalation, however, this increased resistance must be overcome by patient effort and adds substantially to the work of breathing.

SPECIFIC "SUPPORT PHASE" PROBLEMS

Smooth interaction between the patient and machine may be interrupted by malfunctioning of the ventilator system, worsening of cardiopulmonary mechanics, or by factors completely unrelated to ventilation. Malfunctions of the ventilator system prevent adequate ventilation or oxygenation and usually present as altered states of consciousness (agitation or obtundation), worrisome changes in vital signs, or unexplained deterioration in blood gases.

Diagnostic Approach to Agitation During Mechanical Ventilation

When a crisis develops suddenly during mechanical ventilation, the clinician must efficiently diagnose the problem in an organized (even stereotyped) fashion. In many cases, the patient should be ventilated manually until the problem has been diagnosed. The difference between the exhaled versus set tidal volume is crucial data. A major difference unexplained by pressure limiting and "pop-off" leakage indicates a circuit leak or machine dysfunction. Checking the airway pressure manometer and comparing the peak dynamic and static pressures against previous values also provide essential information. Failure to generate or hold pressure during circuit occlusion usually indicates a system leak. A large disparity between P_D and P_S suggests a resistance problem in the tube or airways (bronchospasm, secretions). It is useful to classify these problems as those that usually elevate peak cycling pressure (pressure limiting) and those that usually do not (Table 8.7). Three components of the system must be checked carefully: the patient, the endotracheal tube, and the ventilator system.

TABLE 8–7

SUDDEN CRISES DURING MECHANICAL VENTILATION

Pressure Limiting	Non-Pressure Limiting
Central airway obstruction	Cuff deflation/tube withdrawal
Massive atelectasis	Circuit disruption
Tube occlusion	Machine malfunction
Mainstem intubation	Pneumothorax without tension
Pain, anxiety, or delirium	
Tension pneumothorax	Gas trapping (auto-PEEP)
Irritative bronchospasm	Hemodynamic crisis
Decreased chest wall compliance	Pulmonary embolism
Secretion retention	Pulmonary edema

Patient

The importance of auscultation for signs of pneumothorax, bronchospasm, secretion plugging, and pulmonary edema deserves emphasis. Among the most important distinctions to make is the one between massive atelectasis and tension pneumothorax. Note that a pneumothorax that does not have a tension component may not elevate peak pressure noticeably. Nonpulmonary causes of discomfort (distention of bladder or intestinal tract, unvarying body position, pain, etc.) are overlooked easily. Pulmonary emboli and cardiac ischemia are common.

Problems are unusually frequent among patients with combined cardiac and pulmonary disease. Increased VO_2, heart rate, blood pressure, and left ventricular afterload can cause florid congestive failure ("flash" pulmonary edema), ischemia, or other manifestation of circulatory stress within minutes of onset in a patient with coronary insufficiency or myocardial or valvular dysfunction.

For patients receiving flow-controlled, volume-cycled ventilation (e.g., assist-control or SIMV), the need for increased minute ventilation often causes ventilatory demands to outstrip the ventilator's flow delivery, increasing the work of breathing still further and setting into motion a self-perpetuating cycle of agitation and cardiopulmonary compromise. A boost in ventilatory support and inspiratory flow rate often is required to rectify the situation. Agitated patients often oppose the ventilator, causing dysynchrony and pressure limiting. In the assist-control mode, dysynchrony tends to be self-perpetuating, inasmuch as small (pressure-limited) inflations do not allow adequate ventilation, and dyspnea continues or increases. A vicious cycle is especially likely to develop in patients with airflow obstruction who hyperinflate, causing auto-PEEP with associated muscle dysfunction and hemodynamic stress. Both the work of breathing and dyspnea escalate markedly as the patient struggles to breathe. Temporarily switching to high-level pressure support (sufficient to achieve an effective tidal volume) is a good solution for avoiding patient-ventilator dysynchrony and relieving dyspnea until the situation can be analyzed fully and the underlying cause can be addressed definitively. Disconnecting the ventilator and providing adequate ventilation manually with a resuscitator bag is an alternative strategy that frequently will break the cycle and stop the process.

It must be stressed that once agitation develops, hypoxemia frequently occurs, increasing both the drive to breathe and the dyspnea. Increasing the FiO_2 often reverses hypoxemia and can undo the self-reinforcing process of agitation → hypoxemia → increased drive → agitation → hypoxemia. In fact, increasing FiO_2 is a good first option whenever desaturation accompanies agitation. Although agitation often has a trivial origin, it must never be ignored or suppressed with sedatives until possible serious causes are investigated. Bradycardia is experienced frequently by patients requiring high levels of PEEP and mean airway pressure during temporary machine disconnection for suctioning. Although hypoxemia occasionally is responsible for these episodes of bradycardia, this phenomenon usually is a reflex effect, which is prevented by pretreatment with systemic atropine, "closed circuit" airway suctioning, or the provision of CPAP during secretion removal.

Endotracheal Tube

Modern ventilators are equipped with audible alarms that sense excessive system pressure, failure to exhale a set minimum tidal volume, or disconnection of the patient from the machine. If the cause for distress is not immediately obvious, the caregiver should listen for cuff leaks during inflation (auscultate over the larynx) and palpate the pilot balloon to sense the pressure in the cuff. Endotracheal tubes often kink, block with secretions, or become constricted by the teeth of a biting patient. The physician should then disconnect the patient from the ventilator, oxygenate the patient, and pass a suction catheter to check patency of the ET and aspirate central airway secretions. Vital signs are checked and auscultation is performed quickly for evidence of pneumothorax, massive atelectasis, or bronchospasm as the patient is ventilated manually with 100% oxygen. Tubes that are poorly placed or secured may migrate into the larynx or right main bronchus or may rest on the carina, producing cough and bronchospasm.

Ventilator Circuit

The integrity of the ventilator circuit is then inspected quickly, with special attention given to tubing connections and the settings for tidal volume, frequency, trigger sensitivity, and oxygen fraction. Tubing is inspected for accumulated water, which may increase inspiratory resistance or cause inadvertent expiratory retard or PEEP. If all seems intact, the patient can be reconnected briefly to check delivered versus set minute ventilation. If delivered minute ventilation is too low, all connections should be checked carefully for leaks, especially around the humidifier and the exhalation valve. In a passive patient, the application of an end-inspiratory pause will help detect a circuit leak. If the problem still persists, no cause is detected, and the chest radiograph is negative, judicious doses of morphine or other sedative can be given, as long as gas exchange is well maintained as judged by oximetry or arterial blood gases. Paralysis must never be undertaken until an alert patient is adequately sedated.

Distinction must be made between fighting the ventilator (dysynchrony) and attempting to "breathe around" the ventilator. The first condition may prevent effective ventilation or signal a serious disorder; the second usually is innocuous. Breathing around the ventilator refers to the patient's ineffective attempts to pull additional breaths during the exhalation phase of the ventilator cycle. Often, auto-PEEP is the explanation for impaired triggering. With gas exchange uncompromised, sensitivity appropriately set, and the patient not in distress, such a pattern seems to have little detrimental effect. However, a strong tachypneic patient, especially one intubated for purposes of oxygenation, may attempt to pull breaths deeper than the ventilator is set to deliver. When this happens, gas drawn from the reservoir of the ventilator during inspiration adds to the delivered tidal volume or a second breath is triggered prematurely. As a result, the patient inhales a larger volume of gas than set, but a similar FiO_2 is maintained.

Other Support Phase Problems

Work of breathing during mechanical ventilation, psychological distress, and depression are prevalent during mechanical ventilation and are discussed at length in Chapter 10, Weaning From Mechanical Ventilation.

KEY POINTS

1. Impaired cardiac output is most likely to result from mechanical ventilation when intravascular volume is depleted, vascular reflexes are impaired, and the patient is inflated passively with high mean airway pressure.

2. All forms of alveolar rupture induced by mechanical ventilation—interstitial emphysema, pneumomediastinum, pneumoperitoneum, subcutaneous emphysema, cyst formation, pneumothorax, and systemic gas embolism have been described in both infants and adults. Certain high-pressure ventilatory patterns are strongly suspected to inflict non-rupture damage, such as bronchopulmonary damage and diffuse lung injury.

3. No single cause is responsible for all barotrauma. High peak airway cycling pressure, necrotizing pneumonia, heterogeneity of lung pathology, copious airway secretions, and duration of positive-pressure ventilation are major predisposing factors. Pneumothorax becomes increasingly likely when the patient has been ventilated for more than 1 week at peak cycling pressures that exceed 40 cm H_2O.

4. The pathophysiology of tension pneumothorax involves cardiovascular as well as ventilatory compromise. Tension physiology can develop with only a minor portion of the lung collapsed if the lung is infiltrated or the pleura is adhesed in multiple places.

5. The thoracostomy tube selected should be of such size and location to adequately drain the pleural air and liquid present. The lung must be approximated to the parietal pleura whenever possible. Suction may be needed if an air leak is large and persists on the water seal alone or if fluid drainage is copious.

6. Failure to preserve a crucial minimum level of PEEP in the early phase of ARDS may intensify preexisting alveolar damage, especially when high peak inflation pressures are used. The high shearing forces of each high-peak/low-PEEP tidal cycle may cause small airway damage, capillary stress fractures, and inflammatory changes, as well as overt lung disruption. Later in the disease process, when inflammation has degraded the collagen infrastructure of the lung, minimizing peak pressure helps prevent alveolar rupture, cyst formation, and pneumothorax.

7. Subacute and chronic complications of mechanical ventilation include fluid retention, redistribution of body water, infection, altered ventilatory drive, and respiratory muscle deconditioning.

8. Specific problems encountered after intubation of the critically ill patient include the following: uncontrolled coughing, patient–ventilator dysynchrony, excessive work of breathing, and self-extubation. Agitation during mechanical ventilation demands a systematic search through possible causes relating to the patient, the endotracheal tube and circuitry, and the ventilator itself.

SUGGESTED READINGS

1. Albelda SM, Gefter WB, Kelley MA, et al. Ventilator-induced subpleural air-cysts: clinical, radiographic, and pathologic significance. Am Rev Respir Dis 1983;127:360–365.
2. Bezzant T, Mortensen J. Risks and hazards of mechanical ventilation: a collective review of published literature. Dis Mon 1994;40(11):581–638.
3. Bishop M. Mechanisms of laryngotracheal injury following prolonged tracheal intubation. Chest 1989;96(1):185–186.
4. Brooks-Brunn J. Postoperative atelectasis and pneumonia. Heart Lung 1995;24(2):94–115.
5. Bryan C, Jenkinson S. Oxygen toxicity. Clin Chest Med 1988;9(1):141–152.
6. Deem S, Bishop M. Evaluation and management of the difficult airway. Crit Care Clin 1995;11(1):1–27.
7. Dreyfuss D, Saumon G. Barotrauma is volutrauma, but which volume is the one responsible? Intensive Care Med 1992;18(3):139–141.
8. Dreyfuss D, Saumon G. Role of tidal volume, FRC, and end-inspiratory volume in the development of pulmonary edema following mechanical ventilation. Am Rev Respir Dis 1993;148(5):1194–1203.
9. Dumire R, Crabbe MM, Mapin FG, et al. Autologous "blood patch" pleurodesis for persistent pulmonary air leak. Chest 1992;101:64–66.
10. Estes R, Meduri G. The pathogenesis of ventilator-associated pneumonia: i. Mechanisms of bacterial transcolonization and airway inoculation. Intensive Care Med 1995;21(4):365–383.
11. Fontaine D. Nonpharmacologic management of patient distress during mechanical ventilation. Crit Care Clin 1994;10(4):695–708.
12. Gammon BR, Shin MS, Buchalter SE. Pulmonary barotrauma in mechanical ventilation: patterns and risk factors. Chest 1992;102:568–572.
13. George D. Epidemiology of nosocomial pneumonia in intensive care unit patients. Clin Chest Med 1995;16(1):29–44.
14. Gordon P, Norton J, Merrell R. Refining chest tube man-

agement: analysis of the state of practice. Dimen Crit Care Nurs 1995;14(1):6–12.

15. Hansen-Flaschen J. Improving patient tolerance of mechanical ventilation. Challenges ahead. Crit Care Clin 1994;10(4):659–671.

16. Heffner J. Airway management in the critically ill patient. Crit Care Clin 1991;12(3):533–550.

17. Jantz M, Pierson D. Pneumothorax and barotrauma. Clin Chest Med 1994;15(1):75–91.

18. Kirby T, Ginsberg R. Management of pneumothorax and barotrauma. Clin Chest Med 1992;13(1):97–112.

19. Kollef M, Schuster D. Ventilator-associated pneumonia: clinical considerations. Am J Roentgenol 1994;163(5): 1031–1035.

20. Lachmann B. Open up the lung and keep the lung open. Intensive Care Med 1992;18(6):319–321.

21. Leeper K. Diagnosis and treatment of pulmonary infections in adult respiratory distress syndrome. New Horizons 1993;1(4):550–562.

22. Leijten F, de Weerd A. Critical illness polyneuropathy. Clin Neurol Neurosurg 1994;96(1):10–19.

23. Lockhat D, Langleben D, Zidulka A. Hemodynamic differences between continual positive and two types of negative pressure ventilation. Am Rev Respir Dis 1992; 146(3):677–680.

24. Marcy TW, Marini JJ. Respiratory distress in the ventilated patient. Clin Chest Med 1994;15(1):55–73.

25. Marini JJ. Strategies to minimize breathing effort during mechanical ventilation. In: Tobin MJ, ed. Critical Care Clinics. Philadelphia: WB Saunders, 1990; 635–661.

26. Marini JJ, Culver BH. Systemic air embolism consequent to mechanical ventilation in ARDS. Ann Intern Med 1989; 110(9):699–703.

27. Marini JJ, Rodriguez RM, Lamb VJ. The inspiratory workload of patient-initiated mechanical ventilation. Am Rev Respir Dis 1986;134:902–909.

28. McCulloch T, Bishop M. Complications of translaryngeal intubation. Clin Chest Med 1991;12(3):507–521.

29. McDonald J, Barbieri C. Recurrent pneumothoraces in ventilated patients despite ipsilateral chest tubes. Chest 1995;108(4):1053–1058.

30. Meduri G. Diagnosis and differential diagnosis of ventilator-associated pneumonia. Clin Chest Med 1995;16(1): 61–93.

31. Meduri G. Diagnosis of ventilator-associated pneumonia. Infect Dis Clin North Am 1993;7(2):295–329.

32. Meduri G, Estes R. The pathogenesis of ventilator-associated pneumonia: II. The lower respiratory tract. Intensive Care Med 1995;21(5):452–461.

33. Morris A. Adult respiratory distress syndrome and new modes of mechanical ventilation: reducing the complications of high volume and high pressure. New Horizons 1994;2(1):19–33.

34. Myers E, Carrau R. Early complications of tracheostomy: incidence and management. Clin Chest Med 1991;12(3): 589–596.

35. Parker JC, Hernandez LA, Peevy KJ. Mechanisms of ventilator-induced lung injury. Crit Care Med 1993;21(1): 131–143.

36. Pingleton SK. Complications of acute respiratory failure. Am Rev Respir Dis 1988;137:1463–1493.

37. Quigley R. Thoracentesis and chest tube drainage. Crit Care Clin 1995;11(1):111–126.

38. Roupie E, Dambrosio M, Servillo G, et al. Titration of tidal volume and induced hypercapnia in acute respiratory distress syndrome. Am J Respir Crit Care Med 1995;152: 121–128.

39. Slutsky AS. Barotrauma and alveolar recruitment [editorial]. Intensive Care Med 1993;19(7):369–371.

40. Spencer M, Bird G. Device-related, nonintravascular infections. Crit Care Nurs Clin North Am 1995;7(4): 685–693.

41. Strieter R, Lynch J. Complications in the ventilated patient. Clin Chest Med 1988;9(1):127–140.

42. Sykes MK. Does mechanical ventilation damage the lungs? Acta Anaesthesiol Scand 1991;(Suppl 95)6:35–38.

43. Tocino I, Westcott J. Barotrauma. Radiol Clin North Am 1996;34(1):59–81.

44. Warner L, Beach T, Martino J. Negative pressure pulmonary oedema secondary to airway obstruction in an intubated infant. Can J Anaesth 1988;35(5):507–510.

45. West JB, Mathieu-Costello O. Stress failure of pulmonary capillaries: role in heart and lung disease. Lancet 1992; 340:762–767.

46. Wood D, Mathisen D. Late complications of tracheotomy. Clin Chest Med 1991;12(3):597–610.

47. Woodring JH. Pulmonary interstitial emphysema in the adult respiratory distress syndrome. Crit Care Med 1985; 13(10):786–791.

48. Zochodne DW, Bolton CF, Wells GA, et al. Critical illness polyneuropathy: a complication of sepsis and multiple organ failure. Brain 1987;110:819–841.

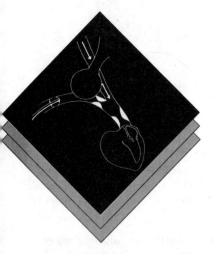

CHAPTER 9

Positive End-Expiratory Pressure

Hypoxemia resulting from alveolar collapse or liquid filling often responds to alveolar recruitment and maintenance of lung unit patency with positive end-expiratory airway pressure (PEEP). Adding PEEP helps keep lung units patent but further distends those that are already open. When PEEP maintains recruited lung volume, it may also reduce the elastic work of expanding the lung or improve the distribution of ventilation. Maintaining adequate end-expiratory lung volume helps prevent ventilator-induced lung injury during the initial stages of the acute respiratory distress syndrome (ARDS) and seems to be useful in avoiding complications after thoracic and upper abdominal surgery. Although PEEP may improve oxygen exchange and allow reduction of the inspired oxygen concentration (FiO_2), it has not been shown conclusively to improve survival.

This chapter focuses primarily on the use of PEEP in hypoxemic respiratory failure; this objective is quite distinct from that of adding PEEP to reduce the work of breathing and improve breath triggering (*without* increasing lung volume) during flow-limiting airflow obstruction. The latter important topic is addressed elsewhere (see Chapter 25, Ventilatory Failure).

"assisted ventilation with PEEP" and "continuous positive pressure breathing" (CPPB, CPPV) are synonymous, referring to mechanically delivered tidal breaths with positive pressure maintained at end expiration (Fig. 9.1). The term "continuous positive airway pressure" (CPAP) refers to spontaneous tidal breathing with a fixed amount of positive pressure applied to the airway opening throughout the ventilatory cycle (including end-exhalation). When two levels of PEEP are alternated, with spontaneous breaths occurring during each phase, the mode is termed "bi-phasic positive airway pressure" or "BiPAP." If the lower level is maintained only transiently (e.g., the span of a single breath), the mode is referred to as "airway pressure release." If only the exhalation line is pressurized, the terms "spontaneous PEEP" and "expiratory positive airway pressure" (EPAP) may be encountered. In this seldom used mode, the patient works much harder to breathe because negative inspiratory pressures must be generated from an elevated pressure baseline. Mean intrathoracic pressure, however, is lower than with other modes that elevate end-expiratory pressure. Several of these PEEP variants are discussed elsewhere in this volume (see Chapters 7 and 10). The discussion here will focus on single levels of end-expiratory alveolar pressure.

DEFINITIONS

Positive end-expiratory alveolar pressure or "total PEEP" ($PEEP_T$) is the sum of PEEP applied intentionally at the airway opening (PEEP or "extrinsic" PEEP) and auto ("intrinsic," "occult," or "inadvertent") PEEP. The expressions

PATHOPHYSIOLOGY

PRIMARY ACTIONS IN ACUTE HYPOXEMIC RESPIRATORY FAILURE (TABLE 9.1)

The normal lung requires no PEEP to maintain full expansion (recruitment)—periodic sighs are

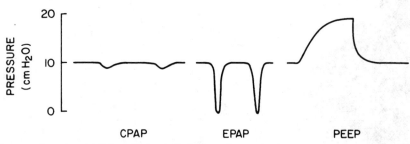

FIG. 9–1. Three modes of maintaining elevated airway pressure at end-exhalation. CPAP and expiratory positive airway pressure (EPAP) require the patient to supply the energy needed to ventilate.

TABLE 9–1

BENEFITS AND PROBLEMS OF PEEP

Benefits	Problems
Improves oxygenation	Predisposes to barotrauma
Reduces work of breathing	
Improves lung compliance	Impedes preload and right ventricular ejection
Aids the left ventricle	Reduces cerebral perfusion
Splints the chest wall	
Mobilizes distal secretions	Weakens the ventilatory pump
	Increases deadspace
	Confounds monitoring

sufficient to prevent or reverse widespread alveolar collapse. When the chest cavity is reduced in size (e.g., after abdominal surgery), the lung is edematous or infiltrated (e.g., pulmonary edema), or the alveoli are inherently unstable (surfactant depletion ARDS), small airways are predisposed to close during the tidal cycle, particularly in dependent regions in which the closing pressures and closing volume thresholds are highest. Evidence for this usually can be detected on the static pressure volume (PV) curve of the respiratory system, which displays a lower inflection region and increased hysteresis relative to the normal PV relationship. Collapsed units require a relatively high trans-alveolar pressure to open—typically > 20 cm H_2O. Once opened, a somewhat lower bias pressure applied to the airway opening (PEEP or CPAP) may then be needed to prevent widespread alveolar collapse and shunting.

PEEP applied to lung units that are already open only serves to increase alveolar dimensions, resting lung volume, and pleural pressure. This tends to redirect blood flow, increase vena caval resistance to venous return, and expand dead-space, even as it translocates alveolar water to the interstitial compartment. The use of PEEP in improving arterial oxygenation, in minimizing ventilator-induced lung injury, and perhaps in preventing pneumonia stems primarily from its ability to impede the recollapse of edematous or compressed alveoli recruited by higher pressures. In a heterogeneous lung with a wide range of unstable alveoli, alveolar opening may occur in different regions throughout inspiration, particularly when PEEP is low and V_T is high. When PEEP is added to an unchanging tidal volume, collapsed lung units are opened by the relatively high alveolar pressures (amplified by interdependence) that occur at the end of the inspiratory cycle; PEEP prevents their reclosure during expiration. Positive end-expiratory pressure also improves the distribution of alveolar liquid and translocates fluid from alveolar to interstitial spaces, lowering the diffusion distance for oxygen exchange. In the presence of alveolar edema, PEEP may prevent airway flooding by expanding the alveolar reservoir. (Conversely, abrupt removal of PEEP may precipitate translocation of alveolar liquid into the airways.) When PEEP reduces cardiac output, blood flow through shunt regions may also decline, reducing venous admixture. Most available data indicate that PEEP redistributes but does not decrease total lung water; in some instances, lung weight may actually increase, because of distention of the interstitial space and raised pulmonary venous and lymphatic pressures.

IMPORTANCE OF CHEST WALL COMPLIANCE

Volume changes resulting from PEEP are shared equally by the lungs and chest wall. Assuming that exhalation occurs passively, the volume recruited by PEEP (ΔV) depends on the compliance of the entire respiratory system,

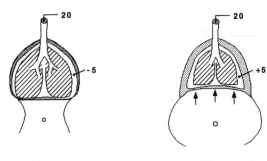

Normal   **Stiff Chest Wall**

FIG. 9–2. Effect of chest wall compliance on lung volume. The effect of positive airway pressure (in this case, 20 cm H_2O) on lung volume is influenced by the compliance of the chest wall. In this example, the distending force across the lung is 25 cm H_2O when the chest wall is normal, but only 15 cm H_2O when the chest wall is poorly compliant. A patient with a stiff chest wall requires a higher PEEP to achieve the same physiologic effect.

which itself is a function of both lung (C_L) and chest wall (C_w) compliances:

$$\Delta V = PEEP \times C_{RS}$$
$$= PEEP \times [(C_L\, C_W)/(C_L + C_W)].$$

As discussed elsewhere (Chapter 5), the pressure distending the lung at end expiration is ($PEEP_T - P_{PL}$), whereas the pressure that distends the passive chest wall is P_{PL} alone. It follows that the effect of PEEP will vary with the compliance of the chest wall (Fig. 9.2). A very obese patient or one with a recently operated abdomen or rib cage requires relatively more PEEP to keep the lung adequately recruited, and although P_{PL} tends to rise disproportionately with each PEEP increment, such patients may also tolerate higher levels of PEEP without cardiovascular compromise (see Cardiovascular Impairment, below).

INTERACTION OF PEEP AND TIDAL VOLUME

Recruitment of lung volume is a joint function of PEEP and tidal volume. Airways open at higher volumes and trans-structural pressures than those at which they close. Therefore, to achieve the same effect on oxygenation and compliance, higher values of PEEP are needed when tidal volumes are small (Fig. 9.3). Moreover, even if calculated tidal (chord) compliance values are identical, failure to maintain sufficient PEEP may result in tidal opening and closure of dependent lung units, a process that produces high shearing stresses believed to damage delicate lung tissues.

REGIONAL EFFECTS OF PEEP

Intrapleural pressure varies from site to site within the pleural space. In the supine position, a ventral-to-dorsal gravitational gradient causes the pleural pressure that surrounds dependent alveoli to be several cm H_2O greater than that in nondependent regions, and the difference increases in the setting of acute lung injury. (Although data are sparse, this gravitational gradient of pleural pressure is believed to be less steep in the prone position.) Because alveolar distention is a function of trans-alveolar pressure, regional alveolar dimensions and propensities to collapse differ, despite a common airway pressure. As progressively higher pressures are applied, individual alveoli pop open and then collapse abruptly as a critical pressure is withdrawn. PEEP sufficient to hold alveoli in the uppermost regions patent throughout the tidal cycle may be insufficient to prevent collapse of gravitationally dependent ones (Fig. 9.4). This gradient of pleural and transalveolar pressures is likely to explain the marked dependency of computed tomographic (CT) densities evident during the initial stages of acute lung injury, as well as the lower "inflection zone" of improving compliance on the pressure–volume curve of the respiratory system early in the course of ARDS. PEEP tends to narrow the pleural pressure gradient if recruitment occurs or alveoli in all regions are open. A PEEP value greater than that which recruits the most dependent alveoli may be needed to avoid tissue-damaging recruitment and recollapse during the tidal cycle. Interestingly, the PEEP value that corresponds to the highest pressure in this lower inflection zone can be predicted from the assumed pleural pressure gradient. With large tidal volumes, nondependent alveoli may be at risk of overdistention by these same PEEP values.

Regional Peep and the Prone Position

In experimental animals, the gradient of alveolar dimensions and pleural pressure is considerably greater in the supine position than in the prone position. Consequently, the prone position alters the distribution of lung volume corresponding to a given airway pressure, with dorsal regions dramatically better expanded (Fig. 9.5). In effect, altering position exerts a differential PEEP-like effect in different lung regions. Ventilation–perfusion matching and arterial oxygenation tend to improve. Available data suggest that a similar phenomenon also occurs in humans. The effect of prone positioning on overall functional residual capacity (FRC) is debated and is likely to be influenced by any positional changes that might occur

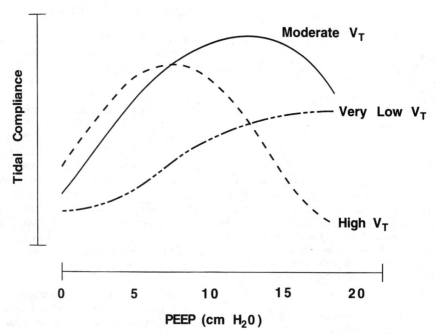

FIG. 9–3. Interaction of PEEP and tidal volume (V_T) in determining tidal compliance. Assuming that the clinical objective is to maximize tidal compliance, there is no single "best PEEP" value relevant to all tidal volumes. Higher values of PEEP are needed to achieve optimal compliance when small tidal volumes are used.

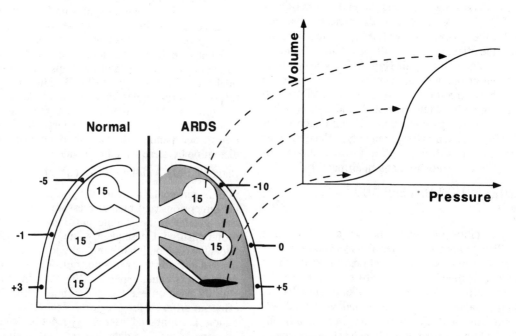

FIG. 9–4. Influence of the gravitational gradient of pressure on regional alveolar mechanics. Dependent alveoli at the base of the lung may remain collapsed at airway pressures that threaten to overdistend those in nondependent regions. Regional mechanics are especially heterogenous in the setting of ARDS. To counterbalance this gradient, higher regional PEEP in dependent areas or modified chest wall compliance in nondependent regions would be needed to improve the uniformity of distention and ventilation.

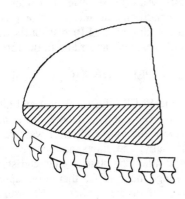

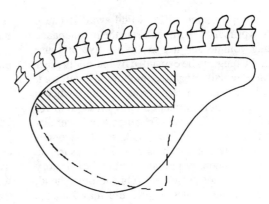

Supine   **Prone**

FIG. 9–5. Lung geometry in supine and prone positions. In the supine position, dorsal regions of the lung (cross-hatched) are subjected to higher pleural (and lower transpulmonary) pressures than they are in the prone position. These dorsal regions tend to expand dramatically in the prone position, whereas sternal regions are only modestly compressed. The prone position increases the overall resting lung volume (FRC) in most patients.

in chest wall compliance due to changes in support. Although the distribution of volume is altered dramatically, FRC increases only modestly or remains unchanged by the turning process.

ACTIVE EXPIRATION

If exhalation occurs passively (as it does during quiet, unstressed breathing), PEEP achieves its desired effect—an increase in end-expiratory lung volume and in the number of open air channels. However, if the resulting lung expansion proves uncomfortable, spontaneously breathing patients may actively oppose PEEP in attempting to limit the volume increase. Active expiration to a volume lower than the equilibrium position that corresponds to the PEEP applied to the passive patient stores potential energy. In this way, PEEP or CPAP may provide a mechanism by which the dyspneic or fatigued patient can use the expiratory muscles to share the inspiratory workload. As the expiratory muscles relax, the outward recoil of the chest wall then provides an inspiratory boost (Fig. 9.6). The expiratory muscles are activated normally during vigorous exercise, hyperpnea, and impeded expiration. Opposition to PEEP occurring in a hypoxemic patient may attenuate volume recruitment. By silencing the expiratory muscles, sedation or paralysis restores the volume recruitment effect of PEEP and can markedly improve oxygenation. The total work of breathing also may

be reduced as the ventilator assumes the task of powering ventilation.

TIME COURSE OF PEEP EFFECT ON GAS EXCHANGE

Although lung recruitment is nearly completed within three to five breaths, the time course is quite variable; several hours may be required to realize the full affect of a given PEEP increment. On the other hand, desaturation usually occurs

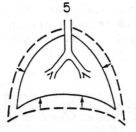 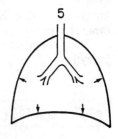

FIG. 9–6. The work-sharing concept. Expiratory muscles may force the lung below the equilibrium volume appropriate to the applied level of PEEP (in this case, 5 cm H_2O). This increases the expiratory work of breathing, reduces functional residual capacity, and tends to impair oxygenation. Thoracic compression against PEEP, however, stores energy for release in early inspiration, thereby sharing the ventilatory workload of the inspiratory muscles.

quite abruptly upon PEEP withdrawal. Because PEEP's primary benefit relates to the maintenance of lung volume and not to the positive pressure itself, the lung can be expanded by internally positive or externally negative pressure. Therefore, it should cause no concern for lost volume when a patient pulls an inspiratory airway pressure lower than the set PEEP level. To generate a lower airway pressure, pleural pressure must have decreased at least as much as alveolar pressure, so that transpulmonary pressure and end-expiratory lung volume are preserved. (On the other hand, such a decline in pleural pressure may indicate significant ventilatory work.)

PEEP AND MEAN AIRWAY PRESSURE

Mean alveolar pressure and its most easily measured analog, mean airway pressure, are discussed at length elsewhere in this text (see Chapters 5 and 24). It is worth noting here, however, that although mean alveolar pressure can be raised in a variety of ways, PEEP has the most predictable effect on oxygenation, raising both mean airway and mean alveolar pressures by the amount of the PEEP applied. Just as $PEEP_T$ corresponds to the end-expiratory alveolar dimension, in a passive patient, the mean airway pressure reflects the average or mean alveolar volume. Most cardiovascular effects of PEEP are mediated by mean alveolar pressure and its effects on mean intrapleural and right atrial pressures. Apart from its effect on mean airway pressure, $PEEP_T$ maintains collapsible alveoli recruited throughout the tidal breath; therefore, it is instrumental in improving oxygen exchange and avoiding ventilator-induced lung injury. (In fact, it has been argued that raising mean airway pressure while holding $PEEP_T$ constant may not help to improve arterial oxygen delivery.)

ADVERSE EFFECTS OF PEEP

CARDIOVASCULAR IMPAIRMENT

PEEP and Venous Return

At the end of passive exhalation, pressure within the central airway approximates alveolar pressure, provided that expiratory flow has stopped (see Auto-PEEP effect). Under these quasistatic conditions, an increment of pressure applied to the airway (PEEP) distributes across the lung and chest wall according to the formula:

$$\Delta P_{pl} = PEEP \times [C_L/(C_L + C_W)]$$

where P_{pl} and PEEP refer to pleural and airway pressures and C_L and C_W denote the dynamic compliances of the lung and chest wall, respectively. Normally, the lungs and passive chest wall have similar compliance characteristics in the tidal range near FRC; therefore, approximately one-half of the applied PEEP transmits to the pleural space. With abnormally stiff lungs, less is transmitted (typically, one-fifth to one-third). With compliant lungs and a stiff chest wall (e.g., in a patient with emphysema, obesity, or massive ascites), the pleural pressure increment is a higher fraction of applied PEEP (Fig. 9.2). Because pressures similar to P_{pl} surround the heart and great vessels, PEEP reduces venous return but tends to raise all intrathoracic vascular pressures. Such pressure changes complicate the interpretation of central venous pressure (CVP) and pulmonary artery occlusion (wedge) pressure.

Depression of cardiac output is seen rarely during the application of modest levels of CPAP to a spontaneously breathing patient. Compared with passive inflation, the magnitude of the CPAP-induced rise of mean intrapleural pressure is routinely small. Moreover, inspiratory descent of the diaphragm boosts intra-abdominal (and therefore upstream) venous pressures relative to their intrathoracic values, improving venous return.

In studies conducted on supine normal dogs, it has been shown that PEEP can also compress the inferior vena cava at the thoracic inlet, increasing the resistance to venous return (Fig. 9.7). Compression is likely to result, in part, from the lifting effect of PEEP on the heart. Lung expansion lifts the supine heart and depresses the diaphragm, thereby stretching the inferior vena cava, which is tethered at the diaphragm, pericardium, and retroabdomen. A relatively high external pressure also is likely to surround the vena cava just inferior to the diaphragm at end-inspiration. Whether caval compression is important when the lungs are stiff (and volume changes small, as they tend to be in ARDS) is an important unanswered question.

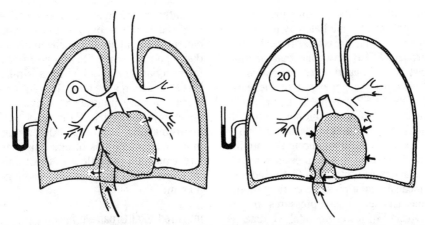

FIG. 9–7. Effects of PEEP on cardiovascular function. As PEEP holds the lungs distended, increased juxtacardiac pressure tends to compress the heart and great vessels, impeding venous inflow to the thorax while raising intracavitary and intravascular pressures. PEEP may also narrow the inferior vena cava at the inlet to the thorax, thereby increasing the resistance to venous return as well. Alveolar overdistention may significantly afterload the right ventricle.

PEEP and Ventricular Afterload

Although PEEP may raise pulmonary vascular resistance, this effect is relatively unimportant when the lung has a normal capacity to accept gas. Right ventricular performance remains little affected unless pulmonary capillary reserve is exhausted, the right ventricle is already failing, or peak and mean alveolar pressures rise to quite elevated levels. It is worth noting that only a small fraction of the lung may remain accessible to gas in the later stages of ARDS—typically one-third or less of the normal amount. The sum of gas, tissue, and liquid in the lung is approximately normal and equal to the volume occupied by the chest wall. Consequently, the cardiovascular consequences of alveolar overdistention, pulmonary hypertension, and right ventricular afterload may predominate over those caused by modest increases of pleural pressure. Even in less compromised lungs, extremely high levels of PEEP can increase right ventricular (RV) afterload sufficiently to cause RV dilation and thereby reduction of left ventricular compliance by the phenomenon of ventricular interdependence.

Left ventricular afterload is decreased by raising intrapleural pressure because the systolic myocardial tension that must developed to achieve any specified systemic arterial pressure is diminished by the extensive compression that results from augmented pleural pressure. Indeed, it has been shown that chest inflation synchronized to systole by a high frequency ventilator can improve cardiac output and blood pressure in patients with cardiac dila-

tation and congestive heart failure. Application of CPAP to patients with pulmonary edema helps reestablish cardiovascular stability through this mechanism, as well as by decreasing central vascular volume and improving arterial oxygenation and the work of breathing. High levels of PEEP have been suggested to cause myocardial dysfunction directly, but such effects, if present at all, are likely to be minor.

Compensation for PEEP-induced reductions in cardiac output may be accomplished by increasing heart rate, by raising venous tone, and by retaining sufficient intravascular fluid to raise the pressure driving venous return. These counterbalancing effects are maximized within hours to days. Cardiac output usually remains stable when moderate levels of PEEP are used in normovolemic patients with good cardiovascular reflexes and myocardial reserves. Repletion of intravascular volume, guided by the PEEP-adjusted wedge pressure, should be the primary treatment for depressed cardiac output resulting from PEEP. When adequate intravascular volume is ensured, vasopressors also may be added to improve the driving pressure for venous return.

BAROTRAUMA

Barotrauma during mechanical ventilation is discussed extensively elsewhere in this volume (see Chapter 8). The extent to which PEEP contributes to the tendency for pneumothorax and other forms of extraalveolar gas accumulation is unclear. When tidal volume remains unchanged, its primary effects may be mediated by increasing peak and mean alveolar pressures. If peak pressure is controlled, PEEP may contribute negligibly to the risk of alveolar rupture. In fact, when high tidal pressures are generated in the early stages of ARDS, PEEP may be instrumental in reducing shear stresses and avoiding ventilator-induced lung edema. It stands to reason that PEEP might accentuate the risk of rupturing alveoli that are weakened by disease if peak pressures are allowed to rise, and once ruptured, a PEEP-induced increase in mean alveolar pressure could promote additional gas leakage. These pressures are reduced effectively by lowering tidal volume as end-expiratory pressure is raised. A lower tidal volume with increased PEEP often results in hypercapnia, which can be either accepted (''permissive hypercapnia'') or offset by increasing the ventilator's cycling frequency.

REDUCED OXYGEN DELIVERY

Although it usually aids tissue oxygenation, PEEP may adversely affect oxygen delivery via three mechanisms: (1) decreased cardiac output, (2) increased venous admixture, and (3) increased intracardiac or noncapillary shunt. Oxygen delivery declines if the drop in cardiac output caused by PEEP outweighs the rise in arterial oxygen content. Assuming that metabolic demands remain unchanged, additional oxygen will then be stripped from arterial blood, dropping the O_2 saturation of mixed venous (pulmonary arterial) blood. In turn, reduced mixed venous O_2 saturation adversely affects arterial O_2 content, unless hypoxic vasoconstriction sufficiently limits admixture. Hence, when the adequacy of tissue oxygen delivery is in question, it is mandatory to follow cardiac output as well as SaO_2 during manipulations of PEEP, supplemented when feasible by determinations of mixed venous saturation, arterial-venous oxygen content difference $\Delta[(a - v)O_2]$, or other indications of tissue O_2 sufficiency.

Positive end-expiratory pressure may adversely alter the distribution of pulmonary blood flow. Positive transpulmonary pressure has its greatest-distending effect on compliant alveoli. As PEEP is raised to high levels, resistance to blood flow through compliant units increases disproportionately, redirecting blood flow toward stiffer, more diseased areas. Fortunately, any such diversion usually does not outweigh the benefits of alveolar recruitment and hypoxic vasoconstriction. PEEP may reduce PaO_2 by this mechanism in certain patients with highly regionalized disease that produces poorly recruitable (but perfused) lung units (e.g., lobar pneumonia). In a similar fashion, PEEP can increase shunt flow in a patient with intrapulmonary or intracardiac right-to-left vascular communications. Pulmonary arteriovenous malformations, atrial septal defects, and the pulmonary shunt vessels of cirrhosis may receive a larger percentage of flow as PEEP raises pulmonary vascular resistance and right heart filling pressure.

Impaired Vital Organ Perfusion

Cerebral Perfusion

PEEP increases cerebral venous and intracranial pressures (ICP) by raising CVP. Predictably, this increment is less when the lungs are stiff or heavily infiltrated and transmit less pressure to the pleural space; conversely, the CVP is higher when chest wall compliance is reduced. Lower arterial pressure (BP) or raised ICP can reduce cerebral perfusion pressure (CPP): CPP = BP − ICP. However, in the setting of intracranial hypertension, PEEP-related arterial hypotension presents a considerably greater risk for precipitating cerebral dysfunction than does central venous hypertension. (When ICP exceeds CVP, increases in CVP caused by PEEP do not transmit fully to the cerebral veins.) Abrupt application of PEEP can raise ICP and precipitate herniation in patients with intracranial mass lesions or seriously elevated ICP. (If CO_2 clearance is impaired by deadspace formation, a rising $PaCO_2$ also can contribute to intracranial hypertension.) Abrupt withdrawal of PEEP also can be dangerous; PEEP withdrawal can cause a surge in venous return, transiently boosting BP and ICP. Despite its potential dangers, PEEP generally can be used safely if high levels are avoided and if it is applied and withdrawn in small increments.

Hepatic and Renal Perfusion

An elevated CVP impedes venous drainage from the liver and thereby reduces hepatic perfusion. As with right heart failure, the resulting passive hepatic congestion can cause mild elevations of bilirubin and hepatic enzymes. Positive end-expiratory pressure also has been reported to interfere with renal function, even when cardiac output

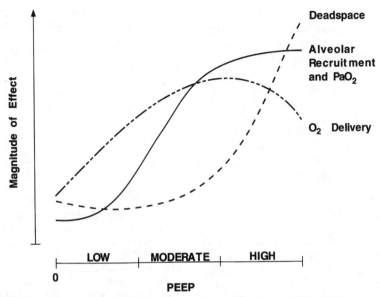

FIG. 9–8. Relationship of PEEP to alveolar recruitment, arterial oxygenation, oxygen delivery, and physiologic deadspace. Alveolar recruitment is marginal at high levels of PEEP, whereas deadspace fraction and cardiovascular compromise (as reflected in declining O_2 delivery) tend to increase.

is well preserved. Although a variety of mechanisms (reflex, humoral) have been proposed, none has been generally accepted. When PEEP contributes to excessive intra-abdominal pressure (e.g., after extensive abdominal surgery), pre-renal oliguria can result.

IMPAIRED CO_2 ELIMINATION

When alveolar recruitment is marginal or nearly maximized ($PEEP_T > P_{flex}$), PEEP impairs CO_2 elimination by overdistending patent and well-ventilated lung units, increasing their vascular resistance, and creating high ventilation/perfusion (V/Q) units (Fig. 9.8). Total pulmonary blood flow also may fall if venous return is seriously impeded. Such changes tend to expand the physiologic deadspace, increasing the ventilation requirement and encouraging CO_2 retention in patients with marginal ventilatory reserves. Fortunately, these effects usually are modest. Alveolar overdistention may be signalled by a widened difference between arterial and mixed expired or end-expiratory values of PCO_2.

ALTERATIONS IN THE WORK OF BREATHING

Although well-designed ventilator circuits maintain airway pressure nearly constant through-

out the spontaneous breathing cycle, many impose substantial external resistance, particularly when PEEP is employed. PEEP itself may either increase or decrease the work of breathing (W_B). Alveolar recruitment tends to reduce the W_B, but overdistention sometimes proves detrimental on two counts. First, lung compliance may worsen as additional volume is forced into a fully recruited lung, increasing the elastic workload. Second, chest distention limits the ability of the inspiratory muscles to perform work by placing them on a disadvantageous portion of their length–tension relationship and altering muscle geometry. When the expiratory muscles oppose volume recruitment, the total (inspiratory plus expiratory) W_B tends to increase. As already discussed, however, PEEP may redistribute the workload by facilitating transfer of inspiratory effort to the expiratory muscles.

CLINICAL USE OF PEEP

GOOD CANDIDATES FOR PEEP

Based on the foregoing discussion, good candidates for a trial of PEEP are those who have: (a) hypoxemia despite an elevated FiO_2, (b) diffuse acute pulmonary disease, (c) a poorly compliant respiratory system, (d) adequate cardiac reserve with normal to increased intravascular volume, (e) a tendency to atelectasis (e.g., after upper abdominal surgery), (f) acute cardiogenic or noncardiogenic pulmonary edema, (g) increased left ventricular afterload, (h) a pressure–volume relationship characterized by a lower inflection zone of rapidly improving compliance, (i) severe airflow obstruction with flow limitation during tidal breathing, characterized by increased work of breathing and inconsistency in triggering the ventilator.

POOR CANDIDATES FOR PEEP

Although there is a good rationale for using at least 3–5 cm H_2O PEEP or CPAP for almost every intubated patient (see below), poor candidates for higher levels have: (a) unilateral or localized lung disease, (b) normally compliant or emphysematous lungs, (c) subacute or chronic lung or chest wall disease, (d) cardiovascular compromise or hypotension resulting from intravascular volume deficit or right ventricular dysfunction, (e) severe intracranial disease or hypertension, (f) pulmonary hyperinflation without tidal flow limitation. Whatever the relative contraindications, a cautious and well-monitored trial of PEEP should not be withheld from apparently poor candidates with refractory hypoxemia.

PHYSIOLOGIC PEEP

Considerable volume loss occurs in moving from the upright to the supine horizontal position in all but severely obstructed patients (Fig. 9.9). (A normal young person loses about 1 L of lung volume in this transition. Because the compliance of the normal respiratory system approximates 100 mL/cm H_2O, this translates into a PEEP effect of approximately 7.5–10 cm H_2O.) Positional volume losses occur disproportionately in juxtadiaphragmatic regions. Other positional changes are also important to consider. Side-to-side turning increases the volume of the upper lung as the shifting abdominal contents alter regional chest wall compliance. Overall, FRC is slightly higher in the lateral decubitus position than in the supine position. The prone position helps dramatically for some patients with diffuse lung injury, presumably because it causes a regionally intense PEEP effect in the dorsal regions that most need it and/or because proning increases overall lung volume. PEEP may reduce the work of breathing and, in the earliest stage of ARDS, also may help

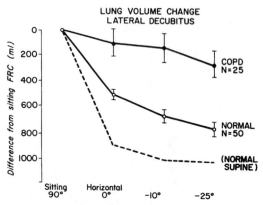

FIG. 9–9. Influence of lateral decubitus and supine postures on resting lung volume. In a normal subject, a volume loss of approximately 900 mL (equivalent to 5–10 cm H_2O PEEP) occurs in the transition from the sitting to the supine horizontal position. Somewhat less volume is lost in assuming the lateral decubitus position. Patients with severe airflow obstruction may lose very little volume but experience positional gas trapping or dramatically increased work of breathing. (Reproduced with permission from Marini JJ, et al. Am Rev Respir Dis 1984;129: 101–105.)

protect against ventilator-induced lung injury, lung infection, and dissemination of lung bacteria and the products of inflammation to the systemic circulation.

CHOOSING THE APPROPRIATE LEVEL OF PEEP

As end-expiratory pressure is raised, the effect is neither smooth nor predictable. Some patients show little response until very high levels (20–25 cm H_2O) are reached, at which point oxygen exchange may (or may not) improve remarkably; others respond adequately at 5 cm H_2O or less. As a rule, diffuse infiltrates are most responsive. Highly regionalized diseases, as demonstrated on CT scans, tend to be relatively refractory to PEEP. Knowledge of where $PEEP_T$ falls on the pressure–volume curve of the respiratory system may help predict the response to a given PEEP increment. Because the beneficial effect of PEEP on transpulmonary oxygen transfer parallels recruitment of collapsed lung units, PEEP responsiveness tends to be greatest during the earliest phase of acute lung injury, when edema and atelectasis are most prevalent. Low levels of PEEP may be insufficient to produce or maintain alveolar patency, especially when used in conjunction with modest tidal volumes. As more PEEP is added, peak inflation pressures rise and collapsed alveoli reinflate.

As a consequence, venous admixture falls and improving arterial oxygenation accompanies improving C_{RS}. After a certain value of PEEP, end-expiratory tangential compliance no longer improves with additional increments. $PEEP_T$ and tidal volume then lie above the P_{flex} zone of the static pressure–volume curve. To this point, adding PEEP usually has not depressed cardiac output and O_2 delivery steadily improves. Although generally less effective than those applied below P_{flex}, additional increments of PEEP above P_{flex} may still improve arterial oxygenation by several mechanisms. When used with a fixed tidal volume, higher values of PEEP boost peak alveolar pressure and thereby may cause end-inspiratory recruitment of units that PEEP can then keep open. More commonly, higher mean airway pressures may reduce cardiac output and shunt flow through diseased units. What happens to total oxygen delivery in this circumstance is unpredictable.

An important distinction should be drawn between *chord* compliance and *tangential* compliance (see Chapter 5). Because recruitment potentially can occur as lung units open at different pressures throughout the tidal cycle, the PEEP level associated with optimal chord compliance varies with tidal volume; smaller tidal volumes are associated with higher optimal PEEP values. There is no single value of PEEP that confers optimal chord compliance for all tidal volumes, and optimizing chord compliance does not guarantee that tidal opening and closure (a potentially injurious process) will not occur. Defining the inflection and deflection points of the pressure–volume relationship is the appropriate procedure.

Alternatives for Choosing "Optimal PEEP"

The effects of PEEP may vary with tidal volume, and the maximal response to a given PEEP increment—although generally rapid—may require 1 hour or more to establish. There is no consensus regarding what constitutes an optimal level of PEEP; however, oxygen saturation, oxygen delivery, venous admixture, lung compliance, and volume recruitment all have been used to guide its selection (Table 9.2). The PEEP values selected by these different strategies often—but not invariably—coincide. Whatever definition is used, it should be understood that, despite its effectiveness in improving O_2 saturation, adding PEEP may prove detrimental if it causes barotrauma or impairs O_2 delivery by reducing cardiac output. Most physicians choose the minimal level of PEEP required to provide acceptable arterial oxygen saturation (85–90%) on an FiO_2 less than

TABLE 9–2

ALTERNATIVE OUTCOME VARIABLES FOR "OPTIMAL PEEP"

O_2 saturation (arterial or mixed venous)
O_2 delivery
Minimal venous admixture
Best tidal compliance
Volume recruitment

0.5. Arterial O_2 saturation alone, however, does not tell the whole story. The mixed venous oxygen saturation (SvO_2) falls when the effects of reduced cardiac output and O_2 delivery outweigh the benefits of improved arterial O_2 saturation. (SvO_2 will fall if O_2 delivery is compromised, even as PaO_2 rises.) A close watch must be kept on peak and mean airway cycling pressures. A marginal boost in PaO_2 or in O_2 delivery may not be worth an increased risk of lung rupture. Many patients with good cardiac function compensate easily for small reductions in O_2 saturation, maintaining O_2 delivery by increasing cardiac output. Two factors are crucial in achieving adequate tissue oxygenation: a PaO_2 sufficient to maintain an appropriate gradient from capillary to mitochondrion and sufficient O_2 flux to satisfy tissue oxygen demands. Rather severe oxygen desaturation can be tolerated without adversity in patients with a healthy heart, a preserved ability to increase oxygen extraction (widen the $\Delta(a - v)O_2$), and an ample time to adapt. If compensatory mechanisms are limited, however, vital tissues may become oxygen deprived unless O_2 delivery is optimized. In this setting, oxygen consumption (CO times the difference between arterial and mixed venous oxygen contents) can provide useful information in gauging the need for added PEEP.

In some centers, an attempt is made to maximize oxygen delivery, even if the airway pressure required is higher than that which achieves 90% saturation. Believing that alveolar inflation improves healing of the injured lung, other clinicians attempt to reduce the shunt fraction below an arbitrary limit, as long as cardiac output can be maintained by fluids and vasopressors. An "optimal" PEEP can be selected without the benefit of wedge pressure or SvO_2 measurements by raising PEEP while monitoring "total thoracic compliance." Advocates of this method believe the level of PEEP, which maximizes (chord) compliance, coincides with the greatest oxygen delivery, lowest alveolar deadspace, and maximal alveolar recruitment. Although this is an attractive

TABLE 9–3

SELECTING PEEP

Define	Least tolerated PaO_2 or SaO_2
	Maximum tolerated FiO_2
	Least tolerated cardiac output
	Maximum tolerated P_{PK}
	Least tolerated tidal volume
Follow	PaO_2
	SaO_2
	Cardiac output (if available)
	Arterial Blood Pressure
	Plateau pressure
Sequence in early ARDS	Begin with PEEP = 7 cm H_2O
	Construct P–V curve or increase PEEP in steps of 2–3 cm H_2O to tolerance or desired effect
	Adjust V_T if peak pressure rises too high (volume-cycled ventilation)
	Consider raising target P_{set} (Pressure controlled ventilation)
	Consider adding recruiting breaths if $V_T < 5$ mL/kg

P_{PK} = End Inspiratory static ("plateau") pressure.

hypothesis, cardiac output may fall independently of changes in total thoracic compliance, and clinical experience suggests that this technique is unreliable. (As already noted, chord compliance varies as a joint function of PEEP and tidal volume. Moreover, for some patients, the peak of the compliance curve is not sharp; in others, total thoracic compliance may continue to rise as PEEP is raised to levels that induce hypotension.) Two other methods are variants of this optimal recruitment concept. The first compares arterial and end-tidal CO_2 tensions. This difference is minimized at the point of maximal recruitment and widens as overdistention increases deadspace. The second variation uses the static airway pressure–volume curve as a guide to identify the point of full lung recruitment.

The "Best PEEP" Trial

Rationale

To determine what level of PEEP is most beneficial, a systematic appraisal should be performed—the PEEP "trial" (Table 9.3). During the trial, PEEP level should be the only variable. Position, level of sedation, FiO_2, tidal volume or pressure control level, and all other ventilator set-

tings remain at fixed, safe levels. Infusions of fluids and cardiotropic and vasoactive drugs also should be maintained at constant levels. The trial should be initiated at the lowest PEEP judged appropriate for that stage of disease. There are two distinct advantages in selecting an FiO_2 as close as possible to that intended for use with PEEP after the trial is completed. First, it is not possible to predict with certainty what PaO_2 will do when FiO_2 is lowered from the trial level to that used for support. The ratio of PaO_2 to FiO_2 (the P/F ratio) serves to estimate what PaO_2 to expect at any given PEEP level, but the actual PaO_2 encountered in response to changing FiO_2 can be variable. Second, if an FiO_2 of 1.0 is selected for the trial, only shunt contributes to hypoxemia; therefore, a beneficial effect of lower levels of PEEP on V/Q mismatching can be missed.

Technique

Before the PEEP trial is started, the airway is suctioned free of secretions and consideration is given to using the prone or lateral decubitus position. After the patient is appropriately sedated, the trial is conducted by raising PEEP in increments of 2–3 cm H_2O every 10–20 minutes, to an arbitrary "upper end" limit (e.g., 15–20 cmH$_2$O) or until a clearly beneficial or detrimental response is seen. Airway pressure, thoracic compliance, O_2 saturation, blood pressure, heart and respiratory rates, and when available, cardiac output and/or SvO_2 should be measured at each level. Timing should be precise. (If arterial blood gases are drawn, changes in PEEP should not be delayed by the tardy return of previous results from the laboratory.) The entire trial should be completed expeditiously to minimize drift in PaO_2 due to factors other than changes in PEEP. However, sufficient time should elapse between increments to allow "slow responders" to improve. (It should be recognized that the PaO_2 values obtained at 20 minutes may underestimate the final response.) Because of such delays in response and because higher PEEP levels may open airways that remain patent at lower levels of PEEP, many clinicians begin at the upper end of the PEEP range and reduce PEEP to find the best value.

The level of PEEP selected will depend on the variable chosen to optimize (see Chapter 24, Oxygenation Failure). Although admittedly arbitrary, one rational method is to adopt the lowest level of PEEP that yields an O_2 saturation greater than 90% at an acceptable FiO_2 without depressing cardiac output or chest compliance. During the first few days of ARDS, many clinicians now insist on applying enough PEEP to position tidal volume above the lower inflection point of the PV curve, usually higher than 10 cm H_2O, even if O_2 exchange is adequate at a lower value.

PEEP WITHDRAWAL

Clinically unstable patients, i.e., those requiring an FiO_2 higher than 0.4 and those with worsening gas exchange, are poor candidates for PEEP withdrawal. However, after the first few days of supporting ARDS, it is important to withdraw PEEP to the lowest well-tolerated level. However, PEEP should be withdrawn cautiously, with oximetry or arterial blood gases monitored before and after each step change. The final reduction of PEEP (from 5 to 0 cm H_2O) should be done with special caution; failure to move successfully to the next lower level most often occurs in this range—perhaps because 3–5 cm H_2O PEEP offset positional reductions of lung volume (see Physiologic PEEP, above). A patient who has shown only marginal PEEP response is a possible exception to these guidelines. Abrupt or premature withdrawal of PEEP can cause deterioration of gas exchange, which may respond slowly to reinstitution of PEEP. Sudden termination of PEEP also can cause cardiovascular overload, increase the work of breathing, result in airway flooding with alveolar fluids, and precipitate dangerous increases in ICP.

"PROPHYLACTIC PEEP"

Some physicians administer low levels of PEEP (3–5 cm H_2O) "prophylactically" to all intubated patients. In the past, the practice of applying PEEP to all intubated patients was defended primarily on the grounds that bypass of the larynx causes FRC to fall. Although there is some documentation of altered FRC post-intubation, its physiologic basis remains unclear. The routine application of PEEP to the airway of patients who require intubation after surgery or trauma rests on firmer ground. As noted earlier, lung volume is reduced by recumbency. Moreover, PEEP could offset the additional fall in FRC known to occur in the first hours to days after thoracic or upper abdominal incisions (a factor contributing to atelectasis and impaired gas exchange). Thus, as long as intubation is required for other reasons and the patient is recumbent, adding 3–5 cm H_2O PEEP seems entirely defensible. At the present time, there is no convincing proof of benefit or danger from this approach. A PEEP of 8 cm H_2O (generally less than P_{flex}) has not been shown to protect routinely against the development of ARDS, whatever benefit PEEP might confer on O_2 exchange or lung mechanics once ARDS is under way.

"SUPER-PEEP"

Occasionally, very high levels of PEEP (>20 cm H_2O) must be applied to achieve acceptable O_2 saturation, especially in patients with massive obesity or ascites and in those who have sustained extensive trauma, burns, or surgery requiring massive fluid resuscitation. Although potentially hazardous, this technique may be justified occasionally if the chest wall compliance is greatly reduced and careful attention is paid to fluid and vasopressor support. Barotrauma is an ever-present risk. When using such high levels of PEEP, the need for it should be frequently re-assessed, and relatively low tidal volumes employed. Aggressive efforts must be made to reduce peak and mean cycling pressures as well as the minute ventilation requirement. Sedation, paralysis, and reducing tidal volume may prove helpful. A trial of "super-PEEP" may be justified in the very small number of desperately ill patients with appropriate anatomy and oxygenation failure that cannot be compensated for by safe concentrations of inspired oxygen and lower end-expiratory pressures. There is clear potential for a self-reinforcing cycle of "fluids $\rightarrow$ PEEP $\rightarrow$ impaired hemodynamics or O_2 delivery $\rightarrow$ fluids." Once initiated, repeated attempts at cautious PEEP withdrawal and fluid restriction or diuresis are prudent.

"AUTO-PEEP" EFFECT

For patients with severe airflow obstruction and high minute ventilation requirements, hyperinflation develops when ventilator cycling occurs before passive expiratory flow ceases. At normal lung volumes, elastic recoil and expiratory flow are inadequate at normal lung volumes to expel the full tidal volume (V_T) at the set frequency; however, active expiration and/or dynamic hyperinflation reestablishes the balance. Patients who trap air above the relaxed volume of the chest maintain positive pressure in the alveoli and small airways at end-exhalation. Hence, alveolar pressure remains continuously positive throughout the ventilatory cycle, raising intrathoracic pressure and often impeding venous return. Monitored pressure in the central airway remains nearly at the set level unless terminal expiratory flow is interrupted. Even then, the value recorded under stopped-flow conditions may seriously underesti-

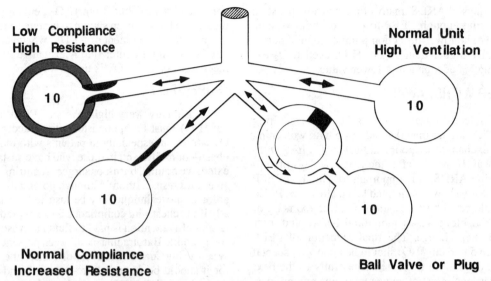

FIG. 9–10. Mechanisms and implications of auto-PEEP. Auto-PEEP can be generated in normal lung units because of increased ventilation (upper right), one-way or ball valving (as by a secretion plug, lower right) or a lengthy expiratory time constant (the product of compliance and resistance, left). As illustrated by the two images on the left, the same auto-PEEP value may or may not be associated with dynamic hyperinflation, depending on the mechanism for time constant prolongation.

mate the alveolar pressure existing in some regional units that are entirely blocked or "ball valved" during tidal ventilation (Fig. 9.10) (see Chapters 5 and 25). The distribution of auto-PEEP is quite heterogeneous, even in the same patient. Many units occluded at end-expiration, for example, seem to be located in dependent regions. Moreover, because the degree of overdistention of individual lung units is a direct function of their

compliance and fragility, the correlation between auto-PEEP and the hazard of barotrauma is imperfect, at best.

Unsuspected, this "auto-PEEP" (AP) effect can seriously reduce true cardiac filling pressures and confound interpretation of pulmonary artery and wedge pressures, raising them by an amount similar to the pressure transmitted to the pleural space (see Chapters 2 and 5). Because AP must

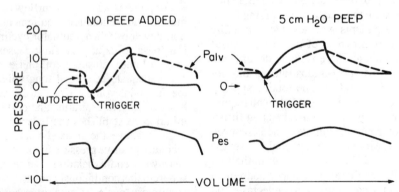

FIG. 9–11. The effect of PEEP on auto-PEEP in a patient with expiratory flow limitation during tidal breathing. Auto-PEEP represents a positive expiratory pressure that must be overcome by inspiratory effort (reflected by esophageal pressure, P_{es}) before the ventilator can be triggered or spontaneous breathing can begin. PEEP similar to the original auto-PEEP added downstream from the site of flow limitation does not slow expiratory airflow significantly. As auto-PEEP is counterbalanced, the inspiratory work of breathing declines. (Reproduced with permission from Smith TC, Marini JJ. Impact of PEEP on lung mechanics and work of breathing in severe airflow obstruction: the effect of PEEP on auto-PEEP. J Appl Physiol 1988;65(4):1488–1499.)

be reversed before inspiratory airflow can begin or the ventilator can be triggered, the ventilatory workload also rises in spontaneously breathing patients. Although AP is most predictable in patients with severe airflow obstruction, it occurs anytime the ventilator cycles automatically before the lung returns to its fully relaxed volume. Thus, auto PEEP can arise in normal lung units if the ventilatory rate is high enough. By adding to total PEEP, AP may have a therapeutic effect in edematous lung disease (e.g., when generated in inverse ratio ventilation). To reduce AP, it is crucial to reduce minute ventilation requirement, improve expiratory flow resistance, and lengthen the percentage of the ventilatory cycle spent in expiration. The cardiovascular consequences of AP can be minimized by increasing the rate of fluid or pressor infusion or by increasing the fraction of

spontaneous breathing efforts (e.g., by reducing intermittent mandatory ventilation frequency or substituting pressure support). The detection, consequences, and management of AP are discussed in greater detail in Chapters 2, 5, and 25.

PEEP on Auto-PEEP

Although PEEP is the sum of applied PEEP and auto-PEEP, adding PEEP to existing auto-PEEP may not raise *total* PEEP proportionately when expiration is flow limited during tidal breathing (Fig. 9.11). Substituting PEEP for auto-PEEP may improve triggering sensitivity, reduce the work of spontaneous breathing, or increase the tidal volume when pressure support is used. Finally, replacing auto-PEEP with PEEP may help even the distribution of ventilation.

KEY POINTS

1. Adding PEEP can help maintain patency of collapsed lung units or further distend those that are already patent. The former action usually is beneficial; the latter may cause alveolar overdistention. Both effects may occur simultaneously in different lung regions at the same level of PEEP.

2. Positive end-expiratory alveolar pressure or total PEEP is the sum of the PEEP applied intentionally at the airway opening (PEEP or extrinsic PEEP) and auto-PEEP ("intrinsic" or "inadvertent" PEEP) that results from dynamic hyperinflation or respiratory muscle activity.

3. Use of PEEP in improving arterial oxygenation, in minimizing ventilator-induced lung injury, and perhaps in preventing pneumonia stems primarily from its ability to impede the recollapse of edematous or compressed alveoli recruited by higher pressures during the tidal inspiratory phase or a sigh maneuver. PEEP also improves the distribution of alveolar liquid, translocating edema fluid from the alveolus to the interstitium. When PEEP reduces cardiac output, it also tends to reduce shunt fraction.

4. The volume recruiting effect of PEEP is influenced by the chest wall compliance, the tidal volume, and the activity of the respiratory muscles. Any benefit from PEEP on oxygen exchange may be offset by expiratory muscle activity and restored by muscle relaxation.

5. A shift to the prone position exerts a selective PEEP-like action in the dorsal regions of the lung.

6. PEEP tends to decrease both preload and

afterload to the left ventricle. Impaired venous return may lower cardiac output in a passive patient who does not have intact vascular reflexes or adequate circulating blood volume. Conversely, reduced left ventricular afterload resulting from PEEP may benefit the patient in acute congestive heart failure. The hemodynamic effects of auto-PEEP are similar to those of external PEEP.

7. Excessive PEEP may produce or extend barotrauma, reduce oxygen delivery, and increase ventilatory deadspace. PEEP may either increase or decrease the work of breathing.

8. Good candidates for PEEP have clinically significant hypoxemia that is refractory to inspired oxygen, diffuse acute pulmonary disease, a poorly compliant respiratory system, a tendency for atelectasis, acute cardiogenic edema with increased left ventricular afterload, a low compliance ("P_{flex}") zone on the pressure–volume curve of the respiratory system, or severe airflow obstruction with flow limitation during tidal breathing. Virtually all intubated patients are candidates for PEEP of 3–5 cm H_2O.

9. Choosing the optimum level of PEEP is a somewhat arbitrary process determined by the response of the variable selected for optimization to a well-monitored PEEP trial.

10. Auto-PEEP can dramatically increase the work of breathing and provoke patient-ventilator dysynchrony. In many patients with flow limitation, this limitation can be offset successfully by the addition of an appropriate level of PEEP that minimizes end-expiratory airflow without raising peak pressure significantly.

SUGGESTED READINGS

1. Brandolese R, Broseghini C, Polese G, Bernasconi M, et al. Effects of intrinsic PEEP on pulmonary gas exchange in mechanically-ventilated patients. Eur Respir J 1993; 6(3):358–363.
2. Brunet F, Jeanbourquin D, Monchi M, Mira JP, et al. Should mechanical ventilation be optimized to blood gases, lung mechanics, or thoracic CT scan? Am J Respir Crit Care Med 1995;152:524–530.
3. Carroll GC, Tuman KJ, Braverman B, Logas WG, et al. Minimal positive end-expiratory pressure (PEEP) may be "best PEEP." Chest 1988;93:1031–1035.
4. Chandra A, Coggeshall JW, Ravenscraft SA, Marini JJ, et al. Hyperpnea limits the volume recruited by positive end-expiratory pressure. Am J Respir Crit Care Med 1994; 150(4):911–917.
5. Dall'ava-Santucci J, et al. Mechanical effects of PEEP in patients with adult respiratory distress syndrome. J Appl Physiol 1990;68:843–848.
6. Gattinoni L, D'Andrea L, Pelosi P, Vitale G, et al. Regional effects and mechanism of positive end-expiratory pressure in early adult respiratory distress syndrome. JAMA 1993;269(16):2122–2127.
7. Kacmarek R, Kirmse M, Nishimura M, Mang H, Kimball WR, et al. The effects of applied vs auto-PEEP on local lung unit pressure and volume in a four-unit lung model. Chest 1995;108(4):1073–1079.
8. Kacmarek RM, Pierson DJ. Positive end-expiratory pressure. Respir Care 1988;33:419–630.
9. Kawagoe Y, Permutt S, Fessler HE. Hyperinflation with intrinsic PEEP and respiratory muscle blood flow. J Appl Physiol 1994;77(5):2440–2448.
10. Mancebo J. PEEP, ARDS, and alveolar recruitment. Intensive Care Med 1992;18:383–385.
11. Marini JJ. Should PEEP be used in airflow obstruction? (editorial). Am Rev Respir Dis 1989;140(1):1–3.
12. Patel H, Yang KL. Variability of intrinsic positive end-expiratory pressure in patients receiving mechanical ventilation. Crit Care Med 1995;23(6):1074–1079.
13. Pelosi P, Cereda M, Foti G, Giacomini M, Presenti A, et al. Alterations of lung and chest wall mechanics in patients with acute lung injury: effects of positive end-expiratory pressure. Am J Respir Crit Care Med 1995;152:531–537.
14. Pepe PE, Marini JJ. Occult positive end-expiratory pressure in mechanically ventilated patients with airflow obstruction. Am Rev Respir Dis 1982;126:166–170.
15. Popple C, Higgins TL, McCarthy P, Baldyga A, Mehta A, et al. Unilateral auto-PEEP in the recipient of a single lung transplant. Chest 1993;103(1):297–299.
16. Ranieri VM, Eissa NT, Corbeil C, Chasse M, et al. Effects of positive end-expiratory pressure on alveolar recruitment and gas exchange in patients with the adult respiratory distress syndrome. Am Rev Respir Dis 1991;144: 544–551.
17. Smith TC, Marini JJ. Impact of PEEP on lung mechanics and work of breathing in severe airflow obstruction: the effect of PEEP on auto-PEEP. J Appl Physiol 1988;65(4): 1488–1499.
18. Suter PM, Fairley HB, Isenberg MD. Effect of tidal volume and positive end-expiratory pressure on compliance during mechanical ventilation. Chest 1978;73:158–162.
19. Suter PM, Fairley HB, Isenberg MD. Optimum end-expiratory pressure in patients with acute pulmonary failure. N Engl J Med 1975;292:284–289.
20. Tobin B, Lewandowski V. Nontraditional and new ventilatory techniques. Crit Care Nurs Q 1988;11:12–18.

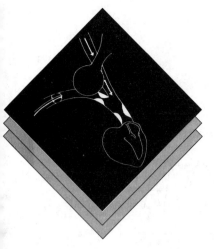

CHAPTER 10

Weaning from Mechanical Ventilation

Many patients tolerate abrupt termination of mechanical breathing assistance without needing to adjust to spontaneous breathing. However, when withdrawing machine support proves to be difficult, a strategy for transferring the respiratory workload to the patient must be developed. Weaning is the graded removal of ventilator support from patients who cannot tolerate immediate conversion to fully spontaneous breathing. The weaning process often takes place in several stages: weaning from positive pressure ventilation, weaning from positive end-expiratory pressure (PEEP), weaning from the endotracheal or tracheostomy tube, and weaning from supplemental oxygen.

PHYSIOLOGIC DETERMINANTS OF VENTILATOR DEPENDENCE

A continuing need for machine assistance may arise from O_2 desaturation of hemoglobin during spontaneous breathing, cardiovascular instability during machine withdrawal, psychologic dependence, or most commonly, imbalance between ventilatory capability and demand. Often, several of these causes operate simultaneously.

PSYCHOLOGICAL FACTORS

Prolonged mechanical ventilation is a harrowing experience that may elicit anxiety, depression, or psychosis. Delirium, manifested by inattentiveness, paranoid behavior, and disorientation, oc- curs very commonly in sleep-deprived and elderly patients receiving many medications that interfere with normal mental functioning (e.g., corticosteroids, benzodiazepines). A careful evaluation of mental status often is fruitful, because cooperation and avoidance of panic reactions during the weaning attempt may depend on control of the delirium. Ensuring sleep and the use of appropriate psychopharmacologic agents (e.g., haloperidol) can speed the process (see Chapter 17).

ARTERIAL HYPOXEMIA

Mechanical ventilation can improve arterial oxygenation by providing large tidal breaths that oppose atelectasis, sealing the airway to allow delivery of high inspired concentrations of oxygen and PEEP, reducing or offsetting the effects of pulmonary edema, improving the output requirements and loading conditions of a compromised heart and improving the balance between tissue oxygen delivery and demand. Under a high breathing workload, the respiratory muscles consume a great deal of oxygen. Stressful breathing may increase the oxygen demand of other body organs by causing agitation or discharge of catecholamines. When cardiac output is compromised, this increased oxygen demand may force greater O_2 extraction. The admixture of the desaturated mixed venous blood that results may then contribute to hypoxemia. Moreover, increased metabolic demands may cause myocardial decompensation, ischemia, or diastolic dysfunction. Mechanical ventilation mitigates these problems by relieving much of the ventilatory workload.

CARDIOVASCULAR INSTABILITY

Resuming a high ventilatory workload often presents a cardiovascular challenge in the setting of ischemic disease, heart failure, or reduced cardiac reserve. Inappropriately low cardiac output can contribute directly to hypoxemia and weakness of the ventilatory pump. Cardiovascular instability overtly limits the pace of ventilator withdrawal when chest pain, diastolic dysfunction, or arrhythmias develop during the reloading of the respiratory system. Hypoxemia, altered cardiac loading, and the stress-related release of catecholamines frequently provoke rhythm disturbances in the transition to spontaneous breathing. The assumption of the spontaneous breathing workload simultaneously increases both preload and afterload of the left heart, as well as increases anxiety and the work of breathing. Overall $\dot{V}O_2$ and cardiac output can easily double at a time when the heart is least well equipped to provide it. Consideration must be given to gradually withdrawing ventilatory support for these patients and to ensuring sufficient diuresis and afterload reduction (e.g., by adding an ACE inhibitor) before the weaning attempt. One interesting and physiologically valid approach may be to titrate nitroprusside to the escalating need of the patient as support is withdrawn.

Oxygen administration, improved electrolyte and pH balance, antiarrhythmic therapy, afterload reduction, antiischemic measures, diuresis, and more gradual conversion to fully spontaneous breathing may be instrumental to the success of machine withdrawal. For patients with coexisting airflow obstruction and left ventricular disease or ischemia, assuming a high ventilatory workload can be associated with a fall (rather than a rise) in mean intrapleural pressure. As forceful inspiratory efforts lower the pressure surrounding the left heart, its effective afterload increases, causing ischemia and/or pulmonary vascular congestion (Fig. 10.1). In such circumstances, it is essential to reduce total ventilatory demands by measures that improve lung mechanics and reduce minute ventilation. The use of continuous positive airway pressure (CPAP) or noninvasive ventilatory support may be strikingly effective. Pharmacotherapy to improve cardiac function or relieve ischemia also can be helpful.

IMBALANCE OF VENTILATORY CAPABILITY AND DEMAND

To sustain spontaneous ventilation, both ventilatory drive and endurance must be adequate. Im-

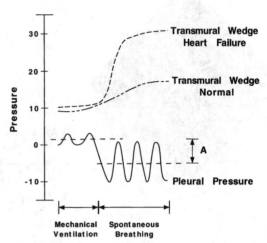

FIG. 10–1. Influence of spontaneous breathing on left ventricular filling pressure in patients with airflow obstruction. After an abrupt transition to spontaneous breathing, the increased effort results in marked decline of pleural pressure. Transmural wedge pressure increases as mean intrapleural pressure falls (A). For patients with left ventricular failure, the increased afterload and oxygen consumption may dramatically elevate transmural wedge pressure, producing pulmonary congestion.

paired ventilatory drive often contributes to CO_2 retention or hypoxemia, especially when excessive sedation or chronic hypercapnia are present. The most common reason for ventilator dependence, however, is the inability to maintain appropriate ventilation without intolerable dyspnea. The total ventilatory workload is determined by the product of minute ventilation requirement ($\dot{V}_E$) and the energy expended per liter of gas flow.

Ventilatory Demand: Minute Ventilation Requirement

Reducing the minute ventilation requirement is an important goal because $\dot{V}_E$ bears a quadratic (rather than linear) relationship to the work of breathing. Three primary factors determine the $\dot{V}_E$ requirement: the CO_2 production, the efficiency of ventilation, and the sensitivity of the central drive mechanism (Table 10.1).

CO_2 Production

Fever, shivering, pain, agitation, increased work of breathing, sepsis, and overfeeding are common causes of increased CO_2 production in the intensive care unit (ICU). In the weaning

TABLE 10–1

FACTORS AFFECTING VENTILATORY DEMAND

CO_2 Production	$\uparrow V_D/V_T$	$\uparrow$ Drive
Fever	Lung disease	Neurogenic
Shivering	Hypovolemia	Psychogenic
Pain/agitation	Vascular occlusion	Metabolic
Trauma/burns	External apparatus	Acidosis
Sepsis	Excessive PEEP	Hypoxemia
Overfeeding		Sepsis
Work of		Hypotension
breathing		

phase, cautious anxiolysis and pain relief can dramatically reduce the ventilatory requirement. Carbon dioxide production is also influenced by underlying nutritional status, as well as by the number and composition of the calories administered. The semistarvation that often precedes critical illness suppresses CO_2 production. Despite the importance of adequate nutrition, patients should not be overfed. Excess calories may be converted to fat, generating CO_2 as a metabolic byproduct unrelated to energy production. Carbohydrate evolves more CO_2 per calorie than fat or protein. However, even though large calorie loads can contribute to ventilatory failure, the importance of calorie composition to ventilator dependence remains to be shown convincingly. Overfeeding also may lead to abdominal distention and discomfort that may adversely impact a patient poised at the boundary of ventilatory failure.

Ventilatory Efficiency

Alveolar ventilation ($\dot{V}_A$), the component of ventilation that is effective in eliminating carbon dioxide, is the total minute ventilation adjusted for the fraction of wasted ventilation. Breathing efficiency can be characterized by the following expression:

$$\dot{V}_A = \dot{V}_E (1 - V_D/V_T)$$

where $\dot{V}_D/\dot{V}_T$ is the physiologic deadspace fraction (see Chapter 5, Respiratory Monitoring). Virtually all of the diverse processes that damage the lung or airways of the critically ill patient increase the wasted fraction of ventilation. Certain reversible factors unrelated to underlying lung pathology also can prove to be important. For example, thromboembolic or vasculitic arterial occlusion or

hypovolemia may reduce perfusion to the ventilated lung, expanding the alveolar deadspace. Small tidal volumes are characterized by a high anatomic deadspace percentage. Adding "apparatus deadspace," disposable heat and moisture exchangers, and other devices or tubing interposed between the endotracheal tube and the "Y" of the ventilator circuit may contribute to ventilatory inefficiency and slow the pace of weaning.

Central Drive

Inappropriately attenuated or enhanced drive to breathe may limit weaning progress. Suppressed ventilatory drive may be explained by advanced age, neurologic impairment, hypothyroidism, excessive sedation, sleep deprivation, and metabolic alkalosis (primary or compensatory). Enhanced central drive arising from neurogenic, psychogenic, reflex, or metabolic stimuli augments ventilatory demand and workload. In conditions such as asthma and acute pulmonary edema, drive-stimulating reflexes arising from the lung or chest wall reverse after correcting the underlying disorder. Hypoxemia, hypotension, developing sepsis, and acidosis also accentuate ventilatory demands. Correction of metabolic acidosis is one of the most important ways to reduce central drive. It is also important not to force $PaCO_2$ below the patient's usual resting value, as the ensuing bicarbonate diuresis redefines the $\dot{V}_E$ needed to maintain (cerebral pH) homeostasis. In fact, a $PaCO_2$ somewhat higher than normal for that patient may help minimize the $\dot{V}_E$ requirement and promote ventilator independence. Anxiety influences ventilatory demand and often can be addressed successfully by counseling, co-opting the patient into the weaning plan, and cautious use of anxiolytics or major tranquilizers (e.g., haloperidol). Supplementing the inspired O_2 fraction is often an effective way to reduce drive and interrupt a panic reaction accompanied by worsening hypoxemia.

Ventilatory Demand: Work per Liter of Ventilation

Intrinsic Factors

Ventilatory power is the product of $\dot{V}_E$ and mechanical work of breathing per liter of ventilation. The quotient of this mechanical workload and neuromuscular efficiency defines how much energy must be expended in breathing. Once tidal

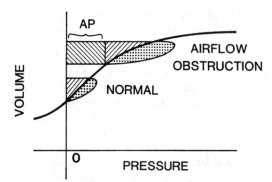

FIG. 10-2. Pressure–volume relationships of the respiratory system for a normal patient and for one with airflow obstruction. The inspiratory work of breathing is increased in patients with airflow obstruction, due to elevated airflow resistance (stippled area), increased elastance at higher lung volume, and auto-PEEP (AP).

volume and inspiratory time are set, the frictional and elastic properties of the respiratory system determine the pressure generated per breath, as well as the external work output per liter of ventilation. The average inspiratory pressure developed by the respiratory system per breath can be approximated as a simple formula:

$$P = R (V_T/t_i) + (V_T/2C_{RS}) + \text{auto-PEEP}$$

where R and C_{RS} are the inspiratory resistance and compliance of the respiratory system, V_T is tidal volume, and t_i is the time required for inspiration (see Chapter 5 and Fig. 10.2). Therefore, for the same level of $\dot{V}_E$, more external work must be done if C_{RS} falls or if V_T, auto-PEEP, mean inspiratory flow (V_T/t_i), or R increase. Bronchospasm, retained secretions, and mucosal edema are the primary reversible factors that increase R. Retained secretions greatly amplify the inspiratory workload in patients with already narrowed airways. Lung edema and infiltration, high lung volumes, pleural effusions, abdominal distention and the supine posture (to a minor extent) reduce C_{RS}. Auto-PEEP is discussed elsewhere in this volume. However, it should be pointed out here that air trapping and auto-PEEP are highly dynamic phenomena influenced powerfully by minute ventilation and the ease with which gas empties from the lungs. Auto-PEEP varies with changes in the breathing impedance (e.g. bronchospasm, secretion retention, minute ventilation, body position, alteration of inspiratory time fraction, and expiratory muscle activity). Auto-PEEP also varies widely in different regions of the lung,

depending on their regional mechanics. Because auto-PEEP distends both lung and chest wall, a given level of auto-PEEP may be associated with very different degrees of alveolar distention at hyperinflation, depending on the relative values of lung and chest wall compliance.

These are not the only factors that determine the energy needed by the respiratory muscles, however. For the same tidal volume, the respiratory muscles consume more oxygen (become less effective) when they begin contraction from a mechanically disadvantageous high lung volume or when the pattern of muscle contraction is poorly coordinated. For example, patients with diaphragmatic weakness may allow the abdominal contents to be drawn upward with each inspiratory effort, so that much of the tension developed by the inspiratory muscles of the chest cage fails to translate into the negative pleural pressure that draws air into the lungs. It is easy to see why patients with chronic obstructive pulmonary disease (COPD), in whom hyperinflation with narrowed airways is combined and a tendency to retain secretions, often have difficulty sustaining spontaneous ventilation.

Extrinsic Factors

The external properties of the ventilator circuit also can play an important role in determining the ventilatory workload. Endotracheal tube resistance exceeds the normal resistance of the upper airway. Frictional pressure losses increase rapidly when high flows are driven through small-caliber tubes. Kinks and encrusted secretions may encroach on an otherwise adequate lumen. In some instances, it may be wise to exchange an orotracheal tube for a larger one (e.g., via a tube changer; see Chapter 6) or replace a nasotracheal tube with an orotracheal one. Tracheostomy is worth considering to reduce resistance and facilitate extraction of airway secretions in particularly difficult patients. As a rule, all applied ventilator pressure (including pressure–support ventilation [PSV] and CPAP) should be withdrawn before extubation to test the marginal patient's ventilatory reserve (see below). Occasionally, however, extubation with some pressure still applied accelerates ventilator withdrawal, especially when the patient bites the tube, the patient experiences extreme discomfort, or a narrow bore tube hinders airflow and impedes (rather than assists) secretion hygiene. Largely for these reasons, many patients tolerate direct extubation or rapid weaning better than gradual removal of pressure support or synchronized intermittent mandatory ventilation (SIMV).

Although the expiratory phase is unaided by the ventilator, expiratory circuit resistance is often severalfold greater than effective inspiratory circuit resistance, primarily due to the unavailability of an expiratory pressure support to overcome tube and expiratory valve resistance. Valving problems become especially important at high breathing frequencies and ventilation levels. High expiratory resistance can result in uncomfortable sensations that stimulate more forceful inspiratory efforts, a consideration that may be important during machine-aided tidal cycles. Although pressure support can help overcome inspiratory resistance, no currently available technique offsets expiratory resistance. Full-cycle tube compensation and control of airway pressure near the carina are promising future options.

Tracheostomy often may be helpful because larger tube diameter, shorter axial length, and improved secretion clearance minimize resistance. The resistance of other circuit components varies widely and can add significantly to the ventilatory burden. Considerable effort may be needed to draw conditioned gas through the ventilator during the spontaneous breaths of SIMV or CPAP. (On the other hand, the addition of low-level CPAP can compensate for microatelectasis or auto-PEEP, thereby reducing the work of breathing.)

Ventilatory Capability

The ability to sustain an acceptable effort is determined by respiratory drive and muscle performance.

Central Drive

Although it is unusual for a patient to remain persistently ventilator-dependent solely because of a lack of breathing effort, multiple interacting factors can suppress the output of the ventilatory drive center. As a rule, old and debilitated patients are the most susceptible to drive suppression. Sedatives and neurologic impairment generally receive adequate clinical attention. However, other important causes of drive suppression may be potentially reversible. For example, chronic loading of ventilation (as during a severe bout of asthma) can condition the ventilatory center to tolerate higher $PaCO_2$. Metabolic alkalosis, hypothyroid-

ism, and sleep deprivation are commonly overlooked as causes of impaired ventilatory drive. Because the output of the ventilatory center tends to parallel metabolic rate and caloric intake, nutritional status is important. Starvation impairs hypoxic and, to a lesser extent, hypercapnic sensitivity. Interestingly, drive is restored rapidly within a few days of reinitiating adequate feeding, perhaps in advance of improved muscle function. Experimentally, the composition of the calories ingested seems to be influential: amino-acid infusion evokes a particularly prompt and convincing enhancement of hypercapnic drive. The drive to breathe is generally higher and the breathing pattern is different in the waking state. Minute ventilation occasionally falls markedly during sleep or sedation and accelerates impressively with the return to alertness. (This pattern often applies to the recovering drug overdose victim.) The administration of pharmacologic stimulants such as doxapram or progesterone has been advocated when depressed drive impedes weaning. These drugs, however, usually are not helpful.

Muscular Performance

Strength With intact ventilatory drive and normal impedance of the respiratory system, carbon dioxide retention is uncommon if the patient can generate more than 25% of the predicted maximum inspiratory pressure against an occluded airway. The strength of the respiratory muscles is determined by muscle bulk, the intrinsic properties and loading conditions of the contractile fibers, and the chemical environment in which the muscle contracts. Poor nutrition causes muscle wasting and thereby limits maximal respiratory pressures. As overall body weight diminishes, the mass and strength of the diaphragm decrease proportionately. Glucocorticoids accelerate the rate of protein catabolism. Optimal concentrations of calcium, magnesium, potassium, phosphate, hydrogen ion, chloride, and carbon dioxide are each important in maximizing muscle performance. Hypoxemia tends to impair endurance more than muscle strength.

Certain commonly used drugs—particularly antibiotics (e.g., aminoglycosides) and antiarrythmics (e.g., calcium channel blockers) also contribute to weakness in the setting of myasthenia gravis or other underlying neuromuscular impairment (see Chapter 17). Conversely, aminophylline and β-sympathomimetic drugs may modestly improve contractility and endurance. Intriguing experimental data suggest that the resting potential of the skeletal muscle membrane may remain abnormal for several days after sepsis and perhaps other critical illnesses. Moreover, a ''critical illness neuropathy'' may help to explain the prolonged and impressive muscle weakness observed in many of these patients after the acute phase has passed. The extended suppression of neuromuscular excitation by paralytic agents may result in very profound weakness for lengthy periods after they are discontinued, especially when corticosteroids have been used concomitantly as in status asthmaticus (see Chapter 17).

Contractile Fiber Properties The contractile force developed by a stimulated muscle fiber relates directly to its resting length at the onset of contraction and inversely to its speed of contraction. Force output is therefore compromised when a patient inhales rapidly from high lung volume, as so often occurs in breathless, hyperinflated patients with COPD or asthma (see Chapter 25, Ventilatory Failure).

Endurance

Endurance, the ability of a muscle to sustain effort, is determined by the balance between the supply and demand of muscular energy. Hypoxemia, anemia, and ischemia are especially important to correct, because working muscles require an adequate flow of well-oxygenated blood for optimal performance. Although the respiratory muscles receive sufficient blood flow under normal circumstances and can access a large recruitable reserve, even this luxuriant supply may be insufficient under conditions of high stress and a failing cardiac pump. Studies of patients in acute respiratory failure indicate that spontaneous breathing routinely consumes approximately 25% of the oxygen used by the entire body and even more during flagrant respiratory distress. (The normal percentage of respiratory oxygen consumption at rest is approximately 1%.) Although current data are inconclusive, inadequate O_2 delivery to vital organs (as gauged by falling gastric mucosal pH) may limit weaning progress in some patients.

Over the years, many attempts have been made to gauge endurance by comparing spontaneous breathing cycles with maximal voluntary efforts. For example, the ability to voluntarily double $\dot{V}_E$ or tidal volume has been considered a positive predictive sign. Unfortunately, such voluntary indices require patient cooperation. Recently, however, indices that do not require full patient cooperation have moved from the physiology laboratory to the bedside. Two such measures are the ratio of average inspiratory pressure to maximal inspiratory isometric pressure ($\overline{PP}_{max}$) and the inspiratory effort quotient (IEQ)—the product of $\overline{P}/P_{max}$ and the inspiratory time fraction (t_i/t_{tot}). $\overline{P}/P_{max}$ ratios greater than 0.4 and IEQs greater than 0.15 indicate that the patient is approaching the threshold of fatigue. $\overline{P}$ can be estimated as already described, and P_{max} is the maximal inspiratory pressure generated during airway occlusion.

The respiratory pattern gives important clues to ventilatory compensation. The respiratory frequency (f) is the most sensitive but least specific indicator of developing problems. Early in the course of respiratory muscle fatigue, f increases. Preterminally, frequency often diminishes—a harbinger of approaching apnea. The respiratory rhythm tends to lose regularity as the fatigue threshold is approached. In responding to an increased ventilatory workload (e.g., increasing exercise), a healthy and well-compensated subject will increase both frequency and tidal volume together. Although tidal volume may reach a plateau value while frequency is still rising, tidal volume does not fall and the ratio of frequency to tidal volume rarely exceeds 50 breaths/minute/L, even during the most vigorously sustained exercise. It has been suggested that a ratio of frequency to tidal volume that exceeds 100 breaths/minute/L indicates a severe and unsustainable workload, as the patient fails to generate sufficient pressure to achieve a tidal volume appropriate to the minute ventilation requirement. The result is inefficient gas exchange and, ultimately, failure to wean from ventilatory support.

Other components of the respiratory pattern, although harder to quantitate, provide equally valuable diagnostic clues. At moderate levels of exertion, pressure in the abdomen rises as the diaphragm contracts, displacing the abdominal contents downward and outward; expiration, which occurs passively at low levels of exertion, often becomes active. Vigorous activity recruits the thoracic musculature, elongating the chest and expanding the rib cage. If diaphragmatic contraction is not forceful enough, the abdomen retracts paradoxically during inspiration. During expiration, the thoracic muscles relax and the abdominal contents return to their original position. When observed in the supine position, this phenomenon, known as paradoxical abdominal motion, indicates a high level of exertion relative to the capability of the diaphragm. Paradoxical abdominal motion may be observed routinely in well-compensated patients with severe airflow obstruction. Some clinicians view the development of this finding as an indicator of established muscle fatigue, but more likely, it is only a sign of high workload that may or may not be tolerable. Much less commonly, the ribcage and abdomen alternate primary responsibility for driving inspiration, a pattern known as respiratory alternans. Overt respiratory alternans is much less commonly observed than paradoxical abdominal motion and, when present, often has a neuropathologic origin.

Importance of Muscle Rest   To reverse fatigue, the primary intervention is to rest the muscles. Total rest certainly is not required, but a substantial fraction of the imposed workload must be relieved. Assisted mechanical ventilation, optimally adjusted to meet patient demands, usually allows the patient to rest sufficiently to achieve this purpose. As a rule, the support level can be assumed to be adequate if the alert patient is made comfortable. How long a skeletal muscle must be rested before it fully recovers from fatigue is not known with certainty. However, physiologic evidence of subnormal performance can be detected in the laboratory setting for 12 to 24 hours after an acutely fatiguing load is applied briefly (<30 minutes). Therefore, a rest period of at least 12 to 24 hours seems appropriate after an episode of acute decompensation. Because recovery may be prolonged, the patient must not be allowed to fatigue by giving insufficient ventilatory assistance during the support phase of ventilation—or even during a failing weaning trial.

Other Considerations

Neural injury and regional neuromuscular dysfunction of the diaphragm are not uncommon in the critical care setting. For example, phrenic nerve dysfunction occurs frequently after cardiothoracic surgery and may be slow to resolve. Transient functional impairment of the diaphragm has been documented after upper-abdominal operations. Such dysfunction of the respiratory muscles tends to resolve over a period of a few days to weeks.

PREDICTING WEANABILITY

Many predictive indices based on ventilatory performance have been suggested to accurately forecast the outcome of the weaning trial (Table 10.2). However, if the patient is ventilator-dependent for reasons unrelated to muscle strength (e.g., hypoxemia, cardiac ischemia, or psychological factors), such indices are of little use. Their predictive performance is equally limited for patients ventilated over the very long term. Even when impaired ventilatory power and endurance are responsible, no single index has been universally successful, perhaps because multiple factors cause the patient to remain ventilator-dependent. One widely used panel of indicators tests $\dot{V}_E$, muscle strength, muscle reserve, and respiratory impedance. Patients who are successfully weaned from mechanical support generally have a $\dot{V}_E$ lower than 10 L/minute, a maximally negative inspiratory pressure exceeding -20 cm H_2O, and an ability to double the baseline $\dot{V}_E$ upon command. In practice, the problem with using such a panel of criteria is twofold: only selected components can be measured in uncooperative patients, and there is uncertainty when only one or two indices lie within the acceptable range. Thus, although these time-honored criteria are reliably predictive when all are satisfied or violated, they are of questionable assistance in difficult cases.

INVOLUNTARY MEASURES

Arterial Blood Gases and Pulse Oximetry

Although not reliable predictive indices per se, arterial blood gases and pulse oximetry are invaluable aids in gauging the progress of a weaning trial, especially when trends are followed. They are of limited value, however, unless the conditions under which they were measured are well documented.

Minute Ventilation

Ventilatory requirement and patient capability can be assessed crudely by $\dot{V}_E$ and the maximal inspiratory pressure (MIP) generated against an occluded airway. Although $\dot{V}_E$ is easy enough to measure, it should be interpreted with regard for body habitus, metabolic rate, and pH. For example, a 50-kg patient with respiratory acidosis at the time of $\dot{V}_E$ measurement, may have a minute ventilation of only 10 L/minute and be unable to resume spontaneous unaided breathing. Conversely, a patient weighing 100 kg with respiratory alkalosis may wean easily at the same level. However, valuable as $\dot{V}_E$ may be, it only tells part

TABLE 10-2

PREDICTORS OF WEANABILITY*

	Measured Values			Clinical Observations	
Ventilation	Strength		Endurance	Neuromuscular	Other
$\dot{V}_E \leq 10-15$ L/minute** $\dot{V}_E \leq 175$ mL/kg/minute	MIP > -20 cm H_2O $V_T \geq 5$ mL/kg VC ≥ 10 mL/kg		MVV $> 2 \times \dot{V}_E$ VC $> 2 \times V_T$ IEQ < 0.15 f < 30/minute f/$V_T < 100$ $P_{0.1} < 6$ cm H_2O	Absence of scalene or abdominal muscle activity Asynchrony Irregular breathing Rapid shallow breathing	$FiO_2 \leq 0.4$ $70 <$ pulse < 120 pH > 7.30 BP > 80 mm Hg

* For abbreviations, see text.
** Depending on body size.

of the story of ventilatory demand; work per liter of ventilation is equally important in this assessment, as already discussed. Just as importantly, demand always must be related to capability.

Spontaneous Breathing Pattern

Patients who are well adjusted to the ventilatory workload usually choose tidal volumes greater than 4 to 5 mL/kg of body weight and breathing frequencies lower than 30/minute. Although each breath taken with a shallow tidal volume is less energy costly than a deeper breath, the total energy expenditure necessary to maintain a given $\dot{V}_E$ may be greater, inasmuch as anatomic deadspace occupies a larger percentage of each breath during shallow breathing. Therefore, patients who must breathe at frequencies greater than 35 per minute usually do so because they are too weak or fatigued to inspire to an appropriate depth. (Some patients with neurologic disease or severe chronic restrictive disease (e.g., massive obesity, kyphoscoliosis, interstitial fibrosis) assume rapid shallow patterns because of disordered ventilatory control or reflex stimulation and may wean successfully at frequencies greater than 40 per minute.) The breathing pattern assumed during a brief (5-minute) trial of spontaneous breathing under direct observation as well as its progression over that interval has proven to be an excellent integrative test of endurance (Fig. 10.3).

VOLUNTARY MEASURES

Maximal Inspiratory Pressure

Maximal inspiratory pressure (MIP) must be measured carefully to be of real value. Although

highly negative numbers encourage a weaning attempt, low values may reflect inadequate measurement technique rather than true patient weakness. For poorly cooperative patients, airway occlusion must start from a low lung volume and continue for at least 8 to 10 efforts before the value is recorded. (A one-way valve that selectively prevents inspiration while allowing unimpeded expiration may be helpful.) The MIP, a good measure of isometric muscle strength, does not yield information regarding endurance. This is better gauged by integrative indices (see below).

Vital Capacity

Considerably less muscular effort is required to approach the vital capacity (VC) than to achieve a valid MIP. Although a one-way valving system can be used effectively to estimate the vital capacity by tidal "breath stacking" without patient cooperation, this involuntary approximation reflects lung mechanics more closely than muscle strength. Although of limited value as an independent weaning parameter, it can be quite helpful. If a cooperative patient achieves a (single effort) vital capacity twofold greater than the tidal volume, the chances are good that ventilatory reserves are sufficient to allow successful resumption of spontaneous breathing.

Cough, Expiratory Pressure, and Maximal Expiratory Flow

Measures aimed at assessing the forcefulness of expiration may be important in gauging the ability to cough and clear secretions and, therefore, the need for continued intubation but have a more limited place in assessing the likelihood

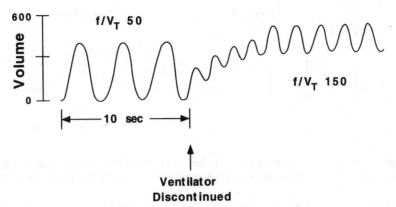

FIG. 10–3. Rapid shallow breathing and the ratio of frequency to tidal volume (f/V_T) in a patient with airflow obstruction. Upon ventilator disconnection, a poorly compensated patient with airflow obstruction tends to increase the work of breathing, develop gas trapping (auto-PEEP), and respond by decreasing tidal volume and increasing respiratory frequency. Although many exceptions exist, a patient recovering from acute illness with an f/V_T ratio exceeding 100 breaths per minute/L during spontaneous breathing is unlikely to be weaned successfully from ventilatory support.

of successful weaning from the ventilator (see below).

Other Measures

Nonrespiratory factors (e.g., coronary ischemia) often predominate in the most difficult weaning cases. In attempting to discontinue mechanical ventilation, some investigators have found that observations apart from standard indices of lung mechanics correlate well with an adverse weaning outcome. Very low or high pulse rates, respiratory rates greater than 30 per minute, forceful abdominal contractions, accessory muscle activity, ataxic breathing patterns, and coma are all negative prognostic factors.

INTEGRATIVE WEANING INDICES

Given the central importance of ventilatory insufficiency to ventilator dependence, it is not surprising that any single prognostic indicator is unlikely to prove successful unless it closely reflects the balance of ventilatory capability and demand. Static measures such as the $\bar{P}/P_{max}$ ratio or inspiratory effort quotient may have some merit. However, analysis of the breathing pattern during a trial of spontaneous breathing is more attractive, in that it allows the brain to integrate the information necessary to relate the workload to work capacity. Among the available options (Table 10.3), the frequency to tidal volume ratio (f/V_T) is perhaps the most useful and readily calculated. A

TABLE 10–3

INTEGRATIVE WEANING INDICES

$\bar{P}/P_{max} < 0.4$
$\bar{P}/P_{max} \times t_i/t_{tot} < 0.15$
$P_{0.1} < 6$ cm H_2O
CO_2-stimulated increase of $P_{0.1} > 4$ cm H_2O
$f/V_T < 100$
$V_T/VC < 0.5$
$\dot{V}_E/MVV < 0.5$

value exceeding 100 breaths/minute/L during the first minute of spontaneous breathing indicates extraordinarily rapid and shallow breathing. Concern has been raised over the accuracy of this index for patients with severe airflow obstruction. It is unclear whether any such index based on respiratory mechanics can reliably reflect cardiac dysfunction or hypoxemia occurring as a consequence of spontaneous breathing effort. However, more complex indexes do not seem to offer major advantages over the f/V_T ratio.

WEANING TRIAL

PREPARATIONS FOR WEANING FROM THE VENTILATOR

Most patients are easily discontinued from mechanical ventilation after the process that initiated

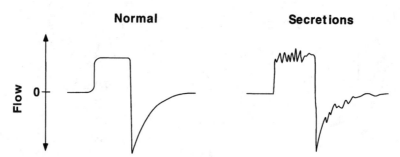

FIG. 10–4. Flow wave forms generated in a patient with retained central airway secretions. Note the highly irregular flow profile. Such a patient may improve airflow and reduce the work of breathing impressively once the secretions are cleared.

the need for this support has improved. Patients who fail require optimal preparation before another weaning trial is undertaken. The inability to discontinue mechanical support often results from failure to correct one or more of the factors that adversely affect strength, capacity for responding to stress, ventilatory requirement, gas exchange, or lung mechanics. The well-prepared patient is in appropriate electrolyte, pH, and fluid balance. Magnesium, potassium, calcium, and phosphate should be checked especially closely. Infection, arrhythmias, cardiac ischemia, and heart failure must be well controlled. Airways should be dilated optimally and kept as clear of retained secretions as possible (Fig. 10.4). Adequate sleep and balanced nutritional support are essential. Psychotropic agents such as haloperidol may be needed to combat delirium, avoid panic reactions, and secure cooperation. Distention of the abdomen must be relieved. Care should be taken not to ventilate patients with chronic CO_2 retention to an artificially reduced $PaCO_2$ before the attempt. If this should happen, the patient may not be able to maintain the lower $PaCO_2$ level during spontaneous breathing, allowing acute acidosis to develop. Indeed, allowing a higher than usual $PaCO_2$ during the support phase may be appropriate, as already noted. The nursing staff should be advised as soon as the physician has decided that a weaning attempt will be undertaken (often the night before). Such warnings can prevent untoward administration of sedatives, nutrients, or procedures that interfere with the trial's success.

WEANING SEQUENCE

The steps in removing mechanical support from the difficult patient are as follows: (a) estimation of the likelihood of success ("parameter" measurement); (b) a trial of spontaneous ventilation; (c) gradual withdrawal of ventilatory power (weaning), if the trial of spontaneous breathing is poorly tolerated; (d) for most patients, a brief period of observation without either pressure support or CPAP before extubation and/or removal of the ventilator; and (e) close follow-up after ventilator discontinuation and extubation. In selected cases (e.g., upper airway obstruction), the patency of the airway above the tube cuff should be evaluated before extubation (see Chapter 6, Airway Intubation). In others, the ability to clear secretions must be tested by measuring expiratory flows or pressures (see below).

Whereas favorable weaning parameters may support a decision to undertake a weaning attempt, poor parameters should not preclude a carefully observed trial of spontaneous breathing or an attempt to wean if clinical judgment otherwise suggests a favorable outcome.

Trial of Spontaneous Breathing

A trial of breathing without inspiratory assistance is a brief but stringent test of the ability to sustain spontaneous ventilation. It is generally undertaken when clinical judgment and a 3- to 5-minute observation period of breathing with only CPAP suggest the likelihood that the patient can breathe spontaneously without ventilator support. For these patients, a longer test period of breathing without pressure support or CPAP (30–120 minutes, depending on the patient) should be conducted. Passing this trial justifies an attempt to withdraw the ventilator quickly; failing either the brief or extended trial indicates that further support and/or more gradual adaptation are necessary.

Such a trial of spontaneous breathing can be conducted either by the classic T-piece method or simply by allowing the patient to breathe through an efficient ventilator circuit without either inspiratory pressure support or significant CPAP. The latter approach allows tidal volume and frequency to be followed, keeps an apnea alarm in place, prevents infections related to frequent circuit breaks, and avoids time and financial costs associated with circuit manipulation. Using pressure support during the trial does not seem advisable because it may mislead the physician into a false sense of optimism. (Even a low level of pressure support may be surprisingly helpful for a marginally compensated patient.) After extubation, upper airway resistance often increases due to glottic edema and narrowing. Breathing through the endotracheal tube without pressure support, therefore, provides an appropriate inspiratory load similar to that which the patient may face postextubation. Similarly, raised end-expiratory pressure (CPAP) can be very helpful in preventing atelectasis or offsetting auto-PEEP—two benefits that are usually forgone during fully spontaneous breathing.

Conducting the Trial

One reasonable method for conducting the trial is as follows.

1. Ideally, the initial trials should be undertaken in the morning when the patient is well rested and a full complement of staff is available. This also allows retesting later in the day when the patient's condition may have improved. If the patient is alert, explain the purpose of the procedure.
2. Place the patient in the sitting or semiupright position for maximal mechanical advantage.
3. Unless PaO_2 is high enough to provide a comfortable margin, increase FiO_2 by at least 10%, because microatelectasis, retained secretions, or mixed venous desaturation may develop during spontaneous breathing.
4. Suction the airway and oropharynx.
5. Monitor heart rate, blood pressure, tidal volume, respiratory rate, pulse oximetry, and level of comfort before starting and every few minutes for the first 20 minutes. Although seldom used, tidal capnometry may be a helpful adjunct, as a steadily rising end-expiratory PCO_2

suggests decompensation. If the outcome is in doubt, arterial blood gases are analyzed. Blood gas analysis may be unnecessary if the patient is monitored continuously by oximetry, with or without end-tidal capnometry.
6. If the patient seems to be doing well, continue. However, if there is any question of tolerance, resume mechanical ventilation immediately. Do *not* let the patient become fatigued or emotionally distressed.
7. Moderate disturbances of vital signs can be seen in successful trials. However, terminate the trial if the patient indicates intolerable dyspnea or if diastolic blood pressure falls or rises by more than 20 mm Hg, pulse rises or falls more than 30 per minute, respiratory rate increases by more than 10 per minute over the initial spontaneous value, arterial blood desaturates sharply, mental status deteriorates, or worrisome arrhythmias or signs of ischemia develop. During trials longer than 15 minutes, periodic suctioning and hyperinflation should be considered.

Very prolonged trials of spontaneous breathing are discouraged for patients who have no continuing need for the airway, inasmuch as the intubated patient cannot cough effectively and the tube may increase airway resistance. In general, the duration of the trial should parallel the duration of pretrial mechanical ventilation and vary inversely with the confidence of the physician in the extubation outcome. It should be noted that the first minutes to hours off the ventilator are often the most stressful because tidal volume and functional residual capacity (FRC) may decrease and changes occur in central vascular volume, respiratory work, and pattern of breathing. When the patient has sustained spontaneous ventilation comfortably for 30 minutes to 2 hours, acute deterioration is less likely and extubation should be considered if no contraindication exists, breathing pattern is stable, and the patient seems to be strong. Preparations for noninvasive ventilation in the immediate postextubation period should be made for the high risk patient with cardiac insufficiency, massive obesity, or marginal weaning parameters. Special caution is indicated for patients who have undergone a prolonged period of ventilatory support. Patients with potentially unstable respiratory drive should be watched for longer periods before removing the tube.

An aerosol of racemic epinephrine should be considered for the patient with postextubation stridor. (Although controversial, moderate-dose steroids also may be justified for 48 hours afterward.) A nasopharyngeal airway inserted immediately postextubation may help to aspirate secretions from the retropharynx and trachea. For cooperative patients, intermittent positive pressure delivered by mouthpiece or face mask can help maintain open airways, as can the sitting position, CPAP, and bilevel positive airway pressure (commercial BiPAP™). Although alertness should be maintained, the patient must be kept as comfortable and free from anxiety as feasible. Despite all precautions, it is distressingly common for marginal patients who apparently have been weaned successfully to require reintubation 12 to 48 hours after extubation (e.g., due to fatigue, sleep deprivation, aspiration, or upper airway obstruction). Therefore, recently extubated patients must be watched very closely for signs of decompensation and not refed until adequate swallowing reflexes have been confirmed.

WEANING STRATEGIES AND METHODS

GENERAL PRINCIPLES

A failed trial of spontaneous breathing in an otherwise viable candidate suggests that a more extended period of rest or gradual weaning is necessary. Care to optimize the physiologic determinants of ventilator dependence is key to the success of the weaning effort, as already described (Table 10.4). Reversal or prevention of heart failure, cardiac ischemia, electrolyte imbalance, hypoxemia, anemia, nutritional deficiencies, and bronchospasm are of particular importance. It should be emphasized that patients undergoing prolonged weaning regimens (of any type) should receive adequate ventilator support at night to permit sleep. Forcing the patient to work continuously may cause fitful sleep and compromise the weaning effort. The patient must be kept fully informed of the weaning plan and most patients should be given absolute authority to terminate the trial if he or she experiences intolerable discomfort. Panic reactions must be avoided, especially in patients with COPD who experience a self-reinforcing cycle of dyspnea, hyperinflation, compromised muscle function, and often pulmonary congestion or chest pain during these episodes. Tracheostomy should be considered after several failed weaning attempts, particularly if rapid recovery of muscle strength is unlikely or impossible. Tracheostomy provides a more stable airway than an endotracheal tube, allows ambulation and oral feeding, improves secretion clearance, and decreases both ventilatory deadspace and the work of breathing.

WEANING PRIORITIES

To successfully withdraw ventilatory support, the problems of the patient that dictate the need for machine assistance must be matched to the methods available to address them. Several principles, however, apply to most patients. First, the added external work of breathing must be minimized. Second, adequate lung volume must be maintained to prevent atelectasis, secretion retention, dysfunctional breathing patterns, and inefficient gas exchange. Third, deep tidal inflations should occur periodically to encourage recruitment of marginal lung units.

METHODS OF WEANING

There are three weaning methods in widespread use at the current time: progressive T-piece trials, intermittent mandatory ventilation (IMV), and PSV (Fig. 10.5). Very recently, other modes of unproven benefit for this application (e.g., volume-assured pressure support [VAPS]) have been introduced to clinical practice (see Chapter 7, Indications and Options in Mechanical Ventilation).

Unsupported ("T-Piece") Weaning

Using the intermittent "T-piece" or "blow by" method, the duration of independent breathing is lengthened progressively, according to patient tolerance. T-piece weaning provides stress periods punctuated by recovery periods of total rest. This time-honored approach can be defended, based on current knowledge of fatigue and muscle reconditioning. Furthermore, the T-piece generally provides conditioned gas at negligible resistive work cost. The main disadvantages of this method are that it requires significant staff time to implement and monitor and fosters abrupt transitions between periods on and off the ventilator. The latter can prove problematic for patients who must assume a high-impedance workload, for those who are anxiety prone, and for those with ischemic or congestive heart failure. Unlike IMV, no apnea alarm is provided during periods of spontaneous breathing on a T piece. Although the "zero-CPAP" option of many older ventilators

TABLE 10–4

THERAPEUTIC MEASURES TO ENHANCE WEANING PROGRESS

Problem	Hypoxemia	↑ Impedance	↑ $\dot{V}_E$
	Positioning	Positioning	Sedation
	↓ Secretions	↑ Secretion clearance	↓ Fever
	Bronchodilation	Bronchodilation	↓ Pain
	Diuresis	Diuresis	↓ V_D/V_T
	CPAP	Relieve cardiac ischemia	Correct acidosis
	↑ F_iO_2	↓ $\dot{V}_E$	Allow ↑ $PaCO_2$
		↓ Circuit resistance	
Problem	↓ Drive	↓ Endurance	Psychological Factors
	↑ Nutrition	Rest periods	Reassure patient
	↓ Loading	Ensure sleep	Convey plan
	↓ Alkalosis	Optimal positioning	Anxiolytics
	↓ Sedatives	Correct electrolytes	Encourage normal activity
	↑ Sleep	↑ Calories	Ambulation/physical R_X
	↑ Thyroid	Optimize heat function	Adjust steroid dose
		Steroid replacement	
		Correct anemia	

↑, increased; ↓, decreased.
* Partial listing.

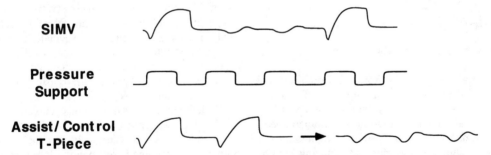

FIG. 10–5. Airway pressure profiles for the three most common modes of partial ventilatory assistance used in weaning: SIMV, pressure support, and intermittently unsupported ("T-piece") breathing. In practice, SIMV and pressure support often are used in combination.

is suboptimal in terms of resistive work, requiring the patient to breathe spontaneously while attached to the ventilator circuit does provide an apnea alarm, enable the application of PEEP, and facilitate rapid interconversion between no support and full support.

Traditionally, the patient is disconnected from the ventilator and attached to a source of humidified conditioned gas for a brief interval. If well tolerated, these periods of spontaneous ventilation are lengthened progressively. Failure to progress to the next interval mandates reinstitution of continuous ventilator support for 12 to 24 hours and a search for correctable problems. If the patient remains comfortable while breathing spontaneously for 30 to 120 minutes, shows no sign of hemodynamic instability or respiratory decompensation, and maintains acceptable blood gases, spontaneous breathing may continue, punctuated by episodic manual hyperinflation and airway suctioning when needed. The time that a patient must be observed during T-piece breathing before the ventilator is entirely discontinued is a matter of clinical judgment but generally should be governed by the length of time the patient has received mechanical ventilation and the apparent tolerance to spontaneous breathing.

CPAP as Ventilatory Assistance

It is well known that PEEP and CPAP (>0 cm H_2O) can improve lung compliance for patients with atelectasis and lung edema. Auto-PEEP presents a significant threshold load to ventilation for patients with a critical limitation of expiratory airflow. CPAP helps to counterbalance auto-PEEP and reduce the ventilatory requirement. For weak patients with severe airflow obstruction, the addition of CPAP may cause tidal volume to increase, as pressure support or the natural force of breathing effort become more effective. For stronger patients, CPAP may be used as a counterspring against which expiratory muscles can store energy for release during the subsequent inspiration—the "work-sharing" phenomenon.

Partial Ventilatory Support

Intermittent Mandatory Ventilation

During SIMV, the machine provides a selected number of positive pressure cycles (volume cycled or pressure controlled) that support 0 to 100% of the total minute ventilation. A clinician-specified number of machine-supported breaths per minute is interspersed among spontaneous breaths in synchrony with patient effort (see Chapter 7, Indications and Options in Mechanical Ventilation). A decelerating flow waveform, which is delivered automatically by pressure control or allowed as a selectable option in volume-cycled ventilation, is a logical choice because it delivers its maximal flow early in the machine cycle, when inspiratory flow demands are greatest. When using volume cycles, the peak flow rate should be increased as frequency is reduced and the patient assumes a progressively greater proportion of the breathing workload. Using pressure-control cycles, such flow adjustments occur automatically.

SIMV provides a method to gradually transfer the work of breathing from the machine to the patient without repeated manipulation of the circuit tubing, thereby reducing the potential for technical error while saving nursing time. Offering a full range of partial ventilatory support is potentially advantageous for patients with congestive heart failure or obstructive lung disease who cannot withstand sudden increments in venous return or the work of breathing and for those who experience anxiety when machine support is withdrawn abruptly. SIMV provides relatively large breaths at a guaranteed backup rate and, when used expertly, may allow the patient to retrain and restrengthen long-rested muscles. Used improperly, however, SIMV can increase the work of breathing, prolong the weaning period unnecessarily, promote chronic "fatigue," or, worse, endanger the patient. Inefficient valving of the IMV circuit can markedly increase the work of spontaneous breathing. Inspiratory resistance of the endotracheal tube can be countered partially by judicious use of pressure support applied in proportion to $\dot{V}_E$ and endotracheal tube resistance. It should be remembered that hypoventilation and respiratory acidosis can develop without a ventilator alarm sounding, especially at low levels of SIMV. In addition, because the respiratory muscles remain continuously active, it is at least theoretically possible that the muscles may never rest sufficiently to enable full recovery from fatigue, even though blood gases and pH might remain within acceptable limits. It is especially important for patients who are stressed significantly by the level of IMV used during the daylight hours to receive increased support with assisted mechanical ventilation (AMV) or a significantly higher IMV level at night. An insidious problem related to IMV is the tendency for clinicians to reduce the machine rate so cautiously that the weaning process is prolonged well beyond the time when machine support can be discontinued successfully.

Pressure Support Ventilation

In the weaning process, PSV offers an attractive option as an alternative or supplement to SIMV. When inspiratory pressure is set high enough, PSV can provide near-total ventilatory support. At low levels, PSV provides enough of a pressure boost to overcome the inspiratory (but not expiratory) resistance of the endotracheal tube. Each breath is aided by the ventilator to the pressure level set by the physician and is flow-cycled by the patient's ventilatory impedance or expiratory effort. Because each breath is machine-assisted, tidal volumes and respiratory rhythms are less variable and more natural than during SIMV weaning (Fig. 10.5). Most importantly, however, inspiratory duration, cycling frequency, and timing of respiratory cycles are influenced by the patient—not set by the machine. In allowing the patient to determine the timing characteristics of the inspiratory cycle, synchrony and patient comfort can improve markedly. Finally, PSV may be a method of training the muscles for endurance or the respiratory center for improved coordination of the respiratory muscles (but this is still unproven). PSV is generally adjusted to keep breathing frequencies lower than 25 to 30 per minute. Unlike SIMV, PSV lends some flexibility to the amount of power available from the machine. The patient can adapt to decreasing PSV by increasing frequency, thereby taking maximal advantage of machine power. In some instances, it is only when PSV falls below some critical value that the patient must work actively to maintain tidal volume (V_T). This flexibility may be particularly important for patients with variable V_E requirements, and therefore, PSV may be an especially helpful adjunct to SIMV weaning.

Potential Problems of Pressure Support Ventilation   Although valuable for overcoming endotracheal tube resistance, in allowing breaths of variable character, and in conferring some flexibility in response to changing power requirements, PSV is not an ideal mode for partial ventilatory support. In providing a fixed rate of rise to a set target pressure, PSV does not tailor its output to the changing character of patient effort. Moreover, for patients with severe airflow obstruction or narrow endotracheal tubes, airway pressurization may need active termination, as inspiratory flow may assume a very slowly decelerating profile (Fig. 10.6). Any machine support must be initiated by the patient, and any backup desired must be provided independently. Tidal volume during PSV is inherently sensitive to changes in frequency, especially during airflow obstruction when muscles are weak, lungs are compliant, auto-PEEP is prevalent, and inspiratory time constants are long.

The threshold between tolerance and intolerance to a decrease in PSV is often quite distinct. A difference of only a few cm H_2O per cycle may separate comfort from overt dyspnea. Furthermore, the level of support offered by PSV varies directly with the impedance to chest inflation. Therefore, patients with variable inflation impedance (e.g., those prone to accumulate secretions or who experience bronchospasm during the weaning trial) are poor candidates for its use. The development of auto-PEEP may partially or completely nullify the contribution of PSV to the inspired V_T. As with any pressure-limited mode, the tidal volume must be monitored closely. Patients with unstable ventilatory drive are also at major risk, unless PSV defaults to an automatic cycling mode when spontaneous efforts cease.

Comparison of SIMV and PSV

At the very onset of the weaning process, SIMV and PSV both support all breathing cycles and provide virtually identical ventilatory assistance for the same tidal volume. Similarly, at the completion of weaning, the patient must eventually breathe without assistance. Unquestionably, however, there are differences in the way that these techniques reload the respiratory muscles as support is withdrawn (Fig. 10.7). The extent of these differences varies from patient to patient. Most patients tend to reload their own ventilatory system later when using pure PSV than when using pure SIMV. SIMV provides a certain number of breaths per minute of preset tidal volume, and in the traditional flow-controlled, volume-cycled configuration, the amount of energy provided per cycle is maximal at the highest levels of machine support. As the patient breathes *more* vigorously, airway pressure falls and *less* ventilator work actually is performed per cycle by the machine. The maximum available ventilatory power is therefore fixed during SIMV, occurs when the patient makes the least effort, and does not respond by increasing flow as SIMV frequency is reduced and patient flow demands rise. Because flow output is greatest in the earliest part of the breath (when the flow demands are maximal), a decelerating waveform may be superior to constant flow that provides the same V_T and inspiratory time. Pressure control may be preferable to flow control during SIMV; pressure-controlled machine breaths are not flow-limited and can therefore respond more adequately to patient demands during vigorous breathing. In contrast to SIMV, the number of pressure assists per minute is patient-variable during PSV, allowing better response to a changing minute ventilation requirement than SIMV. The efficiency of each provided cycle, however, varies with changing impedance to ventilation.

When PSV or SIMV is employed separately, neither is ideal for all patients. The available evidence conflicts regarding their relative merit. A

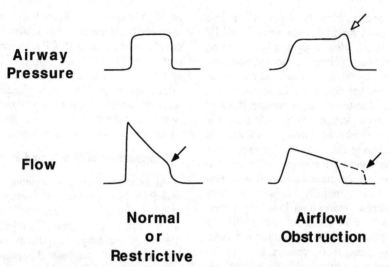

FIG. 10–6. Airway pressure and flow profiles for patients with and without airflow obstruction receiving pressure support. Because inspiratory flow decelerates only slowly when the airway is obstructed, achieving the 25% peak flow off switch criterion (solid arrow) would require an excessive inspiratory time. The patient actively stiffens the chest wall to initiate expiration, as reflected by the end-inspiratory blip in airway pressure (open arrow).

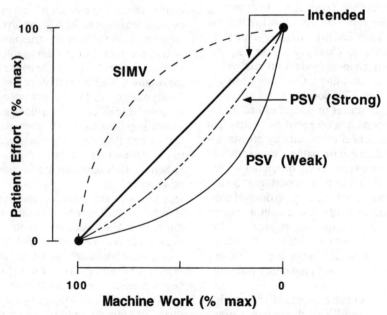

FIG. 10–7. Rate of reloading of the respiratory musculature during weaning by SIMV and PSV. As breathing frequency is reduced from the assist/control (100%) level, the patient receiving SIMV tends to respond by accepting the ventilatory workload relatively early in the machine withdrawal process. In contrast, relatively strong patients tend to reload the musculature linearly as pressure support is reduced, whereas weak patients tend to defer acceptance of the burden until relatively late in the withdrawal process.

multicenter European trial strongly indicated an advantage for PSV, whereas a multicenter Spanish trial failed to demonstrate a difference between them. In another study, a direct comparison of these modes (used alone) for the same patients, no significant differences with regard to dyspnea and anxiety were detected at any level of support.

In PSV, the machine remains well coupled to the patient's breathing rhythm throughout the power withdrawal process. In SIMV, however, the patient and ventilator seem disconnected in the sense that the patient does not respond to the provision of machine cycles by reducing his own energy output. Such independence becomes overt when SIMV falls below approximately 50% of the assist-control frequency.

Other Ventilatory Modes

Certain modes recently introduced to clinical practice (e.g., volume-assured pressure support) have the potential to overcome some of the drawbacks of PSV and SIMV. By targeting maintenance of a certain tidal volume (and/or $\dot{V}_E$) rather than pressure, such modes theoretically could help prevent hypoventilation. Their place in the weaning process is difficult to assess currently, however; the extent to which the patient allows the machine to assist breathing cannot be controlled, and these methods remain untested.

A STRATEGY FOR IMPLEMENTING PARTIAL VENTILATORY SUPPORT AND WEANING

Whenever possible, the electrocardiogram, pulse oximetry, airway pressure, and airflow should be monitored to assess physiologic tolerance. No single mode of ventilatory support is ideal for weaning all patients. The key objectives for weaning are (a) to maintain an adequate end expiratory lung volume (to prevent atelectasis or secretion retention); (b) to provide large breaths intermittently to maintain the lung fully recruited and help reverse atelectasis; (c) to avoid an additional workload related to circuit elements or dyssynchronous breathing; and (d) to withdraw ventilatory support in a timely fashion (Table 10.5). A low level of CPAP helps both to maintain an appropriate lung volume and to compensate for any auto-PEEP. Providing a few SIMV breaths per minute helps to ensure adequate volume maintenance. A low level of pressure support helps

TABLE 10–5

ALTERNATIVE WEANING STRATEGIES

	Primary Power PSV	SIMV
SIMV	0.5–2/min	Assist/control → 0/minute
CPAP	3–5 cm H_2O	3–5 cm H_2O
PSV	PSV_{max} → 0	3–10 cm H_2O

* See text

overcome inspiratory resistance of the endotracheal tube. (The selected level of PSV should vary directly with minute ventilation and inversely with tube diameter.) With these requirements met, either SIMV or PSV can be used to provide the main source of machine power (Table 10.5).

As already noted, SIMV tends to reload earlier and PSV later in the weaning process. It stands to reason, therefore, that special attention should be paid to these particular phases. For marginally compensated patients, SIMV should be withdrawn quite cautiously in the first and middle phases, whereas increased vigilance is required in the middle and later phases of PSV withdrawal. As noted earlier, the decelerating flow waveform, frequent peak flow adjustments, and/or pressure-controlled machine cycles may be indicated to minimize workload and dyspnea.

For patients with severe airflow obstruction or pulmonary congestion, any level of CPAP or pressure support may significantly reduce the breathing workload. As a rule, therefore, marginal patients should be observed during a trial of fully spontaneous breathing (PSV = 0, CPAP = 0) before extubation is attempted. Upper airway resistance may be increased for a variable period after extubation due to glottic edema, inflammation, and secretion retention. Therefore, a higher ventilatory demand may be required postextubation. This guideline for removing all support before extubation occasionally may be relaxed when a patient with apparently good reserve seems to enter a panic cycle at lower levels of machine assistance or when endotracheal tube resistance is extraordinarily high.

PRACTICAL POINTS

General

1. The breathing pattern provides an important and timely indication of tolerance or intolerance to an intended change. Frequency and

tidal volume adapt within seconds to minutes of a change in the breathing workload.

2. The spontaneous breathing pattern during CPAP should be tested once or twice daily for 3 to 15 minutes (depending on tolerance) in almost *all* patients to detect ventilator independence at the earliest possible time and to avoid unnecessarily protracted weaning schedules.

3. Whether PSV or SIMV is elected, enough CPAP (3–5 cm H_2O) is applied to compensate for positional volume losses and/or auto-PEEP and enough PSV is used to overcome ET-tube resistance, considering both tube resistance and minute ventilation. Adding some level of PSV also lends flexibility to the level of support the patient may draw from, even when SIMV is selected (see above).

4. Except in rare instances, both of these supports should be removed entirely in the final stage preextubation to confirm an adequate breathing reserve.

5. Whatever the primary power source, relatively deep breaths should be provided periodically (at least every 30 seconds to 2 minutes) using pressure- or volume-controlled SIMV breaths.

6. The patient must never be allowed to encounter sustained dyspnea and, during weaning efforts extending over days, must be supported adequately at night to allow restful sleep and avoid hypoxemia.

7. If one form of partial ventilatory support (PSV, SIMV) is ineffective, the other should be tried. In selected cases, intermittent T-piece weaning may be the best alternative.

PSV Weaning

With the patient receiving sufficient PSV to seem comfortable with a breathing frequency of less than 20 breaths per minute and a tidal volume of approximately 7–8 ml/kg (PSV max), pressure support is withdrawn in decrements of 2 to 4 cm H_2O every 30 to 120 minutes. Progression to the next decrement is allowed if the breathing frequency does not exceed 30 to 35 breaths per minute and tidal volume remains greater than approximately 3.5 mL/kg. Particular caution may be appropriate as the lowest levels of pressure support are withdrawn. These suggested limits are only guidelines; a dyspneic patient must not be weaned, whereas a comfortable patient may be tested at lower levels of PSV despite violation of these limits.

SIMV Weaning

The patient is supported initially with a $V_T \geq$ 7 mL/kg in the assist/control mode at a low backup rate, and the triggering frequency is noted. SIMV is then initiated at the same tidal volume and frequency as observed during assist/control. Frequency is then reduced by approximately 2 breaths per minute every 30 to 120 minutes, depending on patient fragility and the stage of the withdrawal process. (Longer intervals may be appropriate earlier in the support withdrawal process, when the rate of reloading is disproportionately high.)

WEANING FROM THE ENDOTRACHEAL TUBE

After the patient is weaned from the ventilator, the need for continued endotracheal intubation should be assessed independently. Although virtually all patients have disordered swallowing transiently after extubation, those likely to have a persisting problem of airway protection after tube removal (e.g., deep coma) should not be extubated. Because airway protection reflexes (pharyngeal gag and laryngeal closure) are lost earlier than cough triggered deep within the airway, a patient who fails to cough vigorously upon tracheal suctioning is not likely to protect the airway effectively when the tube is removed. For patients with copious airway secretions and ineffective cough, the tube should be retained to facilitate suctioning. Vital capacity greater than 20 mL/kg, MIP more negative than -40 cm H_2O, a vigorous expulsive effort on tracheal stimulation (secretions coughed into the external circuit), peak expiratory flow greater than 160 L/minute (for patients without severe airflow obstruction), and an expiratory pressure generated against an occluded airway greater than 60 cm H_2O predict effective coughing postextubation.

In a patient with a tracheostomy, the ability to phonate and expectorate with the tube cuff partially deflated (after oropharyngeal suctioning) generally is considered to be a positive predictive sign. Because compromise of coughing and swallowing in the postextubation period generally parallels the duration of translaryngeal intubation, particular attention should be paid to assiduous tracheobronchial hygiene in these cases. Suctioning, corticosteroids, bronchodilators, Bi-PAP, sitting position, antibiotics, and careful regulation of electrolyte, glucose, and cardiovascular status often make the difference between a patient who bridges the period of difficulty and another who must be reintubated.

DELAYED WEANING FAILURES AND REINTUBATION

The 24- to 48-hour period immediately after ventilator disconnection may be highly dynamic, as the patient must readjust to spontaneous breathing and assume responsibility for airway secretion clearance. Stresses arising soon after extubation may result from cardiac ischemia, pulmonary congestion, atelectasis, secretion retention, oropharyngeal aspiration, or temporary swelling of glottic and subglottic tissues. Vigorous attempts to encourage deep breathing, coughing, and mobilization are helpful. In lethargic patients, secretions may pool in the retropharynx and should be aspirated via a nasopharyngeal airway ("trumpet"). Extreme caution should be used when initiating oral feeding after a lengthy intubation. Premature resumption of oral intake is hazardous because temporary swallowing dysfunction and impaired glottic defenses are common. CPAP or noninvasive ventilation during this period may help as a bridge across the immediate postextubation period. Anything that can be done to improve sleep quality (including noninvasive ventilation) is worth implementing to avoid sleep deprivation and eventual exhaustion. Therefore, the potential for excessive mental stimulation by steroids and catecholamines should be considered when selecting doses of these agents. Pulse oximetry, echocardiography, and electrocardiography are helpful monitors during this period as well. A maximum cough flow of approximately 160 L/minute (normal: 360–1,000 L/minute) may be necessary to maintain effective secretion mobilization after decannulation. Manually or mechanically assisted coughing may be helpful in reaching this threshold in the days after extubation.

THE UNWEANABLE PATIENT

The need for continued ventilatory support is often psychological as well as physiologic (Table 10.6). A few points are important to keep in mind.

1. The patient must be "coopted" into the weaning effort and kept fully advised of the treatment plan.

TABLE 10–6

AIDS TO WEAN THE UNWEANABLE PATIENT

Coopt the patient
Confer veto power
Avoid panic reactions
Consider anxiolytics/psychotropics
Fully rest before trial/ensure sleep
Check for "hidden" cardiovascular and endocrine problems
Mobilize and exercise
Respiratory muscle training

2. Most patients must be given full "veto" power to terminate an overly taxing trial.
3. "Panic" reactions are especially detrimental for patients with airflow obstruction. At such times, these patients generate increased volumes of CO_2 and experience discoordinated breathing, hyperinflation, hypoxemia, and extreme dyspnea. Any setback can be mental as well as physical.
4. Nonsedating anxiolytics and psychotropic agents (e.g., haloperidol) may benefit selected patients.
5. The patient must be fully rested. This can best be ensured by 10 to 12 hours of full ventilatory support and a good night of sleep before the trial.
6. Hidden problems such as diastolic dysfunction, coronary insufficiency, endocrinopathy (hypoadrenalism, hypothyroidism), subtle strokes, critical illness polyneuropathy, poststeroid and paralytic neuromyopathy, or Parkinson's disease may explain protracted ventilator dependence and must be sought aggressively in puzzling cases. Large pleural effusions must be drained, and the stomach must be decompressed. Tube feedings should be withheld for 2 or more hours before extubation.
7. Mobilization and exercise aid in general rehabilitation and are often keys to the weaning effort. Prolonged bed rest is attended by multiple adverse physiologic changes related to the changed vector of gravitational forces, including depressed vascular tone, reduced extravascular volume, loss of red cell mass, electrolyte shifts, calcium depletion, aberrations of hormonal balance, and depletion of skeletal mus-

cle mass (see Chapter 18). Prevented from weight bearing, the lower extremities undergo disproportionate atrophy in patients continually at bed rest. Performing arm and leg exercises in bed, standing, and ambulation aid greatly in the rehabilitation effort. From a purely physical standpoint, chronically ventilator-dependent patients demand less nursing attention than other ICU patients. Immobilized and deprived of sensory stimulation, they often become passive, discouraged, or poorly cooperative. Efforts to provide sensory input, to restore the natural diurnal rhythms, normal activities and social interactions, and to provide physical and occupational therapy may improve mental outlook, strength, and prospects for recovery.

Muscle Training

As soon as the crisis period has passed, it makes good physiologic sense to deliberately stress the ventilatory musculature for brief periods several times daily, encouraging spontaneous breathing (CPAP or T piece). After being fully rested, such "wind sprints" may help strengthen and condition the ventilatory muscles in a fashion similar to athletic training for limb muscles. Many patients with good strength but a tendency to panic do best when extubated directly rather than being weaned with low levels of machine support. This is particularly true when a highly resistive endotracheal tube is in place (e.g., a small-caliber nasal tube). Although the precise reason for this response is uncertain, expiratory resistance (which may be disproportionately high in the intubated subject) is unchanged by the use of pressure support. Those who cannot be extubated may benefit from tracheostomy, a procedure that lowers airway resistance and apparatus deadspace, improves secretion hygiene and allows mobilization.

For a patient whose primary problem is ventilatory mechanics (and not respiratory drive), it may be worthwhile to allow $PaCO_2$ to rise slowly over several days, maintaining acceptable oxygenation and pH balance. Higher $PaCO_2$ enables each breath to eliminate CO_2 more efficiently. Furthermore, the higher bicarbonate levels buffer fluctuations in $PaCO_2$ more effectively.

For chronically ventilated patients, improvement in general health and increased activity level are often key interventions. Preparation of the patient is of prime importance. Rehabilitative programs that include physical therapy and ambula-

tion may prove to be the difference between success and failure. It is important to encourage the patient to resume as much normal activity as possible; a useful technique is to have the patient ambulate with assistance for 10- to 15-minute periods one or more times daily. During ambulation, ventilation is provided manually or with a transport or pressure-cycled ventilator. A multifactorial approach based on the answer to the question "What limits withdrawal of machine support?" offers the best hope of ventilator removal at the earliest possible time (Table 10.4). Keeping the patient fully informed and involved in the weaning attempt will help ensure a successful outcome.

TRACHEOSTOMY

Timing for tracheostomy must be considered on an individual basis. Some patients in ventilatory failure (e.g., those with slowly reversible or irreversible neurological problems or upper respiratory pathology) should receive early tracheostomy. For patients with acute lung disorders that are expected to reverse, there is no ironclad rule regarding when tracheostomy should be performed. As a guideline, tracheostomy may be appropriate any time after the first 7 to 10 days. The decision to undertake tracheostomy should consider the pace of improvement; if the patient is progressing sufficiently to be ready for extubation within 3 to 5 days, tracheostomy can be deferred reasonably. It should be emphasized that for some patients endotracheal tubes are kept in place for longer than 3 weeks without permanent laryngeal or tracheal injury.

Importance of Communication

Patients with a tracheostomy who still require ventilatory support often are frustrated in their attempts to communicate with their families, friends, and caregivers. The value of establishing a reliable means of communication frequently is underestimated. Apart from the commonly used but cumbersome writing pads or letter boards, effective devices for communication include vibrators placed over the larynx or cheek, fenestrated tubes, one-way inspiratory valves (Passy-Muir valves), and specialized tubes that direct a manually gated gas flow through the vocal cords ("Pitt" tubes). The speech pathology department often provides helpful consultative advice.

Weaning From Tracheostomy

Consideration should be given to removing the tracheostomy tube when the patient no longer requires suctioning for secretion removal, high fractions of inspired oxygen, or periodic reconnection to the ventilator. Replacement of the standard tracheostomy tube with a fenestrated one facilitates talking and allows easier assessment of true cough effectiveness. The predictors of coughing ability are discussed above. There are essentially three methods for gradually discontinuing a tracheostomy: use of partial plugs, use of progressively smaller tracheostomy tubes, and use of stomal buttons. Plugs that progressively occlude a standard-sized tracheostomy orifice (e.g., $\frac{1}{2}$ to $\frac{3}{4}$ plugs) can be used to assess the need for continued intubation. (The cuff on the endotracheal tube must be deflated during orifice occlusion.) However, it should be remembered that an occluded tracheostomy tube severely narrows the effective tracheal lumen, thereby increasing the work of breathing and the tendency toward secretion retention. For this reason, many physicians prefer to replace the original tracheostomy with progressively smaller uncuffed (or uninflated) endotracheal tubes. Unfortunately, the stomal orifice rapidly adapts to the smaller-caliber tube as well, so that effective ventilation through the tracheostomy might not be possible if an acute need arose. If the ability to sustain spontaneous ventilation, clear secretions, or protect the airway is questionable, a tracheostomy button will maintain the stoma over several days to weeks to allow tube reinsertion, non-invasive nasal or mask ventilation, emergency ventilation, suctioning, and effective administration of inhaled bronchodilators without adding substantially to airway resistance. Noninvasive ventilation often aids in providing adequate nocturnal ventilatory assistance, as well as the power necessary to bridge the period of adaptation that follows decannulation.

For certain difficult patients (e.g., those with advanced weakness, paralysis, or neuromuscular disease), a vigorous program of assisted coughing may be instrumental in achieving airway clearance. This may involve the application of high inflation volumes followed by abdominal thrusts timed to coincide with glottic opening. For patients who cannot maintain glottic closure or for whom abdominal compression is compromised by thoracic cage deformity or extreme obesity, deep spontaneous inspiration and manual abdominal compression may be ineffective; here, a commercially available "insufflation/exsufflation" device (capable of transiently generating 50 cm H_2O of positive and negative pressure when applied to the face mask or endotracheal tube) may be especially useful. A vibratory vest may enhance secretion removal in weakened patients with copious airway secretion who do not respond to other measures (e.g., antibiotics, steroids). For patients with severe obstructive airway disease, however, all assisted coughing techniques may be fruitless.

KEY POINTS

1. A continuing need for ventilator assistance may arise from oxygen desaturation of hemoglobin during spontaneous breathing, cardiovascular instability during machine withdrawal, psychological dependence, or, most commonly, imbalance between ventilatory capability and demand.

2. The minute ventilation requirement bears a quadratic relationship to the work of breathing. Three primary factors determine the V_E requirement: the CO_2 production, the efficiency of ventilation, and the central drive to breathe.

3. Ventilatory power is the product of V_E and the mechanical work of breathing per liter of ventilation. For any specific tidal volume and flow rate, the primary determinants of the work per liter of ventilation are the resistance and elastance of the respiratory system and auto-PEEP, a reflection of dynamic hyperinflation or expiratory muscle activity.

4. Ventilatory capability is determined by the central drive to breathe and the bulk, strength, and endurance of the ventilatory muscles. The induction of fatigue by excessive effort impairs muscular performance for at least 12 to 24 hours afterward. Sleep is essential for optimal neuromuscular performance and for preparing the patient for the weaning attempt.

5. Prediction of success or failure of a weaning trial involves the assessment of oxygen exchange and muscular endurance. Although individual measures of strength, gas exchange, or workload aid in this assessment, "integrative" weaning indices (e.g., f/V_T ratio, inspiratory effort quotient) observed during a brief trial of unaided breathing as well as tests of ventilatory reserve (V_T/V_E, V_E/MVV, tidal/maximum inspiratory pressure) are perhaps the most physiologically sound indicators. Expiratory performance is especially important to evaluate when there is a high secretion load.

6. Persistent failure to wean despite adequate respiratory parameters should prompt consideration of cardiac ischemia, congestive heart failure, psychological dependence, gas exchange deterioration, or other nonrespiratory explanation for the failure.

7. After the patient has had optimal preparation, the weaning sequence involves estimation of the likelihood of success, a trial of spontaneous ventilation, gradual withdrawal of ventilatory assistance (when indicated), a brief period of observation without applied airway pressure of any kind, extubation, and close follow-up after ventilator discontinuance and extubation.

8. Patients experiencing protracted difficulty during removal of ventilatory support should receive adequate ventilator assistance at night to permit sleep. The patient must never be forced to work beyond his or her ability.

9. Three important priorities in weaning are to minimize the external work of breathing, to maintain adequate lung volume (to limit or prevent atelectasis, secretion retention, and ineffectual gas exchange), and to ensure that occasional deep breaths occur (to encourage recruitment of marginal lung units).

10. Three methods are widely practiced during ventilator withdrawal: intermittent unsupported (T-piece) weaning, pressure–support ventilation, and synchronized intermittent mandatory ventilation (SIMV). Various authors, investigators, and practitioners are committed to using one technique exclusively. However, no single method is agreed upon universally as superior to the others for all patients. Recently modified "combination" modes partially address the individual shortcomings of PSV and SIMV.

11. Reintubation occasionally is necessary in the first few days after extubation. These delayed weaning failures usually arise because of an inability to swallow normally (resulting in oropharyngeal aspiration), glottic swelling, inability to clear secretions, or congestive heart failure. Appropriate precautions during this period may avert failure. Noninvasive ventilation may provide a useful bridge across this difficult period.

12. The "unweanable" patient often has unaddressed psychological, cardiovascular, or neuromuscular problems that underlie the difficulty.

13. Weaning from tracheostomy should be considered when the patient no longer requires frequent airway suctioning, high inspired fractions of O_2 or periodic (nocturnal) connection to the ventilator. Conversion to noninvasive ventilation and/or assisted coughing is possible for many patients previously obligated to permanent tracheostomy.

SUGGESTED READINGS

1. Al-Saady N. Does dietary manipulation influence weaning from artificial ventilation? Intensive Care Med 1994; 20(7):463–465.
2. Aldrich TK, Karpel JP, Uhrlass RM, et al. Weaning from mechanical ventilation: adjunctive use of inspiratory muscle resistive training. Crit Care Med 1989;17:143–147.
3. Brochard L, Rauss A, Benito S, Conti G, et al. Comparison of three methods of gradual withdrawal from ventilatory support during weaning from mechanical ventilation. Am J Respir Crit Care Med 1994;150(4):896–903.
4. Crippen D. Pharmacologic treatment of brain failure and delirium. Crit Care Clin 1994;10(4):733–766.
5. Esteban A, et al. A comparison of four methods of weaning patients from mechanical ventilation. Spanish lung failure collaborative group. N Engl J Med 1995;332(6): 345–350.
6. Goldstone J, Moxham J. Assisted ventilation weaning from mechanical ventilation. Thorax 1991;46(1):56–62.
7. Hanneman S, Ingersoll GL, Knebel AR, Shekleton ME, et al. Weaning from short-term mechanical ventilation: a review. Am J Crit Care 1994;3(6):421–441.
8. Heffner J. Timing of tracheotomy in ventilator-dependent patients. Clin Chest Med 1991;12(3):611–625.
9. Knebel AR, Janson-Bjerklie SL, Malley JD, Wilson AG, Marini JJ, et al. Comparison of breathing comfort during weaning with two ventilatory modes. Am J Respir Crit Care Med 1994;149:14–18.
10. LeMaire F. Difficult weaning. Intensive Care Med 1993; 19(Suppl 2):S69–S73.
11. LeMaire F, Teboul JL, Cinotti L, et al. Acute left ventricular dysfunction during unsuccessful weaning from mechanical ventilation. Anesthesiology 1988;69:171–179.
12. Lessard M, Brochard L. Weaning from ventilatory support. Clin Chest Med 1996;17(3):475–490.
13. MacIntyre NR. Respiratory function during pressure support ventilation. Chest 1986;89:677–683.
14. Marini JJ. The physiologic determinants of ventilator dependence. Respir Care 1986;31(4):271–282.
15. Marini JJ. The role of the inspiratory circuit in the work of breathing during mechanical ventilation. Respir Care 1987;32(6):419–430.
16. Marini JJ. Weaning from mechanical ventilation. N Engl J Med 1991;324(21):1496–1498.
17. Marini JJ. Weaning from mechanical ventilation [editorial comment]. N Engl J Med 1991;324(21):1496–1498.
18. Marini JJ, Smith TC, Lamb VJ. External work output and force generation during synchronized intermittent mechanical ventilation. Am Rev Respir Dis 1988;138: 1169–1179.

19. McCartney J, Boland R. Anxiety and delirium in the intensive care unit. Crit Care Clin 1994;10(4):673–680.
20. Murciano D, Boczkowski J, Lecocguic Y, et al. Tracheal occlusion pressure: a simple index to monitor respiratory muscle fatigue during acute respiratory failure in patients with chronic obstructive pulmonary disease. Ann Intern Med 1988;108(6):800–805.
21. Nathan S, Ishaaya AM, Koernen SK, Belman MJ, et al. Prediction of minimal pressure support during weaning from mechanical ventilation. Chest 1993;103(4):1215–1219.
22. Putensen C, Hormann C, Baum M, Lingnau W, et al. Comparison of mask and nasal continuous positive airway pressure after extubation and mechanical ventilation. Crit Care Med 1993;21(3):357–362.
23. Robotham J, Becker L. The cardiovascular effects of weaning: stratifying patient populations. Intensive Care Med 1994;20(3):171–172.
24. Sassoon C, Mahutte C. Airway occlusion pressure and breathing pattern as predictors of weaning outcome. Am Rev Respir Dis 1993;148(4, Pt 1):860–866.
25. Scheinhorn D, Artinian B, Catlin J. Weaning from prolonged mechanical ventilation. The experience at a regional weaning center. Chest 1994;105(2):534–539.
26. Scheinhorn D, Hassenpflug M, Artinian BM, LaBree L, Catlin JL, et al. Predictors of weaning after 6 weeks of mechanical ventilation. Chest 1995;107(2):500–505.
27. Schwab R. Disturbances of sleep in the intensive care unit. Crit Care Clin 1994;10(4):681–694.
28. Tobin M. Weaning from mechanical ventilation. Crit Care Clin 1990;6(3):725–747.
29. Tobin M. Weaning patients from mechanical ventilation using gastric pH. Ann Intern Med 1994;120(5):439.
30. Tobin M. Weaning patients from mechanical ventilation. How to avoid difficulty. Postgrad Med 1991;89(1):171–173.
31. Tobin MJ, Perez W, Guenther SM, et al. The pattern of breathing during successful and unsuccessful trials of weaning from mechanical ventilation. Am Rev Respir Dis 1986;134:1111–1118.
32. Udwadia ZF, Santis GK, Steven MH, Simonds AK, et al. Nasal ventilation to facilitate weaning in patients with chronic respiratory insufficiency. Thorax 1992;47(9):715–718.
33. Weinberger S, Weiss J. Weaning from ventilatory support. N Engl J Med 1995;332(6):388–389.
34. Wolff G. An analysis of desynchronization between the spontaneously breathing patient and ventilator during inspiratory pressure support. Chest 1995;107(5):1387–1394.
35. Yang KL, Tobin MJ. A prospective study of indexes predicting the outcome of trials of weaning from mechanical ventilation. N Engl J Med 1991;324:1445–1450.
36. Zakynthinos S, Vassilakopoulos T, Roussos C. The load of inspiratory muscles in patients needing mechanical ventilation. Am J Respir Crit Care Med 1995;152(4, Pt 1):1248–1255.

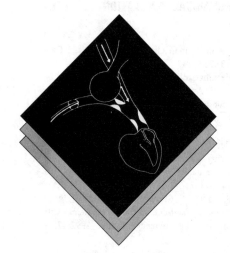

CHAPTER 11

Radiology in the Intensive Care Unit

Conventional and specialized radiographic techniques play key roles in the care of critically ill patients. For example, computed tomography (CT) scanning and magnetic resonance imaging (MRI) are indispensable for neurologic, abdominal, and sinus evaluation. Ultrasound facilitates cardiac, renal, and gallbladder diagnosis, and nuclear medicine techniques help to confirm embolic diseases, gastrointestinal (GI) bleeding, and fistulous communications. These and other specialized applications are discussed elsewhere in this text with the specific diseases they help define. This chapter concentrates on the three studies applied commonly in the critical care setting: the chest radiograph, the chest CT, and the abdominal plain film.

CHEST RADIOGRAPHY

FILMING TECHNIQUE

The usefulness of the portable anterior-posterior (AP) chest x-ray (CXR) is determined largely by positioning and exposure techniques. Orientation of the patient with respect to the radiographic beam is of critical importance. Kyphotic, lordotic, and rotated projections have dramatic affects on the apparent dimensions of intrathoracic structures as well as the detectability of pathology. The use of "gravity-dependent" radiopaque markers on the corners of portable films can help clarify a patient's position if the film is unlabeled. The AP technique blurs and magnifies the anterior mediastinum and great vessels, in some cases by as

much as 20%. When x-rays are obtained in supine patients, cardiovascular structures also appear enlarged, due to augmented venous filling and reduced lung volume. For example, the azygous vein distends in the supine normal subject but collapses in the upright position. Conversely, supine films often render pneumothoraces and pleural effusions imperceptible. Rotation produces artifactual hemidiaphragm elevation ipsilateral to the side of rotation. In diffuse infiltrative processes, lateral decubitus positioning accentuates asymmetry—making the dependent lung appear more affected. Film penetration may emphasize or diminish parenchymal lung markings. Consistency in exposure technique is critical to allow day-to-day comparison of radiographs. A properly exposed CXR should reveal vertebral interspaces in the retrocardiac region. Films on which these interspaces are not visualized are underpenetrated, exaggerating parenchymal markings and making visualization of air bronchograms difficult.

Changes in lung volume influence the appearance of parenchymal infiltrates, especially for mechanically ventilated patients and those receiving positive end-expiratory pressure (PEEP). Infiltrates seen on a radiograph obtained in full inspiration on the ventilator usually appear less dense than when viewed in partial inspiration. Furthermore, roughly one-half of all patients will have a "less infiltrated" appearing chest radiograph after the application of PEEP. Unfortunately, there is no predictable relationship between the level of PEEP applied and its impact on the appearance of the film. To facilitate comparison, serial films should be exposed with the patient in the same position, during the same phase of the respiratory cycle and with comparable tidal volume and end-expiratory pressure. CXR appearance also is influenced by therapeutic interventions and the development of new medical conditions. Infusion of large volumes of fluids, the development of oliguria, or superimposed myocardial dysfunction produce a rapidly deteriorating radiographic picture. Bronchoalveolar lavage may cause the transient appearance of localized infiltrates due to residual lavage fluid and atelectasis.

FILM TIMING

Because of the high likelihood of finding significant abnormalities (e.g., tube malposition, pneumothorax), it is worthwhile to obtain a chest radiograph of almost all patients upon arrival in the intensive care unit (ICU). The frequency with which radiographs are necessary after admission is much more controversial. General agreement exists that chest radiographs should be obtained within 1 hour of invasive procedures, such as endotracheal intubation, transvenous pacemaker insertion, thoracentesis, pleural and transbronchial biopsy, and central vascular catheter placement, to ensure proper tube position and exclude complications. A CXR must also follow failed attempts at catheterization via the subclavian route, especially before contralateral placement is attempted.

Although many ICUs obtain radiographs daily or even more frequently, daily films are probably not necessary for all patients. Despite data indicating that one-quarter to two-thirds of chest radiographs obtained in the ICU demonstrate some abnormality, many of these findings are chronic or inconsequential, and most can be detected by careful examination of the patient before obtaining the radiograph. Prospective study indicates that less than 10% of films demonstrate a new significant finding, and only a fraction of these are not anticipated by clinical examination. A reasonable compromise position is to obtain daily "routine" radiographs of all mechanically ventilated patients who have hemodynamic or respiratory instability (usually for 3–5 days after admission). Additional films should be dictated by changes in the patient's clinical condition. For stable, mechanically ventilated patients, especially those with tracheostomies, films can be obtained safely on a less frequent basis—probably every 2–3 days. Obviously, deterioration should prompt more frequent evaluation.

PLACEMENT OF TUBES AND CATHETERS

Tracheal Tube Position

Radiographic confirmation of tube placement is crucial; positioning the endotracheal tube in the right main bronchus often results in atelectasis or barotrauma. (Left main bronchus intubations are uncommon because the left main bronchus is smaller and angulates sharply from the trachea.) Conversely, if the tube tip lies too high in the trachea (above the level of the clavicles), accidental extubation is likely. When the head is in a neutral position, the tip of the endotracheal tube should rest in the midtrachea, ≈5 cm above the carina. For adult patients, the T5–7 vertebral level is a good estimate of carinal position if it cannot be directly visualized. Endotracheal tubes move with flexion, extension, and rotation of the neck. Contrary to what might be expected, the endotracheal tube tip moves caudally when the neck is flexed, whereas head rotation away from the midline and neck extension elevate the endotracheal tube tip. Total tip excursion may be as much as 4–5 cm.

The normal endotracheal or tracheostomy tube should occupy one-half to two-thirds of the tracheal width and should not cause bulging of the trachea in the region of the tube cuff. Gradual dilation of the trachea may occur during long-term positive pressure ventilation, but every effort should be made to prevent this complication by minimizing ventilator cycling pressure and cuff-sealing pressures.

After tracheostomy, a chest radiograph may detect subcutaneous air, pneumothorax, pneumomediastinum, or malposition of the tube. The T3 vertebral level defines the ideal position of the tracheostomy site. Sharp anterior angulation of the tracheal tube is associated with the development of tracheoinnominate fistulas, whereas posterior erosion can produce a tracheoesophageal fistula. Lateral radiographs are necessary for evaluation of AP angulation.

Central Venous Catheters

For accurate pressure measurement, the tip of the central venous pressure (CVP) catheter must lie within the thorax, well beyond any venous valves. These are commonly located in the subclavian and jugular veins, ~2.5 cm from their junction with the brachiocephalic trunk (at the radiographic level of the anterior first rib). Because CVP catheters positioned in the right atrium or ventricle may cause arrhythmias or perforation, the desirable location for these lines is in the mid-superior vena cava, with the tip directed inferiorly. Radiographically, catheter tips positioned above the superior margin of the right mainstem bronchus are unlikely to rest in the atrium. Stiff catheters, particularly left-sided subclavian hemodialysis catheters, may impinge on the lateral wall of the superior vena cava, potentially resulting in vascular perforation. Complications resulting from vascular puncture include fluid infusion into the pericardium or pleural space, hemopneumothorax, and pericardial tamponade.

Pacing Wires

When transvenous pacing wires are inserted emergently, they are often malpositioned in the coronary sinus, right atrium, or pulmonary artery outflow tract. On an AP view of the chest, a properly placed pacing catheter tip should overlie the shadow of the right ventricular apex. However, it is often difficult to assess the position of the pacing wire on a single film. On a lateral view, the tip of the catheter should lie within 4 mm of the epicardial fat stripe and point anteriorly. (Posterior angulation suggests coronary sinus placement.) For patients with permanent pacemakers, leads commonly fracture at the entrance to the pulse generator, a site that should be checked routinely.

Chest Tubes

The most appropriate position for a chest tube depends on the reason for its placement. Posterior positioning is ideal for the drainage of free-flowing intrapleural fluid, whereas anterosuperior placement is preferred for air removal. When an AP chest x-ray is obtained, posteriorly placed tubes are closer to the film than those placed anteriorly. This proximity of the chest tube to the film results in a "sharp" or focused appearance of the catheter edge and radiopaque stripe. Conversely, anteriorly placed chest tubes often have "fuzzy" or blurred margins. Chest tube location may appear appropriate on a single AP film, even though the tube actually lies within subcutaneous tissues or lung parenchyma. Oblique or lateral films or a chest CT may be necessary to confirm appropriate intrapleural location. On plain film, one clue to the extrapleural location of a chest tube is the inability to visualize both sides of the catheter. Chest tubes are constructed with a "sentinel eye," an

interruption of the longitudinal radiopaque stripe that delineates the opening of the chest tube closest to the drainage apparatus. This hole must lie within the pleural space to achieve adequate drainage and ensure that no air enters the tube via the subcutaneous tissue. After removal of the chest tube, fibrinous thickening stimulated by the presence of the tube may produce lines (the tube track) that simulate the visceral–pleural boundary, suggesting pneumothorax.

Intra-Aortic Balloon

The intra-aortic balloon (IAB) is an inflatable device placed in the proximal aorta to assist the failing ventricle. Diastolic inflation of the balloon produces a distinct, rounded lucency within the aortic shadow, but in systole, the deflated balloon is not visible. Ideal positioning places the catheter tip just distal to the left subclavian artery. Placed too proximally, the IAB may occlude the carotid or left subclavian artery. Placed too distally, the IAB may occlude the lumbar or mesenteric arteries and produce less effective counterpulsation. Daily radiographic assessment of the aortic contour for evidence of IAB-induced dissection is prudent.

Swan-Ganz Catheter

Each of the insertion-related complications of central venous catheterization, including pneumothorax, pleural entry, and arterial injury, can result from the placement of the pulmonary artery catheter. Unique complications of Swan-Ganz catheter placement include knotting or looping and entanglement with other catheters or pacing wires. The most common radiographic finding is distal catheter tip migration, with or without pulmonary infarction. With an uninflated balloon, the tip of the Swan-Ganz catheter should overlie the middle third of a well-centered AP chest radiograph (within 5 cm of the midline). Distal migration is common in the first hours after insertion as the catheter softens and loses slack. If pressure tracings suggest continuous wedging, it is important to look for a laterally positioned catheter tip, a catheter folded on itself across the pulmonic valve, or a persistently inflated balloon (appearing as a 1-cm-diameter, rounded lucency at the tip of the catheter). The width of the mediastinal and cardiac shadows should be assessed after placement of the catheter, because perforation of the free wall of the ventricle may result in pericardial tamponade. Temporary phrenic nerve paralysis due to the lidocaine used in catheter placement rarely precipitates unilateral hemidiaphragm elevation.

SPECIFIC CONDITIONS DIAGNOSED BY CHEST RADIOGRAPHY

Atelectasis

Acute atelectasis is a frequent cause of infiltration on ICU chest radiographs. The wide spectrum of radiographic findings ranges from invisible microatelectasis, through plate and segmental atelectasis, to collapse of an entire lung. The radiographic differentiation between segmental atelectasis and segmental pneumonia is often difficult, particularly since these conditions often coexist. However, marked volume loss and rapid onset and reversal are more characteristic of acute collapse.

Atelectasis tends to develop in dependent regions and, more commonly, in the left rather than the right lower lobe by a 2:1 margin. Radiographic findings of atelectasis include hemidiaphragm elevation, infiltration or vascular crowding (especially in the retrocardiac area), deviation of hilar vessels, ipsilateral mediastinal shift, and loss of the lateral border of the descending aorta or heart. Contrary to popular belief, the ''silhouette sign'' is not always reliable on portable films, particularly in the presence of an enlarged heart or on a film obtained in a lordotic or rotated projection. Air bronchograms extending into an atelectatic area suggest that collapse continues without total occlusion of the central airway and that attempts at airway clearance by bronchoscopy or suctioning are likely to fail.

Pleural Effusion and Hemothorax

Recognition of pleural effusions requires proper patient positioning. On the supine AP CXR, large effusions redistribute—often causing a hazy density to overlie the entire hemithorax without loss of vascular definition. Apical pleural capping is another radiographic sign of large collections of pleural fluid in the supine patient. Upright or lateral decubitus x-rays may help confirm the presence of pleural fluid (Fig. 11.1). If a large collection of pleural fluid obscures the lung parenchyma, a contralateral decubitus film permits visualization of lung parenchyma. Pleural fluid is not ordinarily visible until several hundred milliliters have accumulated. On lateral decubitus films, 1 cm of layering fluid indicates a volume that can usually be tapped safely.

Subpulmonic or loculated fluid may be difficult to recognize. Hemidiaphragm elevation, lateral displacement of the diaphragmatic apex, abrupt transitions from lucency to solid tissue density, and increased distance from the upper diaphragmatic margin to the gastric bubble (on an upright film) are all signs of a subpulmonic effusion (Fig. 11.2). Ultrasound and chest CT are useful adjuncts in detecting the presence of pleural fluid and in guiding drainage.

Extra-Alveolar Gas

Extra-alveolar gas can manifest as interstitial emphysema, cyst formation, pneumothorax, pneumomediastinum, pneumoperitoneum, or subcutaneous emphysema (see Chapter 8, Mechanical Ventilation: Complications).

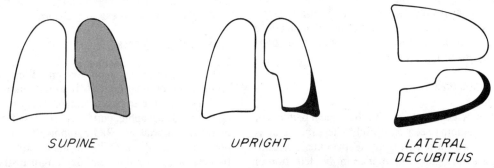

SUPINE   *UPRIGHT*   *LATERAL DECUBITUS*

FIG. 11–1. Appearance of a mobile pleural effusion in three positions. In the supine position, a "ground glass" lateralized diffuse density (with preservation of vascular markings) may be the only sign of layered pleural fluid. A changing appearance with position confirms the diagnosis.

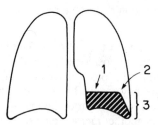

FIG. 11–2. Radiographic signs of a subpulmonic effusion (*1*) hemidiaphragm elevation with separation of lung from gastric bubble, (*2*) lateralization of the diaphragmatic dome, and (*3*) abrupt transition from lucency to soft tissue density.

Pulmonary Interstitial Emphysema

Although long recognized in neonates and young children, radiographic signs of gas in the pulmonary interstitium have been described only recently in adults. These include lucent streaks that do not conform to air bronchograms and cysts at the lung periphery, usually at the bases. Interstitial emphysema may also appear as small target lesions as air surrounds small peripheral pulmonary arterioles viewed en face. These signs, best seen when the parenchyma is densely infiltrated, portend the development of pneumothorax.

Subpleural Air Cysts

Subpleural air cysts, a potential sign of impending pneumothorax for mechanically ventilated patients, are small (3–5 cm diameter), basilar, rounded lucencies. The cysts often present abruptly and may rapidly increase in size (sometimes to as large as 9 cm). Subpleural air cysts frequently progress to tension pneumothorax in the presence of continued mechanical ventilation. The role of prophylactic tube thoracostomy remains unanswered; however, when subpleural air cysts are noted, the clinician should maintain a high level of vigilance and be prepared to emergently insert chest tubes.

Pneumothorax

Few ICU patients exhibit the typical patterns of pneumothorax seen on upright chest radiographs performed on noncritically ill patients. Positioning assumes great importance in the detection of pneumothorax. On supine films or in patients with pleural adhesions, gas may collect exclusively in the basilar (anterior) regions of the thorax. Thus,

gas may outline the minor fissure or may move anteriorly over the heart, mimicking pneumomediastinum or pneumopericardium. Radiographic signs of pneumothorax on the supine CXR include a "deep sulcus sign" and lucency over the upper portions of the spleen or liver (see Chapter 8). An upright expiratory CXR is the best film for detecting a pneumothorax. This view confines a fixed amount of intrapleural air within a smaller volume, accentuating the proportion of thoracic volume it occupies and the separation of lung from chest wall.

The visceral pleura provides a specific marker: a radiodense thin stripe of appropriate curvature with lucency visible on both sides and absent lung markings beyond. Skin folds often mimic the pleural edge but can be distinguished by certain features: lucency present only on one margin, poorly defined limits, and extension beyond the confines of the rib cage. Because pneumothorax reduces blood flow to the collapsed lung, its density may be surprisingly normal, even with an extensive gas collection.

Pneumothoraces often are characterized by the percentage of the hemithorax they occupy. This practice is highly imprecise, both because the CXR is only two-dimensional and because apparent percentage changes occur with variations in breathing depth and position. As with pleural fluid, precise estimation of the size of a pneumothorax is neither possible nor necessary. A tension pneumothorax (of any size) and a "large" pneumothorax both require drainage—the former because of its immediate physiologic effects, the latter because it creates a pleural pocket that is unlikely to reabsorb spontaneously over an acceptable time. The reabsorption rate of a pneumothorax has been estimated to be 1–2% per day, a crude rule that emphasizes the slowness of this process. Thus, a 15% pneumothorax would typically take about 2 weeks to reabsorb.

Tension Pneumothorax

The diagnosis of tension pneumothorax must be made on clinical grounds if serious morbidity and mortality are to be prevented. Delaying therapy for radiographic confirmation significantly increases mortality. Radiographically, tension pneumothorax often shifts the mediastinum and flattens or inverts the hemidiaphragm ipsilateral to the pneumothorax. However, tension usually is difficult to diagnose with confidence on a single film; infiltrated or obstructed lungs fail to collapse completely, and an unyielding mediastinum may not shift noticeably, despite a marked pressure gradient. A comparison of serial films and clinical correlation is most often required.

Pneumothorax occurs in up to 50% of patients receiving mechanical ventilation with peak inflation pressures >60 cm H_2O, and a large fraction of these are under tension. Pneumothorax commonly complicates the course of patients with necrotizing pneumonias, acute respiratory distress syndrome, secretion retention, or expanding cavitary or bullous lesions. Tension pneumothorax can be very difficult to distinguish from bullous disease under tension by plain radiograph. Although a chest CT can be revealing, patients *in extremis* rarely can wait for a diagnostic CT scan. In such emergent settings, erring on the side of chest tube insertion is probably the best course of action, even though rupturing a large bullous lesion can create a bronchopleural fistula.

Pneumomediastinum

After gaining access to the mediastinum, gas normally decompresses into adjacent soft tissues. Thus, unless gas trapping occurs, pneumomediastinum rarely produces important physiologic effects in adults. Mediastinal gas may arise from neck injuries, from rupture of the trachea or esophagus, or (most commonly) from alveolar rupture and retrograde dissection of air along bronchovascular bundles. Pneumomediastinum appears radiographically as a lucent band around the heart and great vessels caused by gas within the space separating the parietal pleura from the mediastinal contents. On the heart's inferior border, this lucency can extend across the mediastinum, linking the two sides of the chest with a "complete diaphragm sign." An unnaturally sharp heart border is the first indicator of pneumomediastinum, a sign that must be distinguished from the "kinetic halo" seen at the heart or diaphragm border of an edematous lung. The mediastinal pleura, defined by gas on both sides of a thin radiodense line, can often be detected. On a lateral film, pneumomediastinum usually appears as a thin crescent of gas outlining the ascending aorta. Not uncommonly, extrapleural gas extends from the mediastinum, lifting the parietal pleura off the diaphragm or outlining the inferior pulmonary ligament.

Subcutaneous Gas

In the adult, subcutaneous gas, also known as subcutaneous emphysema, usually has important diagnostic but limited physiologic significance. Subcutaneous gas produces lucent streaks or bubbles in the soft tissues that outline major muscle groups. During mechanical ventilation, generalized subcutaneous gas usually results from alveolar rupture and medial gas dissection and indicates an increased risk of pneumothorax. Once pneumothorax has occurred, progressive accumulation of gas in the subcutaneous tissue suggests the presence of a bronchopleural fistula or a malfunctioning chest tube, especially if subcutaneous gas is bilateral. Small amounts of subcutaneous gas detected shortly after chest tube placement frequently enter via the tube track itself. Subcutaneous gas detected immediately after blunt chest trauma should raise the possibility of tracheobronchial or esophageal disruption (see Chapter 36, Thoracic Trauma).

PULMONARY EDEMA

Without invasive monitoring, distinguishing between normal permeability (fluid overload and heart failure) and high permeability pulmonary edema, (acute respiratory distress syndrome, ARDS) is difficult. Considerable overlap exists in the radiographic findings of these entities, but certain CXR findings may be helpful in determining the etiology of lung water accumulation. These forms of edema are best distinguished by three features: size of the heart and great vessels, distribution of vascular markings, and the pattern of infiltration (see Table 11.1). Cardiac edema and volume overload are characterized by a widened vascular pedicle, an even or inverted pattern of vascular markings, and a tendency toward a gravitational distribution of edema ("bat wing" or basilar) that may change with position. The vascular pedicle is measured from the point at which the superior vena cava crosses the right main bronchus to a perpendicular dropped from the point of takeoff of the left subclavian artery from the aorta. Kerley's lines are common in established congestive failure (usually of several days to weeks in duration), whereas crisp air bronchograms are unusual. Conversely, the less mobile infiltrates of ARDS are widely scattered, patchy, and often interrupted by distinct air bronchograms. In distinction to the CXR, the CT scan may show marked positioned changes in the distribution of infiltrates. These criteria are better for correctly classifying congestive heart failure and volume overload edema, less accurate for identifying ARDS. Widespread application of these criteria to evaluate the etiology of pulmonary edema

TABLE 11–1

RADIOGRAPHIC FEATURES OF PULMONARY EDEMA

Characteristics	Cardiogenic or Volume Overload Edema	High Permeability Edema
Heart size	Enlarged	Normal
Vascular pedicle	Normal/enlarged	Normal/small
Flow distribution	Cephalad	Caudad/balanced
Blood volume	Normal/increased	Normal
Septal lines	Common	Absent
Peribronchial cuffing	Very common	Uncommon
Air bronchograms	Uncommon	Very common
Edema distribution	Even/Central/gravitational	Patchy/peripheral/nongravitational
Pleural effusion	Very common/moderate-large	Uncommon/small

has shown them to be less successful than originally claimed.

Although pulmonary edema is usually bilateral and symmetric, it may collect asymmetrically when mediastinal tumor, bronchial cyst, or massive thromboembolism diverts flow preferentially to one lung. The recently transplanted lung is also prone to developing unilateral pulmonary edema. Asymmetry may also be observed after unilateral aspiration, reexpansion pulmonary edema, or in the presence of extensive bullous disease. Gravity may redistribute edema fluid to dependent lung regions over brief periods, one mechanism for shifting unilateral edema after patient repositioning.

Because most of the radiographic deterioration seen in ARDS occurs within the first 5 days of illness, worsening infiltrates after this time suggests superimposed pneumonia, fluid overload, sepsis, or the development of heart failure.

NOSOCOMIAL INFECTION IN ARDS

Nosocomial pneumonia affects up to 30% of patients with ARDS but is difficult to detect with certainty because focal parenchymal densities may represent edema, atelectasis, infarction, or infection. Hence, radiographic abnormalities must be interpreted in light of the clinical situation. A new unilateral infiltrate in a patient with a previously stable CXR is the best radiographic indicator of a superimposed infection; however, fever, increased sputum production, and progressive hypoxemia are better indicators than the radiograph. A focal wedge-shaped infiltrate (especially occurring distal to a Swan-Ganz catheter tip or in a patient with hemoptysis) is likely to represent pulmonary infarction.

MEDIASTINAL WIDENING

Mediastinal widening (particularly after chest trauma or an invasive procedure) provides a clue to aortic disruption. Obtaining an upright posterior-anterior CXR is desirable but frequently is not possible because of injuries or hypotension. Radiographic clues to aortic disruption include a widened superior mediastinum (the most sensitive sign), a blurred aortic knob, rightward deviation of the nasogastric tube or aortic shadow, and tracheal deviation to the right and anteriorly. Inferior displacement of the left main bronchus, left-sided pleural effusion (with or without apical capping), and displacement of intimal calcifications of the aorta provide other signs suggestive of aortic disruption (see Chapter 36, Thoracic Trauma). Mediastinal widening with vascular injury frequently is associated with traumatic fractures of the sternum, first two ribs, or clavicle. Widening of the cardiac shadow should prompt careful review of the aortic contour, because blood may dissect from the aorta into the pericardium. If aortic disruption is suspected, angiography is the definitive procedure, although contrast-enhanced CT scanning or echocardiography may be highly suggestive.

PERICARDIAL EFFUSION

Pericardial effusion is recognized radiographically by enlargement of the cardiac shadow. The classic "water bottle configuration" of the cardiac silhouette, although highly characteristic, is unusual. An epicardial fat pad visible on the lateral CXR should raise the suspicion of a pericardial effusion, as should splaying of the tracheal bifurcation. Echocardiography is the procedure of

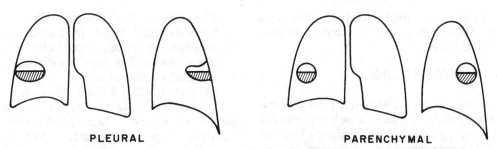

PLEURAL   PARENCHYMAL

FIG. 11–3. Intraparenchymal versus intrapleural fluid collections. Fluid collections within the pleural space usually have a greater horizontal than vertical dimension, do not cross fissure lines, and may have sloping attachments to the pleural surface on one or more views. Furthermore, pleural collections typically have different dimensions on anterior-posterior and lateral views. In contrast, intraparenchymal collections tend to be more spherical, with equal dimensions on anterior-posterior and lateral views.

choice for the detection and evaluation of pericardial effusions and simultaneously affords the opportunity to assess heart chamber size, contractile function, and vena caval diameter.

AIR–FLUID LEVELS (LUNG ABSCESS VERSUS EMPYEMA)

Several guidelines aid in deciding whether an air–fluid level lies within the pleural space or within the lung parenchyma. On an AP film, pleural fluid collections generate wide, moderately dense air–fluid levels, whereas intrapulmonary collections are usually smaller, more dense, and rounded. Lung abscesses and liquid-filled bullae tend to project similar diameters on both AP and lateral films. The air–fluid level of pleural fluid collections must abut the chest wall on either AP or lateral film (Fig. 11.3).

Fluid collections that cross a fissure line on upright films are located within the pleural space. Lung abscesses generally have thick, shaggy walls with irregular contours, unlike liquid-filled bullae and pleural fluid collections. As position is altered, pleural fluid collections frequently undergo marked changes in shape or contour. CT scanning is the technique of choice for sorting difficult cases.

POST-THORACOTOMY CHANGES

After pneumonectomy, fluid accumulates in the vacant hemithorax over days to months. Whereas the absolute fluid level is of little significance, changes in the level of fluid are important. Very rapid postoperative filling of the hemithorax suggests infection, hemorrhage, or malignant effu-

sion. A rapid decline in the fluid level should prompt concern for a bronchopleural fistula, a complication that most commonly develops within 8–12 days of surgery. If a fistula develops earlier, mechanical failure of the bronchial closure should be suspected, prompting consideration of reoperation. Bronchopleural fistulas occurring after thoracotomy may be confirmed by instilling a sterile tracer into the pleural space and inspecting the expectorated sputum immediately afterward, or alternatively, by the inhalation of radioactive gas, followed by imaging of the thorax. Bronchopleural fistulas tend to displace the mediastinum to the contralateral side, an unusual occurrence during uneventful postoperative recovery. Small residual air spaces may remain for up to 1 year after pneumonectomy and do not necessarily imply the presence of a persistent fistula.

FISTULOUS TRACTS

Fistulas between the trachea and innominate artery develop most frequently when a tracheal tube angulates anteriorly and to the right in patients with low tracheostomy stoma, persistent hyperextension of the neck, or asthenic habitus. Because of this association, anteriorly directed tracheal tubes should be repositioned.

Fistulas also may form between the trachea and esophagus during prolonged endotracheal intubation. These usually occur at the level of the endotracheal tube cuff, directly behind the manubrium. Predisposing factors include cuff overdistention, simultaneous nasogastric intubation, and posterior angulation of the tracheal tube tip. The sudden occurrence of massive gastric dilation in a mechanically ventilated patient provides an important clue. A radiographic contrast agent may be introduced into the esophagus after cuff deflation or tube removal in an attempt to confirm the presence of the fistula.

PULMONARY EMBOLISM

Although the plain CXR rarely helps diagnose pulmonary embolism, large emboli may give rise to highly suggestive findings: ipsilateral hypovascularity, enlargement of the pulmonary arteries, and (rarely) abrupt vascular cutoff. Local oligemia (Westermark's sign) may be seen early in the course of pulmonary embolism, usually within the first 36 hours. "Hampton's hump," a pleural-based triangular density due to pulmonary infarction, is seldom seen. About 50% of patients with pulmonary emboli have an associated pleural effusion.

The rarity of a normal CXR diminishes the value of ventilation/perfusion scanning in the critically ill. Nonetheless, normal perfusion scans are very helpful, and abnormal scans help guide the angiographic search for pulmonary emboli. In the absence of a normal perfusion scan, angiography is usually the only way to confirm or rule out pulmonary embolic disease. Angiography can be safely undertaken for most critically ill patients, if: (*a*) care is used in transport; (*b*) pulmonary artery pressures are not excessive at the time of contrast administration; and (*c*) selective injections guided by perfusion scanning are performed. For patients who cannot be moved to the angiography suite, bedside angiography through a flow-directed catheter offers a much less satisfactory option. Because the therapy for deep venous thrombosis (DVT) and pulmonary embolism is usually the same, obtaining a bedside study for DVT (impedance plethysmography or Doppler ultrasound) can eliminate the need for pulmonary angiography in up to 50% of cases. Septic pulmonary embolism should be considered in patients with multifocal cavitary lesions of varying size.

PNEUMONITIS

Although bacterial infection often supervenes, gastric aspiration initially produces a sterile chemical pneumonitis. Massive aspiration, although somewhat position- and volume-dependent, typically appears as bilateral diffuse alveolar and interstitial infiltrates of rapid onset. Aspiration in the supine position usually affects the perihilar regions and superior and basilar segments of the lower lobes. Patients who aspirate in a decubitus position often develop unilateral infiltrates. Foreign objects (teeth, dental appliances, pieces of resuscitation equipment) occasionally are aspirated in patients undergoing resuscitation, trauma, or endotracheal intubation.

Although the CXR is never diagnostic, it may give a clue to the organism producing bacterial pneumonia. Common bacterial pathogens typically produce patchy segmental or lobar involvement. Bulging fissures, although uncommon, suggest *Klebsiella pneumonia.* A diffuse, patchy, "ground glass" appearance suggests *Legionella, Mycoplasma,* or *Pneumocystis.* Small, diffusely scattered nodular densities suggest *Mycobacterium tuberculosis* as the etiologic organism. Larger nodular densities are associated with *Cryptococcoses, Actinomycosis,* or *Nocardiosis. Aspergillus* often gives rise to peripheral wedge-shaped infiltrates caused by vascular invasion and secondary infarction or cavitary formation. Frank cavitation suggests neoplasm, tuberculosis, fungal infection (histoplasmosis, cryptococcoses, coccidiomycosis), lung abscess, or septic pulmonary embolism. Pneumonitis that develops in preexisting areas of bullous emphysema often produces air–fluid levels that can be confused with lung abscess or empyema. The thin contour of the cavity wall, the more rapid pace of development and resolution, and premorbid CXRs demonstrating bullae help to identify this problem.

INTRA-ABDOMINAL CONDITIONS

The upright CXR also helps to diagnose acute intra-abdominal problems. Midline or para-esophageal hiatal hernias usually pose little diagnostic problem. Diaphragmatic disruption may allow abdominal contents to herniate into the chest after abdominal trauma, often displacing a gas containing viscus into the left chest. Oral contrast studies aid in the diagnosis, as does the CT scan, injection of a sterile contrast agent into the pleural space, or diagnostic pneumoperitoneum. The upright CXR also provides the most sensitive method of detecting free air within the abdominal cavity. (A cross-table film of the abdomen taken at least 5 minutes after decubitus positioning serves a similar purpose.) Intubated patients frequently swallow air, producing gastric dilation. In the appropriate setting, massive gastric dilation can suggest the possibility of esophageal intubation or a tracheoesophageal fistula.

CT AND MRI OF THE CHEST

CT scanning and MRI have significant limitations in the critically ill population. Appropriately, concern has been voiced over the risks of moving patients out of the ICU for imaging studies; however, carefully arranged transport typically is performed without incident (see Chapter 18: General Supportive Care). The range of physiologic changes observed in patients transported to the radiology suite is comparable to that of patients who remain in the ICU for a similar time. The most important feature of safe transport is to ensure adequate equipment and personnel are available immediately to cope with a catastrophic emergency (accidental extubation, interruption of critical intravenous infusions, or extraction of venous, arterial, or enteral catheters). Patients with bronchopleural fistulae and those requiring vasopressors or high inspired oxygen concentrations or PEEP are at particular risk.

Metallic appliances create artifact on CT scans and may preclude use of MRI because of the powerful magnetic fields involved. Furthermore, both CT and MRI studies are time consuming, and require the patient to remain immobile. Chest CT scanning often requires the use of potentially toxic, iodinated contrast material, a limitation avoided by MRI. Finally, the financial aspects of imaging cannot be overlooked. A chest CT scan typically costs three to four times as much as a portable chest radiograph in addition to the costs of transport, which can be substantial.

Despite these technical limitations, the chest CT often provides information not otherwise available. It frequently reveals a pneumothorax in trauma patients, even when previous CXRs are unrevealing. Chest CT also aids in the discovery of lung abscess or empyema and can differentiate between the two conditions. For patients with persistent unexplained fever or persistent pneumothorax, the chest CT is invaluable to evaluate the location of thoracic drainage tubes. CT scanning also has added greatly to our understanding of the distribution of lung injury in ARDS. The homogenous-appearing density of the chest radiograph is actually composed of patchy, dependent consolidation when viewed by CT. Within minutes of repositioning a patient, previously normal-appearing lung regions can become infiltrated, a finding that correlates nicely with the clinical observation that positional changes quickly alter oxygenation. CT scanning also demonstrates the severity and distribution of regional barotrauma, offering insight into the potential deleterious effects of excessive airway pressure. Normal-appearing lung is seen immediately juxtaposed with densely infiltrated lung. These normal-appearing and presumably normally compliant lung units are those likely to be overdistended by positive pressure, whereas densely infiltrated lung is likely to remain atelectatic. The physiologic result is shunting of blood past atelectatic alveoli and overdistention of other alveoli, predisposing them to rupture.

In summary, despite technical limitations, the chest CT represents one of the most useful diagnostics tests available. A short list of indications for chest CT scanning includes the following: (a) evaluation of thoracic trauma; (b) searching for occult or persistent sources of fever (empyema, lung, or mediastinal abscess); (c) guiding placement of drainage tubes for loculated or persistent pneumothorax or pleural effusions; and (d) detecting mediastinal pathology (especially in the presence of parenchymal infiltrate). It is also reasonable to perform chest CT scanning in the patient exhibiting "septic" physiology in the absence of a clear source. Considering the potential benefit of precise diagnosis and the costs in terms of time, manpower, and risk involved in transport, an argument could be made to add abdominal or cranial scanning to chest imaging in a single trip if there are any signs of abdominal or cranial pathology.

ABDOMINAL RADIOGRAPHY

SCREENING FILM

Standard examination of the abdomen includes supine kidney–ureter–bladder (KUB) or "flat plate" and upright views. If an upright film cannot be taken, a lateral decubitus view may be substituted. (Cross-table supine x-rays are of little value, except to demonstrate calcification in aortic aneurysms.) Systematic review of the abdominal film may furnish important information, especially after trauma. Fractures of the lower ribs on the left suggest the possibility of a ruptured spleen or lacerated kidney, as does medial displacement of the gastric bubble. Breaks in lower ribs on the right suggest the possibility of renal or hepatic damage. Fractures of the lumbar spine, pelvis, and hips may be seen as "incidental" findings on plain abdominal radiographs in trauma patients. A ground glass appearance, displacement of the retroperitoneal fat stripe, or centralization of gas shadows suggests intra-abdominal ascites or blood. Free air usually indicates a ruptured viscus, gas producing infection, barotraumatic pneumoperitoneum, or postoperative change. Free air is seen much more commonly as the result of upper GI (stomach or duodenum) perforation rather than from colonic perforation (diverticulitis, appendicitis, colon cancer).

Rarely, the KUB view is useful in the setting of undiagnosed coma. Some ingested tablets are radiopaque (e.g., iron, phenothiazines, tricyclics, chloral hydrate). In hydrocarbon ingestion, upright or decubitus films of the abdomen may show a characteristic "fluid–fluid" level of hydrocarbon floating on the gastric contents.

The KUB view is a poor indicator of liver size and should not supplant careful physical examination. The gallbladder is poorly defined on the KUB view unless it is very distended or calcified. Less than 15% of gallbladder calculi are visible. Gas appearing spontaneously in the biliary ducts is highly suggestive of cholangitis. Hepatic calcifications, although rare, may be due to healed infection, hemangioma, or metastatic carcinoma. Films taken in different positions may help to sort out the location of right upper quadrant calcifications. Calcifications within the kidney or liver maintain a relatively fixed position, whereas stones within the gallbladder usually are mobile. Use of the KUB view in the diagnosis of the "acute abdomen" is discussed in Chapter 37.

FINDINGS RELEVANT TO SPECIFIC ORGANS

The use of abdominal ultrasound and abdominal CT scanning is discussed in detail as it relates to specific disease entities in Chapters 37, 38, and 39.

Kidneys and Ureters

The visibility of the nephric shadows on the KUB view depends on the amount of perinephric fat and bowel gas. The combination of kidney enlargement and calcification suggests urinary tract obstruction or polycystic kidney disease. If nephrolithiasis is suspected, the renal outlines and course of both ureters should be inspected carefully for calculi (visible in up to 85% of cases). Gas-producing infections of the bladder also are seen occasionally. Gas in the kidney ("emphysematous kidney") indicates overwhelming infection and the need for urgent surgical intervention.

Pancreas and Retroperitoneum

Asymmetric obliteration of the psoas shadows or retroperitoneal fat lines suggests a retroperitoneal process (most commonly pancreatitis or a ruptured aorta). Similar changes can be seen with spontaneous hemorrhage or traumatic disruption. Although the pancreas is not normally seen on the plain radiograph, calcifications may occur in chronic alcoholic pancreatitis. Localized areas of ileus over the pancreas, such as the "colon cutoff sign" and the "sentinel loop," may also aid in the diagnosis of pancreatic inflammation.

Stomach and Bowel

The stomach normally contains some fluid and air, but massive gastric dilation suggests gastric outlet obstruction, gastroparesis, or esophageal intubation. The small bowel normally contains little air; gaseous distention indicates ileus or small bowel obstruction. Air–fluid levels of different heights within the same loop of small bowel on an upright film usually indicate mechanical small bowel obstruction and imply residual peristaltic activity. Fluid levels at the same height in a loop of bowel do not necessarily indicate mechanical obstruction. Absence of colonic or rectal gas in patients with small bowel air–fluid levels strongly suggests complete obstruction of the small bowel with distal clearing of gas. Conversely, the presence of gas in the colon (except for small amounts of rectal gas) all but excludes the diagnosis of complete small bowel obstruction. (Incomplete obstruction may be present, however.)

Colonic obstruction caused by a sigmoid volvulus may be diagnosed via a KUB view that shows massive sigmoid dilation; the sigmoid forms an inverted "U," the limbs of which rise out of the pelvis. Apposition of the medial walls of these bowel segments produces a midline soft tissue density in which the inferior extent approximates the site of torsion.

Peritoneal Cavity

On the supine abdominal radiograph, ascites is demonstrated by diffuse haze, indistinctness of the iliopsoas stripes, centralization of small bowel segments, and abnormal separation of bowel loops. Increased pelvic density characterizes ascites on the upright film.

Abnormal gas collections are recognized by their nonanatomic location. Therefore, all gas densities on supine and erect films require explanation. Each must be assigned to an anatomic segment of bowel. Gas may collect under the diaphragm or overlie the liver on erect or lateral decubitus films, respectively. Free air also allows visualization of both sides of the walls of gas-filled bowel. In the ICU, a cross-table view in the lateral decubitus position (taken at least 10 minutes later) may be the most sensitive way to diagnose small amounts of free peritoneal gas. "Bubbly," curvilinear, or triangular gas collections between segments of bowel suggest abdominal abscess. Bowel ischemia may produce a characteristic pattern known as pneumatosis cystoides that represents gas within the bowel wall. Rarely, pneumatosis may rupture to produce free intraperitoneal air, simulating a perforated viscus.

KEY POINTS

1. The value of a portable chest radiograph is critically dependent on obtaining an appropriatedly penetrated, upright exposure in full inspiration.

2. Although certain signs may be suggestive, the chest radiograph does not reliably distinguish high permeability from low permeability pulmonary edema.

3. Parenchymal infiltrates have many common potential etiologies (including atelectasis, embolism, edema, and hemorrhage). Only a minority of infiltrates represent infection; the diagnosis of nosocomial pneumonia requires strong clinical correlation.

4. Chest CT is safe and often reveals conditions that were not suspected by plain radiograph; therefore, a low threshold should be maintained for its use in patients with difficult-to-interpret radiographs and those who are deteriorating despite seemingly adequate therapy.

5. CT is the single best imaging modality for evaluating the abdomen unless the primary working diagnosis is cholelithiasis, ureteral obstruction, or ectopic pregnancy, in which case ultrasound is equal or superior.

SUGGESTED READINGS

1. Federle MP, ed. Symposium on CT and ultrasonography in the acutely ill patient. Radiol Clin North Am 1983; 21(3):423–606.
2. Goodman LR, Putnam CE. Intensive care radiology: imaging of the critically ill. 2nd ed., vol. 20. Philadelphia: WB Saunders, 1983.
3. Milne EN, Pistolesi M, Miniati M, Giuntini C, et al. The radiologic distinction of cardiogenic and noncardiogenic edema. Am J Roentgenol 1985;144:879–894.
4. Putman CE. Symposium on cardiopulmonary imaging. Radiol Clin North Am 19833;21(4):607–826.
5. Wegenius G, Erickson U, Borg T, Modig J. Value of chest radiography in adult respiratory distress syndrome. Acta Radiol 1984;25:177–184.
6. Greenbaum DM, Marschall KE. Value of routine daily chest x-rays in intubated patients in the medical intensive care unit. Crit Care Med 1982;10:29–30.
7. Henschae CI, Pasternak GS, Schroeder S, et al. Bedside chest radiography: diagnostic efficacy. Radiology 1983; 149:23–26.
8. Janower ML, Jennas-Nocera Z, Mukai J. Utility and efficacy of portable chest radiographs. Am J Radiol 1984; 142:265–267.
9. Harris RA. The preoperative chest film in relation to postoperative management: some effects of different projection, posture and lung inflation. Br J Radiol 1980;5: 196–201.
10. Zimmerman JE, Goodman LR, Shahvari MB. Effect of mechanical ventilation and positive pressure on chest radiograph. Am J Roentgenol 1979;133:811.
11. Gattinoni L, Mascherroni D, Torresin A, et al. Morphological and functional changes induced by PEEP in ARF. Intensive Care Med 1986;12:136–142.
12. Aberle DR, Wiener-Kronish JP, Webb WR, et al. Hydrostatic versus increased permeability pulmonary edema: diagnosis based upon radiographic criteria in critically ill patients. Radiology 1988;168:73–79.
13. Miniati M, Pistolesi M, Paoletti P, et al. Objective radiographic criteria to differentiate cardiac, renal, and lung injury edema. Invest Radiol 1988;23:433–440.
14. Smith RC, Mann H, Greenspan RH, et al. Radiographic differentiation between different etiologies of pulmonary edema. Invest Radiol 1987;22:859–863.
15. Weiner-Kronish JP, Matthay MA. Pleural effusions associated with hydrostatic and increased permeability pulmonary edema. Chest 1988;93:852–858.
16. Peruzzi W, Garner W, Bools J, Rasanen J, Mueller CF, Reilley T. Portable chest roentgenography and computed tomography in critically ill patients. Chest 1988;93: 722–726.
17. Snow N, Bergin KT, Horrigan TP. Thoracic CT scanning in critically ill patients. Chest 1990;97:1467–1470.
18. Maunder RJ, Shuman WP, McHugh JW, Marglin SI, Butler J. Preservation of normal lung regions in the adult respiratory distress syndrome: analysis by computed tomography. JAMA 1986;255:2463–2466.

19. Gattanoni L, Pesenti A, Torresin A, et al. Adult respiratory distress syndrome profiles by computed tomography. J Thorac Imaging 1986;1:25–31.

20. Bombino M, Gattinoni L, Pesenti A, Pistolisi M, Miniati M. The value of portable chest radiography in adult respiratory distress syndrome: comparison with computed tomography. Chest 1991;100:762–769.

21. Woodring JH. Pulmonary interstitial emphysema in the adult respiratory distress syndrome. Crit Care Med 1985; 13:786–791.

22. Unger JM, England DM, Bogust GA. Interstitial emphysema in adults: recognition and prognostic implications. J Thorac Imaging 1989;4:86–94.

23. Rohlfing BM, Webb WR, Schlobotim RM. Ventilator related extra alveolar air in adults. Radiology 1976;121: 25–30.

24. Tocino IM, Miller MH, Fairfax WR. Distribution of pneu-

mothorax in the supine and semi-recumbent critically ill adult. Am J Roentgenol 1985;144:901–905.

25. Chiles C, Ravin CE. Radiographic recognition of pneumothorax in the intensive care unit. Crit Care Med 1986;16: 677–680.

26. Gobien RP, Reines HD, Schabel SI. Localized tension pneumothorax: unrecognized form of barotrauma in adult respiratory distress syndrome. Radiology 1982;142: 15–19.

27. Albeda SM, Gefter WB, Kelley MA, et al. Ventilator-induced subpleural air cysts: clinical, radiographic and pathologic significance. Am Rev Respir Dis 1983;127: 360–365.

28. Gagliardi PD. Correlative imaging in abdominal infection: an algorithmic approach using nuclear medicine, ultrasound, and computed tomography. Semin Nucl Med 1988; 18:320–334.

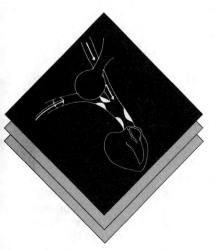

CHAPTER 12

Acid–Base Disorders

Disturbances of acid–base balance can be suggested by the clinical findings of altered mental status or respiratory rate and by laboratory studies revealing an abnormal serum bicarbonate or elevated anion gap. Despite suspicions raised by these findings, only the combination of a properly obtained arterial blood gas, electrolyte profile, and clinical examination can accurately diagnose the cause of an acid–base disorder.

ARTERIAL BLOOD GASES

OBTAINING ARTERIAL BLOOD GASES

Arterial blood gases (ABGs) are valuable only if obtained properly and measured carefully. Patients should have a stable FiO_2 for at least 10 minutes before sampling to allow the PaO_2 to equilibrate. Patient position should be noted, because PaO_2 may change significantly with varying body position. (Saturation usually is worse in the supine position.) Ventilatory pattern (breath-holding or hyperventilation) also should be noted. Changes in breathing rate or depth may significantly alter the $PaCO_2$ and cause milder changes in the PaO_2. Prolonged attempts to obtain an ABG often result in mild hyperventilation as pain and anxiety build in the patient.

The patient's body temperature should be recorded. For any given O_2 content, the measured PaO_2 increases as blood is warmed. An increased PaO_2 occurs both because of rightward shifts in the oxyhemoglobin dissociation curve and because the solubility of gases decreases in warmer fluids. Hypothermia shifts the oxyhemoglobin dissociation curve leftward; therefore, as cold blood is warmed to the standard analysis temperature (37°), O_2 solubility decreases (resulting in an artificially high measured PaO_2). The $PaCO_2$ also will rise as blood is warmed, producing modest declines in the pH. Thermal correction usually is unnecessary, except at temperature extremes, and the physiologic relevance of temperature ''correction'' remains debatable (see Appendix).

When sampling from the radial artery, it is important to assess collateral blood flow to the hand. Patency of the alternate blood supply, the ulnar artery, is confirmed by the Allen test, which is performed by elevating the hand, occluding both ulnar and radial arteries, and releasing compression of the ulnar artery. If adequate collateral circulation is present, the hand should flush pink within 5 to 7 seconds. For arterial puncture, the wrist is positioned in mild extension and the skin is cleansed—first with an iodophor solution and then with alcohol. Lidocaine (approximately 0.5 mL of 1% solution) may be used but is rarely necessary; furthermore, excessive anesthetic volume may obliterate normal landmarks and arterial pulsations. Now, a commercially prepared ABG syringe usually is used; however, in its absence, a heparin-coated 3-mL syringe tipped with a 21-gauge needle will suffice. The artery is approached from a 45° angle. Immediately upon vessel entry, pulsatile blood will fill the syringe. (Aspiration is not necessary in most cases.) Blood flow will cease if the needle penetrates the posterior arterial wall, but flow often may be reestablished merely by retracting the needle. After sam-

209

pling is complete, the needle should be removed and firm pressure should be applied to the puncture site for 5 minutes (or longer if coagulation disorders exist). The syringe should be capped or the needle should be inserted into a cork and the blood and heparin should be mixed by a rolling motion. Prompt analysis is required to obtain accurate results.

PITFALLS IN COLLECTION, ANALYSIS, AND INTERPRETATION

Timing of Analysis

Accuracy depends on prompt analysis. Under most circumstances, the $PaCO_2$ rises approximately 3 to 10 mm Hg/hr in un-iced specimens, causing a modest fall in pH. Conversely, the PaO_2 usually is stable in an iced sample for 1 to 2 hours. Samples of body fluids that do not contain as much hemoglobin or other protein buffers as blood (e.g., pleural or joint fluid) demonstrate more rapid pH changes if analysis is delayed.

Pseudohypoxemia

The PaO_2 may dramatically decrease if significant O_2 is consumed *in vitro* after the blood is sampled—a problem that is most common with marked leukocytosis or thrombocytosis. Leukocyte counts higher than $10^5/mm^3$ or platelet counts higher than $10^6/mm^3$ usually are required to produce significant changes. Addition of cyanide to ABGs and/or immediate icing of the sample decreases the likelihood of "pseudohypoxemia." Diffusion of O_2 through the wall of plastic syringes may lead to false reductions in measured PaO_2 (particularly in samples with high O_2 tensions), because plastic syringes are much more permeable than glass to oxygen.

Pseudoacidosis

"Pseudoacidosis" may occur when incubating, metabolically active leukocytes generate large quantities of CO_2, causing an acidosis to develop *in vitro*. This problem is most likely to occur with delayed analysis of warm samples containing high numbers of leukocytes. Excessive amounts of acidic heparin in the sampling syringe also may cause pseudoacidosis by diluting and/or neutralizing serum bicarbonate. (The potential magnitude of heparin-related change is small, however.)

Air Bubbles

The PO_2 of room air is approximately 150 mm Hg and the PCO_2 is near 0 mm Hg. Therefore, when large air bubbles are mixed with arterial blood, usually the PaO_2 rises and the $PaCO_2$ falls. (If the PaO_2 in the blood exceeds that in the bubble, however, the measured PaO_2 could decline.) A small air bubble in a relatively large sample usually has little effect, but when the ratio of bubble to blood volume is large, increases in PaO_2 of up to 30 mm Hg may occur. It is uncommon for bubbles to significantly reduce the $PaCO_2$ unless the baseline CO_2 tension is very high.

Contamination of Arterial Samples with Venous Blood

Normally, the $PaCO_2$ is higher and PaO_2 is lower in venous blood than in arterial blood as oxygen is extracted and carbon dioxide is added by metabolically active tissues. The degree of oxygen extraction varies greatly among organ systems; the heart is a near complete extractor of oxygen, whereas venous blood from the kidney still contains large amounts of oxygen and less added CO_2. Furthermore, the degree of O_2 extraction can vary substantially over time for any specific organ. This heterogeneity of venous gas tensions explains why a peripheral venous sample, predominantly reflecting skin and muscle oxygen extraction, cannot serve as an accurate indicator of total body oxygen extraction or consumption. Because of the presence of effective buffering systems described below, however, pH changes little in venous blood, even with increases in $PaCO_2$.

Because gas tensions in venous blood differ from those in the arterial circuit, addition of any venous blood to an arterial sample tends to produce an artifactual hypoxemia and hypercarbia but does little to measured pH. Thus, peripheral venous samples may be useful to gauge pH but are not valuable in the analysis of PaO_2 or $PaCO_2$ and cannot be used to assess global oxygen supply:demand ratios, an analysis that requires a true "mixed venous blood sample" (see below).

RISKS

Risks of arterial puncture are very low for single sticks but increase when persistent cannulation is used (see Chapter 2, Hemodynamic Monitoring). Infection is very rare unless infected tissue is traversed en route to the artery. Arterial occlusion can be avoided by varying sampling sites, using the smallest needle that produces good blood flow, and confirming collateral flow before puncture. (Approximately 3% of hospitalized patients have inadequate collateral circulation.) Even when all appropriate precautions are taken, ischemic complications can occur as a result of thrombosis, systemic hypotension, vasopressor use, or an underlying vascular disorder (e.g., Raynaud's disease). Occult bleeding into large adjacent soft tissue spaces may occur after femoral or brachial arterial punctures. (Large quantities of blood can be lost into the thigh with only subtle physical signs.) Nerve trauma usually is due to direct nerve puncture by an inexperienced phlebotomist but also may result from a compressive hematoma if coagulopathy is present or if inadequate pressure is held at the puncture site.

MIXED VENOUS BLOOD SAMPLES

Occasionally, it is desirable to measure PaO_2 and hemoglobin saturation in the mixed venous blood in an attempt to evaluate the overall balance between oxygen supply and demand or to determine the cause for arterial hypoxemia. (The concept and practice of this analysis is discussed in detail in Chapter 2, Hemodynamic Monitoring.) The normal mixed venous sample has a PO_2 near 40 mm Hg, equating to a saturation of approximately 75%. Although convenient to obtain, peripheral venous blood is inadequate for evaluation because, unlike systemic arterial blood, which has a uniform PaO_2 the O_2 saturation of venous blood sampled at different sites varies greatly (see above). For this reason, mixed venous oxygen saturation must be measured using thoroughly mixed pulmonary artery blood, not blood from a peripheral vein, the vena cava, or even the right ventricle. Technique is important in obtaining the mixed venous sample—if obtained with the catheter in the "wedged" position, an artificially high mixed venous oxygen tension (saturation) will result as oxygenated blood is sucked retrograde past functioning alveoli into the syringe.

BASICS ABG CONCEPTS

NORMAL VALUES

Normally, arterial pH, the negative common logarithm of the hydrogen ion (H^+) concentra-

tion, varies between 7.35 and 7.45. When breathing room air, normal $PaCO_2$ varies between 35 and 45 mm Hg, and PaO_2 values greater than 80 to 90 mm Hg are considered normal, depending on age. Venous blood gases have a lower pH than arterial gases (normal, approximately 7.35), a lower PaO_2 (normal, approximately 40 mm Hg), and a slightly increased $PaCO_2$ (normal, approximately 45 mm Hg). Values for $PaCO_2$, PaO_2, and pH are measured directly. In contrast, the reported HCO_3^- concentration usually is not measured but rather is calculated from pH and $PaCO_2$, using a nomogram derived from the Henderson-Hasselbalch equation. Direct automated determinations of serum HCO_3^- (total CO_2 content) are more accurate than nomograms for determining HCO_3^- content. In a similar fashion, the reported arterial oxygen saturation (SaO_2) usually is not measured but is calculated from the PaO_2.

GAS TENSION VERSUS SATURATION AND CONTENT

The partial pressure of a gas in blood—its tension—reflects the rapidity with which gas molecules move in the serum. Gas content depends not only on its partial pressure but also on the storage capacity for that gas in blood. CO_2 is carried in dissolved form, as well as bound to hemoglobin and other protein buffers, and its content parallels its tension across a wide range. However, transport of O_2 is more complex, so that the relationship between tension and saturation (content) is highly alinear. ABGs provide the data necessary to calculate indices of the efficiency of oxygenation such as the alveolar-arterial oxygen gradient (A-aDO_2), the alveolar:arterial ratio (A/a ratio), and the PaO_2/FIO_2 ratio. The advantages and limitations of each of these indices is discussed in detail in Chapter 5, Respiratory Monitoring.

ALTERATIONS IN OXYGENATION

Oxygen Tension Versus Saturation

At ambient pressure, oxygen content of blood is determined predominantly by the quantity of O_2 bound to hemoglobin (Hgb), with a minor contribution from dissolved O_2. The O_2 carried in a volume of blood (mL/dL) is influenced by PaO_2 (mm Hg), Hgb concentration (gm/dL), pH, and by the characteristics of the Hgb itself: O_2 content $= 1.34$ (Hgb)(%Sat) $+ (0.003)(PaO_2)$. Under most circumstances, the quantity of dissolved oxygen is negligible but becomes significant when pure oxygen is administered under hyperbaric conditions. In such circumstances, PaO_2 can exceed 2000 mm Hg.

ABG analysis determines the partial pressure of dissolved O_2 directly but provides only an indirect (and often inaccurate) indicator of O_2 content. Anemia has a direct and obvious effect on this relationship. More subtly, abnormal hemoglobins (e.g., methemoglobin, carboxyhemoglobin) may bind O_2 with lower affinity than normal, or they may have their O_2 binding sites occupied, producing a lower O_2 content than the relationship between PaO_2 and normal Hgb would predict.

Hypoxemia

With regard to tissue needs, both the quantity of oxygen delivered per unit of time (the product of cardiac output and oxygen content per unit volume) and the arterial partial pressure of O_2 (PaO_2) are important. Tolerance for hypoxemia depends not only on the extent of desaturation but also on compensatory mechanisms available and the sensitivity of the patient to hypoxia. Apart from increased O_2 extraction, the major mechanisms of compensation are increased cardiac output, improved perfusion (due to capillary recruitment and changes in distribution of resistance), and manufacture of red cells (erythrocytosis). Other adaptations, such as improved unloading of O_2 by tissue acidosis and increased anaerobic metabolism, assume importance when failure of the primary methods calls them into action (e.g., circulatory arrest).

If an individual without cardiac limitation or anemia is made hypoxic over a short period of time, no important effect will be noted until PaO_2 falls below 50 to 60 mm Hg. At that level, malaise, lightheadedness, mild nausea, vertigo, impaired judgment, and incoordination generally are the first symptoms noted, reflecting the preferential sensitivity of cerebral tissue to hypoxia. Although minute ventilation increases, little dyspnea develops unless hyperpnea uncovers underlying mechanical lung problems, as in chronic obstructive pulmonary disease (COPD). Confusion resembling alcohol intoxication appears as PaO_2 falls into the range of 35 to 50 mm Hg, especially in older individuals with ischemic cerebrovascular disease. (Such patients also are prone to heart rhythm disturbances.) As PaO_2 falls below 35 mm Hg, renal blood flow decreases, urine output slows, and atropine-refractory bradycardia and

conduction system blockade develop. Lactic acidosis also appears at this level, even with normal cardiac function. The patient becomes lethargic or obtunded and minute ventilation is maximal. At a PaO_2 of approximately 25 mm Hg, the normal unadapted individual loses consciousness, and minute ventilation begins to fall due to respiratory center depression. This sequence of events occurs at higher O_2 tensions if any of the major compensatory mechanisms for hypoxemia are defective. Even mild decreases in O_2 tension are tolerated poorly by anemic patients with impaired cardiac output or coronary insufficiency. In addition, critically ill patients may have impaired autonomic control of perfusion distribution, due to either endogenous pathology (e.g., sepsis) or vasopressor or vasodilator therapy. Because the pulmonary vasculature constricts when alveolar O_2 tension falls, hypoxemia may provoke decompensation of the right ventricle in patients with preexisting pulmonary hypertension or cor pulmonale.

Hyperoxia

At normal barometric pressures, venous and tissue O_2 tensions rise very little when pure O_2 is administered to healthy subjects. Hence, nonpulmonary tissues are little affected. However, high concentrations of O_2 eventually replace nitrogen in the lung, even in poorly ventilated regions. Oxygen replacement of nitrogen eventually causes collapse of poorly ventilated units as O_2 is absorbed by venous blood faster than it is replenished. Atelectasis and diminished lung compliance result. More importantly, high O_2 tensions may accelerate the generation of free radicals and other noxious oxidants, injuring bronchial and parenchymal tissue. Although O_2-induced lung injury certainly occurs in experimental models using healthy animals, oxygen toxicity in patients with injured lungs is much less certain. In fact, the very processes that commonly incite lung dysfunction (e.g., sepsis, alveolar hemorrhage, etc.) may protect against hyperoxia.

EVALUATING VENTILATION

Hypercapnia

In addition to its key role in regulation of ventilation, the clinically important effects of CO_2 relate to changes in cerebral blood flow, pH, and adrenergic tone. Hypercapnia dilates cerebral vessels, and hypocapnia constricts them, a point of particular importance for patients with raised intracranial pressure. Acute increases in CO_2 depress consciousness, probably a combined result of intraneuronal acidosis, excessive cerebral blood flow, and increased intracranial pressure. Slowly developing hypercapnia is better tolerated, presumably because buffering has time to occur. Nonetheless, if CO_2 production is constant, a higher $PaCO_2$ signifies alveolar hypoventilation, which tends to decrease alveolar and arterial PO_2. Patients with renal insufficiency tolerate hypercapnia especially poorly because of their inability to adequately buffer the carbonic acid generated. The adrenergic stimulation that accompanies acute hypercapnia causes cardiac output to rise and peripheral vascular resistance to increase. During acute respiratory acidosis, these effects may partially offset those of H^+ on cardiovascular function, allowing better tolerance of the low pH than of metabolic acidosis of a similar degree. Hypercapnia-induced constriction of glomerular arterioles may produce oliguria in some patients. Muscular twitching, asterixis, and seizures can be observed at extreme levels of hypercapnia in patients made susceptible by electrolyte or neural disorders.

As a practical matter, for mechanically ventilated patients, many practitioners permit a modest respiratory acidosis (pH of 7.15–7.20) resulting from gradual increases in $PaCO_2$ (<10 mm Hg/hour) if the alternative is markedly elevated airway pressures to achieve normocapnia. With little controlled data to suggest either safety or efficacy, the practice of "permissive hypercapnia" has become widely accepted or at least tolerated. Because patients with hypoxemia, pulmonary hypertension, or increased intracranial pressure and those receiving β-blocking drugs may develop significant side effects from the hypercapnia-induced acidosis, permissive hypercapnia may not be wise for these individuals.

Hypocapnia

The major effects of acute hypocapnia relate to alkalosis and diminished cerebral perfusion. Abrupt lowering of $PaCO_2$ reduces total cerebral blood flow, raises neuronal pH, and reduces available ionized calcium, causing disturbances in cortical and peripheral nerve function. Lightheadedness, circumoral and fingertip paresthesias, and muscular tetany can result. Alkalosis caused by sudden reduction of $PaCO_2$ (e.g., shortly after ini-

tiating mechanical ventilation) can produce life-threatening seizures or arrhythmias.

EVALUATING HYDROGEN ION CONCENTRATION

Generation and Excretion of H^+ Ion

For mammalian cells to function optimally, hydrogen ion concentration (as reflected in pH) must be controlled rather rigidly. Free hydrogen ion (H^+) has a potent effect on tissue enzyme systems. To keep H^+ within physiologic limits, generation and elimination rates must be equal. H^+ ion is generated in two ways: (a) by hydration of CO_2 to form "volatile" acid according to the reaction:

$$CO_2 + H_2O \lor H_2CO_3 \lor H^+ + HCO_3^-$$

and (b) by production of "fixed" acids (sulfates and phosphates) as chemical by-products of metabolism. Ventilation eliminates volatile acid while the kidney excretes the bulk of the fixed acid load. If excretion of CO_2 speeds or slows inappropriately when compared to its rate of production, the result is a respiratory derangement of acid–base balance. If the excretion rate of fixed acid speeds or slows disproportionately in relation to its production rate, or if abnormal metabolic loads of acid or alkali develop, metabolic acidosis or alkalosis occurs. In clinical practice, the concentration of free H^+ ion is tracked by $pH = -\log [H^+]$.

BUFFER SYSTEMS

Carbonic Acid

Chemical and protein buffer systems oppose changes in free H^+. The CO_2/HCO_3^- (carbonic acid) and hemoglobin systems are quantitatively the most important. Clinical attention usually is focused on the carbonic acid system because each of its components is measured readily and because CO_2 and HCO_3^- determinations allow clinical judgments to be made concerning the respiratory or metabolic origin of the problem at hand. To maintain pH at 7.40, the ratio of HCO_3^- to ($0.03 \times PaCO_2$) must remain in the 20:1 proportions dictated by the Henderson-Hasselbalch equation: $pH = 6.1 + \log [(HCO_3^-)/(0.03 \times PaCO_2)]$.

Noncarbonic (Protein) Buffers

Hemoglobin and other protein buffers also bind or release H^+ ion, minimizing pH changes while allowing the hydration reaction for CO_2 to continue to run in either direction.

$$CO_2 + H_2O \ v \ [H^+] + HCO_3^-$$

$$\downarrow$$

$$[H^+] + Hgb \ v \ H^+ Hgb$$

For this reason, if $PaCO_2$ changes acutely, there will be a small associated change in HCO_3^- in the same direction (approximately 1 mEq/L per 0.1 pH unit). Such automatic changes in HCO_3^- do not imply a metabolic disturbance, and the "base excess" attributable to this mechanism is zero (see below). Anemic blood fails to buffer fluctuations in H^+ concentration with normal efficiency.

Base Excess

Clinically, it is important to recognize and quantitate metabolic acid–base derangements. At pH = 7.40, simple inspection of the HCO_3^- suffices to detect a metabolic component, whether primary or compensatory. For a chronic respiratory disturbance, however, the presence of noncarbonic buffers complicates interpretation as pH deviates from 7.40. The "base excess" is a number that quantitates the metabolic abnormality. It hypothetically "corrects" pH to 7.40 by first "adjusting" $PaCO_2$ to 40 mm Hg, thus allowing a comparison of the "corrected" HCO_3^- with the known normal value at that pH (24 mEq/L). As a quick rule of thumb, base excess (mEq/L) can be calculated from the observed values for HCO_3^- and pH: base excess = HCO_3^- + 10 (pH − 7.40) − 24.

A "negative" base excess means that HCO_3^- stores are depleted. However, the base excess does not indicate whether retention or depletion of HCO_3^- is pathologic or compensatory for long-standing respiratory derangements; that judgment must be made by an analysis of the clinical setting. Likewise, it does not dictate the need for bicarbonate administration. Calculation of base excess is especially helpful when the observed HCO_3^- is nearly normal (24 ± 3 mEq/L). The base excess calculation is unlikely to provide new insights at more extreme HCO_3^- deviations.

Compensatory Mechanisms

As physiologic stresses on pH balance persist, adjustments in the excretion rate of CO_2 and H^+ counterbalance the effect of these disturbances on pH. In general, renal compensation for a respiratory disturbance is slower (but ultimately more successful) than respiratory compensation for a metabolic disturbance. Thus, although quick to respond initially, the respiratory system will not eliminate sufficient CO_2 to completely offset any but the mildest metabolic acidosis. Furthermore, the respiratory compensatory response is not developed fully until 24 to 48 hours after initial activation. The lower limit of sustained compensatory hypocapnia in a healthy adult is approximately 10 to 15 mm Hg. Once that limit is reached, even small additional increments in H^+ ion have disastrous effects on pH (and often, on survival).

Patients with disordered lung mechanics, such as those with COPD or neuromuscular weakness, are highly vulnerable to metabolic acid loads because they lack the normal ability to compensate by hyperventilation. CO_2 retention in response to alkalosis is very limited—only rarely exceeding 60 mm Hg. (The hypoxemia resulting from hypoventilation helps limit the rise in CO_2 by eventually triggering increased ventilatory effort.) Although the kidney cannot respond effectively to abrupt respiratory acidosis or alkalosis, renal compensation may eventually (3–7 days) totally counterbalance a respiratory alkalosis of even moderate severity. The kidney also compensates well for chronic respiratory acidosis but cannot compensate completely for a $PaCO_2$ above 65 mm Hg unless another stimulus for HCO_3^- retention (e.g., volume depletion) is present.

Acidemia

Although all organs malfunction to some extent during profound acidemia, cardiovascular function is among the most impaired. By stimulating ventilation, acidemia often exacerbates dyspnea. Myocardial fibers contract less efficiently, systemic vessels react sluggishly to vasoconstrictors, vasomotor control deteriorates, blood pressure falls, and arrhythmias develop. Because H^+ ions are readily exchanged for K^+ across cell membranes, hyperkalemia frequently accompanies acidosis unless K^+ is lost concurrently (e.g., diabetic ketoacidosis). As a result of these cardiovascular and electrolyte abnormalities, defibrillation and cardiopulmonary resuscitation become more difficult in a markedly acidotic patient. In addition, acidemia impairs neuronal conduction and mental status, acts synergistically with alveolar hypoxia to cause pulmonary vasoconstriction, and blunts the action of adrenergic bronchodilators. Each of these effects is more pronounced as pH falls below 7.20.

Respiratory acidosis has particularly profound effects on mental status, perhaps because of the independent central nervous system (CNS) effects of hypercapnia (e.g., increased intracranial pressure) and the direct effects of accompanying hypoxemia. A pH value between 7.20 and 7.40 is not a major concern and should not prompt therapy aimed solely at pH correction. (In fact, the rightward shift of the oxyhemoglobin curve may improve tissue O_2 delivery if cardiovascular performance remains adequate.) However, the pH scale is logarithmic; therefore, when pH falls below 7.20, H^+ rises dramatically. Mild acidemia is less alarming for its physiologic effects than for what it signifies—seriously decompensated ventilatory, metabolic, or cardiovascular systems in need of urgent attention.

Alkalemia

Alkalemia causes less apprehension among physicians than acidemia of similar magnitude for several reasons. First, the root cause of metabolic alkalosis usually is less life threatening. Second, elevated pH does not exert the same depressant influence on myocardium and blood vessels seen with similar degrees of acidemia. Finally, unless very abrupt and severe, the effects of raised pH on the brain are limited to confusion and encephalopathy. These facts do not imply that alkalosis is entirely benign—the major risks of extreme alkalosis seem to relate to lowering of the seizure threshold and provocation of cardiac arrhythmias, effects caused in part by electrolyte shifts (Ca^{+2}, K^+) and diminished oxygen delivery. Alkalosis exerts detrimental effects with regard to release of O_2 to the tissues, shifting the oxyhemoglobin dissociation curve leftward. As a general rule, a pH higher than 7.60 warrants vigorous measures for reversal. Metabolic alkalemia may cause compensatory CO_2 retention that, when severe, results in alveolar hypoxemia.

ACID–BASE DERANGEMENTS

TERMINOLOGY OF ACID–BASE DISORDERS

The terms "acidemia" and "alkalemia" refer to blood pH. Systemic pH lower than 7.35 defines acidemia. A pH higher than 7.45 defines alkalemia. In contrast, acidosis and alkalosis do not refer to pH but rather to basic pathophysiologic processes or tendencies favoring the development of acidemia or alkalemia. For example, a patient with diabetic ketoacidosis (a primary metabolic acidosis) and hypocapnia stimulated by pneumonia (a primary respiratory alkalosis) may exhibit acidemia, alkalemia, or a normal pH depending on the relative changes in $PaCO_2$ and HCO_3^-. Uncomplicated metabolic acidosis is characterized by a decline in HCO_3^-, whereas a primary increase in HCO_3^- denotes metabolic alkalosis. Conversely, respiratory acidosis is defined as a primary increase in $PaCO_2$, whereas respiratory alkalosis occurs when the central feature is a decrease in $PaCO_2$.

Stepwise ABG Analysis

Because no set of ABG values has a unique interpretation, concomitant analysis of serum electrolytes and the review of the clinical situation is essential to reach the correct diagnosis in an acid–base disorder. Three specific factors (pH, $PaCO_2$, and the ratio of $PaCO_2$ to HCO_3^-) must be analyzed in a logical stepwise fashion to come to a correct diagnosis. Interpretation of the pH and $PaCO_2$ rapidly provides a definitive diagnosis in most cases. The remaining disorders can be classified by examining the relationship of the measured $PaCO_2$ to the $PaCO_2$ expected based on the measured bicarbonate level. Consideration of the anion gap often lends supportive information.

The pH is analyzed first. Values below the normal range indicate acidemia (elevated H^+). pH values above the normal range (reduced H^+) define alkalemia. A pH within the normal range has three possible interpretations: (*a*) no acid–base disorder exists; (*b*) two or more acid–base disorders with perfectly offsetting pH effects exist (rare); or (*c*) near-complete physiologic compensation has occurred for one or more primary disorders. Deviations of pH from normal usually are quickly acted upon by compensatory mechanisms in an attempt to restore the pH to a normal value. When the primary disorder is respiratory, the kidney attempts to compensate. When metabolic consumption or wasting of buffer base is the primary problem, the lung attempts to return the pH to normal.

In the acidemic patient, an elevated $PaCO_2$ indicates that some component of respiratory acidosis is present. In such patients, the bicarbonate concentration can be used to decide whether appropriate metabolic compensation is occurring or if a concurrent metabolic disorder is present. If the measured HCO_3^- concentration has increased over baseline by 0.1 to 0.35 unit for each 1-mm Hg change in $PaCO_2$, appropriate metabolic compensation for a respiratory acidosis is taking place. Lesser increases in HCO_3^- are indicative of a complicating metabolic acidosis or suggest that insufficient time has elapsed for the kidney to compensate for the rapidly changing $PaCO_2$. Greater rises in HCO_3^- indicate a superimposed metabolic alkalosis.

Conversely, a reduced $PaCO_2$ in an acidemic patient indicates metabolic acidosis. In the case of a metabolic acidosis, the ultimate diagnosis is reached by comparing the observed $PaCO_2$ to that predicted by directly measuring the serum HCO_3^- content. For any given HCO_3^- value, the expected $PaCO_2 = (1.5 \times HCO_3^-) + 8\,(\pm 2)$. This equates to roughly a 1- to 1.3-mm Hg change in $PaCO_2$ for each mEq change in bicarbonate. (Typically, respiratory compensation for a metabolic acidosis is more rapid but less complete than the converse.) If the observed $PaCO_2$ equals the expected value, a simple metabolic acidosis with appropriate respiratory compensation is present. If the $PaCO_2$ exceeds the expected value, the patient has both a respiratory and metabolic acidosis. When the observed $PaCO_2$ fails to reach the expected level, the patient has both a metabolic acidosis and respiratory alkalosis.

In the alkalemic patient, a low $PaCO_2$ diagnoses respiratory alkalosis. Determination of whether the disorder is simple or mixed results from examining a concurrently measured HCO_3^- concentration. Reductions in HCO_3^- concentration of 0.2 to 0.5 times the change in $PaCO_2$ will occur slowly to provide the compensation necessary. Failure to lower HCO_3^- by at least 0.2 times the change in $PaCO_2$ suggests a superimposed metabolic alkalosis (or insufficient compensatory time), whereas a HCO_3^- that declines by more than 0.5 times the change in $PaCO_2$ suggests a component of metabolic acidosis (see Table 12.1).

The ultimate diagnosis of the alkalotic patient with an elevated $PaCO_2$ is made by comparing the measured $PaCO_2$ value with that expected (calculated) based on the measured serum HCO_3^- concentration. In the presence of a simple compensated metabolic alkalosis, the expected $PaCO_2 = (0.7 \times HCO_3^-) + (20 \pm 1.5)$. A higher observed $PaCO_2$ indicates the presence of a simultaneous respiratory acidosis. A value lower than that expected indicates a concomitant respiratory alkalosis.

SIMPLE ACID–BASE DISORDERS

METABOLIC ACIDOSIS

Mechanisms

Metabolic acidosis is the consequence of one of three basic mechanisms: bicarbonate consumption from decreased H^+ excretion, bicarbonate consumption from increased H^+ production, or bicarbonate loss.

Bicarbonate Consumption

H^+ normally is excreted renally as titratable acid (phosphates and sulfates) and ammonia. Renal failure, adrenal insufficiency, distal renal tubular acidosis (RTA), and hypoaldosteronism all impair this excretion. Patients with renal failure due to a reduced number of functioning nephrons cannot adequately filter and excrete the H^+ load. In distal (type I) RTA, proximal tubular glomerular filtration and HCO_3^- reabsorption are normal but distal tubular H^+ secretion is impaired.

TABLE 12–1

EXPECTED COMPENSATION FOR ACID-BASE DISORDERS

Primary Disorder	Primary Change	Compensatory Change	Expected Compensation
Metabolic acidosis	$\downarrow HCO_3^-$	$\downarrow PaCO_2$	$\Delta PaCO_2 = 1.2\,\Delta HCO_3^-$
Metabolic alkalosis	$\uparrow HCO_3^-$	$\uparrow PaCO_2$	$\Delta PaCO_2 = 0.9\,\Delta HCO_3^-$
Respiratory acidosis	$\uparrow PaCO_2$	$\uparrow HCO_3^-$	
Acute			$\Delta HCO_3^- = 0.10\,\Delta PaCO_2$
Chronic			$\Delta HCO_3^- = 0.35\,\Delta PaCO_2$
Respiratory alkalosis	$\downarrow PaCO_2$	$\downarrow HCO_3^-$	
Acute			$\Delta HCO_3^- = 0.2\,\Delta PaCO_2$
Chronic			$\Delta HCO_3^- = 0.5\,\Delta PaCO_2$

Because H^+ excretion in the distal tubule depends on exchange of sodium ions, volume depletion worsens the tendency for acidosis. Through a similar mechanism (reduced tubular sodium delivery), adrenal insufficiency or selective hypoaldosteronism also impairs H^+ excretion. The later condition may be recognized by the association of metabolic acidosis, hyperkalemia, hyponatremia, and hypercalcemia.

Hydrogen Ion Load and the Anion Gap

An increased H^+ load also may cause metabolic acidosis. In such cases, the disparity between the measured concentrations of serum cations and anions—the anion gap—will widen beyond the normal range of 9 to 13 mEq/L. The unmeasured anions are composed of serum proteins (predominantly albumin), phosphate, sulfate, lactate, ketoacids (beta hydroxybutyrate, acetoacetate), and other unmeasured compounds (e.g., drugs). Knowledge of the anion gap, calculated as anion gap = $Na^+ - (Cl^- + HCO_3^-)$, may be quite valuable in distinguishing the etiology of metabolic acidosis. The addition of unmeasured anions elevates the anion gap (e.g., HCl administration does not increase the anion gap because Cl^- is a measured anion). The most common causes of an elevated anion gap can be recalled using the mnemonic "S.L.U.M.P.E.D.D." (see Table 12.2). The anion gap should be adjusted for hypoalbuminemia, which tends to reduce it by ≈ 2.5 meq/L per gm/DL reduction in albumin concentration.

As a rule, the larger the anion gap, the easier it is to determine the cause of the acidosis. A wide anion gap acidosis usually can be diagnosed rapidly with a clinical history and a limited number of serum tests (i.e., serum creatinine, lactate, and ketone levels). Lactic acidosis generated by anaerobic glycolysis is the most common cause of an elevated anion gap; however, lactic acidosis often

TABLE 12–2

ETIOLOGY OF ANION GAP ACIDOSIS

Salicylate

Lactate

Uremic toxins

Methanol

Paraldehyde

Ethanol/ethylene glycol

Diabetic ketoacidosis

Drugs (e.g., iron, isoniazid)

is mixed with another form of acidosis. For example, very high serum levels of anionic salicylate molecules may directly elevate the anion gap, but salicylates also raise the anion gap by interfering with carbohydrate metabolism and O_2 use, thereby inducing a lactic acidosis. Similarly, diabetic ketoacidosis produces a mixed anion gap/metabolic acidosis by increasing the concentration of unmeasured ketones and by inducing a lactic acidosis, usually from hypoperfusion (see Chapter 32, Endocrine Emergencies). Uremia commonly leads to accumulation of titratable acids, producing an anion gap/metabolic acidosis.

If the creatine, ketone, and lactate levels are all normal in the setting of a high anion gap, a toxic ingestion becomes the most likely etiology. In such patients, comparing the calculated osmolality to measured serum osmolality proves particularly helpful. (An osmolal gap usually indicates some form of alcohol toxicity: ethylene glycol, ethanol, or methanol.) Other drugs that can cause an anion gap acidosis include isoniazid, iron, and paraldehyde (see Chapter 33, Drug Overdose and Poisoning).

Bicarbonate Loss

Bicarbonate loss may produce metabolic acidosis but does not elevate the anion gap because HCO_3^- loss results in compensatory hyperchloremia. Although renal failure usually impairs H^+ excretion, renal failure may also induce direct HCO_3^- loss. In renal failure, the HCO_3^- usually plateaus at 12 to 20 mmol/L, as further H^+ accumulation is blunted by tissue (bone) buffers. Three conditions decrease HCO_3^- disproportionately to reductions in glomerular filtration rate: renal medullary tubular disorders (e.g., proximal renal tubular acidosis), low renin/aldosterone states, and renal failure, in which there is decreased HCO_3^- resorption (due to a constant filtered Na^+ load and an increased filtration fraction through a few remaining nephrons). The mild metabolic acidosis of proximal (type II) RTA usually is an incidental finding resulting from an inability to fully resorb filtered HCO_3^-. In this self-limited disease, the impaired reabsorptive capacity for HCO_3^- renders pH correction difficult and produces an alkaline urine. In such patients, exogenous $NaHCO_3$ increases the filtered HCO_3^- load, raising urine pH, but rarely affects serum pH. In addition to metabolic acidosis and alkaline urine, ancillary features characteristic of proximal RTA are as follows: decreased serum urate, $PO4^-$, and potassium; glycosuria; and amino aciduria.

The gastrointestinal (GI) tract provides a route for HCO_3^- loss in patients with chronic diarrhea. Diarrhea related to human immunodeficiency virus (HIV) or laxative abuse are common. In such patients, urinary pH can be a helpful diagnostic test—a normal kidney will increase acid excretion (and reclaim HCO_3^-) resulting in a urine pH lower than 5.0. Cholestyramine also may cause metabolic acidosis by exchanging HCO_3^- for Cl^-. Because the ileum and colon have ion pumps that reabsorb HCO_3^- in exchange for Cl^-, hyperchloremic (nongap) acidosis frequently develops in patients with ureterosigmoidostomy.

Signs and Symptoms

Unlike those with respiratory acidosis, patients with metabolic acidosis usually have an increased depth and rate of respiration unless ventilatory drive is depressed. If the acidosis is severe, lethargy or coma may occur. Neurologic changes are less prominent with metabolic than with respiratory acidosis, perhaps because hypercapnia and hypoxemia of respiratory acidosis exert independent effects. The fact that CO_2 is freely permeable to the brain is also a likely factor. In the most severe cases (e.g., pH < 7.1), hypotension may result from cardiovascular depression.

Compensation

There are four compensatory mechanisms for metabolic acidosis. Initially, extracellular buffers (predominantly HCO_3^-) blunt the falling pH. Rapidly thereafter, the respiratory system increases minute ventilation to reduce $PaCO_2$. The $PaCO_2$ declines at a rate of approximately 1.2 mm Hg per mEq/L reduction in serum HCO_3^- but rarely falls below 10 mm Hg. The $PaCO_2$ expected in response to an established metabolic acidosis may be predicted from the following equation: expected $PaCO_2 = 1.5 \times$ measured $HCO_3^- + 8$ (± 2).

As a rule of thumb, in chronic metabolic acidosis, the expected $PaCO_2$ approximates the last two digits of the pH value (e.g., the expected $PaCO_2$ for a pH of 7.25 is 25). Although respiratory compensation is relatively prompt (fully developed within 24–48 hours), it is rarely complete. If the $PaCO_2$ is above that expected for a given HCO_3^-, either the time for compensation has been too short or respiratory acidosis is present. If the $PaCO_2$ is less than expected, concomitant respiratory alkalosis is present. Buffering of H^+ by intracellular protein and fixed buffers in bone (calcium salts) represents a third major mechanism for blunting the decrease in pH. Finally, the kidney may enhance H^+ excretion, but this function requires the active excretion of H^+ in combination with phosphate and ammonium. Such losses of H^+ are limited to approximately 50 to 100 mEq/day, a rate that approximates the normal pace of mineral acid production.

Treatment

If pH disturbances are severe, therapeutic measures may be necessary to alter the PCO_2 or bicarbonate content directly. However, the treatment of acid–base disorders usually should be directed at the underlying cause. Mistakenly, the lack of definitive evidence proving efficacy of bicarbonate therapy in some forms of metabolic acidosis has been interpreted to mean that base therapy is futile in all situations. Potential indications for direct treatment of metabolic acidosis are: (a) pH < 7.20, (b) overt physiologic compromise attributable to acidosis, and (c) excessive work of breathing required to maintain an acceptable pH (>7.20).

If bicarbonate therapy is used, calculation of the HCO_3^- dose assumes a distribution into total body water. Total body water (in liters) is approximately 0.6 to 0.7 times the lean body weight (in kg). The following expression HCO_3^- deficit = (total body water) $\times$ (24 − HCO_3^-) approximates the HCO_3^- deficit in mEq. Larger bicarbonate doses may be required with very profound reductions in serum bicarbonate levels, as the apparent volume of distribution for bicarbonate increases. Because $NaHCO_3$ has potentially adverse effects and because the effectiveness of a given dose is not entirely predictable, it is customary to replace one-half the calculated HCO_3^- deficit over several hours while following the pH response closely. $NaHCO_3$ partially equilibrates in total body water within 15 minutes of administration; however, cellular equilibration requires approximately 2 hours to complete.

$NaHCO_3$ administration entails many potential problems. In large doses, hypertonic hypernatremia and fluid overload may occur. (An ampule of $NaHCO_3$ contains approximately as much Na^+ as $\frac{1}{2}$ L of normal saline.) Bolus injection of $NaHCO_3$ may elicit a biphasic ventilatory response. Immediately after administration, peripheral pH rises and the drive to breathe falls. However, soon thereafter, rising CO_2 (due to both metabolic load and buffered H^+ ion) diffuses across the blood–brain barrier to reduce intracerebral pH and stimulate breathing ("paradoxical CNS acidosis"). Rapid bolus injection of $NaHCO_3$ is potentially dangerous—it may cause a rapid leftward shift of the oxyhemoglobin dissociation curve, alter cerebral hemodynamics, or induce life-threatening hypokalemia. A pH higher than 7.10 usually is sufficient to maintain near-normal vascular tone and myocardial contractility and can almost always be obtained using small doses of $NaHCO_3$. Furthermore, some types of acidosis (e.g., proximal RTA) are very difficult to correct with exogenous bicarbonate. In organic acidosis (diabetic ketoacidosis or lactic acidosis), $NaHCO_3$ therapy eventually may lead to an alkalosis as the organic acids (ketones, lactate) are recycled to HCO_3^- by the liver. (There is no loss of potential bicarbonate in these disorders; therefore, bicarbonate therapy is rarely necessary.)

METABOLIC ALKALOSIS

Metabolic alkalosis, a pH higher than 7.45 with a normal or elevated $PaCO_2$, usually is generated and maintained by two distinct pathophysiologic mechanisms. Metabolic alkalosis is always due to the gain of HCO_3^-, loss of H^+ ions, or loss of body fluid rich in chloride compared to plasma concentrations. In the first situation, exogenous base may accumulate when excess bicarbonate, citrate, lactate, or acetate is administered. The second mechanism for establishing metabolic alkalosis occurs when H^+ is lost. Loss most commonly occurs in gastric juice from nasogastric suctioning or vomiting, but this is much less common with the widespread use of H_2 blockers. Rarely, H^+ loss may result from a renal disorder in which losses may be mediated by excess mineralocorticoids, increased distal tubule Na^+ delivery, or excessive filtration of nonreabsorbable anions (e.g., calcium, penicillin). Interestingly, renal mechanisms almost never generate metabolic alkalosis but are almost always responsible for its perpetuation. The normal kidney rapidly excretes an alkaline urine in response to a HCO_3^- load, provided that serum Cl^-, K^+, and Mg^{+3} are normal. However, hypokalemia, hypomagnesemia, and hypochloremia all inhibit the excretion of excess HCO_3^-. Hypokalemia augments proximal tubular HCO_3^- resorption and increases distal tubular H^+ secretion, perpetuating the alkalosis. The volume depletion that almost always accompanies

Cl^- deficiency (commonly the result of diuretic therapy) stimulates renin and aldosterone secretion, promoting H^+ excretion. In turn, hyperaldosteronism increases H^+ secretion, an effect potentiated by high tubular flow rates, the presence of nonreabsorbable anions, and K^+ deficiency.

Diagnostic Criteria

Metabolic alkalosis is characterized by an elevated pH, elevated HCO_3^-, and often a compensatory increase in $PaCO_2$ if the disorder is chronic. The anion gap may increase because of the increased "charge equivalency" of albumin and stimulation of organic anion synthesis.

Signs and Symptoms

Metabolic alkalosis impairs neural transmission and muscular contraction, especially when accompanied by hypokalemia and hypophosphatemia—two commonly coexisting abnormalities. Indeed, metabolic alkalosis mimics hypocalcemia in its symptomatology. Changes in mental status and thirst due to volume depletion are common.

Precipitants of Metabolic Alkalosis

Severe hypokalemia ($K^+ < 2.0$) causes generalized intracellular acidosis, an effect that impairs the function of the renal tubule. This effect favors HCO_3^- retention and perpetuates metabolic alkalosis. Nasogastric suctioning or vomiting can deplete circulatory volume as well as H^+, Mg^{+3}, and Cl^- concentrations. In replacing these H^+ losses, HCO_3^- is generated and retained. Volume depletion causes hyperaldosteronism (HCO_3^- retention, K^+ loss). Aldosterone also promotes maximal Na^+ resorption, leading to high rates of tubular Na^+ for H^+ exchange, which further worsens the alkalosis.

Relief of longstanding respiratory acidosis (e.g., with institution of mechanical ventilation) results in a rapidly evolving metabolic alkalosis from the HCO_3^- previously retained in compensation. For unknown reasons, chronic respiratory acidosis promotes urinary Cl^- wasting, which further helps to perpetuate alkalosis. Mineralocorticoid excess (primary or secondary) is commonly accompanied by K^+ loss and impaired renal tubular HCO_3^- excretion. When loop diuretics are given to volume-depleted patients, increased amounts of Na^+ are presented to the distal renal tubule, and the resulting intensified exchange of Na^+ for H^+ perpetuates metabolic alkalosis. If Na^+ is administered along with a nonresorbable anion (e.g., penicillin) to volume-depleted patients, the Na^+ will be reabsorbed in the renal tubule and H^+ will be secreted to maintain electroneutrality. The weak aldosterone-like properties of glucocorticoids may cause metabolic alkalosis in Cushing's syndrome or with exogenous administration of corticosteroids. Excess HCO_3^- retention may occur after therapeutic administration, but if circulating volume and K^+ are normal, the kidney has a remarkable ability to excrete excess HCO_3^-. Iatrogenic metabolic alkalosis often complicates therapy of acidosis due to diabetic ketoacidosis (DKA) or lactate because HCO_3^- is regenerated in the recovery period. Blood transfusion also delivers citrate, an HCO_3^- equivalent; however, metabolic alkalosis is rare unless more than 8 to 10 units of blood are given. Overt alkalosis rarely complicates antacid administration, because most such agents are nonabsorbable. Contraction alkalosis is a state in which losses of intravascular volume, K^+, and Cl^- act in conjunction with hyperaldosteronism to deplete extracellular fluid around a near-constant amount of HCO_3^-. This effectively "shrinks" the volume of distribution of bicarbonate, increasing its concentration.

Maintenance of the Alkalosis

Metabolic alkalosis can be maintained by the same four mechanisms responsible for its development: Cl^- deficiency, mineralocorticoid excess, and depletion of circulating volume or K^+. However, in a given patient, metabolic alkalosis often is maintained by a different mechanism from that which established it. For example, nasogastric removal of Cl^- and H^+ may generate a metabolic alkalosis, but it is the intravascular volume and Cl^- depletion that maintains it, even after nasogastric (NG) suction is discontinued. Cl^- and volume must be administered for reversal. Given a choice, the body chooses to maintain circulating volume status at the expense of Cl^- and pH homeostasis.

Compensation for Metabolic Alkalosis

In metabolic alkalosis, the $PaCO_2$ normally rises approximately 0.6 mm Hg per mmol increase in HCO_3^-. (Lower $PaCO_2$ values indicate a superimposed respiratory alkalosis.) It is rare to see a compensatory increase in $PaCO_2 > 60$ mm Hg

when breathing room air, because at this level of hypercarbia, the PaO_2 falls to approximately 60 mmHg and hypoxemia begins to drive respiration.

Diagnosis

As already indicated, the clinical history, the medication profile, serum chemistries, and intravascular volume status are keys to the differential diagnosis. The laboratory evaluation should be directed at differentiating chloride-responsive from chloride-resistant alkalosis (see below). A chloride-responsive alkalosis usually can be identified by measuring urine electrolytes. Such measurements are useful provided that they are not obtained within 24 hours of diuretic administration, because most diuretics result in Cl^- and K^+ losses. Urine Na^+ and Cl^- concentrations lower than 10 to 15 mEq/L characterize a chloride-responsive condition, suggesting volume depletion or posthypercapnic alkalosis as potential mechanisms. If the urine Cl^- and Na^+ concentrations exceed 20 mEq/L, mineralocorticoid excess, diuretic use, and severe hypokalemia or hypomagnesemia are common causes. Marked disparity between urinary Cl^- and Na^+ concentrations strongly suggests mineralocorticoid excess.

Treatment

Metabolic alkalosis often is considered in two general categories—"salt" (NaCl)-responsive or salt-unresponsive (Table 12.3). NaCl frequently reverses volume contraction and secondary hyperaldosteronism. The "chloride dose" required to correct a chloride-responsive alkalosis can be approximated as the desired change in chloride concentration times 25% of body weight. NaCl also provides Cl^- ions for reabsorption, with Na^+ obviating the need for H^+ secretion. (The effective-

TABLE 12–3

CLASSIFICATION OF METABOLIC ALKALOSIS BASED ON CHLORIDE RESPONSIVENESS

Cl^- Responsive	Cl^- Resistant
Volume depletion	Hyperaldosteronism
Vomiting/diarrhea	Exogenous steroids
NG suction	Glucocorticoids
Diuretics	Mineralocorticoids
Post-hypercapnia	Cushing's syndrome
Cationic drugs (e.g., penicillin)	

ness of NaCl replacement may be determined by measuring urinary pH—if Na^+ replacement is sufficient, urinary pH will rise above 7.0.) Chloride, the only absorbable anion, is the critical component in NaCl administration. For example, administration of other sodium salts (e.g., sodium sulfate) will not improve metabolic alkalosis, even though Na^+ is provided and the volume is corrected. Because K^+ depletion contributes to maintenance of metabolic alkalosis by preventing adequate HCO_3^- excretion, potassium chloride replacement is the preferred therapy.

Chloride-resistant alkaloses (adrenal disorders, corticosteroid administration, excess alkali ingestion, or administration) usually are due to mineralocorticoid excess. Therefore, in most such disorders, hypokalemia (sometimes severe) is a predictable feature. Therapy of mineralocorticoid excess may be directed at removal of the hormonal source (tumor control, withdrawal of steroids) or blockade of mineralocorticoid effect (spironolactone). K^+-sparing diuretics or the combination of Na^+ restriction and K^+ supplementation also are effective. Rarely, metabolic alkalosis is sufficiently protracted or severe to warrant the administration of intravenous HCl. This therapy should be reserved for patients with normal volume status and potassium but refractory severe symptomatic alkalosis. HCl may be infused as a 0.1- to 0.2-M solution but must be given directly into a central venous catheter at a rate not exceeding 0.2 mEq/kg/hour. In a similar manner as calculating bicarbonate deficit, the appropriate HCl dose may be approximated from the product of the desired change in HCO_3^- and 50% of the total body weight. Ammonium chloride may be used instead of HCl but should not be administered to patients with renal or hepatic failure.

RESPIRATORY ALKALOSIS

Inciting Mechanisms

Respiratory alkalosis—primary or compensatory—is defined by hypocapnia, a finding that implies alveolar hyperventilation. Central neurologic disorders, agitation, pain, inappropriate mechanical ventilation, hypoxemia, and alterations in thoracic and lung compliance all may produce primary respiratory alkalosis.

Symptoms

Acute respiratory alkalosis usually is manifest by tachypnea and often dyspnea; however, when chronic, this disorder may be associated with large tidal volume breaths at near-normal respiratory rates. The symptoms of respiratory alkalosis, "the hyperventilation syndrome," vary only in intensity from those of any alkalosis—most notably impaired neuromuscular function (e.g., parasthesias, tetany, tremor). A constellation of symptoms have been described with respiratory alkalosis, including chest pain, circumoral paresthesias, carpopedal spasm, anxiety, and lightheadedness.

Compensatory Mechanisms

Protracted respiratory alkalosis induces renal HCO_3^- wasting to offset hypocapnia. When the stimulus for hyperventilation is removed, hyperpnea tends to continue, driven by CNS acidosis until intracerebral HCO_3^- and pH are corrected.

MIXED ACID–BASE DISORDERS

Complex (mixed) acid–base disorders occur most frequently when there is concurrent lung and renal disease, when compensatory mechanisms are rendered inoperative, or when mechanical ventilation is used. For example, sedatives or narcotics can blunt the compensatory hyperpneic response to metabolic acidosis, producing a mixed acidosis. Acetazolamide, when given to patients with compensated chronic hypercapnia, can promote bicarbonate wasting and induce a complex acid–base disorder. Even by itself, aspirin overdosage can cause a combined respiratory alkalosis and metabolic acidosis. The presence of a complex or mixed acid–base disorder is discovered by applying the rules of expected compensation given above and in Chapter 5.

One particular situation, the "triple acid base disorder," deserves special mention. It should be recognized that the term "triple acid–base disorder" has no unique interpretation. It could represent three simultaneous metabolic acidoses or alkaloses or any combination of metabolic processes. However, because respiratory acidosis and respiratory alkalosis cannot coexist, a so-called triple acid–base disorder usually is the result of two metabolic derangements and a ventilation abnormality.

The diagnosis of a mixed or complex acid–base disorder is made by applying the rules of expected compensation. When observed values of $PaCO_2$ or HCO_3^- fall outside the expected ranges, a complex disorder is present.

KEY POINTS

1. No particular ABG has a unique interpretation; each blood gas must be evaluated in light of clinical information and electrolyte status. The technique for obtaining blood gases is critically important for accurate diagnosis.

2. Acid–base balance is finely tuned within a narrow range using complex buffering systems and compensatory responses. Usually, the respiratory system is more rapid to respond to metabolic derangements but achieves less complete compensation. In contrast, the kidney slowly compensates for respiratory abnormalities but eventually is much better able to achieve and sustain the compensatory response.

3. The anion gap provides a valuable tool to determine whether a metabolic acidosis is the result of loss of bicarbonate or the result of titration of bicarbonate with excess hydrogen ion equivalents. It makes good sense to calculate the anion gap when evaluating every set of electrolytes. The anion gap further provides a useful framework for the differential diagnosis of metabolic acidosis. A short list of common conditions usually is responsible for elevation of the anion gap (Table 12.2).

4. Nonanion gap acidosis usually is the result of administration of large volumes of chloride containing fluid, frequently to patients with gastrointestinal loses of bicarbonate.

5. The rules of compensation for primary acid–base disorders in Table 12.1 are important for the accurate evaluation of acid–base disorders. They must be memorized or kept closely at hand.

SUGGESTED READINGS

1. Brenner M. Clinical significance of the elevated anion gap. Am J Med 1985;79:289–296.
2. DuBose TD. Clinical approach to patients with acid-base disorders. Med Clin North Am 1983;67:799–813.
3. Garella S, Chang BS, Kahn SI. Dilution acidosis and contraction alkalosis: review of a concept. Kidney Int 1975; 8:279–283.
4. Hruska KA, Ban D, Avioli LV. Renal tubular acidosis. Arch Intern Med 1982;142:1909–1913.
5. Kreisberg RA. Pathogenesis and management of lactic acidosis. Ann Rev Med 1984;35:181–193.
6. Laski ME. Normal regulation of acid-base balance: renal and pulmonary response and other extrarenal buffering mechanisms. Med Clin North Am 1983;67:771–780.
7. Mitchell JH, Wildenthal K, Johnson RL. The effect of acid-base disturbances on cardiovascular and pulmonary function. Kidney Int 1973;1:375–389.
8. Narins RG, Emmett M. Simple and mixed acid-base disorders: a practical approach. Medicine 1980;59:161–187.
9. Riley LJ Jr, Ilson BE, Narins RG. Acute metabolic acid-base disorders. Crit Care Clin 1987;5(4):699–724.
10. Preuss HG. Fundamentals of clinical acid base evaluation. Clin Lab Med 1993;13:103–116.
11. Haber RJ. A practical approach to acid base disorders. West J Med 1991;155:146–156.
12. Bank N. Acid base balance and acute renal failure. Miner Electrolyte Metab 1991;17:116–123.
13. Brenner M. Pulmonary acid-base assessment. Nurs Clin North Am 1990;25:761–770.
14. McLaughlin ML. Practical treatment of acid-base disorders. Drugs 1990;39:841–855.
15. Brewer ED. Disorders of acid base balance. Pediatr Clin North Am 1990;37:429–447.

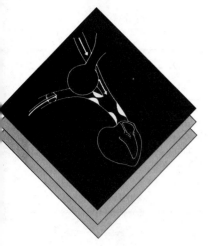

CHAPTER **13**

Fluid and Electrolyte Disorders

DISORDERS OF SODIUM AND OSMOLALITY

Despite great variability in sodium and water intake, the circulating intravascular volume, serum sodium, and serum osmolality remain remarkably constant in health. Increases in serum osmolality result in thirst and augmented antidiuretic hormone (ADH) secretion by the pituitary hypothalamic axis. ADH then acts on the medullary collecting duct of the kidney to stimulate water resorption. ADH, in combination with the renin-angiotensin-aldosterone system, restores circulating volume in response to depletion. The combined effects of ADH and the renin system result in balanced retention of sodium and water. When plasma osmolality declines, ADH release is inhibited and excess water is lost in an attempt to return osmolality toward normal.

HYPONATREMIA

Disorders of fluid and sodium balance are a daily occurrence in the intensive care unit (ICU) because patients often have multiple coexisting organ system failures, are usually denied self-regulation of water balance, and are administered medications that disturb fluid and electrolyte status. Hyponatremia, defined as a serum sodium lower than 125 mEq/L, is one of the most common electrolyte disorders.

In approaching disorders of sodium and osmolality, answers to seven questions provide useful clues to the cause of the disorder.

1. What is the intravascular volume status?
2. What are the serum concentrations of sodium, albumin, and lipids?
3. What is the serum osmolality?
4. What is the urinary volume, osmolality, and electrolyte composition?
5. What medications and fluids is the patient receiving?
6. Is there evidence of renal disease?
7. Is the patient edematous?

The manifestations of hyponatremia range from the subtle to the profound but generally are proportional to the magnitude of the abnormality and the speed with which it develops. Symptoms of hyponatremia span the spectrum from muscle cramps, nausea, vomiting, and anorexia to confusion, lethargy, coma, and seizures.

Laboratory Evaluation

In combination with a thorough history and physical examination, the urine sodium concentration, serum glucose, and the serum and urine osmolality provide essential data to determine the etiology of hyponatremia. Because sodium is the predominant osmotically active extracellular cation, serum osmolality is determined largely by the relative proportions of water and sodium. Measurements of serum osmolality help to separate hyponatremic disorders into three distinct categories, thereby guiding appropriate intervention. The diagnostic categories and causes of hyponatremia are summarized in Table 13.1. Apart from disturbances in sodium/water balance, marked elevations of glucose, blood urea nitrogen (BUN),

TABLE 13–1
_____
HYPONATREMIA: DIAGNOSTIC CATEGORIES AND CAUSES

Hypertonic Hyponatremia	Hypotonic Hyponatremia			Isotonic Hyponatremia
Osmotic agents:	Hypovolemic:	Isovolemic:	Hypervolemic:	Hyperproteinemia
Glucose	Hemorrhage	Water intoxication	Heart failure	Hyperlipidemia
Mannitol	Vomiting	Reset osmostat	Chronic renal	Isotonic infusions:
Starch	Diarrhea	Inappropriate ADH	failure	Glucose
	Diuretics		Hypoproteinemia	Mannitol
	Third-space loss (with			Glycine
	hypotonic fluid			Starch
	replacement)			

or exogenous substances (alcohols and complex carbohydrates) can elevate serum osmolality. Conversely, reductions in osmolality virtually always are reflected in the sodium concentration. The serum osmolality can be approximated by using the following equation:

Osmolality = 2 [Na$^+$] + glucose/18 + BUN/2.8 + [serum ethanol]/4.6 + ("unmeasured" osmoles)

Subclasses of Hyponatremia

Isotonic Hyponatremia

Hyponatremia with normal serum osmolality occurs when osmotically active solutes such as proteins, like those seen in myeloma or Waldenstrom's macroglobulinemia, expand the plasma volume, thereby diluting the serum sodium concentration. This reduction in serum sodium can be viewed as a form of "pseudohyponatremia." Serum protein concentrations higher than 12–15 g/dL usually are required to produce noteworthy hyponatremia. Dilution of serum sodium results not only from the osmotic drag of the serum proteins but also from the need to maintain electroneutrality. As positively charged proteins enter the circulation, chloride is retained and sodium is excreted to prevent charge imbalance. (Hyperlipidemia also may artifactually increase apparent serum volume, decreasing the measured sodium concentration; however, lipid removal before analysis normalizes the sodium.) Isotonic hyponatremia also may occur during the administration of large volumes of isotonic, non–salt-containing solutions (glucose, hydroxyethyl starch, mannitol, glycine). Before their solutes are metabolized or

excreted, these fluids are restricted to the extracellular space, where they expand the circulating volume and dilute sodium. (After solute excretion or metabolism, free water distributes proportionally among intracellular and extracellular sites.) "Isotonic hyponatremias" are reported when less specific methods of sodium analysis are employed, but true serum sodium levels can be determined using flame photometry.

Hypertonic Hyponatremia

Hypertonic hyponatremia results from the infusion or generation of (nonsodium) osmotic substances predisposed to extracellular partitioning. Nonketotic hyperglycemia and therapeutic administration of hypertonic glucose, mannitol, or glycine can cause hypertonicity as they depress sodium levels. (Although urea also increases osmolality, it fails to affect sodium concentration because it easily traverses cell membranes, dissipating any potential osmotic gradient.) Extracellular hypertonicity draws cellular water to the extracellular space in an attempt to reduce the osmotic gradient. This effect partially corrects the hyperosmolality, but it lowers the sodium concentration and causes cellular dehydration. The cause of hypertonic hyponatremia usually can be diagnosed by measuring serum glucose concentration and by reviewing a list of the patient's drugs. When hyperglycemia is the etiology, sodium concentration falls approximately 1.6 mEq/L per 100 mg/dL rise in serum glucose. Thus, hyperglycemia is rarely of consequence for sodium levels until the plasma glucose exceeds 200–300 mg/dL.

Hypotonic Hyponatremias

Hypotonic hyponatremia is the most common type of hyponatremia. Hypotonic hyponatremia can be subclassified rapidly into one of three categories. Knowledge of the patient's circulating volume status is key to determining etiology and treatment. Hypotonic hyponatremia almost never develops unless the patient has unrestricted access to water or is administered a hypotonic fluid.

Hypovolemic Hypotonic Hyponatremia Hypovolemic hyponatremia with low serum osmolality results from replacing losses of salt-containing plasma with hypotonic fluid. Volume depletion is a potent stimulus for antidiuretic hormone (ADH) release that overwhelms competing osmotic stimuli (hypotonicity) for ADH suppression. Intake of hypotonic fluid, when combined with the decreased free water clearance that results from ADH release, causes hyponatremia. Physical examination reveals signs of volume depletion. Thirst and postural hypotension (the hallmark of hypovolemia in patients with intact vascular reflexes) are more objective and reliable signs than are skin turgor, absence of axillary sweating, sunken orbits, or mucous membrane dryness.

Causes Hypovolemic hypotonic hyponatremia may result from renal or nonrenal causes. Bleeding, diarrhea, and vomiting, which are common nonrenal mechanisms of circulating volume loss, are usually apparent. Third-space losses (pancreatitis, gut sequestration, or diffuse muscular trauma) are less obvious. Renal causes of volume depletion and hyponatremia include salt-wasting nephropathy, diuretic use, mineralocorticoid deficiency, and osmotic diuresis from ketones, glucose, urea, or mannitol. Partial urinary tract obstruction and bicarbonaturia from renal tubular acidosis or metabolic alkalosis may also deplete volume and produce hyponatremia.

Laboratory Examination Because hypovolemia reduces renal blood flow and slows tubular flow, urea may "back-diffuse" into the bloodstream. Conversely, because creatinine cannot back-diffuse, its excretion is less severely impaired and the BUN/creatinine ratio rises. For patients with functioning kidneys and normal levels of mineralocorticoid hormones, small volumes of hypertonic urine with a very low sodium concentration reflect intense conservation of sodium and water. If urine sodium concentration is high and urine osmolality normal, renal salt wasting is the probable etiology of volume depletion. In primary adrenal insufficiency, the urine sodium concentration is high and the urine osmolality is elevated.

Hypervolemic Hypotonic Hyponatremia Edema is the hallmark of hypervolemic hypotonic hyponatremia, a syndrome in which water is retained in excess of sodium. Because approximately 70% of total body water is intracellular, a 12- to 15-L excess of total body water must be present before sufficient interstitial fluid accumulates to cause detectable edema (unless hypoalbuminemia or vascular injury is present). Despite increases in both total body water and sodium, effective intravascular volume usually is modestly decreased.

Causes The basic problem in this condition is that the kidney cannot excrete sodium and water at a rate sufficient to keep pace with intake. This reduced sodium and water clearance can be the result of intrinsic renal disease or conditions that limit kidney blood flow. Nonrenal causes include conditions that decrease effective renal perfusion (congestive heart failure) and diseases characterized by hypoproteinemia and decreased colloid osmotic pressure (cirrhosis, hepatic failure, and nephrotic syndrome). Renal causes include almost any form of acute or chronic renal failure.

Laboratory Evaluation If the cause is extrarenal, there is intense conservation of salt and water with very low urinary sodium concentrations (<10 mEq/L), low urine volumes, and high urine osmolality. Urine electrolytes and osmolality are more variable (and less helpful) in renally induced hypervolemic hyponatremia. Because diuretics impair the ability to conserve sodium and water, at least 24 hours must elapse between the last dose of diuretic and determinations of urinary electrolytes and osmolality.

Isovolemic Hypotonic Hyponatremia Isovolemic hypotonic hyponatremia is a misnomer. In patients with isovolemic hypotonic hyponatremia, a slight (clinically undetectable) excess of total body fluid (approximately 3–4 liters) is maintained. Inappropriate secretion of antidiuretic hormone (SIADH) and water intoxication are the two most frequent causes. When renal function is normal and ADH can be inhibited, free water loads are rapidly cleared (>1 L/hour). Because of this impressive capacity, most cases of water intoxication occur in patients with impaired ability to clear free water or ADH excess. For example, water intoxication occurs with increased frequency in renal disease (decreased clearance) and schizophrenia (increased ADH and increased water intake). Diuretics commonly cause isovolemic hyponatremia. When normal circulating volume is maintained by diuretics, natriuresis impairs free water clearance and sensitizes to ADH. A "reset" of the serum osmostat may be seen in patients with a variety of underlying problems. (For example, cirrhosis and tuberculosis frequently cause chronic hyponatremia by this mechanism.) The "reset" phenomenon may be distinguished from inappropriate ADH secretion by normal responses to water loading or deprivation, despite hypo-osmolality.

Inappropriate ADH syndrome (SIADH) is often misdiagnosed in hospitalized patients. A diagnosis of exclusion, SIADH requires normal volume status, normal cardiac and renal function, and a normal hormonal environment (exclusive of ADH). SIADH is most frequently associated with malignant tumors, particularly of the lung; however, central nervous system (CNS) or pulmonary infections, drugs (Table 13.2), and trauma also may be the cause. SIADH is characterized by an inappropriately concentrated urine, with urinary excretion of sodium that matches the daily intake. Urine osmolality usually exceeds plasma osmolality. Urine sodium concentrations are higher than 20 mEq/L, and the urine cannot be diluted appropriately in response to water loading. (When water-challenged, patients with most other types of hyponatremia completely suppress ADH release and excrete maximally diluted urine <100 mOsm/L.) Excessive ADH or ADH-like compounds decrease free water clearance, resulting in modest expansion of the extracellular and intravascular volumes. Volume expansion increases cardiac output and glomerular filtration rate (GFR), eventually depleting the stores of total body sodium. (Because a constant fraction of filtered sodium is resorbed, there is obligatory renal loss of sodium.) Serum values of sodium, creatinine, and uric acid are all subnormal because of the expanded circulating volume and increased GFR. The treatment of SIADH is to restrict free water and correct the underlying disorder.

Treatment of Hyponatremia

Regardless of etiology, hyponatremia primarily affects the CNS. As the sodium concentration drops below 125 mEq/L, changes in cognition and motor function are common. Confusion and seizures often occur at a serum sodium value lower than 120 mEq/L, particularly if the decline occurs acutely. The severity of the complications increase rapidly with a declining sodium: half of all patients with severe hyponatremia (sodium level < 105 mEq/L) die. Unfortunately, rapid correction of hyponatremia also is associated with serious neurologic sequelae—central pontine myelinolysis (CPM) may result. CPM is a demyelinating syndrome of central nervous system damage characterized by weakness, dysarthria, dysphagia, coma, and potentially death. Risk factors include not only the rate of hyponatremia correction but also advanced age, preexisting liver or CNS disorders, diuretic use, and alcoholism.

Correction of hyponatremia must be skillful, balancing the competing risks of cerebral edema from too slow restoration and of central pontine myelinolysis from too rapid repair. In general, the rate of correction should be proportional to the speed with which the disorder developed. Practically speaking, most hyponatremic patients should have the sodium corrected to an initial level of 120–130 mEq/L over a 12- to 24-hour period, at an hourly rate not to exceed 2 mEq/L. Slower correction (i.e., 0.5 mEq/L/hour) is prudent in patients with chronic hyponatremia.

The specific treatment of hyponatremia de-

TABLE 13–2

CAUSES OF INAPPROPRIATE ADH SYNDROME

CNS Disorders	Cancers	Pulmonary Disorders	Drugs
Trauma	Lung carcinoma	Tuberculosis	Narcotics
Stroke	Pancreatic carcinoma	Pneumonia	Chlorpropamide
Infections			Tolbutamide
			Cyclophosphamide
			Vincristine
			Carbamazepine

pends on cause and severity. In hypervolemic hyponatremia, salt and fluid restriction are the mainstays of therapy. However, diuretics or dialysis may be required when renal function is impaired. In hypovolemic hyponatremia, normal or hypertonic (3%) saline should be used to restore circulating volume. In isovolemic hyponatremia, free water restriction and treatment of the underlying disorder are preferred. Patients with severe hyponatremia may require hypertonic saline and diuretics to achieve a safe serum sodium with adequate speed. In less acute cases of SIADH, hyponatremia may respond to demeclocycline (600–1200 mg/day).

HYPERNATREMIA

Etiology and Pathophysiology

Hypernatremia, defined as a serum sodium level higher than 150 mEq/L, is rare in patients with intact ADH secretion, a sensitive thirst mechanism, and access to free water. Although hypernatremia theoretically may result from water loss or sodium gain, water loss or deprivation is, by far, the most common mechanism. Hypernatremia is primarily a disease of patients who are unable to obtain and drink water (infants, elderly, and bedridden), particularly those simultaneously sustaining increased water losses. Hence, hypernatremia is relatively common in the ICU setting. Enteral feedings given without adequate free water are often contributory. Furthermore, because many elderly patients have defective osmoregulation, they are more likely to develop hypernatremia when faced with a provocative stimulus. Hypernatremia implies hyperosmolarity, the major mechanism of toxicity. Dehydration may result solely from increased insensible losses due to burns, tachypnea, or hyperthermia (high fever, heat stroke, neuroleptic malignant syndrome, malignant hyperthermia). Tachypnea does not cause dehydration in mechanically ventilated patients, however, because fully humidified gas is employed. But even with increased water losses, the development of hypernatremia usually requires water deprivation. Renal losses of free water may occur from intrinsic kidney diseases or from deficient or ineffective ADH. Osmotic diuretics such as glucose, mannitol, or glycerol may exaggerate free water clearance. Salt loading (primary hyperaldosteronism, hypertonic saline, sodium bicarbonate therapy, or oral sodium ingestion) is a rare

cause of hypernatremia. For patients with impaired sodium clearance, the sodium–potassium exchange ion resin, Kayexalate, can raise serum sodium by transferring significant sodium loads across the bowel wall. Diabetes insipidus produces hypernatremia by preventing appropriate water handling by the kidney. Central diabetes insipidus results from insufficient hypothalamic–pituitary release of antidiuretic hormone (ADH) secondary to CNS trauma, surgery, tumor, stroke, or granulomatous diseases. The kidney may also fail to respond fully to secreted ADH in the setting of chronic renal insufficiency, hypercalcemia, hypokalemia, or sickle cell disease, or in the presence of some drugs such as lithium, loop diuretics, or demecyclocine.

Diagnosis

Regardless of cause, the common symptoms of hypernatremia are thirst, nausea, vomiting, agitation, stupor, and coma. Unfortunately, all of these symptoms are nonspecific, and often go unrecognized or are attributed to another cause. The history and physical examination typically lead to the correct diagnosis, which is usually water deprivation–dehydration. The impressive urine output of the volume-replete patient with full-blown diabetes insipidus (up to 1–2 L/hour) is almost always noted, but the correct diagnosis may still be overlooked. It is important to note that the diagnosis of diabetes insipidus may be missed if free water losses have progressed to the point that profound intravascular volume depletion has occurred. In such cases, the classic "tip off" of massive urine output usually is absent. Caution must be exercised in the diagnosis of diabetes insipidus. In the unstable, volume-depleted patient in the ICU, the often recommended "water deprivation test" may prove harmful. A better strategy is to replete circulating volume and provide an empiric trial of ADH. When hemodynamically stable, additional elective endocrine testing, including a water deprivation test, may be safely performed. Although hypernatremia usually does not provide a diagnostic challenge, the urinary osmolarity can be a particularly helpful diagnostic test if the etiology is unclear (see Table 13.3).

Treatment

Treatment of hypernatremia consists of the replacement of free water, (either given enterally or

TABLE 13-3

URINARY OSMOLALITY IN HYPERNATREMIA

Urine Osmolarity	Differential Diagnosis	Therapy
>800	Dehydration	Free water replacement
	Hypodipsia	
	Sodium intoxication	
300-800	Osmotic diuretics	Free water replacement
	Partial or mild diabetes insipidus	Trial of ADH
<300	Central or nephrogenic diabetes insipidus	Free water replacement and ADH therapy

as D_5W), with frequent evaluation of electrolytes and osmolality. Correction of the defect at a rate of approximately 2 mEq/L/hour is an appropriate target. Like hyponatremia, very rapid correction, especially of longstanding hypernatremia can precipitate central pontine myelinolysis. If endogenous ADH is deficient or ineffective, it may be replaced with DDAVP, an ADH analog (see Chapter 32, Endocrine Emergencies).

POTASSIUM DISORDERS

HYPOKALEMIA

Because obligatory potassium losses are only 5-15 mEq/day in healthy patients with normal kidneys, potassium depletion virtually always occurs when there are excessive potassium losses or impaired potassium intake. Once hypokalemia (a serum potassium < 3.5 mEq/L) manifests, the average potassium deficit approximates 250-300 mEq (approximately 5-10% of the total body potassium stores). However, systemic pH influences extracellular potassium during acidosis as hydrogen ions move into cells in exchange for potassium, raising extracellular potassium. Therefore, hypokalemia in the face of acidosis suggests a large total-body deficit. Ninety-five percent of total body potassium is intracellular, but despite the small size of the extracellular compartment, its potassium concentration critically influences neuromuscular function. As a general rule, the large intracellular pool effectively maintains serum potassium concentration until total body potassium depletion occurs. Conversely, hyperkalemia does not always signify excess total body potassium. Even relatively small potassium loads may induce hyperkalemia as slow cellular uptake

of potassium occurs from the small intravascular space.

Etiology

Hypokalemia may result from decreased intake, increased losses, or redistribution of potassium. Measurement of urinary potassium and chloride concentrations and systemic acid–base status is very helpful in determining the etiology of hypokalemia (Table 13.4). If urinary potassium levels are low (<20 mEq/L), either decreased dietary intake or excessive gastrointestinal losses are to blame; however, hypokalemia rarely results from decreased intake alone. The healthy kidney can reduce potassium excretion to less than 10 mEq/day, a level that is almost always less than dietary intake. Furthermore, although the potassium content of liquid stool may reach 60 mEq/L, with the exception of cholera like illnesses, gastrointestinal (GI) losses are rarely severe enough to produce symptomatic hypokalemia. Losses of potassium directly from gastric fluid are minimal. Thus, vomiting induces hypokalemia—not through direct losses, but by promoting renal potassium wasting as a result of volume depletion and hypochloremic metabolic alkalosis.

If the urinary potassium is high (>20 mEq/L), measurement of systemic acid–base status helps determine the correct diagnosis. High urinary potassium excretion with systemic acidosis usually is caused by renal tubular acidosis or diabetic ketoacidosis. If high urinary potassium losses are accompanied by a systemic alkalosis, urinary chloride becomes key to diagnosis. A low value (<10 mEq/L) is indicative of diuretic use, vomiting, or nasogastric suction, all of which can be discovered by history. Diuretic use constitutes the most common cause of hypokalemia. Diuretics

TABLE 13–4

CAUSES OF HYPOKALEMIA DETERMINED BY EVALUATING URINE ELECTROLYTES

If urinary potassium concentration > 20 mEq/L

Acid–base status normal:	Acidemic patient:	Alkalemic patient:	
Drug or electrolyte disorder likely	Diabetic ketoacidosis	Urine Cl^- < 10 mEq/L	Urine Cl^- > 10 mEq/L
Amphotericin B	Renal tubular acidosis	Diuretics	Mineralocorticoid excess
Penicillin		Vomiting	
Aminoglycosides		Gastric suction	
Platinum compounds			
Hypomagnesemia			

If urinary potassium concentration < 20 mEq/L

Extrarenal mechanism is the etiology:
Decreased dietary intake
Diarrhea

increase distal tubular flow, promoting the exchange of sodium for potassium (an effect that may be profound in edematous patients), induce secondary hyperaldosteronism, and encourage alkalosis resulting in a shift of potassium from the extracellular to intracellular compartment. Simultaneous use of two or more diuretics having actions at different sites in the nephron, especially a thiazide/loop diuretic combination, can produce massive potassium losses.

A high urinary loss of potassium accompanied by alkalosis and a high urinary chloride concentration (>10 mEq/L) usually is due to mineralocorticoid excess (e.g., hyperaldosteronism, Cushing's syndrome, cirrhosis, or intravascular volume depletion).

Patients with a high rate of presentation of salt to the distal renal tubule also are predisposed to develop hypokalemia because high filtered sodium loads accentuate tubular exchange of sodium for potassium. In such patients, the acid–base status and urinary chloride concentration are variable but are often normal. Examples include high-dose sodium penicillin therapy, aminoglycoside administration, cisplatin therapy, and use of amphotericin B. For uncertain reasons, magnesium deficiency also is associated with high renal potassium losses.

A number of mechanisms may facilitate potassium entry into cells to produce hypokalemia. High insulin levels, whether exogenous or induced by continuous alimentation (e.g., total parenteral nutrition [TPN] or tube feedings), increase cellular uptake. Metabolic alkalosis also causes potassium to enter cells in exchange for H^+. In turn, hypokalemia increases renal bicarbonate absorption, perpetuating the alkalosis. (Potassium levels decline 0.1–0.4 mEq/L for each 0.1-unit

increase in pH.) Hypokalemia often occurs within 48 hours of treating vitamin B12 or folate deficiency, as potassium is massively incorporated into newly formed red cells and platelets. Such patients routinely experience reduction in serum potassium of approximately 1 mEq/L—a potentially life-threatening change.

Pathophysiology

Hypokalemia impairs muscle contractility and, when severe (potassium < 2.5 mEq/L), may cause profound, life-threatening respiratory muscle weakness. The severity of the muscular effects of a given potassium level depends on pH, calcium, and the rapidity with which hypokalemia developed. Hypokalemia increases the resting membrane potential of neuromuscular tissue, reducing excitability. Severe hypokalemia can cause cell membrane disruption, resulting in rhabdomyolysis. The muscles of the lower extremities usually are the first to be affected by hypokalemia, followed by those of the trunk and the respiratory system. Profound hypokalemia can even produce quadriplegia. Even moderate degrees of hypokalemia may impair smooth muscle function, producing ileus, pseudo-obstruction, or decreased ureteral motility. Severe hypokalemia also impairs the vascular smooth muscle response to catecholamines and angiotensin, influencing blood pressure stability. Hypokalemia may cause polyuria and polydipsia by injuring the renal tubular epithelium or diminishing responsiveness to ADH. Furthermore, hypokalemia results in increased ammonia production by the kidney and serves as one mechanism for worsening encephalopathy in patients with hepatic failure. Although

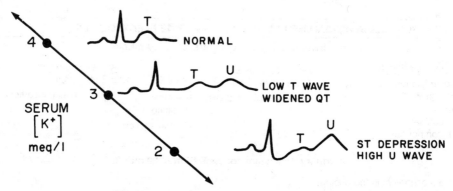

FIG. 13–1. ECG manifestations of hypokalemia.

focal neurologic findings rarely result from hypokalemia, lethargy and confusion are common in severe potassium depletion. Virtually any arrhythmia may surface during hypokalemia, especially in the presence of digitalis. Hypokalemia significantly increases the incidence of life-threatening arrhythmias in patients with acute myocardial ischemia, lowers the threshold for ventricular fibrillation, and promotes the re-entry phenomenon. Mild hypokalemia delays ventricular repolarization and is manifest by ST segment depression, diminished or inverted T waves, heightened U waves, and a prolonged Q-U interval. When hypokalemia is severe (potassium < 2.5 mEq/L), P-wave amplitude, PR interval, and QRS duration increase (Fig. 13.1).

Treatment

Total body deficits of potassium usually exceed 200 mEq in patients with hypokalemia. However, because the intracellular space must be accessed via the small extracellular compartment, potassium therapy (especially intravenous replacement) must be cautious and closely monitored to avoid potentially lethal hyperkalemia. Special care must be exercised when replacing potassium in patients with renal disease or diabetes and in those receiving drugs that block renin, angiotensin, or prostaglandin activity (e.g., angiotensin-converting enzyme [ACE] inhibitors, potassium-sparing diuretics, nonsteroidal anti-inflammatory drugs [NSAIDs]) because of the limited reserve to excrete excess potassium. Because hypomagnesemia aggravates the physiologic effects of hypokalemia and renders deficit correction difficult, checking serum magnesium levels is reasonable, especially for patients who are resistant to potassium replacement therapy. Possibly the most difficult situation occurs when hypokalemia and acidosis coexist. Correction of the acidosis aggravates the hypokalemia and often requires very aggressive potassium administration. In this somewhat unusual case, consideration should be given to use of potassium bicarbonate rather than the more common potassium chloride.

As a general rule, potassium should not be infused more quickly than 40 mEq/hour, and only then in dire emergencies. Infusion into a peripheral vein is often painful, occasionally induces chemical phlebitis, and if extravasated into soft tissue, can lead to tissue necrosis. Rapid infusion of potassium into central venous catheters can result in arrhythmias as the cardiac tissue is exposed transiently to high potassium concentrations not reflected by peripheral samples. It is best to administer intravenous potassium diluted in non–glucose-containing solutions. (When glucose solutions are used, insulin release is stimulated and the subsequent rapid incorporation of potassium into cells can further aggravate hypokalemia.) When possible, potassium deficits should be replaced with oral (enteral) preparations. Enteral administration provides an effective, safe alternative to intravenous infusion at substantially lower cost and actually allows larger doses to be administered. One note of caution: if potassium chloride solutions are repeatedly placed directly into the small bowel via feeding tube, irritation and ulceration may develop. In addition, many liquid potassium preparations contain sorbitol, a poorly absorbed sugar, which often precipitates diarrhea.

HYPERKALEMIA

It is difficult for healthy subjects to develop hyperkalemia because even minimally functional kidneys efficiently excrete excess potassium. In addition, adaptation to chronic potassium administration even further increases the ability of the kidney to excrete it. Furthermore, when renal clearance decreases, the colon may increase potassium excretion. Cellular buffering (particularly by muscle and liver) acutely blunts the impact of a potassium load while the kidneys eliminate the excess. Insulin deficiency inhibits cellular buffering, whereas excretion requires functioning kidneys. Therefore, potassium handling is greatly impaired in patients with diabetes and renal insufficiency. Potassium-sparing diuretics, angiotensin-converting enzyme inhibitors, and, less commonly, nonsteroidal anti-inflammatory agents can induce hyperkalemia, especially in patients with baseline reductions in glomerular filtration rate or intrinsic renal disease.

Diagnosis

Pseudohyperkalemia may occur if venous blood is analyzed after exercise or prolonged tourniquet application. Hemolysis also may cause artifactual elevation of potassium, especially when blood is withdrawn rapidly through a small needle (smaller than 22 gauge). Serum potassium is normally 0.5 mEq/L higher than plasma potassium because potassium is released from platelets during clotting. However, marked hemolysis, severe leukocytosis ($>100,000/mm^3$), or thrombocytosis ($>10^6/mm^3$) also may raise the potassium of the clotted specimen to extraordinary levels. The diagnosis of clot-related "pseudohyperkalemia" is confirmed by detecting a disparity between simultaneous determinations of plasma and serum potassium.

Mechanisms

Three basic mechanisms contribute to hyperkalemia: (*a*) increased potassium intake, (*b*) translocation of potassium from the intracellular to the extracellular compartment, and (*c*) decreased excretion.

Increased Potassium Intake

Even with the wide distribution of potassium supplements, hyperkalemia from excessive intake alone is very rare in the normal patient, perhaps with the exception of intentional overdose. Conversely, iatrogenic potassium overloading often is seen in hospitalized patients with limited excre-

tory power. The potassium source may be an unmodified standing order for potassium replacement or other unsuspected therapy (e.g., potassium-containing intravenous fluids, potassium penicillin G, blood products, or salt substitutes). Ringer's lactate contains 4 mEq/L of potassium per liter and therefore should only be administered carefully to patients with renal insufficiency. Potassium penicillin G contains 1.6 mEq of potassium for each 10^6 units of penicillin, constituting a significant potassium load in patients receiving high penicillin doses. Packed red cells, stored for long periods, may deliver as much as 7 mEq/unit. Renal transplant recipients receive significant intraoperative potassium loads when donor kidneys perfused with Collins' solution (140 mEq of potassium per liter) are implanted.

Potassium Shifts

Acidosis is the most common cause of shift-related hyperkalemia. Changes in serum potassium are more sensitive to changes in serum bicarbonate than to pH itself. Therefore, respiratory acidosis has relatively little effect on potassium, whereas metabolic acidosis exerts a potent effect. Potassium shifts are more marked when mineral acids (e.g., HCl) than when organic acids (e.g., lactate) are the etiology of acidosis. A 0.1-unit decrease in pH produces an average 0.6-mEq/L increase in potassium (range, 0.4–1.3 mEq/L). Hypertonic solutions (mannitol or hypertonic saline) also may increase the serum potassium by uncertain mechanisms. Hyperkalemia may follow the breakdown of red blood cells in large hematomas or following injury that produces extensive tissue necrosis with subsequent potassium release (particularly rhabdomyolysis, crush injuries, burns, and tumor lysis). Digitalis toxicity poisons the cellular sodium/potassium pump and may produce severe refractory hyperkalemia. (Potassium levels exceeding 5.5 mEq/L are associated with poor survival rates in digitalis toxicity.) β-adrenergic blockers also can increase the serum potassium by blocking adrenergic-receptor-mediated cellular uptake of potassium. Hemolytic transfusion reactions and other forms of acute hemolysis also cause life-threatening hyperkalemia. Succinylcholine (a depolarizing neuromuscular blocker) predictably produces a small rise in plasma potassium (approximately 0.5 mEq/L) but may precipitate a striking hyperkalemia in patients with burns, tetanus, or other neuromuscular diseases. These effects are minimized by pretreatment with a subparalyzing dose of a nondepolarizing neuromuscular blocking drug (see Chapter 17, Analgesia, Sedation and Therapeutic Paralysis).

Decreased Potassium Excretion

Even though 80 to 90% of renal function must be lost before the kidney noticeably fails to excrete potassium, renal insufficiency remains the most common cause of hyperkalemia. Among patients with renal insufficiency, concomitant drug therapy often is a complicating factor (see Table 13.5). Acidosis induced by renal failure further impairs the ability of the kidney to excrete potassium and promotes the shift of potassium from cellular stores into the circulation. In renal failure of abrupt onset, serum potassium tends to rise before the BUN or creatinine, especially when exogenous potassium is given; low tubular flow rates immediately prevent exchange of sodium for potassium, whereas creatinine and BUN require time to build to noteworthy concentrations. However, even when complete renal shutdown occurs, the serum potassium seldom rises by more than 0.5 mEq/L/day in response to natural loads. (When normal potassium intake is exceeded or excessive relapse of potassium from damaged cells occurs, this rate may be surpassed.)

Aldosterone is required to maintain circulating volume and to enable tubular sodium/potassium exchange. Therefore, serum potassium may rise in primary adrenal failure and adrenal insufficiency should be strongly considered in patients with hyperkalemia and prominent fluid deficits. Even with primary adrenal failure, hyperkalemia usually is not significant in the absence of another confounding factor (e.g., increased potassium intake or renal failure). Drugs that interfere with the formation or action of aldosterone (e.g., potassium-sparing diuretics and heparin) also may produce overt hyperkalemia. Finally, by virtue of the frequency of their use, NSAIDs and ACE inhibitors are relatively common causes of hyperkalemia.

TABLE 13–5

DRUGS ASSOCIATED WITH DECREASED RENAL POTASSIUM EXCRETION

Angiotensin-converting enzyme (ACE) inhibitors
Cyclosporine
Heparin
Nonsteroidal anti-inflammatory agents (NSAIDs)
Potassium-sparing diuretics

Signs and Symptoms

Hyponatremia, hypocalcemia, hypermagnesemia, and acidosis potentiate the neuromuscular effects of hyperkalemia. Therefore, levels of sodium, calcium, and magnesium ions should be evaluated and corrected concurrently. Obvious functional impairment of skeletal muscle rarely occurs at potassium levels lower than 7.0 mEq/L. Proximal lower extremity weakness is the most common symptom. Hyperkalemia usually spares the respiratory muscles, cranial nerves, and deep tendon reflexes. The most devastating effects of hyperkalemia are cardiac arrhythmias. The pump-impairing and vasodilatory effects of severe hyperkalemia may cause refractory hypotension.

Electrocardiogram

An electrocardiogram (ECG) should be obtained for every patient with a potassium level higher than 5.5 mEq/L (Fig. 13.2). Widening of the QRS complex (due to delayed depolarization) follows early narrowing and peaking of T waves and QT interval shortening. Atrial activity usually is lost shortly before the characteristic sine wave hybrid of ventricular tachycardia/fibrillation appears.

Treatment

The aggressiveness with which hyperkalemia is treated should parallel the severity of the clinical manifestations of the disorder—largely the electrocardiographic manifestations. Before initiating therapy, the diagnosis should be certain because of the potential risk of inducing hypokalemia if the ''hyperkalemia'' is artifactual. When an elevated potassium is the culmination of a progressive process in a patient with risk factors for hyperkalemia (e.g., renal insufficiency) and significant clinical or ECG manifestations are present, immediate treatment is indicated. Conversely, the unexpected discovery of an isolated, elevated potassium value in an asymptomatic patient should be approached with some skepticism and caution. In such cases, the assay should be repeated before treatment is undertaken. A second serum sample and a separate plasma specimen both should be drawn slowly through a large needle. Leukocyte and platelet counts also should be obtained, and an ECG should be recorded. The ECG is a key diagnostic test in determining the urgency with which hyperkalemia should be ad-

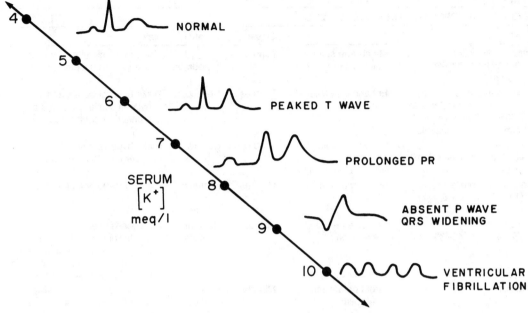

FIG. 13–2. ECG manifestations of hyperkalemia.

dressed. If the ECG is normal, elective treatment may await repeat confirmatory potassium determinations. If the ECG is diagnostically abnormal, muscle weakness is present, or the reported potassium exceeds 7 mEq/L, immediate action probably is indicated. Continuous ECG monitoring should be initiated, followed by specific treatment on five fronts as outlined in Table 13.6: (a) stop all potassium; (b) begin replenishing circulating volume in dehydrated patients; (c) administer drugs to shift potassium into the cellular compartment; (d) stabilize neuromuscular and cardiac function with calcium, if indicated; and (e) remove potassium from the body.

Shifting potassium from serum into muscle rapidly lowers the serum concentration, but this maneuver only temporizes. Sodium bicarbonate (NaHCO$_3$) causes an exchange of H$^+$ for potassium across all membranes, lowering the serum potassium within minutes and lasting for up to 12 hours. Two ampules of NaHCO$_3$ ($\approx$ 100 mEq) usually suffice. However, in the face of ongoing acidosis, sufficient HCO$_3^-$ should be given to correct the pH. The hypertonicity of bicarbonate solution may lower potassium independently of its pH effect. Insulin also enhances cellular uptake. A 10-unit intravenous bolus of regular insulin usually is sufficient to produce at least transient reduction in glucose levels. Hyperglycemic pa-

tients require only insulin; patients with normal blood sugar levels should receive glucose concurrently to prevent hypoglycemia (2–3 g of glucose is required for each unit of regular insulin). Insulin produces a reduction in serum potassium of 1–3 mEq/L within minutes, an effect that may last for hours. Calcium, in the form of 1–2 g of intravenous calcium chloride, rapidly stabilizes cardiac conduction by lowering the depolarization threshold. Although calcium acts within minutes, its effect usually persists less than 2 hours. Because precipitates form when HCO$_3^-$ and calcium are admixed, each drug must be given through a separate intravenous catheter or sequentially through a single well-flushed line. Calcium should be administered with extreme caution in patients receiving digitalis preparations. Dialysis is most often required for patients with renal insufficiency, severe hyperkalemia, or high potassium loads that result from multiple trauma or tumor lysis. Hemodialysis may remove up to 40 mEq/hour of potassium, whereas peritoneal dialysis removes only 5–10 mEq/hour. Loop diuretics promote potassium excretion but are only useful for patients with good urine output and modest hyperkalemia. Ion exchange resins lower potassium by trading sodium for potassium across the bowel wall. (More sodium is gained than potassium is lost, and electroneutrality is maintained by additional

TABLE 13–6

THERAPEUTIC OPTIONS FOR HYPERKALEMIA

Treatment	Action	Onset	Duration	Notes
Intravenous saline (0.9% NaCl, 200–300 mL/hour)	Membrane stabilizer Volume expander	Minutes	Several hours	May induce circulating volume overload or hypernatremia.
Glucose and insulin (10 U regular insulin, add D50W 1–2 ampules in normoglycemic patients)	Enhances cellular uptake	Minutes	Several hours	Risks hyperglycemia and hypoglycemia. Requires careful monitoring of glucose.
NaHCO$_3$ (1–2 ampules over 5–10 minutes)	Enhances cellular uptake Membrane stabilizer	Minutes	Several hours	Risks hypervolemia, hypernatremia, and alkalosis.
Calcium gluconate (10–20 mL over 5 minutes)	Membrane stabilizer	Minutes	Minutes to hours	May induce hypercalcemia.
Diuretics (Furosemide 40–80 mg)	Enhances renal excretion	Minutes	Several hours	High doses needed in renal insufficiency. Ineffective in frank renal failure. Risks circulating volume depletion. Loop diuretic plus thiazide may enhance effect.
Dialysis	Direct potassium removal	Minutes	Hours to days	Hemodialysis most effective. Risks all complications of dialysis.
Potassium-binding resins (Kayexalate 50 g p.o. or rectally in 100 mL sorbitol)	Enhances GI excretion	Hours	Hours to days	Risks hypernatremia, volume overload. Slow effect. Sorbitol necessary to promote GI motility.

losses of magnesium and calcium.) Resultant sodium retention may produce volume overload in oliguric or anuric patients. A typical 50-mg dose of resin decreases serum potassium by 0.5–1 mEq/L. When given orally, ion exchange resins require a vehicle to prevent constipation (usually 20% sorbitol solution). Such resins also may be given rectally if oral dosing is not tolerated or advisable. Rectal dosing may prove more efficient than oral dosing at potassium removal. Volume expansion with normal saline will rapidly lower potassium in dehydrated patients.

CALCIUM DISORDERS

HYPERCALCEMIA

Etiology

The long list of possible causes of hypercalcemia (see Table 13.7) may be narrowed significantly by careful history taking, review of medications, and a limited number of basic laboratory tests. Relatively few disorders are responsible for most cases of hypercalcemia in most hospitals:

neoplasia and hyperparathyroidism each account for approximately 45% of cases. All other causes constitute the remainder. Furthermore, the hypercalcemia associated with hyperparathyroidism is usually mild and uncommonly associated with significant intravascular volume depletion. Thus, most cases of significant hypercalcemia encountered in the ICU will be the result of malignancy.

TABLE 13–7

CAUSES OF HYPERCALCEMIA

Paget's disease
Adrenal insufficiency
Malignancies
    Squamous cell lung carcinoma
    Breast carcinoma
    Leukemia
    Lymphoma
    Multiple myeloma
Thiazide diuretics
Sarcoidosis
Hyperparathyroidism
Milk–alkali syndrome
Immobilization
Vitamin D or A intoxication
Hyperthyroidism

Interestingly, when neoplasia is the cause, as many as one-half of patients have no evidence of bony metastases.

Signs and Symptoms

The signs and symptoms of hypercalcemia are nonspecific but most commonly result from the two major pathophysiologic derangements—dehydration and depressed neuromuscular function. Hypercalcemia induces an osmotic diuresis resulting in complaints of polyuria and polydypsia, but if fluid intake is unrestricted, severe calcium elevations are unlikely. Unfortunately, the decreased gut motility of hypercalcemia often produces nausea, vomiting, abdominal pain, and constipation, negating this potential mode of compensation. The most common manifestations of hypercalcemia are neuromuscular disturbances (lethargy, agitation, coma, fatigue, and weakness). Although symptoms are correlated poorly with calcium levels, severe manifestations of toxicity (e.g., coma) are rare unless levels exceed 14 mg/dL. The ECG reflects the altered cellular electrical potential when it demonstrates a truncated QT or increased PR interval. Calcium salts form and are deposited in tissue when a critical calcium-phosphate product (usually > 60) is reached. In the kidney, renal stones and renal insufficiency may result; skin deposits may induce pruritus. Muscle and other soft tissue also may be affected by this "metastatic" calcification. Pancreatitis or peptic ulcer disease are rare GI presentations. Hypercalcemia may produce hypertension by increasing peripheral vascular resistance, an effect that is usually offset by significant volume depletion.

Laboratory Evaluation

Calcium is predominately an extracellular cation present in the plasma in three forms: free, ionized (as sulfate or phosphate salts), and bound to serum proteins. Because as much as one-half of the total serum calcium is bound to serum proteins (predominately albumin), calcium levels must be evaluated in light of the serum protein level. Even "normal" levels of total calcium may represent relative hypercalcemia in patients with severe hypoproteinemia. Conversely, hyperproteinemic states such as myeloma can raise total serum calcium levels. Normally, an inverse relationship exists between the serum phosphate and calcium. Vulnerable to dietary influences, the serum phosphate level is a highly labile measurement—unlike serum calcium. Alkaline phosphatase may be elevated by any cause of hypercalcemia and, therefore, is not diagnostically helpful. Urinary calcium usually is very high in hypercalcemic disorders that are not dependent on parathyroid hormone (PTH) activity (i.e., sarcoid or vitamin D intoxication). Vitamin D levels are useful in confirming suspected toxicity but are not diagnostic in any other form of hypercalcemia. Although frequently assayed, PTH levels are not helpful diagnostically unless markedly elevated in a patient with severe hypercalcemia and normal renal function. Even mild renal insufficiency severely limits the use of PTH assays, because it decreases the clearance of the commonly assayed carboxy-PTH fragment. For this reason, midmolecule or aminoterminal assays are superior.

Treatment

As with hyperkalemia, the simplest and most rapid method to begin reducing calcium in the dehydrated patient is to expand the circulating volume with isotonic saline. Although the absolute magnitude of this intervention is usually small (reductions of 1–3 mg/dL), such corrections often are critical in reducing symptoms. After volume expansion, loop diuretics, like furosemide, are rapidly effective in lowering serum calcium concentration if good urine flow is established. By blocking calcium reabsorption in the kidney, furosemide can reduce serum calcium levels as much as 4–5 mg/dL each day. A reasonable goal for saline and diuretic therapy is to establish and maintain a urine output of 200 mL/hr. Because immobilization worsens hypercalcemia, ambulation is helpful when feasible. Phosphate therapy is effective immediately but generally is not recommended because of its many side effects, which include soft-tissue calcification, "overshoot" hypocalcemia, and acute renal failure. Oral phosphates are safer than intravenous preparations, but GI intolerance (predominately diarrhea) limits their use. The antimetabolite mithramycin inhibits osteoclast function to prevent reabsorption of bone calcium. Although, mithramycin (25 μg intravenously) is helpful in acute severe cases of hypercalcemia associated with malignancy, side effects (hepatic, renal, and marrow toxicity) usually prohibit chronic use. Mithramycin rarely has an immediate effect, usually requiring 1–2 days to achieve any reduction in serum calcium levels. Because of these delays, mithramycin is usually a second-line therapy. Glucocorticoids are most useful in the hypercalcemia of malignancy (especially breast carcinoma and lymphoma). By inhibiting gut absorption of calcium, steroids also are effective in sarcoidosis and vitamin D intoxication. Calcitonin inhibits osteoclast function and promotes incorporation of calcium into bone but is expensive, unpredictable, and prone to tachyphylaxis. In symptomatic, severe hypercalcemia, doses as high as 8 units given every 12 hours (intravenously or subcutaneously) can produce prompt (4–6 hours) reductions in serum calcium levels. When used, calcitonin is more effective when administered in combination with glucocorticoids. Diphosphonates, such as etidronate and pamidronate, prevent osteoclast-mediated bone resorption. They currently are used for the treatment of Paget's disease and malignancy-related hypercalcemia but are effective only in a minority of patients. In the truly emergent setting, serum calcium levels of the hypercalcemic patient can be reduced rapidly by hemodialysis.

HYPOCALCEMIA

Mild hypocalcemia is a common finding in patients in the ICU but rarely is symptomatic. Overt hypocalcemia is less common than symptomatic hypercalcemia but is just as life threatening. The urgency of evaluation and treatment depends on the severity of symptoms.

Clinical Manifestations

Hypocalcemia usually is asymptomatic if ionized calcium remains normal despite low total calcium levels or if hypocalcemia develops slowly. Alkalosis, however, lowers the fraction of ionized calcium at any given total calcium, aggravating symptoms. The threshold at which symptoms develop in hypocalcemia is highly variable; most of the symptoms are due to neuromuscular irritability. The most common complaints are paresthesia, cramps, or tetany. Dyspnea or stridor may occur if ventilatory or upper airway muscles are affected. Although usually a consequence of hypocalcemia, tetany also may develop in acute respiratory alkalosis and acute hyperkalemia. Rare but more specific signs of neuromuscular irritability, including carpopedal spasm (Trousseau's sign) or facial muscle hyperreflexia (Chvostek's sign), may be elicited in patients with hypocalcemia. Other potential CNS effects include seizures, papilledema, hallucinations, confusion, and depression. In humans, the relationship between hypocalcemia and impaired circulatory system performance is spec-

ulative, but in experimental models, hypocalcemia may compromise perfusion by lowering the systemic vascular resistance and decreasing cardiac contractility. The QT prolongation seen with hypocalcemia may result in a variety of arrhythmias (most significantly, Torsades de Pointes).

Causes

There are four recognized mechanisms of hypocalcemia: (*a*) decreased calcium intake or absorption; (*b*) binding and sequestration of calcium; (*c*) inability to mobilize bone calcium; and (*d*) decreases in serum protein concentration. Because most calcium is bound to serum protein, reductions in protein concentration result in hypocalcemia. A reduction in albumin of 1 gm/dL reduces the serum calcium by approximately 0.8 mg/dL. The globulin fraction of serum protein has less influence. Calcium may be removed from the circulation by binding to other drugs or chemicals such as phosphate, chelating agents (e.g., ethylenediaminetetraacetic acid [EDTA]), or the citrate anticoagulant in transfused blood. Calcium may also bind inflamed intra-abdominal fat in victims of pancreatitis. Hyperphosphatemia induces hypocalcemia in patients with renal failure or in those who are otherwise unable to excrete PO_4^{-3} normally. Reductions in calcium intake or impaired absorption resulting from reduced activity of vitamin D also may induce hypocalcemia. Anticonvulsants and glucocorticoids impair calcium absorption (probably by inhibiting vitamin D action). Prolonged hospitalization (particularly among patients receiving TPN) may also cause vitamin D deficiency. Although renal failure decreases vitamin D production, symptomatic hypocalcemia usually is prevented by the development of secondary hyperparathyroidism. PTH deficiency and resistance to PTH are rare causes of hypocalcemia, except in patients undergoing thyroid or parathyroid surgery. For such patients, life-threatening hypocalcemia may develop within hours of surgery. Therefore, monitoring postoperative calcium assumes added importance after surgical procedures in the neck, which have the potential to injure the parathyroid glands. Very rarely, protracted, severe hypotension may result in parathyroid infarction and subsequent hypocalcemia. Magnesium levels should be obtained in hypocalcemic patients because magnesium is necessary, for both PTH secretion and action. Hypocalcemia secondary to hypomagnesemia is particularly common in alcoholics and in patients receiving chronic TPN or diuretics. The causes of hypocalcemia are outlined in Table 13.8.

TABLE 13–8
CAUSES OF HYPOCALCEMIA

Hypoparathyroidism
Hypomagnesemia
Systemic alkalosis
Pancreatitis
Chronic renal failure
Sepsis
Massive transfusion
Fat embolism syndrome
Burns
Vitamin D deficiency
Anticonvulsant use

Treatment

The first step in the treatment of hypocalcemia is to ensure airway patency and adequate ventilation and perfusion. Serum levels of potassium, magnesium, vitamin D, and PTH should be obtained. Alkalosis should be corrected to raise the ionized calcium fraction. In nonemergent settings, hyperphosphatemia should first be corrected with phosphate buffers (aluminum-containing antacids) and a low phosphate diet preferably before administering calcium. Calcium administration in the setting of profound hyperphosphatemia is unlikely to correct the defect, because calcium phosphate salts will rapidly deposit in tissues. Calcium replacement is always empiric because deficits are impossible to calculate accurately. Symptomatic patients should be given intravenous calcium preferably via a large central vein because of the tendency of calcium solutions to induce chemical phlebitis or tissue necrosis when given in peripheral veins. Intramuscular injection should be avoided for this same reason. Slow infusion of 10–20 mL of 10% calcium gluconate is the preferred method of supplementation. Such dosing provides approximately 10 mg of elemental calcium per milliliter. Maintenance of calcium administration must be guided by serial determinations of serum calcium. Concomitant vitamin D deficiency should be treated. Therapy with the costly, 1,25-OH vitamin D analog may be required if renal and liver function are compromised, but for patients with preserved hepatic and renal function, nonhydroxylated vitamin D preparations will suffice. Because thiazides increase renal tubular calcium reabsorption, they are useful adjuncts to increase serum calcium.

MAGNESIUM DISORDERS

HYPERMAGNESEMIA

Under normal circumstances, the gut and kidney work in concert to tightly regulate serum magnesium levels. When deficient, gut absorption of magnesium increases and excretion decreases. When a larger magnesium load is presented, the gut absorbs a smaller fraction and the kidney excretes a greater proportion. Therefore, hypermagnesemia is uncommon unless very large intravenous doses of magnesium sulfate are infused (e.g., during eclampsia) or patients with renal insufficiency are given dietary magnesium supplements. However, for patients with severe renal insufficiency or ileus, unintentional gut absorption of magnesium-containing cathartics also may overload the excretory capacity. Hypermagnesemia also has been described after extravasation of renal "stone dissolving" drugs that contain high concentrations of magnesium.

Clinically, hypermagnesemia presents as hyporeflexia and hypotension when levels exceed 4 mEq/dL, somnolence presents at levels higher than 7 mEq/dL, and heart block and paralysis present at levels higher than 10 mg/dL. Hypermagnesemia prolongs the PR interval on ECG, impairs conduction, and may produce heart block. Initially, calcium gluconate (1–2 grams intravenously) should be administered to reverse the effects of hypermagnesemia. If feasible, administration of isotonic saline and loop diuretics can facilitate magnesium excretion. Emergent dialysis should follow.

HYPOMAGNESEMIA

Hypomagnesemia is one of the most common electrolyte abnormalities in hospitalized patients. Its common causes are presented in Table 13.9. Hypomagnesemia almost always results from excessive renal or GI losses. Because magnesium is predominately absorbed in the small bowel, inflammatory bowel disease, chronic diarrhea, and malabsorption are common precipitants. Malnutrition (particularly in alcoholics) decreases magnesium by limiting intake and predisposing to chronic diarrhea. The problem of hypomagnesemia may be particularly acute in alcoholic patients because magnesium is a required cofactor for the effective action of thiamine. Pancreatitis also causes hypomagnesemia through uncertain mech-

TABLE 13–9

CAUSES OF HYPOMAGNESEMIA

Starvation, malnutrition

Diarrhea

Inflammatory bowel disease

Alcoholism

Diabetes

Medications:
  Loop diuretics
  Digitalis
  Aminoglycosides
  Amphotericin
  Cyclosporine
  Cisplatinin
  Pentamidine

anisms. Although any form of renal disease may produce magnesium wasting, it most commonly results from the use of diuretics (thiazides, loop, and osmotic). "Forced saline diuresis" also may waste magnesium during chemotherapy or treatment of hypercalcemia. Aminoglycosides, cyclosporine, amphotericin, and platinum compounds all aggravate renal magnesium losses. Perhaps more importantly, by encouraging potassium egress from cells and calcium egress from bone, over the long run, hypomagnesemia may induce hypokalemia and hypocalcemia. Because of the frequency of concurrence of the disorders, magnesium deficiency should be considered in patients with hypokalemia, hypocalcemia, and hypophosphatemia.

Hypomagnesemia's most frequent clinical effects are neuromuscular and cardiac. Like hypocalcemia, hypomagnesemia causes neuromuscular irritability manifest as altered mentation, seizures, tremor, and Chvostek's and Trousseau's signs. Hypomagnesemia seems to predispose patients to almost all types of arrhythmias (particularly Torsades de Pointes and those of digitalis toxicity); however, large clinical studies have been unable to confirm beneficial antiarrhythmic and survival effects of magnesium in patients suffering from myocardial infarction. Hypomagnesemia should be suspected when the ECG demonstrates prolonged QT and PR intervals and long flat T waves.

Plasma levels imperfectly reflect total body magnesium stores and correlate even less well with ionized plasma levels. Therefore, magnesium deficits, like calcium deficits, are hard to estimate, making the treatment of hypomagnesemia largely empiric. For patients with normal renal function, magnesium is safe, even in large doses. For asymptomatic hypomagnesemic patients, oral magnesium compounds usually are effective at raising the magnesium but sometimes produce such severe diarrhea that hypomagnesemia actually worsens. If the oral route is chosen, doses of 0.5 mEq/kg represent a good starting dose. In life-threatening hypomagnesemic crises, magnesium can be administered as magnesium sulfate (1–2 g) intravenously over 2–3 minutes. Rapid intravenous magnesium infusions can produce hypotension and, therefore, should be avoided except in emergent circumstances.

PHOSPHATE DISORDERS

HYPERPHOSPHATEMIA

In the ICU, high levels of phosphate (PO_4^{-3}), (>5 mg/dL) usually reflect impaired PO_4^{-3} excretion (i.e., renal insufficiency with GFR < 20 mL/minute) or increased cellular release of PO_4^{-3} (e.g., chemotherapy, rhabdomyolysis, sepsis). Symptoms, however, are few, apart from those of concurrent hypocalcemia induced by excess phosphate levels. In treating hyperphosphatemia, attention should first be directed to the primary cause of PO_4^{-3} elevation. When symptomatic hypocalcemia urges treatment, PO_4^{-3} binders (30–45 mL of aluminum hydroxide every 6 hours), volume expansion with intravenous saline, acetazolamide, and restricting intake usually are effective. Dialysis may be required in severe or refractory cases.

HYPOPHOSPHATEMIA

As the major intracellular anion, PO_4^{-3} plays a crucial role in phospholipid, phosphoprotein, and phosphosugar metabolism. It is the depletion of the intracellular PO_4^{-3} store that produces clinical symptomatology, imperfectly reflected by depressed serum values. Although PO_4^{-3} is easily depleted from skeletal muscle and erythrocytes, levels tend to be well preserved in most other tissues, such as cardiac muscle. Factors predisposing total body phosphate depletion include malnutrition, alcoholism, hypomagnesemia, renal tubular dysfunction (diuresis, nonoliguric acute tubular necrosis), and gastrointestinal losses (antacid binding, malabsorption, nasogastric suctioning, emesis, diarrhea). It is important not to equate hypophosphatemia with intracellular PO_4^{-3} depletion. Extracellular to intracellular transfer of PO_4^{-3} occurs during anabolism, insulin administration, correction of metabolic acidosis, and the acute phase of respiratory alkalosis. Hypophosphatemia is therefore commonly observed in alcohol-dependent patients, during refeeding or caloric loading, during recovery from diabetic ketoacidosis, and during hyperventilation. In many such patients, hypophosphatemia does not reflect pathologic PO_4^{-3} depletion. Profound hypophosphatemia has been reported among patients with pernicious anemia treated with vitamin B12 replacement. As erythrocyte synthesis rapidly gears up, huge amounts of phosphate are incorporated into the formed red blood cells.

As a rule, serum PO_4^{-3} must fall below 1.0 mg/dL before overt symptoms develop. Dysfunction of the cellular elements of the blood, muscle weakness, GI upset, neural dysfunction, and (rarely) tissue breakdown are the major clinical consequences. Depletion of 2,3-diphosphoglyceric acid (2,3-DPG) diminishes the ability of erythrocytes to unload oxygen to the tissues. Thrombocytopenia, platelet dysfunction, and impaired leukocyte killing have been shown experimentally. Skeletal muscle dysfunction is of major clinical interest in the setting of ventilatory failure, in which PO_4^{-3} depletion contributes to weakness and ventilator dependence. A PO_4^{-3}-related sensorimotor neuropathy is occasionally observed 4–7 days after PO_4^{-3}-poor hyperalimentation is started. Very rarely, severe PO_4^{-3} depletion can produce hemolysis, rhabdomyolysis, or congestive cardiomyopathy especially when generous re-feeding is abruptly initiated.

Although PO_4^{-3} should be a component of all nutritional regimens, urgent correction should be reserved for situations in which clinical symptoms accompany a serum PO_4^{-3} level less than 1.0 mg/dL. As with potassium repletion, PO_4^{-3} must traverse the small extracellular compartment to reach its intracellular target, so repletion must be cautious. An intravenous infusion of 2.5–5.0 mg/kg as potassium or sodium phosphate over 6 hours should not cause the calcium-phosphate product to climb to dangerous levels (>60 mg/dL). Oral PO_4^{-3} supplementation (125 mg twice daily, as potassium phosphate or equivalent) usually will suffice when the serum PO_4^{-3} is only modestly reduced (>1.0 mg/dL). Concurrent hypomagnesemia must be corrected. Oral PO_4^{-3} supplementation should continue for 5–10 days after reestablishing a normal serum level.

KEY POINTS

1. The diagnosis of the etiology of hyponatremia relies on an accurate assessment of fluid status of the patient. In most cases, the etiology can be determined by history and physical examination. For cases in which the diagnosis is uncertain after examination, urine sodium and osmolality measurements are useful.

2. Severe hyponatremia (serum sodium < 120 mEq/L) defines an urgent clinical situation in which levels of the ion should be raised to 120 mEq/L or above. The rate of correction should be approximately 1–2 mEq/L/hour—sufficiently rapid to reduce the risk of seizures but slow enough to avoid the potential for central pontine myelinolysis. Water restriction or isotonic or hypertonic saline is used when hypervolemic or hypovolemic hyponatremia is present, respectively.

3. Hypernatremia usually is the result of restricted access to free water or absence of the sensation of thirst. Rarely, central diabetes insipidus (DI), a fatal condition unless recognized and treated with antidiuretic hormone, is the etiology. DI can be recognized by noting large volumes of dilute urine in a patient with hyperosmolar serum.

4. Because a small minority of the body's potassium is in the extracellular compartment, hypokalemia signals total body depletion of potassium, usually exceeding 200 mEq. Because of the importance of potassium in maintaining normal neural and muscular function, correction of the deficit is prudent in the critically ill. When possible, oral replacement avoids the rapid swings of intravenous dosing. When intravenous replacement is used, dosing should probably be limited to 40 mEq/hour.

5. Significant hyperkalemia usually is the result of renal insufficiency. Hyperkalemia sufficient to cause symptoms or induce electrocardiographic changes should be treated aggressively. Combined therapy with bicarbonate, calcium, insulin, glucose, volume expanders, and loop diuretics constitutes initial therapy. Clearance of potassium with dialysis or potassium binding resins may then be required.

6. Both calcium and magnesium depend on their ionized forms for biologic action; therefore, total serum concentrations do not accurately reflect bioactivity. Acid–base status can dramatically alter the fraction of ionized ions. Total calcium and magnesium levels, and possibly ionized forms of each, should be measured when unexplained neuromuscular disorders occur in the ICU.

SUGGESTED READINGS

1. Arief A. Management of hyponatremia. Br Med J 1993; 307:305.
2. Ayus JC, Krothapalli RK, Arieff AI. Treatment of symptomatic hyponatremia and its relationship to brain damage. N Engl J Med 1987;317:1190–1195.
3. Balestri FJ. Magnesium metabolism in the critically ill. Clin Crit Care Med 1985;5:217.
4. Baldwin TE, Chernow B. Hypocalcemia in the ICU: coping with the causes and consequences. J Crit Illness 1987; 2:9.
5. Brown RS. Extrarenal potassium homeostasis. Kidney Int 1986;30:116.
6. Cooke CR, Turin MD, Walker WG. The syndrome of inappropriate antidiuretic hormone secretion (SIADH): pathophysiologic mechanisms in solute and volume regulation. Medicine 1979;58:240–251.
7. Desai TK, Carlson RW, Geheb MA. Hypocalcemia and hypophosphatemia in acutely ill patients. Crit Care Clin 1987;5:927.
8. Fassler CA, Rodriguez RM, Badesch DB, Stone WJ, Marini JJ. Magnesium toxicity as a cause of hypoventilation in patients with normal renal function. Arch Intern Med 1985;145:1604–1606.
9. Felig P, McCurdy DV. The hypertonic state. N Engl J Med 1977;297:1444–1454.
10. Geheb M, Carlson R, eds. Renal failure and associated disturbances (symposium). Crit Care Clin 1987;3(4): 699–955.
11. Kamel KS, Bear RA. Treatment of hyponatremia: a quantitative analysis. Am J Kid Dis 1993;21:439.
12. Kamel KS. Urine electrolytes and osmolality: when and how to use them. Am J Nephrol 1990;10:89–102.
13. Knocher JP. The pathophysiology and clinical characteristics of severe hypophosphatemia. Arch Intern Med 1977; 137:203–220.
14. Kruse JA, Carlson RW. Rapid correction of hypokalemia using concentrated intravenous chloride infusions. Arch Intern Med 1990;3:529.
15. Kunau RT, Stein JH. Disorders of hypo and hyperkalemia. Clin Nephrol 1977;7:173–190.
16. Laureno R, Arieff AI. Rapid correction of hyponatremia: cause of pontine myelinolysis? Am J Med 1981;71: 846–847.
17. List A. Malignancy hypercalcemia: choice of therapy. Arch Intern Med 1991;151:437.
18. Mettaurer B, Rouleau JL, Bichet D, et al. Sodium and water excretion abnormalities in congestive heart failure. Ann Intern Med 1988;105:161.
19. Newman JH, Neff TA, Ziponin P. Acute respiratory failure associated with hypophosphatemia. N Engl J Med 1977;296:1101–1102.
20. Oh MS, Carroll HJ. Disorders of sodium metabolism: hypernatremia and hyponatremia. Crit Care Med 1992;20:94.
21. Nolph KD, Schrirer RW. Sodium, potassium and water metabolism in the syndrome of inappropriate hormone secretion. Am J Med 1970;49:534.
22. Oster JR, Epstein M. Management of magnesium depletion. Am J Nephrol 1988;8:349.
23. Reinhart RA. Magnesium metabolism: a review with special reference to the relationship between intracellular content and calcium levels. Arch Intern Med 1988;148: 2415.
24. Rhyzen E, Wagers PW, Singer FR, Rude RK. Magnesium deficiency in a medical ICU population. Crit Care Med 1985;13:19.
25. Roswell RH. Severe hypercalcemia: causes and specific therapy. J Crit Illness 1987;2:14.
26. Schrier RW. Pathogenesis of sodium and water retention in high-output and low-output cardiac failure, nephrotic syndrome, cirrhosis and pregnancy. N Engl J Med 1988; 319:1065.
27. Singhal PC, Abramovici M, Venkatesan J, Mattana J, et al. Hypokalemia and rhabdomyolysis. Miner Electrolyte Metab 1991;17:335.
28. Smithline N, Gardner KD. Gaps-anionic and osmolal. JAMA 1976;236:1594–1597.
29. Solomon R. The relationship between disorders of K^+ and Mg^{+2} homeostasis. Semin Nephrol 1987;7:253.
30. Sterns RH. Severe hyponatremia: the case for conservative management. Crit Care Med 1992;2:534.
31. Sterns RH. Severe symptomatic hyponatremia: treatment and outcome. A study of 64 cases. Ann Intern Med 1987; 107:656.
32. Van Hook JW. Hypermagnesemia. Crit Care Clin 1991; 7:215.
33. Votey SR, Peters AL, Hoffman JR, et al. Disorders of water metabolism: hyponatremia and hypernatremia. Emerg Med Clin North Am 1989;7:749–769.
34. Whang R. Magnesium deficiency: pathogenesis, prevalence and clinical implications. Am J Med 1987;82:22.
35. Whang R, Flink EB, Dyckner T, et al. Magnesium depletion as a cause of refractory potassium repletion. Arch Intern Med 1985;145:1686.
36. Wrenn KD, Slovis CM, Slovis BS. The ability of physicians to predict hyperkalemia for the ECG. Ann Emerg Med 1991;20:1229.
37. Zaloga GP, Chernow B. Calcium and calcium channels: implications in intensive care. Crit Care Med 1989;10:79.

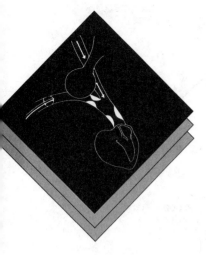

CHAPTER 14

Transfusion and Blood Component Therapy

INDICATIONS FOR BLOOD TRANSFUSION

There are three major reasons for administration of blood products: (*a*) to increase oxygen-carrying capacity; (*b*) to restore circulating volume; and (*c*) to reverse deficiencies of clotting proteins or platelets.

Tissue oxygen delivery can remain adequate in the face of anemia if reductions in hemoglobin are offset by proportional increases in tissue perfusion or oxygen extraction. Unfortunately, these compensatory mechanisms often are impaired in critically ill patients. For this reason, hemoglobin concentration generally is maintained above 10 g/dL (packed cell volume [PCV] > 30%). This level of oxygen-carrying capacity is especially important for patients with coronary or carotid occlusive disease, refractory hypoxemia, or limited cardiac reserve. Conversely, the lower acceptable limit for hemoglobin can be relaxed somewhat for patients with longstanding anemia and for those whose tissues and cardiac performance accommodate to chronically reduced O_2 delivery (e.g., chronic renal failure). However, even healthy patients rarely can sustain blood loss of 1–1.5 L without transfusion. Boosting PCV to levels above 40% produces diminishing returns in oxygen delivery. As the PCV rises, increases in viscosity eventually reduce overall oxygen delivery (Fig. 14.1).

DETERMINING THE SOURCE OF BLOOD LOSS

Each time a hematocrit is measured or clotting abnormality is considered, a more fundamental question must be asked: might this laboratory determination be in error? But, if the abnormality is real, where did the blood, clotting factors, or platelets go? With few exceptions, it is difficult to lose substantial quantities of red blood cells rapidly without external evidence of blood loss. In the intensive care unit (ICU), the most common sources of visible blood loss will be through the gastrointestinal tract or surgical and traumatic wounds. Because blood is a gastric irritant and cathartic, rarely will large quantities of blood be "concealed" in the gut for long. For stable patients with no "visible" site of blood loss, an acute decline in hematocrit of nine points or more (the equivalent of 3 units of red blood cells) should make the laboratory result suspect. The sudden development of apparent "pancytopenia" is likely to indicate that the blood sample for determination was drawn from an indwelling intravenous catheter and was diluted by infusate. Obviously, for unstable patients, simultaneous replacement of blood products should accompany a search for a source of bleeding.

When a true acute drop in PCV is not accompanied by obvious bleeding, alveolar hemorrhage, retroperitoneal or thigh (soft tissue) bleeding, and hemolysis should be suspected. Alveolar hemorrhage is most common in immunocompromised thrombocytopenic patients and is seen less commonly with Goodpasture's Disease, Wegener's granulomatosis, or systemic lupus. Retroperitoneal bleeding may occur spontaneously in patients with thrombocytopenia or soluble factor deficiencies but, more commonly, anticoagulation and trauma (including angiography or placement of

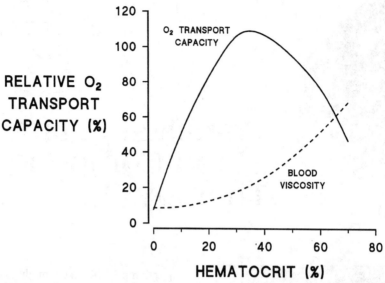

FIG. 14–1. Relationship between hematocrit, oxygen transport capacity, and serum viscosity. At low hematocrit values, oxygen transport capacity (solid line) is impaired because of anemia. Oxygen transport increases with a rising hematocrit, reaching a maximum value when hematocrit nears 35–40%. Transport capacity declines after this peak because of nonlinear increases in blood viscosity (broken line).

venacaval filters) are causes. Soft tissues of the thigh can clandestinely harbor large amounts of blood after femoral artery or vein puncture. Hemolysis may occur spontaneously but, in the ICU, is more commonly drug or transfusion induced.

When production of platelets is diminished but consumption is not excessive, platelet counts usually decline slowly over 3–5 days. Therefore, sudden (less than 1 day) decreases in circulating platelet counts usually are indicative of a consumptive process, often disseminated intravascular coagulation (DIC) or a drug-associated (heparin, penicillin) thrombocytopenia.

Similar to the situation with platelets, when production of soluble clotting factors is curtailed but consumption is not excessive, changes in the prothrombin and partial thromboplastic times occur over several days. Rapid development of a coagulopathy is most likely related to accelerated consumption of DIC, especially that caused by sepsis or resulting from dilution of clotting factors by massive transfusion.

BLOOD CONSERVATION

Many red blood cell transfusions performed in the ICU can be averted if the volume and frequency of blood drawing are minimized. The in-

sertion of central venous and arterial catheters can encourage blood sampling more frequently than clinically necessary. Whenever possible, alternative monitoring methods should be used to minimize the volume of blood removed from patients. Such techniques include bedside finger stick sampling of blood glucose and the use of pulse oximetry and capnography to determine arterial oxygen and carbon dioxide tensions, respectively. The emerging technology of bedside small-volume multichannel chemistry and blood gas analyzers will further reduce the volume of blood necessary for laboratory monitoring. Use of "cell savers" for trauma victims and for patients undergoing bloody surgical procedures is also prudent. Attention to these details during a protracted ICU stay reduces cost, the risk of transfusion complications, and the workload for nurses and laboratory personnel.

THE COMPONENT SYSTEM

Most patients needing transfusion do not require all of the components available in fresh whole blood (Table 14.1). Component therapy "stretches" the blood supply by allowing prolonged storage of stable factors and by permitting several patients to receive the specific compo-

TABLE 14–1

WHOLE BLOOD COMPONENTS

Erythrocytes
Factor VIII concentrate
Platelets
Factor IX concentrate
Fresh frozen plasma
Cryoprecipitate
Plasma protein fraction
Albumin
Leukocytes
Immunoglobulin
Antithrombin III

nents they need from a single blood donation. By limiting administered volume, component therapy also reduces the risk of fluid overload, the amount of transfused anticoagulant, and the risk of infection. When elective surgery necessitates transfusion, every effort should be made to use autologous blood or directed donations from low risk individuals.

RED BLOOD CELL COMPONENTS

Whole Blood

Whole blood is increasingly difficult to obtain and is of questionable advantage over use of individual components. Its use is often more based on emotional rather than rational arguments. Whole blood can be used in the emergent restoration of circulating volume and oxygen-carrying capacity, but it is a poor source of clotting factors and platelets if more than 24 hours old. (By that time, Factors V and VIII are present only in reduced amounts.) Furthermore, transfusion of whole blood may produce circulatory overload in the euvolemic patient who requires only red blood cells (RBCs). (The volume effects of whole blood are particularly risky for patients with renal failure or congestive heart failure.) A 500-mL "unit" of whole blood contains ~60 mEq of sodium and has a PCV averaging 35–40%. Whole blood also is more likely to contain microaggregates of leukocytes and platelets, which may be detrimental. The only major indication for whole blood is in support of massively bleeding patients in whom fresh whole blood is preferred. Even then, whole blood usually must be supplemented by transfusions of platelets, plasma, or plasma volume expanders.

"Fresh" Whole Blood

Fresh whole blood is less than 6–8 hours old and is useful for patients needing simultaneous replacement of circulating volume, red cells, platelets, and clotting factors. Platelets become nonfunctional within 24 hours of collection. After 48 hours, essentially all factor VIII is depleted. Within 1 week, even the longer-lived factor V is depleted. Furthermore, RBCs become less pliable and lyse as blood ages, reducing the PCV and increasing the plasma potassium concentration. (Thirty percent of RBCs may be lost after 3 weeks of storage.) Reductions in adenosine triphosphate (ATP) and diphosphoglyceric acid (2,3-DPG) produce a leftward shift of the oxyhemoglobin dissociation curve, inhibiting oxygen release to the tissues.

Fresh blood is used to prevent dilutional coagulopathy in massively transfused patients who require 10 or more units of whole blood within a 24-hour period. In actively hemorrhaging patients, repletion of clotting proteins and platelets with fresh whole blood or component therapy should begin after approximately 6–10 units of packed RBCs have been given.

Packed Red Blood Cells

Removing plasma from whole blood leaves a 200- to 300-mL unit of packed red blood cells (PRBCs) having a PCV of 65–75%. PRBCs are used to restore oxygen-carrying capacity. A unit of transfused PRBCs should raise the PCV of an adult patient by approximately 3%. (Continued bleeding or excessive volume expansion blunts the expected increase.) PRBCs contain few platelets, clotting factors, or leukocytes and are not effective as volume expanders when used alone. PRBCs can be infused as rapidly as whole blood when viscosity is reduced by adding ~75 mL of normal saline per unit.

PRBCs offer several advantages: (*a*) less volume expansion than whole blood for a given increase in oxygen-carrying capacity (each unit of PRBCs contains only 8–20 mEq of sodium, a particularly helpful feature for patients with heart or kidney failure); (*b*) less anticoagulant than whole blood, reducing the potential risk of anticoagulant-preservative (citrate) toxicity; and (*c*) lower plasma volume, reducing the risk of viral hepatitis, immunologic reactions from transfused antibodies, and anaphylaxis.

Leukocyte-Poor Components

Leukocyte-poor components are indicated for patients who have experienced white cell or leukoagglutinin reactions and are particularly useful for patients with anti-IgA or IgE antibodies. Leukocyte-poor red blood cells are produced by removing the leukocyte-rich buffy coat by repeated washing, spin filtering, or freezing. Each method destroys platelets while reducing the white blood cells (WBCs) and plasma by approximately 75–90%. Because of the loss of RBCs in processing, a unit of leukocyte-poor RBCs contains less hemoglobin than a unit of PRBCs. Even leukocyte-poor RBCs contain limited numbers of viable WBCs; therefore, blood products transfused into immunosuppressed patients must be irradiated to prevent graft-versus-host disease (GVHD).

WHITE BLOOD CELL COMPONENTS

Granulocyte Transfusions

Granulocyte transfusions are indicated only for neutropenic patients with overwhelming infections who fail conventional antimicrobial therapy. Because of the risk, expense, and limited benefit of granulocyte transfusions, they are rarely used.

Many problems exist in the transfusion of WBCs. Allergic reactions are nearly universal and, because WBCs have a circulating half-life of only 6 hours, frequent transfusion is required. WBCs also must be ABO-compatible. Several types of hepatitis commonly are transmitted in WBC components. For patients with severe bone marrow depression, WBC transfusion also carries a nearly certain risk of GVHD. WBCs often aggregate, a tendency that precludes the use of transfusion filters and frequently leads to pulmonary dysfunction. No laboratory measure of effectiveness exists because peripheral WBC counts usually do not rise for most patients receiving WBCs (presumably secondary to sequestration and consumption). Concurrent administration of WBCs and amphotericin B may cause acute respiratory distress syndrome (ARDS).

PLATELET COMPONENTS

Random Donor Platelets

The risk of thrombocytopenia-associated hemorrhage increases as functional platelet concentrations decline. The risks of bleeding are amplified at any given platelet concentration by concomitant abnormalities in humoral clotting factors and vascular damage. Commonly used platelet counts to guide the need for transfusion are illustrated in Table 14.2. Platelet counts of $>100,000/mm^3$ rarely are associated with significant bleeding, even for trauma or surgical patients. Therefore, it is uncommon to provide platelet transfusions to such patients unless they are actively bleeding. Functional platelet counts $>50,000/mm^3$ usually are sufficient to provide hemostasis for patients undergoing invasive procedures, and such levels rarely permit spontaneous hemorrhage. Platelet counts $<20,000/mm^3$ are associated with spontaneous hemorrhage (especially if counts fall below $5,000/mm^3$). Therefore, platelet transfusions sometimes are performed for counts of $20,000–50,000/mm^3$, are often undertaken with platelet counts $5,000–20,000/mm^3$, and almost always are tried when counts fall below $5,000/mm^3$. For patients with ongoing hemorrhage and for those scheduled to undergo invasive procedures, higher platelet counts are desirable.

Regardless of number, platelet transfusions often are undertaken for therapy of platelet dysfunction. Uremia, liver disease, and nonsteroidal anti-inflammatory drugs are the most common reasons for platelet dysfunction.

A unit of pooled random donor platelets (RDPs) contains 40–70 mL of platelet concentrate and large numbers of WBCs that may be removed by spin filtration. For each 5–6 units of transfused RPDs, patients receive roughly the equivalent of 1 unit of plasma. The usefulness of RDPs is limited by many factors: (a) repeatedly transfused patients develop antibodies to common platelet surface antigens and eventually require human lymphocyte antigen (HLA)-matched platelets to prevent rapid immune destruction of the transfused platelets; (b) platelets often produce minor allergic reactions, including chills, fever, and rash; (c) WBCs contained in platelet transfusions may produce GVHD in the pancytopenic patient; (d) platelet transfusions are unlikely to be helpful for "immune thrombocytopenias" (idiopathic thrombocytopenic purpura [ITP] or thrombotic thrombocytopenic purpura [TTP]) because of rapid platelet destruction. In such cases, corticosteroids and intravenous immunoglobulin preparations may extend the circulating half-life of transfused platelets.

Platelets may be administered as rapidly as they will infuse (5–10 minutes/unit). The normal life span of circulating platelets is 3–4 days; therefore,

TABLE 14–2

PLATELET TRANSFUSION GUIDELINES

Platelet Count (Number/mm^3)	Risk of Spontaneous Bleeding	Platelet Transfusion Given?
<5,000	High	Almost always
5,000–20,000	Moderate to high	Usually given to boost counts >20,000
20,000–50,000	Moderate to low	Occasionally. More likely if soluble factors are abnormal or invasive intervention is planned.
50,000–100,000	Low	Transfused only if patient is actively bleeding, an invasive procedure is planned, or a second coagulation abnormally is present.
>100,000	Low	Rare unless platelets are dysfunctional, soluble factors are abnormal, or invasive procedures are planned.

platelet transfusions usually are needed every 2–3 days if production is reduced without accelerated destruction. Each unit increases the count by 5,000–10,000 platelets/mm^3, unless destruction is ongoing. When assessed 1 hour after transfusion, an increment of <2,000/mm^3 per unit confirms platelet destruction. Platelets usually are administered as "six packs," which raise the platelet count by ~25–50,000 platelets/mm^3. A blunted increment is common for patients with burns, splenic sequestration, fever, infection, and/or platelet antibodies. Because young (large) platelets have enhanced hemostatic function, the presence of many large platelets may indicate a lower risk of bleeding at any given total count.

ABO-compatible platelets minimize formation of antiplatelet antibodies and survive longer in the circulation. Because of the very small volume of plasma present in transfused platelets, incompatibility between donor plasma and recipient RBCs usually is insignificant. However, if multiple units of platelets and incompatible plasma are transfused, a positive Coombs' test or overt hemolysis may occur. The small number of RBCs transfused in platelet concentrates makes RBC cross-matching unnecessary. (However, 10% of massively transfused patients will develop ABO sensitization.) Platelets do not contain Rh antigens, and therefore, Rh sensitization is not a problem. Although platelets should be administered through a filter to prevent aggregation, filtration lengthens infusion time and decreases the number of viable platelets transfused.

Single-Donor Platelets

For patients refractory to RDPs, single donors may be pheresed as often as two or three times weekly to provide large numbers of platelets for transfusion. Administration of these pheresed concentrates commonly produces a rise of 30–60,000 platelets/mm^3. Single-donor pheresed platelets often, at least transiently, raise platelet counts even if not HLA matched. For patients failing to respond to RDP or single-donor pheresed platelets, HLA-matched pheresed platelets usually will boost platelet counts. The effective survival of HLA-matched platelets can be nearly normal if used for patients alloimmunized to platelet antigens in random donors, but if accelerated destruction is caused by non-HLA antigen mechanisms (e.g., DIC), HLA-matched platelets will not offer a substantial advantage over RDPs. Single-donor platelets have the advantage of reducing transfusion-related infection risk.

CLOTTING FACTOR CONCENTRATES AND PLASMA PRODUCTS

Fresh Frozen Plasma

Fresh frozen plasma (FFP) contains fibrinogen; clotting factors II, V, VII, VIII, IX, X, XI, XIII; and von Willebrand's factor. Factors V and VIII and fibrinogen are present in the highest functional concentrations. A unit of FFP contains 180–300 mL of plasma. Indications for transfusing FFP include the following: (a) dilutional coagulopathy for the massively transfused patient; (b) excessive anticoagulation with warfarin; (c) congenital or acquired coagulation factor deficiencies; and (d) von Willebrand's disease. FFP should not be used primarily for intravascular volume expansion because less costly, equally effective alternatives exist. In addition, FFP carries a real risk of allergic and infectious complications.

FFP usually is used to replete deficiencies of multiple factors, and dosing commonly is guided by the degree of prothrombin time (PT) or partial thromboplastic time (PTT) prolongation. When used to replete a single missing factor, administration usually is reserved for factor levels below 25% of normal. (When possible, use of specific factor concentrates are preferred to FFP.) PTs less than 18 seconds and PTTs below 55 seconds usually are not treated unless patients are actively bleeding. For cases in which hemorrhage is ongoing, the endpoint of FFP administration usually is "normalization" of the PT and PTT. PTs greater than 18 seconds and PTT greater than 55 seconds often are treated with 2 units of FFP initially before reassessment of in vitro clotting times, even for patients who are not currently bleeding.

FFP has several disadvantages: (a) each milliliter of transfused plasma contains only 1 unit of each clotting factor (therefore, relatively large volumes of FFP are needed to correct deficiencies compared to factor concentrates); (b) the risk of allergic reactions is high due to residual platelets and leukocytes; (c) although FFP need not be ABO compatible with recipient plasma, it should be compatible with the recipient's RBCs.

Cryoprecipitate

Cryoprecipitate forms when plasma separated from fresh whole blood is rapidly frozen and then allowed to rewarm. The precipitate contains most of the factor VIII (about 80–100 units), fibrinogen (250 mg), and 40–60% of the von Willebrand's factor present in the original unit of plasma. Cryoprecipitate may be used to treat: (a) hypofibrinogenemic states (e.g., thrombolytic therapy, congenital deficiency, and consumptive coagulopathy); (b) hemophilia A (factor VIII deficiency); and (c) von Willebrand's disease.

In hypofibrinogenemic states, one bag of cryoprecipitate/5 kg of body weight is a usual dose. When used for von Willebrand's disease, one bag/10 kg is usually adequate. Because infection risk is now minimized by product formulation, factor VIII concentrates are favored over cryoprecipitate for the treatment of von Willebrand's disease and hemophilia A.

Factor VIII Concentrate

Factor VIII concentrate, a component used in the treatment of hemophilia A, is prepared from the plasma of many donors (frequently hundreds). For the bleeding hemophiliac, factor VIII activity

TABLE 14–3

CALCULATION OF FACTOR VIII DOSES

Blood volume (mL) = wt in kg × 70

Plasma volume (mL) = blood volume × (1 − PCV fraction)

Units of factor VIII = plasma volume × (desired factor VIII % − current factor VIII %)

is negligible and should be increased to >50% of normal levels to arrest hemorrhage. The dose of factor VIII may be calculated by replacing 1 unit of factor VIII per milliliter of calculated plasma volume per percent of desired factor VIII activity (Table 14.3). Alternatively, the factor VIII requirement may be roughly approximated:

$$\text{Dose (units)} = 40 \times (\text{wt in kg}) \times (\%\text{factor VIII activity desired}).$$

Because administered factor VIII has a half-life of only 8–12 hours, close monitoring of clinical signs of bleeding and factor VIII level is necessary. Historically, factor VIII concentrates have carried a much higher risk of viral infections than cryoprecipitate; however, institution of heat treatment and serologic testing have reduced the risk of hepatitis and acquired immune deficiency syndrome (AIDS).

Antithrombin III Supplements

Antithrombin III (AT III) concentrate recently has become available for treatment of congenital AT III deficiency and represents a preferable alternative to the use of large volumes of fresh frozen plasma. The role of this drug in acquired AT III deficiency states (especially sepsis) is under investigation.

Intravenous Immunoglobulin

Intravenous immunoglobulin (IVIG), a pooled immunoglobulin fraction from multiple donors, is useful in three basic situations: (a) replacement therapy of humoral immune deficiency states such as congenital agammaglobulinemia and chronic lymphocytic leukemia; (b) control of selected infections such as neonatal group B streptococcal disease, disseminated cytomegalovirus infection in transplant recipients, and *Pseudomonas* infections in burn victims; (c) treatment of ITP, TTP, and refractory thrombocytopenia due to repeated platelet transfusions. IVIG is not without risk—patients with immunoglobulin A deficiency may develop anaphylactic reactions from preformed anti-IgA antibodies, and antibody aggregates in IVIG may cause other allergic reactions. IVIG preparations also may transmit infections such as non-A and non-B hepatitis; however, the risk of human immunodeficiency virus (HIV) is low.

PROBLEMS ASSOCIATED WITH MASSIVE TRANSFUSION

EXSANGUINATION AND CROSS MATCHING

A formal cross-match procedure requires 45–60 minutes. Therefore, when the patient's condition does not allow completion of a formal cross-match, O-negative (universal donor) or type-specific (ABO- and Rh-compatible) blood may be given. The small amount of plasma in O-negative blood often contains antibodies to the recipient's red blood cells and can provoke "minor" transfusion reactions. ABO determination alone usually takes less than 10 minutes. Therefore, type-specific blood is preferred, except in cases in which transfusion must occur even more urgently.

MASSIVE TRANSFUSION

The rate at which blood products can be administered is proportional to the driving pressure for delivery and the fourth power of the i.v. catheter radius and is inversely proportional to the length of the i.v. catheter and viscosity of the fluid to be infused. Therefore, using multiple, rapidly inserted (usually peripheral), short, large-bore i.v. catheters usually will be more efficient than smaller, longer, centrally placed catheters, except when large-bore "introducer" sheaths are already in place. Obviously, flow rates will be augmented by increasing the driving pressure for delivery through use of pressure bags. Fluid viscosity is rarely a limiting factor, except when transfusing cold packed red blood cells. The viscosity can be dramatically reduced by warming the blood or by adding 100–200 mL of sterile isotonic saline to the PRBCs before infusion.

Massive transfusion usually is defined as the administration of >10 units of blood per 24 hours. Problems resulting from massive transfusion include: (a) dilutional thrombocytopenia and coagulopathy; (b) acute respiratory distress syndrome (ARDS); (c) hypokalemic alkalosis as HCO_3^- is generated from transfused citrate; (d) hypocalcemia; (e) hypothermia; and (f) transfusion-related infection. The risk of viral hepatitis approximates 1% per unit of transfused blood product even after institution of testing for hepatitis B.

Dilutional clotting disorders begin to emerge when one blood volume equivalent (5 units of blood) has been replaced. Clotting factor levels then commonly drop below 30% of normal activity, and platelet counts fall below 100,000/mm³. After 5–10 units of blood have been transfused, platelet counts, prothrombin time, and partial thromboplastin time should be monitored. To maintain a normal clotting profile, 2 units of FFP and 6 units of platelets should be transfused per 6–10 units of PRBCs.

ARDS may result from hemorrhage-related hypotension in conjunction with the transfusion of component microaggregates. Although it is not certain that blood filters reduce this risk, they probably should be used during massive transfusion. Even during massive transfusion, the incidence of citrate-induced hypocalcemia is very low; although it is prudent to monitor calcium levels, replacement is rarely necessary.

COMPLICATIONS OF TRANSFUSION

IMMEDIATE HEMOLYTIC REACTIONS

Hemolytic reactions can be immediate or delayed. If immediate, they usually are due to major ABO incompatibility. The most common cause of major transfusion reaction is misidentification of the patient sample or transfusion of blood into the wrong patient. These mistakes essentially are always due to clerical errors and usually occur at the bedside. As a result, stringent rules have been instituted in most hospitals to prevent these occurrences. When notified by the blood bank that an improperly labeled tube has been received, repeat sample collection is indicated.

Most severe reactions occur as the first 50–100 mL of blood product are infused. For this reason, frequent vital signs should be taken in the initial period of transfusion. Major reactions are potentially fatal because they produce intravascular hemolysis, coagulopathy, shock, renal failure, and pulmonary dysfunction. Transfusion reactions may be difficult to recognize, particularly in the unconscious critically ill patient. New-onset dyspnea, fever, bone pain, or diffuse bleeding are all clues to transfusion reaction. Primary treatment of a major reaction is to stop the transfusion. Using sterile technique, donor blood and blood tubing should be returned to the blood bank. Clotted and anticoagulated samples of the recipient's blood and a urine sample also should be sent to the blood bank with notification of a suspected transfusion reaction. Fluids and vasopressors should be administered as required to maintain perfusion of vital organs. Intravenous sodium bicarbonate may be given to alkalinize the urine, in an effort to prevent precipitation of hemoglobin in the renal tubules and subsequent acute renal failure. Loop and osmotic diuretics also may be useful to preserve urine flow and avert renal failure.

DELAYED HEMOLYTIC REACTIONS

Low titer antibodies (often undetectable by Coombs' test) can cause delayed hemolysis in multiply transfused or multiparous patients. RBC transfusion recalls an immune response that produces IgG antibodies directed against donor cells. During the subsequent 10–14 days, the direct Coombs' test becomes positive and transfused RBCs are lysed. This problem usually presents as a sudden (but often asymptomatic) drop in the PCV about 2 weeks after transfusion. Although usually benign, falling hematocrit and rising bilirubin levels in a postoperative patient often raise concerns of hepatic failure or occult bleeding.

OTHER CAUSES OF HEMOLYSIS

Blood always should be administered through a needle larger than 19 gauge to prevent mechanical shredding of RBCs. Heating above 38°C or freezing will also cause hemolysis. Normal saline is the only suitable solution for the transfusion of RBCs. Solutions containing calcium (e.g., Ringer's lactate) lead to clumping, and iso-osmotic glucose solutions (D5W) may produce cell lysis and aggregation.

INFECTIONS

Bacterial infections transmitted through transfused blood are most frequently caused by breaches in sterile technique at the time of the transfusion and prolonged infusion time. *Listeria monocytogenes* is capable of growing at the usual storage temperature of blood and may cause transfusion-related bacteremia.

Because of the large number of donors required for their preparation, the risk of infection, in the past, has been greatest from pooled blood products (e.g., factor VIII concentrate and activated factor complexes). Viral infections occur in up to 10% of all transfused patients and include cytomegalovirus (CMV), hepatitis B, and non-A and non-B hepatitis. Because of donor testing, the risk of acquiring hepatitis B is less than 1 in 200,000 whereas risks of hepatitis C infection remain substantial, at approximately 1 in 3,000. Up to 50% of the general population demonstrates serologic evidence of prior CMV infection; therefore, the high rate of transfusion-related CMV infection is not surprising. Other infections transmitted via blood include malaria, syphilis, brucellosis, toxoplasmosis, and Epstein-Barr virus.

Depending on the region of the country, screening tests for HIV have lowered the risk of transfusion-acquired AIDS infection to between 1 in 50,000 and 1 in 500,000 for each unit of transfused blood component.

OTHER RISKS OF TRANSFUSION

Febrile, nonhemolytic transfusion reactions may occur due to surface antigens on WBCs or platelets and represent the most common cause of transfusion-related fever. For patients with previous febrile reactions, the use of leukocyte-poor RBCs and HLA-matched components reduce the risk.

Allergic reactions range from urticaria to anaphylaxis and usually occur in IgA-deficient patients with preformed IgG antibodies directed against IgA in the donor blood. Stopping the transfusion and administering antihistamines usually are sufficient to abort the reaction. Full-blown anaphylaxis should be treated with intravenous epinephrine and volume expansion. Inhaled β-adrenergic agonists and theophylline may moderate bronchospasm. Despite widespread use of diphenhydramine and corticosteroids, their effectiveness is uncertain.

RBCs, WBCs, platelets, and cryoprecipitate all should be administered through standard blood filters to prevent transfusing aggregates of these components. All filters reduce the maximal infusion rate and should be changed after every 2–4 units because of filter plugging.

Hyperkalemia may occur in massively transfused patients given PRBCs stored for long periods of time (especially patients with renal dysfunction). Potassium concentration in the transfused plasma may rise as high as 20 mEq/L in PRBCs stored longer than 3 weeks. Hyperkalemia may be prevented by using "fresh" whole blood or by using RBC products containing little plasma, such as washed or packed RBCs.

Systemic hypothermia has numerous adverse effects (see Chapter 28), but fortunately, hypothermia rarely is seen outside the setting of massive transfusion. Blood warming has not been shown clearly to be beneficial but is reasonable with (*a*) massive transfusion, (*b*) transfusion rates exceeding 50 mL/minute, or (*c*) cold agglutinin disease. Caution should be used because RBCs may hemolyze if heated above 38°C.

Citrate-induced hypocalcemia has been touted as a problem for massively transfused patients but is a rare event even in these patients. Prophylactic administration of calcium is not recommended, but if patients exhibit signs of hypocalcemia, determination of ionized calcium is warranted.

Because citrate is used to anticoagulate most blood components, alkalemia may develop as the liver converts citrate to bicarbonate. Patients with normal liver function are able to metabolize massive amounts of citrate (up to 20 units of PRBCs per hour). Therefore, metabolic alkalosis of citrate infusion usually is clinically insignificant and self-correcting.

BLOOD SUBSTITUTES

Extracted, purified, and stabilized hemoglobin and genetically engineered hemoglobin solutions are being investigated as blood substitutes but are not ready for clinical use. In the past, hemoglobin solutions have carried substantial risk of renal tubular damage. Newer products have surmounted this problem. Limited application of oxygen-carrying perfluorochemical solutions in coronary reperfusion has shown promise, but there is no evidence supporting the safe and effective systemic use of these solutions.

KEY POINTS

1. Many blood transfusions can be avoided if careful thought is given to blood conservation measures, including limiting laboratory determinations to only those necessary.

2. Use of blood components effectively targets specific patient deficiencies and is a much more efficient use of the limited blood supply than use of "whole" blood.

3. Reasonable target levels are 30–40% for hematocrit and 50,000/mm^3 for platelets. Higher levels may be appropriate for patients actively bleeding or those at particularly high risk from anemia or hemorrhage.

4. Massive transfusion of the actively bleeding patient should be guided by frequent measurements of PCV, coagulation parameters, and platelet counts. An empiric ratio of 6 units of packed cells to 2 units of fresh frozen plasma to 6 units of platelets is a good starting plan for transfusion.

5. Despite many safeguards, transfusion still has a substantial risk of transmitting infection or causing an allergic reaction.

SUGGESTED READINGS

1. American Red Cross. Circular of information for the use of human blood and blood components. ARC Publication No. 1751. American Red Cross, 1984.
2. Berkman SA, Lee ML, Gale RP. Clinical uses of intravenous immunoglobulin. Ann Intern Med 1990;112: 278–292.
3. Boral LI. Platelet transfusion therapy. Lab Med 1985; 16(4):221–227.
4. Collins JA. Recent developments in the area of massive transfusion. World J Surg 1987;11:75–81.
5. Consensus Conference. Fresh-frozen plasma. Indications and risks. JAMA 1985;253(4):551–553.
6. Greenwalt TJ. Pathogenesis and management of hemolytic transfusion reactions. Semin Hematol 1981;18(2): 84–121.
7. Hewson JR, Neame PB, Kumar N, et al. Coagulopathy related to dilution and hypotension during massive transfusion. Crit Care Med 1985;13:387–391.
8. Insalaco SJ. Massive transfusion. Lab Med 1984;15(5): 325–330.
9. Isbister JP. Blood component therapy in the critically ill. In: Vincent JL, ed. Update in intensive care and emergency medicine. Berlin: Springer-Verlag, 1989; 411–422.

10. Menache D, Grossman BJ, Jackson CM. Antithrombin III: physiology, deficiency, and replacement therapy. Transfusion 1992;32:580–588.
11. Rosenberg RD. Role of antithrombin III in coagulation disorders: state of the art review. Am J Med 1989; 87(Suppl 3B):1S–67S.
12. Rudowski WJ. Evaluation of modern plasma expanders and blood substitutes. Br J Hosp Med 1980;23:389–397.
13. Solanki D, McCurdy PR. Delayed hemolytic transfusion reactions. An often-missed entity. JAMA 1978;239(8): 729–731.
14. Taylor BL, Collins C. The management of massive hemorrhage. Br J Hosp Med 1988;40:104–110.
15. Thompson AR, Harker LA. Manual of hemostasis and thrombosis. 3rd ed. Philadelphia: FA Davis Co., 1983.

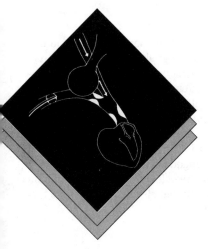

CHAPTER 15

Medication Administration

BASIC PHARMACOKINETICS

Although many physicians have little enthusiasm for studying pharmacokinetics (the science of drug absorption, distribution, and clearance) or pharmacodynamics (the practical application of pharmacokinetics to the patient), understanding these concepts is essential to providing quality critical care. For the critically ill patient, drug absorption is altered: pharmacologic agents often have abnormal distribution patterns, and impaired or accelerated drug clearance is common. Ignorance of such alterations predisposes patients to side effects, adverse drug interactions, and the potential for ineffective therapy. Four major concepts are key to understanding drug dosing: bioavailability, volume of distribution (V_d), clearance, and half-life ($t_{1/2}$).

BIOAVAILABILITY

When a drug is administered intravenously, the entire dose is made available to body tissues. All other routes of administration reduce bioavailability, i.e., the fraction of unmetabolized drug reaching the circulation, compared to the total dose given. For enterally administered drugs, impaired absorption and hepatic metabolism are the most important determinants of bioavailability. The severely ill patient often has reduced peristalsis and gut blood flow, which both alter absorption. Furthermore, many enterally administered drugs have reduced bioavailability because splanchnic blood flows first through the liver (possibly the major ultimate drug-clearing organ) en route to the systemic circulation. Severe liver damage commonly increases available concentrations of orally administered medications because of hepatocellular dysfunction and portal-to-systemic shunts (particularly in cirrhosis). Administration of some medications like fentanyl transcutaneously avoids the hepatic first pass effect, allowing much lower analgesic doses to be effective.

Dose, concentration, route of administration, solubility, rate of dissolution, absorptive area, gastrointestinal motility, and drug–drug interactions all influence bioavailability. Problems of altered bioavailability abound in the intensive care unit (ICU). For example, some drugs, (e.g., ketoconazole, tetracycline, sucralfate) require an acidic gastric environment for absorption or effect. Therefore, concurrent use of histamine blocking agents or antacids can significantly reduce bioavailability. The formation of inactivated drug complexes is also very common among patients receiving antacids, activated charcoal, or bile-acid-binding drugs. Although all the drugs in which absorption is limited by these agents is too long to list, warfarin, theophylline, digoxin, n-acetylcysteine, isoniazid, tetracycline, valproate, phenobarbital, carbamazepine, and phenytoin exhibit impaired absorption.

Alterations in gastrointestinal motility have unpredictable effects on drug absorption. For example, the increased motility induced by metoclopramide increases the absorption of acetaminophen and lithium but decreases the absorption of cimetidine and digoxin. Circulation to the site of drug deposition (intramuscular or subcutaneous injections) or to the gut mucosa (enteral route) also affects absorption and bioavailability, which is a key consideration in states of hypoperfusion. After absorption, bioavailability can be increased by certain drug interactions. For most drugs, the free or nonprotein-bound form of the drug is the active moiety. Therefore, coadministration of any two highly protein bound drugs can result in enhanced activity of one or both compounds. Common examples include the potentiated effects of warfarin, diazepam, phenytoin and tolbutamide by salicylates.

VOLUME OF DISTRIBUTION

Drugs distribute unevenly among the intracellular and extracellular compartments, in accordance with serum protein binding, cardiac output, vascular permeability, and tissue solubility. The V_d relates the total amount of drug in the body to its plasma concentration. Knowledge of V_d is most useful in determining loading doses of drugs, particularly those that distribute in multiple compartments (such as lidocaine). Distribution effects may account for such phenomena as ultrarapid buildup and termination of drug effects and prolongation of drug action with repeated dosing (e.g., narcotics). The critically ill patient often has an abnormally large volume of distribution for hydrophilic drugs because of the accumulation of large amounts of extracellular water. This large "compartment" can require a massive loading dose of medication initially to become saturated. Later in the course, this same reservoir of drug must be metabolized to fully terminate a drug's effect. This alteration can explain why it can be difficult to achieve a drug effect at first but that same effect can be prolonged in duration.

CLEARANCE

In simplest terms, clearance reflects the rate at which drug is eliminated from the circulation. Drug clearance may occur either through chemical conversion and subsequent excretion of metabolites or through excretion of unchanged drug. Although other tissues may participate, the liver is the central site of most drug metabolism. Hepatic metabolites are secreted into bile and are then either eliminated directly in the stool or, alternatively, reabsorbed across the gut wall, assimilated into the bloodstream, and eliminated by the kidney. Because the liver is the most common site of metabolism, the administration of one hepatically metabolized drug can adversely affect bioavail-

ability or clearance of another. The most common examples involve drugs that rev-up hepatic metabolism (e.g., phenobarbital, phenytoin, rifampin, ethanol), thereby accelerating the clearance of other hepatically metabolized drugs (e.g., oral contraceptives, warfarin, phenytoin, theophylline, glucocorticoids). Occasionally, drug-induced enhanced bioavailability or reduced clearance can be used to therapeutic advantage. For example, administration of even low doses of some calcium channel antagonists can elevate cyclosporine levels dramatically.

HALF-LIFE

After administration, most drugs exhibit a two-phase concentration profile corresponding to distribution and elimination. The serum half-life ($t_{1/2}$) is the time required for drug concentration to decrease by 50% without further supplementation. The $t_{1/2}$ incorporates distribution and clearance effects to give a useful index for predicting the time required to achieve steady-state concentration and determine dosing interval. With repeated intermittent dosing, most drugs accumulate and wash out exponentially to their final concentrations (first-order kinetics). Usually, five half-lives are required before drugs administered in constant dosage achieve a steady-state concentration—a delay that may compromise treatment. Therapeutic drug levels may be achieved more rapidly by the use of loading doses, but loading doses will not shorten the time to reach the steady state. Drug level monitoring before five half-lives have elapsed will underestimate the eventual steady-state peak and trough concentrations (see Fig. 15.1). Unfortunately, the half-lives of drugs are determined in relatively healthy individuals and seldom reflect the kinetics in the critically ill patient. Commonly, chronic dosing and dysfunction of several organ systems leads to a prolonged half-life. In fact, the practitioner should be wary of a claim of a "short half-life" for any drug administered repeatedly to ICU patients. Examples include the "expanding" half-life seen with chronic midazolam or fentanyl infusions. Furthermore, the plasma half-life may not accurately portray the duration of biologic effect: if a drug is highly tissue bound, prolonged effects can be observed, even when plasma drug levels approach zero.

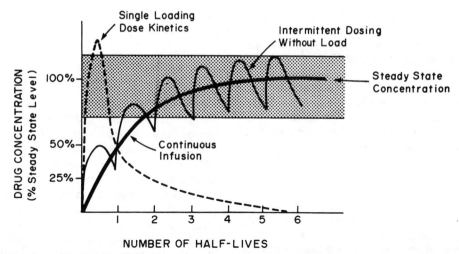

FIG. 15–1. Dosing and elimination kinetics. After a single dose, drug concentration falls exponentially to undetectable levels after more than five half-lives (dashed line). During continuous infusion or intermittent administration of smaller maintenance doses (without load), a steady-state concentration is not achieved until five half-lives have elapsed (solid line). The therapeutic range can be achieved and maintained quickly by combining a large initial loading dose with a maintenance schedule of either type.

PHARMACOKINETICS IN DISEASE

To a greater or lesser extent, the dysfunction of each major organ system alters the distribution, metabolism, and clearance of medications. Specific organ system failures and their effects on drug metabolism are discussed below.

CIRCULATORY FAILURE

In circulatory failure, blood flow is diverted from the skin, splanchnic bed, and muscle to maintain cerebral perfusion. Depressed cardiac output impairs drug absorption from subcutaneous, intramuscular, and gastrointestinal sites. Although intravenous dosing averts the problem of absorption, the smaller V_d often results in high blood levels immediately after injection. For example, usual doses of lidocaine commonly cause central nervous system (CNS) toxicity after bolus injection. Circulatory failure compromises the clearance of many drugs by diminishing renal function and hepatic metabolism. Reduced clearance increases the steady-state drug level for any given dosage and prolongs the time required to reach equilibrium. These two facts help explain why circulatory failure frequently results in the delayed expression of toxicity of slowly accumulating drugs like lidocaine, quinidine, and theophylline.

HEPATIC FAILURE

As the primary organ of drug metabolism and serum protein formation, the liver plays a key role in pharmacokinetics. Hepatic failure depresses the synthesis of albumin and other serum proteins, causing the total serum levels of highly protein-bound drugs to fall. On the other hand, serum concentrations of free drug may be normal or increased. (Phenytoin is a classic example.) Reduced liver blood flow impairs hepatic drug clearance. Specifically, portosystemic shunts (as in cirrhosis) decrease "first pass" metabolism, thereby increasing bioavailability. Unstable patients with vacillating hepatic blood flow or parenchymal function can be difficult to manage with medications subject to extensive first-pass metabolism (e.g., diltiazem, morphine, nifedipine, propranolol). To avoid the vagaries of fluctuating liver function, it is often useful to use renally metabolized and excreted drugs for patients with impaired hepatic function. (For example, oxacillin is a logical substitute for nafcillin, and pancuronium is a reasonable replacement for vecuronium.) As a rule for the ICU, the half-life of a chosen drug should parallel the duration of the desired effect.

Biliary obstruction impairs the ability of the liver to concentrate drugs (particularly antibiotics) in the bile. Even drugs that normally enter the bile (e.g., ampicillin) fail to do so in the setting of complete biliary obstruction. Drug therapy may cause artifactual elevations in liver-related laboratory tests; tetracycline and intravenous lipid preparations may elevate reported values of serum bilirubin, and hydroxy ethyl starch may spuriously elevate serum amylase. Metronidazole and para-aminosalicylic acid cause artifactual elevations in serum glutamic-oxaloacetic transaminase (SGOT).

RENAL FAILURE

For many drugs (e.g., aminoglycosides, acyclovir, cyclosporine), dosages must be modified to prevent accumulation of the parent drug or its metabolites. Often, a nonrenally excreted compound may be substituted successfully for one dependent upon the kidney for removal (e.g., quinolones for aminoglycosides). Renal failure is accompanied frequently by reduced albumin concentration and diminished protein binding. As in hepatic failure, these changes may result in low total serum drug concentrations but normal free drug levels. The clearance of most renally excreted drugs is proportional to the glomerular filtration rate (GFR), which in turn parallels creatinine clearance. At steady state, drug dose (as a percentage of normal) can be calculated by estimating creatinine clearance, expressed as a percentage of the normal value (see Chapter 29, Acute Renal Failure). Cefoxitin and flucytosine can produce artifactual elevations of creatinine levels.

LUNG DISEASE

Although lung disease very rarely affects drug metabolism (one exception may be prostacyclin infusions), cor pulmonale, positive pressure ventilation, and positive end-expiratory pressure may reduce hepatic and renal blood flow, predisposing to drug toxicity.

BURNS

Beginning immediately after injury in burn patients, fluid is translocated from the intravascular to the extravascular space, changing V_d and reducing renal and hepatic blood flows. Later (more than 1 week after injury), the GFR and metabolic rate accelerate and the concentrations of serum albumin and protein-bound drugs decline. Consequently, larger doses of many drugs (e.g., cimeti-

dine, aminoglycosides) are needed to achieve therapeutic levels.

ACID–BASE DISORDERS

Acid–base status plays a significant role in the absorption, distribution, and elimination of drugs. Ionized drugs traverse cell membranes poorly. Systemic acidosis inhibits the ionization of weak acids (e.g., salicylates, phenobarbital), thereby promoting their translocation to target tissues. For similar reasons, weak bases (e.g., amphetamines, quinidine) enter cells more readily under alkalemic conditions. These same acid–base properties can be used to bolster drug excretion. Urinary alkalinization traps weak acids in the urine, increasing the renal excretion of salicylates and phenobarbital, whereas acidosis promotes excretion of amphetamines, quinidine, and phencyclidine (PCP). pH also affects the binding of certain drugs to serum proteins. Therefore, manipulation of acid–base status can rapidly influence drug activity—a principle that should be kept in mind during crisis intervention. (One example is the use of bicarbonate to sequester free tricyclic antidepressant in protein complexes in the treatment of overdose.)

GOALS OF DRUG ADMINISTRATION

The aim of drug therapy is to rapidly achieve and maintain effective and nontoxic tissue drug concentrations. For critically ill patients, these goals are met by combining appropriate loading and maintenance regimens. During intermittent dosing, drug levels may demonstrate peaks and troughs that potentially expose patients to toxicity and subtherapeutic levels (Fig. 15.1).

In an attempt to avoid these fluctuations, many drugs used in the ICU are infused at a constant rate. Unfortunately, even constant infusions do not guarantee constant drug levels. Highly lipid-soluble drugs, drugs with long half-lives, and those with a large V_d may accumulate for long periods of time before toxic side effects emerge. Deterioration of renal or hepatic function may impair drug excretion. The addition of new drugs to an established regimen may also alter metabolism, compete for protein binding, or alter absorption.

INHALATION (AEROSOLS)

Endobronchial administration normally achieves high local drug concentrations without adverse systemic effects. β-agonist bronchodilators, inhaled corticosteroids, and pentamidine serve as examples. However, certain inhaled solutions reaching the pulmonary parenchyma can be absorbed rapidly across the massive surface area of the capillary bed (e.g., isoproterenol, lidocaine).

INTRATRACHEAL INSTILLATION

The intratracheal route may be used to produce therapeutic drug levels rapidly in settings in which intravenous access is limited or denied (e.g., cardiopulmonary resuscitation). Drugs given via the intratracheal route must be delivered in at least 10 mL of liquid to permit most of the dose to access the alveolar compartment, where absorption occurs.

The intratracheal route has been demonstrated to be effective for emergent use of lidocaine, epinephrine, naloxone, and atropine (Table 15.1). Interestingly, intratracheal administration may prolong the duration of action of certain drugs (lidocaine, atropine).

It is unwise to mix drugs when dosing via the intratracheal route. Furthermore, some commonly used drugs should never be given intratracheally (norepinephrine and calcium chloride, for example, may cause pulmonary necrosis). Because sodium bicarbonate depletes surfactant, massive atelectasis may result from intratracheal use.

INTRAVENOUS INJECTION

Intravenous injection is the most reliable route of drug administration. Intravenous infusions avoid problems of bioavailability and eliminate

TABLE 15–1

INTRATRACHEAL DRUGS

Drug	Dose (mg)
Lidocaine	50–100
Atropine	1–12
Naloxone	2–5
Epinephrine	1 (1 : 10,000 dilution)

delays associated with absorption. Therapeutic levels can be obtained immediately. Intravenous injection also allows the administration of drugs that otherwise would be too caustic, unstable, or poorly absorbed to dose via other routes. At steady state, an uninterrupted, continuous intravenous infusion sustains drug levels, limits peaks and troughs, and avoids the associated problems of subtherapeutic levels and toxicity. It should be noted, however, that fluctuating drug clearance may cause important changes in drug concentrations—even at an unchanging rate of infusion. Unfortunately, constant intravenous infusion is the most costly method of drug administration and may not be necessary. Many medications achieve a similar blood concentration, whether given by the enteral or intravenous route. When enteral absorptive function is intact, oral doses of fluconazole, clindamycin, tetracycline, metronidazole, doxycycline, trimethoprim-sulfa, and ofloxicin produce comparable blood levels as after intravenous dosing.

INTRAMUSCULAR INJECTIONS

Because uptake of drug from muscle into the intravascular compartment is a gradual process, the duration of action of an intramuscular injection is usually longer than that of an equivalent intravenous bolus. Under normal circumstances, aqueous solutions are more promptly absorbed than oily or viscous preparations. Drug absorption may be erratic if local perfusion is impaired, as during shock or cardiopulmonary arrest.

Problems occurring with intramuscular injections include pain or abscess formation at the injection site and hematoma formation for patients with clotting disorders. Intramuscular injections also cause fever, raise the serum creatinine phosphokinase, and may interfere with the diagnosis of myocardial infarction and rhabdomyolysis.

SUBCUTANEOUS INJECTIONS

Subcutaneous injections (particularly of insulin, epinephrine, or heparin) may be appropriate if the drug is nonirritating and administered in a small volume (<1 mL). Rates of absorption vary widely, depending on the drug given and local blood flow. For example, subcutaneous epinephrine is absorbed with sufficient speed to be a mainstay of therapy in anaphylactoid reactions. Conversely, insulin must not be given subcutaneously to the hypotensive diabetic. Delayed absorption of some drugs (e.g., heparins) may be useful to allow prolonged low-level drug effects.

INTRA-ARTERIAL INJECTIONS

Direct injection into peripheral arteries delivers massive concentrations of drug to a local region and may produce serious complications (tissue ischemia and necrosis), particularly if vasoactive drugs are infused. Consequently, the only common use of intra-arterial therapy is the deliberate, selective, and closely metered administration of vasoconstrictors by catheterization of mesenteric vessels in the treatment of gastrointestinal bleeding or vasodilators in mesenteric ischemia. Rarely, selective infusions of antineoplastic agents into visceral arteries may be performed.

INTRATHECAL THERAPY

Intrathecal therapy is rarely employed, except when high CNS concentrations of drugs that cross the blood–brain barrier poorly must be obtained. Refractory CNS infection (i.e., fungal meningitis, gram-negative meningitis, or abscess) constitutes one such indication. Intraventricular or spinal access to the cerebrospinal fluid may be appropriate, depending on the organism and clinical condition of the patient. Rarely, intrathecal antineoplastic drugs may be used for leukemic meningitis.

INTRAPERITONEAL THERAPY

Intraperitoneal antibiotics are often used to treat peritonitis developing in patients undergoing peritoneal dialysis. (Gram-positive coverage usually is provided by a cephalosporin or vancomycin, and gram-negative coverage is provided by an aminoglycoside.) Intravenous loading doses are given initially, but serum levels are sustained by absorption of drug given via the intraperitoneal route. Because intraperitoneal concentrations of drug equilibrate with those in the serum, the concentration of drug in the dialysate should equal that desired in the serum. For example, if a serum level of 7 mg/dL is desired, the dialysate concentration of drug should be maintained at 7 mg/dL.

TRANSCUTANEOUS ADMINISTRATION

Cutaneous drug absorption depends on skin permeability, blood flow, moisture content, and the presence of skin disorders. The highest penetration of transcutaneously administered drugs is for lipid-soluble preparations applied to moist skin. At the current time, nitroglycerin, clonidine, fentanyl, and scopolamine are the only systemic drugs commonly administered transcutaneously. Because diffusion of drug through the skin often requires a significant period of time, onset of action commonly is delayed. Because the skin acts as a reservoir, removal of medications (e.g., fentanyl patches, nitroglycerin paste) does not immediately terminate the action of the drug.

SYSTEMIC ABSORPTION OF DERMATOLOGIC PREPARATIONS

High concentrations of topical corticosteroids applied over large areas occasionally may result in significant systemic absorption. Chronic use of long-acting (fluorinated) topical corticosteroids can suppress the pituitary–adrenal axis, particularly if applied to inflamed skin under occlusive dressings. Certain topical antibiotics used in burn therapy may also produce metabolic acidosis (mafenide) or salt wasting (sodium nitrate) (see Chapter 41).

INTRAOCULAR DRUGS

Even eye drops may be absorbed systemically in significant concentrations if given frequently, if given in high doses, or if there is significant corneal inflammation or trauma. Corticosteroids and β blockers (e.g., timolol) both have the potential for producing systemic effects when administered intraocularly. (Intraocular β blockers are contraindicated for asthma or congestive heart failure.)

ORAL DRUG ADMINISTRATION

Bioavailability of orally administered drugs is limited by acid digestion, poor absorption across the gut wall, and first-pass metabolism by the liver. Effective oral therapy requires gut motility, adequate mucosal perfusion, and epithelial integrity. Patients with ileus, gut hypoperfusion, or atrophic or injured gut epithelium are poor candidates for oral dosing. Drugs given in aqueous solutions are more rapidly absorbed than those given in oily solutions, and nonionized drugs are absorbed more readily than ionized drugs. A few poorly absorbed drugs (e.g., vancomycin, polymyxin) are given orally by design to act locally in the gastrointestinal tract. Drugs destroyed by an acidic pH may be protected partially by enteric coating. Conversely, some drugs require acid for activation or absorption (e.g., sucralfate, ketoconazole, and iron), a point that deserves consideration for patients receiving antacid therapy.

Although not often considered, significant fluid overload may result from giving such fluid-intensive oral preparations as sodium–potassium exchange resin (Kayexalate) or bowel preparations, e.g., saline or polyethylene glycol.

SUBLINGUAL ADMINISTRATION

Because only minute quantities of drug are absorbed across intact oral epithelium, an effective sublingual drug must be potent and lipid soluble. Nitroglycerin is one of the few drugs that fits this description. If swallowed and absorbed enterally, nitroglycerin is eliminated rapidly by first-pass liver metabolism. However, because drugs absorbed from the sublingual plexus drain directly to the superior vena cava, such first-pass clearance is bypassed, increasing bioavailability.

RECTAL ADMINISTRATION

Rectal administration of certain drugs occasionally can be useful in children, combative patients, and patients with problematic venous access or refractory vomiting and/or ileus. Hepatic first-pass metabolism is less extensive with rectally administered drugs than with orally administered drugs, but it is still significant. Unfortunately, rectal administration results in erratic and incomplete absorption and, therefore, is less desirable than either oral or parenteral dosing. Rectal dosing is best confined to sedatives, antiemetics, antipyretics, laxatives, and theophylline compounds.

INTRAVESICULAR ADMINISTRATION

Amphotericin bladder lavage is employed commonly when yeast is found in the urine, but it is of limited usefulness. Intravenous amphotericin should be employed if invasive *Candida* or *Aspergillus* infection of the bladder is suggested by evidence of hyphal forms or clumps of fungus and urine or by histologic evidence of bladder wall invasion. Yeast in the urine of an asymptomatic patient rarely requires treatment (particularly for patients with indwelling urinary catheters), and when treatment is necessary, oral imidazoles are highly effective. Intravesicular therapy may result in hyponatremia if aqueous solutions are used, and

fluid overload may result from isotonic saline. Bladder lavage with glycine-containing solutions often is used to control bleeding after urinary tract surgery.

COST-CONTROL STRATEGIES

Critical care is very expensive, and medication charges can account for 20–30% of a patient's ICU bill. Although the cost of any "life-saving" drug may be justified and no one advocates using less expensive, less effective therapies, careful consideration often reveals that equally effective, less expensive alternatives exist. Medication costs can be lowered in at least five basic ways: (*a*) eliminating unnecessary (often redundant) medications; (*b*) using the least expensive course of therapy when several equally effective alternatives exist (note that the least expensive drug does not always translate into the least expensive course of therapy); (*c*) converting parenteral medications to an oral route as soon as patient condition allows; (*d*) reducing the frequency of administration; (*e*) avoiding drugs that require frequent, expensive, laboratory monitoring.

Daily review of pharmacotherapy often reveals use of redundant, unnecessary, or competing medications. Common examples of these three problems include the following: concomitant use of antacids or sucralfate with a histamine blocker; administration of subcutaneous heparin to patients treated with intermittent pneumatic compression devices; and inhibition of quinolone absorption by antacid therapy.

In most cases, more than one drug alternative exists. For example, the same uncomplicated, *Escherichia coli* urinary tract infection could be treated with oral trimethoprim-sulfa for several dollars or with an intravenous extended-spectrum penicillin for several hundred dollars. Amazingly, however, the cost of a course of therapy often depends more on the route and frequency of administration than it does on the cost of purchasing the drug itself. Another "hidden" and often forgotten cost is that of monitoring drug effects (e.g., drug levels, creatinine monitoring). In general, the oral cost of an equivalent dose of any medicine is 1/10–1/100 that of the same drug given intravenously. This vast discrepancy exists because intravenous preparations usually are more expensive to purchase, some drug is wasted, and there are substantial labor costs associated with stocking, retrieving, mixing, transporting, and administering an intravenous preparation. Any time an intramuscular or intravenous preparation can be changed to an oral route, substantial savings can be achieved (antibiotic therapy offers the best example). Another area of pharmacotherapy not often considered for route switching is that of sedatives and analgesics. Even mechanically ventilated patients can receive enteral sedatives and analgesics if they have a functioning gut. Benzodiazepines and narcotics are both available in liquid form and can be used effectively. Even switching from a continuous intravenous infusion to intermittent intravenous dosing is sometimes cost effective. A constant infusion of a short-acting agent usually requires a dedicated intravenous line and pump for precise control. In contrast, intermittent dosing of a longer-acting agent can avoid the charges for dedicated infusion apparatus.

Because patient charges for preparation of a dose of any intravenous medication average $20–40, it is apparent that patient charges for a drug that costs $1 per dose but must be given six times daily will exceed those for a drug that costs $80 per dose but can be given once daily. In most cases, the most cost-effective measure is to minimize the number of times a drug is given per day, even if that requires using a more expensive drug. The same sort of logic may be applied to drugs that require monitoring. Although aminoglycosides are very inexpensive to purchase, their cost to the patient can be enormous: peak and trough serum levels must be tested on multiple occasions (at about $100 per determination) and frequent creatinine determinations must be made. Another example is the use of warfarin or low-molecular-weight heparin for deep venous thrombosis prophylaxis. At $0.01 per tablet, compared to approximately $10 per injection, warfarin seems to be the clear choice. Interestingly, however, the costs of prothrombin and partial thromboplastic and hematocrit determinations typically performed on patients treated with warfarin, but not on patients treated with low-molecular-weight heparin, rapidly outstrip the savings for the drug itself.

KEY POINTS

1. The multiple organ dysfunction present in most patients in the ICU dramatically alters the pharmacokinetics of most drugs. Experience with any drug's actions in healthy patients is difficult to translate to patients in the ICU.

2. The volume of distribution and half-life of most medications are increased in the critically ill.

3. Drugs generally should be selected for use based on their putative duration of action and method of clearance.

4. Avoiding continuous infusions, ultra-short-acting compounds, and frequent intermittent dosing are the best methods of reducing drug costs.

5. In choosing a cost-effective course of therapy, consider not only the cost of the drug but also the costs associated with administration and monitoring of its effect.

SUGGESTED READINGS

1. Bennett WM, Aronoff GR, Morrison G, et al. Drug prescribing in renal failure: dosing guidelines for adults. Am J Kidney Dis 1983;3:155–193.
2. Friedman H, Greenblatt DJ. Rational therapeutic drug monitoring. JAMA 1986;256:2227–2233.
3. Greenblatt DJ, Koch-Weser J. Drug therapy: intramuscular injection of drugs. N Engl J Med 1976;295:542–546.
4. Pentel P, Benowitz N. Pharmacokinetic and pharmacodynamic considerations in drug therapy of cardiac emergencies. Clin Pharmacokinet 1984;9:273–308.
5. Pond SM, Tozer TN. First-pass elimination. Basic concepts and clinical consequences. Clin Pharmacokinet 1984;9:1–25.
6. Richard C. The effect of mechanical ventilation on hepatic drug pharmacokinetics. Chest 1986;90:837–841.
7. Sellers EM, Frecker RC, Romach MK. Drug metabolism in the elderly. Drug Metab Rev 1983;14:225–250.
8. Trujillo MH, Arai K, Bellorin-Font E. Practical guide for drug administration by intravenous infusion in intensive care units. Crit Care Med 1994;22:1049–1063.
9. Williams RL. Drug administration in hepatic disease. N Engl J Med 1983;309:1616–1622.

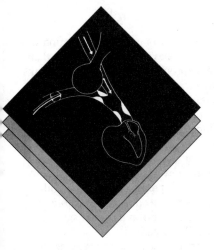

CHAPTER 16

Nutritional Assessment and Support

WHY FEED CRITICALLY ILL PATIENTS?

In the intensive care unit (ICU), the more pressing concerns of hemodynamic and respiratory instability often divert attention from nutritional support. However, suppressing malnutrition may prove decisive by potentially impairing immune function, reducing plasma oncotic pressure, reducing muscle strength, respiratory drive, and delaying wound healing. Studies demonstrating improvement in surrogate endpoints of nutritional status (e.g., serum protein concentrations or lymphocyte counts) and the visceral appeal of providing "food" has promoted an entire industry of nutritional support. Despite the inherent appeal of providing nutritional supplementation, there is surprisingly little credible evidence that any single nutritional regimen improves outcome in the critically ill, and there are significant complications associated with providing nutritional support, especially when instituted after long periods of starvation.

WHY WITHHOLD NUTRITIONAL SUPPORT FROM CRITICALLY ILL PATIENTS?

The gastrointestinal tract is commonly dysfunctional or inaccessible in critically ill patients; therefore, "feeding" often necessitates intravenous nutritional support, which can be fraught with complications and expense. It should be noted that the "food" patients receive in enteral or parenteral preparations bears little resemblance to a usual diet. This is especially true for total parenteral nutrition (TPN), in which fiber, some vitamins, nucleic acids, some proteins, and trace elements are missing. Thus, TPN falls short of being "total nutrition." Furthermore, hemodynamically unstable, hypoxemic, or catabolic patients, especially those with sepsis, ineffectively use nutrients provided in any form. Even if nutritional substrate could be fully used by the tissues of seriously ill patients, the generally high likelihood of survival and brief stay of most ICU patients (average, 3–4 days) raises serious doubt about the ability of any form of nutrition to improve survival or shorten length of stay. Current practice allows critical care physicians to delay the institution of nutritional support for 2 to 4 days. The controversy surrounding who should receive nutritional support and when it should be initiated cannot be resolved using the available scientific data; therefore, therapeutic guidelines must be flexible and based on reason, rather than fact.

SELECTING CANDIDATES FOR SUPPLEMENTAL NUTRITION

CLINICAL HISTORY

Given glucose, thiamine, and water, most patients can safely tolerate protein and calorie deprivation for 1 week or more before supplementation becomes necessary. However, there are patients who probably should be considered for "earlier" support, even in the absence of proven benefit. Nutritional support should not be delayed inordinately for patients who: (*a*) are clearly malnourished at the time of ICU entry; (*b*) have an abnormal dietary history; (*c*) will be deprived of food for long periods of time; (*d*) have massive calorie requirements (e.g., burns, sepsis, major surgery, or trauma); and (*e*) sustain high protein losses (e.g., corticosteroid or tetracycline usage, nephrotic syndrome, or draining fistulas).

Patients anticipated to have short stays in the ICU almost always can do without nutritional support. Such patients include those with simple drug overdoses, patients with asthma exacerbations, and patients admitted for postoperative monitoring. Although controversial, it makes little sense to provide full nutritional support to a moribund patient.

PHYSICAL AND LABORATORY EXAMINATION

Complex scales for nutritional assessment include anthropomorphic measurements, clinical nutrition history, and analytical laboratory criteria. Whereas precise indices of nutritional status may occasionally be helpful, simple clinical and dietary evaluation—history of weight loss, dietary history, and knowledge of underlying disease—provides a good working assessment. Of the widely available clinical measures of nutritional status, clinical history probably is the most useful.

Malnutrition is almost certain in patients losing 5% of their body weight in 1 month or more than 10% of body weight in the 6 months preceding admission. Absolute lymphocyte counts <1200 cells/mm^3 and <800/mm^3 signify moderate and severe malnutrition, respectively, but obviously the lymphocyte count is invalidated as a nutritional index for patients with human immunodeficiency virus (HIV) or hematologic malignancy and for patients receiving chemotherapy. It is widely believed that because albumin normally has a long half-life (~18 days), weeks of nutritional deficiency are needed to produce hypoalbuminemia. This is not true for patients in the ICU because vascular permeability for albumin is often increased dramatically, the liver ceases to produce albumin during severe illness, and extracellular water is often expanded. The net effect of these processes is to cause hypoalbuminemia within days. Even faster declines in serum protein concentrations may occur during intense catabolic stress. Transferrin and thyroid-binding globulin (TBG) prealbumin may be more sensitive acute

indicators of response to nutritional depletion or therapy because they have shorter half-lives than albumin, but these proteins also are subject to leak from the vascular space and dilution by crystalloid volume resuscitation. Complement levels and anthropomorphic measurements are not reliable indices of nutritional status. In the absence of hypothyroidism or nephrotic syndrome, severe depressions of serum cholesterol reliably indicate calorie deprivation. Fever, sepsis, tumors, HIV infection, and immunosuppressant drugs invalidate the antigenic skin test response. Therefore, no good laboratory indicator of nutritional status exists for the critically ill patient.

After a decision has been made to provide supplemental nutrition, four basic questions must be answered:

1. What will be the route of feeding?
2. How many calories are required?
3. How much protein is needed?
4. Are there any special considerations related to the patient's underlying disease?

ESTIMATING NUTRITIONAL REQUIREMENTS

ENERGY/CALORIES

The first step in calculating the nutritional prescription is to estimate the energy or caloric needs of the patient. Three basic methods exist to accomplish this estimation: (*a*) use of a standardized predictive formula based on patient gender, height, and weight; (*b*) direct measurement of oxygen consumption and carbon dioxide production; and (*c*) simple guessing, based on body weight.

Formulas for calculating calorie requirements (basal energy expenditure [BEE]) are often complicated, as exemplified by the Harris–Benedict equation:

$$BEE \text{ (men)} = 66 + (13.7 \times wt) + (5 \times ht) - (6.8 \times age)$$

$$BEE \text{ (women)} = 655 + (9.6 \times wt) + (1.8 \times ht) - (4.7 \times age)$$

Weight (wt) and height (ht) are expressed in kilograms and centimeters, respectively.

Despite their complexity, the Harris–Benedict formulas still require adjustment for additional stress. A well-nourished, minimally active patient should receive 1.25 times the BEE. A severely anabolic patient may require up to 1.75 times the BEE.

Bedside indirect calorimetry (metabolic cart study) provides a direct measure of caloric expenditure while the test is performed (usually 15–20 minutes). Resting energy expenditure (REE) is determined using the Weir equation (below) by measuring oxygen consumption ($\dot{V}O_2$), carbon dioxide production ($\dot{V}CO_2$), and minute ventilation ($\dot{V}_e$).

$$\text{Daily REE} = [(\dot{V}O_2)\,(3.94) + (\dot{V}CO_2)\,(1.11)] \times 1440$$

$\dot{V}O_2$ and $\dot{V}CO_2$ are expressed in liters per minute.

Accuracy of REE determinations are highly dependent on proper setup and calibration of the measuring device and on the patient's being sedated. These calculations are substantially less reliable for patients receiving $FiO_2 > 0.5$. Calorimetry provides only a brief snapshot of caloric expenditure, often disrupts the patient care routine, is expensive, and is not universally available. REE measurements occasionally may be helpful for difficult-to-wean patients, who may be overfed, and for obese or edematous patients, for whom current body weight may not provide an accurate estimation of caloric requirements.

Although such detailed calculations as outlined above occasionally may prove helpful, adequate caloric requirements usually can be estimated by assessment of the patient's general condition and lean body weight. Simply providing 25 to 35 kcal/kg/day will be close to the mark for most patients. For the severely stressed patient, two to three times that number of calories may be required (see Fig. 16.1).

Calorie Sources

Approximately 80% of all calories should be supplied by nonprotein sources. Typically, glucose provides ½ to ¾ of this total (2–4 gm/kg/day), with the remainder coming from lipids. The precise proportions of glucose and lipid are not of crucial importance. However, at least 100 to 150 nonprotein calories per gram of nitrogen (25–35 calories/gram protein) must be provided

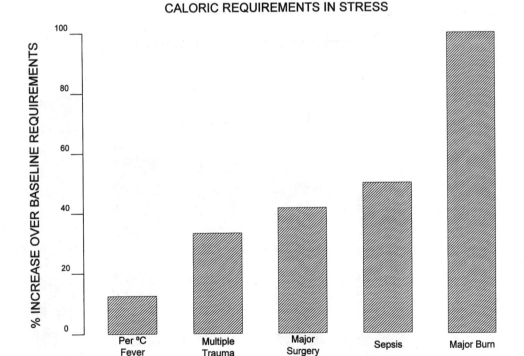

CALORIC REQUIREMENTS IN STRESS

FIG. 16–1. Caloric requirements in stress.

to avoid using amino acids as an energy source. Some glucose is required for protein-sparing effects and to supply tissues with an obligate requirement for glucose (e.g., brain). However, when given in excess of 7 mg/kg/min, glucose is largely converted to fat, leading to potential complications of overfeeding (volume overload, hyperglycemia, increased CO_2 production, and fatty liver).

PROTEIN

After caloric requirements are estimated, protein needs should be calculated. As with energy calculations, a simple or complex method can be used to arrive at a protein estimate. The most difficult and precise method involves measuring daily urinary nitrogen excretion. This is accomplished by performing a 24-hour urine collection for excreted nitrogen and then adding an estimate of nonurinary nitrogen losses. (Calculation of nitrogen balance is outlined below under Indices of Adequate Nutrition.) Obviously, this method is time consuming, expensive, and difficult to perform in the ICU, where patients often do not produce urine or the collection is lost, spilled, or mistimed.

Fortunately, a much simpler approximation is adequate for most patients. Normal adults require 0.5—1.0 gm/kg/day of protein and the average ICU patient requires 1.5 gm/kg/day (see Fig. 16.2). The corresponding amount of nitrogen supplied may be calculated by dividing grams of protein by 6.25. Nutritional supplements provide amino acids capable of being reassembled intracellularly to form structural proteins and enzymes. Providing excess quantities of amino acids is not likely to be beneficial because amino acids themselves cannot be stored. Thus, overfeeding requires the oxidation and excretion of these compounds as urinary nitrogen wastes. (For most patients, anabolism or protein-sparing effects are not enhanced by administration of protein in amounts greater than 1.5 gm/kg/day.) In addition to the normal routes of catabolism, important protein losses may also occur in the urine (e.g., nephrotic syndrome), surgical drains, or chest tubes (especially chylothorax).

The classical distinction between "essential" and "nonessential" amino acids is artificial. His-

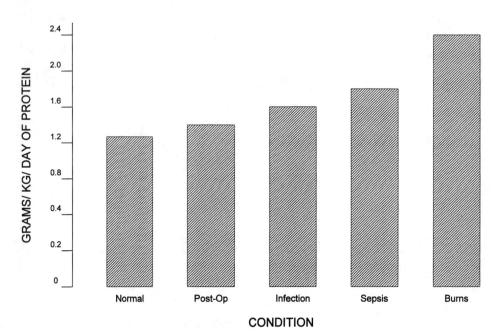

PROTEIN REQUIREMENTS IN STRESS

CONDITION

FIG. 16—2. Protein requirements in stress.

tidine, isoleucine, leucine, lysine, methionine, phenylalanine, threonine, tryptophan, and valine have been considered essential, but for critically ill patients, probably all amino acids are ''conditionally essential.'' Glutamine, alanine, and aspartate are possibly the only nonessential amino acids.

LIPIDS

Some lipid intake is required to prevent the eventual occurrence (over several weeks) of essential (linoleic) fatty acid deficiency. Minimal daily linoleic acid requirements are estimated to be between 3 and 20 grams, an amount easily supplied by providing as little as 5% of calories in the form of lipid. Usual lipid doses are in the range of 0.5 to 2.0 gm/kg/day. Lipids also provide a rich source of calories in a small volume. The lower respiratory quotient observed from the oxidation of fats as compared to carbohydrates indicates that fats generate a lower CO_2 burden for any given caloric intake. Effective lipid metabolism requires a functioning liver; therefore, lipids may not represent the best caloric choice for patients with hepatic dysfunction.

VITAMINS AND TRACE ELEMENTS

Vitamins and trace elements serve as antioxidants and play key roles as intracellular cofactors for enzymatic and energy-generating reactions. More than a dozen different vitamins and trace minerals have been identified as essential for normal physiologic function. It is well recognized that plasma levels of these substances are often abnormal in the plasma of critically ill patients.

In general, fat-soluble vitamins (K, E, D, A) are less prone to acute changes induced by critical illness by virtue of their relatively large storage pool in most patients. Fat-soluble vitamin levels can be reduced in patients suffering from prolonged starvation or malabsorption and in patients treated with broad-spectrum antibiotics, warfarin compounds, or bile-sequestering drugs. In contrast, the water-soluble vitamins (C, folate, and other B complex vitamins) are prone to rapid declines when patients are subjected to dietary deprivation. (Vitamin B_{12} is an exception to this rule.) Table 16.1 is a list of clinical conditions associated with specific vitamin deficiencies.

Isolated deficiencies of the trace minerals copper, zinc, selenium, chromium, manganese, and molybdenum all have been associated with spe-

TABLE 16–1

CLINICAL SYNDROMES RESULTING FROM VITAMIN DEFICIENCIES

Vitamin Deficiencies	Clinical Syndrome/Symptoms
A	Decreased vision, dermatitis
B1 (Thiamine)	Peripheral neuropathy, Wernicke–Korsakoff syndrome
B2 (riboflavin)	Glossitis, cheilosis, pruritus
B3 (niacin)	Pellagra (dermatitis, diarrhea, dementia)
B6 (pyridoxine)	Calcium oxalate urinary stones
B12 (cyanocobalamin)	Pernicious, macrocytic anemia
Biotin	Alopecia, myalgia, paraesthesia, dermatitis
C	Scurvy (anemia, hemorrhage, gum swelling, muscle weakness) poor wound healing
D	Osteomalacia
E	Hemolytic anemia
Folic acid	Macrocytic anemia
K	Bleeding diathesis (warfarin-like effect)
Pantothenic acid	Paresthesia, abdominal cramping/pain

cific syndromes. A full discussion of these syndromes is well beyond the scope of this text. Significant clinical deficiencies of these elements is rare, given even meager nutritional support. Luckily, all commercially available tube-feeding products, and now essentially all parenteral nutrition solutions, contain at least the daily minimum requirements of vitamins and trace minerals, making clinical deficiencies of these nutrients uncommon.

ADVERSE EFFECTS OF MALNUTRITION

Chronic malnutrition depresses the immune system by reducing immunoglobulin levels and by decreasing T-cell function. Deficiencies of glutathione and other antioxidant compounds (vitamin E, beta-carotene) induced by starvation may be associated with impaired resistance to the oxidative stress of sepsis, cancer chemotherapy, or high levels of inspired oxygen. Low colloid osmotic pressure caused by hypoalbuminemia predisposes to pulmonary and peripheral edema at a lower-than-normal hydrostatic pressure. Poor nutrition may impair wound healing and increase rates of infection in burns, trauma, and postoperative states. Starvation impairs ventilatory capacity by decreasing drive and diaphragm bulk. Severe nutritional deficiencies may be fatal for otherwise healthy persons. (Even under optimal conditions, otherwise healthy adults die from subacute losses >40% of lean body mass.)

INDICES OF NUTRITION

As discussed above, laboratory "indices of nutrition" are of very limited value because of their lack of specificity. However, even with these limitations, rising serum protein concentrations and lymphocyte counts are probably good signs. Because albumin is slowly repleted, leaks from the vessels, and can be diluted rapidly by intravenous fluid administration, it is not a useful index of acute improvement or deterioration in nutritional status. With much shorter half-lives, both prealbumin and transferrin may be more helpful, but as acute-phase reactants, levels of both can be raised by inflammatory processes independent of nutritional status. (Note that iron deficiency can also increase transferrin levels independent of nutritional status.) Weight gain clearly is not a dependable sign for patients in the ICU; edema may produce rapid weight increases without any improvement in nutritional status.

Nitrogen balance is possibly the best indicator of nutritional homeostasis. Because nonurinary (skin and stool) losses of nitrogen are usually small (~2 gm/day), the 24-hour urine collection effectively quantitates nitrogen losses. Urine urea nitrogen (UUN) accounts for 80% of total urinary N_2 losses, and acute illness promotes urinary excretion of nitrogen as a result of catabolism. Therefore, unless excessive nonurinary nitrogen losses occur (e.g., through fistulas or open surgical wounds), the balance between nitrogen intake and loss can be approximated using this formula:

$$N_2 \text{ balance} = [\text{Protein intake}/6.25] - [(\text{UUN} + 20\%) + \text{nonurinary losses}]$$

ROUTES OF NUTRITIONAL SUPPLEMENTATION

ENTERAL THERAPY

The numerous advantages of enteral feeding almost always make it preferable to the parenteral

TABLE 16–2
ADVANTAGES OF ENTERAL NUTRITION

Maintains gut mucosa
Promotes enteric hormone secretion
Eliminates need for central catheter
  Reduced risk of sepsis and line-related complications
Buffers gastric acid
Less likely to induce hyperglycemia
Provides unique and complex nutrients not in TPN
  glutamine
  dietary fiber
  medium- and short-chain fatty acids
Dramatically reduces cost

feeding (Table 16.2). Enteral feeding is less expensive, impedes gastrointestinal (GI) tract ulceration, and preserves mucosal integrity and small bowel function better than intravenous nutrition. Because enteral feeding stimulates insulin secretion, hyperglycemia is a less likely complication than during TPN. Furthermore, stimulation of the release of cholecystokinin and gastrin by enteral feeding preserves normal gastrointestinal hormonal responses, promoting emptying of the gallbladder and pancreatic secretion. Enteral feeding also provides iron and trace elements more effectively than TPN. Although the importance of any individual component found in enteral feedings is uncertain, nucleic acids, medium and short-chain amino acids, fiber, glutamine, and intact proteins are not present in TPN solutions.

The GI tract often is not used for nutrition in favor of TPN because of concerns that the gut is immotile. Because small bowel function is often preserved, even when gastric peristalsis is lost, air may not move from the stomach into the small bowel, but food introduced into the small bowel may be well tolerated. This is why patients without the characteristic vigorous gurgling "bowel sounds" usually tolerate enteral feeding. Obviously, patients receiving continuous gastric suction or neuromuscular blocking drugs do not swallow the air or fluid necessary to produce bowel sounds. Neither mild abdominal distention nor reduced bowel sounds should deter a trial of enteral feeding. In fact, it is often only after feeding is begun that bowel sounds return.

When the upper GI tract must be bypassed, soft small-bore (6–8 French) feeding tubes passed through the nose or larger Salem tubes passed through the mouth are both acceptable conduits.

The risk of nosocomial sinusitis is minimized by inserting feeding tubes through the mouth rather than the nose of orotracheally intubated patients. (For the orotracheally intubated patient, there is no disadvantage to having the feeding tube pass through the mouth.) For most patients with ileus, peristalsis of the small bowel returns before gastric and colonic motility; therefore, it may be advantageous to deliver nutrients directly to the small bowel. Feeding tubes should migrate to a final position in or beyond the duodenum for optimal function, a process that may require 12 hours or longer to complete. For some patients, the short-term use of metoclopramide, erythromycin, or cisapride can facilitate migration of the tube past the duodenum.

Before instituting nasogastric (NG) feeding, it is important to ensure proper tube placement by radiograph. Neither the aspiration of what appears to be stomach contents nor characteristic gurgling with air insufflation indicates satisfactory positioning. Feeding tubes malpositioned in the airway may produce similar sounds. (Clinical hints to intratracheal placement of a feeding tube include persistent coughing in an alert patient or, in mechanically ventilated patients, a reduction in exhaled tidal volume, as gas insufflated by the ventilator is vented through the feeding tube.) Initiating feeding before confirming that the tube is in the GI tract invites disaster. For patients who require long-term enteral support, endoscopic placement of a percutaneous gastrostomy (PEG) tube or surgical placement of a jejunostomy feeding catheter may be advantageous.

Continuous feedings are preferable to bolus feedings because they constantly buffer gastric acid, reduce the aspiration risk, produce less bloating, and generate smaller residual volumes. Gastric residual volumes may be checked to ensure that the stomach is not overfilling, but the clinician should not become fixated on the gastric residual if all other clinical indicators are acceptable. As a rule, gastric residuals approximate one to two times the hourly infusion rate of continuous tube feeding and are usually <200 mL. Large (>200 mL) gastric residuals present before initiation of feeding should discourage, but not prohibit, a cautious trial of enteral feeding. A measured gastric residual that increases hourly by exactly the volume of tube feeding infused suggests that the eventual failure of enteral feeding is likely. Vomiting of tube feeding is a clear sign of intolerance that should prompt temporary interruption of enteral feeding, but simple reflux is not.

Almost all patients will exhibit some reflux of tube feedings into the mouth if maintained absolutely supine. The key to combating reflux is elevation of the head of the bed to 30°. Even when delivered to the duodenum, tube feeding stimulates additional gastric secretion (sometimes up to 3–4 L/day). For patients with depressed gastric motility, metoclopramide or cisapride may aid in normal gastric egress of food.

Selection of Feeding Formulas

Certain modular products are available to supplement oral diets and enteral feedings. A calorie boost can be provided by complex carbohydrates (Polycose, 2 kcal/mL) or oils (MCT oil, Microlipid, 4.5 kcal/mL). Certain protein supplements may be particularly helpful for patients on liquid or fat restriction diets (Citrotein or Promod, 5 gm protein per scoop). Puddings made from complete formulas are ideal for fluid-restricted patients.

Nutritionally balanced feedings may be obtained either in polymeric form, in which protein, fat, and carbohydrates are all present as complex molecules, or as elemental diets, in which amino acids provide nitrogen and oligosaccharides serve as the carbohydrate source. Polymeric tube feedings are useful when the gut digestion of fat and protein is normal. The most commonly used formulations (Isocal, Ensure, Ultracal, Osmolite, Precision LR) can provide adequate protein, fat, and 1 to 2 kcal/mL. The high fat content of polymeric feedings enhances palatability if taken orally. The potential for diarrhea from polymeric feedings is low because they have a small lactose content, a low residual, and low osmolarity. Formulations containing fiber (e.g., Enrich, Ultracal, Jevity, Complete B) may help to regularize bowel evacuation. Characteristics of commonly available enteral formulas are provided in Table 16.3.

Elemental diets consisting of oligosaccharides as the carbohydrate source and amino acids as the nitrogen source (Vivonex, Vital-HN, and Travasorb) contain virtually no fat or lactose and have little residual material. Therefore, they require minimal digestion, making them ideal for patients with short bowel syndrome, inflammatory bowel disease, and pancreatic insufficiency. The low viscosity of these preparations renders them useful for catheter-needle jejunostomy feeding. Unfortunately, such preparations are quite expensive, and their high osmolarity predisposes diarrhea despite their low residual content. Essential fatty acids

TABLE 16-3

CATEGORIES OF ENTERAL NUTRITION PRODUCTS

Formula Type/Characteristics	Patient Uses	Examples
Polymeric, nutritionally complete tube feeding, 1 kcal/mL	General purpose, normal digestion	Osmolite, Isocal
Polymeric, nutritionally complete concentrated tube feeding, 2 kcal/mL	Normal digestion, fluid restricted	Magnacal, Isocal-HCN
Polymeric, nutritionally complete oral supplement, 1–1.5 kcal/mL	Oral supplement	Sustacal, Ensure Plus
Elemental, nutritionally complete tube feeding, 1 kcal/mL	Malabsorption (short bowel, pancreatic insufficiency)	Vivonex TEN, Vital-HN
Fiber containing, nutritionally complete tube feeding, 1 kcal/mL	Diarrhea or constipation	Enrich, Ultracal, Jevity
Peptide-based, nutritionally complete tube feeding, 1–1.2 kcal/kg	Hypoalbuminemia with malabsorption	Reabilan, Peptimen

also must be supplemented. Although specific advantages of individual products have not been demonstrated convincingly in specific disease states, Table 16.4 provides a listing of enteral supplements that may have niche indications.

When initiating hypertonic (550–850 mOsm) tube feeding, a half strength solution usually is begun at 25 to 50 mL/hr. At this rate, discomfort, bloating, and diarrhea are seldom encountered. If diarrhea occurs, reduction in the rate of infusion rather than further dilution is the preferred remedy. However, prolonged continuation of such a protocol delays full calorie and protein supplementation. Isotonic formulas are best started at full strength but at a rate one-half of the projected

target. After 12 to 24 hours, it is reasonable to advance the infusion rate to the usual 100 to 150 mL/hr volumes required for full support.

Tube Types

Gastrostomy tubes offer the advantages of stable position and large caliber. The large-bore gastrostomy tube allows administration of pulverized medications, an advantage over jejunostomy or NG tubes, which frequently obstruct. Although gastrostomy tubes enter the stomach directly through the abdominal wall, they do not prevent regurgitation and aspiration. Endoscopic placement of percutaneous gastrostomy tubes, the

TABLE 16-4

DISEASE SPECIFIC NUTRITIONAL SUPPLEMENTS

Disease Condition	Solution Characteristics	Examples
Acute renal failure (without dialysis)	Low protein and electrolyte, 2 kcal/mL	Amin-aid, Suplena
Acute renal failure (with dialysis)	Moderate protein and electrolytes, 2 kcal/mL	Nepro
Hepatic failure (with encephalopathy)	Increased branched-chain AAs, low aromatic AAs, 1.1 kcal/mL	HepaticAid, Travasorb-Hepatic
Respiratory failure (with CO_2 retention)	Increased fat, decreased carbohydrate, 1.5 kcal/mL	Pulmocare, Nutrivent
Diabetes (glucose intolerance)	Increased fat, decreased carbohydrate, 1 kcal/mL	Glucerna
Immunocompromised (trauma, burns, AIDS?)	Enhanced arginine, omega-3 fatty acids, nucleotides, beta carotene, 1–1.3 kcal/mL	Impact, Immun-Aid, Perative
Physiological stress states (burns, trauma, sepsis) (long-term NPO, stress)	Increased branched-chain AAs, high protein, or both, 1–1.2 kcal/mL, enhanced glutamine	Stresstein, Traumacal Alitraq

"PEG" tube, has recently gained popularity, avoiding expense and risks of open surgery. Jejunostomy feeding requires direct surgical placement of a small-bore catheter. Jejunostomy prevents regurgitation and may be withdrawn later (without reoperation) to leave a self-closing fistula.

Problems and Complications of Enteral Nutrition

The most common problem encountered in the use of enteral nutrition is putative "intolerance." Often, "intolerance" equates to reluctance to initiate a trial of tube feeding for a patient with mild abdominal distention or minimal bowel sounds. On other occasions, intolerance represents excessive concern over an arbitrary "gastric residual volume" or abdominal distention as the result of an excessively rapid initial infusion rate. Sometimes, tube feedings are interrupted for gastric residuals as low as 90 mL 6 tablespoons). In general, less reliance should be placed on the gastric residual. More liberal volume limits should be allowed for gastric residuals, with greater emphasis placed on the trend in residual rather than any absolute value. Obviously, a residual that increases every hour by exactly the amount of feeding infused suggests that eventual regurgitation is likely.

Aspiration, the most important and life-threatening complication of enteral alimentation, may be reduced by feeding continuously at a well-tolerated infusion rate, ensuring that the feeding tube is in the duodenum, preventing large gastric residuals, and elevating the head of the bed to 30° from horizontal.

Diarrhea occurs in 30 to 40% of patients in the ICU and is a common reason that tube feedings are interrupted. (Interestingly, diarrhea occurs in a similar percentage of patients in the ICU not receiving tube feedings.) Most cases of diarrhea in enterally fed patients are not due to tube feeding but the concurrent use of other medications, hypoalbuminemia, underlying disease (e.g., hyperthyroidism) or enteral infection (see Table 16.5). In cases in which another cause of diarrhea cannot be determined, reductions in feeding volume, solution osmolarity, and carbohydrate content can reduce the frequency of diarrhea. (Because lactose intolerance is common, the clinician should check to be sure that the nutritional supplement is lactose free.) The addition of pectin to the feeding solution may be a useful countermeasure. Antibiotic-related colitis and *Clostridium difficile* infection

TABLE 16–5

COMMON CAUSES OF DIARRHEA IN PATIENTS RECEIVING TUBE FEEDING

Medications
  Antibiotics
  Antacids (especially magnesium-containing)
  Histamine blockers
  Peristalsis-promoting drugs (metoclopramide, cisapride)
  Cholinergic agents (physostigmine)
  Sorbitol-containing oral medicines (KCl, metoclopramide, theophylline elixirs)
  Quinidine
  Alpha methyl dopa
Colonic infections
  Clostridium difficile
  Enteric pathogens (toxogenic *Escherichia coli, Salmonella, Shigella, Campylobacter*)
Hypoalbuminemia
Colonic impaction (overflow diarrhea)
Lactose intolerance
Underlying diseases (hyperthyroidism)

are common causes of diarrhea for patients in the ICU (see Chapter 26, Severe Infections). For patients receiving tube feedings, diarrhea may result from bacterial overgrowth; therefore, tube feeding preparations should not dwell at ambient temperature for more than a few hours. Although unproven to prevent diarrhea, it is reasonable to rinse feeding infusion bags and administration tubing with clear water on a regular basis and to use good handwashing practices in the preparation and administration of tube feedings.

Nasogastric tubes often become obstructed and require replacement. Obstruction may be avoided if pill fragments are not administered and if the lumen is flushed with water several times daily. Placement of small-bore feeding tubes using a metallic stylet can be dangerous and should be avoided when possible. Esophageal perforation and translaryngeal introduction of the catheter into the lung or pleural space are possible complications.

The pH-neutralizing effect of enteral feedings may encourage overgrowth of pathogenic bacteria, predisposing to gastrointestinal and pulmonary infections. Paradoxically, fiber-containing tube feedings may occasionally cause fecal impaction due to colonic hypomotility and the undigestible nature of fiber. The correct diagnosis is often missed because patients often demonstrate "overflow" diarrhea and have impaction in the transverse or ascending colon (beyond the reach of the rectal examination). Cathartics usually are effective after the diagnosis is confirmed by abdominal radiograph.

TOTAL PARENTERAL NUTRITION

TPN is sometimes necessary but certainly is a less than ideal method of providing nutritional support. The cost of TPN often reaches $150/day for hospitalized patients before costs of monitoring are included and, contrary to its name, TPN does not provide total support. Intravenous nutrition lacks proteins, nucleic acids, some vitamins, glutamine, and other proteins available through the enteral route. TPN solutions may be delivered into peripheral or central veins, with each route having specific advantages and disadvantages.

Peripheral TPN

Peripheral TPN alone is an expensive way to supplement patients with minimal requirements; however, it is not acceptable for catabolic patients requiring protracted total support. Similar protein solutions are used in both central and peripheral TPN mixtures; however, to avoid osmolality-induced phlebitis, the glucose concentration of peripheral TPN is lower than that of central TPN. Consequently, fewer calories are available in a given infused volume. If lipid is not used as a major calorie source, up to 7 L/day of peripheral TPN may be needed to fully satisfy calorie and protein requirements. Even when ~60% of calories are derived from intravenous lipid, 3 to 3.5 L of fluid is needed to deliver 2100 calories (3 L of glucose plus amino acids and 500 mL of 20% lipid solution). Consequently, underfeeding is common when peripheral TPN is used as the sole means of nutritional support.

The corrosive nature of the TPN solution presents another major problem for peripheral administration. Venous inflammation results from the high osmolarity of glucose and amino acid mixtures as well as from the high potassium content of TPN solutions. Up to 50% of patients receiving 600-mOsm (standard) TPN solutions develop phlebitis within 2 days. Therefore, peripheral intravenous sites should be changed at least every other day. The concurrent infusion of a low-osmolality lipid solution through a Y connector reduces the risk of chemical phlebitis. Because of numerous practical problems, peripheral TPN is rarely used.

Central TPN

Central administration of TPN incurs all of the risks of large-vessel cannulation. Catheter tip position must be checked before starting feeding to prevent inadvertent infusion of fluids into the pericardium or pleural space. To minimize the risk of infection, a fresh, dedicated central venous line should be inserted to initiate therapy. Clearly, a balance exists between the risk of repeated catheter insertions and the risk of infection if catheter sites are not changed on a regular schedule. For multiuse catheters (those inserted or used for fluids other than TPN), catheter changes at approximately 5-day intervals probably best balances these two competing risks. A 10- to 14-day interval between catheter changes is probably acceptable for cleanly inserted, dedicated catheters. When a skin-tunneled catheter is placed exclusively for TPN, it is not clear that the catheter ever needs changing unless it malfunctions or becomes persistently infected. TPN catheters should not be used for medication delivery or non-TPN solutions if at all possible. (Multiuse triple lumen catheters are less than ideal, because multiple catheter entries increase the risk of infection.) To prevent bacterial growth in TPN solutions, individual bottles should not hang longer than 24 hours. Controversy surrounds the optimal management of the patient with a TPN catheter who develops fever without another obvious source. The safest course of action in such patients is removal of the catheter (culturing the catheter tip and blood) with reinsertion at a new clean site. Changing catheters over a guidewire is a much less acceptable alternative.

After a central catheter is positioned properly, a highly concentrated (usually 1400–1800 mOsm/L) solution of 5 to 10% amino acids mixed with 40 to 50% glucose is administered. An 8.5% amino acid solution usually is mixed with an equal volume of D50W or D25W to yield a solution containing 150 to 200 kcal/gmN$_2$. Normal electrolyte composition of TPN solution includes sodium (40–50 mEq/L), potassium (30–45 mEq/L), chloride (40–220 mEq/L), phosphate (14–30 mEq/L), magnesium (25 mEq/L), calcium (20 mEq/L), plus an anion (usually acetate) needed to electrically balance the solution. Within broad ranges, these electrolytes can be varied to fit the needs of individual patients. The specific vitamins and trace metals added to standard TPN solutions vary on a hospital-to-hospital basis.

Soy bean (Intralipid) or safflower (Liposyn) oil

mixtures provide extra calories and prevent essential fatty acid deficiency. These iso-osmolar lipid solutions normally provide all essential fatty acids (linoleic, linolenic, and oleic acids). As little as 500 mL of 10% lipid solution given weekly will prevent essential fatty acid deficiency. Lipid solutions also serve as a concentrated source of calories, providing 1.1 kcal/mL for 10% solutions. Under most circumstances, no more than 60% of total daily calories should be provided as fat. Lipids are contraindicated in patients with profound hyperlipidemia. Rapidly administered large-volume infusions of lipid may produce pulmonary dysfunction or thrombocytopenia. Adding small amounts of heparin to lipid solutions (up to 1000 U/L) may accelerate triglyceride clearance by activating lipoprotein lipase. It should be noted that the vehicle used to solubilize the sedative anesthetic agent, propofol, provides substantial lipid and caloric supplementation.

Monitoring TPN

Careful monitoring is required to prevent complications and to ensure that TPN accomplishes its goal. Daily weights should be obtained to monitor fluid status. (Weight gains in excess of 1 lb/day are likely to result from accumulating fluid.) Frequent sampling of glucose during the initiation of TPN therapy is necessary to avoid hyperglycemia and hyperosmolarity. Gross examination of the serum for lipemia 3 to 6 hours after fat infusion or ingestion may confirm hyperlipidemia induced by lipid supplements. Electrolytes (including magnesium, calcium, phosphorus), liver function tests, creatinine, protein, and albumin should be monitored at least twice weekly. Each week, a 24-hour determination of urine urea aids in assessing nitrogen balance.

Complications of TPN

Complications of parenteral nutrition are reduced by an experienced team versed in all aspects of TPN, including the local care of infusion catheters. Insertion of a central TPN catheter carries all of the potential complications of central venous catheter insertion (e.g., pneumothorax and arterial cannulation). Fortunately, complications related to catheter insertion occur at a very low (<5%) rate in most series. Catheter-related sepsis occurs in <3% of patients when proper precautions are taken.

Metabolic complications are more likely to occur in starved and severely malnourished patients and those with diabetes or impaired hepatic or renal function. Sudden refeeding, especially with concentrated carbohydrate loads, can trigger a severe and sometimes fatal refeeding syndrome. In this condition, dextrose challenge stimulates excessive insulin secretion, which in turn, decreases distal renal tubular excretion of sodium and water. Profound hyperinsulinemia promotes the intracellular migration of phosphate, potassium, and magnesium, occasionally resulting in dramatic disturbances of muscular function and cardiac conduction.

Certain free fatty acids (linoleic, linolenic, and arachidonic acids) are considered essential because they cannot be synthesized by the body. Essential fatty acid requirements are met easily by 500-mL lipid emulsion (10%) given once or twice weekly. Deficiency of essential fatty acids also may be avoided by giving 15 to 30 mL corn oil orally each week. Vitamin deficiencies are common during TPN use because many hospitals do not include vitamins K, B_{12}, or folic acid in parenteral solutions. In general, these specific vitamin deficiencies are easy to avoid: B_{12} injections are not required more than monthly, and weekly injections usually are adequate to prevent vitamin K deficiency. Folate requirements do not exceed 1 mg/day, except for patients undergoing dialysis. During prolonged use, deficiencies of trace elements including zinc, iron, cobalt, iodine, copper, selenium, and chromium may produce skin disorders, immunologic defects, and other metabolic problems.

Bone pain and increased alkaline phosphatase may occur with the chronic use of TPN, but the mechanism is unknown. (Both are usually associated with normal vitamin D levels and decreased serum phosphorus.) Hypophosphatemia occurs in approximately one-third of patients started on TPN and is particularly likely when markedly elevated serum glucose levels induce an osmotic diuresis. Hypophosphatemia shifts the oxyhemoglobin dissociation curve leftward and decreases glycolysis but does not produce obvious weakness until levels fall below 1 mg/dL. Hemolysis, impaired phagocytosis, and rhabdomyolysis all may be seen with severe phosphate depletion. Hypomagnesemia may present as refractory hypocalcemia, hypokalemia, or both. Hypomagnesemia is particularly common in patients with pancreatitis and underlying alcoholism.

Mild increases in serum glucose (to <250 mg/dL) are desirable because they produce protein-sparing effects. More profound hyperglycemia, however, causes hyperosmolality (seizures and coma), osmotic diuresis, and depressed immune function. Hyperosmolarity is a common complication of TPN when glucose is infused at rates >0.5 mg/kg/hr, particularly for dehydrated patients. Problematic hyperglycemia occurs most commonly in infants, patients with diabetes or cirrhosis, elderly patients, and patients receiving corticosteroids. To avoid hyperglycemia, glucose infusions should be limited to 5 g/kg/day. If this proves ineffective, insulin should be added to TPN if the serum glucose remains >250 mg/dL for more than 1 day. It is best to add insulin directly to the TPN bottle to match insulin dosing to the rate of TPN infusion. (Hypoglycemia is likely when separate insulin and TPN infusions are used.) To prevent hypoglycemia as TPN is stopped, the infusion rate may first be tapered slowly to ~1 L per 24 hours. D10W can then be substituted for an additional 24 hours. (The need for tapering TPN, however, is debated.)

Acalculous cholecystitis and cholelithiasis are seen with increased frequency in patients receiving TPN, probably secondary to diminished gallbladder secretion and emptying. Symptomatic gallbladder disease may occur in one in four patients receiving TPN for more than 12 weeks. It is especially high in patients with impaired small bowel absorption (e.g., Crohn's disease).

Lipid administration encourages cholestasis by inhibiting hepatic bilirubin excretion. Restricting lipid intake to <2 gm/kg/day and keeping a 200:1 ratio of calories to protein may help prevent this problem. Rapid infusion of amino acids (particularly histidine, alanine, and glycine) may cause hyperchloremic acidosis. The addition of acetate to TPN solution can prevent these changes. Amino acid infusions also promote gastric and pancreatic secretion and stimulate ventilatory drive.

Mild, selective increases in liver function tests (LFTs) are almost universal in patients receiving TPN for more than 10 days. Approximately one-half of all patients experience a 50% rise in alkaline phosphatase and serum glutamic oxaloacetic transaminase (SGOT) levels. Serum glutamic pyruvic transaminase (SGPT) is affected less commonly. Fatty infiltration is the presumed cause. High insulin levels produced by continuous glucose infusion may inhibit lipolysis and favor triglyceride synthesis. Decreases in the glucose infusion rate usually correct the problem. LFT abnormalities may be decreased or prevented by giving less than 60% of nonprotein calories as glucose. Patients who remain normoglycemic rarely develop hepatic function test abnormalities. Even when TPN solutions are continued, LFT abnormalities usually revert to normal in 3 weeks.

NUTRITIONAL SUPPORT IN SPECIAL SETTINGS

CANCER

TPN improves the weight and nutritional parameters of many patients with cancer; however, a survival benefit has yet to be demonstrated. The catabolic mediators (e.g., tumor necrosis factor) released in response to many neoplasms often blunts the anabolic effects of TPN. Protein gain is not as rapid for cancer patients as for other TPN candidates, but fat gain is similar. TPN may improve the tolerance to chemotherapy for some patients; one study of TPN for patients undergoing bone marrow transplantation suggests that both short- and long-term outcomes are improved. Enteral nutrition is often avoided for patients with neoplasms and those receiving chemotherapy because of the high incidence of mucositis and presumed enteritis. It remains unproven that enteral feeding cannot be accomplished successfully in the population.

CHRONIC OBSTRUCTIVE LUNG DISEASE

Malnutrition is common for patients with chronic obstructive lung disease (COPD) because of reduced food intake and increased caloric expenditure. Most patients with COPD requiring nutritional support can have their needs met through the enteral route. One specific problem that often complicates enteral support for these patients is an infusion rate that is too rapid. Because patients with COPD have depressed diaphragms from lung hyperinflation, early satiety and gastric distention are common. Simply reducing the infusion rate slightly usually cures complaints of gastric distention. COPD patients with respiratory failure can devote massive energy expenditure to power ventilation when respiratory failure supervenes. Even after the institution of mechanical ventilation, caloric requirements remain elevated by an average of 10%.

Rarely, respiratory failure is precipitated or prolonged by overfeeding or excessive carbohydrate intake. Overfeeding causes excessive CO_2 production, further stressing a limited excretory capacity for CO_2. Overfeeding is particularly likely to result in hypercapnia when carbohydrates are the predominant energy source, because oxidation of sugars generates 30% more CO_2 than that produced by burning the amount of fat necessary to supply an equal amount of calories. To avoid the problem of carbohydrate overfeeding, carbohydrates should be limited to no more than 50% of the total caloric load and should be administered no faster than 4 mg/kg/minute. Commercial preparations that reduce the fraction of calories provided by carbohydrates and boost the fat content are not without their problems—the high fat content often induces diarrhea.

After a prolonged period of starvation, patients with lung disease are particularly prone to refeeding syndrome. When nutritional support is reinstituted after a prolonged absence, profound hypophosphatemia, hypokalemia, and hypomagnesemia may occur, resulting in glucose intolerance, impaired respiratory muscle function, and myocardial contractility. Special nutritional formulations rich in omega-3 fatty acids or branched-chain amino acids have been tried experimentally for patients with lung disease, but their benefits remain unproven.

RENAL FAILURE

Studies reveal that acute renal failure, by itself, has little affect on resting rates of energy expenditure. In contrast to the benefits noted in early studies, a beneficial effect of parenteral nutrition on outcome in acute renal failure is uncertain. Goals of nutritional support (regardless of route) in acute renal failure are to provide 2000 to 3000 calories and 0.6 to 1.5 gm/kg of protein with high biologic value daily. (Protein requirements should be guided by urinary losses.) Reaching this goal often requires administration of sufficient fluid, sodium, and protein to necessitate earlier institution of maintenance dialysis than might be necessary in the starved state.

When TPN is employed, high glucose concentrations are used to minimize administered volume. Some evidence suggests that although TPN does not hasten recovery of renal function, it may improve uremic symptoms by limiting catabolism. Use of essential amino acids and histidine

as protein sources may stimulate hepatic protein synthesis and anabolism more effectively than standard TPN formulations in such patients. The recycling of nitrogen into nonessential amino acid synthesis theoretically can decrease urea production, hence reducing the need for dialysis. Some amino acids, such as glutamine, may be essential conditionally for patients with severe catabolism. TPN solutions low in sodium and potassium are used unless volume depletion or sodium wasting is a problem. Determinations of urine sodium may help guide the TPN sodium concentration.

In chronic renal failure, an appropriate goal is to provide 0.5 to 1.0 g/kg/day of high-grade protein; intake should seldom be restricted to <20 g/day. Because losses can be massive in the nephrotic syndrome, protein intake should not be limited in this group. Patients with end-stage renal disease should be dialyzed at a rate sufficient to allow nearly normal protein ingestion. Vitamin depletion is a potential problem for patients with renal failure because almost all low-protein diets are vitamin deficient and water-soluble vitamins are lost during dialysis.

HEPATIC FAILURE

The nutritional prescription must be altered radically in cases of hepatic failure. Because fat metabolism is impaired (long-chain triglycerides are metabolized by the liver), hyperlipidemia may result when a large fraction of nonprotein calories are provided as lipid. Carbohydrate intolerance is also common, and high carbohydrate loads may lead to fatty liver. Heightened aldosterone secretion and depressed free-water clearance require low sodium and low volume when TPN is used. Encephalopathy may be precipitated by large protein loads, particularly when aromatic amino acids (e.g., phenylalanine, tyrosine, tryptophan) are the major nitrogen source. Although controversial, the substitution of intravenous branched-chain amino acids for their aromatic counterparts probably reduces ammonia formation and improves mental status in hepatic encephalopathy but offers no benefit to patients with liver disease lacking encephalopathy. Therefore, efficacy and cost considerations dictate use of branched-chain amino acid preparations only in the setting of encephalopathy.

KEY POINTS

1. For patients with preexisting nutritional deficiencies, profound hypermetabolic states, or prolonged ICU stays, nutritional support is important and probably should be initiated as soon as hemodynamic stability is achieved. In contrast, for patients with normal nutritional status and brief ICU stays, nutritional support is much less critical.

2. Detailed nutritional assessments and metabolic cart studies are expensive and offer little benefit for most patients in the ICU over a simple nutritional history.

3. Both enteral and parenteral nutrition are associated with significant complications: the potential for aspiration in the former, and risk of metabolic and septic complications in the latter.

4. The enteral route of nutrition with a small-bore nasal or oral tube is preferred over parenteral TPN in essentially all circumstances in which the gut is functioning. Even among patients with gastric distention, diarrhea, and absence of bowel sounds, enteral feeding can be accomplished successfully.

5. If intravenous nutritional support is required, central TPN delivered through a freshly placed dedicated catheter is the best option. The TPN prescription should be customized to meet patient requirements and limitations based on underlying organ failures.

SUGGESTED READINGS

1. Alverdy J, Chi HS, Sheldon GF. The effect of parenteral nutrition on gastrointestinal immunity. Ann Surg 1985; 202:681–684.
2. Apelgren KN, Wilmore DW. Nutritional care of the critically ill patient. Surg Clin North Am 1983;63(2):497–507.
3. Askanazi J, Weissman C, Rosenbaum SH, et al. Nutrition and the respiratory system. Crit Care Med 1982;10(3): 163–172.
4. Barrocas A, Tretola R, Alonso A. Nutrition and the critically ill pulmonary patient. Respir Care 1983;28(1): 50–61.
5. Berger R, Adams L. Nutritional support in the critical care setting (parts 1 and 2). Chest 1989;96:139–150, 372–380.
6. Bower RH, Talamini Ma, Sax HC, et al. Postoperative enteral versus parenteral nutrition: a randomized controlled trial. Arch Surg 1986;121:1040–1045.
7. Edes TE, Walk BE, Austin JL. Diarrhea in tube-fed patients: feeding formula not necessarily the cause. Am J Med 1990;91:91–93.
8. Grant JP, James S, Grabowski V, et al. Total parenteral nutrition in pancreatic disease. Ann Surg 1984;125: 223–227.
9. Hamaoui E, Leftkowitz R, Oleander L, et al. Enteral nutrition in the early post-operative period: a new semi-elemental formula versus total parenteral nutrition. J Parenter Enteral Nutr 1990;14:501–507.
10. Keohane PP, Attrill H, Love M, et al. Relation between osmolality of diet and gastrointestinal side effects in enteral nutrition. Br Med J 1984;288:678–680.
11. Kittingert JW, Sandler RS, Heizer WD. Efficacy of metoclopramide as an adjunct to duodenal placement of small-bore feeding tubes: a randomized, placebo controlled, double-blind study. J Parenter Enteral Nutr 1987;11: 33–37.
12. Koretz RL. Nutritional support in the ICU: how critical is nutrition for the critically ill? Am J Resp Crit Care Med 1995;151:570–573.
13. Laaban JP, Kouchakji B, Dore MF, et al. Nutritional status of patients with chronic obstructive pulmonary disease and acute respiratory failure. Chest 1993;103:1362–1368.
14. McMahon MM, Farnell MB, Murray MJ. Nutritional support of critically ill patients. Mayo Clin Proc 1993;68: 911–920.
15. Mizok BA. Nutritional management of hepatic failure. Acute Care 1998–89;14–15:71–90.
16. Moore FA, Feliciano DV, Andrassy RJ, et al. Early enteral feeding, compared with parenteral, reduces postoperative septic complications. Ann Surg 1992;216:172–183.
17. Nussbaum MS, Fischer JE. Pathogenesis of hepatic steatosis during total parenteral nutrition. Surg Annu 1991;23:1–11.
18. Ormes JF, Clemmer TP. Nutrition in the critical care unit. Med Clin N Am 1983;67(6):1295–1304.
19. Pingleton SK. Nutritional support in the mechanically ventilated patient. Clin Chest Med 1988;9(1):101–112.
20. Pingleton SK, Harmon GS. Nutritional management in acute respiratory failure. JAMA 1987;257(22): 3094–3099.
21. Raguins H, Levenson SM, Singer R, et al. Intrajejunal administration of an elemental diet at neutral pH avoids pancreatic stimulation. Am J Surg 1973;126:606–614.
22. Rochester DF, Esau SA. Malnutrition and the respiratory system. Chest 1984;85(3):411–415.
23. Shelly MP, Church JJ. Bowel sounds during intermittent positive pressure ventilation. Anaesthesia 1987;42: 207–220.
24. Solomon SM, Kirby DF. The refeeding syndrome: a review. J Parenter Enteral Nutr 1990;14:90–97.
25. Weinsier RL, Krumdieck CL. Death resulting form overzealous total parenteral nutrition: the refeeding syndrome revisited. Am J Clin Nutr 1981;34:393–399.

26. Weissman C, Hyman AI. Nutritional care of the critically ill patients with respiratory failure. Crit Care Clin 1987; 3:185–203.

27. Wilson DO, Rogers RM, Hoffman RM. Nutrition and chronic lung disease. Am Rev Respir Dis 1985;132: 1347–1365.

28. Wolfe RR. Carbohydrate metabolism in the critically ill patient: implications for nutritional support. Crit Care Clin 1987;3:11–24.

29. Zaloga GP. Bedside method for placing small bowel feeding tubes in critically ill patients. Chest 1991;100: 1643–1646.

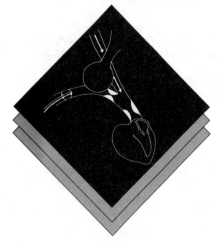

Analgesia, Sedation, and Therapeutic Paralysis

GOALS OF THERAPY

The relief of pain and anxiety is often overlooked while efforts focus on lifesaving therapies. A growing awareness of the stress imposed by the intensive care unit (ICU) and the increasing popularity of some modes of mechanical ventilation that are poorly tolerated without sedation have highlighted the need for effective pharmacotherapy. The goal of such therapy is to provide analgesia and anxiolysis without adversely affecting cardiopulmonary function—a goal best accomplished using a balanced multidrug approach. Nonparalyzed patients should be comfortable but sufficiently awake to communicate their needs and cooperate in their care. Sedation to unconsciousness is mandated during paralysis in all but the most extreme circumstances. Excessive sedation causes respiratory depression, hypotension, and gastrointestinal hypomotility and masks the presence of intercurrent illnesses. Unfortunately, concerns about these side effects often result in insufficient analgesia and sedation being administered to patients. Reluctance to sedate nonintubated patients is understandable but has its own liabilities: it can result in unrelieved pain and anxiety, causing splinting, atelectasis, and increased O_2 consumption; it discourages activity; it promotes venous thrombosis and deconditioning; and it adversely affects immune function.

CORRECTABLE FACTORS CAUSING AGITATION

Agitation should not be regarded solely as a "sedative deficiency" but rather as a potential sign of unrelieved pain or physiologic distress. Hence, before sedating or paralyzing agitated patients, especially those being mechanically ventilated, it is critical that common correctable problems be excluded (Table 17.1). Often, nonpharmacologic actions can enhance patient comfort. Difficulty interfacing with the ventilator shortly after intubation is often improved by varying ventilatory mode, tidal volume, flow rate, and trigger sensitivity (see Chapters 7 and 8, Mechanical Ventilation).

CHOOSING PHARMACOLOGIC AGENTS

The choice of an analgesic, sedative, or paralytic drug, its dosage, and the route of administration should be based on properties of the drug and individual patient requirements. The most common errors in sedative analgesic selection are insufficient sedative/analgesic doses given too infrequently and use of short-acting agents when long-term sedation is desired. Whereas use of "short-acting" agents offers the theoretical advantage of titration of drug effect, rapid reversal is rarely necessary. Furthermore, undersedation is common with short-acting drugs, and prolonged infusions of "short-acting" drugs often result in drug accumulation and prolonged effects. Finally, use of short-acting drugs for long-term sedation is often very costly (sometimes thousands of dollars per day).

ANALGESICS

Opioids

Opioids (narcotics) are potent, predictable, and reversible analgesics but are poor amnestic

TABLE 17–1
CORRECTABLE FACTORS CAUSING AGITATION

Endotracheal tube malposition or obstruction

Hypoxemia

Pneumothorax

Ventilator malfunction

Stomach/bladder distension

Pain

Impaired communication

agents. When analgesic doses of opiates are used alone, few hemodynamic or respiratory effects are observed; however, when large "anesthetic-range" doses (often 10 times the analgesic dose) are used or when narcotics are combined with neuromuscular blockers or other sedatives, the risk of cardiopulmonary instability is greatly magnified. Opioid complications are minimized by (a) ensuring that intravascular volume is adequate; (b) using the lowest effective dose; and (c) using slow administration rates. The histamine-releasing (vasodilating) potential of narcotics is minimal unless rapid, large intravenous doses are given (meperidine and morphine are the most common offenders). Histamine effects can be attenuated by pretreatment with H_1 and H_2 blockers. A feature common to all narcotics is blunting of the hypercapnic and hypoxic respiratory drives. Although usually considered a liability, reduction in respiratory drive often benefits mechanically ventilated patients by reducing their sense of dyspnea and minute ventilation.

Unfortunately, opiates and their metabolites accumulate in patients with hepatic and/or renal failure and in patients receiving prolonged treatment. Hepatic biotransformation typically precedes renal excretion of parent drugs and their metabolites. Initially, the synthetic, highly lipid-soluble opiates (e.g., fentanyl, sufentanil, alfentanil) have their actions terminated by redistribution, not metabolism. With chronic use, however, patients become "saturated" with drug, requiring metabolism for termination of drug effect. Narcotics complicate attempts at enteral feeding by reducing gastrointestinal motility and inciting nausea and vomiting. Rarely, biliary spasm may be precipitated by opiate use. Reluctance to use narcotics for long-term pain relief for fear of dependence and addiction is unfounded; addiction is rare among patients with real pain who lack a history of substance dependence. Epidural narcotic delivery and patient-controlled analgesia are signifi-cant advances in pain control, providing superior pain relief with a lower total narcotic dose and risk of oversedation.

Morphine is an inexpensive drug with a rapid onset of action and a 1- to 3-hour half-life. Intermittent doses of 2 to 10 mg i.m. or i.v., or 1 to 3 mg/hr (0.03 to 0.15 ml/kg/hr) by constant infusion usually are adequate for relief of moderate pain in the average adult. Intravenous administration at rates less than 10 mg/minute minimizes the risk of hypotension. Although morphine is an excellent analgesic, high doses or the addition of a benzodiazepine is required to produce unconsciousness. Morphine's action is prolonged by both renal and hepatic failure because a fraction of each morphine dose is directly excreted unchanged by the kidney but most is metabolized hepatically before renal excretion.

Meperidine offers no substantial advantage over other opioids, and its myocardial depressant effect and vagolytic and histamine-releasing tendencies often cause tachycardia and hypotension. The perceived superiority of meperidine over morphine for patients with ureteral or biliary colic is questionable. Meperidine's major metabolite, normeperidine, is active, accumulates in renal failure, and causes seizures when present in high concentrations.

Fentanyl is a very potent, highly lipid-soluble, synthetic opioid possessing a very rapid onset and brief duration of action—at least with initial use. With repeated injections or when given by continuous infusion, large stores of drug may accumulate in lipophilic tissues that then must be metabolized to terminate the drug's action. Because of this accumulation, fentanyl's effective half-life after chronic use may exceed that of morphine. Initial analgesic doses of 0.5 to 10 μg/kg i.v. may be titrated upward as necessary. Interestingly, because fentanyl cannot be prepared in highly concentrated aqueous solutions, it is one of the few medications that can present a "volume" challenge. With chronic use, it is not uncommon to require several hundred milliliters of fluid each day to administer the analgesic dose. Fentanyl's perceived chief advantage is its minimal hemodynamic effect for a given level of analgesia. Very rarely, fentanyl causes seizures or a bizarre syndrome of profound chest wall rigidity (most common when large i.v. doses are given rapidly to elderly patients). Thoracic rigidity may be so severe that intubation, neuromuscular paralysis, and mechanical ventilation are necessary. Transdermal administration bypasses the substantial first-pass hepatic clearance seen with i.v. dosing, offering a useful alternative method of administration. Unfortunately, the skin slows diffusion, resulting in a long lag time between patch application and effective analgesia, and removal of the patch fails to rapidly terminate the drug's effect because the skin serves as a "reservoir." For patients with modest analgesic requirements but intolerance of intravascular volume required to administer fentanyl, the patch delivery system is especially worth considering. In addition, a very high incidence of nausea has been reported with transdermal dosing.

Alfentanil is a nonionized, short-acting, lipid-soluble, synthetic opiate that is more potent than morphine but less than fentanyl. Consciousness returns rapidly after high-dose alfentanil, making this drug useful for brief but painful procedures. Absence of active metabolites results in minimal drug accumulation unless hepatic failure is present. Sufentanil is 400 to 1000 times as potent as morphine but, except for a potentially smaller volume requirement, does not offer any significant advantages over fentanyl. Both alfentanil and sufentanil present a substantial financial challenge without unique therapeutic effect.

Reversing Narcotic Effects

In the event of inadvertent narcotic overdose, the antagonist naloxone promptly reverses excessive sedation. Intravenous doses of 0.4 to 2 mg are usually sufficient, at least transiently. Naloxone's duration of action is not as long as many commonly used narcotics, necessitating close observation and sometimes repeated administration to prevent recurrence of sedation.

Nonsteroidal Anti-Inflammatory Agents

Nonsteroidal anti-inflammatory agents (NSAIDs) are often discounted for use in the ICU because of their antiplatelet activity and reputation of causing bleeding and renal insufficiency. The frequency and severity of these adverse events are overestimated by many clinicians. Whereas the cyclooxygenase and platelet-inhibiting activities make NSAIDs less than ideal choices for patients with impaired renal function, coagulation disorders or active bleeding, the antiplatelet activity of NSAIDs may be advantageous for patients with coronary or cerebral ischemia. These simple, potent, inexpensive compounds (e.g., aspirin and ibuprofen) often suffice for pain

relief alone and act synergistically with narcotics. Their major drawback is that most NSAIDs can only be given through the alimentary tract. Only ketorolac (Toradol) is currently available in parenteral form, and it does not offer properties sufficiently unique to justify its substantial cost.

SEDATIVE-ANXIOLYTIC AGENTS

Benzodiazepines

Benzodiazepines are sedative, anxiolytic, amnestics with a wide therapeutic range. Because pain and anxiety are synergistic and often indistinguishable to the patient or caregiver, benzodiazepines often reduce analgesic requirements even though they have no intrinsic analgesic properties. Benzodiazepines also induce amnesia and provide anticonvulsant and muscle-relaxant properties. Although not as potent as barbiturates, benzodiazepines reduce cerebral O_2 consumption, intracranial pressure, and cerebral blood flow. Although they may induce unconsciousness, this state is not equivalent to normal slumber. Sleep fragmentation occurs without the full range and depth of normal sleep stages. When sleep is the primary objective, a hypnotic (e.g., zolpidem or triazolam) may be a better choice than a benzodiazepine intended for sedation (e.g., midazolam or diazepam). Paradoxically, benzodiazepines also can excite patients by "disinhibition" of normal social-behavioral control. In similar fashion, amnestic and dissociative effects may linger after consciousness returns, resulting in an agitated, confused, dream-like state that prompts additional doses of the very medication that produced it—a potentially vicious cycle. Haloperidol is a particularly effective agent to break this cycle.

Unless used in large doses or combined with narcotics or neuromuscular blockers, benzodiazepines have few cardiovascular effects. Although they are not direct suppressants of gastrointestinal smooth muscle function, gastrointestinal motility may slow if therapeutic coma is induced. Mild tachycardia and minimal reductions in blood pressure are most commonly observed in elderly patients, dehydrated patients, patients using β-blockers, and patients with underlying cardiac disease. Benzodiazepines exhibit mild dose-dependent respiratory depression but rarely cause apnea. (Apnea is most common after rapid administration of large i.v. doses to chronically ill patients, elderly patients, or patients receiving concomitant narcotics.) The highly lipid-soluble

TABLE 17–2
COMPARISON OF THE PROPERTIES OF PARENTERAL BENZODIAZEPINES

Compound	Duration of Action	Hepatic Metabolism Required?	Metabolites Active?	Relative Hourly Cost
Diazepam	long	yes	yes	$
Lorazepam	long	no	no	$$
Midazolam	variable	yes	yes	$$$

benzodiazepines (e.g., midazolam) accumulate in fat after repeated or prolonged use, resulting in delayed recovery. The avid protein binding of all benzodiazepines leads to frequent interactions with other protein-bound drugs and exposes hypoproteinemic patients to high concentrations of free (active) drug. Most benzodiazepines require hepatic metabolism and/or excretion; therefore, liver disease can prolong the action of these drugs (lorazepam and oxazepam are exceptions). Conversely, patients with highly activated liver enzyme systems (e.g., alcoholics) may require enormous doses for therapeutic effect. The properties of the three most commonly used parenteral benzodiazepines are contrasted in Table 17.2.

Diazepam is an inexpensive, long-acting sedative-amnestic-anxiolytic agent that is available in oral or parenteral forms. Unpredictable absorption from muscle usually limits use in the ICU to the intravenous route. Unfortunately, phlebitis is common after i.v. injection in a peripheral vein (Midazolam shares this liability to a lesser degree). Diazepam's high lipid solubility and large volume of distribution result in a rapid onset and prolonged action. Doses of 2 to 10 mg (0.04–0.2 mg/kg i.v.) given every 5 to 10 minutes are reasonable to initiate therapy.

Because of its solubility and high receptor affinity, lorazepam has a slower onset and longer duration of action than midazolam or diazepam. Prolonged action generally is a desirable characteristic for an ICU sedative because of the common requirement for long-term sedation. Minimal cardiovascular effects and excellent amnestic properties make lorazepam a good choice for performing "awake" endotracheal intubation and as a premedicant for procedures. Initial i.v. doses of 1.0 to 2.0 mg (0.03–0.04 mg/kg) may be repeated every few minutes until the desired degree of sedation is achieved. Predictable absorption with oral or intramuscular dosing permits an easy transition from intravenous therapy not possible with midazolam. Lorazepam is comparable to diazepam in hourly cost for equal effect.

Midazolam is an expensive, potent, "short-acting" benzodiazepine. The high lipid solubility of midazolam and its ability to cross the blood–brain barrier produce a rapid onset of action (2–3 minutes). A steep dose–response curve dictates that, initially, low doses of midazolam and close observation are indicated to avoid excessive sedation. Starting doses of 0.5 to 1.0 mg (0.01–0.1 mg/kg) given intravenously at 5- to 15-minute intervals are customary. Whereas isolated doses of midazolam are eliminated rapidly by hepatic extraction and metabolism, the effective half-life of midazolam is prolonged after extended i.v. infusion as the drug accumulates in fat. Accumulation of midazolam can produce an effective duration of action that exceeds diazepam or lorazepam. When combined with topical or local anesthetics, midazolam is a good agent to provide sedation and anxiolysis during brief procedures. Cost often prohibits use of midazolam as a long-term sedative.

Chlordiazepoxide is limited to oral use but is a very popular choice for the prophylaxis of delirium tremens. Despite its popularity, chlordiazepoxide has no unique properties distinguishing it from the other available benzodiazepines.

Benzodiazepine Antagonism

Flumazenil is an expensive competitive receptor antagonist capable of reversing the respiratory and central depressant effects of benzodiazepines in approximately 80% of patients. Chronic or high-dose benzodiazepine use lowers the success rate of reversal. Flumazenil has no beneficial effect on ethanol, barbiturate, narcotic, or tricyclic antidepressant-induced central nervous system depression. Because flumazenil is cleared rapidly by the liver, its duration of action is substantially shorter than that of most of the compounds it antagonizes. As with the naloxone opioid combination, up to 10% of patients given flumazenil relapse into a sedated state, making close observation essential. Doses of 0.2 mg at 1-minute intervals (up to 1 mg total) are customary. Flumazenil should be used cautiously because it may precipitate withdrawal symptoms (agitation, vomiting, and seizures), especially for chronic benzodiazepine users. For patients with suspected combined (benzodiazepine and tricyclic antidepressants) drug overdose, flumazenil can precipitate seizures, presumably as a result of unmasking tricyclic effects. Flumazenil is seldom needed in the ICU. Although it may confirm a diagnosis of benzodiazepine overdose, it rarely alters patient management.

Barbiturates

The most lipid-soluble barbiturates (e.g., thiopental, thiamalyl, and methohexital) have a rapid onset of action because the luxuriously perfused lipophilic brain becomes saturated rapidly with drug after dosing. By achieving high brain concentrations, barbiturates depress the reticular activating system. Occurring almost as rapidly as the onset of action, redistribution terminates these drug effects. Less lipid-soluble barbiturates, (e.g., phenobarbital) have a slower onset of action and longer recovery time. The nearly immediate onset of action of ultrashort-acting barbiturates makes them useful for "rapid sequence intubation" of carefully selected patients. Barbiturates have a limited role in the ICU because of their narrow therapeutic margin and propensity to cause hypoventilation, cardiac depression, and vasodilation. Hypotension is most common in patients with underlying cardiovascular disease, elderly patients, and volume-depleted patients. Barbiturates do not produce muscle relaxation nor analgesia. In fact, they may paradoxically enhance the perception of pain. Tolerance and physiologic dependence occur rapidly, and withdrawal symptoms occur frequently. Because most barbiturates are highly protein bound and alter hepatic metabolism of other compounds, drug interactions are common. Diseases that reduce the serum protein concentration (e.g., sepsis, nephrotic syndrome, cirrhosis) may potentiate the effect of barbiturates by increasing the free fraction of drug in plasma. After hepatic metabolism, barbiturates are renally excreted; therefore, liver or kidney dysfunction potentiates these agents as metabolites. Reduced intracranial pressure and cerebral O_2 consumption account for the neuroprotective effects of barbiturates; however, fluid and vasopressor therapy is almost always required to maintain blood pressure. In the ICU, barbiturate use should probably be limited to: (a) second-line anticonvulsant therapy; (b) induction of coma for cerebral preservation; and (c) rapid-sequence induction/intubation.

MISCELLANEOUS AGENTS

Phenothiazines (e.g., Phenergan) are sedative antiemetics that may be used to potentiate the analgesic and sedative effects of narcotics. With the exception of their antiemetic effects, the combination of phenothiazines and narcotics offers no substantial advantage over the more commonly used benzodiazepine–narcotic combination. Phenothiazines have the disadvantage of inducing dystonic (extrapyramidal) reactions in a small minority of patients.

Haloperidol

Haloperidol, a butyrophenone tranquilizer, has gained substantial popularity for control of severely agitated patients in the ICU, particularly when psychosis or delirium are prominent features. Initial i.v. doses of 1 to 2 mg commonly are doubled every 15 to 30 minutes until behavioral control is obtained. For the patient with agitated delirium, a combination of a benzodiazepine and haloperidol is superior to either agent alone. Although few adverse effects have been reported, haloperidol has α-blocking effects and anticholinergic properties. Haloperidol also lowers the seizure threshold and may precipitate torsades de pointes, neuroleptic malignant syndrome, transient extrapyramidal reactions, and potentially permanent tarditive dyskinesia. Because of these risks, haloperidol should be used with caution.

Propofol

Propofol is an i.v. anesthetic mixture of the alkylphenol drug in an egg and soybean oil emulsion. (Because of its fat content, the vehicle provides 1.1 calories/mL). Initial doses of 1 to 2 mg/kg result in profound sedation (but not analgesia) that may be maintained using similar hourly doses. For some patients, however, drug requirements have been impressively high. Although useful because it can be titrated easily and is neither hepatically nor renally metabolized, propofol has limitations. Potent cardiovascular depressant effects cause hypotension in up to one-third of patients, especially when a loading dose is administered. Propofol also has a propensity to cause seizures. The drug vehicle may also cause allergic reactions, and users should not be surprised by the green-tinged urine produced by excretion of the phenol compound. The vehicle's composition supports the growth of bacteria, and epidemics of nosocomial bacteremia have been associated with contaminated infusions. For these reasons, strict sterile precautions must be used when infusing this drug, and the duration of infusion of an individual vial should be limited to a few hours.

NEUROMUSCULAR PARALYTIC AGENTS

Mechanism of Action

Normally, electrical impulses reach the neuromuscular junction, causing calcium-mediated release of acetylcholine into the junctional cleft. Acetylcholine binding to muscle receptors then causes a sodium–potassium flux (depolarization). Through a combination of acetylcholine reuptake and local degradation by "true or specific" acetylcholinesterase, muscle repolarization occurs and the opportunity for subsequent contraction is restored. A second nonspecific plasma enzyme, pseudocholinesterase, metabolizes acetylcholine and acetylcholine-like molecules.

Depolarizing neuromuscular blockers stereochemically resemble acetylcholine and mimic its action at the neuromuscular junction resulting in Na^+–K^+ flux across the muscle. Depolarizing blockers are not metabolized in the neuromuscular junction by acetylcholinesterase; therefore, persistent depolarization occurs until the neuromuscular blocker diffuses out of the synaptic cleft, where it is metabolized by plasma or pseudocholinesterase. Nondepolarizing blockers act by passively occupying acetylcholine binding sites or sodium–potassium ion channels, thereby competitively blocking acetylcholine's depolarizing action.

Indications

Controversy surrounds the use of paralytic agents in the ICU. Many practitioners contend that there is no role for these drugs in appropriately sedated patients. Although paralytic agents rarely are needed when adequate sedation is employed, carefully selected patients can benefit. Unless absolutely necessary to preserve life, awake paralysis is never an acceptable alternative to sedation. Experience with these inherently dangerous agents must come from carefully supervised use and cannot be learned safely by only reading

TABLE 17–3

POTENTIAL INDICATIONS FOR PARALYSIS

Endotracheal intubation

Muscle relaxation during surgery

Facilitation of mechanical ventilation

Reduction of oxygen consumption

Injury prevention (e.g., electroconvulsive therapy)

Termination of tetanus/convulsive activity

about them. Because of the potential for numerous complications, paralytic agents should be used in the lowest possible doses and for the shortest possible time.

Commonly accepted indications for paralytic drug use are given in Table 17.3. Facilitation of endotracheal intubation is probably the most common indication, but extreme caution is indicated; as a rule, the hazards of paralysis for intubation parallel the perceived need for muscle relaxation. For example, use of paralytics for morbidly obese patients or those with spinal instability can precipitate complete upper airway obstruction. Provisions to secure the airway surgically must always be available when using paralytic drugs.

Diseases in which muscular contraction is itself harmful (e.g., tetanus and hemodynamic instability resulting from intractable convulsions) may benefit from neuromuscular blockade. It is important to remember that although paralytics terminate the muscular convulsive activity, they do *nothing* to terminate chaotic cerebral electrical activity or protect the brain. Because paralytics obscure clinical assessment of seizure activity, continuous electroencephalographic monitoring must be provided if they are used for a seizing patient.

High levels of positive end expiratory pressure (PEEP) and modes of ventilation with prolonged inspiratory times (e.g., extended ratio or airway pressure release ventilation) are sometimes actively opposed by patients. The practice of "permissive hypercapnia" also drives ventilation. In these settings, sedation alone usually is sufficient to provide comfort, aid ventilation, and lower peak airway pressures. Neuromuscular blockers, however, are occasionally useful to facilitate ventilation. Neuromuscular paralysis also can reduce oxygen consumption in patients with marginal oxygenation, but there is little evidence that paralysis is superior to deep sedation in this situation.

Cautions

Neuromuscular blockade has many dangers—the most problematic of which is the potential for paralysis of inadequately sedated patients. Insufficient sedation is difficult to recognize: hypertension, tachycardia, diaphoresis, and lacrimation are the only possible physiologic manifestations. Paralyzed patients are helpless—unrecognized extubation, ventilator malfunction, or arterial line disconnection can be fatal. Paralysis also predisposes patients to developing decubitus ulcers, nerve compression syndromes, corneal erosions, deep venous thrombosis, and muscle atrophy. By preventing patient communication and concealing physical signs (e.g., abdominal rigidity, rigors) paralysis obscures the diagnosis of intercurrent conditions (e.g., intra-abdominal disasters, myocardial ischemia, hypoglycemia, seizures, and strokes). Essentially all data on paralytic drugs come from their short-term use in the operating room; therefore, actions, interactions, and side effects for critically ill patients in the ICU after long-term administration are unknown. For example, it took substantial time before reports emerged regarding prolonged muscle weakness after use of corticosteroid-derived neuromuscular blockers.

Profound, prolonged weakness can develop with continuous long-term use of any neuromuscular blocker. However, the combined use of high-dose corticosteroids and nondepolarizing neuromuscular blockers is of particular concern. Numerous instances of myopathy or neuromyopathy, often associated with marked elevation of creatine phosphokinase (CPK), have been reported among patients with obstructive airway disease. The particular neuromuscular blocker, the total paralytic dose, the duration of therapy, the presence of renal failure, and the quantity and duration of corticosteroids all may be risk factors for development of this syndrome.

The potency and duration of paralytic agents are affected by the duration of therapy and by the presence of concomitant medications and medical conditions. Burns and use of methylxanthines, phenytoin, lithium, corticosteroids, and carbamazepine all reduce or antagonize the effectiveness of paralytics (Table 17.4). Edematous states produce more complex problems: by increasing the volume of distribution, edema makes initial paralysis more difficult to achieve; however, the large reservoir of drug that accumulates in edema fluid may prolong recovery. Tachyphylaxis is often seen with long-term use.

Respiratory acidosis and metabolic alkalosis, hypokalemia, hyponatremia, hypocalcemia, hypermagnesemia, and hypothermia all potentiate the

TABLE 17–4

CONDITIONS INFLUENCING THE INTENSITY OF NEUROMUSCULAR BLOCKADE

Conditions That Potentiate Blockade	Conditions That Interfere With Blockade
Respiratory acidosis	Edematous states
Metabolic acidosis	Prolonged paralytic use
Hyponatremia	Burns
Hypocalcemia	Drug interactions
Hypermagnesemia	Methylxanthines
Hypothermia	Phenytoin
Neuromuscular diseases	Lithium
Myasthenia gravis,	Corticosteroids
Guillain-Barre	Carbamazepine
Drug interactions	
β blockers	
Calcium channel blockers	
Cyclosporine	
Aminoglycosides	
Tetracycline	
Clindamycin	
Procainamide	
Quinidine	

neuromuscular blockade. Patients with "de-innervation hypersensitivity" caused by diseases such as myasthenia gravis and Guillain-Barre syndrome are particularly sensitive to depolarizing paralytic agents. β-blockers, calcium channel blockers, cyclosporine, aminoglycosides, tetracycline, clindamycin, and the antiarrhythmics procainamide and quinidine also potentiate neuromuscular blockade.

Specific Blockers

Depolarizing Neuromuscular Blockers

Succinylcholine is the drug of choice for many intubations because it has a very rapid onset of action (seconds) and a brief duration (<10 minutes). Because it is degraded rapidly by plasma cholinesterase, most of an administered dose never reaches the neuromuscular junction (see also Chapter 6, Airway Intubation). Succinylcholine causes fasciculations (depolarizations) in skeletal muscle but does not affect smooth muscle action. Despite its brief duration of action, succinylcholine is not without side effects. Most adult patients develop a sympathomimetic response; however, hypotension may occur, especially when succinylcholine is combined with barbiturates. Succinylcholine is not suited for repeated injection or constant infusion because, when given in this manner, it causes vagal stimulation and bradycardia. If more than one dose of succinylcholine is required, atropine should be given before the second dose.

Depolarization causes muscle contraction and, hence, the release of potassium from muscles. Plasma potassium increases of 0.5 to 1 meq/L are common; but among patients with peritonitis, burns, multiple trauma, or rhabdomyolysis, hyperkalemia may be severe. Patients with increased numbers of acetylcholine receptors due to the deinnervation hypersensitivity of neuromuscular disease are especially prone to hyperkalemia. Vomiting caused by abdominal muscle contraction and postparalysis muscle pain commonly result from succinylcholine use but may be attenuated by pretreating with a subparalyzing dose (10–15% of the usual dose) of a nondepolarizing blocker. Succinylcholine raises intraocular pressure and should be avoided in patients with glaucoma or ocular injuries.

Nondepolarizing Neuromuscular Blockers

Nondepolarizing neuromuscular blockers act by preventing the action of acetylcholine at its receptor. Nondepolarizing blockers may be grouped conveniently by several basic properties: duration of action, route of metabolism and excretion, propensity to release histamine, and the tendency to cause vagal blockade (Table 17.5). Many of these compounds (e.g., pancuronium, vecuronium, pipecuronium) chemically resemble corticosteroids. Each of the nondepolarizing blockers has a slower onset of action than succinylcholine

but produces paralysis of a longer duration than that of succinylcholine. The duration of action ranges from 20 minutes for mivacurium to often more than 1 hour for pipecuronium, pancuronium, doxacurium, metocurine, and tubocurarine.

Pancuronium is the least expensive and longest acting of the nondepolarizing agents. Pancuronium falls short of being the perfect paralytic drug for the ICU because it requires renal excretion, like tubocurarine, metocurine, doxacurium, and pipecuronium. Pancuronium also undergoes substantial (~20%) hepatic metabolism yielding active metabolites and complicating its use in hepatic failure. Pancuronium also has modest histamine-releasing properties and vagolytic effects that may cause tachycardia and hypotension. Vecuronium is used widely because of its intermediate duration of action and paucity of cardiovascular effects. Because vecuronium is removed in large part (~80%) by hepatic metabolism and biliary excretion, it is a poor choice for patients with liver disease. Although not cleared directly by the kidney, vecuronium has two active metabolites that are cleared renally. Hence, reports of prolonged paralysis after vecuronium administration in patients with renal insufficiency are not necessarily surprising. Paralysis using vecuronium is more expensive than that produced by pancuronium but less so than atracurium.

Atracurium, cis-atracurium, and mivacurium have theoretical advantages for patients with hepatic or renal failure because these drugs undergo extensive plasma degradation. Mivacurium is broken down by pseudocholinesterase, whereas atracurium undergoes esterase degradation and spontaneous breakdown at the physiologic pH and

TABLE 17–5

PROPERTIES OF COMMONLY USED NON-DEPOLARIZING NEUROMUSCULAR BLOCKERS

Drug	Onset (min)	Duration	Histamine Release	Vagal Blockade	Metabolism	Excretion
Mivacurium	1–2	short	+	0	extensive	minimal
Vecuronium	1–2	intermediate	0	0	moderate	hepatic ≫ renal
Atracurium	1–2	intermediate	+	0	mostly nonenzymatic	minimal
Doxacurium	2–3	long	0	0	minimal	renal
Pancuronium	1–2	long	0 to +	+	moderate	renal ≫ hepatic
Pipecuronium	1–2	long	0	0	moderate	renal
Tubocurarine	1–2	long	+ + +	0	minimal	renal ≈ hepatic

temperature called "Hoffman elimination." Because of its metabolism, atracurium is probably least affected by the presence of renal failure. Atracurium's metabolism yields laudanosine, a renally cleared excitatory tertiary amine that may precipitate seizures. Its clinical importance is uncertain. Breakdown of atracurium is delayed by hypothermia and acidosis, but unlike most other neuromuscular blockers, its termination is not impaired by advanced age.

General Recommendations

Intubation

The rapidity of onset and brief duration of action make succinylcholine the drug of choice for most ICU intubations, unless neuromuscular diseases or electrolyte disorders dictate otherwise. Mivacurium's nondepolarizing properties, short duration of action, and plasma metabolism make it an attractive alternative for patients with contraindications to succinylcholine.

Long-acting, nondepolarizing neuromuscular blockers may be used as well. The onset of paralysis is hastened by administration of large doses or subparalytic "priming doses" given several minutes before the paralytic dose. Vecuronium and mivacurium represent good alternate choices for rapid-sequence intubation because both drugs exhibit a priming effect and have an intermediate duration of action and even large doses have minimal side effects. Although atracurium and vecuronium can be used for intubation, their long duration of action can be problematic if difficulty is encountered in passing the endotracheal tube.

Long-Term Paralysis

For patients with reasonable hemodynamic reserves and near-normal hepatic and renal function, paralysis for longer than 1 hour can be accomplished safely and most economically with pancuronium. Patients with extremely tenuous hemodynamic status may be less likely to experience adverse cardiovascular effects if paralyzed with atracurium or vecuronium. Hepatic failure would be an additional consideration favoring atracurium. Renal failure may favor a choice of vecuronium. Doxacurium, pipecuronium, and vecuronium do not offer any substantial advantage over pancuronium with respect to cost, duration of action, or side effect or elimination profiles. Tubocurarine and metocurine do not seem

to have a niche in the ICU because they require intact renal function for clearance and are potent histamine releasers. Despite the limitations of pancuronium, it can be used safely even for patients with advanced hepatic and renal insufficiency if care is taken to avoid massive overdose through close clinical monitoring.

Complications of Paralysis

Pseudocholinesterase Deficiency

Pseudocholinesterase is the plasma enzyme that metabolizes acetylcholine, succinylcholine, and mivacurium. Genetic or acquired reductions in levels of this enzyme increase the duration of paralysis when using these drugs. Up to 5% of patients are heterozygous for plasma cholinesterase, resulting in prolongation of paralysis by several minutes. Approximately 1 in 2500 persons has a homozygous pseudocholinesterase deficiency, extending the duration of the paralysis to 6–8 hours. Because the goal of therapy in the ICU, unlike the operating room, is usually to produce paralysis that lasts for hours, prolongation of paralysis usually is of little consequence. There is no certain clue to pseudocholinesterase deficiency short of a clear history of prior prolonged paralysis; however, cholinesterase levels tend to decrease in patients with liver disease, renal failure, advanced age, pregnancy, marked anemia, and organophosphate toxicity.

Malignant Hyperthermia

Malignant hyperthermia is a calcium-mediated genetic disorder that is rarely precipitated by use of neuromuscular blockers, usually in combination with an inhalational anesthetic (see Chapter 28, Thermal Disorders). Clinical features include the rapid development of muscular rigidity, high fever, and enormous increases in metabolic rate resulting in metabolic acidosis with massive CO_2 production and O_2 consumption. Untreated, lethal cardiac ischemia and ventricular arrhythmias are common. Treatment consists of removing the offending agent(s) and administering intravenous dantrolene.

Assessment of Neuromuscular Blockade

Approximately 75% receptor occupancy is required to cause any muscle weakness, with 95% percent blockade needed for complete muscular relaxation. Interestingly, the diaphragm is one of the muscles most resistant to paralytic drugs, requiring 90% or more of receptors to be blocked to develop paralysis. It can be difficult to clinically assess the degree of neuromuscular blockade in the ICU, but as a practical bedside test, the ability to sustain a head lift for several seconds indicates reversal of paralysis and is more reliable than tests of negative inspiratory force, vital capacity, tongue protrusion, or grip strength.

A peripheral nerve stimulator provides the best objective index of the intensity of neuromuscular blockade but commonly is not used effectively in practice. The goal in using a peripheral nerve stimulator is to prevent complete obliteration of a "train of four" electrical stimulus. If patients are able to produce one to three muscular contractions per four electrical stimuli, paralytic overdose is presumed to have not occurred. Unfortunately, appropriate monitoring sites can be difficult to find and maintain, and it is possible to have complete obliteration of "train of four" stimulus but to maintain diaphragm function. The practical implication of this observation is that patients may still exhibit ventilator dyssynchrony despite profound peripheral skeletal muscle blockade; or, the

desired obliteration of diaphragm function may require excessive peripheral blockade.

A more commonly used monitoring strategy is to allow blockade to lapse before subsequent doses of a paralytic agent are given. This practice has several practical advantages: (a) it does not require special equipment or training or induce patient discomfort, (b) it allows early discovery of patients who are inadequately sedated, (c) it permits assessment that may discover new intercurrent conditions, and (d) it often reveals that continued paralysis is not necessary, thereby reducing duration of paralysis and expense.

Reversal of Neuromuscular Blockade

The reversing agents (e.g., neostigmine, pyridostigmine, and edrophonium) act by raising acetylcholine levels in the neuromuscular junction and therefore will not reverse blockade of succinylcholine or the profound (ion channel) blockade due to nondepolarizing blockers. Reversal of paralysis is rarely necessary in the ICU, and use of these agents risks muscarinic stimulation (severe bradycardia, bronchorrhea, and salivation). Muscarinic effects may be countered by pretreatment with the anticholinergic atropine or glycopyrrolate.

KEY POINTS

1. Agitation is often a manifestation of discomfort or physiologic distress that can be resolved without the use of pharmacologic agents. Ventilator adjustments, repositioning, relief of gastrointestinal and bladder distention, and reassurance are essential nonpharmacologic methods of agitation control.

2. When pharmacotherapy is deemed necessary, drug selection should be based on desired effect, duration of action, and cost. In general, long-acting compounds are preferred to smooth peak and trough effects and to reduce costs.

3. Pharmacodynamics in the ICU often differ greatly from those of less ill patients. Most drugs have longer durations of action and larger volumes of distribution when given to ICU patients than to less ill patients.

4. A narcotic (morphine or fentanyl) with a benzodiazepine (diazepam or lorazepam) offers a safe, effective, economical analgesic–sedative package for most ICU patients.

5. Haloperidol (often given with a benzodiazepine) represents an excellent choice for treatment of the extremely agitated or delirious patient not experiencing pain.

6. Neuromuscular blockers should be used sparingly because of numerous risks, which include: awake paralysis, hemodynamic instability, prolonged muscle weakness, and obscuration of intercurrent illnesses. When necessary for long-term paralysis, pancuronium is a safe, economical choice for most patients.

SUGGESTED READINGS

1. Wheeler AP. Sedation, analgesia and paralysis in the intensive care unit. Chest 1993;104:566–577.

2. Freeman JW, Hopkinson RB. Therapeutic progress in intensive care sedation and analgesia. Part I: principles. J Clin Pharm Ther 1988;13:33–40.

3. Freeman JW, Hopkinson RB. Therapeutic progress in intensive care sedation and analgesia. Part II: drug selection. J Clin Pharm Ther 1988;13:41–51.

4. Crippen DW. The role of sedation in the ICU patient with pain and agitation. Crit Care Clin 1990;6:369–392.

5. Bodenham A, Park GR. Reversal of prolonged sedation using flumazenil in critically ill patients. Anesthesia 1989; 44:603–605.
6. Shelly MP, Mendel L, Park GR. Failure of critically ill patients to metabolize midazolam. Anesthesia 1987;42: 619–626.
7. Partridge BL, Abrams JH, Bazemore C, Rubin R. Prolonged neuromuscular blockade after long-term infusion of vecuronium bromide in the intensive care unit. Crit Care Med 1990;18:1177–1179.
8. Parker MM, Schubert W, Shelhamer JH. Perceptions of a critically ill patient experiencing therapeutic paralysis in an ICU. Crit Care Med 1984;12:69–71.
9. Loper KA, Butler S, Nessly M, Wild L. Paralyzed with pain: the need for education. Pain 1989;37:315–316.
10. Rouby JJ, Eurin B, Glaser P, Guillosson JJ, Guesde R, Viars P. Hemodynamic and metabolic effects of morphine in the critically ill. Circulation 1981;64:530–539.
11. Dundee JW, Johnston HM, Gray RC. Lorazepam as a sedative-amnestic in an intensive care unit. Curr Med Res Opin 1976;4:290–295.
12. Driessen JJ, Crul JF, Vree TB, Van Egmond J, Booij HDJ. Benzodiazepines and neuromuscular blocking drugs in patients. Acta Anesthesiol Scand 1986;30:642–646.
13. Malacrida R, Fritz ME, Suter PM, Crevoisier C. Pharmacokinetics of midazolam administered by continuous intravenous infusion to intensive care patients. Crit Care Med 1991;20:1123–1126.
14. Buck ML, Reed MD. Use of non-depolarizing blocking agents in mechanically ventilated patients. Clin Pharmacol 1991;10:32–48.
15. Fiamengo SA, Savaraese JJ. Use of muscle relaxants in intensive care units. Crit Care Med 1991;19:1125–1130.
16. Coggeshall JW, Marini JJ, Newman JH. Improved oxygenation after muscle relaxation in adult respiratory distress syndrome. Arch Intern Med 1985;145;1718–1720.
17. Hansden-Flaschen JH, Brazinsky S, Basile C, Lanken PN. Use of sedating drugs and neuromuscular blocking agents in patients requiring mechanical ventilation for respiratory failure. JAMA 1991;266(Suppl):2870–2876.
18. Sokoll MD, Gergis SD. Antibiotics and neuromuscular function. Anesthesiology 1981;55:148–159.
19. Gronert GA, Theye RA. Pathophysiology of hyperkalemia induced by succinylcholine. Anesthesiology 1975;43:89.
20. Whittaker M. Genetic aspects of succinylcholine sensitivity. Anesthesiology 1970;32:143.
21. Gramstad L, Lilleahsen P. Neuromuscular blocking effects of atracurium, vercuronium and pancuronium during bolus and infusion administration. Br J Anaesth 1985;57: 1052–1059.
22. Nelson TE, Flewellen EH. The malignant hyperthermia syndrome. N Engl J Med 1983;309:416–418.
23. Ali HH, Savarese JJ. Monitoring of neuromuscular function. Anesthesiology 1976;45:216.
24. Cronnelly R, Morris RB. Antagonism of neuromuscular blockade. Br J Anaesth 1982;54:183–194.

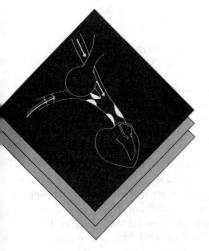

CHAPTER 18

General Supportive Care

INTRODUCTION

Certain aspects of management are important to consider, independent of the precipitating cause for admission to the intensive care unit (ICU) and the sophistication of monitoring or treatment. Attention to the background details of day-to-day nursing and respiratory care often determines the rate of adverse events and the eventual success or failure of specific management approaches leveled at the primary problems. This chapter reviews the basic elements of evaluation and therapy that apply to most patients in an ICU environment.

BEDSIDE EVALUATION OF THE CRITICALLY ILL PATIENT

Receiving care in the ICU implies an ongoing problem with or a perceived threat to the integrated cardiorespiratory system. Therefore, although individual decisions must be guided by the specific pathophysiology at hand, central principles of daily evaluation apply to most critically ill patients. Individual practice styles need not be identical to be equally effective. However, in this complex, high-stakes arena, an element of compulsiveness serves the clinician well; failure to systematically review the available database relevant to vital organ performance and prescribed therapy often leads to misinterpretation, inappropriate care plans, or ineffective communications among caregivers that translate into adverse outcomes or protracted hospital stays.

THERAPEUTIC PERSPECTIVE

The term "intensive" care implies the potential for rapid changes in clinical status. Therefore, the patient must be monitored carefully and the lines of communication among caregivers must be kept open. To care for the most critically ill, a knowledgeable and responsive physician must be continuously accessible and committed to reevaluating the patient at the bedside as often and as long as required. Except under exceptional circumstances, vital communications are too severely strained by long-distance discussions for complicated decision-making.

Although isolated data points are unquestionably important, trends in the data stream are often of equal or greater value. For many variables, the trend interval should be extended to include the prehospital period. (What is the patient's chronic blood pressure, weight, cardiac rhythm, $PaCO_2$, etc.?)

The ICU practitioner must intercede quickly and decisively when action is clearly necessary to avert disaster. In most circumstances, however, the clinician's prime objective should not be to reestablish "normal physiology" as quickly as possible, but rather to encourage smooth resolution or adaptation to the pathophysiologic insult. A working diagnosis and updated plan of action must be clearly formulated and communicated. Because the clinician cannot always foresee the consequences of intervention, it is important to question data quality and to consider alternative explanations before intervening—what really is known for certain and what must be better established?

ELEMENTS OF THE BEDSIDE EVALUATION

To be maximally effective, the intensivist must quickly probe and organize extensive information flowing from verbal and written communications, monitored data, laboratory output, and imaging studies (Table 18.1). Using the available database and his/her own observations at the time of evaluation, the physician formulates a listing of current problems, ranks their urgency and relative priority, and thoughtfully devises a plan of action. When things become hectic, 5 or 10 minutes spent away from the bedside in a quiet setting to reflect on the database, identify problems, and decide on the management approach is nearly always time well spent.

Caution is indicated whenever the bedside evaluation is inconclusive. Conducting a closely observed "therapeutic mini-trial" is a key element in the successful management of fragile or unstable patients, especially when the physician is uncertain regarding the outcome of a planned intervention. After the evaluation has been completed and a course of action has been decided upon, the patient and physician are often well served by implementing the proposed change under direct observation for a brief interval, before formalizing the order. This approach is particularly helpful when making ventilator adjustments, position changes, or alterations in the infusion rates of fluids or rapidly acting drugs, the effects of which can be monitored directly (see "Volume Challenge" in Chapter 2, Hemodynamic Monitoring).

Verbal Communications

As most experienced practitioners realize, the ICU tends to function best with a team approach in which caregivers of varied descriptions (physicians, nurses, therapists) are professionally well acquainted, mutually respected, and equally committed. The day-to-day routines and the expectations for the unit must be well understood, ideally with an awareness of the work schedules and priorities of all involved. Despite the unquestioned value of "hard data," overreliance on "the numbers" to guide decision-making fosters an incomplete, immature, and dangerous style of practice. Drawing from moment-by-moment observations made over extended periods, a well-trained nurse or therapist is often the caregiver with the best insight regarding the relation of events and medications to evolving problems, tolerance of current therapy, and the probable effects of intended interventions (weaning from mechanical ventilation, mobilization, transport, reaction to medication, mental status, airway secretion volume, and character, etc.). The skillful clinician seeks their active involvement and advice in the planning process. For the team to operate with maximum effectiveness, the nurse, respiratory therapist, and unit pharmacologist (if available) should make formal rounds with the physician to share observations and advise, as well as to be kept abreast of the doctor's current thinking and care plan. The specific objectives of therapy and conditions or developments for which the doctor desires to be contacted should be communicated explicitly. Uncertainty regarding the appropriateness and dosage of certain medications often can be addressed, valuable time can be saved, and prescription errors can be avoided by communicating intent of treatment and writing goal-oriented orders when possible. The latter strategy lends flexibility and allows timely dosage adjustment, (e.g., for fluids and/or diuretics).

Family Communications

It is difficult to overestimate the importance of direct, unambiguous communication with the family. The ICU environment holds undeniable potential for miscommunication, as the concerned family member may seek or receive information and advice from many caregivers with differing perspectives, knowledge, and attitudes. One or two physicians must be identified as the primary contact(s). Clearly, the family must be allowed to visit the patient as soon as appropriate after admission or in an unanticipated emergency. However, although some caregivers with the best intentions maintain unrestricted access to the pa-

TABLE 18–1

ELEMENTS OF THE BEDSIDE EVALUATION

Verbal communication	Laboratory record
Caregivers	Imaging studies
Patient	Physical examination
Family	Vital signs
Referring physician or	Systems review
institution	Directed examination
Written communication	Monitored information
Chart record	Ventilator
Nursing notes	Hemodynamics
Current orders	Electrocardiogram
Medication/therapy lists	Other apparatus
Data board	

tient, it seems wisest to restrict routine visiting hours to two or three predictably "quiet periods" in the work day (e.g., late morning, late afternoon, early evening), especially in high-acuity ICUs. More frequent contact eventually confuses and exhausts the worried family, seldom benefits the comatose or sedated patient, and interferes with caregiving.

Whatever the local policy, it is wise to set aside a fixed time in the day when the physician reliably communicates progress and plans and receives vital feedback from family members. Some well-functioning units reserve a specific hour each day (e.g., $11:00-12:00$ AM) during which the intensivist can be scheduled (by the unit clerk) to discuss progress and plans with relatives of long-term patients. To reduce the emotional strain on both family and staff in an inherently unstable environment, it is important to emphasize that monotonic improvement (albeit desirable) seldom occurs, that minor setbacks and complications are to be anticipated, and that it is often most appropriate to view the general trend over days to weeks, not minutes to hours. Clearly conveying the likely diagnoses and plausible alternatives, the team's approach, the strategy for action, and contingency plans helps instill confidence and trust.

Written Communications and Records

In addition to discussions with other caregivers, the physician must review the chart record, nursing notes, orders, medication and therapy lists, bedside databoard, ventilator sheet, and laboratory record. The nursing record often provides an overlooked and valuable source of information. Puzzling entries with the potential to influence decision-making should be clarified by direct verbal communication. Calculations required to synthesize the clinical picture and formulate revisions to the care plan (e.g., anion gap, systemic vascular resistance, respiratory compliance, airway resistance) should be automated or made quickly. Specific attention should be directed to the patient's weight, intake, urinary and fecal output ("I's and O's"), diet, and drugs (those scheduled and given as needed). Sedatives, antibiotics, vasoactive agents, and diuretics tend to be of special interest. The volume and description of expectorated or suctioned airway secretions and gastric aspirates should be noted.

Laboratory Data

The most recently obtained values for arterial blood gases, hemoglobin concentration, leukocyte and platelet counts, serum glucose, blood urea nitrogen (BUN), creatinine, and electrolytes, as well as urinalysis, must be reviewed in every patient for whom they are available. Serial tests for liver or cardiac enzymes, leukocyte differential, coagulation profile, drug levels, renal function tests, etc. may be of unusual interest in specific patients. As already noted, trends in such data often are more meaningful than individual test results.

Physical Examination and Monitoring

The contribution of the physical examination has become undervalued as our technical abilities to image noninvasively, to electronically monitor cardiorespiratory function, and to use laboratory data have improved. However, certain key bits of information that are impossible to gather quickly by other means should be assessed by physical examination one or more times daily for virtually every patient with cardiorespiratory instability or compromise. Although the directed physical examination is the practical standard, outstanding clinicians are sufficiently self-disciplined to quickly but systematically assess certain aspects of the physical examination each day to develop the background against which to gauge any future changes.

Vital Signs

Review of the vital signs record is a frequent starting point in the bedside evaluation. What are often overlooked, however, are telling relationships among them. For example, heart rate may not parallel the height of fever or may be inappropriately slow for the clinical setting of congestive failure, as suggested by a disjunction between elevations of heart rate and respiratory rate. Extreme respiratory variation evident on an arterial pulse tracing suggests the paradox associated with severe airflow obstruction, severe left heart failure, or pericardial disease. Vital signs may change abruptly with sleep or level of alertness.

Mental Status and Neuromuscular System

The categories of the Glasgow Coma Scale serve as a reminder of the gross characteristics to be screened and followed: best verbal, motor, and eye opening (and pupillary) responses. Muscle tone and strength, facial appearance, eye movements, alignment, reflexes, and asymmetry should be noted. Signs of fear, anxiety, depression, and delerium should be elicited actively by attempting to engage the patient in meaningful conversation as well as light banter. (A well-preserved sense of humor generally indicates a high level of integrative mental capacity.) It is important to question the nursing staff regarding how well the patient has been sleeping, especially if delerium is suspected, dyspnea is questioned, or weaning is contemplated.

Cardiovascular System

Sequential cardiovascular examinations can reveal a new gallop, murmur, rhythm disturbance, paradoxical pulse, neck vein distention, basilar rales, dryness of the mucous membranes, diaphoresis, edema, impaired capillary refill, and other signs that provide clues to underlying pathophysiology. This knowledge should be interpreted in conjunction with an examination of electrocardiographic and arterial pressure tracings, echocardiographic and radiographic information, and Swan-Ganz data, where available. Serial examinations are especially important in the setting of myocardial infarction, acute valvular endocarditis, or other potentially life-threatening, rapidly changeable conditions.

Respiratory System

Consecutive physical examinations of the respiratory system should focus on the quality, intensity, and symmetry of breath sounds, the presence or absence of regional percussion dullness, the breathing pattern, the audibility and distribution of wheezes, rales, rubs, ronchi, and bronchial breath sounds, and the vigor and effectiveness of breathing efforts. Pulse oximetry can be extremely helpful when adjusting inspired oxygen fraction (FiO_2), positive end-expiratory pressure (PEEP), position, or ventilator settings. Mechanically ventilated patients require a careful review of the record documenting minute ventilation, oxygen, and pressure requirements (peak, plateau, mean, and end-expiratory), gas exchange efficiency, patient–ventilator synchrony, integrity of the breathing circuit, and machine mode and settings (as detailed in Chapter 5, Respiratory Monitoring).

Renal and Electrolyte Status

Although urine output and composition often should be followed closely, not every patient in the ICU requires an indwelling bladder catheter. However, because the urinary output of the healthy kidney tends to parallel fluid volume status and serves as a useful indicator of vital organ perfusion, patients with questionable cardiovascular status often benefit from continuous urimetry. The clinician should allow a trend to evolve over 1 to 3 hours before making radical interventions based primarily on urinary output, because oliguria may be transient or may respond only slowly to corrective action. Moreover, it is prudent to keep in mind recent changes in therapy, cardiovascular status, sleep–wake cycles, serum electrolytes, etc. in making the interpretation. The color, pH, specific gravity, glucose and electrolyte concentrations, results of tests for leukocyte esterase, erythrocytes, hemoglobin, and a review of sediment characteristics and pending urine cultures aid in assessing fluid status as well as in determining the etiology and severity of many common disorders. BUN and creatinine should be compared with previous values. This data should be considered in conjunction with the I&O record, the daily weight trend, and the listing of medications in assessing the fluid balance. Weight should be compared with that of previous hospital days, as well as those recorded previously in clinic or prior admissions. Arterial blood gases and serum electrolytes should be reviewed, and anion gap and serum osmolality should be estimated.

Gastrointestinal/Nutritional

Daily assessments should include a review of nutritional intake. The volume and character of gastric aspirates and stool output also must be tracked. To evaluate motility, the physical examination of the abdomen always should include auscultation. Persistently active bowel sounds without stool or gas output may suggest bowel obstruction. When confronting a quiet abdomen, it is especially important to palpate deeply and to elicit signs of peritoneal inflammation. Ascites, excessive bowel gas, gastric distention, and gut edema may explain a visibly distending abdomen. A "tight belly" may explain high ventilator cycling pressures or, if extreme, a dwindling urinary output.

Apparatus

Extensive use of equipment and devices helps characterize the care delivered to critically ill patients. Intravascular lines and pumps should be inspected quickly, and their sites of entry should be examined for evidence of phlebitis, local cellulitis, or purulence. The dressings that cover suspicious points of catheter insertion must be taken down and the wound beneath must be examined carefully, preferably at the time of routine dressing changes. When specialized life-support equipment is used (e.g., balloon pump), the key variables relevant to its operation and the level of support must be noted. The essential data provided by the bedside cardiac monitor and ventilator display are reviewed with each visit to the bedside.

Imaging Data

Radiographs, computed tomographs (CT), and radioisotopic and ultrasonic images have become integral to the evaluation of the critically ill patient. Rounds should incorporate a review of such data, which often redirect thinking or confirm diagnoses made by other means.

THERAPEUTIC SUPPORTIVE CARE

Intensive life support has no evolutionary precedent. Before modern civilization, our primate ancestors were at constant risk of predatory attack and disease. Survival required foraging and continuous vigilance; our predecessors seldom remained off their feet or motionless for longer than a few hours at a time. Most conditions that currently prompt admission to the ICU previously would have resulted in a quick demise. Deprived of food and water and unable to take shelter from the elements and natural enemies, the sick individual became vulnerable to many of the traumatic, infectious, and environmental problems that now are easily manageable. A philosopher or anthropologist could argue effectively that evolutionary pressures have encouraged elimination (rather than survival) of those weak enough to fall prey to catastrophic disease or severe trauma. Because recumbency is central to extended life support but is inherently unnatural, a working knowledge of the consequences of sustained bed rest and immobility is fundamental to understanding the rationale and consequences of ICU nursing practice.

PHYSIOLOGY OF BED REST

Noncardiorespiratory Effects of Recumbency

Certain consequences of protracted bed rest are well known to most practitioners, whereas other,

more subtle repercussions are either unknown or ignored. Physiologic adaptations to gravity affect nearly all organ systems, and release from gravitational stress may set in motion changes that impede recovery.

Neuromuscular

While under the influence of gravity, contracting skeletal muscles compress the veins and lymphatics, counteracting the gravitational forces that would otherwise cause body fluids to pool in the legs and lower abdomen. Contraction of muscles used in maintaining the upright posture and locomotion preserves muscle bulk and strength. Moreover, muscular traction and gravitational stresses help the bones retain calcium. It is not known what fiber tension or duration of contraction is necessary to sustain these benefits. It is clear, however, that release of the skeletal muscles from their diurnal activity for longer than 24 to 48 hours initiates metabolic processes that eventually culminate in tissue atrophy and impressive physiologic changes.

Aerospace science and experiments in healthy volunteers have yielded impressive data on the effects of bed rest in healthy individuals (Table 18.2). Skeletal muscles quickly lose tone when not called upon to support the body's weight. After only 72 hours, the loss of myofibrillar protein is under way—even in a well-nourished, physiologically unstressed subject. The greatest protein losses occur in the muscle groups that normally bear the greatest postural burden—legs and dorsal trunk. The rates at which bulk and strength diminish are believed to be functions of the length at which the muscle fiber is immobilized, as well as the completeness of relaxation. Judging from the devastating weakness that may result from extended neuromuscular paralysis, neural excitation may be a crucial factor in preserving muscle function. Intense stimulation may not be required to dramatically slow the pace of sarcomere depletion, and although active movement is clearly better than passive manipulation of resting muscle, physical therapy of the immobilized patient aids significantly in preventing contractures.

As any sleepless physician understands, periodic rest in the recumbent position is essential for optimal cerebral functioning. Even during sleep, however, the healthy adult turns or makes a significant positional adjustment on an average of five times per hour. As noted below, there may be important physiologic advantages to such fre-

TABLE 18–2

PHYSIOLOGIC EFFECTS OF BED REST

Noncardiorespiratory effects	Cardiovascular effects
Reduced muscle bulk and strength	Pulmonary vascular congestion
Altered biorhythms	Impaired vasomotor tone and reflexes
Decreased glucose tolerance	Increased preload and stroke volume
Endocrine dysfunction	Altered autonomic activity
Fluid shifts and diuresis	Respiratory effects
Calcium, potassium, and sodium depletion	Reduced functional residual capacity
Immunologic impairment	Altered distribution of lung volume
Nasal congestion/impaired sinus drainage	Altered airway drainage
Reduced gastrointestinal motility / esophageal reflux	

quent repositioning. Moreover, most adults do not prefer to sleep in the supine horizontal position that is used routinely in the ICU. Many individuals express great difficulty in falling asleep in this position or awaken quickly if they inadvertently shift into it. In fact, all nonarboreal four-footed mammals—including the primates—ambulate prone, with vulnerable vital structures protected by proximity to the ground. Most animals sleep in that position as well.

With the development of modern intensive care and the need to cannulate blood vessels and access the various orifices of the respiratory, gastrointestinal, and urinary systems, the recumbent critically ill patient was kept oriented in the supine position for extended periods, often immobilized by sedation or paralyzed pharmacologically by muscle relaxants. Periodic turning is known to be important in the avoidance of pressure trauma (decubitus ulcers, see below), which is most likely to develop over points of high contact pressure—especially when the patient is cared for on a firm traditional bed. (Perhaps this helps explain the need for frequent movement during sleep.)

Endocrine and Metabolic

Release of many hormones normally is timed to a diurnal cycle. For example, cortisol and epinephrine normally vary in a circadian fashion, with trough levels occurring in the early morning hours. Cholinergic (vagal) tone also increases at night. The unnatural activity, lighting, and noise within many ICU environments disrupt these cycles. Moreover, bed rest itself alters certain biorhythms; cycles for insulin and growth hormone (and consequently glucose) often demonstrate multimodal patterns, time-shifted peaks, and other perturbations in normal healthy subjects, even when feeding schedules remain unchanged. The

activity of the pancreas gradually declines, and glucose intolerance may develop after as little as 3 days of enforced bed rest. These changes usually reverse within 1 week of resuming normal activity. Thyroid hormones tend to rise as bed rest continues beyond a few weeks, whereas androgen levels fall. Oxygen consumption declines significantly during recumbency.

Fluid and Electrolyte Shifts

Recumbency shifts about 10% of the total blood volume ($\approx$500 mL) cephalad, away from the legs. Almost 80% of the shifted volume migrates to the thorax; the remainder translocates to the head and neck. The nasal mucosa swells, and the patient may experience nasal congestion. Diuresis begins on the first day of recumbency for the normal subject, who loses approximately 600 mL of extracellular fluid by the second day (more if edema was present initially). Bed rest initiates losses of sodium and potassium but reduces the amplitudes of the diurnal excretory cycles for water, sodium, potassium, and chloride. Weight bearing seems to be an important stimulus to osteoblastic activity and, during prolonged bed rest, $\approx$0.5% of total body calcium stores are leached per month from the bones and muscles. Rarely, impaired renal excretion of the increased calcium load results in hypercalcemia.

Gastrointestinal Changes

Well-known gastrointestinal responses to inactivity include anorexia and constipation. Recumbency impairs the efficiency of swallowing and may precipitate esophageal reflux in those with lax esophageal sphincter function. The gut may lose all but a vestige of its natural motility if food is not provided, gastric secretion is pharmacologically suppressed, and air swallowing is inhibited—even if opiates are not prescribed (see Chapter 17, Analgesia, Sedation, and Therapeutic Paralysis).

Immunologic Defenses

Bed rest impairs the body's resistance to infection, even when no catheters enter the vascular, urinary, respiratory, or gastrointestinal compartments. The normal rate of catabolizing immunoglobulin G doubles and neutrophilic phagocytosis slows. The mucosal colonization rate for certain pathogens, such as the staphylococcus, may increase. An adverse gravitational bias results in stasis, secretion pooling, and bacterial overgrowth within the maxillofacial sinuses and tracheobronchial tree, further predisposing patients to infection.

Blood Components and Coagulation

It generally is understood that patients on protracted bed rest are vulnerable to thrombosis—largely because of venostasis and unrelieved compression of the leg veins. Subtle changes also occur in the coagulation profile; procoagulant synthesis and fibrinolytic activity increase, and the thromboplastin time shortens. Independent of any coexisting disease process, the red blood cell mass tends to decline during the first several weeks of inactivity, primarily due to a decrease in erythropoesis.

Cardiovascular Effects of Recumbency

Vasomotor changes in arterial resistance both maintain blood pressure relatively constant and regulate the distribution of blood flow. In the active and fully conscious normal individual, fluctuations in regional tissue blood flows occur naturally and spontaneously. In the immobile supine patient, these fluctuations gradually disappear over the first hour of recumbency. Alert subjects may then experience sufficient discomfort to impel a change in position.

Many significant cardiovascular changes occur in the normal individual during the transition to the supine position (Table 18.2). In the conscious subject, heart rate declines as stroke volume increases. Cerebral, renal, and hepatic blood flows increase, whereas blood pressure and systemic and pulmonary vascular resistances tend to decline. Sympathetic tone decreases, and parasym-

pathetic tone increases. The renin–angiotensin axis down-regulates, promoting diuresis. The baroreceptive reflexes that are instrumental in adapting to the upright position are blunted after sustained bed rest; therefore, chronic orthostatic stress seems necessary, both for the preservation of an adequate blood volume, as well as for maintaining adaptive cardiovascular reflexes.

The Trendelenburg ("head down") position offers no significant hemodynamic benefit over that provided by the supine position, and despite its widespread use, has no confirmed place in the management of shock. The gravitational bias of the Trendelenburg position increases intracranial arterial and venous pressures equally and, therefore, leaves cerebral perfusion unimpaired in normal individuals. However, elevated intracranial pressures may compromise cerebral perfusion in the patient with preexisting head injury. Head inversion also increases the tendency for esophageal reflux. These drawbacks do not mean that the Trendelenburg position is never indicated; airways drain more effectively, and distention of neck veins facilitates insertion of central venous catheters while helping to avoid air embolism.

In the lateral and prone positions, gravitational effects on hydrostatic pressure are of less importance, but venous obstruction occasionally may pose significant problems. Extreme truncal flexion in infants, obese adults, and advanced pregnancy may not only result in hypoxemia but also may impede venous return. For a woman in the advanced stages of pregnancy, lying in the supine position may cause compression of the vena cava and hypotension that is relieved by lying on her left side. Increased abdominal pressure leading to inferior vena cava obstruction also has been associated with the prone position, especially when there is exaggerated knee–chest positioning or noncompliant abdominal support.

Respiratory System

Conversion from the upright to the supine position is accompanied by important changes in ventilation, perfusion, secretion clearance, muscle function, gas trapping, and tendency for lung collapse. In normal subjects, reclining decreases functional residual capacity (FRC), primarily due to the upward pressure of the abdominal contents on the diaphragm and to a lesser extent on declining lung compliance. The functional residual volume declines by approximately 30% (or 800 mL) in shifting from the sitting to the horizontal supine position and by about half as much in the sitting to lateral decubitus transition. Head-down tilting causes only a marginal additional volume loss. The magnitude of these reductions is somewhat less in older than in younger patients. Conversion from the supine to the prone position is accompanied by an increase of resting lung volume of approximately 15%, with most of this change occurring in dorsal regions. Patients with airflow obstruction generally lose much less volume in supine recumbency (Fig. 18.1) (see Chapter 25).

Pulmonary hemodynamics also are influenced by position. Hydrostatic pressures and blood flows tend to distribute preferentially to the dorsal regions in the supine position. Recumbency redistributes lung volume, because it alters the geometry of the thorax. The heart tends to compress the left lower lobe bronchi and is supported partially by the lung tissue beneath. This anatomy helps account for the tendency for atelectasis to develop so commonly in the left lower lobe in postoperative and bedridden patients—especially those with cardiovascular disease. The pleural pressure adjacent to the diaphragm is considerably less negative than at the apex. The vertical gradient of transpulmonary pressure (alveolar minus pleural pressure) is $\approx$0.25 cm H_2O per cm of vertical height for normal subjects in the erect position

and $\approx$0.17 cm H_2O per cm for normal subjects in recumbency; alveolar volumes are greatest in the nondependent regions. For patients with edematous lungs, an intensified gravitational gradient of pleural pressure accentuates dorsal atelectasis and consolidation.

Available data indicate that the gradient of pleural pressure is considerably less in the prone than in the supine position, perhaps in part because of the shifting weight of the heart and mediastinal contents. The prone position also favors drainage of most airways. The lateral decubitus position causes the upper lung to assume a resting volume nearly as large as it has in the sitting position and to undergo better drainage, whereas the lower lung tends to pool mucus and is compressed to a size similar to or less than it has in the supine position. Positional losses of lung volume are considerably less in patients with airflow obstruction, in part due to gas trapping in dependent regions.

Distribution of Ventilation   During spontaneous breathing, ventilation distributes preferentially to the dependent lung zones in the supine, prone, and lateral positions. The normal subject also takes "sigh" breaths two to four times deeper than the average tidal volume approximately eight to ten times per hour. Postural changes occur frequently. Microatelectasis and arterial O_2 desatura-

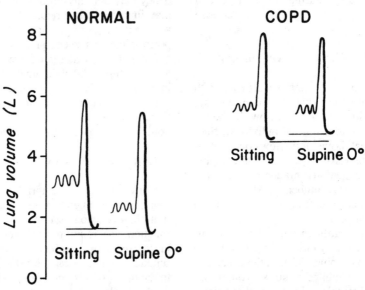

FIG. 18–1. Influence of recumbency on the spirograms of the normal subject and the patient with chronic obstructive pulmonary disease (COPD). Note that the marked positional drop in functional residual volume (FRV) is not matched by the change in residual volume in either instance. Patients with COPD may lose very little volume in the transition to the supine position.

tion tend to develop if breathing remains shallow and uninterrupted by these periodic sighs or variations of position. In contrast to spontaneous breathing, the nondependent regions receive the most ventilation when the patient is inflated passively by a mechanical ventilator. Dependent regions not only have the least end-expiratory (resting) lung volume but also receive less ventilation, further promoting atelectasis in those areas.

Positional Dyspnea Certain positions may relieve or exacerbate dyspnea. Orthopnea, although most emblematic of congestive heart failure, also characterizes severe airflow obstruction, pregnancy, extreme obesity, and diaphragmatic weakness. Conversely, patients with quadriplegia or extreme orthostatic hypotension and those who experience abdominal or back pain accentuated by the upright position may not tolerate sitting without breathlessness.

IMMOBILITY: PREVENTATIVE AND THERAPEUTIC MEASURES

Against the physiologic background just described, it is clear that prolonged immobility must be avoided. In profoundly weak or pharmacologically immobilized patients, range-of-motion exercises and high-top tennis shoes or foot boards may help prevent foot drop. As a rule, bedridden patients must be repositioned every 2 hours unless there is an important contraindication (e.g., hemodynamic instability). Inclining the upper torso above the horizontal plane (Fowler's, reverse Trendelenberg, sitting position) helps preserve vascular reflexes, limits the risks of esophageal reflux and aspiration, and reduces the tendency for peridiaphragmatic (basilar) atelectasis. The lateral decubitus and prone positions effectively stretch and drain the uppermost lung regions. Certain automated beds can effectively rotate the patient about the craniocaudal axis, in an attempt to ensure such benefits and preserve skin integrity (see Specialty Beds, below).

Skin Breakdown and Pressure Ulcers

Etiology

When local surface pressures exceed capillary pressure, the resulting ischemia can cause necrosis of the integument. Breakdown of the skin over pressure points is a common and costly problem for critically ill patients. Pressure ulcers tend to prolong hospitalization and increase morbidity.

The toll that skin breakdown takes is not easily measured, but it has been estimated that each year more than one million patients receiving treatment in an ICU are affected with pressure sores at a financial cost that may exceed five billion dollars. Although decubitus ulcers develop primarily in elderly patients, any patient with one or more of the major risk factors (high local pressure, increased shear force, friction, reduced capillary perfusion, anemia, malnutrition, tissue edema, or prolonged moisture exposure) can develop a pressure ulcer. Because mechanically ventilated patients often are sedated or paralyzed, malnourished, edematous, hypotensive, or confined to bed for lengthy periods, they are especially vulnerable.

Pressure ulcers are most likely to develop over bony prominences as compressive forces exceed the normal capillary filling pressure of ≈ 30 mm Hg for an extended period. Reduced perfusion pressure promotes ischemic injury. Relieving local pressure is especially important for patients in the prone position, when the nose, chin, shoulders, knees, and hips are the contact points rather than the broad surface of the back and upper legs. Pressure ulcers also can develop without sustained compression when the skin is subjected repeatedly to friction or shear or becomes macerated due to prolonged exposure to urine or feces.

Prevention and Treatment

Varied measures can be used to interrupt and reverse progression toward pressure ulceration (Table 18.3). Frequent repositioning and mobilization relieve local pressure and forestall skin breakdown. Massage of reddened skin and areas of bony prominence improves local circulation. Prevention of decubitus ulcers is one reason to avoid deep sedation or paralysis whenever possi-

---

TABLE 18–3

PREVENTION OF CUTANEOUS PRESSURE SORES

Avoidance of high local pressure

Avoidance of:
  Malnutrition
  Edema
  Maceration
  Ischemia

Mobilization

Topical coverings

Specialty mattresses and beds

ble. As already noted, adjustments of position occur frequently during sleep. Motionless patients should be repositioned no less frequently than every 2 hours, unless such manipulation disrupts wounds or other injuries, impairs oxygenation, or promotes hemodynamic instability. When frequent repositioning is not possible, careful padding of bony prominences can help prevent injury. Oscillating beds continually vary the gravitational forces applied to specific high-risk areas, decreasing the likelihood of skin breakdown (see below).

Preventing the development of pressure ulcers is much easier than treating established lesions. Once established, however, more than 100 topical products can be brought to bear. These are organized into several categories: wet gauze, ulcer-covering films (e.g., Tegoderm), foams (e.g., LYOfoam), hydrocolloids (e.g., DuoDerm), hydrogels (e.g., Carrington) and alginates (e.g., Sorbsan). Each product group claims superiority in specific settings and, because of the complexity of this topic, it is best to consult a wound care specialist for significant problems. In the healing process, the importance of optimizing nutritional status, of avoiding extended moisture exposure (especially that due to incontinence) and of early mobilization cannot be overemphasized.

For patients whose decubitus ulcers fail to heal despite these measures, infection of soft tissue or underlying bone is often responsible. To optimize healing, devitalized tissue should be debrided and appropriate antibiotics administered. Although the site of ulceration may influence the spectrum of flora recovered, infected wounds often contain a mixture of gram-positive cocci and gram-negative rods and anaerobes, making blanket antibiotic recommendations difficult. In non–life-threatening infections, cefazolin used in combination with gentamicin or ofloxicin may suffice. However, in most cases of serious infection, an extended-spectrum penicillin and an aminoglycoside or quinolone—with or without metronidazole—are necessary for complete coverage. Vancomycin usually is indicated when methicillin-resistant *Staphylococci* are likely.

Prevention of pressure sores for the comatose or immobilized patient emphasizes frequent turning, early mobilization, and avoidance of deep sedation or paralysis whenever possible. Prophylactic use of thick or quilted foam ("egg carton") or air-flotation mattresses should be considered for high-risk patients; they are effective preventative devices when used for short periods in patients exhibiting some spontaneous movement.

Adjunctive measures include maintenance of an adequate tissue perfusion pressure (avoidance of hypotension), prevention of malnutrition, and elimination of tissue edema. When pressure sores develop, consultation with a wound care specialist for appropriate topical treatment can help prevent the devastating complications of cellulitis and systemic sepsis.

Specialty Beds

Specialized beds such as the air-fluidized (Clinitron) bed and the low-air-loss (KinAir) bed have gained great popularity. Although both effectively prevent decubitus ulcers, neither has shown efficacy in healing established lesions. Air-fluidized beds rely on heated air circulated around glass beads covered by a polyester sheet. Although the circulating air may help evaporate edema, water loss and heating may be disadvantageous for febrile patients and those with impaired temperature regulation. Air-fluidized beds are unwieldy (weighing nearly one-half ton) and expensive (rental fees usually exceed $100 per day). Low-air-loss beds composed of inflatable pillows are available at roughly half of this cost. Because these beds are cooler, lighter, and less expensive, they have become used widely for patients at higher risk. To ensure that the high-risk patient receives decubitus prevention while simultaneously avoiding unnecessary use of this expensive technology, each ICU should establish specific guidelines for specialized bed use. Indications should be developed in consideration of the major risk factors already outlined.

Although costly to implement and still of unproven benefit, a variety of specialty beds seem to have a clear rationale, depending on the clinical setting. In addition to their capability to turn the patient automatically, many also enable fluoroscopy. Certain rotational beds percuss and vibrate as well as turn the patient, aiding in edema resolution and secretion clearance. Beds with segmented air cushion capability can help in a variety of settings in which skin breakdown is well established or imminent. Soft beds of this type are particularly helpful for patients who must be positioned prone for extended periods, as they both cushion the contact points and facilitate the "flipping" process. Massively obese patients may not be candidates for many of the specialty beds but can benefit from "chair beds," which allow easy transitions between the supine and upright postures.

ISOLATION PRECAUTIONS

In a busy ICU, transfer of communicable pathogens is facilitated by the variety and multiplicity of the interactions that occur between patient, family, and caregivers. Certain principles of infection prevention in the individual patient are detailed in Chapter 26. Frequently, patients will require special attention to avoid transmitting infections to themselves or to others. To protect staff and fellow patients, the need for isolation should be reconsidered frequently and ICU nursing staff should be notified immediately of isolation plans. Visitors as well as staff must adhere to hygienic guidelines.

Several levels of protection are used in most ICUs (Table 18.4): *Universal Precautions* require use of gloves with any direct patient contact, including handling of body fluids. They generally are recommended as the basal level of care for all patients in the ICU, but in reality, these standards are sometimes violated. Handwashing between patient contact is mandatory when gloves are not employed, because it is among the most effective simple measures for avoiding spread of communicable pathogens. The use of gloves does not entirely eliminate the need for handwashing; the warm, moist environment of the tight-fitting glove can serve as an effective incubator for small innocula of pathogens trapped beneath the fingernails, under rings, and between fingers. Relatively large innoculae can then be transferred via fomites, coworkers, visitors, or subsequent ungloved contact with patients.

Strict isolation demands the donning of gowns, gloves, and masks whenever entering a patient's room and removal of these items before exiting.

Respiratory isolation is observed in cases in which there is potential for airborne transmission of a dangerous, communicable pathogen. Well-fitting masks that meet a rigorous filtration standard (HEPA) are mandated or recommended in most hospitals for pathogens such as tuberculosis.

TABLE 18–4

CATEGORIES OF PROTECTION AND ISOLATION

Universal precautions
Isolation
  Strict
  Respiratory
  Contact
  Reverse

Isolation rooms for respiratory pathogens are designed for one-way (outside to inside) airflow to prevent dissemination of airborne pathogens to corridors and public areas.

Contact isolation requires the practitioner to take appropriate precautions (gloves, mask, and/or gown) when dealing with the affected area. Handwashing should follow glove removal.

Reverse isolation is employed for immunocompromised patients or at any time the clinician may transfer a communicable pathogen to the patient.

AMBIENT ENVIRONMENT

Modern ICUs recognize the need for critically ill patients to be cared for in a pleasant, temperature-controlled environment that encourages a normal sleep–wake cycle. Many units are required to provide visual access to the outdoors and appropriately ventilated and temperature-conditioned rooms. However, equipment and external temperatures during peak summer hours may cause even well-designed rooms to overheat. Such simple measures as drawing the shades during times of sunlight exposure and use of fans to improve air circulation can moderate any resulting discomfort.

Noise levels should be reduced whenever possible; gentle music provided via headphones or bedside radio may comfort the conscious patient. Earplugs should be considered for use during sleeping hours in unusually noisy (e.g., multipatient) rooms. In many instances, the volume of certain alarms can be muted safely at the bedside or "remoted" to the nursing station. Attempts to encourage a normal sleep–wake lighting and activity cycle may include "batching" of routine monitoring observations and patient manipulations, as well as the systematic use of hypnotics, analgesics, and anxiolytics when appropriate. The importance of adequate high-quality natural sleep cannot be overrated. Providing adequate sleep markedly diminishes the incidence of disorientation and delirium.

COMFORT MEASURES

Anxiety and pain occur almost universally in the ICU setting. The skillful team blends the use of anxiolytics with psychotropics, analgesics, physical measures, and concerted attempts to communicate. Vigilance to prevent or treat bladder and bowel distention, muscular skeletal discomfort, and pain arising from medication infusions (e.g., potassium, amphotericin, diazepam, bicarbonate, erythromycin) are essential. Slowing the rate of administration, coadministration with a more swiftly flowing diluent, local use of lidocaine, hydrocortisone (e.g., for amphotericin, ≈1 mg/mg of drug), or heparin (≈0.5–1.0 U/mL), and administration of the irritating fluid via a central vein are helpful strategies to minimize local pain. For certain medications, e.g., amphotericin, premedication with an antipyretic and antihistamine (e.g., diphenhydramine) can blunt the chills and fever that predictably accompany its administration.

Although benzodiazepines and opiates are used universally to reduce ongoing discomfort, haloperidol has been recognized as a valuable adjunct. Anxiety and pain reinforce each other; early intervention can pay high dividends in aborting a spiraling pain–anxiety cycle (see Chapter 17, Analgesia, Sedation, and Therapeutic Paralysis). Such simple measures as variation of body position, back rubs, and heating pads may make an important difference. It has been shown that directing a stream of air over the patient's face (using a fan) may reduce the sense of dyspnea even in intubated, mechanically ventilated patients.

GASTROINTESTINAL CARE

Impairment of gastrointestinal motility occurs frequently in critically ill patients, even in the absence of primary gastrointestinal disease. Prolonged abstinence from oral intake, dehydration, nasogastric suctioning, bed rest, opiates, and sedation slow gastrointestinal motility, especially in elderly patients. Simultaneously, air swallowing and/or fixed-rate enteral feedings encourage abdominal distention and impaired diaphragmatic excursion. On the other hand, mucosal atrophy, edema of the bowel wall, antibiotics, and alterations of the native gut flora encourage malabsorption and diarrhea. Strategies to cope with these disturbances emphasize mobilization and the institution of oral intake as soon as feasible. Enteral feedings given at a well-tolerated rate generally are preferred to parenteral nutrition. Bedside commodes are preferred to bedpans by many patients who otherwise would voluntarily retain and tend to obstipate. Appropriate hydration, stool softeners, bulk-forming agents, gentle enemas, laxatives, motility stimulants (e.g., metaclopromide, cisapride) and manual disimpaction are helpful options for problematic patients.

Copious diarrhea is a difficult management problem that carries the potential for nutritional depletion, electrolyte disturbances, and skin maceration (see Chapter 16, Nutritional Assessment and Support). Ointments and coverings serve as an effective barrier when skin breakdown is imminent. Although theoretically appropriate, fecal bags seldom work well, usually leak, and may be difficult to remove. When diarrhea is profuse and thin, rectal tubes may be inserted for brief periods. To avoid serious complications due to erosion of the rectal mucosa, the tube should be removed once per nursing shift. Balloon inflation generally is inadvisable.

BLADDER CARE

Although invaluable for precisely monitoring urinary output, Foley catheters should not be viewed as innocuous or inserted merely as a convenience. Periodic bladder drainage via a straight catheter and external collection apparatus are useful options when they are feasible to employ and continuous urinometry is not required.

DRESSING AND WOUND CARE

Dressings around central lines and arterial catheters should be changed every other day unless required earlier. These routine procedures usually are undertaken in the morning in conjunction with other hygienic maneuvers. (Dressings should not be allowed to remain soaked in wound drainage [blood, serum, pus].) Communication with the nursing staff will enable the interested physician to examine the wound at the time it is scheduled to be exposed, obviating unnecessary dressing changes.

TRANSPORTATION ISSUES

Transportation of the critically ill patient to a site outside the intensive care unit tends to be a complicated and somewhat hazardous process that requires coordination among multiple caregivers. Patients requiring studies outside the ICU (most commonly the central radiology department) must be well monitored, and all vital life support systems must be functional. Emergency drugs and supplies should be taken with the patient. Available transport monitors allow display of all important variables tracked at the bedside. As a rule, at least one ICU nurse is needed to observe the patient, to monitor cardiorespiratory function and to intervene rapidly if a difficulty arises. Two or more additional persons generally are required to maintain appropriate ventilation and move the bed, pumps, and ancillary equipment. Consequently, the nursing staff must know as early as possible about the need for and time of the intended transport.

Because of the considerable risk and resource commitment, it is wise to consolidate studies and interventions that take place outside the ICU if feasible. For example, a CT scan performed in search of an abscess or loculated effusion also should serve to guide catheter insertion by a radiologist or physician who is standing by, prepared to intervene. Sequential imaging procedures should take place during the same visit, whenever possible; it is not unreasonable to conduct CT scans in a predetermined exploratory sequence during the same transport episode when the patient is critically ill and several diagnostic possibilities are at hand. To judge the wisdom of proceeding to the next step, the physician must be available to make the appropriate decision to proceed with, extend, or abort the planned studies.

Unstable patients are not good candidates for transport, especially when extended elevator and hallway exposure is required. Stable patients can be manually ventilated successfully, with the help of oximetry and cardiovascular monitoring. A "mini-trial" of manual ventilation should be conducted at the bedside for several minutes before the actual move is attempted. More seriously ill, mechanically ventilated patients may require a specialized transport ventilator capable of maintaining the required ventilatory pattern.

With modern drainage systems, thoracostomy (chest) tubes present little difficulty in transport if no suction is required to keep the lung adequately inflated. If a reliable transport suction system is not available, for patients who are suction-dependent (e.g., those with large bronchopleural fistulae) a water seal should be attempted at the bedside for a duration similar to that projected for the transport before its execution during the "mini-trial" of transport ventilation—manual or automated. Prior arrangements should be made to reestablish suction drainage at the remote site.

COMMUNICATION

The experience of receiving intensive care is simultaneously isolating, frightening, and disorienting. Intubated patients cannot verbally express needs, sensations, or emotions. Familiar photographs, a clock plainly visible to the patient, and a readable calendar help maintain proper orientation. Although no strategy works effectively for all patients, caregivers should remain sensitive to the possibility of hearing or sight impairment. The fact that the patient normally wears a hearing aid or uses glasses may be forgotten in the highly charged, technology driven setting of the ICU. Alert patients may be able to express basic needs or pose questions via note writing, lip-reading or letter boards, or graphic charts. Close friends and family members may interpret gestures more effectively than the medical staff, especially if the patient has been chronically disabled. For patients with tracheostomies, cuff deflation or specialized tracheostomy tubes may permit adequate flow over the vocal cords. Vibrating devices that can be held over the hyoid region may allow the motivated patient to communicate effectively, but these instruments generally require a level of concentration and practice that cannot be elicited from the acutely ill patient. Communication with family members has been discussed previously in this chapter.

GASTROINTESTINAL ULCER PROPHYLAXIS

Before the availability of histamine antagonists of gastric acid production, aggressive enteral nutrition, and sucralfate, gastrointestinal bleeding resulting from stress ulceration frequently presented an annoying and occasionally a life-threatening problem (see Chapter 39, Gastrointestinal Bleeding). Fortunately, these complications currently are encountered much less frequently. Patients receiving effective enteral feeding seldom experience erosive stress ulcers and may not require special measures to forestall them. Whether acid inhibition encourages the overgrowth of bacteria within the stomach and thereby predisposes patients to aspiration pneumonia remains an unsettled and hotly contested issue.

LEG-CLOTTING PROPHYLAXIS

Trauma, recent surgery, sepsis, dehydration, immobility, venostasis, procoagulants, clotting factor aberrations, and a variety of other predisposing factors accentuate the tendency to form lower-extremity clots. Prophylactic interventions—both mechanical and pharmacologic—to prevent venous thrombosis in the lower extremities are indicated in most patients placed on bed rest in the ICU setting. Support stockings are used for otherwise mobile patients. Unusually high-risk patients may be given subcutaneous heparin or low-molecular-weight heparin unless there is an overriding contraindication (e.g., ongoing blood loss or coexisting risk of bleeding complication) (see Chapter 23, Venous Thrombosis and Pulmonary Embolism). Compressive "pneumo boots" are more effective than support stockings and do not present the risks of anticoagulants. They may, however, be uncomfortably warm or may result in skin breakdown in poorly nourished, edematous patients with circulatory insufficiency.

RESPIRATORY CARE

Few hospital services are as valuable to patient care as respiratory therapy (RT). However, RT often is applied indiscriminately, at substantial discomfort, morbidity, and financial cost. Respiratory care services are now under extraordinary pressure to become optimally cost effective, as hospitals face the constraints of prospective payment and managed care. Because the physician determines treatment type and intensity, understanding the indications and contraindications for RT procedures is vital to appropriate patient management (Table 18.5).

Procedures

Assisted Coughing

Encouraging the reluctant patient to cough productively is among the most effective services a therapist provides. Gentle external vibration of the cricoid cartilage may stimulate cough, as may deep breathing alone in patients with airways irritated by edema or inflammation. An ultrasonic aerosol of distilled water or hypertonic saline often is effective when other methods fail but must be administered cautiously and preceded by a bronchodilator to prevent bronchospasm.

Cooperative patients with cuffless or fenestrated tracheostomy tubes can be taught to cough

TABLE 18–5

RESPIRATORY CARE SERVICES

Assisted coughing

Deep breathing

Incentive spirometry

CPAP / Bi-PAP / IPPB

Chest percussion and postural drainage

Airway suctioning and hygiene

Bronchodilator administration

Oxygen therapy

effectively by momentarily occluding the tube orifice as a forceful effort is made against a closed glottis. Pressure can then build to a level sufficient to expel secretions through the pharynx upon glottic release. Many patients can be assisted by applying a pillow to splint painful areas of the abdomen or chest. Exhalation pressure can be increased in patients with quadriplegia by abdominal compression coordinated with the patient's spontaneous efforts. Mechanical devices are available to encourage effective coughing by pressurizing and depressurizing the air column.

Deep Breathing

Healthy individuals spontaneously take breaths that are two to three times greater than the average tidal depth multiple times per hour. Sighs to volumes approaching total lung capacity occur less often but are by no means unusual. Animated, uninterrupted speech also requires deep breathing. Many influences, including sedatives, coma, and thoracoabdominal surgery, abolish this pattern, encouraging atelectasis and secretion retention. Although the main purpose of deep breathing ("hyperinflation") is to restore prophylactic lung stretching, stimulation of a productive cough is an additional benefit for some patients. Useful deep breathing starts from FRC, ends at total lung capacity (TLC), and sustains inflation at a high lung volume for several seconds. Maneuvers that encourage exhalation rather than inhalation actually may be counterproductive.

Positioning of the patient is the most effective means of sustaining a higher lung volume in the nonintubated patient. In moving from the supine to the upright posture, a normal lung may experience a 500- to 1000-mL increase in volume, a change equivalent to 5 to 10 cm H_2O PEEP. Changing position of patients with unilateral disease may notably affect both gas exchange and secretion clearance. Turning is especially important for patients immobilized by trauma, sedation, or paralysis.

Incentive Spirometry, IPPB, CPAP, and Biphasic Airway Pressure

Several methods are used to encourage sustained deep breathing in nonintubated patients. An incentive spirometer is a device that gives a visual indication of whether the inhalation effort approaches the targeted volume. The frequency of deep breathing also may be tabulated. Unlike intermittent positive pressure ventilation (IPPB; described below), an incentive spirometer can be used by the cooperative, unattended patient. Furthermore, the distribution of ventilation tends to be more uniform than with IPPB. Although some devices measure inspiratory flow rate, it is better to measure inhaled volume. Units that reward flow are prone to misuse, because a high inspiratory flow rate can be achieved by low-amplitude, unsustained effort begun from a low lung volume.

IPPB aids the patient in deep inspiration by applying positive pressure via mask or mouthpiece (with nose clips). Although costly and formerly overprescribed, IPPB can be a useful intervention when employed in well-selected patients for brief periods. One valid use is to provide multiple deep breaths to a cooperative patient otherwise too weak to inhale a similar volume. (Effective IPPB is difficult to deliver to an uncooperative patient.) Unaccompanied by a meaningful increase in lung volume, positive pressure alone does little to forestall or reverse atelectasis. Recently, IPPB has yielded to noninvasive ventilation (e.g., biphasic or bi-level airway pressure [Bi-PAP]) and continuous positive airway pressure (CPAP; see Chapter 7, Indications and Options for Mechanical Ventilation).

Intermittent use of CPAP applied by a tight-fitting mask often succeeds in improving gas exchange. Its primary advantages are that little patient cooperation or personnel time are required and that the increment in lung volume is sustained, improving efficacy. Unfortunately, many patients most in need of CPAP and Bi-PAP cannot tolerate its sustained application. In these cases, the application of IPPB by a trained nurse or therapist may be worthwhile.

Bronchodilator Administration

Another reasonable use of IPPB is to administer an aerosolized bronchodilator to a nonintubated patient who cannot breathe deeply. For stronger, cooperative patients, a compressor-driven nebulizer provides a more effective method. Although suboptimal, a nebulizer used with a mouthpiece or simple face mask can be used to deposit a small amount of drug on the airways if no other method is feasible. Metered-dose canisters do not deliver the intended dose unless the patient coordinates the puff with the breathing cycle or a spacing chamber attachment is used. The latter is essential for marginally cooperative or maladroit hospitalized patients and may be comparable in efficacy to the compressor-driven method when a sufficient number of puffs are given through a spacing inhalation chamber. If the patient is mechanically ventilated, medication delivery is accomplished by nebulization into the inspiratory limb of the circuit. For patients with severe airflow obstruction, continuous nebulization may be more effective than episodic administration of the same total dose over the same interval.

Chest Percussion and Postural Drainage

The objectives of chest percussion and postural drainage (chest physiotherapy [CPT]) are to dislodge secretions from peripheral airways and to aid in clearance of sputum retained in the central airways. Vibration or hand percussion of the involved region is performed for 5 to 15 minutes, optimally with the involved segment(s) in the position of best gravitational drainage and with the postural drainage position maintained for an additional 5 to 15 minutes afterward. For well-selected patients with diffuse airway disease and copious secretions (e.g., cystic fibrosis or bronchiectasis), a vibrating inflatable vest powered by a compressor may be effective as an aid in secretion clearance. Bronchodilator administration should precede CPT, and deep breathing and coughing should be encouraged before, during, and after the 10 to 15 minutes of posturing.

These resource-intensive and intrusive methods are best reserved for patients with unusually copious secretions who can safely undergo them and empirically demonstrate unequivocal benefit. Patients who probably improve after treatment are those who retain secretions because of impaired clearance mechanics (e.g., airflow obstruction, neuromuscular weakness, or postoperative pain). Although CPT may benefit patients with acute lobar atelectasis, patients with a vigorous cough experience little benefit. CPT may be helpful for patients with pneumonia who are unable to clear secretions pooled in the central airways. Chest physiotherapy is appropriate in the intensive care unit setting, provided that hypotension, cardiac arrhythmias or ischemia, thoracic incisions, tubes, position limitation, rib fractures, or other mechanical impediments do not contraindicate its use.

Many patients experience dyspnea during chest physiotherapy, presumably due to increased venous return, positional hypoxemia, increased work of breathing, or decreased muscular efficiency in head-dependent positions. Available data warrant prophylactic oxygen supplementation and oximetric monitoring during and shortly after treatment.

TABLE 18–6
METHODS OF OXYGEN ADMINISTRATION

Nasal cannulae and catheters
Masks
  Open
  Closed
    Simple
    Partial rebreather
    Nonrebreather
    Venturi
  Tracheostomy dome
Sealed airway (endotracheal tube or tracheostomy)

Airway Suctioning

Nasotracheal suctioning serves two purposes: (*a*) to stimulate the coughing efforts that bring distal secretions to more proximal airways, and (*b*) to aspirate secretions retained in the central bronchi. Traumatic and uncomfortable, the airway must be suctioned sparingly, especially in patients with heart disease; associated vagal stimulation and hypoxemia can be arrhythmogenic. Inherently traumatic, hazardous, and less effective than a productive cough, tracheal suctioning should be performed only when a sputum specimen must be obtained or when ventilation or oxygenation is compromised by secretions retained in the central airways. A blindly placed suction catheter usually reaches the lower trachea or right main bronchus and recovers sputum from more distal airways only if cough propels sputum forward. Soft nasal "trumpets" facilitate retropharyngeal clearance and act as guiding channels to the glottic aperture (see Chapter 6, Airway Intubation). Shaped catheters favor cannulation of the left main bronchus. For mechanically ventilated patients, closed systems allow the simultaneous provision of PEEP.

Proper technique emphasizes hygienic but not rigidly sterile precautions. "Preoxygenation" is first accomplished by several deep inflations of pure oxygen. After the trachea is entered, the catheter is advanced 4 to 5 inches and then is withdrawn as intermittent suction is applied and released for no longer than 5 seconds. Several "hyperinflations" of oxygen are given before resuming the usual ventilatory pattern.

Methods of Oxygen Administration

Most patients admitted to the ICU will require supplementation of inspired oxygen. To apply this vital treatment most effectively, the clinician must be aware of the advantages, drawbacks, and limitations of each available technique (Table 18.6).

Nasal Cannulae (Prongs) and Nasal Catheters

Nasal prongs are perhaps the best choice for most applications requiring moderate oxygen supplementation. Continuous flow fills the nasopharynx and oropharynx with oxygen. These reservoirs empty into the lungs during each tidal breath, even when breathing occurs through a widely open mouth. One of the two prongs can be taped flat (or cut off and the hole sealed) without a notable change in FiO_2 allowing effective supplementation to continue despite the presence of an occlusive nasogastric tube, nasotracheal suction catheter, or bronchoscope in the other nostril. Nasal prongs allow an uninterrupted flow of oxygen while eating or expectorating and during procedures involving the oropharynx (such as suctioning and orotracheal intubation). Prongs taped in place reliably deliver oxygen to patients who tend to remove their face masks.

Rates of nasal oxygen administration vary from 0.5 to 8 L per minute, depending on clinical situation, duration of application, patency of the nasal canals, and size of the patient. At a fixed oxygen flow rate, the FiO_2 achieved depends on minute ventilation. Therefore, a "low-flow" rate of 2 L per minute may correspond to a low or moderately high FiO_2 depending on whether it is diluted with a large or small quantity of ambient air. For an average patient, 0.40 approximates the upper limit of FiO_2 achievable by this method.

The jet of oxygen dries the nasal mucosa, encourages surface bleeding, and may invoke pain in the paranasal sinuses at high flow rates. Oxygen must be humidified if given faster than 4 L per minute with two prongs or 2 L per minute with one prong. A non–petroleum-based lubricating jelly applied to each nostril is a useful prophylactic measure against local irritation.

A nasal catheter is a single perforated plastic tube advanced behind the soft palate. Somewhat more secure than nasal prongs, catheters deliver similar concentrations of oxygen. They are less popular than prongs because of greater irritation to nasal tissues, because location must be checked frequently and because the catheter must be alternated between nostrils every 8 hours.

Oxygen-conserving devices that inject gas only during inspiration have been introduced successfully to outpatient practice. Whether similar units will prove cost-effective in the hospital setting has not yet been determined.

Face Masks

Face masks can provide higher oxygen concentrations than are available with open tents and nasal devices but are inherently uncomfortable and less stable than other methods that deliver similar inspired fractions of oxygen (Fig. 18.2). Masks must be removed when eating and expectorating, allowing the oxygen concentration to fall during these activities. Unrestrained patients often dislodge them when agitated, dyspneic, or sleeping.

There are five common types of face mask: simple, partial rebreathing, nonrebreathing, open tent, and Venturi. Simple masks have an oxygen inlet at the base and 1.5-cm-diameter holes at the sides to allow unimpeded exhalation. Because the peak inspiratory flow rate usually exceeds the set inflow rate of oxygen, room air is entrained around the mask and through the side holes. Therefore, the FiO_2 actually delivered depends not only on the oxygen flow rate but also on the patient's tidal volume and inspiratory flow pattern. In an "average" patient, the oxygen percentage delivered by a simple mask varies from approximately 35% at 6 L per minute to 55% at 10 L per minute. The addition of short lengths of circuit tubing to each hole of the mask creates the appearance of "tusks," which act as T-piece oxygen reservoirs. At low flow rates, CO_2 can collect in the mask, effectively adding dead space and increasing the work of breathing.

The structure of the partial rebreather (reservoir) mask is virtually identical to the simple mask, but oxygen flows continuously into a collapsible reservoir bag attached to the base. If the mask is well sealed, the patient inspires from the bag when demand exceeds the constant line supply. Peak efforts draw less air from the room and a higher FiO_2 is achieved. The reservoir must be kept well filled; if the bag is allowed to collapse, the partial rebreather converts to a simple mask. Although these masks may make more efficient use of oxygen, the highest FiO_2 usually achievable with this device is approximately 0.65.

Nonrebreather masks are identical to partial rebreather masks, except for two sets of one-way valves. One valve set is placed between the reservoir and the breathing chamber so that exhaled gas must exit through the side ports or around the mask. The second valve set seals one or both side ports during inspiration in such fashion that nearly

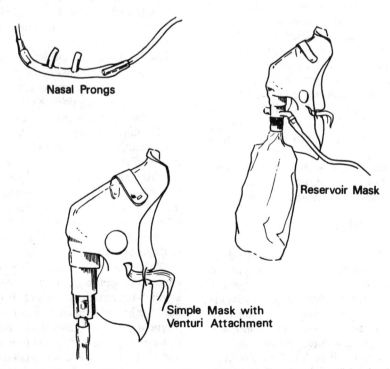

Nasal Prongs

Reservoir Mask

Simple Mask with Venturi Attachment

FIG. 18–2. Three types of oxygen delivery devices. (From: Marini JJ. Respiratory medicine for the house officer. Baltimore: Williams & Wilkins, 1987; 95.)

all inhaled gas is drawn directly from the oxygen reservoir. With a tightly fitting mask, inspired oxygen concentrations exceeding 80% can be delivered. Oxygen inflow must be high enough to prevent collapse of the reservoir bag. If collapse occurs, oxygen delivery rate would be insufficient to meet ventilation requirements, causing the patient to struggle against the one-way valves to entrain additional room air. Masks without a safety release mechanism could conceivably allow a weak or restrained patient to suffocate. Therefore, patients on nonrebreather masks should remain under direct observation.

Open-face tents can deliver either oxygen or mist and can serve a useful purpose for patients who will not tolerate tight-fitting masks or nasal cannulae. They allow the patient to communicate and expectorate easily but impede eating. The FiO_2 varies widely with the set flow rate, tent position, and minute ventilation. Inspired oxygen fractions cannot be boosted above approximately 0.6 because of entrainment of ambient air. With all of the methods of oxygen delivery discussed thus far, FiO_2 can vary depending on the patient's breathing pattern. In certain clinical situations, such as decompensated chronic obstructive pulmonary disease (COPD) with CO_2 retention, more precise control of FiO_2 may be desired.

Venturi masks provide a concentration of oxygen no higher than that specified. Oxygen is directed into a jet that entrains room air to flood the facial area with a gas mixture of fixed oxygen concentration. If the patient's peak inspiratory flow rate does not exceed the combined flow of the oxygen–air mixture, the FiO_2 will be the nominal value, provided that the mask fits snugly. Venturi masks are available to deliver selected oxygen percentages varying from 24 to 50%. Some masks allow rapid switching of the delivered concentration by adjustment of a collar selector, which changes the entrainment ratio.

Endotracheal Tubes

Any inspired fraction of oxygen can be delivered when a cuffed endotracheal tube prevents access to room air. If the patient is not connected to a ventilator circuit, humidified gas is administered either by a T-piece adapter or a tracheostomy tent. If no "tail" (wide-bore tubing) is attached to the T-piece adapter, the concentration of oxygen delivered will be less than that in the afferent tubing because of dilution by room air. A length of tubing attached downstream from the endotracheal tube orifice provides an inspiratory reservoir to counteract this effect without adding dead space. The length needed depends on the source flow rate and the patient's peak flow demand.

A tracheostomy mask is a small, open-domed hood that creates a tent-like area over the tracheostomy orifice. Some room air entrainment occurs, tending to reduce both humidity and FiO_2. The latter usually can be overcome by increasing the FiO_2. The tracheostomy mask is less unwieldly than a T piece and does not produce traction on the tracheostomy tube.

Humidification

During spontaneous normal breathing, humidification is accomplished by the well-vascularized mucosa of the nasal and oral passages. At normal rates of breathing, the nose is an efficient air conditioner, filtering out particles greater than 10 μm in size and completing the warming and humidifying process before gas enters the larynx. The mouth is somewhat less effective, especially at high minute ventilation. If humidification is not completed in the upper airway, water must be drawn from the tracheobronchial mucosa, causing desiccation, impaired mucociliary clearance, and thickened sputum.

Unlike ambient air (which is, on average, 50% saturated), medical gases contain no water vapor, so that the entire amount must be supplied. Unhumidified gas rapidly dries the nasal and oral mucosae. If the upper airway is bypassed, as by endotracheal intubation, drying of the sensitive lower tract occurs, with the attendant risk of infection and ventilatory impairment. The object of external humidification is to provide gas containing acceptable amounts of water vapor to the respiratory tract. Gas introduced at the tracheal level must be fully prewarmed and saturated. If the upper tract is not bypassed, humidity and temperature similar to those of ambient air suffice.

Without the upper airway bypassed, low flow rates of oxygen (e.g., up to 3 L by nasal prongs) admix with sufficient ambient air to preclude the need for humidification, unless the ambient environment is exceptionally dry. External humidification is required with higher flow rates by prongs and with masks that deliver moderate to high oxygen concentrations. For intubated patients, humidification can be accomplished by units that fully saturate the inspired airstream as it is warmed to near body temperature (32–37°C) (see Chapter 7, Indications and Options for Mechanical Ventilation). Heated wire circuits often are employed to maintain a nearly uniform temperature within the inspiratory tubing and thereby prevent airstream cooling and excessive "rain-out" of supersaturated water vapor.

In recent years, disposable hygroscopic filters placed in the common limb of the ventilator circuit have supplanted sophisticated mechanical humidifiers for many less demanding applications.

These "artificial noses" are designed to recover much of the exhaled moisture that otherwise would be lost to the atmosphere, releasing it to the inspirate. Such units economically serve the needs of patients without severe illness who have adequate breathing reserve and modest ventilation requirements. However, because they clog easily, impose dead space, and exhibit declining efficiency at high levels of ventilation, hygroscopic filters are less well suited to severely ill patients and those who have a high secretion burden or marginal ventilatory reserve.

KEY POINTS

1. Failure to systematically review the available database relevant to vital organ performance and prescribed therapy often leads to misinterpretation, inappropriate care plans, or ineffective communications among caregivers that translate into adverse outcomes or protracted hospital stays.

2. Although the ICU practitioner must intercede quickly and decisively when action is clearly necessary to avert disaster, in most circumstances, however, the clinician's prime objective should not be to reestablish "normal physiology" as quickly as possible but rather to encourage smooth resolution or adaptation to the pathophysiologic insult.

3. In the presence of uncertainty, conducting a closely observed "therapeutic mini-trial" is a key element in the successful management of fragile or unstable patients. After the evaluation has been completed and a course of action has been decided, the patient and physician are often well served by implementing the proposed change under close observation for a brief interval, before formalizing the order.

4. Uncertainty regarding the appropriateness and dose of certain medications (e.g., diuretics) often can be addressed, valuable time can be saved, and prescription errors can be avoided by communicating intent and writing goal-oriented orders when possible to do so.

5. Concerned family members may seek or be offered information from multiple caregivers with differing perspectives, knowledge, and attitudes, one or two physicians must be identified as the primary contact(s). It is wise to restrict routine visiting hours to no more than two predictably "quiet periods" in the day, especially in high-acuity ICUs. More frequent contact eventually confuses and exhausts the worried family, seldom benefits the comatose or sedated patient, and interferes with caregiving. Some well-functioning units reserve a specific hour each day during which the intensivist can be scheduled (by the unit clerk) to discuss progress and plans with interested family members.

6. Although certain consequences of protracted bed rest are well known to most practitioners, other more subtle repercussions are either unknown or ignored. Physiologic adaptations to gravity affect nearly all organ systems, and release from gravitational stress may set in motion changes that impede the recovery process. Unrelieved recumbency has particularly adverse implications for the respiratory, cardiovascular, and neuromuscular systems.

7. Bedridden patients must be repositioned every 2 hours unless there is an important contraindication. Motion about the gravitational plane (Fowler, reverse Trendelenberg, sitting positions) helps preserve vascular reflexes and reduces the tendency for peridiaphragmatic (basilar) atelectasis. The lateral decubitus and prone positions effectively stretch and drain the nondependent lung. Certain automated beds can effectively rotate the patient around the craniocaudal axis, in an attempt to ensure such benefits and preserve skin integrity.

8. Anxiety and pain occur almost universally in the ICU setting. The skillful team blends the use of anxiolytics with psychotropics, analgesics, physical measures, environmental modification, and concerted attempts to establish two-way communication. Attempts to encourage a normal sleep–wake lighting and activity cycle may include "batching" of routine monitoring observations and patient manipulations, as well as the systematic use of hypnotics, analgesics, and anxiolytics where appropriate. Early intervention and the synergistic use of psychotropics help alleviate pain and disorientation.

9. Aggressive respiratory therapy is essential to the care of patients with impaired lung expansion, retained secretions, and broncho-spasm.These techniques, which include reposi-tioning, deep breathing, coughing, inhalation of a bronchodilator, and chest physiotherapy, must be targeted to the specific problem at hand and employed only as long as they are unequiv-ocally indicated—either as prophylaxis or as a treatment of demonstrated benefit.

10. Oxygen supplementation can be accom-plished by nasal prongs and catheters, closed and open face masks, or a sealed airway (endo-tracheal tube). The selection is influenced by the range and precision of the FiO_2 required, patient tolerance, and the empirical response. The need for external humidification and the ef-ficiency of humidifier required is determined by the flow of oxygen delivered relative to the total minute ventilation, the proximity of the injector to the respiratory mucosa, and the need to by-pass the upper airway. Because disposable hygroscopic units clog easily, impose dead space, and exhibit declining efficiency at high levels of ventilation, they may be unsuitable for severely ill patients and for those who have a high secretion burden or marginal ventilatory reserve.

SUGGESTED READINGS

1. Allen V, Ryan D, Murray A. Potential for bed sores due to high pressures: influence of body sites, body position, and mattress design. Br J Clin Pract 1993;47(4):195–197.
2. Anonymous. Preoxygenation: physiology and practice (editorial). Lancet 1992;339(8784)t.
3. Guidelines Committee. Guidelines for the transfer of criti-cally ill patients. Am J Crit Care 1993;2(3):189–195.
4. Guidelines Committee of the American College of Critical Care Medicine. Guidelines for the transfer of critically ill patients. Crit Care Med 1993;21(6):931–937.
5. Arens R, Gozal D, Omlin K, et al. Comparison of high frequency chest compression and conventional chest physiotherapy in hospitalized patients with cystic fibrosis. Am J Resp Crit Care Med 1994:150(4):1154–1157.
6. Bach J. Update and perspective on noninvasive respiratory muscle aids. Part 1: the inspiratory aids. Chest 1994; 105(5):1230–1240.
7. Bach J. Update and perspective on noninvasive respiratory muscle aids. Part 2: the expiratory aids. Chest 1994; 105(5):1538–1544.
8. Barker A, Burgher L, Plummer A. Oxygen conserving methods for adults. Chest 1994;105(1):248–252.
9. Bernauer E, Yeager M. Optimal pain control in the inten-sive care unit. Int Anesthesiol Clin 1993;31(2):201–221.
10. Bone R, Hayden W, Levine R, et al. Recognition, assess-ment, and treatment of anxiety in the critical care patient. Dis Mon 1995;41(5):293–359.
11. Broccard A, Marini JJ. Effect of position and posture on the respiratory system. In: Vincent JL, ed. Yearbook of intensive care and emergency medicine. Berlin: Springer-Verlag, 1995; 165–184.
12. Carroll P. Bed selection: help patients rest easy. RN 1995; 58(5):44–51.
13. Ciesla N. Chest physical therapy for patients in the inten-sive care unit. Phys Ther 1996;76(6):609–625.
14. Day S. Intra-transport stabilization and management of the pediatric patient. Pediatr Clin North Am 1993;40(2):263–274.
15. Dealey C. Mattresses and beds. A guide to systems avail-able for relieving and reducing pressure. J Wound Care 1995;4(9):409–412.
16. Doering L. The effect of positioning on hemodynamics and gas exchange in the critically ill: a review. Am J Crit Care 1993;2(3):208–216.
17. Fenelon L. Protective isolation: who needs it? J Hosp In-fect 1995;30 (Suppl):218–222.
18. Ferrell B, Osterweil D, Christenson P. A randomized trial of low-air-loss beds for treatment of pressure ulcers. JAMA 1993;269(4):494–497.
19. Forshap M, Cooper A. Postoperative care of the thoracot-omy patient. Clin Chest Med 1992;13(1):33–45.
20. Fortney SM, Schneider VS, Greenleaf JE. The physiology of bed rest. In: Fregley MJ, Blatteis CM, eds. Handbook of physiology. New York: Oxford University Press, 1996; 889–939.
21. Garner J. Guideline for isolation precautions in hospitals. Part I: evolution of isolation practices. Hospital infection control practices advisory committee. Am J Infect Control 1996;24(1):24–31.
22. Gattinoni L, Pelosi P, Valenza F, Mascheroni D. Patient positioning in acute respiratory failure. In: Tobin MJ, ed. Principles and practice of mechanical ventilation. New York: McGraw-Hill, 1994; 1067–1076.
23. Gross N, Jenne J, Hess D. Bronchodilator therapy. In: Tobin MJ, ed. Principles and practice of mechanical venti-lation. New York: McGraw-Hill, 1994; 1077–1124.
24. Harris C, Wilmott R. Inhalation-based therapies in the treatment of cystic fibrosis. Curr Opin Pediatr 1994;6(3):234–238.
25. Hospital Infection Control Practices Advisory Committee. Guidelines for isolation precautions in hospitals. Part II: recommendations for isolation precautions in hospitals. Am J Infect Control 1996;24(1):32–52.
26. Inman K, Sibbald W, Rutledge F, Clark B. Clinical utility and cost-effectiveness of an air suspension bed in the pre-vention of pressure ulcers. JAMA 1993;269(9):1139–1143.
27. Jensen D, Justic M. An algorithm to distinguish the need for sedative, anxiolytic, and analgesic agents. 1995;14(2):58–65.
28. Jiricka M, Ryan P, Carvalho M, Bukvich J. Pressure ulcer

risk in an ICU population. Am J Crit Care 1995;4(5): 361–367.

29. Johnson C, Gonyea M. Transport of the critically ill child. Mayo Clin Proc 1993;68(10):982–987.

30. Levine J, Totolos E. Pressure ulcers: a strategic plan to prevent and heal them. Geriatrics 1995;50(1):32–37.

31. Mancinelli-Van Atta J, Beck S. Preventing hypoxemia and hemodynamic compromise related to endotracheal suctioning. Am J Crit Care 1992;1(3):62–79.

32. Marini JJ, Tyler ML, Hudson LD, Davis BS, Huseby JS. Influence of head-dependent positions on lung volume and oxygen saturation in chronic airflow obstruction. Am Rev Respir Dis 1984;129:101–105.

33. Martin JT. The Trendelenburg position: a review of current slants about head down tilt. AANA Journal 1995; 63(1):29–36.

34. O'Connor B, Vender J. Oxygen therapy. Crit Care Clin 1995;11(1):67–78.

35. O'Donohue W. Postoperative pulmonary complications. When are preventive and therapeutic measures necessary? Postgrad Med 1992;91(3):167–170.

36. Ostrow C, Hupp E, Topjian D. the effect of Trendelenburg and modified Trendelenburg positions on cardiac output, blood pressure, and oxygenation: a preliminary study. Am J Crit Care 1994;3(5):382–386.

37. Peruzzsi W, Smith B. Bronchial hygiene therapy. Crit Care Clin 1995;11(1):79–96.

38. Pierson DJ, Kacmarek RM. Foundations of respiratory care. New York: Churchill Livingstone, 1992.

39. Pontieri-Lewis V. Therapeutic beds: an overview. Medsurg Nursing 1995;4(4):323–324.

40. Reynolds M, Thomsen C, Black L, Moody R. The nuts and bolts of organizing and initiating a pediatric transport team. The Sutter Memorial experience. Crit Care Clin 1992;8(3):465–480.

41. Shannon M, Lehman C. Protecting the skin of the elderly patient in the intensive care unit. Crit Care Nurs Clin North Am 1996;8(1):17–28.

42. Sing R, O'Hara D, Sawyer M, Marino P. Trendelenburg position and oxygen transport in hypovolemic adults. Ann Emerg Med 1994;23(3):564–567.

43. Stannard C, Jones J. Neuromuscular blockade, sedation, and pain. In: Tobin MJ, ed. Principles and practice of mechanical ventilation. New York: McGraw-Hill, Inc., 1994; 1125–1148.

44. Szem J, Hydo L, Fischer E, Kapur S, Klemperer J, Barie P. High-risk intrahospital transport of critically ill patients: safety and outcome of the necessary "road trip." Crit Care Med 1995;23(10):1660–1666.

45. Takiguchi S, Myers S, Yu M, Levy M, McNamara J. Clinical and financial outcomes of lateral rotation low air-loss therapy in patients in the intensive care unit. Heart Lung 1995;24(4):315–320.

46. Terai C, Anada H, Matsushima S, Shimizu S, Okada Y. Effects of mild Trendelenburg on central hemodynamics and internal jugular vein velocity, cross-sectional area, and flow. Am J Emerg Med 1995;13(3):255–258.

47. Todres I. Communication between physician, patient, and family in the pediatric intensive care unit. Crit Care Med 1993;21(9 Suppl):S383–S386.

48. Traver G, Tyler M, Hudson L, Sherrill D, Quan S. Continuous oscillation: outcome in critically ill patients. J Crit Care 1995;10(3):97–103.

49. Venkataraman S, Orr R. Intrahospital transport of critically ill patients. Crit Care Clin 1992;8(3):525–531.

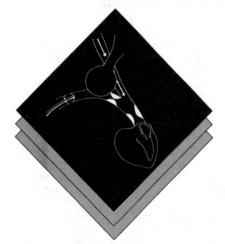

CHAPTER **19**

ICU Utilization and Cost Control

To many, "intensive care" equates with "expensive care." Unarguably, critical care is costly; a critically ill patient's life savings can be spent in hours, with costs now averaging thousands of dollars per day. The 5 to 10% of hospital beds used for critical care generate nearly one-third of all hospital charges; astonishingly, critical care expenses approach 1 to 2% of the gross national product. With the trend toward more care delivered in the outpatient setting, hospitals probably will become smaller with an even higher fraction of beds devoted to the care of critically ill patients.

Critical care is expensive for a variety of reasons, some influenced by patients and their families, some influenced by physicians, and some the result of the shear volume and complexity of the treatments provided. The aging population brings more problems to the hospital with each acute illness, making intensive care unit (ICU) admission ever more likely. It is not just elderly patients who are incurring ICU costs, however; the increasing frequency of traumatic injury and incidence of human immunodeficiency virus (HIV), predominately in the young, account for increasing demand for ICU care. Expanding numbers of middle-aged patients suffering the effects of lifelong smoking, alcohol, and obesity represent a large segment of the coronary care unit (CCU) and medical ICU populations. Finally, complications of aggressive immunosuppression for cancer

and transplant therapy place patients of all ages in the ICU.

Against the backdrop of increasing severe illness, the population has shown little restraint in their desire for critical care. The public perceives that miracles occur regularly in the ICU, and it seems that everyone wants their miracle if the need arises. This perception is not without some basis in fact: most large ICUs have mortality rates well under 20% despite a gravely ill patient group. Undoubtedly, a more realistic view of critical care by the public would help allocate the limited resources most effectively, but there is little evidence that the public perception is changing. Physicians who are not trained in critical care occasionally have unrealistic perceptions of the capabilities of the ICU.

Physicians and nurses also contribute to the high costs of critical care. Some of these costs are the result of well-intentioned desires to provide the best care possible; others are the result of inflexibility or ignorance. Some members of the medical profession share the view, along with much of the rest of society, that more is better. More diagnostic tests, more monitoring, more medicines, and longer stays all have been (consciously or unconsciously) equated with quality care. Furthermore, physicians have been rewarded financially, rather than penalized, for increasing use of ICU resources. Times are changing; we now recognize that more is not always better. More blood sampling eventually causes anemia, requiring transfusion with its attendant risks and costs. "Unnecessary" tests are likely to yield false-positive results, which then prompt more, expensive, and potentially dangerous tests. Higher numbers of radiographic studies expose patients and staff to more radiation, and all such studies are expensive. More medications increase the risk of an adverse drug reaction requiring diagnostic or therapeutic intervention. In particular, imprudent use of antibiotics increases the risk of an antibiotic-resistant infection, not only for the treated patient but for subsequent patients admitted to the ICU.

By focusing only on providing critical care, the medical profession generally has ignored its costs. Many practitioners have no idea what tests and treatments cost; and, even when aware of costs, some believe that no amount is too much to spend, provided that there is even the smallest chance of recovery. Although charges vary widely by region and hospital, Table 19.1 presents a realistic picture of the potentially staggering bill that can accrue on only the first day in the ICU. Moreover, this illustration does not include charges for emergency services, transportation, or physicians' professional fees.

The ICU, like the emergency department, must be constantly prepared to accept a nearly unlimited number of admissions at any time and must be prepared to provide a full range of services for these admissions. Most ICUs operate at approximately 85% capacity to satisfy this requirement for flexibility. In business terms, this excess capacity and its accompanying technology is

"wasted." Moreover, a perverse competition occurs as the hospital with the greatest range of services and amenities entices doctors to hospitalize patients in that facility, promoting geographic duplication of services. Regionalization of ICU care represents one solution to this problem of excess capacity, but without strong financial incentives, it is not likely to occur.

Tests and interventions are performed at a greater rate in the ICU than anywhere else in the hospital. Selecting which of these events are appropriate and reducing the rate at which unneeded interventions occur reduce cost. Thus, much of the discussion that follows focuses on methods of reducing use and eliminating waste. Unfortunately, rapid deployment of new operations, devices, and drugs, many of which have not been demonstrated to be sufficiently useful to justify their cost, inflate the price of care. It should be the role of the intensivist to be certain that new technology passes muster for safety, efficacy, and cost-effectiveness in well-designed clinical studies before being embraced. To fully grasp cost-control strategies, it is important to be able to distinguish costs from charges and to know the source of ICU expenditures.

DIFFERENCES BETWEEN COST AND CHARGE

Charges are easy to measure and are undoubtedly important. They are what patients and insurance companies pay and, at the hospital level, are the major determinant of the success or failure of attempting to secure contractual relationships to care for groups of patients. Charges do not track costs for several reasons. First, the cost of providing care for a specific diagnosis has multiple components, many of which, like utility or capital equipment costs, cannot be itemized but must be passed along to patients. Hence, arbitrary charges are set that vastly exceed the true "cost." Second, a large fraction of patients do not pay all or any of their bills, and these business losses are recovered from private paying or insured patients. Third, some treatment options are so costly or used so rarely that no patient could bear his or her true share of the cost. Therefore, charges are distributed, or "shifted," to other patients who do not receive the service to ensure that the treatment remains available. For example, helicopter/air ambulance service is so expensive that users of the service cannot bear the cost by themselves.

TABLE 19–1

ITEMIZED TYPICAL ICU FIRST-DAY CHARGES*

Item	Charge
Room	$ 800.00
"Routine" admission laboratories	500.00
Blood, sputum, and urine cultures	225.00
Electrocardiogram	50.00
Portable chest radiograph	150.00
Foley catheter, urine meter	50.00
Mechanical ventilator	700.00
Noninvasive monitors (oximeter, blood pressure cuff)	100.00
Intravenous pump, tubing, and maintenance fluid	225.00
One intravenous antibiotic	150.00
Pulmonary artery monitoring catheter, insertion sets, tubing, fluids	900.00
Simple sedative, analgesic regimen	100.00
	~$4000.00

* Exclusive of physician fees.

This cost shifting is manifest as inflated charges for more commonly used therapies (e.g., "the $5 aspirin"). Moreover, certain high-volume services may be targeted as high revenue generators. Finally, over time, insurers and hospitals have come to agreement on "reasonable and customary charges" for services that do not even remotely reflect cost.

Patient charges for a service, especially drug treatment, can differ greatly from the hospital's acquisition cost for that drug because of the introduction of labor costs. For example, ampicillin is a very inexpensive antibiotic to purchase; the cost for a day's supply of the intravenous form is probably less than $10.00. Why then is the daily patient charge likely to exceed $100.00? How could this drug be more expensive per day than an antibiotic costing 50 times as much per dose? The answers lie in the dosing schedule and costs of drug preparation. The less expensive compound may require more frequent administration and laboratory monitoring. In the end, the patient is charged much more for this "less expensive" drug because of the labor costs associated with repeatedly measuring, mixing, transporting, infusing, and monitoring the drug. The bottom line is that in today's environment, costs do not equate with charges, and many hidden charges exist in prescribing a course of drug therapy; therefore, the cost of the entire therapeutic package must be considered.

WHERE THE MONEY GOES

Fertile targets for cost reduction come from examining the pattern of ICU spending (Fig. 19.1). Well more than half of the money spent goes to labor costs (the largest portion of which are nursing salaries). About 10 to 15% of expenditures pay physicians; a similar amount is divided among other support personnel. It would be easy to say that fewer or less well trained nurses (or physicians) is the answer, but generally you get

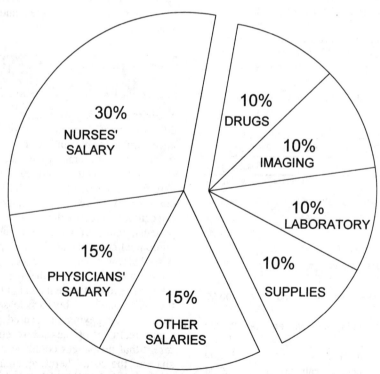

FIG. 19–1. Typical distribution of intensive care unit spending. The majority (approximately 60%) of expenses are labor costs—in large part those necessary for constant bedside nursing. Costs for drugs, imaging procedures, laboratory studies, and supplies vary by individual patients, but each category averages about 10% of total expenses. This figure highlights the difficulty associated with significant cost reduction—substantial saving usually requires reducing personnel and risks lowering the quality of care.

what you pay for. Lower pay usually means less experience, and few believe that quality care can be delivered with much fewer nurses or physicians or a less well qualified staff. Using lower paid physician assistants or primary care physicians to provide critical care does not seem tenable, considering the complexity of the patient population and time requirements. As highly skilled and paid nurses are replaced with less expensive "care extenders," quality of certain essential ICU features may deteriorate. This process may have an unforeseen effect on professionalism, morale, and other difficult-to-quantify factors that reduce the efficacy and efficiency of care delivery. Furthermore, forcing health care professionals to undertake tasks for which they have little interest, training, or experience is demoralizing and accelerates staff turnover. These problems can offset any potential cost saving and, over time, staff retraining becomes necessary. "Cross-training" ICU employees to perform a variety of tasks (e.g., food service, transport, phlebotomy, bathing, inventory, maintenance, housekeeping) can reduce the total number of employees, but the reduction of lower paying jobs results in little net cost savings. For the near future, major reductions in the single largest area of expenditure, labor costs, seem unlikely.

A portion of ICU charges pass to the hospital to maintain the physical plant, durable equipment, required infrastructure (radiology, laboratory, etc.), and administrative staff and to provide a profit. The extensive administrative structure of managed care organizations and hospitals raises concerns that *real* cost savings will not happen; instead, funds will be redirected from patient care to administration. Although many methods of hospital-wide cost reductions are possible, they are well beyond the scope of this text.

RADICAL COST CONTROL MEASURES

Sadly, most cost control measures that do exist have been arbitrary and externally imposed, rather than being thoughtfully, internally fashioned. Regardless of the source of the spending restraint, quality will suffer if cost becomes the major determinant of care. The most effective way to reduce overall hospital costs is to reduce length of stay; the same is true for the ICU. The most obvious, radical, and possibly effective cost-control strategies (rationing admission, limiting duration of support, or prohibition of certain therapies) are

not now, and may never be, palatable to the public or to conservative physicians. Ideally, improved therapeutics would shorten the ICU stay, resulting in a salutary effect on cost without such policies. Unfortunately, few dramatic therapeutic advances have occurred; success has come haltingly. In the absence of dramatic advances in care, we are left with less grand cost-control strategies: making optimal use of available beds, minimizing labor costs, improving efficiency of care delivery, and reducing equipment, imaging, laboratory, and drug expenditures.

ICU ORGANIZATION STRATEGIES

THE ICU DIRECTOR

The first step in a quality improvement/cost reduction plan is to provide a respected, competent, experienced leader devoted to providing high-quality care. An absentee "figurehead," who is uninvolved and uninterested in the internal daily workings of the ICU, is an extremely costly employee in terms of direct compensation and lost opportunity to the ICU itself. The director plays a vital role in smoothing patient admission, discharge, and transfer; in establishing standard policies and procedures; and in assembling a competent, effective, and efficient team. Ideally, cost reduction is a byproduct of improved quality and efficiency. For cost reduction to succeed, the ICU director must remain open to cost-control solutions and must have the authority to change practice by establishing policy.

ADMISSION AND DISCHARGE CRITERIA

To ensure that adequate resources are available to treat salvageable critically ill patients while costs are minimized, admission and discharge criteria must be established. These criteria should minimize the number of "unnecessary" admissions and minimize safe length of stay. Admissions only for "observation," in which no specific ICU intervention occurs, are probably most wasteful. Despite being at very low risk, patients who are admitted for observation still consume substantial resources and block access to the ICU for more seriously ill patients. This group, although fully deserving of close observation, should not occupy beds better used for those requiring treatment. Furthermore, it is intuitively obvious that such low-risk patients cannot experience an incremental benefit in outcome from ICU care because their prognosis is excellent to begin with. Stable postoperative patients and patients with nonserious drug ingestion comprise most of this group. The propriety of ICU admission for moribund patients or patients of very advanced age who choose not to undergo intubation, invasive monitoring, or resuscitation because of personal, family, or physician preference is also questionable. Clearly, not all patients destined to die must do so in an ICU.

Interestingly, cost reduction is not always best achieved by keeping patients out of the ICU. Early admission of seriously ill, deteriorating patients can avert costly complications. For example, delaying ICU transfer until a patient with pneumonia experiences a cardiopulmonary arrest on the floor is bad medicine and ends up costing *more* to reverse multiple postarrest complications. Likewise, premature discharge from the ICU can result in a "bounce back"—a clinical event that is often costly or fatal. Moreover, there obviously are times when patients not requiring the "technology" of the ICU are appropriately admitted for intensive nursing care or pain control.

TRIAGE

There never seem to be enough beds in the ICU to meet peak demand, and a policy of "first-come first-served" rarely provides an equitable solution to the problem of limited resources. Because each physician views (and should view) his or her own patient to be the most deserving of an ICU bed, someone must prioritize need and adjudicate disputes. Thus, when the ICU is at 100% occupancy, it is important to have a triage officer to judge the severity of illness of both current ICU occupants and potential admissions. The triage function is best performed by an experienced critical care physician, because although nurses usually have more than sufficient medical knowledge, they rarely have the political clout necessary to say "No." Triage problems are minimized when only a small number of trained critical care physicians admit patients to the ICU (a "closed unit") and maximized when physicians with little ICU training or experience control the process. When the triage feature is absent, the most powerful, belligerent, or persistent physician's patient usually gets the bed—not necessarily the patient who needs it most. In some hospitals, the emergency department physician determines the destination of each

emergency room (ER) admission, but obviously this practice is flawed because the ER physician cannot be intimately familiar with the condition of all other patients in the ICU. Furthermore, possibly the worst-case scenario occurs when a patient at another hospital is directly admitted "sight unseen," by any physician accepting the transfer.

THE ROLE OF THE INTENSIVIST

Physicians who admit patients to the ICU must be thoroughly trained, experienced, and available. Fewer than one in 20 ICUs has a senior physician present around the clock, and less than one-third of all ICUs have continuous "resident"-level coverage. Despite the popularity of having all services provided by a "primary care practitioner," critical care is not just internal medicine, pediatrics, or general surgery "plus some procedures." The ICU poses a wide range of potentially lethal problems and employs sophisticated technology to which the primary care provider has limited exposure. Furthermore, a busy office practice or operating room schedule is incompatible with providing quality critical care. Intensive care cannot be delivered "long distance" or by a "which doctor" (i.e., an off-site practitioner who knows "which doctor" to call for a particular problem). When critical care is practiced by such consultation, each consultant responds at a pace dictated by his or her schedule and communication between consultants and the primary physician is often poor.

Limited studies to date indicate that a closed unit and the presence of a trained critical care physician (staffed) reduces length of stay, mortality, *and* cost. The reason(s) for these findings are speculative but probably relate to several factors. First, ICU physicians are on site and have a breadth of experience allowing them to anticipate and preempt serious problems before they are morbid, fatal, or costly. For example, subtle increases in airway pressures and modest declines in saturation or blood pressure at the bedside may signal the presence of an early pneumothorax that can be successfully treated long before it results in serious injury. But these same findings are not likely to be recognized by a "long distance" physician.

Second, the dedicated intensivist provides important standardization of care among patients. Examples abound: when no standards exist, deep venous thrombosis prophylaxis is inconsistent in method and application. When a different method is ordered for every patient, it is likely that the therapy will be overlooked in some and ineffective in others. There, usually, is a "best" way to treat the "average" patient. Furthermore, a strong case can also be made that a dedicated intensivist is more likely to be consistent in the care of each patient over time. Knowledge of what treatments have succeeded or failed recently leads to more efficient and less costly care. In an era in which both patient and staff turnover is rapid, well-crafted policies and protocols are essential to maintain a consistent level of quality care.

Finally, with little supporting data, it is likely that the on-site critical care physician is less likely to summon multiple, possibly unnecessary, consultants. Excessive consultation may be inefficient, costly, and potentially dangerous when care is directed by a physician who "practices" by consultation. In this setting, it is possible for numerous, often redundant, diagnostic tests to be ordered as subspecialists attempt to justify their involvement by searching for obscure conditions. An even worse situation occurs when the therapeutic goals of the consultants are at odds or when one consultant is oblivious to the recommendations and thoughts of another. In this situation, competing or potentially harmful combinations of therapy are prescribed. For example, for a febrile cirrhotic patient with ascites, the surgical consultant orders a contrasted computed tomography (CT) scan, the infectious disease specialist initiates an aminoglycoside, and the cardiologist institutes aggressive diuresis and volume restriction. All too often, the result is not good care but renal failure.

One experienced physician should make the decisions and direct therapy with the input of necessary consultants. The intensivist best fits this role and the essential function of communicating with the physicians who provide ongoing care of the patient outside the hospital. Because of the nature of the ICU, decisions must be made quickly and often with incomplete information. An intensivist's experience in the stressful ICU environment tends to provide a greater level of comfort with the inevitable diagnostic uncertainty that can avoid excessive consultation, diagnostic tests, and unnecessary therapy.

Perhaps no one is better attuned to the potential and limits of the ICU than the intensivist, the person who is most likely to identify patients who cannot benefit from ICU care because they either are not sufficiently ill or are not salvageable. Un-salvageable patients are not well served by staying in the ICU, where they often suffer isolation from family and friends and pay a high financial price. Even with all of the difficulty in determining what is "futile" care, reasonable limits can be developed. The bounds of support are best developed on a case-by-case basis. The intensivist is the best person to guide the patient and family in developing these limits by having honest, open, and recurring discussions of expectations. Regular, preferably daily, consultation with the patient and family are important to maintain common goals. Ideally, the discussions of prognosis are initiated early in the ICU stay. Such consultations often require 30–60 minutes per patient each day, a level of additional work that few physicians with responsibilities outside the ICU can accomplish.

THE TEAM APPROACH

An automobile journey would prove to be long and expensive if there were no clear destination or defined route and numerous people took turns driving. In the same way, successfully negotiating the route through the ICU becomes expensive if all of the potential "drivers" do not understand the route or destination. For most of the day, the bedside nurses "drive," and if the plan and priorities are not clear, a wandering route is likely. For the ICU patient, this confusion is manifest as redundant or irrelevant laboratory testing, inappropriate therapeutic interventions, or missed critical opportunities. Examples include: sending a serum pregnancy test for a patient with an intrauterine pregnancy previously determined by ultrasound; giving diuretics to an oliguric patient with a right ventricular myocardial infarction to "reduce" the high central venous pressure; or missing a small window of opportunity for weaning from a ventilator because a patient receives a paralytic drug or does not have tube feeding discontinued. The only solution to such problems is to have an involved senior physician, acting in concert with all members of the ICU team, execute a carefully constructed plan. One good way to make this happen is to require participation of all team members (physicians, nurses, pharmacists, social workers, case managers, and respiratory, occupational and physical therapists) in daily work rounds. New problems and major organ system function should be reviewed. Diagnostic information gained since the previous day and its implications should be discussed. Changes in therapy should be agreed upon (not just what to do, but in what order to do it, with contingency plans for unexpected events). Appropriate information to be communicated to the patient, family, and referring physicians should be discussed, and plans for transfer or discharge should be finalized. Following these steps all but guarantees that members of the team move efficiently in the same direction. This cooperative process offers the physician in charge the most information upon which to make decisions; and, as a major benefit, the staff becomes more cohesive, educated, happy, and respectful of one another.

SPECIFIC COST-CONTROL SUGGESTIONS

REDUCING IMAGING COSTS

Imaging studies account for 10 to 20% of an ICU patient's hospital charges. Thus, reducing the number of radiologic studies can dramatically affect cost; this reduction can be accomplished in several ways: (*a*) eliminating inappropriate portable studies that are essentially never diagnostic because of their poor technical quality (e.g., sinus studies, bone films); (*b*) for stable patients, reducing the frequency of "routine" studies, especially the portable chest radiograph; (*c*) when two options of comparable quality and cost exist, using the one that can be performed in the ICU; (*d*) optimizing scheduling to minimize the number of trips to the radiology department; (*e*) using required visits to the radiology department as an opportunity to substitute higher quality images for less optimal portable studies; (*f*) when a diagnostic study is performed in the radiology suite, it should be interpreted immediately so that additional views, complementary imaging studies, or therapeutic intervention can be performed without a second visit to the department. (This mandates the ready availability of a physician decision-maker.)

Overall, the portable chest radiograph is the most common and costly radiographic procedure for most ICU patients. As discussed in Chapter 11, the portable chest radiograph provides vital information but has many limitations. Unless imaging guidelines are established, most ICU patients undergo one to two portable chest radiographs each day at a charge of $200 to $400. Although the chest radiograph usually is abnormal

in ICU occupants, in stable patients, abnormalities are often insignificant or are equally evident through other less costly means and the monitoring that nearly all receive, such as the physical examination. When hemodynamic and respiratory status is stable, typically 2 to 3 days after admission, the practice of ordering "routine" daily chest radiographs should be reconsidered. A justification commonly given for daily chest radiographs is the necessity to evaluate endotracheal tube position. However, because the chest radiograph images less than 1 second of each day, that argument rings hollow and obviously loses validity for patients with a much more stable nasotracheal or tracheostomy tube in place. Paradoxically, the very act of obtaining the radiograph may displace the tube as the patient is repositioned (see Chapter 6, Airway Intubation). A policy of not performing "routine" daily chest radiographs for stable patients (even those on mechanical ventilators) seems to be safe and can reduce imaging costs by up to one-third for the average patient. Obviously, a significant change in cardiopulmonary status should prompt consideration of a chest radiograph, as should insertion or manipulation of tubes or catheters. Practically, even when "routine" films are not obtained, patients are likely to have at least one chest radiograph each day because of changing physiology or insertion of monitoring devices.

Other potential cost savings can be realized when patients must leave the ICU for an imaging study. Substantial manpower and charges and some risk are associated with transporting patients to the ICU—at least one report suggests savings of $300 to $500 per trip for transport charges alone. Regardless of the true cost, it makes sense to make this trip as few times as necessary. When a diagnostic study can be performed in the ICU using portable equipment with comparable quality to that performed in the radiology department, opting for the portable examination avoids transport cost, risk, and inconvenience. One common example would be the search for gallstones or biliary obstruction, in which portable ultrasound and department-based CT scan are both viable options but the portable study offers substantial cost advantage. Arranging several studies to be performed in the radiology department during the same visit is also cost effective. For example, if plans exist to perform an elective chest CT today and head CT tomorrow, it is reasonable to consider rescheduling to accomplish both in a single trip.

DISPOSABLE EQUIPMENT SAVINGS

Equipment savings can be substantial if stocking is well planned. Almost all disposable equipment (e.g., sutures, dressings, sterile trays, intravenous catheters, suction catheters) has an expiration date. None of these items are inexpensive, and careful inventory will often reveal that much is discarded because it "expired" without ever being used. The justification for continued stocking of seldom-used items is often "we needed it once." Don't do away with immediately essential equipment, but reconsider all materials stocked. Limit the variety and quantity of supplies to a safe level that minimizes waste. For example, many different sizes and types of tracheal suction catheters or pulmonary artery monitoring catheters are not necessary. Likewise, it is not necessary to have immediately available every type and size of suture and needle. Take stock of what is used regularly, and what is rarely used but must be available immediately. Stock only those items, and stock them in reasonable quantities. In some cases, expanding the inventory can be cost effective. For example, the guidewires used to insert central venous catheters frequently become contaminated during line insertion. If individual replacement wires are available, an entire new "central line kit" does not have to be opened. For the average ICU, annual savings of tens of thousands of dollars can be realized with no decrement in quality of care.

RESPIRATORY THERAPY STRATEGIES

Some types of respiratory care equipment are ineffective or obsolete. "Room humidifiers" do not augment the water content of tracheal gas and provide little if any benefit for patients with sinus disease. They do, however, generate a substantial patient charge and, more importantly, present a potential source of nosocomial infection.

Another simple, effective cost-control measure involves the process of weaning and extubation. For many patients, "weaning" is not a complex or prolonged process—mechanical support is removed temporarily and, if well tolerated, extubation is performed. Three simple measures can decrease the cost.

1. Avoid "T-piece" weaning unless absolutely necessary. Charges for the T-piece equipment and labor charges for setup are often substantial; instead, use the continuous positive airway pressure (CPAP) mode of the ventilator. When necessary, CPAP can be combined with a low level of pressure support to overcome intrinsic resistance of the ventilator circuitry. For most patients, no significant increase in work of ventilation is realized in breathing through well-adjusted ventilator circuitry, and the machine provides the advantage of an "apnea alarm."

2. At the time of extubation, charges can be reduced further by immediately placing patients on nasal cannula oxygen rather than some variety of mask or face tent. In common practice, the mask is discarded within minutes or hours in favor of a nasal cannula anyway. Going directly to the cannula avoids the cost of the equipment and the respiratory therapist's time. Obviously, patients extubated from high FiO_2 and those with conditions that would impede oxygen flow through the nose would be poor candidates for such a strategy.

3. Finally, once the patient is extubated, remove the ventilator from the room if safe to do so. When not connected to the patient, the ventilator offers little more than expensive psychological comfort. Many hospitals charge ventilator fees in 12- or 24-hour blocks, and if the ventilator is still in the room, the patient probably will be charged (often several hundred dollars) for unneeded equipment.

DRUG COST-REDUCTION STRATEGIES

Medications represent a large potential area for cost savings. Numerous cost-control strategies are outlined in Chapter 15 (Medication Administration), but a few specific suggestions will be reviewed briefly here.

1. Review the Medications List on a Daily Basis

Discontinue unneeded medicines and alter therapy to avoid adverse drug reactions. Regular systematic review of medication lists usually is revealing. Very commonly, patients are receiving more medications than the physician realizes, and one or more of these drugs may no longer be necessary. This problem is magnified greatly when multiple consulting physicians are allowed to write orders for medications. Not uncommonly, review of the medication list reveals a drug or drug interaction responsible for a major therapeutic problem. It is also likely that several drugs, probably prescribed at different times and often in suboptimal doses, are being used to treat the same problem. (Sedatives, analgesics, and antibiotics are the most common offenders.) Daily medication review also prompts the adjustments in dosage necessary to cope with the constantly changing organ function of the critically ill patient. Including a pharmacist in daily rounds is helpful to suggest alternative, less costly strategies and to point out potential drug interaction problems.

2. Use Generic Medications Whenever Possible

Generic equivalents are always less expensive, and the good business practice of competitive bidding further reduces costs. Establishing an automatic substitution program in which the least expensive therapeutically equivalent compound is substituted for a brand name medication also dramatically reduces costs. Excellent areas in which to realize these savings are with some antibiotics (e.g., quinolines, third-generation cephalosporins), histamine blockers, sedatives (especially the benzodiazepines), and the nondepolarizing neuromuscular blockers. The process of therapeutic substitution requires involvement of a proactive pharmacy committee and consensus of local experts that the substitutions are truly "equivalent."

3. Establish a Restricted Formulary

Reducing the number of medications stocked in the pharmacy and the number of staff members who can prescribe expensive or possibly dangerous medications has numerous benefits. Pharmacy size is reduced, fewer personnel are necessary to track and stock medications, and waste is reduced as fewer expired drugs need to be discarded. Costs and complications of medications (especially those particularly dangerous or expensive) are reduced when used by experienced physicians. In this restrictive process, however, a multidisciplinary pharmacy committee must remain open to well-reasoned arguments for formulary additions or exceptions. A mechanism must exist for waiver of formulary rules under exceptional (emergency) circumstances. Common examples of drugs that can be restricted rationally to especially qualified practitioners include cancer chemotherapeutic agents, thrombolytic drugs, inhala-

tional anesthetics, and neuromuscular blocking drugs.

4. Establish Specific Recommendations for Use of Expensive or Dangerous Medications

Excellent areas for drug practice guidelines include use of sedatives, paralytic agents, some antiemetics, and antibiotics. Examples include the following: generally encouraging the use of diazepam or lorazepam over midazolam or propofol for sedation; promoting the use of pancuronium for most situations in which long-term paralysis is needed. (As pointed out in Chapter 17, paralytic agents constitute a class of drugs in which limiting physician access to some of the "niche" drugs can prevent physical and economic damage.)

Development of hospital-specific antibiotic guidelines that include appropriate initial choices and suggestions for duration of therapy is prudent. Requiring infectious disease consultation for decisions regarding side effect prone, or expensive antimicrobial therapies (e.g., gancyclovir, intravenous fluconazole) also makes sense.

5. Switch Parenteral Drugs to an Oral Route for Patients with a Functioning Gastrointestinal Tract

Equivalent doses of oral medications usually are between one-tenth to one-hundredth the cost of the same medication given parenterally. Essentially all patients eating or successfully receiving tube feeding can receive enteral medications. In fact, many medications (including benzodiazepines, narcotics, and some antibiotics) achieve equal blood concentrations when given orally or by the i.v. route (see Chapter 15, Medication Administration).

6. Avoid Continuous Infusion of Medications Whenever Possible

The belief that giving medications by continuous i.v. infusion automatically confers precise control over drug effects is fallacious, even when the practice achieves precise regulation of plasma drug levels. Exact titration of a plasma drug level is rarely necessary or achievable, and drug levels often do not correlate with effects. Critically ill patients commonly have such altered pharmacodynamics that "short-acting drugs" have prolonged actions. Accumulation of medications given by continuous infusion is frequent enough to be considered routine (lidocaine, fentanyl, theophylline, and midazolam are prime examples). Continuous i.v. infusion is the most expensive method of administration, because a dedicated i.v. line, infusion pump, and specialized cassettes and tubing, all of which are expensive, are required. Also, each i.v. line increases the risk of infection, and the mere presence of an i.v. line in a patient with fever is likely to prompt an expensive fever evaluation and empiric antibiotic therapy. Furthermore, if a central venous line must be inserted to maintain an infusion, the risk of infection persists, and the risks of arterial puncture and pneumothorax are incurred.

8. Avoid Parenteral Nutrition Unless Enteral Feeding is Impossible

Enteral feeding offers many advantages over parenteral nutrition, as outlined in Chapter 16, Nutritional Assessment and Support. Physiologically, preservation of gut mucosal integrity is perhaps most important, but another advantage is a dramatic, 10- to 100-fold reduction in total nutrition cost. Moreover, risks of catheter-related sepsis also are reduced. Despite reluctance on the part of some practitioners, almost all appropriate candidates will tolerate enteral feeding. Even patients with abdominal distention or absent bowel sounds usually can be fed successfully by the enteral route. The most notable exceptions are patients with recent bowel surgery and severe ileus. With an assertive program, almost all patients can be fed promptly using the gut at a modest cost.

9. Establish Criteria for Prophylactic Treatments

Deep venous thrombosis (DVT) is so frequent in the critically ill population that it makes sense to use some form of preventative therapy in almost all appropriate candidates. The annual costs of DVT prophylaxis for an entire ICU probably are dwarfed by the costs of treating one case of established DVT or pulmonary embolism. Low-dose heparin is generally safe and so inexpensive that it probably should be the prophylactic agent of choice unless contraindications to anticoagulation are compelling (noncompressible bleeding sites, recent trauma or surgery, thrombocytopenia,

heparin allergy). For patients who are unable to receive heparin, a combination of graded compression stockings and intermittent pneumatic devices is a reasonable alternative. This issue is discussed in detail in Chapter 23, Venous Thrombosis and Pulmonary Embolism.

Likewise, patients at high risk for developing gastric ulceration and upper gastrointestinal bleeding should receive prophylactic therapy. Because of the costs, ease of therapy, and effectiveness, a generic histamine blocker represents the best therapeutic option. Acid-suppressive therapy can be discontinued safely after oral feeding or enteral nutrition is established. This topic is discussed in detail in Chapter 39, Gastrointestinal Bleeding.

In similar fashion, preventing skin breakdown averts a costly, potentially lethal complication. Either frequent repositioning or specialized beds are necessary for patients at high risk. Each method of prevention can be expensive in its own way; rental or purchase of beds incurs direct expense, whereas the labor-intensive and unpopular repetitive turning can result in staff injuries and dissatisfaction. In this way, the decision to forgo use of specialized beds may be "penny-wise and pound foolish."

10. Preferentially Use Crystalloid Over Colloid

Extensive study has failed to demonstrate superiority of colloid over crystalloid in almost all clinical situations. (Exceptions may include plasmapheresis and priming of the cardiopulmonary bypass pump for infants.) Although an absolute larger volume is necessary, crystalloid rapidly and effectively restores circulating volume at a small fraction of the cost of colloid. Furthermore, colloid (i.e., albumin) represents an ineffective and expensive method of "nutritional therapy." Avoidance of colloid in general, and albumin specifically, results in dramatic cost reductions without decrement in quality of care.

LABORATORY STUDIES

Legitimate concern over physiologic and chemical abnormalities is a major factor driving laboratory use for the critically ill patient. Unfortunately, the frequency of laboratory use is determined in large part by a physician's comfort and experience in the care of critically ill patients. For example, less experienced physicians often order chemistry and hematology profiles and blood gases daily. In addition, standing orders for blood, sputum, and urine cultures are often written to evaluate temperature elevations. Frankly, there

is little justification for such rigid practices; more flexibility and thought are required. Although laboratory use should be customized for each patient, reasonable guidelines for major areas of laboratory use for the "average" patient can be proposed (Table 19.2).

MICROBIOLOGY LABORATORY

Fever evaluations are most fruitful when performed for new-onset fever in the absence of antibiotic therapy. A temperature threshold for obtaining cultures of <96° or >101°F is rational in the absence of other alarming indicators. For patients with continuous or near continuous fever, it is reasonable to repeat cultures every 3 days. A 3-day interval offers sufficient time for full evaluation of previously obtained cultures and a period of time to evaluate empiric antibiotic choices. An obvious exception includes patients with suspected endocarditis or septic thrombophlebitis in whom bacteremia may be continuous and patients who have dramatic physiologic deteriorations associated with worsening of fever. Some studies have reported that one-half of all "positive" blood cultures grow organisms ultimately deemed to be "contaminants." These false-positive cultures prove costly, as they prompt additional diagnostic studies (more cultures and imaging studies) and antibiotic therapy, as well as prolonging hospital stay. Meticulous technique in obtaining blood cultures will minimize the problem of contamination.

CHEMISTRY LABORATORY

Evaluation of electrolytes is often useful several times a day during the period of initial instability after admission. During this time, provision or removal of large amounts of fluid often leads to dramatic changes in sodium, chloride, and potassium concentrations. Likewise, changes in acid–base status alter bicarbonate and potassium levels in these unstable patients. After 2 to 3 days in the ICU, however, daily chemistry evaluations are rarely needed. Granted, patients with acute renal failure, especially those undergoing dialysis, and patients with severe hypokalemia or hyperkalemia warrant more frequent monitoring. Although very reasonable upon admission, extensive automated blood chemistry profiles (e.g., SMA12) are rarely needed more than once or twice weekly. If specific components of the profile are necessary (e.g., liver function tests, albu-

---

TABLE 19–2

ONE SCHEME FOR ICU LABORATORY MONITORING

All Patients on Admission:
1. 12-lead electrocardiogram
2. Portable chest radiograph
3. Urinalysis
4. Complete blood count with platelet count and white cell differential
5. Automated chemistry profile
   - Electrolytes Na$^+$, K$^+$, Cl$^-$, HCO$_3^-$
   - Liver function tests: serum glutamic-oxaloacetic transaminase, serum glutamic-pyruvic transaminase, bilirubin, alkaline phosphatase
   - Renal function tests: creatinine, blood urea nitrogen
   - Nutritional indices: cholesterol, total protein, albumin
   - Glucose
6. Prothrombin time

Individualized Studies:
  Arterial blood gas
  Partial thromboplastin time
  Magnesium
  Creatinine phosphokinase
  Blood, urine, sputum cultures

Daily Assessment for Patients with Hemodynamic or Respiratory Instability:
1. Portable chest radiograph
2. Electrolytes
3. Creatinine, blood urea nitrogen
4. Glucose
5. White blood cell count, hematocrit

After Stabilization (tests to be done once or twice weekly):
1. Electrolytes and renal function tests
2. Complete blood count
3. Portable chest radiograph
4. Automated profile of nutritional status and liver function
5. Arterial blood gas

Indications for Cultures:
1. New onset fever or hypothermia
2. Reculture approximately every 3 days for persistently febrile patients
3. New, unexplained hemodynamics or respiratory deterioration

min, etc.), it is often more cost effective to order the individual components. When such automated chemistry profiles are used to track the status of nutrition, evaluation at more than weekly intervals is probably wasteful; the slow pace at which nutritional parameters change rarely makes more frequent monitoring necessary.

HEMATOLOGY LABORATORY

Like chemistry measurements, with some notable exceptions, daily or more frequent monitoring of hematocrit, platelet count, and white blood cell count is probably not necessary after the initial period of instability. Patients undergoing therapeutic anticoagulation are prone to declines in hematocrit and possibly the thrombocytopenic effects of heparin. Thus, once-daily monitoring of each parameter is reasonable. Similarly, patients with active hemorrhage (especially trauma victims, patients with active gastrointestinal bleeding, and others receiving transfusion) probably should be monitored on at least a daily basis. But even for these patients, there is potential for cost reduction: white blood cell, particularly differential, counts are not necessary for patients in whom the purpose is to track hemorrhage. Furthermore, differential counts are seldom helpful after admission, except for patients with neutropenia from sepsis or chemotherapy.

COAGULATION LABORATORY

Tests of coagulation frequently are abused at great expense. At the time of admission, it is very reasonable to assay the prothrombin time (PT) and international normalized ratio (INR) once. Measuring the partial thromboplastin time (PTT) is less likely to yield useful information unless hereditary coagulopathy is suspected. The combination of normal PT and PTT at admission all but excludes hereditary coagulopathy, consumptive coagulopathy, and profound nutritional deficiency. After admission, the PT is subject to change by consumption, dilution, or decreased production of vitamin-K-dependent clotting factors. Hence, disseminated intravascular coagulation, dilutional coagulopathy, progressive liver disease, or warfarin anticoagulation would be clear indications for monitoring the PT or INR over time. The PT will not respond quickly to warfarin therapy and is essentially useless as an indicator of the effect of heparin. Although frequently done, it is wasteful to obtain repeated PT determinations from patients receiving heparin alone. The PTT is increased by dilution, consumption, heparin therapy, or congenital coagulopathy. Therefore, it is reasonable to obtain PTT measurements for patients being treated for disseminated intravascular coagulopathy (DIC) or dilutional coagulopathy and it is essential for patients being treated with continuous infusion heparin therapy. There is no indication for repeated PTT determinations in a patient receiving warfarin alone.

BLOOD GAS LABORATORY

Before wide application of pulse oximetry, arterial blood gases (ABGs) were recommended after every ventilator change and frequently were performed routinely on a daily basis for chronically ventilated patients. Daily ABGs are not necessary in the absence of a change in clinical status or noteworthy ventilator parameter change. Furthermore, changes in administered oxygen concentrations do not routinely require ABGs if saturation is monitored. Unfortunately, capnography has not lived up to expectations, so that ABGs are still necessary for evaluation of arterial carbon dioxide content in most cases. Likewise, the technology for on-line arterial pH monitoring has not yet matured sufficiently to recommend routine use. Thus, it is only suspected changes in pH or arterial carbon dioxide content that require ABG determinations. Obviously, ABGs prove most useful in the initial period of hemodynamic and ventilatory instability, in the weaning process, or when metabolic acid–base disorders are suspected (see Chapter 5, Respiratory Monitoring).

SUMMARY

In summary, a dedicated and experienced leader, a team approach to care, a defined procedure for admission, discharge, and transfer, restriction of attending privileges, and comprehensive guidelines for the use of drugs, imaging studies, and laboratory tests can produce substantial cost savings while simultaneously improving the quality of care. In the end, the best hope for cost containment and quality care lies in the education of caring physicians so they can choose wisely from the bewildering and ever-expanding set of diagnostic therapeutic alternatives.

KEY POINTS

1. Salary expenses comprise most ICU spending; therefore, profound reductions in charges will almost certainly be associated with fewer or less-well-trained staff.

2. Patient charges for critical care services bear little relationship to actual costs because of high inflexible "overhead," inherent excess capacity of the ICU, use of expensive and rarely needed services, and arbitrary price fixing by hospitals and payers.

3. Quality, cost-efficient care requires a dedicated, open-minded, well-trained ICU director with the power to establish unit policy.

4. Critical care is best delivered by on-site, critical-care-trained physicians using well-reasoned standardized care plans in a unit in which all patients are treated primarily by intensivists.

5. The entire ICU staff must work as a team toward well-defined, patient-directed goals. Daily morning multidisciplinary rounds are an essential feature of team building and quality care.

6. Wise use of diagnostic laboratory, radiology, and pharmacy services can dramatically reduce cost and charges. Protocols or pathways for using these services must be crafted individually to meet the needs of each ICU and patient population.

SUGGESTED READINGS

1. Bone RC, McElwee NE, Eubanks DH. Analysis of indications for early discharge from the intensive care unit. Chest 1993;104:1812–1817.
2. Carson SS, Stocking C, Podsadeki T, et al. Effects of organizational change in the medical intensive care unit of a teaching hospital: a comparison of "open" and "closed" formats. JAMA 1996;276:322–328.
3. Durbin CG, Kopel RF. A case control study of patients readmitted to the intensive care unit. Crit Care Med 1993; 21:1547–1553.
4. Fisher M. Intensive care: do intensivists matter? Int Care World 1995;12:71–72.
5. Gyldmark M. A review of cost studies of intensive care units: problems with the cost concept. Crit Care Med 1995;23:964–972.
6. Groeger JS, Guntupalli KK, Strosberg M, et al. Descriptive analysis of critical care units in the United States: patient characteristics and intensive care unit utilization. Crit Care Med 1993;21:279–293.
7. Halpern NA, Bettes L, Greenstein R. Federal and nationwide intensive care units and healthcare costs: 1986–1992. Crit Care Med 1994;22:2001–2007.
8. Koch KA, Rodeffer HD, Wears JR. Changing patterns of terminal care management in an intensive care unit. Crit Care Med 1994;22:233–243.
9. Lanken P. Critical care at the crossroads: the intersection of economics and ethics in the intensive care unit. Am J Respir Crit Care Med 1994;149:3–5.
10. Montazeri M, Cook D. Impact of a clinical pharmacist in a multi-disciplinary intensive care unit. Crit Care Med 1994;22:1044–1048.
11. Oye RK, Bellamy PE. Patterns of resource consumption in medical intensive care. Chest 1991;99:685–689.
12. Pollack MM, Katz RW, Ruttimann UE, et al. Improving the outcome and efficiency of intensive care: the impact of an internist. Crit Care Med 1988;16:11–17.
13. Rappaport J, Gehlbach S, Lemeshow S, et al. Resource utilization among intensive care patients. Arch Intern Med 1992;152:2207–2212.
14. Roberts DE, Bell DD, Ostryznuik T, et al. Eliminating needless testing in intensive care: an information-based team management approach. Crit Care Med 1993;21:1452–1458.
15. Smythe Ma, Melendy S, Jahns B, et al. An exploratory analysis of medication utilization in a medical intensive care unit. Crit Care Med 1993;21:1319–1323.
16. Snider GL. Allocation of intensive care: the physician's role. Am J Respir Crit Care Med 1994;150:575–580.
17. Society of Critical Care Medicine Ethics Committee. Attitudes of critical care medicine professionals concerning forgoing life-sustaining treatments. Crit Care Med 1992; 20:320–326.
18. Szem JW, Hydo LJ, Fischer E, et al. High risk intrahospital transport of critically ill patients: safety and outcome of the necessary "road trip." Crit Care Med 1995;23:1660–1666.
19. Teres D. Civilian triage in the intensive care unit: the ritual of the last bed. Crit Care Med 1993;21:598–606.
20. Varon AJ, Hudson-Civetta J, Civetta JM, et al. Preoperative intensive care unit consultations: accurate and effective. Crit Care Med 1993;21:234–239.
21. Zimmerman JE, Shortell SM, Rousseau DM, et al. Improving intensive care: observations based on organizational case studies in nine intensive care units: a prospective, multi center study. Crit Care Med 1993;21:1443–1451.

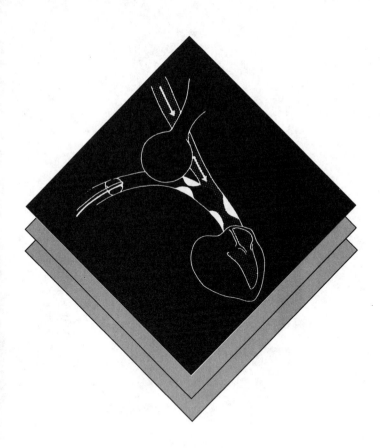

SECTION **2**

Medical Crises

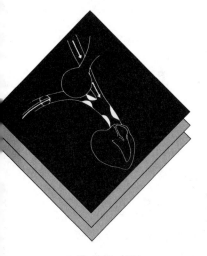

CHAPTER 20

Cardiopulmonary Arrest

Outside the hospital and the coronary care unit, most cardiopulmonary arrests are cardiac in origin and occur in patients with underlying heart disease. In contrast, primary respiratory events (respiratory failure, pulmonary embolism, airway obstruction) are more common in hospitalized patients, especially those in medical and surgical intensive care units (ICUs)—a principle that must be kept in mind during resuscitative efforts and prophylaxis. For example, because an arrhythmia is so likely to be the cause of sudden death in the coronary care unit, a patient in cardiopulmonary arrest should be treated immediately with unsynchronized direct current (DC) cardioversion. In contrast, arrest situations on a general hospital ward are much more likely to be managed successfully if initial attention is devoted to airway management and oxygenation.

PRIMARY PULMONARY EVENTS (RESPIRATORY AND PULMOCARDIAC ARREST)

Patients found unresponsive without respirations but with an effective pulse have suffered a respiratory arrest. Failure to rapidly achieve effective ventilation results in progressive acidosis and hypoxemia that culminates in cardiovascular dysfunction, hypotension, and eventual circulatory collapse. Although the etiology of many respiratory arrests remains uncertain even after thorough investigation, the cause often can be traced to respiratory center depression (due to excessive sedation) or to failure of the respiratory muscle pump (due to excessive workload, impaired mechanical efficiency, or muscle weakness). Tachypnea usually is the first response to stress. As overloading continues, the respiratory rhythm then disorganizes, slows, and eventually ceases.

The partial pressure of arterial oxygen (PaO$_2$) plummets shortly after ventilation ceases. Body stores of oxygen are restricted and consumed rapidly, unlike carbon dioxide, which has a huge storage pool and an efficient buffering system. On the other hand, if effective circulation is maintained, PaCO$_2$ builds rather slowly, at a rate of 6–9 mm Hg in the first apneic minute and 3 to 6 mm Hg/ minute thereafter (Fig. 20.1). After the apneic patient develops metabolic acidosis, however, H$^+$ combines with HCO$_3^-$ to generate carbon dioxide and water, dramatically increasing the rate of CO$_2$ production. Thus, life-threatening hypoxemia occurs long before significant respiratory acidosis.

Initially, hypoxemia enhances the peripheral chemical drive to breathe and stimulates the heart rate. Profound hypoxemia, however, depresses neural function and produces bradycardia refractory to sympathetic and parasympatholytic influences. At this point, cardiovascular function usually is severely disturbed, not only because cardiac and vascular smooth muscle function poorly under conditions of hypoxia and acidosis but also because cardiac output is the product of stroke volume and heart rate. The result of this process is a pulmocardiac arrest. Nearly one-half of hospitalized cardiac arrest victims exhibit an initial bradycardic rhythm, strongly suggesting a primary respiratory etiology.

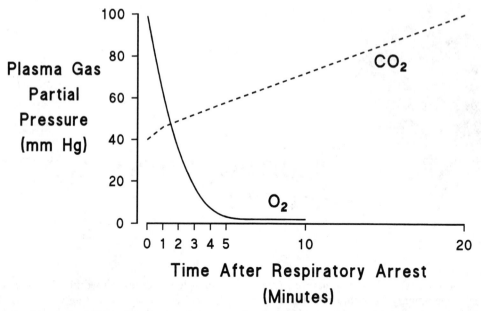

FIG. 20–1. Change in arterial partial pressure of oxygen and carbon dioxide in patients after respiratory arrest. Oxygen concentrations fall precipitously to dangerously low levels within minutes. In contrast, the rise in carbon dioxide tensions is much slower, requiring 15 to 20 minutes to reach levels sufficient to produce life-threatening acidosis.

PRIMARY CARDIOVASCULAR EVENTS (CARDIOPULMONARY ARREST)

The heart may abruptly fail to achieve an effective output because of a new dysrhythmia or suddenly impaired pump function resulting from diminished preload, excessive afterload, or decreased contractility. The normal heart compensates for changes in heart rate over a wide range through the Starling mechanism. Thus, cardiac output normally is maintained by compensatory chamber dilation and increased stroke volume despite slowing of rate. Patients with dilated or stiff hearts lose this reserve and are highly sensitive to rate changes. Thus, bradycardia is tolerated especially poorly by patients with impaired ventricular function.

Decreases in preload sufficient to cause cardiovascular collapse usually are the result of venodilation, massive hemorrhage, pericardial tamponade, or tension pneumothorax. In contrast to the left ventricle, which is constantly adapting to a widely changing afterload, the right ventricle is not adept at adjusting quickly to increased afterload. Therefore, abrupt increases in afterload sufficient to cause catastrophic cardiovascular collapse usually affect the right (rather than left) ventricle. These often result from embolism to the pulmonary circuit by clot or air. Acute dysfunction of the cardiac muscle fiber itself can result from hypoxemia, sepsis, acidosis, electrolyte disturbance, or myocardial infarction. Regardless of the precipitating event, patients with narrowed coronary arteries are particularly susceptible to the adverse effects of a reduced perfusion pressure.

Neural tissue is disproportionately susceptible to reductions in blood flow. Circulatory arrest always produces coma within seconds, and respiratory rhythm ceases very rapidly thereafter. Thus, ongoing respiratory efforts indicate very recent cardiovascular collapse or the continuation of effective blood flow below the palpable pulse threshold. (In a person of normal body habitus, a systolic pressure of approximately 80 mm Hg, 70 mm Hg, or 60 mm Hg must be present for a pulse to be detected at radial, femoral, or carotid sites, respectively.)

CARDIOPULMONARY RESUSCITATION

Cardiopulmonary resuscitation (CPR) was developed as a temporary circulatory support procedure for use in otherwise healthy patients suffering sudden cardiac death. In most cases, acute

TABLE 20–1

COMMON CLINICAL SCENARIOS OF CARDIOPULMONARY ARREST

Setting	Likely Etiology	Appropriate Intervention
Early during mechanical ventilation	1. Misplaced ET tube	Confirm proper location by direct visualization and auscultation
	2. Tension pneumothorax	Physical examination, consider chest tube placement
	3. Hypovolemia	Consider fluid bolus
	4. Auto PEEP	Reduce V_E, increase expiratory time, consider bronchodilator
	5. Profound hypoxemia	Check ET placement, confirm oxygenation with oximeter or ABG administer 100% O_2
During chronic mechanical ventilation	1. ET tube displacement	Confirm proper ET placement by auscultation and chest radiograph
	2. Hypoxemia	Confirm oxygenation with oximeter or ABG, increase FiO_2
	3. Tension pneumothorax	Physical examination, consider chest tube placement
	4. Hyperinflation/auto-PEEP	Reduce V_E, increase expiratory time, consider bronchodilator
Post central line placement/ attempt	1. Tension pneumothorax	Physical examination, consider chest tube placement
	2. Tachyarrhythmia	Withdraw intracardiac wires or catheters, try cardioversion/antiarrhythmic
	3. Bradycardia/heart block	Withdraw intracardiac wires or catheters, try chronotropic drugs, temporary pacing
During dialysis or plasmapheresis	1. Hypovolemia	Fluid therapy
	2. Transfusion reaction	Stop transfusion; treat anaphylaxis
	3. IgA deficiency:allergic reaction	Stop transfusion, treat anaphylaxis
	4. Hyperkalemia	Check K+, treat empirically if ECG suggests hyperkalemia
Acute head injury	1. Increased intracranial pressure (especially with bradycardia)	Lower Intracranial pressure
	2. Diabetes insipidus: hypovolemia (especially with tachycardia)	Administer fluid
Pancreatitis	1. Hypovolemia	Fluid administration
	2. Hypocalcemia	Calcium supplementation
After first dose of a new medicine	1. Anaphylaxis (antibiotics)	Stop drug, administer fluid, epinephrine, corticosteroids
	2. Angioedema (ACE inhibitors)	
	3. Hypotension/volume depletion (ACE inhibitors)	Volume expansion
Toxin/drug overdose (tricyclic antidepressants, β-blocker/ Ca^{+2} blocker MAO inhibitor CO, cyanide)	1. Seizures/tachyarrhythmias	Sodium bicarbonate
	2. Severe bradycardia	Chronotropic agents, pacing, glucagon
	3. Hypertension	Drug removal
	4. Hypoxia	Oxygen, sodium nitrite + sodium thiocyanate
After myocardial infarction	1. Tachyarrhythmia/VF	DC countershock, lidocaine
	2. Torsade de pointes	Cardioversion, Mg^{+3}, isoproterenol, pacing Stop antiarrhythmic and phenothiazine
	3. Tamponade, cardiac rupture	Pericardiocentesis, fluid, surgical repair
	4. Bradycardia, AV block	Chronotropic drugs, temporary pacing
After trauma	1. Exsanguination	Fluid/blood administration, consider laparotomy–thoractomy
	2. Tension pneumothorax	Physical examination, consider chest tube placement
	3. Tamponade	Pericardiocentesis/thoracotomy
Burns	1. Airway obstruction	Intubate
	2. Hypovolemia	Massive fluid administration
	3. Carbon monoxide, cyanide	100% O_2, sodium nitrite–thiosulfate

ABG, arterial blood gases; ACE, angiotensin-converting enzyme; AV, atrioventricular; DC, direct current; ECG, electrocardiogram; ET, endotracheal; PEEP, positive end-expiratory pressure; VF, ventricular fibrillation.

myocardial infarction or primary arrhythmia was the inciting event. Since its inception however, the use of CPR has been expanded to include nearly all patients who suffer cessation of circulatory function. Understandably, its success rate has declined. Now, less than one-half of all patients undergoing CPR will be resuscitated initially, and well less than one-half of these initial survivors will be alive at hospital discharge. Even more discouraging, at least one-half of the discharged patients suffer significant neurologic damage, often sufficiently severe to prohibit independent living. Thus, unlike the popular image portrayed on television, as few as 5% of all CPR recipients enjoy even a near-normal postdischarge life.

The likelihood of successful CPR (hospital discharge without neurologic damage) depends on the population to whom the procedure is applied, the time elapsing before resuscitation is started, and to the duration of CPR needed before circulation is restored. Brief periods of promptly instituted CPR are highly successful when applied to patients with sudden cardiac death, but when CPR is used as a "last rite" in the course of progressive multiple organ failure, the likelihood of benefit is exceedingly small.

Although it is useful to consider cardiac arrest situations as primarily cardiac or pulmonary in origin, the occurrence of a cardiopulmonary arrest in certain hospital settings should raise suspicion of a specific (potentially treatable) etiology. The multiplicity of potential specific causes for arrest mandates a methodical, nearly reflex, approach to analysis and management in these settings. Probable causes of cardiopulmonary arrest in common clinical settings and appropriate initial considerations are listed in Table 20.1.

BASIC PRINCIPLES OF RESUSCITATION

Because survival declines exponentially with time after arrest (Fig. 20.2), most successfully resuscitated patients are revived within 5 to 10 minutes. Because of the urgency of resuscitation, the first responder to a cardiopulmonary arrest should summon help, begin artificial ventilation, and deliver unsynchronized DC cardioversion as quickly as possible. Most patients who can be resuscitated will be resuscitated rapidly using these basic measures. If these initial attempts at resuscitation are unsuccessful, institution of more prolonged, "advanced" resuscitation measures may or may not be indicated.

The primary activities of resuscitation include

(*a*) airway management and ventilation; (*b*) cardioversion/defibrillation; (*c*) circulatory support; (*d*) establishing and maintaining intravenous access; (*e*) preparation and administration of drugs; and (*f*) performance of specialized procedures (e.g., pacemaker and chest tube placement). Managing a complete cardiopulmonary arrest, therefore, usually requires four persons in addition to the team leader. Additional personnel may be needed for specialized tasks such as chart review and communicating with the laboratory, pharmacy, or other physician specialists, but limiting the number of people involved in the resuscitation to only those who are essential avoids confusion.

Principle 1: Define the Team Leader

A single person must take charge of the resuscitation team because chaos often surrounds initial resuscitative efforts. This person should integrate all pertinent information and establish priorities for response. The team leader should monitor the electrocardiogram (ECG), order medications, and direct the action of the other team members but should avoid distraction from the leadership role by performing procedures.

Principle 2: Maintain Oxygenation, Establish Circulation and Ventilation

Establishing Effective Oxygenation and Ventilation

Basic support of the airway and circulation should not be interrupted for long periods to perform adjunctive procedures. For almost all pulseless apneic patients, establishing an airway and achieving effective oxygenation (and ventilation if possible) is the initial priority. (The most common exception to this rule is the witnessed or monitored occurrence of a pulseless tachyarrhythmia, in which DC cardioversion should be the initial priority.) Except in unusual circumstances, ventilation can be accomplished with mouth-to-airway or bag-mask ventilation. Because position, body habitus, and limitations of available equipment often compromise either upper airway patency or the seal between the mask and face, effective use of bag-mask ventilation often requires two people. Although cricoid pressure (Sellick maneuver) may help seal the esophagus, gastric distention and vomiting may still occur if inflation pressures are excessive. To minimize the risk of these complications, breaths should be delivered

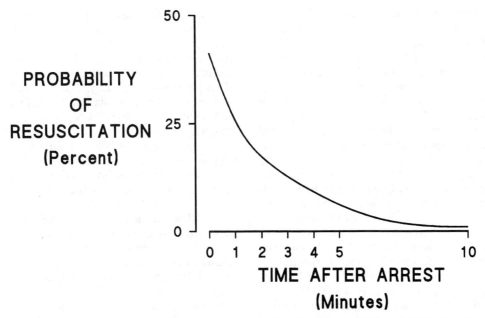

FIG. 20–2. Probability of successful initial resuscitation after cardiopulmonary arrest. Exponential declines in survival result in success rates well under 5% after 6 to 10 minutes of full arrest conditions.

slowly, avoiding excessive inflation pressures and allowing complete lung deflation between breaths. Inflation pressures generated by bag-mask ventilation are sufficient to cause barotrauma and impede venous return.

When the airway is patent, the chest should rise smoothly with each attempted inflation. After effective chest compression and ventilation have been achieved, the most experienced person should intubate the airway (see Chapter 6, Airway Intubation). Intubation attempts should not interrupt ventilation or chest compression for longer than 15 to 30 seconds. Therefore, all materials, including laryngoscope, endotracheal tube, and suction equipment, should be assembled and tested before any attempt at intubation. Inability to establish effective oral or bag-mask ventilation should prompt an immediate intubation attempt. When neither intubation nor effective bag-mask ventilation can be accomplished because of abnormalities of the upper airway or restricted cervical motion, temporizing measures should be undertaken while preparations are made to create a surgical airway. Insufflation of oxygen (1–2 L/minute) via a large bore (14–16 gauge) needle puncture of the cricothyroid membrane can temporarily maintain oxygenation in this critical situation. Phasic delivery of higher flows of oxygen by the transtracheal route also can promote CO_2

clearance, but CO_2 removal is of much lower priority.

Direct visualization of the endotracheal tube entering the trachea, symmetric chest expansion, and auscultation of phasic airflow distributed equally across the chest are the most reliable clinical indicators of successful intubation in the arrest setting. Colorometic CO_2 detectors attached to the endotracheal tube may support impressions of proper tracheal tube placement; however, because circulation is severely compromised during CPR, detectors will fail to change color on as many as 25% of properly placed endotracheal tubes. Furthermore, esophageal intubation can produce a temporary false–positive color change if carbonated beverages are present in the stomach.

Esophageal obturator airways have no use in resuscitation of hospitalized patients because they are less effective than endotracheal intubation at providing ventilation or preventing aspiration and are prone to produce life-threatening complications. Complications include (a) tracheal intubation (quickly fatal); (b) esophageal and gastric rupture; (c) hypoventilation; and (d) vomiting and aspiration.

During CPR, ventilation should attempt to restore arterial pH to near-normal levels and provide adequate oxygenation. Unfortunately, the adequacy of ventilation and oxygenation is difficult to judge during resuscitation because blood gas data are rarely available in a timely fashion. Furthermore, blood gases alone are poor predictors of the outcome of CPR, making their use in decisions to terminate resuscitation of questionable value. The cornerstone of pH correction is adequate ventilation during effective circulation—not sodium bicarbonate administration. Carbon dioxide in mixed venous blood returned to the lung during CPR freely diffuses into the airway for elimination; however, reductions in pulmonary blood flow profoundly limit the capacity for CO_2 excretion. Consequently, hypocapnia seldom is produced at the tissue level during ongoing CPR. Conversely, excessive bicarbonate administration can produce hyperosmolality and paradoxical cellular acidosis. Because end-tidal CO_2 measurements integrate the effectiveness of both ventilation and circulation during CPR, they predict outcome. Higher end-tidal levels of CO_2 (>17 mm Hg) indicate good perfusion and portend a better prognosis, whereas persistently low end-tidal CO_2 concentrations (<7 mm Hg) portend a dismal prognosis.

Establishing Effective Circulation

Blood flow during (closed-chest) CPR is theorized to occur by two basic mechanisms: cardiac compression and thoracic pumping. Both mechanisms probably contribute to circulatory output during CPR.

The cardiac compression theory proposes that chest compression generates positive intraventricular pressure, simulating cardiac muscle contraction. According to this scheme, the heart valves function normally to achieve a forward blood flow with each compression. The thoracic pump theory proposes that the heart serves only as a passive conduit for blood flow. This mechanism currently is believed to predominate in adults. Chest compression creates a positive pressure relative to extrathoracic structures and flow is valved at the thoracic inlet. Retrograde vena caval flow is prevented by jugular venous valves and functional compression of the inferior vena cava at the diaphragmatic hiatus. Upon relaxation of chest compression, falling intrathoracic pressure causes increased blood flow into the pulmonary artery. This theory may account for augmented flow with phasically increased intrathoracic pressure and for improved flow observed during simultaneous chest compression and positive pressure inflation of the lungs.

At best, closed chest compression provides approximately one-third of the usual output of the beating heart. Thus, when CPR is performed for any significant period of time (>15 minutes), hypoperfusion will predictably result in tissue acidosis. If performed improperly, CPR is not only ineffective but potentially injurious. Several points of technique deserve emphasis. Short-duration chest compressions simulate the low stroke volume of heart failure, whereas failure to fully relax chest compression simulates pericardial tamponade or excessive levels of positive end-expiratory pressure. Maximal blood flows occur when approximately 60% of the cycle is in the compression phase. (Unfortunately, even the higher outputs produced by optimal CPR technique do not guarantee increased cerebral perfusion; some blood seems to flow into the external carotid circulation.) When a 60% compression ratio is used, the compression rate becomes much less critical. For most patients, a compression rate of 70 to 100 beats per minute is about right. Open chest cardiac compression may provide double the cardiac output of the closed chest technique but has obvious practical logistical problems and has not been demonstrated to improve survival. Although experimental data suggest that phasic increases in intrathoracic pressure improve blood flow during CPR, currently there is no evidence that interposed abdominal compressions or simultaneous ventilation and chest compression improves survival. Similarly, although theoretically attractive, abdominal binding, military antishock ("MAST") trousers, and volume loading have not been proven to be beneficial.

During CPR, it is difficult to determine whether blood flow is adequate, because pulse amplitude does not directly parallel blood flow (i.e., pressure does not equal flow) and because important organ systems may derive optimal blood flow from different pressures. For example, brain flow is determined by differences between mean aortic pressure and right atrial pressure, assuming normal intracranial pressure. Therefore, increasing right atrial pressure may decrease blood flow to the brain. A similar situation exists for the heart, in which the driving pressure for myocardial blood flow most closely relates to the diastolic aortic/right atrial pressure gradient.

Although the α-adrenergic activity of high-dose epinephrine augments aortic perfusion pressure and initial resuscitation rates, high-dose catecholamines have not been shown to reduce the risk of neurologic damage or improve the probability of hospital discharge. Notwithstanding, there is little risk in trying high-dose epinephrine if conventional doses are not rapidly successful.

Principle 3: Correct Systemic Acidosis

Adequate ventilation is key to pH correction. No data support the early routine use of sodium bicarbonate for improving the ability to defibrillate patients or to improve outcome of resuscitation. When used, bicarbonate should be administered cautiously, guided by blood gas analysis. Sodium bicarbonate is rarely necessary if circulation and ventilation are restored promptly. The inability to restore pH toward normal is an ominous sign indicating some combination of failed ventilation and circulatory support. An arterial pH higher than 7.15 usually is adequate for cardiovascular function when the heart is actively beating. However, the appropriate pH target for the arrested circulation is highly controversial. Previously recommended doses of sodium bicarbonate (1 mg/kg) may produce unwanted side effects, including (a) arrhythmogenic alkalemia, (b) increased CO_2 generation, (c) hyperosmolarity, (d) hypokalemia, (e) paradoxical central nervous system (CNS) and myocardial intracellular acidosis, and (f) a leftward shift in the oxyhemoglobin dissociation curve, limiting delivery of O_2 to tissues. Exceptional circumstances in which bicarbonate may be useful are hyperkalemia, tricyclic antidepressant overdose, and protracted hypoperfusion-induced acidosis.

Principle 4: Create an Effective Cardiac Rhythm

Asystole

Any rhythm is better than asystole, which is the complete absence of electrical activity (a flat ECG). Therefore, a key aim is to stimulate any electrical activity and then modify that activity to a rhythm with a pulse. Asystole usually indicates extended interruption of perfusion and carries a grave prognosis. It makes little sense to countershock the truly asystolic patient because there is no "rhythm" to modify. However, low-amplitude ventricular fibrillation may go unrecognized unless searched for using a full 12-lead ECG. Ventricular fibrillation may be best distinguished from "asystole" in leads II and III.

Epinephrine (1 mg i.v., q 3–5 minutes) and atropine (1 mg i.v., q 3–5 minutes to a total dose of 2–4 mg) sometimes can restore a vestige of electrical activity, even if disorganized. Manipulation of electrolyte balance (Ca^{+2}, K^+) also may be useful in refractory cases. Use of transcutaneous pacing should be instituted early in patients with asystole to attempt ventricular capture (see also Chapter 4, Arrhythmias, Pacing, and Cardioversion). Sodium bicarbonate also may be useful if severe acidosis, hyperkalemia, or tricyclic antidepressant overdose is the cause of asystole.

Ventricular Fibrillation

Blind DC countershock should be administered immediately to all pulseless unresponsive adult patients; ventricular fibrillation (VF) is the most common rhythm in victims of sudden death, and the success of defibrillation declines exponentially with each passing minute. A series of rapidly delivered, unsynchronized cardioverting shocks of increasing intensity (200, 300, 360 J) is recommended. The goal of cardioversion is to abolish all chaotic ventricular activity, allowing an intrinsic pacemaker to emerge. Many defibrillators allow a "quick look" at the cardiac rhythm before countershock is attempted, but careful inspection of the rhythm is not mandatory before proceeding. Blind cardioversion will not harm adult patients with bradyarrhythmias or asystole and usually benefits those with pulseless tachycardias or VF. Conversely, because respiratory arrest is much more common than VF as a cause of sudden death in children, blind countershock without examining the rhythm is not recommended.

The success of cardioversion is influenced by the amplitude of VF, which correlates inversely with the duration of fibrillation (success rates decline approximately 5% per minute). The success rates vary from less than 5% when "fine" (low amplitude) VF is the initial rhythm to more than 30% when coarse VF is the rhythm. When fine VF is cardioverted, the most likely resulting rhythm is asystole, whereas coarse VF is more likely to be converted to a supraventricular tachycardia or sinus rhythm. After an organized rhythm has been reestablished, epinephrine can increase vascular tone, improving brain and heart perfusion. On the other hand, inappropriately high doses of adrenergic agents may be deleterious by increasing myocardial oxygen consumption. If three initial attempts at defibrillation prove unsuccessful, use of the antiarrhythmic agent lidocaine or "coarsening" the rhythm and increasing vascular tone with epinephrine (1 mg i.v. q 3–5 minutes) may be helpful. In cases of refractory VF, bretylium or intravenous magnesium sulfate may prove useful. Each drug intervention should be followed approximately 1 minute later by maximal current defibrillation.

Defibrillation Technique

Defibrillators are calibrated to discharge through a 50-ohm impedance, a value that often is less than the electrical impedance of the adult chest (range, 14–140 ohms). Therefore, the delivered energy usually is somewhat lower than is indicated by the nominal machine settings. There is no consistent relationship between body weight and the energy required for defibrillation, but most optimally prepared patients have a defibrillation threshold of 100 to 150 J. Although higher energy levels are often needed, defibrillation with the least-effective energy level reduces cardiac damage and the risk of high-grade atrioventricular (AV) block. Although the mechanism is uncertain, thoracic impedance declines with repeated shock. Therefore, if defibrillation fails initially, patients should be reshocked rapidly at the same or increased electrical dosage.

Improper paddle positioning dissipates energy and reduces the rate of successful defibrillation. Using the anterolateral technique, paddles are placed at the cardiac apex and just below the clavicle to the right of the sternum. Because bone and cartilage are poor conductors of electricity, paddles should not be located over the sternum. For some patients, anterior–posterior paddle placement delivers energy to the heart more efficiently than the anterior–lateral approach. For patients requiring open chest defibrillation, epicardial shocks of 10 to 20 J are almost always sufficient.

Defibrillator paddles should not be placed over ECG monitor leads or transcutaneous drug patches because of the possibility of electrical arcing, equipment damage, and explosion. Contact between the defibrillator and chest wall should be maximized by use of conducting gels or gauze pads soaked in saline, but conducting fluids must not bridge the chest paddles. (Note: ultrasound gel is a poor electrical conductor.)

Standard-sized (8–13 cm in diameter) paddles on adult defibrillators provide optimal electrical impedance matching between machine and chest wall. Because thoracic impedance decreases during expiration, defibrillation during the expiratory cycle of ventilation is more likely to be successful. After cardioversion has been accomplished, ventricular irritability should be suppressed with intravenous lidocaine (or procainamide) unless contraindicated by high-grade conduction disturbances or medication allergy (see Chapter 4, Arrhythmias, Pacing, and Cardioversion). Attention is then turned to normalizing blood pressure, arterial blood gases, and electrolytes.

Refractory Ventricular Fibrillation

For patients who are resistant to defibrillation, the following should be done.

1. Confirm effective oxygenation and ventilation by chest auscultation or arterial blood gas analysis if available immediately.
2. Ensure that the defibrillator is working. One of the most common reasons for failure of the defibrillator to discharge in the setting of VF is for the machine to be set in the synchronized cardioversion mode. (If there is no QRS complex, there is no signal to trigger a "synchronized" discharge of the defibrillator.)
3. Correct severe acidemia (pH < 7.2) by improving circulation and ventilation, if possible. Be cautious of overcorrection through the use of sodium bicarbonate; a pH higher than 7.5 also may render the heart resistant to defibrillation.

If defibrillation consistently produces a bradycardic rhythm that degenerates to VF, try to increase heart rate with epinephrine, isoproterenol, atropine, or pacing. If countershock returns any tachycardia that repeatedly degenerates to VF or ventricular tachycardia, consider the possibility of excessive catecholamine stimulation and decrease infusion rates of adrenergic agents, or try administering antiarrhythmics (lidocaine, procainamide, bretylium). Hypokalemia, a frequent cause of refractory VF, is found in approximately one-third of all patients suffering sudden death. In this desperate setting, up to 40 mEq of potassium may be administered rapidly but cautiously. Hypomagnesemia also may result in refractory VF, but magnesium levels are unlikely to be measured during the time span of a resuscitative effort. Thus, it makes some sense to administer magnesium sulfate empirically (1–2 g over several minutes). Hypomagnesemia is a cause of both hypokalemia and hypocalcemia and should be considered in patients who exhibit these electrolyte abnormalities.

Ventricular Tachycardia

The primary therapy of hemodynamically compromising ventricular tachycardia (VT) is immediate electrical shock. A precordial "thump" may create a small electrical discharge that occasionally cardioverts witnessed VT or VF but is rarely effective. For pulseless patients, wide complex tachycardia of uncertain origin should be treated as VT with countershock or drug therapy, depending on the hemodynamic status of the patient. Progressively more powerful countershocks of (200, 300, 360 J) should be administered sequentially as quickly as possible. Intravenous lidocaine generally is considered the drug of choice for patients with VT and a stable blood pressure (see Chapter 4, Arrhythmias, Pacing, and Cardioversion). VT that is unresponsive to lidocaine may respond to procainamide or bretylium. The latter drug has a biphasic action that initially produces adrenergic discharge, followed by adrenergic blockade. Bretylium has a long delay between administration and peak action (15–45 minutes) and can produce severe postural hypotension when effective circulation is restored. Advantages of bretylium include its ability to lower the defibrillation threshold, making cardioversion easier and occasionally producing "chemical defibrillation." Magnesium sulfate (1–2 g i.v.) may be beneficial in Torsades de Pointes or in refractory ventricular tachycardia and ventricular fibrillation. Repeated defibrillation attempts should shortly follow administration of each antiarrhythmic. Verapamil may cause asystole in patients with VT; therefore, for cases in which a supraventricular origin of tachycardia is uncertain, verapamil probably should be withheld.

Electromechanical Dissociation (Pulseless Electrical Activity)

Electromechanical dissociation (EMD), also known as pulseless electrical activity, is characterized by the inability to detect pulsatile activity after coordinated ECG complexes. When cardiac in origin, EMD carries a dismal prognosis because it usually is a sign of massive pump destruction or free wall rupture. Additionally, mechanical obstructions to the normal transit of blood through the heart may cause EMD. Hence, atrial myxoma, mitral stenosis, and critical aortic stenosis may cause refractory EMD (Table 20.2). Other reversible conditions that can produce this syndrome include (a) hypovolemia, particularly from acute

---

TABLE 20–2

CAUSES OF ELECTROMECHANICAL DISSOCIATION

Hypovolemia
Hypoxemia
Cardiac tamponade
Tension pneumothorax
Dynamic hyperinflation (auto-PEEP)
Hypothermia
Massive pulmonary embolism
Drug overdose
   Tricyclic antidepressants
   Digitalis
   β blockers
   Calcium channel blockers
Severe acidosis
Extensive left ventricular infarction

---

blood loss (vasopressors are relatively ineffective in the setting of hypovolemia; hence, adequate circulating volume must be ensured); (b) pericardial tamponade suspected on the basis of venous engorgement, a history of cardiac trauma, or preexisting pericardial disease, for which pericardiocentesis should be attempted; (c) tension pneumothorax; (d) dynamic hyperinflation (auto-PEEP) from overly zealous ventilation; and (e) massive pulmonary embolism by clot or air. Thromboembolism may fragment and migrate during CPR, opening the central pulmonary artery and reestablishing effective output. Air embolism can be treated by positioning the patient (left side down, Trendelenburg position) and/or transvenously aspirating air from the right heart.

Pharmacologic therapy of EMD includes epinephrine or atropine in doses identical to those used for asystole. Recent controversy has arisen regarding the use of calcium in EMD. Calcium benefits only a few patients (particularly those with hypocalcemia or extreme hyperkalemia) and has the potential for serious complications. Nonetheless, it is probably worth trying when other measures (e.g., epinephrine and bicarbonate) have failed.

Bradyarrhythmias

Bradyarrhythmias that cause sudden death have a particularly bad prognosis. In adults, these are often a manifestation of prolonged hypoxemic,

TABLE 20–3

COMMON CAUSES OF BRADYCARDIA

Hypoxemia

Intense vagal stimulation

β blockade

Sinus/atrioventricular node ischemia

Calcium channel blocker use

Drug overdosage (cholinergic effects)

Digitalis

Increased intracranial pressure

---

hypercarbic respiratory failure (Table 20.3). Indeed, the most important measure to undertake first in treating a patient with hypotensive bradycardia is ensuring adequate ventilation and oxygenation—not administering sympathomimetic or vagolytic drugs. In general, the slower the rate and wider the ventricular complex, the less effective the myocardial contraction. The vagolytic action of atropine is most useful in narrow complex bradycardias resulting from sinoatrial node failure or AV blockade. Doses of at least 1 mg of atropine should be administered and can be repeated every 3 to 5 minutes to a total dose of 4 mg. (Lower doses may paradoxically increase AV block.) Isoproterenol, dopamine, or epinephrine also may be helpful for their chronotropic action. (Isoproterenol may be counterproductive, however, because of its peripheral vasodilating properties.) Although useful for symptomatic bradycardia, transvenous ventricular pacing is difficult to achieve in the arrest situation and rarely proves effective in asystole due to massive myocardial infarction. Transthoracic pacing now has advanced to the point where it can provide sufficient temporary support while definitive pacing is established.

DRUG ADMINISTRATION

Intravenous Administration

Central venous catheters can deliver higher concentrations of drugs directly to the heart and are therefore desirable during CPR but are not required if peripheral venous access is adequate. Saphenous or femoral venous access is less desirable than a jugular or subclavian route. When medications are administered through peripheral intravenous tubes, they should be followed by at least 20 mL of a compatible fluid bolus.

Because of the association of a poor neurologic outcome with hyperglycemia in the setting of cardiac arrest, current recommendations emphasize the use of nonglucose-containing isotonic saline or Ringer's lactate as resuscitation fluid, although no cause-and-effect relationship has been established between glucose and neurologic damage.

Intracardiac Injections

Intracardiac injections, although dramatic, are rarely necessary, offer no greater likelihood of successful resuscitation, and are fraught with complications. Many such attempts fail to puncture the heart. Complications include coronary laceration, pneumothorax, and cardiac tamponade. Intracardiac injection may expose the myocardium to massive concentrations of vasoactive drugs, destabilizing its electrical properties. Inadvertent injection of medication into the myocardial wall may result in intractable ventricular arrhythmias. There is little if any indication for intracardiac injection because most drugs used for resuscitation may be given as effectively and in more appropriate concentrations via the intravenous or endotracheal routes.

Intratracheal Instillation

The intratracheal route may be used to produce therapeutic drug levels rapidly during cardiopulmonary resuscitation. Drugs given via the intratracheal route must be delivered in at least 10 to 20 mL of liquid to permit most of the dose to access the alveolar compartment, where absorption occurs. The doses of all drugs given by an endotracheal route should be increased at least 2 to 2.5 times that used with intravenous dosing. The intratracheal route has been demonstrated to be effective for emergent administration of lidocaine, epinephrine, naloxone, and atropine. Interestingly, intratracheal administration may prolong the duration of action of lidocaine and atropine.

It is unwise to mix drugs (administer more than one) when dosing via the intratracheal route. Furthermore, some commonly used drugs should never be given intratracheally. Norepinephrine and calcium chloride, for example, may cause pulmonary necrosis. Because sodium bicarbonate depletes surfactant, massive atelectasis may result from intratracheal use.

Use of Calcium in Cardiac Resuscitation

Until fairly recently, calcium was used widely during cardiac resuscitation. Although contractility may improve in patients with low circulating levels of ionized calcium, excessive calcium exacerbates the arrhythmic tendency of unstable ischemic myocardium, impairs cardiac relaxation, and may hasten cellular death. Furthermore, extremely high calcium levels may occur with indiscriminate dosing. Calcium also exacerbates digitalis toxicity, enhances coronary artery spasm, and forms insoluble precipitates when administered with sodium bicarbonate. When indicated, 1 g of calcium chloride usually is sufficient for maximal therapeutic effect. (However, even at these doses, potentially toxic levels of calcium may result.) Calcium administration seems warranted when there has been a prolonged period of arrest and absent or ineffective pump activity. Outside the setting of CPR, the use of intravenous calcium should be restricted to symptomatic patients with hypocalcemia, calcium channel blocker overdose, and hyperkalemia.

COMMON ARRHYTHMIA PROBLEMS

Post-resuscitation Arrhythmias

A low threshold for the treatment of dysrhythmia should be maintained in recently resuscitated patients. Chapter 4 provides a discussion of arrhythmias, but two specific types of rhythm disturbances deserve emphasis here.

Digitalis-Related Arrhythmias

In the setting of digitalis toxicity, the cardiac rhythm should be stabilized by stopping the drug and by correcting hyperkalemia and hypomagnesemia. Digitoxic arrhythmias may be exacerbated by the administration of calcium. Cardioversion (with the lowest effective wattage) is indicated if ventricular arrhythmias cause symptomatic hypotension. Phenytoin, lidocaine, and procainamide are especially useful drugs for the treatment of digitalis-induced arrhythmias. Pacing usually is required for high-grade AV block. Use of the specific digitalis neutralizing antibody fragment preparation, Digibind®, is safe and highly effective therapy for digitalis/glycoside-induced arrhythmias.

Torsades de Pointes

Torsades de Pointes is a form of polymorphic VT that is frequently associated with prolongation of the QT interval. Torsades de Pointes is characterized by a constantly changing QRS axis that produces an apparent "twisting of points" about the isoelectric axis (Fig. 20.3). A host of reversible precipitating factors has been identified, including hypokalemia, hypomagnesemia, tricyclic antidepressants, haloperidol, and type Ia antiarrhythmics (quinidine, procainamide, and disopyramide), astemazole, sotalol, and cisapride. Cardioversion is almost always effective in pulseless patients, but Torsades de Pointes frequently returns within a short time. Lidocaine also may be transiently beneficial, but the most effective measures include those that correct the underlying stimulus and shorten the QT interval, usually by increasing the heart rate with atropine, isoproterenol, or pacing. Type 1a antiarrhythmics are contraindicated.

DECIDING WHEN TO FORGO OR TERMINATE RESUSCITATION

Certain clinical disorders are associated with a virtually hopeless long-term prognosis (e.g., refractory widely metastatic carcinoma, late-stage acquired immune deficiency syndrome [AIDS],

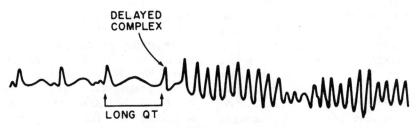

FIG. 20–3. Torsades de Pointes.

multiple organ failure following bone marrow transplantation), and in such cases, it often is appropriate to forgo CPR. Each case must be considered individually with regard for the physical condition of the patient, the wishes of the patient and family, and the likelihood that CPR can succeed if performed. CPR is rarely successful if cardiac arrest ensues as the final manifestation of days or weeks of multiple organ failure. The importance of clarifying the "code status" of all seriously ill patients early in the course of an illness should be emphasized. Ideally, the code status is included as part of the admission order sent to the ICU. When doubt exists regarding the propriety of resuscitative efforts, CPR should be initiated. A single set of guidelines regarding termination of effort cannot be applied to all clinical situations.

During ongoing CPR, neurologic signs and arterial blood gases are unreliable predictors of outcome and should not be used in the decision to terminate resuscitative efforts. With that caveat, however, resuscitation seldom is successful when more than 20 minutes are required to establish coordinated ventricular activity. Several studies have reported that, with rare exception, failure to respond to 30 minutes of advanced life support predictably results in death. Best results occur when sudden electrical events are corrected promptly with cardioversion. Prolonged resuscitation with a good neurologic outcome may occur, however, when hypothermia or profound pharmacologic central nervous system (CNS) depression (e.g., barbiturates) precipitates the arrest.

SEQUELAE OF RESUSCITATION

IMMEDIATE POST-RESUSCITATIVE PERIOD

CPR initially returns circulatory function in 40 to 50% of patients to whom it is applied. (The fraction is lower in out-of-hospital cardiac arrests and higher in hospitalized patients, especially those who suffer arrest in the ICU.) Of these early "successes," 60 to 80% survive 24 hours, but at best, only 25% of CPR recipients survive to hospital discharge and many of these survivors suffer neurologic impairment. Poor pre-arrest health, out-of-hospital location of the arrest, and presence of hyperglycemia all are associated with a poor outcome. Although a prompt response improves the chance for cardiac and neurological recovery, antecedent sepsis, renal failure, and pneumonia are predictors of poor outcome. Long-term survival of severe anoxia is unusual in patients with underlying vital organ dysfunction, perhaps because further organ injury occurs or because neural centers critical to autonomic control and maintenance of protective reflexes are damaged by the event. Interestingly, age alone is not a powerful predictor of the success of CPR. Duration of ischemia longer than 4 minutes, initial rhythms of asystole or bradycardia, prolonged resuscitative efforts, a low exhaled CO_2 concentration, and the need for vasopressor support after resuscitation all are poor prognostic factors.

TABLE 20–4

COMPLICATIONS OF CPR	APPROXIMATE %
Rib fractures and cartilage separation	20%
Bone marrow emboli	15%
Fractured sternum	10%
Mediastinal bleeding	5%
Liver laceration	<5%
Subcutaneous emphysema	<5%
Mediastinal emphysema	<5%

Iatrogenic alkalosis, hypokalemia, and other electrolyte abnormalities are extremely common after resuscitation. Hepatic and aortic lacerations, pneumothorax, flail chest, and flail sternum may occur as a result of CPR but are especially common when improper chest compression technique is used (Table 20.4). Aspiration pneumonitis is frequent, and seizures from cerebral ischemia or lidocaine toxicity often emerge. Gastrointestinal bleeding from stress ulceration affects as many as one-half of all resuscitated patients. After resuscitation, impressive elevation of hepatic (and/or skeletal muscle) enzymes frequently is seen, although frank ischemic necrosis and failure of the liver rarely occur. Creatine phosphokinase (CPK) is routinely elevated in patients receiving high-dose countershock. However, noteworthy elevation of the myocardial band (MB) isoenzyme of CPK is unusual unless repeated high-energy electrical shocks have been delivered.

LONG-TERM PROGNOSIS

The primary goal of CPR is full cerebral resuscitation. The best current strategy is to provide early CPR and defibrillation. After "successful" CPR, approximately one-half of patients do not awaken. Of the patients who recover consciousness, about 50% suffer a serious permanent neurologic deficit. The probability of awakening after cardiac arrest is greatest in the first day after resuscitation and declines exponentially thereafter to a very low stable level. (Almost all awakening occurs within 96 hours of resuscitation. Nonetheless, recovery from comatose or vegetative states has been reported after 100 days.) Pupillary response to light, cephalic reflexes, and patterns of motor response to stimulation are valuable clues to eventual outcome. In the initial post-CPR period, absence of pupillary and oculomotor responses are the best single predictors of an adverse outcome, whereas defective motor responses predict nonfunctional recovery best after 24 hours of observa-

tion. For uncertain reasons, glucose levels higher than 300 mg/dL during the immediate post-CPR period seem to correlate inversely with meaningful neurologic recovery. The effect of glucose may relate to excessive production of lactate during cerebral ischemia.

"Brain resuscitation" with calcium antagonists, steroids, or barbiturates is experimental and cannot be advocated on the basis of the currently available evidence. The diagnosis of irreversible brain damage or brain death is made by using the specific clinical and electroencephalographic criteria outlined in Chapter 34.

KEY POINTS

1. The goal of CPR is to preserve neurologic function by rapidly restoring oxygenation, ventilation, and circulation to patients with arrested circulation.

2. The success (hospital discharge without neurologic impairment) of CPR is highly variable among patient populations. CPR is very effective when applied promptly to patients with sudden cardiac death due to electrical instability but is exceedingly ineffective when used in chronically debilitated patients and those suffering arrest as part of the natural progression of multiple organ failure.

3. Most successful resuscitations require only 2 to 3 minutes. Establishing a patent airway and promptly applying DC cardioversion are the only actions necessary in most successful cases. It is rare to successfully resuscitate a patient after more than 20 to 30 minutes of effort. The most notable exception to this rule occurs in patients with hypothermia who are occasionally successfully resuscitated after hours of CPR.

4. In most cases, creating an effective rhythm

involves cardioverting either ventricular fibrillation or ventricular tachyarrhythmias or accelerating the ventricular rate of bradyarrhythmias.

5. Although widely published guidelines provide a framework for resuscitation, cardiopulmonary arrest in a hospitalized patient often has a specific cause; therefore, resuscitative efforts should be individualized. The most common situations are outlined in Table 20.1.

6. Although the systemic acidosis seen in patients with arrested circulation can be buffered with sodium bicarbonate, a better strategy is to optimize ventilation and circulation. Sodium bicarbonate should not be used routinely but retains a role for specific arrest circumstances such as tricyclic antidepressant overdose and prolonged resuscitation.

7. The code status of every patient admitted to the ICU should be considered at the time of admission. When a clear decision regarding code status cannot be made by reasoned deliberation with appropriate participants, the physician generally should err on the side of resuscitation. There are obvious exceptions to this guideline, where CPR is not indicated because it cannot produce successful results.

SUGGESTED READINGS

1. Auerbach PS, Geehr EC. Inadequate oxygenation and ventilation using the esophageal gastric tube airway in the prehospital setting. JAMA 1983;250:3067–3071.
2. Baskett PJ. Advances in cardiopulmonary resuscitation. Br J Anaesth 1992;69:182–193.
3. Lo B, Strull W. Survival after cardiopulmonary resuscitation. N Engl J Med 1984;310:463.
4. Eisenberg MS, Hallstrom A, Bergner L. Long-term survival after out-of-hospital cardiac arrest. N Engl J Med 1982;306:1340–1343.
5. Gonzalez ER. Pharmacologic controversies in CPR. Ann Emerg Med 1993;22:317–323.
6. Grillo JA, Gonzalez ER. Changes in the pharmacotherapy of CPR. Heart Lung 1993;22:548–553.
7. Hebert P, Weitzman BN, Stiell IG, Stark IG. Epinephrine in cardiopulmonary resuscitation. J Emerg Med 1991;9:487–495.
8. Jaffee AS. The use of antiarrhythmics in advanced life support. Ann Emerg Med 1993;22:307–316.
9. Levy DE, Caronna JJ, Singer BH, et al. Predicting outcome from hypoxic-ischemic coma. JAMA 1985;253:1420–1426.
10. Linder KH. Adrenergic agonist drug administration dur-

ing cardiopulmonary resuscitation. Crit Care Med 1993; 21:S324–S325.

11. Longstreth WT, Inue TS. High blood glucose level on hospital admission and poor neurological recovery after cardiac arrest. Ann Neurol 1984;15:59–63.

12. Niemann JT. Cardiopulmonary resuscitation N Engl J Med 1992;327:1075–1080.

13. Ornato JP. Use of adrenergic agonists during CPR in adults. Ann Emerg Med 1993;22:411–416.

14. Paradis NA, Martin GB, Rosenberg J, et al. The effect of standard and high-dose epinephrine on coronary perfusion pressure during prolonged cardiopulmonary resuscitation. JAMA 1991;265:1139–1144.

15. Paradis NA, Koscove EM. Epinephrine in cardiac arrest: a critical review. Ann Emerg Med 1990;19:1288–1301.

16. Ornato JP. Hemodynamic monitoring during CPR. Ann Emerg Med 1993;22:289–295.

17. Pepe PE, Zachariah BS, Chandra NC. Invasive airway techniques in resuscitation. Ann Emerg Med 1993;22: 393–403.

18. Safar P. Cerebral resuscitation after cardiac arrest: research initiatives and future directions. Ann Emerg Med 1993;22:324–349.

19. Stacpoole PW. Lactic acidosis. The case against bicarbonate therapy. Ann Intern Med 1986;105:276–278.

20. Urban P, Scheidegger D, Buchmann B, et al. Cardiac arrest and blood ionized calcium levels. Ann Intern Med 1988;109:110–113.

21. von Planta M, Bar-Joseph G, Wiklund L, et al. Pathophysiologic and therapeutic implications of acid base changes during CPR. Ann Emerg Med 1993;22:404–410.

22. Weaver WD, Cobb LA, Dennis D. Amplitude of ventricular fibrillation waveform and outcome after cardiac arrest. Ann Intern Med 1985;102:53–55.

23. Weil MH, Rackow EC, Trevino R, et al. Difference in acid-base state between venous and arterial blood during cardiopulmonary resuscitation. N Engl J Med 1986;315: 153–156.

24. Weil MH, Noc M. Cardiopulmonary resuscitation: state of the art. J Cardiothorac Vasc Anesth 1992;6:499–503.

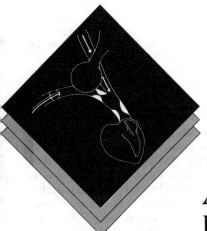

CHAPTER 21

Angina and Myocardial Infarction

UNSTABLE ANGINA

PATHOPHYSIOLOGY

Myocardial ischemia results from an imbalance between oxygen supply and demand. Anginal chest pain is the clinical expression of this imbalance. Because the left ventricle (LV) comprises most of the cardiac muscle mass and faces the greater afterload, it is at higher risk for ischemia. Myocardial oxygen delivery may be limited by (*a*) coronary atherosclerosis, (*b*) plaque rupture with thrombosis, (*c*) coronary artery spasm, (*d*) anemia, (*e*) hypoxemia, (*f*) limited diastolic filling time (tachycardia), and (*g*) hypotension.

In addition to a limited oxygen supply, four major factors increase cardiac oxygen demand: (*a*) tachycardia/exercise; (*b*) heightened LV afterload causing increased transmural wall tension (e.g., hypertension, heart failure, aortic stenosis); (*c*) increases in LV mass (hypertrophy); and (*d*) increases in contractility. Despite the proclivity of the LV to ischemia, conditions that cause hypertrophy or increased afterloading of the right ventricle (RV) also can put its muscle mass at risk. For example, pulmonary embolism may precipitate RV ischemia–a phenomenon that is most common in patients with underlying right coronary artery narrowing or cor pulmonale.

Unstable angina is synonymous with preinfarction angina, crescendo angina, intermediate coronary syndrome, or acute coronary insufficiency. Unstable angina is caused by the presence of complex intimal plaques with or without subocclusive thrombus, whereas stable angina is caused by smooth intracoronary plaques without overlying thrombosis. Almost all patients with unstable angina have demonstrable coronary narrowing; however, most of these structural lesions obstruct far less than 50% of the vessel lumen until rupture of an atherosclerotic plaque results in an overlying occlusive thrombus. This clot, composed of platelets and thrombin, not only produces a fixed vessel occlusion but also promotes reversible vasoconstriction. Unstable angina represents a high-risk transition period during which most patients undergo accelerated myocardial ischemia. If unchecked, this transition culminates in acute myocardial infarction (MI) or sudden cardiac death in up to 15% of patients within just a few weeks.

DIAGNOSIS

History and Physical

The term "unstable angina" denotes new pain or a departure from a previous anginal pattern. Unstable angina occurs at rest, more frequently, or with less exercise than stable angina. Angina occurring in the early post-MI period or within weeks of an interventional coronary procedure also is best termed "unstable." Pain lasting longer than 15 minutes also suggests unstable angina. Commonly, the pain is described as a "tightness," "heaviness," or "squeezing" in the substernal region. Unstable angina may awaken patients from sleep or present as pain at a new site such as the jaw or arm. Autonomic manifestations (nausea, vomiting, or sweating) also favor "instability." Blood pressure frequently rises "before"

335

the onset of pain, even in resting patients. Rising blood pressure boosts afterload, increasing the wall tension and myocardial O_2 consumption. Less commonly, the onset of congestive heart failure (CHF) may be the only manifestation of unstable angina.

Laboratory

During episodes of ischemic chest pain, electrocardiogram (ECG) features may include: (*a*) ST segment elevation or depression; (*b*) T-wave flattening or inversion; (*c*) premature ventricular contractions (PVCs); or (*d*) conduction disturbances, including bundle branch block. (Reversible ST depression or T wave inversion is seen in most patients if continuous Holter monitoring is employed, but ST/T-wave changes are often missed on a single 12-lead ECG.) Even with intensive monitoring, ECG findings are absent in up to 15% of symptomatic patients with unstable angina. Therefore, a normal ECG does not exclude a diagnosis of unstable angina or MI. Furthermore, up to 70% of all ECG-documented episodes of ischemia are clinically silent. In unstable angina, the total creatine phosphokinase (CPK) and myocardial band (MB) fraction may be elevated to the upper limits of normal, but it is unclear whether these elevations reflect true myocardial necrosis.

PROGNOSTIC FACTORS

The serious complications of unstable angina (e.g., MI and sudden death) are most likely in patients with (*a*) a recent history of MI, (*b*) ST segment depression on ECG, (*c*) a history of diabetes mellitus, (*d*) age greater than 65 years, (*e*) a requirement for intravenous nitroglycerin to relieve pain, and (*f*) omission of β-blocker therapy from the treatment regimen.

THERAPY OF UNSTABLE ANGINA

Patients with unstable angina should be monitored and should receive aggressive antithrombotic and antianginal treatment. Most patients with unstable angina can be stabilized medically and rarely require immediate coronary angiography or other invasive procedures. Only a small percentage of appropriately treated patients presenting with unstable angina will progress to subendocardial or transmural MI or experience sudden cardiac death. The two basic principles in the treatment of unstable angina are to reduce myocardial O_2 demand and improve O_2 supply.

Reducing Myocardial Oxygen Consumption

The principal measures to decrease myocardial oxygen consumption are to limit heart rate and afterload. These goals are first accomplished by curtailing physical activity; therefore, exercise studies are contraindicated because frank infarction may ensue. Arrhythmias (particularly tachycardias) should be controlled to reduce O_2 consumption and to optimize diastolic filling time, thereby maximizing cardiac output and coronary perfusion. Controlling hypertension and congestive heart failure decreases myocardial wall tension and therefore facilitates perfusion (see Chapter 22, Hypertensive Emergencies). Underlying conditions that increase heart rate (e.g., excessive calcium channel blocker therapy) or both heart rate and total body oxygen consumption (e.g., thyrotoxicosis or stimulant drug intoxication) should be corrected. β-blockers effectively reduce myocardial oxygen consumption by decreasing heart rate and cardiac contractility and improve supply by lengthening diastolic filling time. β-blocking drugs are particularly useful in reducing oxygen consumption in the hypertensive patient with unstable angina but are contraindicated in acute heart failure, coronary artery spasm, or severe bronchospasm.

Increasing Myocardial Oxygen Supply

Myocardial oxygen supply can sometimes be increased simply by boosting hemoglobin saturation or elevating hemoglobin concentration to levels higher than 10 gm/dL. More often, however, pharmacotherapy is necessary to optimize myocardial perfusion. Nitroglycerin (TNG) is used commonly and may be administered sublingually, orally, transcutaneously, or intravenously. (For unstable patients, the intravenous route is most reliable.) In addition to dilating coronary vessels, TNG also decreases wall tension of the LV by reducing preload and, to a lesser extent, afterload. Acting through these mechanisms, TNG also reduces the risks of life-threatening arrhythmias in acute ischemia. Nitrates are effective both for classic and variant angina because of their direct coronary vasodilating properties. TNG is titrated to relieve chest pain or to reduce blood pressure by 10 to 20%. Usually, intravenous doses of 0.7 to 2 μg/kg/minute suffice. Intravenous TNG usually is begun at 5 to 15 μg/minute and titrated upward as necessary in increments of 5 μg/minute every 5 minutes. Headache is a common side effect but usually responds to simple oral analgesics. When the dose is excessive or the patient is dehydrated, hypotension and tachycardia result from TNG-induced vasodilation. These adverse effects usually can be offset by volume expansion or α-agonist therapy. Because ethanol is used as a vehicle for TNG infusions, violent adverse reactions may occur in patients taking Antabuse®. Obviously, use of high doses of TNG for prolonged periods may also produce intoxication. Within 48 to 72 hours of initiating TNG therapy, tolerance is often observed, necessitating higher infusion rates. Rare problems induced by TNG therapy include increased intraocular and intracranial pressure and methemoglobinemia.

Coronary spasm, a major contributor to myocardial ischemia in certain settings, may be ameliorated by nitrates or calcium channel blockers. Blockers of slow calcium channels (e.g., nifedipine, nicardipine) can be rapidly effective in reversing coronary spasm. In unstable angina, these drugs should be viewed as adjuncts to nitrate, β-blocker, and antithrombotic therapy. Because calcium antagonists have vasodilating, negative inotropic, and positive chronotropic actions, they may have beneficial or detrimental effects for certain patients. If coronary vasodilating effects predominate, the myocardial oxygen supply–demand balance is benefited. Conversely, if systemic vasodilation, hypotension, and reflex tachycardia predominate, myocardial oxygen demand can outstrip supply and ischemia can worsen. Therefore, caution must be exercised to avoid hypotension or excessive tachycardia when using calcium channel antagonists.

Antithrombotic Therapy

Aspirin   Most patients with unstable angina have an ulcerated atherosclerotic plaque covered by a subocclusive accumulation of platelets, thrombin, and red blood cells. Therefore, anticoagulants and antiplatelet drugs are effective therapies. Aspirin (160–325 mg daily) should be initiated immediately for all patients with unstable angina unless compelling contraindications exist. Cyclooxygenase-mediated platelet aggregation is inhibited within 15 minutes of aspirin administration, if nonenteric coated tablets are chewed and swallowed. Aspirin reduces the risk of death and acute MI by 50% by irreversibly acetylating plate-

lets, thereby inhibiting their aggregation. The benefits of aspirin may persist for years with continued therapy. At the low doses needed for platelet inhibition, few hemorrhagic or gastrointestinal side effects occur. Although inhibition of platelet aggregation may complicate subsequent coronary artery surgery, aspirin-related clotting defects are reversible with platelet transfusions. Dipyridamole does not enhance the protective effect of aspirin in coronary ischemia.

Ticlodipine   For patients who are allergic to aspirin, ticlodipine, an inhibitor of the glycoprotein IIb/IIIa receptor complex, is an alternative antiplatelet agent. Unfortunately, ticlodipine is substantially more expensive than aspirin, requires 3 to 5 days of therapy for full effect, and carries a small risk of agranulocytosis. Because ticlodipine takes days to maximally inhibit platelet function, heparin is the first-line therapy for a patient with unstable angina who is allergic to aspirin. The usual dosage of ticlodipine is 250 mg by mouth twice daily.

Heparin   Rapid administration of adequate doses of intravenous heparin reduces mortality and morbidity of acute MI and unstable angina up to fivefold by immediately interrupting clotting on the coronary endothelium. Conversely, warfarin takes days to achieve full anticoagulation and therefore should not be used alone for the acute treatment of unstable angina. The combination of heparin and aspirin is superior to aspirin alone in preventing the early complications of unstable angina. Superiority of the combination probably results from the different mechanisms of the two treatments: heparin inhibits soluble clotting factors and thrombin-mediated platelet aggregation, whereas aspirin inhibits cyclooxygenase-mediated platelet aggregation. Even though the addition of heparin to aspirin raises the bleeding incidence slightly, the risk:benefit ratio almost always favors combination therapy. The goal of heparin therapy is to rapidly achieve and maintain a partial thromboplastin time (PTT) of 1.5 to 2.0 times the patient's baseline or laboratory control value for 3 to 5 days. This goal is best achieved using a continuous intravenous heparin infusion. Thereafter, use of aspirin alone can result in a 50% reduction in the incidence of angina recurrence.

Thrombolytic Therapy   Probably because a completely occlusive coronary thrombus is present in fewer than 50% of unstable angina patients, thrombolytic agents have not been demonstrated to be effective in reducing the risk of MI or death in unstable angina, even though they can reduce the size of an intraluminal clot. This is in contrast to acute MI, in which a totally occlusive thrombus is nearly universal and the benefit of thrombolytic therapy is proven. Thrombolytic therapy carries substantial risk of hemorrhage compared to aspirin or anticoagulant therapy and has a dramatically higher cost. Because existing data do not support routine use of thrombolysis in unstable angina, a reasonable compromise is to reserve thrombolytics for patients who have unstable angina with persistent pain and ECG changes that are unresponsive to nitrates, aspirin, and full-dose heparin. Patients fitting this clinical description are more likely to have a true MI than unstable angina and, therefore, are more likely to benefit from thrombolytic therapy.

Angioplasty Because subocclusive thrombus superimposed on atherosclerotic coronary narrowing is the mechanism for unstable angina, coronary angiography with angioplasty (PTCA) theoretically could be beneficial. However, because the precipitating lesion is an ulcerated and unstable plaque, angioplasty can be detrimental. Although PTCA usually is successful (80 to 90%) in acutely opening the occluded coronary arteries in unstable angina, the rates of early (5 to 10%) and late acute coronary reocclusion (40 to 60%) are much higher than when PTCA is used as a treatment for stable angina. (The smooth, nonulcerated coronary narrowing of stable angina is much less thrombogenic). The risk of coronary reocclusion in unstable angina is substantially reduced by treatment with heparin, aspirin, nitrates, and β-blockers for 3 to 7 days before attempting PTCA. One reasonable strategy is to reserve coronary angiography for patients who do not stabilize with medical therapy within 48 hours. Then, based on the angiographic results, the best decision can be made regarding the use of angioplasty or coronary bypass grafting. Because solid scientific data are lacking, indications for use of angioplasty vary widely. In general, however, severe, proximal anatomically amenable lesions (usually in the coronary artery distribution associated with ECG evidence of ischemia) are candidates for PTCA. In contrast, patients with multivessel disease or complex lesions and those with valvular heart disease or congestive heart failure usually are viewed as better candidates for coronary bypass grafting.

Coronary Bypass Surgery Coronary bypass grafting (CABG) performed urgently in the setting of unstable angina has not improved overall mortality or infarction rates. Medical control of angina before elective CABG results in a better outcome when compared to urgent bypass. Therefore, CABG probably should be reserved for patients who cannot be stabilized medically and who are unsuitable for PTCA (poor LV function, concomitant valvular disease, multivessel disease, or left main coronary disease).

Aortic Balloon Pump An intra-aortic balloon pump (IABP) may prove useful for hemodynamic stabilization while awaiting PTCA or CABG, particularly for patients with proximal coronary occlusion, hypotension, or acute mechanical defects (e.g., mitral regurgitation or ventricular septal defect). Balloon inflation during diastole augments coronary perfusion, and deflation during systole decreases LV afterload. Unless a rapidly correctable mechanical defect is present, the use of IABP does not improve outcome.

Risk Factor Modification For the patient who is stabilized medically, or with PTCA or CABG, risk factor modification is essential in preventing further stenosis, infarction, and sudden death. Smoking cessation, correction of abnormal lipid patterns, and weight reduction are critical factors. Establishing a regular program of exercise is pivotal in achieving these goals and improving exercise tolerance.

MYOCARDIAL INFARCTION

MECHANISMS

Myocardial infarction usually results from extension of the same processes responsible for unstable angina–thrombosis superimposed on an area of atherosclerosis. If angiography is performed promptly, a fresh occlusive coronary thrombus may be demonstrated in most cases (approximately 90%). Nonthrombotic spasm of the coronary arteries in an area of atherosclerosis is responsible for a small fraction of acute MIs. Rarely, coronary flow may be interrupted by embolism in patients with endocarditis, prosthetic valves, or rheumatic valvular disease. Only 5 to 10% of patients sustaining an MI have normal coronary arteries. (Although spontaneous thrombolysis of clot is suspected, the mechanism of infarction remains unknown.) Now, cocaine is responsible for an alarming number of myocardial infarctions. Because cocaine enhances platelet aggregation, vasoconstricts, and increases heart rate through catecholamine-mediated mechanisms, it can produce infarction even in patients with normal coronary arteries.

DIAGNOSIS

History

A classic history of unstable angina precedes myocardial infarction in only one of four patients with MI. More typically, MI is characterized by the abrupt onset of squeezing or heavy substernal chest pain radiating to the neck and/or medial aspect of the left arm. It must be emphasized that the pain description may be highly atypical (burning, stabbing, sharp) or may be localized only to the arm or neck. Autonomic symptoms (nausea, vomiting, and sweating) are more common than in unstable angina. Up to 20% of MIs are painless (more likely in diabetics and the elderly). A history of palpitations is not helpful. Young age, paucity of classic risk factors, and atypical chest pain character are more common in patients with cocaine-induced infarction.

Physical Examination

Blood pressure and pulse rate usually are mildly increased. (Tachycardia is more common in anterior or lateral MIs than in inferior or posterior MIs, in which bradycardia is more likely.) Fever may accompany uncomplicated MI but rarely exceeds 102° or persists beyond 1 week. An S4 gallop is very common, whereas an S3 suggests congestive failure, especially if accompanied by pulmonary rales. A paradoxically split S2 indicates increased LV ejection time. A systolic murmur at presentation should raise the suspicion of acute papillary muscle dysfunction. A pericardial friction rub commonly appears in the first 48 hours after MI and may be easily confused with a murmur. Although possible in classic MI, findings of a hyperadrenergic state (mydriasis, agitation, hypertension, diaphoresis, and/or tachycardia) should raise suspicion of cocaine-induced infarction.

Laboratory

Cardiac Enzymes

Although CPK is the most sensitive test for MI in patients presenting within 24 hours of the onset of symptoms, total CPK may be mildly elevated by trivial skeletal muscle injury (e.g., severe exercise or intramuscular injection). Electrical cardioversion may increase total CPK levels, but unless multiple high-wattage shocks are given, the myocardial or MB fraction of CPK (CPK-MB) should not rise significantly. CPK-MB is relatively specific for cardiac muscle but also may be released during massive skeletal or smooth muscle damage (e.g., rhabdomyolysis, polymyositis, and small bowel surgery). The CPK begins to rise within 6 hours of the onset of coronary occlusion and peaks at 24 to 36 hours. Because of the time course of release, serial CPK determinations rarely are necessary for more than 24 hours after the onset of symptoms and, during this period, are not necessary more than every 8 hours. CPK peaks earlier in non–Q-wave infarctions and in patients who have received thrombolytic therapy to abort an acute infarction. The rapid washout of CPK associated with thrombolysis may produce peak enzyme levels as early as 30 minutes after reperfusion. Typically, CPK returns to normal within 3 to 4 days. The MB fraction peaks earlier and resolves more quickly than total CPK. An elevated total CPK with an MB fraction higher than 5% is diagnostic, although an MB fraction exceeding 5% may occur with a normal CPK. Peak CPK activity correlates with the degree of muscle loss.

Although sensitive, the serum glutamic oxaloacetic transaminase (SGOT) is not sufficiently specific for diagnosis. Similarly, total lactic dehydrogenase (LDH) rises in most cases of MI but has a low specificity. Levels of the LDH-2 isoenzyme normally exceed those of the LDH-1 isoenzyme. Reversal of the ratio suggests MI. LDH begins to rise 12 to 24 hours after coronary occlusion, peaking at 2 to 4 days and resolving in 7 to 10 days. Because LDH rises later than CPK, it may be used to diagnose infarction in patients presenting more than 24 hours after onset of symptoms. Initial experience is now being gathered with troponin-I, believed to be a sensitive and specific serum marker of myocardial damage.

Electrocardiogram

A single ECG cannot be used to exclude a diagnosis of angina or MI. Often, the ECG remains normal early in infarction and damage to certain portions of the heart (particularly the high lateral wall) may be electrocardiographically silent. Furthermore, in patients with an abnormal baseline ECG (particularly left bundle branch block), the tracing may be uninterpretable for infarction. As an MI evolves, injury proceeds from the endocar-

TABLE 21–1

ANATOMIC PATTERNS OF MYOCARDIAL INJURY

Location of injury	Affected Leads
Inferior	II, III, F
Anterior/septal	V2–V4
Anterolateral	V3–V6
Lateral	I, AVL, occasionally V6
Apical	II, III, F, V5–V6
Posterior*	V1 and V2

* ST segment depression with R waves; T wave is inverted initially and then becomes upright.

dial to the epicardial surface. When damage does not extend to the epicardial surface, a "subendocardial infarction" pattern, characterized by ST segment depression and T-wave inversion, is the rule. Conversely, transmural MIs reflect the epicardial damage pattern of ST segment elevation and delayed Q-wave development in leads overlying the infarcted region (Table 21.1). Although Q-wave formation is highly specific for transmural MI, it is not a sensitive marker. The T waves invert within hours after coronary occlusion and usually remain so for 24 to 48 hours. (Occasionally, T-wave inversion fails to reverse.) The ST segment in MI usually is flattened and elevated above the isoelectric baseline. The typical ECG evolution of transmural MI is illustrated in Figure 21.1. For anatomic reasons, the posterior epicardium cannot be monitored directly by leads placed on the anterior surface of the chest. Therefore, true posterior transmural infarctions differ in their ECG presentation, producing ST depression (rather than elevation) and R waves (rather than Q waves) in leads V1 and V2. ST segment elevation of pericarditis or cardiac contusion usually may be distinguished from acute MI by a "nonstereotyped" ECG pattern failing to correspond to distributions typical for the coronary circulation.

Unlike in MI, reciprocal ST segment changes seldom occur in opposing leads. Elevated leukocyte counts, glucose levels, and erythrocyte sedimentation rates in the appropriate clinical setting are suggestive but not diagnostic of acute MI.

Echocardiography

Although echocardiography cannot be considered a definitive test for ischemia, it is a helpful adjunctive technique. Echocardiography offers suggestive evidence for ischemia when focal dyskinesis is demonstrated and effectively rules out alternative diagnoses (e.g., pericarditis with effusion). Echocardiography also can explain hypotension or congestive symptoms (e.g., valvular disease, aortic dissection) and proves instrumental in diagnosing complications of infarction (e.g., chordal disruption, papillary muscle dysfunction, septal perforation, ventricular aneurysm, mural thrombus). The addition of transesophageal echocardiography to the diagnostic armamentarium has substantially increased the ability to detect subtle mitral regurgitation, small ventriculoseptal defects, papillary muscle damage, and posterior wall infarction (see Chapter 2, Hemodynamic Monitoring).

Nuclear Scans

Infarct-avid scanning (technetium) is most useful in detecting infarction in patients with abnormal baseline ECGs or those with non–Q-wave infarcts, chest pain after cardiac surgery, and previous infarcts. Technetium pyrophosphate concentrates in areas of myocardial damage, producing scintigraphic "hot spots" over recently infarcted regions. This test may be positive as early as 10 to 12 hours after MI, and reaches peak sensitivity at approximately 72 hours. Pyrophosphate scanning is highly sensitive in transmural

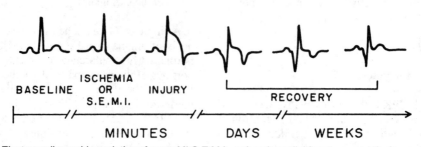

FIG. 21–1. Electrocardiographic evolution of acute MI.S.E.M.I., subendocardial (nontransmural) myocardial infarction.

MI, but approximately 50% of all patients with subendocardial injury fail to demonstrate localized uptake. Technetium scans rapidly become positive (hours) if thrombolytic therapy reestablishes perfusion to an infarcted area. Four days after infarction, more than half of positive pyrophosphate scans revert to normal.

Thallium scanning demonstrates scintigraphic "cold spots" in nonperfused areas of myocardium. Thallium has a lower specificity than technetium because "cold" spots occur in patients with reversible areas of impaired perfusion or infarcts of any age. Thallium scans are most useful in demonstrating areas of reversible ischemia. (Injection of the radionuclide during peak exercise will demonstrate a cold spot in ischemic areas that becomes perfused at rest.) Thallium is difficult to obtain and delivers a relatively high radiation dose, both of which are disadvantages to its use. Other potentially useful diagnostic tests (e.g., radionuclide ventriculogram, echocardiography) are reviewed elsewhere (see Chapter 2, Hemodynamic Monitoring).

TREATMENT

During the last 30 years, aggressive treatment of coronary ischemia and arrhythmias has reduced the mortality of acute MI from 30% to less than 10%. Recently, the major therapeutic goal has been to limit infarct size, primarily by achieving early reperfusion. Reperfusion is achieved by pharmacologic or mechanical measures and is performed in conjunction with measures to minimize myocardial oxygen demand. The early therapy of acute MI has now evolved to a five-armed attack: (*a*) relieve pain and anxiety; (*b*) achieve reperfusion using thrombolytic therapy or PTCA in appropriate candidates; (*c*) improve the balance between myocardial oxygen supply and demand by using supplemental oxygen, nitrates, and β-blockers; (*d*) initiate antithrombotic therapy (aspirin and heparin) to prevent reformation of a second occlusive thrombus; and (*e*) improve ventricular function and limit infarct expansion using angiotensin-converting enzyme (ACE) inhibitors. These initial steps are followed by critically important secondary prevention efforts, which include continued use of β-blockers and aspirin, and modification of cardiac risk factors.

Initial Steps

Patients with a chest pain history suggestive of acute MI should be placed on bed rest, undergo immediate ECG testing, receive oxygen (2–3 L nasal cannula), and have two peripheral intravenous catheters inserted, at which time blood samples should be obtained for electrolyte, hematocrit, and CPK enzyme analysis. Unless absolutely necessary, central venous catheters and arterial punctures should be avoided because of the potential for hemorrhage if thrombolytic therapy is administered. (Oxygenation usually can be sufficiently assessed by oximetry without arterial blood gases.) If the ECG is diagnostic of (and the history is compatible with) MI, aspirin and nitrates should be administered to almost all patients while thrombolytic therapy is prepared. Unless presentation to medical care is seriously delayed following the onset of chest pain or a clear contraindication exists, thrombolytic therapy is administered to all suitable acute MI victims within 1 hour of diagnosis. Morphine and/or benzodiazepines should be considered for control of pain and anxiety. Unless contraindications exist, β-blockers should be administered to most patients with acute MI.

Aspirin

Because it is safe, fast, effective at preventing recurrent thrombosis and inexpensive, aspirin (160–325 mg) should be given promptly to all patients with acute MI without contraindications (e.g., history of aspirin allergy) and should be continued on a daily basis. Aspirin alone achieves an average 20% reduction in mortality and, when combined with thrombolytic agents, an amazing 40% reduction in death rate is observed. For patients who are allergic to aspirin, ticlodipine (250 mg orally twice a day), an inhibitor of the glycoprotein IIb/IIIa receptor complex, is an alternative antiplatelet agent but requires 3 to 5 days of therapy for full effect. Regardless of the suitability of the patient for thrombolytic therapy or angioplasty, an aspirin tablet once or twice daily reduces mortality and reinfarction rates for essentially all subgroups of patients with MI. Aspirin can be continued safely for years while providing continued benefit. Aspirin alone is as effective as its combination with sulfinpyrazone or dipyridamole.

Nitrates

Nitroglycerin probably should be tried for all patients with acute ischemic symptoms and an ECG suggesting MI. If a portion of the affected coronary artery remains patent, nitrates can promote flow through the narrowed segment. If the coronary occlusion is complete, however, nitrate therapy is unlikely to offer much, if any, boost in flow. Nitrates improve myocardial oxygen supply by reducing preload and afterload and by directly dilating coronary arteries. Intravenous nitrates may reduce infarct size and probably reduce mortality of acute MI by 10 to 30%. Except for hypotension or profound tachycardia, few contraindications to nitrate therapy exist. Nitrates should be used cautiously in inferior MI because of the potential to aggravate bradycardia and with great caution for patients with RV infarction in which small reductions in venous return can produce profound hypotension. Initially, sublingual dosing makes sense because it is fast, is titrated easily, and can help alleviate symptoms while definitive (thrombolytic) therapy is prepared and administered. If pain relief is achieved temporarily with sublingual nitroglycerin, administration by continuous intravenous infusion often proves useful for longer relief. Long-acting oral nitrates should be avoided because of the inability to easily reverse or titrate their effects. Headache is common but easily treated with acetaminophen. Alcohol intoxication (from the intravenous preparation) and methemoglobinemia are uncommon complications of therapy.

Analgesia and Anxiolysis

Relief of pain and anxiety are important in the treatment of acute MI. Ideally, ischemic pain is reversed by achieving reperfusion of the hypoxic cardiac muscle; however, direct analgesia may be necessary. Morphine, given in carefully measured doses, is the drug of choice. In addition to providing direct pain relief, morphine serves to reduce preload and, to a lesser degree, afterload, both potentially improving the balance in myocardial oxygen supply–demand. Furthermore, morphine inhibits anxiety-induced catecholamine release, further reducing myocardial oxygen consumption. Despite fears on the part of physicians, morphine-induced bradycardia and hypotension occur rarely; when they do occur, they usually respond promptly to fluids and/or atropine. When analgesic range doses of morphine (2 to 10 mg) are given slowly, the risk of respiratory depression or any other complication is minimized. For the extremely anxious patient, especially one experiencing MI from cocaine use, benzodiazepines are very useful anxiolytic agents.

β-Blockade

Intravenous β-blockade given soon after the onset of MI reduces infarct size and lowers the risk of cardiac arrest, reinfarction, and death. These benefits are achieved predominantly by lowering myocardial oxygen consumption through reductions in heart rate, blood pressure, and contractility; however, β-blockers also provide independent antiarrhythmic effects. In addition to the early protective effects, continued therapy also lowers the long-term risk of sudden cardiac death, for as long as 1 to 2 years. With these proven benefits, it is curious that so few patients with MI receive β-blocker therapy. Possibly, concerns over the potential side effects of therapy or lack of enthusiasm over a "low-tech" treatment are responsible.

Prompt administration of metoprolol, atenolol, timolol, or carvedilol, first intravenously and then orally, provides the greatest benefit. (Suggested dosing regimens are listed in Table 21.2.) Absolute contraindications to β-blockade include known drug hypersensitivity, severe active bronchospasm, type I or type II second-degree atrioventricular (AV) block, complete heart block, sinus bradycardia (pulse <60), hypotension (systolic blood pressure <100 mm Hg), or overt LV failure (i.e., cardiogenic shock or pulmonary edema). Relative contraindications include insulin-dependent diabetes, concurrent use of a calcium channel antagonist, a history of obstructive lung disease, bibasilar rales, heart rates of approx-

---

TABLE 21–2

β-BLOCKER REGIMENS

Atenolol
  i.v. load: 5 mg repeated once after 10 minutes if pulse rate >60.
  Oral maintenance: 50 mg b.i.d. or 100 mg daily.

Metoprolol
  i.v. load: 5 mg every 5 minutes, to total dose of 15 mg.
  Oral maintenance: 50–100 mg b.i.d.

Timolol
  i.v. load: 1-mg bolus, then 0.6 mg/hr for 24 hours.
  Oral maintenance: 10 mg b.i.d.

Carvedilol
  i.v. load: 2.5 mg.
  Oral maintenance: 12.5 to 25 mg b.i.d.

Propranolol
  i.v. load 0.1 mg/kg times 3 at 15-minute intervals (hold for pulse <50–60).
  Oral maintenance: 10–80 mg p.o. every 6 hours.

imately 60 beats per minute, systolic blood pressure near 100 mm Hg, and a wedge pressure higher than 20 mm Hg. If the history or physical examination suggests that the patient is prone to complications of β-blocker therapy, a short-acting intravenous agent such as esmolol (0.5 mg/kg load followed by 0.05 mg/kg/min infusion) can be tried. If adverse events occur, the drug's effects can be terminated rapidly. Despite the benefits of β-blockers, many patients are unable to tolerate their most common side effects: bronchospasm, heart failure, and conduction system disturbances. Potential side effects must be monitored closely and the drug must be discontinued if they develop.

Thrombolytic Therapy

Mechanism

If angiography is performed promptly, most (approximately 85%) patients sustaining acute MI have coronary thrombosis. Streptokinase, antistreptlase (APSAC), urokinase, and tissue plasminogen activator (TPA) all have been shown to limit infarct size, improve LV function, and reduce the mortality of groups of patients with acute MI by dissolving intracoronary clot and restoring myocardial blood flow. All four agents accelerate conversion of plasminogen to plasmin, an enzyme that attacks fibrin. This accelerated thrombolysis usually produces a hypocoagulable state by reducing circulating levels of most clotting proteins (especially fibrinogen). Unfortunately, none of these drugs can distinguish a "good" from a "bad" clot; therefore, all are associated with some increased risk of hemorrhage. Despite claims of "superiority" of one drug over another in individual trials, there are no convincing clinical differences in efficacy or safety of these four agents as currently used in clinical practice. Even though there are clear protective effects on groups of treated patients, perhaps only half of those suffering acute MI are candidates for thrombolysis; among those treated, the obstructed artery is reperfused in only 50 to 75% of patients.

Patient Selection

Thrombolytic agents benefit all anatomic locations of infarction; but proportionately, the greatest benefits are experienced by patients at greatest risk: those with larger and anterior infarctions. Overall, thrombolytic therapy reduces mortality rates by 20 to 50% compared to conservative ther-

apy, and as might be expected, the greatest benefits are enjoyed by patients treated within 1 to 3 hours of the onset of pain. The magnitude of benefit derived from therapy administered more than 6 hours after the onset of pain is controversial; however, it is clear that little benefit comes from treatment given 24 or more hours after the onset of infarction. To achieve maximum salvage of ischemic myocardium, time is of the essence. In theory, direct intracoronary dosing could offer the potential for reduced drug requirements, fewer hemorrhagic complications by avoiding a systemic lytic state, and the opportunity to immediately define the coronary anatomy. In practice, however, inherent delays in performing cardiac catheterization and the incremental risk introduced by the procedure itself offset these potential advantages. Therefore, unless a patient can immediately undergo catheterization, intravenous thrombolytic administration is the standard of care. Intracoronary therapy does offer the option of "rescue" angioplasty if thrombolytic therapy is not rapidly successful or if residual high-grade coronary obstruction remains (see discussion of angioplasty below).

Contraindications

All patients with MI without contraindications to thrombolytic therapy or an excessive delay in presenting to medical care should receive thrombolysis. (Unfortunately, this group represents less than half of all patients with MI.) Absolute and relative contraindications to thrombolytic therapy are summarized in Table 21.3. Absolute contraindications include: (*a*) active bleeding; (*b*) history of central nervous system (CNS) disease (stroke, arteriovenous malformation, surgery, tumor, or head trauma) within 6 months; (*c*) underlying coagulopathy, including thrombocytopenia; (*d*) severe diastolic hypertension (diastolic blood pressure >110); (*e*) recent (2–4 weeks) trauma, deep tissue biopsy, or operation; and (*f*) pregnancy. Relative contraindications to thrombolytic therapy include (*a*) systolic blood pressure higher than 180; (*b*) remote history of stroke or transient ischemic attack; (*c*) recent prolonged (>10 minutes) cardiopulmonary resuscitation; (*d*) needle puncture of a noncompressible vessel; and (*e*) intracardiac thrombus. Some conditions that were once considered to be contraindications, such as advanced age or diabetic retinopathy, have been found to be insignificant.

TABLE 21–3

CONTRAINDICATIONS TO THROMBOLYTIC THERAPY

Absolute contraindications
  Active bleeding
  History of CNS disease (stroke, arteriovenous malformation, surgery, tumor, or head trauma) within 6 months
  Underlying coagulopathy, including thrombocytopenia
  Severe diastolic hypertension (diastolic blood pressure >110 mm Hg)
  Recent (2–4 weeks) trauma, deep tissue biopsy, or operation
  Pregnancy
Relative contraindications
  Systolic blood pressure >180 mm Hg
  Remote history of stroke or transient ischemic attack
  Recent prolonged (>10 minutes) cardiopulmonary resuscitation
  Needle puncture of a noncompressible vessel
  Intracardiac thrombus

Specific Agents

Streptokinase is a naturally occurring plasminogen activator extracted from streptococci. A standard adult dose of 1.5 million units given intravenously over 30 to 60 minutes produces thrombolysis in most patients. The chief advantage of streptokinase is its substantially lower cost (10-fold less) than TPA. Although anaphylaxis is extremely rare, approximately 5% of patients treated with streptokinase, or the related compound APSAC, experience some allergic reaction presumed to be caused by preformed antistreptococcal antibodies. APSAC, an isolated plasminogen–streptokinase activator complex, has an activity and side effect profile identical to streptokinase. The usual adult dose is 30 units intravenously over 5 to 10 minutes.

Urokinase is a naturally occurring human-derived thrombolytic agent that, like streptokinase and APSAC, activates both circulating and bound plasminogen. A standard dose is 2 to 3 million units given IV over 45 to 90 minutes.

TPA activates only plasminogen bound to fibrin, therefore providing "specificity." Although TPA's short circulating half-life and a local mechanism of action result in less marked reductions in serum fibrinogen than those seen with streptokinase, urokinase, or APSAC, this property does not translate into improved efficacy or a reduced frequency of hemorrhagic complications. An initial intravenous bolus dose of 15 mg is followed by a 0.75-mg/kg infusion over 30 minutes and then a 0.5-mg/kg infusion given over the next hour. The total maximum dose should be limited to 100 mg.

Almost certainly, selection of a specific thrombolytic drug is not as important as timely administration. We can anticipate continued clinical trials using accelerated or "front-loaded" therapy in an attempt to optimally salvage myocardium and improve survival.

Complications

Although thrombolysis transiently reperfuses the occluded coronary artery in 50 to 75% of patients, the therapy suffers from many limitations. Streptokinase and APSAC are foreign proteins that occasionally precipitate allergic or anaphylactic reactions. Because of the risk of allergic reaction, streptokinase and APSAC are contraindicated for patients with a known history of recent streptococcal infection. Allergic risk is minimized by using TPA or urokinase. All four thrombolytic agents suffer from the tendency to induce bleeding. Bleeding is most common in patients given high doses for prolonged periods and in those with impaired platelet numbers or function or breached vascular integrity. Over all, the risk of hemorrhage averages 4 to 5%, but thrombocytopenia ($<100,000$ platelets/mm^3) can raise the risk 8- to 10-fold. The most devastating complication, intracranial hemorrhage, occurs in approximately 0.5% of patients receiving thrombolytic agents. This risk is marginally higher for patients receiving a combination of TPA and heparin as compared to the other thrombolytic agents.

In summary, the available thrombolytic agents are essentially indistinguishable in efficacy. Although TPA and urokinase carry a lower risk of allergic reaction, they do so at a substantially higher cost. TPA also has a slightly higher rate of intracerebral hemorrhage than other available drugs. Because efficacy and safety of these drugs are so similar, selection of a specific agent should be driven by side-effect profiles and cost.

Heparin

Even after successful reperfusion with thrombolytic therapy, a substantial number of patients (5 to 10%) experience abrupt coronary reocclusion from thrombus within 7 days. Aspirin substantially reduces this risk, but in certain settings, heparin provides additional protection. Large clinical studies have shown that heparin (given either subcutaneously or intravenously) does not improve survival or artery patency when added to a combination of streptokinase and aspirin therapy. Likewise, subcutaneous heparin therapy has not improved patency of infarct-related arteries or survival in patients given TPA and aspirin. In contrast, intravenous heparin therapy has shown a beneficial effect on coronary artery patency if given after successful TPA therapy, regardless of whether or not aspirin is used. Unfortunately, the benefits of intravenous heparin on coronary patency after TPA have not been proven to improve survival. (Mortality has been lower in heparinized patients.) Addition of heparin to TPA probably does increase the overall risk of hemorrhage, including that of intracranial bleeding; however, the benefits outweigh the risks for most patients. Heparin has the additional benefit of reducing the risk of deep venous thrombosis and systemic embolism from mural thrombus formation.

Based on current data, heparin is not indicated after streptokinase but should be used after TPA. When given, heparin should be administered intravenously in doses sufficient to prolong the PTT to 1.5 to 2 times a control value (generally 60–70 seconds) and should be continued for 24 to 48 hours. Heparin can be initiated before, during, or at the termination of thrombolytic infusion but should be stopped if significant or life-threatening bleeding occurs. The decision to use heparin should be weighed carefully for patients at higher risk for bleeding (e.g., patients who are elderly, female, hypertensive, or have renal insufficiency or underlying coagulation disorders).

Percutaneous Coronary Angioplasty

Because thrombosis usually involves portions of the coronary circulation previously narrowed by atherosclerosis, mechanical measures (e.g., PTCA, coronary artery bypass) often are required to ensure long-term patency, even when thrombolysis is successful initially. Angioplasty has been studied in four specific settings: "primary angioplasty," in which balloon dilation is attempted before or in the absence of thrombolytic therapy; "immediate angioplasty," in which dilation is attempted as soon as possible after thrombolytic administration; "rescue angioplasty," in which PTCA is attempted after failed thrombolytic therapy; and "deferred angioplasty," in which catheterization and dilation are attempted in the first week after the ischemic episode. The

safety and efficacy of each of these procedures differ sufficiently to warrant discussion.

Primary PTCA probably is the most rapid and reliable method of restoring coronary flow through an amenable (noncomplex, proximal) coronary occlusion. Successful coronary opening is very likely (>90%), and mortality rates are low. After successful dilation, an acute reocclusion rate of 10 to 15% is typical; however, long-term follow-up of successfully dilated patients has suggested excellent survival rates. Unfortunately, few patients present promptly enough (<6 hours) to benefit from primary PTCA. Because patients often delay going to the hospital and because few hospitals can assemble an experienced team and perform PTCA rapidly, patients almost must suffer coronary occlusion during daylight hours while in the hospital to have prompt successful reperfusion. Curiously, rates of hemorrhage after primary PTCA are similar to those seen with thrombolytic therapy; up to 15% of patients require transfusion. Bleeding complications probably occur with similar frequency because systemic anticoagulation follows PTCA.

Primary PTCA should be considered for patients who are not candidates for thrombolytic therapy and those with a history suggesting progressive ischemia ("stuttering pain"). Although the benefit is less certain, data suggest that patients with infarct-induced cardiogenic shock who undergo successful PTCA within 12 hours of the onset of pain derive a survival benefit. In contrast, primary PTCA rarely is indicated for patients presenting more than 12 hours after the onset of pain or for patients with coronary lesions in arteries not responsible for the ischemic symptoms. Insufficient data exist to allow conclusions about the value of primary PTCA for patients seen 6 to 12 hours after the onset of pain.

Immediate angioplasty was conceived as a procedure to prevent reocclusion of a coronary artery recently opened by thrombolytic therapy. Immediate PTCA has been studied in several large clinical studies. Because the procedure is associated with no improvement in ventricular function, a twofold to threefold increased risk of complications, and a trend toward higher short-term and long-term mortality, it has no role in treating patients with MI who have been reperfused with thrombolytic drugs.

Rescue PTCA is an attempt to reperfuse an infarct-related artery that is not recanalized using thrombolytic therapy. When the infarct-related artery is reperfused successfully, rescue PTCA results in a mortality rate of approximately 10%; however, when it is unsuccessful, mortality rates approach 40%. The high mortality in failed attempts probably is due to the underlying nature of the coronary disease rather than morbidity of the PTCA procedure itself. The biggest problem in performing rescue PTCA is identifying appropriate candidates. Although resolution of symptoms and normalization of the ST/T-wave changes on surface ECG suggest reperfusion, such clinical findings are neither sensitive nor specific. Therefore, to truly identify those with persistent occlusion after thrombolytic therapy, all patients would require coronary angiography; present data do not support such a practice. Rescue angioplasty probably should be reserved for patients clearly failing thrombolytic therapy with continued pain and classic ECG findings and for patients with ischemia-induced cardiogenic shock.

Delayed angioplasty was designed to identify and correct residual coronary stenosis within 1 week after MI to prevent recurrent thrombosis. Current data indicate that "routine" delayed PTCA is associated with an increased risk of emergency CABG, similar rates of infarction, similar LV function, and unchanged short-term and long-term mortality when compared to a more conservative approach in which catheterization and PTCA is reserved for patients with symptoms of recurrent ischemia.

Regardless of its timing, there are logistical problems of accomplishing PTCA and the procedure risks reocclusion, hemorrhage, and coronary dissection, as well as incurring substantial cost. Such limitations make intravenous thrombolytic therapy the preferred option for most patients. Furthermore, there are no convincing data indicating improvement in LV function or survival provided by PTCA if thrombolytic therapy is successful. Despite its limitations, emergency PTCA retains a role for patients who cannot receive or who have failed to improve under thrombolytic therapy and for those experiencing cardiogenic shock. Additionally, coronary reocclusion occurring after initially successful thrombolytic therapy often is treated with PTCA. For patients with evolving transmural infarction, angioplasty still may be the preferred procedure if it can be performed expertly within a similar time frame as that for thrombolytic therapy (1–3 hours).

Coronary Artery Bypass Grafting

It is difficult to make conclusions about the value of CABG in acute MI because there are no randomized trials comparing it to other forms of therapy. It is reasonable to conclude, however, that, like other methods of reperfusion, surgery must reestablish blood flow within 6 hours of the onset of symptoms if it is to provide maximal benefit. Because CABG requires preoperative coronary angiography, many patients can be reperfused at that time with PTCA, alleviating the need for acute surgery. However, for patients demonstrating multivessel high-grade stenosis, CABG often is the better option. Patients with cardiogenic shock as a result of proximal coronary occlusion (usually left main or left anterior descending) who require intra-aortic balloon assistance also are candidates for CABG. Therefore, for patients with single-vessel occlusions, acute CABG usually is reserved for patients failing both thrombolysis and PTCA and for whom adequate time remains to revascularize the ischemic area. In such a setting, CABG may be complicated by thrombolytic drug-induced coagulopathy. After 4 to 6 hours, CABG is unlikely to salvage myocardium and is associated with higher morbidity and mortality.

Angiotensin Converting Enzyme Inhibitors

By decreasing preload and afterload, ACE inhibitors favorably influence ventricular remodeling after acute MI, thereby reducing the risk of congestive heart failure. The greatest benefits have been observed in patients at highest risk (e.g., patients with large anterior wall infarctions, patients who are older than 70 years of age, and women). Ideally, an oral ACE inhibitor is started within 24 to 48 hours of the onset of the infarction. Intravenous dosing and use of "loading doses" is not only unnecessary, but may prove harmful. Several examples of potential ACE inhibitor regimens are presented in Table 21.4. Contraindications to ACE therapy include known hypersensitivity, cardiogenic shock, and renal artery stenosis. The duration of ACE therapy must be tailored individually; low-risk patients derive benefit for only the first few weeks and can have these agents discontinued shortly after hospital discharge. In contrast, high-risk patients (such as those with ejection fractions below 40%, overt heart failure, or clinical evidence of a large infarction) benefit from long-term (potentially permanent) therapy. Large trials have failed to substantiate fears that ACE inhibitors could worsen outcome by precipitating hypotension.

TABLE 21–4

ACE INHIBITOR REGIMENS

Captopril
    6.25 mg p.o., followed 2 hours later by:
    12.5 mg p.o., followed 12 hours later by:
    25 mg p.o., then:
    50 mg p.o. b.i.d.
Lisinopril
    5 mg p.o. daily for 2 days, then:
    10 mg p.o. daily.
Enalapril
    2.5 mg p.o. b.i.d. titrated upward to:
    10 mg p.o. b.i.d. as tolerated.
Ramopril
    2.5 mg p.o. b.i.d. for 2 days, then:
    5 mg p.o. b.i.d.

Calcium Channel Blockers

Although they are effective for controlling acute hypertension, reversing coronary spasm, and relieving pain of coronary thrombosis, calcium channel antagonists have not improved survival in several clinical trials; in at least one study, these agents adversely affected survival. Therefore, the routine use of calcium channel antagonists cannot be advocated. In settings in which severe hypertension complicates acute MI or unstable angina, however, use of a short-acting intravenous calcium channel blocker (e.g., nicardipine) can be beneficial.

General Support

Close monitoring for electrical and mechanical complications and direct control of pain and stress are basic measures applied for all MI victims. A liquid diet usually is provided for 24 hours after infarction. Temperature extremes of foods are avoided in an attempt to minimize the risk of arrhythmias. Sedation and stool softeners to prevent anxiety and straining also may decrease the risk of arrhythmias. Subcutaneous heparin is indicated for the prevention of deep venous thrombosis for patients with MI on strict bed rest if systemic anticoagulation is not performed. Despite numerous large scale clinical trials, several commonly used therapies remain of unproven benefit (Table 21.5).

TABLE 21–5

UNPROVEN INTERVENTIONS IN ACUTE MI

Antiarrhythmic agents
Calcium channel antagonists
Magnesium sulfate therapy

OUTCOME OF MYOCARDIAL INFARCTION

Overall, MI carries a mortality of approximately 10 to 20%. Most deaths are the result of prehospital arrhythmias, which, to a large degree, cannot be prevented. Conversely, most deaths in patients reaching the hospital result from refractory pump failure. Therefore, survival is maximized by limiting infarct size and by promptly treating mechanical and electrical complications. Survival is best predicted by the patient's age and degree of left ventricular impairment (a reflection of the volume of lost myocardium).

COMPLICATIONS OF MYOCARDIAL INFARCTION

Half of all patients sustaining MI have no significant complications. Of those with a complicated course, most serious events occur within the first 5 days. Complications generally fall into one of two categories—electrical or mechanical. With the advent of specialized coronary care units able to immediately treat arrhythmias, mechanical complications have assumed greater importance.

Electrical Complications

A detailed discussion of arrhythmias, heart block, and the use of cardiac pacing is presented in Chapter 4 (Arrhythmias, Pacing, and Cardioversion). Tachyarrhythmias are very common within the first 3 days after MI as a result of the electrical instability from ischemic or dying cells. Fortunately, most early tachyarrhythmias are self-limited. These early arrhythmias have little prognostic import if they receive appropriate treatment when symptomatic. A major change in the philosophy of caring for patients with MI has occurred in the practice of arrhythmia treatment. Whereas essentially all patients with MI once received prophylactic antiarrhythmic therapy (lidocaine) to suppress ventricular arrhythmias, the use of routine arrhythmia prophylaxis is now rare. Similarly, results of the cardiac arrhythmia suppression trials over the last decade have led to a dramatic reduction in the use of antiarrhythmic therapy after hospital discharge.

Premature Ventricular Contractions

Premature ventricular contractions (PVCs) occur in almost all patients with MI, but their incidence declines rapidly with time. (Baseline levels usually are restored within 24 to 72 hours.) Isolated unifocal PVCs are of little importance. However, in the setting of acute ischemia, consideration should be given to treating PVCs if they are frequent, multifocal, coupled, or clearly precipitate angina. "Prophylactic" lidocaine rarely is indicated for patients without arrhythmias because its use is not associated with a reduction in death rate for MI but is associated with frequent complications. If used at all, lidocaine prophylaxis probably should be reserved for patients at high risk for ventricular tachycardia or ventricular fibrillation who have a low risk of toxicity (e.g., younger patients with good pump function). For patients with hepatic disease or high-grade AV block and for elderly patients, the risks of prophylactic lidocaine usually exceed the benefits. In the skillfully monitored critical care unit, the development of early ventricular tachycardia or ventricular fibrillation is of little import because it is corrected rapidly by electrical cardioversion.

Ventricular Tachycardia

For patients with acute ischemia, ventricular tachycardia (VT) occurs commonly and usually should be suppressed. Lidocaine is the drug of choice for control. Initially given as a 1-mg/kg bolus and then followed by 0.5-mg/kg doses (at 10- to 15-minute intervals) to a maximum total dose of 4 mg/kg, lidocaine rapidly achieves a therapeutic concentration. (It is important to use lean body weight in calculating lidocaine doses to avoid toxicity.) After loading, a continuous infusion of 1 to 3.5 mg/minute is used for continued control. Because lidocaine is eliminated by the liver, patients with hepatic disease, congestive heart failure with passive hepatic congestion, and advanced age can have a reduced rate of clearance. Toxicity usually is manifest as either a CNS alteration (e.g., agitation, somnolence, seizures, confusion, muscle twitching) or cardiac effect (hypotension, bradycardia, sinus arrest). Plasma lidocaine levels probably should be monitored on a daily basis in patients at highest risk for lidocaine toxicity and should be spot checked in all patients who exhibit CNS alterations compatible with lidocaine toxicity. For patients who are refractory to the effects of lidocaine in therapeutic doses, procainamide (a 1-g intravenous loading dose, in 1- to 2-mg/kg doses given every 5–10 minutes) should be considered.

One particular form of VT, idioventricular rhythm (IVR), deserves special mention. Usually self-limited, IVR is a series of wide QRS complexes of ventricular origin. When IVR occurs at a rate of 60–100 beats per minute, it is termed "accelerated." This rhythm most commonly occurs after reperfusion of ischemic myocardium or as an escape mechanism for patients with high-grade AV block. If perfusion is adequate, no treatment is indicated. Indeed, suppression may cause asystole.

Ventricular Fibrillation

Ventricular fibrillation (VF) occurs in up to 10% of all cases of MI and is responsible for 65% of all deaths. Most deaths occur in the prehospital phase of care, usually within the first hour of ischemia. An additional 15 to 20% of patients suffer VF after hospitalization. If applied promptly, DC cardioversion can correct more than 50% of episodes of acute VF due to acute MI. VF carries little prognostic import if defibrillation is successful and if the disturbance occurs as an isolated electrical event early in the course of a small MI. However, VF occurring as a result of an extensive LV infarction or resulting from refractory shock carries a dismal prognosis. Reversible factors increasing the risk of VF should be addressed. Reversible factors include electrolyte imbalances, anemia, hypoxemia, excessive catecholamine stimulation, or presence of pulmonary artery catheters or pacemakers in the heart. Lidocaine given in similar doses to those used to suppress ventricular tachycardia can suppress ventricular fibrillation. Magnesium sulfate has been advocated as a safe, prophylactic antiarrhythmic agent. Although magnesium is almost certainly safe in patients with normal renal function, commonly used doses (2–4 grams intravenously over 1–2 hours) are of questionable efficacy.

Bradycardia

Bradyarrhythmias occur more commonly in inferior and posterior MIs because of intense vagal stimulation and a higher incidence of sinoatrial (SA) and AV nodal ischemia resulting from occlusion of the right or circumflex coronary arteries. AV block and use of pacemakers is described in detail in Chapter 4 (Arrhythmias, Pacing, and Cardioversion).

Mechanical Complications

Pericarditis/Tamponade

Post-MI pericarditis can be divided conveniently into two distinct types: acute early pericarditis and delayed pericarditis (Dressler's syndrome). The pain of pericarditis may be distinguished from that of continued or recurrent myocardial ischemia by its failure to radiate to distant sites, its poor response to antianginal therapy, the presence of a friction rub, and its sharp, pleuritic, or positional nature. The ECG usually exhibits diffuse ST segment elevation not typically seen after occlusion of a major coronary artery. Histologic evidence of pericarditis occurs in almost all transmural MIs but usually is mild and clinically insignificant. Symptoms typical for pericarditis occur in only a small proportion of such cases. In the 10% of patients affected by acute pericarditis, symptoms usually emerge 2 to 4 days after the MI. Nonsteroidal anti-inflammatory drugs (e.g., aspirin, ibuprofen, or indomethacin) are helpful in controlling the inflammation and pain. Although effective as analgesic/anti-inflammatory agents, corticosteroids increase the risk of free ventricular wall rupture. Large pericardial fluid accumulations occur in fewer than 10%. Rarely, pericardial fluid may become hemorrhagic and accumulate sufficiently to cause tamponade in anticoagulated patients.

Delayed episodes of immunologically mediated febrile pleuropericarditis (Dressler's syndrome) may complicate either MI or pericardiotomy any time within 3 months. Dressler's syndrome is much less common than acute pericarditis, occurring in only 1 to 3% of patients with MI. Leukocytosis and an elevated sedimentation rate are associated laboratory features. Pleural effusions are common in Dressler's syndrome but rare in acute pericarditis. Because of the substantial risk of hemorrhagic pericarditis and tamponade in Dressler's syndrome, anticoagulants are contraindicated.

Pump Failure

Most in-hospital deaths from MI occur within 96 hours of admission secondary to shock resulting from LV failure. Clinical evidence of heart failure develops when more than 20% of the LV sustains damage. (Persistent sinus tachycardia may be a hint of incipient heart failure if present longer than 48 hours after infarction.) Fatal pump failure usually ensues when more than 40% of the LV mass is infarcted or dysfunctional. The muscle mass lost during infarction is a much more powerful determinant of outcome than the anatomic location of the infarct. Therefore, rapid myocardial

reperfusion is the key to optimal outcome. Contractility of ischemic but salvageable muscle may return after a period of hours to days ("stunned myocardium"). Ischemia-induced decreases in LV compliance usually require increased filling pressures to maintain stable cardiac output. Under most circumstances, a pulmonary capillary wedge pressure near 18 mm Hg is optimal.

Pulmonary edema should be treated with oxygen, mechanical ventilation, diuretics, vasodilators, and inotropic drugs as dictated by hemodynamics and ventilatory parameters. For most patients with pump failure secondary to LV infarction, reduction of afterload represents a preferred alternative—relieving pulmonary congestion while usually increasing cardiac output. Because a substantial portion of the limited cardiac output must be diverted to the respiratory pump, mechanical ventilation can boost oxygen delivery to deprived vital organs and should be considered whenever respiratory distress becomes evident. Treatment of severe heart failure and cardiogenic shock are detailed in Chapter 3 (Support of the Failing Circulation). Unfortunately, the prognosis for cardiogenic shock remains dismal, with in-hospital mortality exceeding 80%.

Right Ventricular Infarction

Some degree of right ventricular (RV) infarction is seen in up to 40% of all inferior MIs. Hypotension, jugular venous distention, Kussmaul's sign, and clear lung fields are key diagnostic characteristics. An important feature distinguishing RV infarct from pulmonary embolism is the rarity of dyspnea in the former condition. RV infarction may be confirmed electrocardiographically by ST segment elevation in right precordial leads (V_3R and V_4R). Pulmonary artery catheterization may be confirmatory when right atrial pressures are disproportionately elevated in relation to a wedge pressure. (Hemodynamic monitoring is also useful to exclude the presence of pericardial tamponade or constriction, which may have similar clinical appearance.)

RV infarction, usually the result of right coronary artery occlusion, rarely occurs as an isolated event. Inferior LV infarction almost always accompanies RV infarct because LV wall thickness and afterload exceed those of the RV and because the RV, posterior interventricular septum, and inferior LV wall share a common blood supply.

The physiologic derangements of RV infarction

closely parallel those of constrictive pericarditis and tamponade. As the right ventricle fails, it dilates, restricting LV filling. This combination of reduced RV systolic function, RV dilation, and limited LV filling occurring within the relatively nondistensible pericardial sac results in dramatic reductions in cardiac output. The presenting symptom of RV infarction is hypotension, not pulmonary edema. Therefore, the treatment of the RV infarct differs in several important respects from symptomatic LV infarction. As a priority, the filling pressure of the right ventricle must be optimized. This may require mean right atrial pressures higher than 20 mm Hg to maintain an acceptably high wedge pressure and cardiac output. Once adequate RV filling has been ensured, cautious trials of inotropic drugs and/or afterload reduction also may prove helpful.

Conduction disturbances are very common in RV infarction and are often refractory to ventricular pacing. Because of the difficulty in achieving successful ventricular pacing and because of the substantial contribution of the atria to cardiac output during RV infarction, sequential atrioventricular pacing is often more successful than ventricular pacing alone. Atrial fibrillation occurring during RV infarction is particularly detrimental because of reduced ventricular compliance and should be treated aggressively with electrical or chemical cardioversion.

Atrial infarction occurs rarely, usually in combination with infarction of the inferior wall of the left ventricle. Fed by branches of the right coronary artery, the right atrium is the most commonly affected chamber. Ischemia of the SA node and conduction pathways accounts for its most common manifestations: bradycardia, atrial arrhythmias, and heart block. Thrombi formed within the infarcted right atrium may embolize to the pulmonary artery.

Mitral Regurgitation

Papillary muscle dysfunction or rupture is the most common mechanical complication of MI. In most cases, mitral regurgitation (MR) is mild and transient as the result of papillary muscle ischemia or changes in LV geometry. MR has a wide range of presentations, from minimal malfunction to frank rupture. Mitral regurgitation most commonly results from malfunction of the posterior papillary muscle because it is fed by the single posterior descending artery, whereas the anterior papillary muscle is supplied by branches of both the left anterior descending and circumflex arteries. Frank papillary muscle rupture is a rare but highly lethal event that carries a 24-hour mortality near 70%. Mitral regurgitation typically occurs 2 to 10 days after posterior or inferior MI and should be suspected in any patient with MI developing a new murmur (often at the cardiac apex).

The murmur of mitral regurgitation is often unimpressive; therefore, a high degree of suspicion should be maintained anytime a patient rapidly develops symptoms of left ventricular failure, especially when normal systolic function seems preserved. Regurgitant flow is greatest after papillary muscle rupture and less intense when dysfunction is caused by ischemia without structural damage. The diagnosis may be confirmed by echocardiography or pulmonary artery catheterization. Echocardiography (especially transesophageal studies) may reveal a hyperdynamic (unloaded) LV and flail mitral leaflet. (The surface echocardiogram may fail to detect small valvular defects.) Doppler studies may demonstrate the regurgitant left atrial jet. Invasive monitoring is indicated in almost all patients with MI who develop a new murmur, particularly if pulmonary congestion is present. Although pulmonary artery pressure tracings usually reveal large V waves produced by retrograde flow of blood across an incompetent mitral valve, V waves are much more sensitive than specific. Ventricular septal defect, mitral stenosis, or severe heart failure occasionally mimic mitral regurgitation by producing large V waves.

The primary objective in treating acute mitral regurgitation is to reduce left ventricular impedance (afterload). For stable patients with mild MR, LV afterload reduction may be sufficient. However, when florid pulmonary edema follows papillary muscle rupture, vasodilators (nitroprusside, nicardipine, or nitroglycerin) and intra-aortic balloon pumping should be followed immediately by surgery.

Ventriculoseptal Defect (VSD)

The ventricular septum ruptures in approximately 2% of all MIs. Predisposing factors for postinfarction VSD include an anterior–septal MI, hypertension, female gender, advanced age, and first infarction. Ventriculoseptal defect-related, left-to-right shunting reduces effective output and causes pulmonary edema. The anterior portion of the interventricular septum is supplied predominantly by a single vessel (the left anterior descending), whereas the posterior portion is fed collaterally by several sources. Therefore, postinfarction VSD usually is a consequence of an anterior MI that involves the left anterior descending artery (LAD). Conversely, VSD developing after a (true) posterior MI is a marker of diffuse multivessel disease and carries a worse prognosis.

For most patients, physical examination reveals biventricular heart failure and a new murmur. The new murmur usually is loud, harsh, holosystolic, and of maximal intensity at the left lower sternal border. An accompanying thrill is common. Pulmonary artery catheterization demonstrates a step-up in hemoglobin saturation between the right atrium and pulmonary artery (usually >10%). Diagnosis also can be made by left heart catheterization demonstrating movement of contrast from the LV to the RV. Hemodynamic compromise and magnitude of the left-to-right shunt parallel the size of the defect. Echocardiography may demonstrate a VSD, particularly if Doppler techniques and transesophageal imaging are used. A "bubble" echocardiogram occasionally shows bidirectional ventricular flow.

Therapy for a VSD depends on systemic and pulmonary capillary wedge pressures. Hypotensive patients with a low wedge pressure should receive fluids initially. If the blood pressure is maintained adequately and the wedge pressure is lower than 18 mm Hg, semielective surgical repair should be undertaken. If blood pressure is adequate with a low cardiac output and an elevated wedge pressure, vasodilators are useful. If the patient is hypotensive with a high wedge pressure, temporary support by balloon pumping, ionotropes, and vasodilators should precede immediate surgical correction.

The outcome of post-MI VSD is very poor, with mortality mounting to approximately 90% at 2 months. However, the long-term results in patients undergoing successful early repair are excellent. Therefore, surgical repair at the earliest possible time after hemodynamic stabilization is desirable.

Free Wall Rupture

Almost invariably, rupture of the ventricular free wall is rapidly fatal as the patient succumbs

TABLE 21–6

THERAPY OF ACUTE MI

Confirm Diagnosis	
Acute therapy	Aspirin, 325 mg p.o.
	Sublingual TNG p.r.n. for pain
	Morphine sulfate, 2–10 mg i.v. p.r.n. for pain
	Oxygen 2–3 L by nasal cannula
	i.v. β-blocker (see Table 27.2)
	Consider thrombolytic therapy, PTCA
	Continue ECG monitoring, daily aspirin, and β-blocker.
Day 1	Oral ACE inhibitor for high risk patients
	Begin risk factor modification
During hospitalization	Consider starting ACE inhibitor and β-blocker if not started on admission.
6-weeks postdischarge	Discontinue ACE inhibitor for low-risk patients with ejection fraction >40%, without CHF.
1 year postdischarge	Discontinue β-blocker if low risk and no other indications exist for its use.
Indefinitely	Continue aspirin and risk factor modification.

to tamponade physiology. Although unusual (incidence between 2 and 8%), ventricular rupture occurs more commonly than either papillary muscle rupture or VSD; 10% of MI deaths result from free wall rupture. Most myocardial ruptures are early events; half occur within 4 days and almost all occur within 2 weeks after acute MI. Hypertension accentuates wall stress and contributes to muscle disruption at the border of the normal and infarcted tissue. Ventricular rupture is most likely in elderly patients with extensive transmural damage and little collateral flow. The clinical presentation of wall rupture usually is one of recurrent chest pain without ECG changes, rapidly followed by neck vein distention, paradoxical pulse, shock, and death. Differential diagnosis includes pericardial tamponade, tension pneumothorax, and massive muscle damage. Immediate thoracotomy must follow temporary stabilization with volume expansion, transfusion, and pericardiocentesis. If immediately available, echocardiography may visualize a defect of the LV wall, free pericardial fluid, and diastolic right-sided cardiac collapse. Cardiac catheterization is not feasible for most patients, and delays definitive surgical therapy.

Systemic Embolism

The incidence of mural thrombi and arterial embolism may reach 30% in selected subsets of patients with MI. Large infarctions, particularly those involving the anterior and apical segments of the left ventricle, predispose systemic embolism. Systemic embolism is less common now that many patients receive heparin and aspirin (with or without thrombolytic therapy) for acute MI therapy. Patients with large infarctions, mural thrombi, or overtly dyskinetic segments on echocardiography should be anticoagulated unless compelling contraindications exist.

KEY POINTS

1. In ischemic heart disease, survival and ventricular function are maximized by rapidly reestablishing sufficient myocardial blood flow to prevent myocardial necrosis.

2. Reducing myocardial oxygen consumption by limiting heart rate (avoidance of exercise and use of β-blockade), reducing afterload (controlling hypertension and normalizing ventricular filling pressures), and reducing contractility (alleviation of excessive catecholamine stimulation and use of β-blockers) are important steps to optimize myocardial supply and demand.

3. Myocardial oxygen supply can be quickly and simply boosted with nitrates, supplemental oxygen, and optimization of hemoglobin concentration.

4. As summarized in Table 21.6, all suitable MI candidates should receive antithrombotic therapy (aspirin with or without heparin) and thrombolytic therapy as quickly as possible in an attempt to open thrombosed coronary arteries.

5. Early administration of an ACE inhibitor should be considered to reduce infarct expansion and minimize the risk of ventricular dysfunction.

6. For patients who fail to respond to thrombolytic therapy, those with contraindications to thrombolytic therapy, and those with cardiogenic shock due to persistent ischemia, consideration should be given to immediate coronary angioplasty.

SUGGESTED READINGS

1. Gossage JR. Acute myocardial infarction: reperfusion strategies. Chest 1994;106:1851–1866.
2. ACC/AHA Task Force Report. Guidelines for the early management of patients with acute myocardial infarction. J Am Coll Cardiol 1990;16:249–292.
3. Reeder GS. Adjunctive therapy in the management of patients with acute myocardial infarction. Mayo Clin Proc 1995;70:464–468.
4. Yusuf S. The use of beta-adrenergic blocking agents, I.V. nitrates and calcium channel blocking agents following acute myocardial infarction. Chest 1988;93:25S–28S.
5. Simari RD, Berger PB, Bell MR, et al. Coronary angioplasty in acute myocardial infarction: primary, immediate adjunctive, rescue, or deferred adjunctive approach? Mayo Clin Proc 1994;69:346–358.
6. SOLVD Investigators. Effect of enalapril on mortality and the development of heart failure in asymptomatic patients with reduced ventricular ejection fractions. N Engl J Med 1992;327:685–691.
7. Held P. Calcium channel blockers in acute myocardial infarction and unstable angina: an overview. BMJ 1989;299:1187–1192.
8. Yusuf S, Wittes J, Friedman L. Overview of results of randomized clinical trials in heart disease. I: treatments following myocardial infarction. JAMA 1988;260:2088–2093.
9. Yusuf S, Sleight P, Held P, McMahon S. Routine medical management of acute myocardial infarction: lessons from overviews of recent randomized controlled trials. Circulation 1990;82(Suppl II):II-117–II-134.
10. Yusuf S, Collins R, MacMahon S, Peto R. Effect of intravenous nitrates on mortality in acute myocardial infarction: an overview of the randomized trials. Lancet 1988;2:1088–1089.
11. The Cardiac Arrhythmia Suppression Trial (CAST) Investigators. Preliminary report: effect of encanide and flecanide on mortality in a randomized trial of arrhythmia

suppression after myocardial infarction. N Engl J Med 1989;321:406–412.

12. Greene H, Roden DM, Kutz RJ, et al. The cardiac arrhythmia suppression trial: first CAST . . . then CAST II. J Am Coll Cardiol 1992;19:894–898.

13. Siegel D, Grady D, Browner WS, Hulley SB. Risk factor modification after myocardial infarction. Ann Intern Med 1988;109:213–218.

14. Deedwania P, Nelson J. Pathophysiology of silent myocardial ischemia during daily life: hemodynamic evaluation by simultaneous electrocardiographic and blood pressure monitoring. Circulation 1990;82:1296–1304.

15. Sharpe N, Smith H, Murphy L, Hannan S. Treatment of patients with symptomless left ventricular dysfunction after myocardial infarction. Lancet 1988;1:255–259.

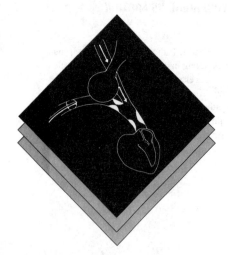

Hypertensive Emergencies

DEFINITIONS

Historically, the term "malignant hypertension" was defined by severe elevations of blood pressure and advanced retinopathy (grade 3 or 4 Keith-Wagner) and papilledema. For patients meeting this definition, accompanying organ dysfunction is common but not universal. "Accelerated hypertension" was traditionally defined by comparable elevations of blood pressure (BP) with lesser degrees of retinopathy in patients not exhibiting organ damage.

Unfortunately, this historical distinction is artificial and not very clinically useful. A better approach is to classify hypertensive crises by the presence or absence of life-threatening organ damage and, hence, the urgency for treatment. When organ failure accompanies severe hypertension, interventions to reduce blood pressure toward normal should be accomplished within minutes, whereas in cases of hypertension without organ failure, more gradual blood pressure reduction over hours to days is prudent.

PATHOPHYSIOLOGY

Organ damage in hypertension is caused, in large part, by a small vessel (arteriolar) necrotizing vasculitis that results in platelet and fibrin deposition and loss of vascular autoregulation. In most cases, the pathophysiology is elevated systemic vascular resistance, not volume overload or elevated cardiac output. Therefore, the most efficacious hypertension treatments reduce afterload.

Although hypertension with a specific etiologic cause is rare in the general population, as many as half of all patients presenting for the first time with hypertension-induced organ failure are discovered to have a secondary cause of hypertension. Young patients (30 years of age or younger) and black patients are most likely to have one of these secondary (usually renovascular or endocrine) causes. Most recurrent hypertensive crises occur in patients with known hypertension who have been prescribed inadequate therapy or who discontinue their own medications. Regardless of the etiology, hypertension-induced organ failure is a serious problem. Of untreated patients with malignant hypertension, 90% are dead within 1 year of the diagnosis, most commonly from uremia, heart failure, or stroke.

HISTORY AND PHYSICAL EXAMINATION

The goals of the history and physical are to distinguish hypertension that requires immediate treatment from that to be corrected more gradually and to define the reason for the crisis. Obtaining a history of hypertension, antihypertensive drug use, or illicit or over-the-counter drug use is critical. Knowledge of preexistent organ failures also helps define the urgency of therapy. (Patients with well-established chronic renal failure do not require the same haste for blood pressure control as patients acutely developing a similar elevation in serum creatinine.)

Most patients with hypertensive crises are symptomatic but have nonspecific complaints.

Headache occurs in approximately 85% of patients and blurred vision occurs in more than 50%. Cardiac symptoms (angina, congestive heart failure) are frequent, whereas nausea, vomiting, and focal neurologic deficits are distinctly uncommon.

Physical examination should devote special attention to inspection of the ocular fundus and to examination of the neurologic and cardiopulmonary systems. Retinopathy is a rather sensitive monitor of hypertension-induced organ injury. Papilledema, exudates, flame hemorrhages, and arteriolar constriction characterize the retinopathy traditionally associated with "malignant hypertension" and correlate well with renal involvement. After control of BP, retinal hemorrhages and papilledema resolve or heal over weeks to months. Detection of an abdominal bruit, suggestive of renal artery stenosis, is an uncommon but critical physical finding. Laboratory examination should include urinalysis, electrocardiogram, chest radiograph, blood smear, and determinations of electrolytes and creatinine. Evidence of ventricular enlargement or renal insufficiency (i.e., serum creatinine > 3.5 mg/dL) is present in about one-fourth of cases. In patients with an elevated creatinine, urinalysis commonly shows albuminuria, hematuria, and cast formation. The peripheral blood smear may demonstrate microangiopathic hemolysis. Hypokalemic alkalosis frequently occurs as a result of secondary hyperaldosteronism consequent to diuretic usage.

TREATMENT PRINCIPLES

HYPERTENSION WITH ORGAN FAILURE (HYPERTENSIVE EMERGENCIES)

The aggressiveness of antihypertensive therapy should be guided by chronicity of the condition and evidence for organ damage, not by BP values alone. Patients requiring immediate treatment should be admitted to an intensive care unit for closely monitored therapy. If there are doubts regarding the accuracy of noninvasive BP monitoring, an arterial catheter should be inserted. A potent, titratable, and rapid but short-acting intravenous agent should be the initial therapy for most hypertensive emergencies. Sodium nitroprusside, nicardipine, and nitroglycerin fit this description. The advantages and disadvantages of parenteral drug therapy for severe hypertension

are listed in Table 22.1. Whenever possible, oral therapy should be initiated concurrently to minimize the duration of intravenous therapy and ICU stay.

When myocardial infarction, aortic dissection, pulmonary edema, cerebral hemorrhage, or hypertensive encephalopathy complicate severe hypertension, steps should be taken to lower the mean BP to approximately 120 mm Hg within minutes. Slowly progressive renal insufficiency, borderline left ventricular failure, or recent myocardial infarction present less threatening problems and mandate less urgent treatment. In such cases, the goal should be to reduce the BP more gradually, usually over 6 to 12 hours.

HYPERTENSION WITHOUT ORGAN FAILURE (HYPERTENSIVE URGENCY)

Although important to normalize BP over days, hypertension occurring in the absence of organ failure does not present the same therapeutic crisis as that when organ failure is present. In this setting, a reasonable goal is reduction in mean arterial BP by approximately 25%, usually to a diastolic value near 100 to 110 mm Hg over several (6–12) hours. Subsequent normalization of BP over days to weeks is safe and averts complications associated with rapid or excessive BP reductions.

An elevated BP alone does not always require invasive monitoring or parenteral treatment; for less ill patients, several oral regimens can be successfully employed (Table 22.2). Oral clonidine and nifedipine have been used effectively for this purpose. With nifedipine, BP usually starts to fall quickly, with peak action occurring at approximately 30 minutes. The effects of oral or sublingual nifedipine are primarily due to gastric absorption; therefore, "squirt and swallow" or "chew and swallow" techniques that accelerate gastric absorption result in the most rapid action. Patients with the highest BP usually show the largest declines in response to nifedipine. It has long been believed that nifedipine's coronary dilating properties may help prevent myocardial ischemia as BP is lowered, but occasionally disastrous results occur when BP plummets to dangerous levels after nifedipine use. Headache, tachycardia, flushing, and dizziness are common side effects after all calcium channel antagonists.

Orally administered clonidine promptly reduces BP in most cases of moderate hypertension, but because of its propensity to cause sedation and

TABLE 22–1

PARENTERAL DRUG THERAPY FOR SEVERE HYPERTENSION

Drug	Site of Vasodilation	Advantages	Side Effects/Problems
Nitroprusside	Direct dilator (balanced)	Immediate action Easy to titrate No CNS effects	Hypotension, reflex tachycardia, vomiting Methemoglobinemia thiocyanate/cyanide toxicity Light-sensitive drug
Nicardipine	Ca^{++} blocker, arterial dilator	Rapid onset Easy to titrate Coronary dilator	Rare reflex tachycardia Headache
Nitroglycerin	Direct dilator (venous–arterial)	Coronary dilator Rapid onset	Headache, ETOH vehicle Absorbed into some i.v. tubing
Labetolol	α-blocker and β-blocker	No "overshoot" hypotension Maintained cardiac output, heart rate	Exacerbates CHF, asthma, causes AV block Tolerance with prolonged use
Enalaprilat	ACE inhibitor	Very effective in high-renin states	Profound hypotension in volume depleted May exacerbate renal failure
Hydralazine	Direct dilator (arterial–venous)	No CNS effects	Reflex tachycardia, overshoot hypotension Headache, vomiting, lupus syndrome (chronic use)
Diazoxide	Direct dilator (arterial and venous)	Rapid action Not sedating	Imprecise dosing, reflex tachycardia Hyperuricemia, hyperglycemia
Trimethaphan	Ganglionic blocker (balanced)	Aortic aneurysm Subarachnoid bleed	Anticholinergic effects (urinary retention, ileus, cycloplegia) Decreased cardiac output
Phentolamine	Alpha blocker + direct vasodilator (balanced)	Pheochromocytoma MAO crisis	Tachycardia/angina Tachyphylaxis

ETOH, alcohol; MAO, monoamine oxidase; AV, atrioventricular.

potential for severe bradycardia and high-grade atrioventricular block, many physicians are reluctant to use it.

SPECIFIC HYPERTENSIVE PROBLEMS

A summary of preferred therapy for various hypertensive emergencies is presented in Table 22.3; however a brief discussion of the most common hypertensive crises is needed to emphasize the unique aspects of pathophysiology and treatment.

HYPERTENSIVE ENCEPHALOPATHY

Hypertensive encephalopathy is diffuse brain dysfunction caused by cerebral edema resulting from the loss of central nervous system (CNS) vessel autoregulation. The rate at which the BP increases probably is as important as the absolute level achieved. In chronic hypertension, changes in cerebral autoregulation tend to reduce the risk of hypertensive encephalopathy, even with marked elevations in BP. In contrast, an acute BP rise during pregnancy or an episode of glomerulo-

TABLE 22–2

ORAL REGIMENS FOR MODERATE HYPERTENSION

Drug	Initial Dose	Subsequent Doses	Duration
Clonidine	0.1–0.2 mg orally	0.1 mg every 1 hr to maximum dose of 0.7 mg	8–12 hours
Nifedipine	10 mg orally	10–20 mg every 15 minutes	3–6 hours
Captopril*	12.5–25 mg	25 mg every 8 hours	6–8 hours

* Use with extreme caution for patients with renal insufficiency or intravascular volume depletion.

TABLE 22-3

ANTIHYPERTENSIVE CHOICES IN SPECIFIC CONDITIONS

Condition	Preferred drugs	Drugs to avoid
Dissecting aneurysm	Trimethaphan, nitroprusside + β-blocker Nicardipine, labetolol	Direct vasodilators alone (nitroprusside, diazoxide, hydralazine)
Pulmonary edema	Nitroprusside, nitrates, nicardipine Morphine, diuretics	β-blockers,* trimethaphan, labetolol
Angina/MI (no CHF)	β-blockers,* nitrates, nicardipine Calcium blockers, labetolol	Direct vasodilators, phentolamine
Cerebral hemorrhage	No treatment?/nitroprusside	Trimethaphan, methyldopa, clonidine diazoxide, β-blockers
Hypertensive encephalopathy	Nitroprusside, nicardipine Labetolol, diazoxide	Methyldopa, clonidine, reserpine, β-blockers
Catecholamine excess	Phentolamine, trimethaphan Nitroprusside + β-blocker	β-blockers alone, diazoxide, labetolol
Postoperative HTN	Nitroprusside, nicardipine Nitrates	Long-acting agents

* Contraindicated in patients with CHF.

nephritis may cause hypertensive encephalopathy with a BP as low as 160/100 mm Hg.

Hypertensive encephalopathy must be distinguished from the much more common mental-status-altering disorders, including ischemic or hemorrhagic stroke, hypoglycemia, subarachnoid hemorrhage, meningitis, encephalitis, brain tumors, and seizures. The distinction may be difficult because many of these conditions may be accompanied by secondary elevations of BP. Headache is the most common complaint in hypertensive encephalopathy, followed by nausea, vomiting, blurred vision, and confusion. Focal neurologic deficits, including hemiparesis and cranial nerve palsies (particularly of the facial nerve), may occur. Arteritis of the vessels nourishing the optic nerve (not increased intracranial pressure) produces the papilledema seen in most cases of hypertensive encephalopathy. There are no specific laboratory findings in hypertensive encephalopathy; the electroencephalographic features are nondiagnostic, and although the opening pressure recorded during a lumbar puncture may be elevated, the fluid analysis usually is unremarkable.

The sine qua non of hypertensive encephalopathy is mental clearing within hours of BP control. Therefore, the goal of therapy in hypertensive encephalopathy is to lower the BP to "safe" levels as quickly as possible with nitroprusside, nicardipine, diazoxide, or trimethaphan. A diastolic blood pressure of 100 mm Hg (mean arterial pressure near 120 mm Hg) is an appropriate initial

target that must not be undershot. Normally, cerebral blood flow (CBF) is autoregulated to maintain constant perfusion over a wide range of mean arterial pressures (Fig. 22.1). Failure of cerebral autoregulation may allow excessive perfusion (resulting in cerebral edema) or transient periods of hypoperfusion and ischemia. Normal autoregulatory mechanisms are modified by the presence of chronic hypertension, making mean arterial pressures of 100 to 120 mm Hg necessary for adequate cerebral perfusion. Therefore, it is important not to lower perfusion pressure excessively in any hypertensive CNS syndrome.

CEREBRAL ISCHEMIA AND HEMORRHAGE

Hypertension predisposes three specific "stroke syndromes:" bland cerebral infarction, subarachnoid hemorrhage, and intracerebral hemorrhage. In all three situations, vascular autoregulation is lost in areas of acute bleeding or infarction. Sudden onset of focal neurologic deficits, obtundation, headache, and vomiting are the most frequent symptoms of these disorders. (Focal deficits are uncommon with subarachnoid hemorrhage.)

The role for BP reduction in patients with bland cerebral infarction remains unknown, but in the absence of effective autoregulation, reducing severe hypertension (diastolic BP > 130 mm Hg) may salvage areas bordering the infarct. On the other hand, excessive reductions in BP may worsen CNS deficits. Therefore, cautious reduc-

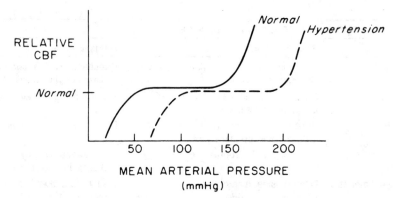

FIG. 22–1. Effects of mean arterial pressure on CBF. Although CBF normally is autoregulated in the range of 50 to 150 mm Hg, chronic hypertension shifts this curve rightward and necessitates a higher minimal pressure for adequate flow.

tion in diastolic BP to 100–120 mm Hg range is the accepted goal.

Without a predisposing anatomic abnormality, hypertension alone rarely results in subarachnoid hemorrhage. Arterial vasospasm, a process that further reduces perfusion, is common after subarachnoid hemorrhage. Experimental use of calcium channel blockers has proven efficacious in subarachnoid hemorrhage, even in the absence of blood pressure reductions. Because no clear benefit of BP reduction has been shown in subarachnoid bleeding, therapy is usually withheld unless severe hypertension is present.

Hypertension is a major predisposing factor for intracerebral hemorrhage, especially in patients with cerebral aneurysms and those receiving systemic anticoagulation. In patients with intracerebral hemorrhage, blood often enters the subarachnoid space (mimicking subarachnoid hemorrhage) by dissecting through the internal capsule or putamen into the lateral ventricles. Although it makes some sense to reduce blood pressure to near normal levels, the benefit of reducing BP is unproven, except for diastolic pressures > 130 mm Hg.

When reduction in blood pressure is indicated in any of three conditions discussed above, the short-acting agents nitroprusside and nicardipine are the drugs of choice. The sedative effects of clonidine, methyldopa, and reserpine impair monitoring of mental status and should be avoided. Diazoxide also is a poor choice, because it decreases cerebral blood flow disproportionately. Indeed, except for hypertensive encephalopathy, diazoxide is contraindicated in all cerebral disorders complicating hypertension.

AORTIC DISSECTION

Aortic dissection should be suspected in the setting of profound malignant hypertension when there are characteristic signs or symptoms. "Tearing" chest or back pain and an arm/leg BP difference, absent pulses in the lower extremities, or asymmetry in BP between arms are all suggestive. Artifactual hypotension may result if BP is checked only in the left arm of a patient with aortic dissection as blood flow to the left subclavian artery is compromised. The diagnosis of aortic dissection is supported by finding a widened mediastinum on chest radiograph. Confirmation may be sought by chest computed tomography (CT), magnetic resonance imaging (MRI), or aortography. The goal of BP reduction is to immediately decrease both mean BP and the rate of increase in systolic pressure (dp/dt) while preserving vital organ perfusion. A target diastolic BP of approximately 100 mm Hg usually is appropriate. Reducing dp/dt decreases the shear force on the aortic wall, helping to limit dissection and can be achieved by β-adrenergic or ganglionic blockade. Unfortunately, β-blockade alone usually does not provide a sufficiently rapid reduction in BP. Therefore, β-blockers often are used in conjunction with nitroprusside or nicardipine. Alternatively, labetolol or trimethaphan alone are appropriate regimens. Although trimethaphan has been recommended as the drug of choice in this condition, unfamiliarity with its use often leads to therapeutic misadventure. Because hydralazine and diazoxide increase heart rate, cardiac output, and dp/dt, they represent poor choices for therapy.

RENAL FAILURE

Renal failure may be the cause of hypertension as in glomerulonephritis, vasculitis, or renal artery stenosis or may be the result of a hypertensive crisis. When hypertension is the cause of renal insufficiency, reversible perfusion-related increases in creatinine and blood urea nitrogen (BUN) frequently follow BP reduction. In this setting, reestablishing a safe BP is the main priority. Although other reversible causes of renal insufficiency (volume depletion, renal artery occlusion, lower tract obstruction) should be sought, an increasing BUN or creatinine should not dissuade the clinician from continuing antihypertensive therapy. For patients presenting with a serum creatinine > 3.5 mg/dL, progressive renal failure is a likely and often unavoidable consequence of therapy. In renal insufficiency, nitroprusside is a good drug for BP control, even though thiocyanate toxicity occurs more commonly than when normal renal function is present. Labetolol and the calcium channel blocker nicardipine represent good alternatives.

PULMONARY EDEMA

In most cases of malignant hypertension, pulmonary edema primarily is the result of excessive left ventricular afterload, not circulatory volume overload, and usually responds rapidly when systemic vascular resistance is lowered. Heightened afterload is most likely to cause pulmonary edema in patients with preexisting left ventricular dysfunction or aortic insufficiency. Effective therapy focuses on reduction of afterload, making nitroprusside, nicardipine, and nitroglycerin the most useful agents. In clearly volume-overloaded patients, morphine sulfate, diuretics and dialysis are useful adjuncts.

ANGINA AND MYOCARDIAL INFARCTION

In acute myocardial ischemia, reductions in BP preserve endangered myocardium by reducing afterload, decreasing wall stress, and increasing myocardial perfusion. In severe hypertension with myocardial ischemia, unopposed use of arterial vasodilators that produce tachycardia and increase myocardial oxygen consumption (hydralazine, diazoxide, minoxidil) should be avoided. Caution also should be exercised when using nitroprusside, a drug that tends to divert blood away from the most ischemic areas of myocardium. Labeto-

lol, nicardipine, and β-blockers are attractive therapeutic options because they improve the ratio of oxygen supply to demand. Nitroglycerin, primarily a venodilator, affects both peripheral and coronary circulations, thereby reducing preload and decreasing BP.

CATECHOLAMINE EXCESSES

Conditions resulting in catecholamine-induced hypertension include (*a*) pheochromocytoma, (*b*) sympathomimetic drug (cocaine, lysergic acid diethylamide [LSD], phencyclidine, amphetamine) overdose, (*c*) monoamine oxidase (MAO) inhibitor crisis, and (*d*) antihypertensive withdrawal (rebound) syndrome. Patients with these disorders commonly present with tachycardia, diaphoresis, pallor, pounding headache, and vomiting.

Pheochromocytoma is a rare cause of hypertensive crisis, but should be considered in patients with hypertension induced by performance of angiography or the induction of anesthesia and in patients with a history of hyperparathyroidism or a family history of pheochromocytoma. MAO inhibitor crisis is also rare, occurring when tyramine-containing foods (cheese, beer, wine, chocolate) or other sympathomimetic agents are ingested by patients receiving MAO inhibitors. The problem of rebound hypertension is especially common in postoperative patients and those in the intensive care unit after abrupt discontinuation of antihypertensive drugs. Although this syndrome is most frequently associated with the centrally acting α-agents (e.g., clonidine, methyldopa, and guanabenz), withdrawal of β-blockers also may produce rebound hypertension. Such drugs probably should be avoided for noncompliant patients and, when discontinued, should be tapered over several days.

Treatment for all of these syndromes is similar. α-adrenergic blockers (e.g., phentolamine) or direct vasodilators (e.g., nitroprusside) are the mainstays of therapy. Used alone, β-blockers are contraindicated in catecholamine excess, because unopposed α-effects may paradoxically worsen hypertension. The same problem may be encountered with labetolol because its β-blocking effects are substantially more prominent than its α-blocking actions. Many patients will have severe hypertension but exhibit orthostatic symptoms due to hypertension-induced diuresis. In such patients, administration of isotonic saline is indicated in addition to antihypertensive agents.

ECLAMPSIA

Eclampsia is defined as the occurrence of hypertension, edema, proteinuria, and seizures in the last trimester of pregnancy. Although the specific cause of eclampsia is unknown, the syndrome responds to delivery of the infant. Hydralazine and α-methyldopa have been the traditional choices for drug treatment. All other antihypertensives are controversial because of potential adverse effects on uterine contractility, uterine blood flow, or the fetus itself. For severe cases of hypertension, labetolol or nitroprusside may be necessary to preserve the life of the mother and fetus.

THERAPY FOR HYPERTENSIVE EMERGENCIES

COMMONLY USED AGENTS

Diuretics

Because most patients with severe hypertension have normal or reduced circulating blood volume, diuretics should be avoided in the emergency setting unless overt signs of heart failure, pulmonary edema, or fluid overload are present. Although not intuitive, volume supplementation with isotonic saline often is necessary when using potent vasodilators to correct hypertensive crises. (With more chronic use, however, most antihypertensive agents tend to cause sodium retention and, thus, should be used in conjunction with a diuretic.) Intravenous furosemide is the most commonly used diuretic. Furosemide is potent, rapidly acting, inexpensive, and has the added benefit of providing mild vasodilation. Bumetanide is essentially equivalent in its actions.

Nitroprusside

Nitroprusside is a direct-acting arteriovenous dilator with an immediate onset of action (usually <1 minute) and the potential for rapid termination of action (1–3 minutes). Nitroprusside's effects probably are mediated by the release of the endogenous vasodilator (nitric oxide). The photo-instability of nitroprusside mandates frequent changes of solutions and use of light-protected containers. Infusion typically is initiated at a dose of 0.5 μg/kg/minute and titrated upward to produce the desired BP. Doses required for hypertension often are higher than those needed for the treatment of

congestive heart failure but generally do not exceed 10 μg/kg/minute. Because of its potency, controlled administration by pump infusion is mandatory. At low dosage rates, reductions in systemic resistance are compensated for by increases in cardiac output. Therefore, BP may remain stable initially despite a beneficial action; actual reduction of BP often requires dosing in the higher range. The effects of nitroprusside are most pronounced in patients taking multiple other antihypertensive drugs and those who are volume depleted.

Nitroprusside is metabolized hepatically to cyanide and then thiocyanate, which is then cleared renally. Therefore, renal failure may result in thiocyanate toxicity. Levels higher than 10 mg/dL may cause hepatic failure, metabolic acidosis, dyspnea, and vomiting. Cyanide may accumulate in hepatic failure, but toxicity is very rare when nitroprusside is administered at the usual doses of less than 3 μg/kg/minute for less than 72 hours. Nitrates, cyanocobalamin, and thiosulfate are useful in the treatment of thiocyanate toxicity.

Calcium Channel Blockers

All calcium channel blockers produce systemic and coronary vasodilation as a result of their inhibition of the slow calcium channel. Nicardipine, the newest parenterally available calcium channel blocker, rapidly reduces BP when administered by continuous infusion at rates of 5 to 15 mg/hour. Unlike its parenteral predecessor, verapamil, cardiac contractility and conduction rarely are adversely affected. Increases in ejection fraction and stroke volume are responsible for the rises in cardiac output observed in most patients. Reflex tachycardia stemming from vasodilation rarely is a problem, making this drug an excellent alternative to nitroprusside in cases of hypertension associated with myocardial ischemia of congestive heart failure.

Verapamil, the first parenterally available calcium channel blocker, causes myocardial depression and conduction blockade in a substantial number of patients, even though it promptly but briefly lowers BP after a single intravenous dose. Because of its negative inotropic action and because cardiac conduction is so often impaired, resulting in a slower heart rate, increased PR interval, and occasionally second-degree and third-degree atrioventricular block, verapamil represents a relatively poor choice for most patients with acute hypertension.

Labetolol

Labetolol is a combined α- and β-blocker with rapid onset but a long and variable duration of action (1–8 hours). The β-blocking properties of labetolol are substantially more potent than its α-blocking effects, occasionally resulting in paradoxical hypertension in high catecholamine states. An advantage of labetolol is the rarity of "overshoot hypotension." An initial bolus of 20 mg is almost always effective in lowering BP, whereas doses of 20 to 80 mg at 20- to 40-minute intervals provide continued BP control. Labetolol also is available in tablet form, facilitating conversion from intravenous to oral therapy. The primary disadvantages of labetolol lie in its potential to exacerbate heart failure and bronchospasm and its long duration of action.

Nitrates

Nitroglycerin is an arterial and venous vasodilator having an immediate onset of action but a brief duration. Nitroglycerin is particularly useful in the setting of myocardial ischemia or congestive heart failure associated with hypertension. Liver disease reduces the hepatic metabolism of nitrates potentiating their effects. The side effects of nitrates include headache, tachycardia, and flushing but rarely are dose-limiting.

Angiotensin Converting Enzyme Inhibitors

Angiotensin-converting enzyme (ACE) inhibitors antagonize the conversion of angiotensin I to the extremely potent vasoconstrictor angiotensin II. Reductions in systemic vascular resistance with stable pulmonary capillary wedge pressures and cardiac outputs usually are seen after administration of ACE inhibitors. Patients with congestive heart failure may have a fall in filling pressures and a rise in cardiac output. Captopril and enalapril, when given orally, are absorbed within 30 to 90 minutes, providing blood pressure reduction for 8 and 24 hours, respectively. Few side effects are associated with these drugs if their dose is reduced in renal insufficiency and if they are not given to profoundly volume-depleted patients. Hyperkalemia may be seen in patients with renal artery stenosis and those receiving potassium supplements or nonsteroidal anti-inflammatory drugs.

The parenteral preparation, Enalaprilat®, is an active form of enalapril that produces rapid BP reduction by inhibiting angiotensin II formation. Enalaprilat may produce severe hypotension in volume-depleted patients. Equally potent hypotensive effects are observed at almost all doses; increasing the dose only extends the duration of action. A long duration of action represents a potential disadvantage in cases of overshoot hypotension.

RARELY USED AGENTS

Diazoxide

Diazoxide, a direct arteriolar vasodilator, frequently induces hypotension when given suddenly in large (5 mg/kg) doses. Use of small intravenous boluses of 1 to 2 mg/kg (given at 10-minute intervals) or a constant infusion (at rates of up to 15 mg/minute) are alternative methods of administration that reduce the risk of hypotension. With an onset of action of 1 to 2 minutes and a mean duration of action of 8 hours, diazoxide is useful for patients who cannot be monitored on a minute-to-minute basis.

Nausea and vomiting are common side effects of diazoxide, limiting its usefulness in patients with altered levels of consciousness. Furthermore, cerebral perfusion may be reduced disproportionately to BP by this drug. Reflex increases in heart rate make diazoxide alone a poor choice for patients with ischemic heart disease or aortic aneurysm. The potent fluid-retaining properties of diazoxide almost always require the concurrent use of diuretics after BP has been controlled. Hyperglycemia, hyperuricemia, and potentiation of warfarin anticoagulation are other common side effects.

Trimethaphan

Trimethaphan, a ganglionic blocker, exerts direct peripheral vasodilating effects. Although its rapid onset (1–2 minutes) is desirable, the sustained (10-minute) duration of action may be problematic for patients who develop hypotension in response to an excessive dose. Like nitroprusside, trimethaphan must be administered by an infusion pump because of its potency. Severe orthostatic hypotension is seen in almost all patients receiving the drug, and positional sensitivity should be considered when difficulty is encountered in obtaining precise BP control. Tachyphylaxis limits its efficacy to 3 to 4 days. Trimethaphan routinely reduces cardiac output and renal blood flow and rarely causes apnea. Furthermore, parasympathetic blockade may result in such distressing symptoms as dry mouth, blurred vision, constipation, and abdominal distention. With the possible exception of dissecting aortic aneurysm and catecholamine excess, equally efficacious and less toxic alternatives have generally supplanted the use of trimethaphan.

Hydralazine

The action of hydralazine, a direct vasodilator, begins within 10 minutes if given intravenously and within 30 minutes if given intramuscularly. Unfortunately, its prolonged duration of action (3–6 hours) may cause persistent overshoot hypotension. Because hydralazine is not consistently effective at lowering BP, it is a poor choice for acute treatment of life-threatening hypertension. Unless counteracted by a β-blocker, the arteriolar dilating effects of hydralazine often result in reflex tachycardia and contractility, thereby worsening coronary ischemia and aortic dissection. By reducing its clearance from the body, renal failure potentiates the effects of hydralazine.

Methyldopa

Methyldopa is a long-acting central sympatholytic with a delayed onset of action (2–4 hours). Its delayed action and tendency to cause sedation make it undesirable for use in hypertensive emergencies; however, for patients with non–life-threatening hypertension, methyldopa has the advantage of lowering BP gradually (over several hours). Overshoot hypotension is uncommon, but long-term use is associated with drug-induced fever, hepatocellular inflammation, and hemolytic anemia.

Phentolamine

Phentolamine is an α-adrenergic blocking drug with an abrupt onset of action (1–2 minutes). Its twin effects of α-blockade and non–α-mediated vasodilation precipitate hypotension, tachycardia, nausea, and vomiting in a large percentage of patients who receive it. Unfortunately, reflex tachycardia induced by phentolamine may worsen coronary ischemia, even when beneficial reductions in afterload are achieved. Again, because of the development of equally effective and less toxic therapies, phentolamine use has largely fallen out of favor.

KEY POINTS

1. Most cases of severe hypertension in the ICU do not stem from an exotic cause but are the result of patients interrupting previously efficacious treatment for essential hypertension. Initial episodes of severe hypertension clearly should be investigated for a secondary cause, especially for young patients and black patients, in whom such secondary causes are much more common.

2. Immediate parenteral therapy is indicated for hypertensive crises with associated organ failure. In most cases, sodium nitroprusside is the initial drug of choice.

3. For most hypertensive crises with organ failure, a mean arterial pressure of 120 mm Hg represents a good initial BP target.

4. When organ failure accompanies severe hypertension, BP generally should be reduced within minutes; in the absence of organ failure, reduction over hours is not only acceptable but desirable.

5. Patients with chronic severe hypertension often do not tolerate rapid, profound BP reductions, because cerebral autoregulation is reset by chronic hypertension.

6. Oral therapy should be initiated early in the hospitalization to minimize the duration of parenteral therapy and ICU stay.

SUGGESTED READINGS

1. Huysmans FT, Thien TA, Sluiter HE, et al. Acute treatment of hypertensive crisis with nifedipine. Br J Clin Pharmacol 1983;16:725–727.
2. Huysmans FTM, Thien TA, Koene RAP. Combined intravenous administration of diazoxide and beta-blocking agent in acute treatment of severe hypertension or hypertensive crisis. Am Heart J 1982;103:395–400.
3. Lavin P. Management of hypertension in patients with acute stroke. Arch Intern Med 1986;146:66–68.
4. Ram CVS. Hypertensive encephalopathy-recognition and management. Arch Intern Med 1978;138:1851–1853.

5. Calhoun DA, Oparil S. Treatment of hypertensive crisis. N Engl J Med 1990;323:1177–1183.
6. Danish Multicenter Study. Emergency treatment of severe hypertension evaluated in a randomized study: effect of rest and a randomized evaluation of chlorpromazine, dihydrazine and diazoxide. Acta Med Scand 1980;208: 473–480.
7. Garcia JY, Vidt DG. Current management of hypertensive emergencies. Drugs 1987;34:263–278.
8. Wikson DJ, Wallin JD, Vlachakis ND, et al. Intravenous labetolol in the treatment of severe hypertension and hypertensive emergencies. Am J Med 1983;75(Suppl 4): 95–102.
9. Bertel O, Conen D, Radu EW, et al. Nifedipine in hypertensive emergencies. BMJ 1983;286:19–21.
10. Houston M. Hypertensive emergencies and urgencies: pathophysiology and clinical aspects. Am Heart J 1986; 111:205–210.
11. Strandgaard S, Olesen J, Shinhoj, et al. Autoregulation of brain circulation in severe arterial hypertension. BMJ 1973;1:507–510.
12. Houston M. Pathophysiology, clinical aspects, and treatment of hypertensive crises. Prog Cardiovasc Dis 1989; 32:99–148.
13. Britton M, de Faire U, Helmers C. Hazards of therapy for excessive hypertension in acute stroke. Acta Med Scand 1980;207:253–257.
14. Wallace JD, Levy LL. Blood pressure after stroke. JAMA 1981;246:2177–2180.
15. Vidt DG, Gifford RW. A compendium for the treatment of hypertensive emergencies. Cleve Clin Q 1984;51: 421–430.
16. McRae RP, Liebson PR. Hypertensive crisis. Med Clin North Am 1986;70:749–767.
17. Cumming AM, Davies DL. Intravenous labetolol in hypertensive emergency. Lancet 1979;1:929–930.
18. Silver HM. Acute hypertensive crisis in pregnancy. Med Clin North Am 1989;73:623–638.
19. Houston MC. Treatment of hypertensive emergencies and urgencies with oral clonidine loading and titration: a review. Arch Intern Med 1986;146:586–589.
20. Halpern NA, Goldberg M, Neely C, et al. Postoperative hypertension: a multicenter, prospective, randomized comparison between intravenous nicardipine and sodium nitroprusside. Crit Care Med 1992;20:1637–1643.
21. MacGregor GA. Blood pressure, angiotensin-converting enzyme (ACE) inhibitors, and the kidney. Am J Med 1992;92:20S–27S.

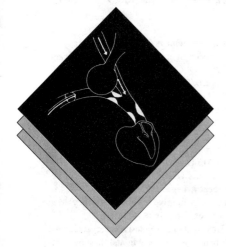

CHAPTER 23

Venous Thrombosis and Pulmonary Embolism

DEFINITIONS AND MECHANISMS

Pulmonary embolism (PE) may result when any insoluble substance gains access to the systemic veins. Because blood filtering is a natural function of the lung, small and asymptomatic embolism may occur periodically, even in healthy persons. Distinctive syndromes have been described for embolism of air, oil, fat, tumor cells, amniotic fluid, foreign objects, and injected particulates, as well as for bland and infected fibrin clots. In critical care, air embolism, fat embolism, septic embolism, and bland thrombotic embolism are the major syndromes of interest. Air embolism is discussed in Chapter 8 (Practical Problems and Complications of Mechanical Ventilation).

Oil or fat embolism (during lymphangiography or trauma to long bones) does not directly impede blood flow. Instead, symptoms develop because the fatty acid products of lipid digestion produce bronchoconstriction, vasoconstriction, and vascular injury with capillary leak and edema (acute respiratory distress syndrome [ARDS]) (see Chapter 24, Oxygenation Failure).

Similarly, the major threat to life in septic embolism is not vascular obstruction but septic physiology. Small, friable fragments of infected material embolize to cause fever, toxicity, and a characteristic radiograph: multiple ill-defined infiltrates or nodules of varied sizes that frequently cavitate and usually display soft, irregular outlines. Perfusion defects on lung scan are typically unimpressive compared to the radiograph. Pelvic inflammation, venous catheters or right-sided heart valves, phlebitis, and nonsterile injections

(related to drug abuse) are common sources of infected material. After identification, the source must be isolated surgically or removed and the infection treated vigorously with antibiotics directed at the offending organism(s).

Among the most frequent preventable causes of death in hospitalized patients, bland thrombotic pulmonary embolism is a disease that mandates skillful integration of clinical and laboratory data. Its subtlety requires considerable judgment regarding the need for invasive pursuit of the diagnosis.

DEEP VENOUS THROMBOSIS

DIAGNOSIS

Predisposing Factors

Essentially all victims of PE and deep venous thrombosis (DVT) have clearly defined risk factors: stasis of venous blood, injury to the vascular intima, or hypercoagulability. Thus, bed rest, the later stages of pregnancy, immobilization, chronic venous disease, trauma (especially to the lower extremities), sepsis, and heart failure are common predisposing factors. In some settings (hip or knee surgery), DVT may occur in up to 70% of patients who do not receive prophylactic therapy. Primary hypercoagulable states are uncommonly diagnosed. Hypercoagulability associated with factor V Leiden disease, anticardiolipin antibodies, homocystinuria or deficiencies of antithrombin III, or proteins C or S should be suspected in young patients, patients without other recognized risk factors, and in patients with a personal or family history of recurrent thrombosis (see Chapter 30, Clotting and Bleeding Disorders and Anticoagulation Therapy).

In the general hospital population, most (approximately 90%) of pulmonary emboli are believed to result from deep venous calf thrombi that propagate above the knee. Clots confined to the calf are of little physiologic importance. Unfortunately, approximately one-half of calf thrombi extend above the knee, and approximately one-half of these eventually produce symptomatic PE. Therefore, as many as 10 to 20% of patients with calf thrombus will develop PE without prophylaxis. Not all of these patients will be symptomatic. Patients in the intensive care unit (ICU) differ in that they often have other nontraditional sources for thrombus formation. Indwelling central venous catheters provide a constant nidus for thrombus formation: embolization is particularly likely to occur upon catheter removal, as the encasing thrombus is stripped away. Heparin-treated catheters may be protected temporarily from thrombosis until the heparin is leached out over a period of 24 to 36 hours.

Physical Examination

Superficial thrombophlebitis manifest by erythema, tenderness, and a palpable "venous cord" poses little embolic risk unless it extends to the deep system. Such extension is suggested strongly by generalized and asymmetric leg swelling, a highly unusual feature of uncomplicated superficial inflammation.

The physical examination is poor for detecting DVT and distinguishing DVT from conditions that commonly mimic it. The signs of DVT relate to venous inflammation and obstruction. Unilateral lower extremity erythema, heat, swelling, and pain suggest DVT, as do unilateral ankle and leg edema. Unfortunately, neither inflammation nor obstruction may be present or obvious, and other processes unrelated to thrombosis may cause the same findings. At least half of large vessel clots go unsuspected on physical examination. Homans' sign is a nonspecific indicator of calf inflammation that is seldom present in documented DVT.

Several common conditions mimic DVT. A ruptured Baker's cyst presents as a mass in the calf with pain and erythema, usually in patients with rheumatoid arthritis. An accurate diagnosis

must be made to avoid the use of potentially dangerous therapies (e.g., thrombolytic drugs) that could provoke bleeding into the cyst. Rupture of the plantaris tendon also may mimic DVT on examination, but the history is key, revealing recent exertion with the acute onset of excruciating pain. Crystalline arthritis (gout or pseudogout) may produce intense joint space inflammation that extends into the calf. Cellulitis seen in the setting of direct trauma or chronic fungal infection of the feet or after coronary bypass surgery often is confused with DVT. It is frequently so difficult to distinguish DVT from cellulitis that concomitant antibiotic therapy and heparin are begun empirically until the diagnosis of DVT is confirmed or excluded. Although sometimes confused with DVT, pulmonary osteoarthropathy presents with pain, tenderness, and swelling over the *anterior* tibia, with or without clubbing, and can be confirmed radiographically. In patients with hemophilia or those taking anticoagulants, hematoma formation in the muscles of the calf also may produce a syndrome clinically similar to DVT. Postphlebitic syndrome usually presents with recurrent painless calf swelling after an episode of DVT.

DIAGNOSTIC TESTING

Even though most emboli originate in the legs, a negative imaging study for DVT does not exclude the possibility of a pulmonary embolism. Non-occlusive thrombi may be missed by screening techniques. In up to one-third of angiographically proven cases of pulmonary embolism, imaging studies of the legs are negative. (Often because all detectable clots have moved to the lung.) For this reason, a negative leg study cannot be used as evidence of the absence of pulmonary emboli.

Duplex ultrasound scanning is capable of directly imaging veins and probing venous flow rates. When ultrasound visualizes intravenous, noncompressible clot, the diagnosis is certain. Doppler flow studies also accurately identify large vein obstruction, unless flow is compromised by low cardiac output or central venous congestion. Because Doppler studies sense large-vein obstruction, ultrasound is not as sensitive as contrast venography or fibrinogen scanning in detecting calf clot or nonobstructive thigh clots. Although its predictive value in young, symptomatic, ambulatory patients is near perfect, ultrasound is less sensitive and specific than contrast venography among the critically ill. Portability, low cost, and unquestioned safety make ultrasound the preferred test in the ICU population despite these limitations.

Impedance plethysmography (IPG) detects changes in the electrical conductance of the leg occurring as the venous circulation is obstructed and then released. If large veins are significantly obstructed, the slower changes in conductance are observed as the obstruction to venous outflow is released. IPG has the same low rate of false–positive results in acute DVT as ultrasound. Unfortunately, like ultrasound, IPG cannot reliably diagnose pelvic disease and is insensitive to calf vein thrombosis. Also similar to ultrasound, attractive features of the IPG include portability, low cost, and the ability to repeat studies daily if necessary to detect the progression of calf thrombus above the knee.

The contrast phlebogram (venogram) is simultaneously the most sensitive, definitive, time-consuming, and potentially injurious method for defining clots of the deep veins. Unfortunately, vein patency neither ensures that emboli will not occur in the future nor guarantees that an intraluminal clot did not break free or recanalize before the study. Furthermore, contrast may precipitate renal insufficiency, allergic reactions, and local phlebitis. Venography is most useful in distinguishing large-vessel occlusion from cellulitis or other causes of swelling and inflammation in the lower extremities. Rarely diagnostic, the radionuclide venogram is all but useless because of its low sensitivity and specificity.

Iodine-131 fibrinogen scanning is a sensitive technique for detecting active fibrinogen turnover in the calf veins. Unfortunately, its sensitivity is diminished by heparin therapy and it is expensive and time consuming, requiring 12 to 24 hours from injection to diagnosis. Radiofibrinogen scanning is a poor test for clot in the iliac veins or pelvis because the signal emitted by the incorporated fibrinogen is low compared with that of the background blood pool. Because of the associated technical problems and risk of viral hepatitis transmission, radiofibrinogen scanning currently is rarely performed.

PREVENTION

Primary prevention is the most important treatment of DVT. In fact, DVT prevention is so important that it makes sense to have unit-wide recommendations for prophylaxis for essentially all patients in the ICU. A major step toward DVT prevention is early ambulation. A corollary is the avoidance of excessive sedation and unnecessary paralysis, because both actions prolong the period of bed rest for the critically ill patient. Although considered by some practitioners to be impractical, it is clearly possible to have some mechanically ventilated patients ambulate with portable ventilatory support. When early ambulation is not possible, mechanical or pharmacologic prophylaxis should be instituted.

Well fitting, graded compression elastic stockings and sequential pneumatic compression devices both promote venous flow and may decrease stasis in patients who must avoid anticoagulation (e.g., trauma, vascular surgery, or coagulopathy). Alone, each type of device has been shown to reduce the risk of DVT, but even lower rates of DVT have been observed when graded compression stockings and intermittent pneumatic compression devices are used together. Although controversial, it seems that neither of these mechanical devices is as effective as pharmacologic prophylaxis.

Prophylactic subcutaneous heparin is a highly effective method of preventing DVT but is inadequate treatment for existing clot. Heparin can reduce the risk of DVT by as much as 50 to 75% in selected populations but does not entirely eliminate the risk of DVT or PE. Subcutaneous fixed dose (''minidose'') heparin (5,000 units every 8–12 hours) is of proven benefit in medical and general surgery patients; however, patients undergoing hip, knee, or prostatic surgery do not seem to enjoy the same level of protection. These high-risk patients require oral warfarin; heparin in a dose adjusted to prolong the partial thromboplastin time (PTT) (typically 5,000–10,000 units subcutaneously every 8–12 hours); or low-molecular-weight heparin (LMWH) for maximal protection. Fixed low-dose therapy does not predictably prolong the PTT or cause hemorrhagic complications; however, symptomatic thrombocytopenia may occur (see Chapter 30, Clotting and Bleeding Disorders and Anticoagulation Therapy).

In some studies, the newer LMWHs equal or surpass the effectiveness of conventional heparin for DVT prophylaxis and have a lower incidence of hemorrhagic complications. When used for lower extremity orthopedic procedures, LMWH is as effective or more effective than standard heparin or warfarin. A reduction in the risk of bleeding complications probably is the result of less intense interaction of the drug with the platelet-associated von Willebrand's factor than that occurring with traditional, nonfractionated heparins.

For some orthopedic procedures (e.g., hip or knee replacement), low-dose preoperative warfarin reduces the risk of DVT without increasing bleeding complications. Because of the relatively long time between beginning warfarin therapy and when effective prophylaxis is achieved, warfarin is most useful for elective procedures, not emergent ICU cases. Dextran also reduces the risk of DVT, but frequent side effects, including aggravation of bleeding tendency, limit its use. Aspirin and dipyridamole have not been shown to be as effective as warfarin or the heparins for prophylaxis.

TREATMENT

The goals of treatment in DVT are to prevent clot extension, preserve the venous architecture, and relieve pain. Although desirable, even optimal anticoagulation does not guarantee that PE will not occur in patients with established DVT. (Up to 15% of ideally anticoagulated patients with DVT will develop a PE.) Patients with DVT and active ongoing thrombosis can require large doses of heparin initially. As the thrombotic process is inhibited and the clot undergoes endogenous thrombolysis, daily heparin requirements usually decline. Although a point of frequent speculation, it is not possible to accurately predict the "clot burden" or precise heparin requirements. Luckily, because the treatment of DVT and pulmonary embolism is essentially the same, the diagnosis of either usually obviates the need to search for the complementary condition.

For the time being, continuous heparin infusion remains the standard treatment for established DVT, unless contraindications to anticoagulation are compelling. It is likely, however, that intermittently dosed LMWHs will soon replace continuous infusion heparin because of their equivalent efficacy, relative ease of administration, and potentially reduced cost of therapy. The "target" for continuous infusion heparin therapy is a PTT of 1.5 times the laboratory control or the patient's baseline PTT if known. PTT values less than 1.5 times the control value are associated with an increased likelihood of clotting recurrence; however, there is no certain advantage of maintaining more intense anticoagulation.

Excessive prolongation of the PTT (>100 seconds) may increase the risk of bleeding, but the relationship between the PTT and bleeding complications remains controversial. Over all, approximately 1% of anticoagulated patients will suffer some bleeding complication each day of treatment, accounting for the overall 7 to 15% incidence of hemorrhage during in hospital anticoagulant therapy. Spontaneous hemorrhage is rare in the absence of breached vascular integrity, impaired platelet function, or massive heparin overdose. Therefore, bleeding is most common among alcoholics, elderly patients, postoperative patients, and patients receiving drugs that impair platelet aggregation. Heparin should be continued for approximately 5 days while establishing oral anticoagulation and allowing the thrombus to organize and attach to the vessel wall.

LMWHs have equal or superior efficacy to standard heparin in treating established DVT. The ability of LMWH to be administered safely by intermittent subcutaneous injection without PTT monitoring promises to reduce cost and shorten hospital stay. (Perhaps the therapy of uncomplicated DVT will move entirely to the outpatient setting.) Fewer platelet-inhibiting effects of these compounds may reduce the risk of hemorrhagic complications.

Warfarin should be initiated shortly after beginning heparin to maintain effective anticoagulation without a therapeutic break and to minimize hospital stay. A prothrombin time (PT) maintained at 1.2 to 1.5 times control (international normalized ratio [INR] = 2–3) usually will prevent clot recurrence; however, patients with inherited or acquired coagulopathies often require more intense anticoagulation. For example, patients with anticardiolipin antibody syndrome often require INRs higher than 3 for effective prophylaxis. Warfarin usually is continued for 3 to 6 months after an uncomplicated episode of DVT or until the precipitating risk factors are reversed. Shorter periods of anticoagulation are associated with higher rates of recurrence, but a lower risk of bleeding complications. The duration of anticoagulation must be individualized, balancing the risks of bleeding against the risk of recurrent thrombosis. Extensive or recurrent DVT episodes are often treated for longer periods of time.

Thrombolytic therapy reduces the incidence of postphlebitic syndrome among patients with DVT but has not been shown to reduce the risk of PE or death. Because of the rare but potentially devastating risks of thrombolytic therapy (e.g., central nervous system [CNS] hemorrhage) it is not often used for uncomplicated DVT. If thrombolytic therapy is contemplated, little data suggest superiority of one agent over another in either DVT or PE.

PULMONARY EMBOLISM

PE is a complication of the root disease, DVT. Many critically ill patients die with PEs, if not from them. Perhaps as many as one-third of patients with untreated, symptomatic PE succumb to a fatal recurrence; the estimated mortality of treated PE averages 10 to 15%. This overall mortality rate may underestimate the risk to the critically ill. The diagnosis of PE for the critically ill patient is often elusive because of the nonspecificity of symptoms, physiologic disturbances, physical findings, and radiographic features.

SYMPTOMS AND PHYSICAL FINDINGS

Signs and symptoms of PE are modified in severity and duration by underlying cardiopulmonary status. No symptom or physical finding is either universal or specific. Therefore, when PE is suspected, the patient must be treated empirically or the diagnosis must be confirmed by specialized diagnostic testing. The symptoms of embolism resolve at least in part quite rapidly, usually in the first few hours or days after the event. Signs disappear more slowly. Among patients with massive and submassive emboli, the following signs and symptoms are observed: dyspnea and tachypnea (90%); pleuritic pain (70%); apprehension, rales, and cough (50%); and hemoptysis (30%). Tachycardia (>100/minute) and fever occur in a significant minority of cases. Pleural pain (presumably caused by pulmonary infarction) is most likely to be caused by emboli of moderate size occurring in patients with preexistent heart or lung disease. When syncope occurs, it usually is the result massive embolism.

Pulmonary artery pressures do not rise markedly unless the embolism obstructs more than 50% of the capillary bed or the capillary bed was compromised previously. Therefore, a right-sided gallop, increased pulmonic component of the second heart sound (P_2), or pulmonary hypertension documented by echocardiography or pulmonary artery catheterization correlate with massive acute obstruction or lesser acute obstruction in a patient with underlying pulmonary vascular disease. Detection of a pleural effusion may be suggestive: among patients with pleuritic chest pain, PE is a more likely diagnosis than infectious pleurisy when effusion is present.

ROUTINE DIAGNOSTIC TESTS

Routine diagnostic tests (chest radiograph, electrocardiogram [ECG], blood gases, leukocyte count) are most useful to exclude alternative diagnoses (e.g., pneumonia, pneumothorax, myocardial infarction, and pulmonary edema) rather than to make a certain diagnosis of PE.

Electrocardiogram

The ECG is sensitive but nonspecific. Even in patients without prior cardiopulmonary disease, the ECG is normal in only a small proportion (approximately 10%). Nonspecific ST and/or T-wave changes occur in most patients. Except for moderate sinus tachycardia, rhythm disturbances are unusual. Atrial fibrillation and flutter seldom occur in patients without preexisting cardiovascular compromise. Similarly, bundle branch block is highly unusual. Left and right bundles are affected equally often. ECG evidence of acute cor pulmonale (S_1, Q_3, T_3 pattern or acute right bundle branch block) appears rarely and then only in patients with severe vascular obstruction.

Blood Studies

Although hypoxemia is the rule, pulmonary emboli frequently are found in patients with normal values for PaO_2, $PaCO_2$, and A-a gradient. Even a normal arterial blood gas (ABG) result does not exclude the diagnosis of PE, especially in young, otherwise healthy patients. (A normal ABG is seen in up to 40% of young healthy patients with documented PE.) As a general rule, the more profound the underlying cardiovascular disease, the less likely the ABG is to be normal when a PE occurs. Although lactic dehydrogenase (LDH), serum glutamic oxaloacetic transaminase (SGOT), and bilirubin each are occasionally elevated, this classic triad is both unusual and nonspecific.

Fibrinogen and fibrin-split-product assays are not helpful in diagnosis. Recently, claims that a normal plasma d-dimer level can exclude a diagnosis of DVT or PE have been made. These data are provocative but unproven. It should be noted that several different types of d-dimer assays are available, some of which have dismal sensitivity and specificity. Experience with numerous blood tests that are claimed to "simplify" the diagnosis of PE suggests that it is not prudent to bet a patient's life on a negative d-dimer assay and exclude other clinical, radiographic, and laboratory data. DVT and PE are sufficiently difficult diagnostic problems; it is unlikely any single laboratory test can make or exclude the diagnosis.

Chest Radiograph

Nonspecific findings, including consolidation, elevated hemidiaphragm, small pleural effusion, and atelectasis, are common. Indeed, the chest radiograph remains unchanged from the pre-event film in fewer than half of all patients. Small or moderate-sized effusions occur in approximately half of all cases; most (but not all) are exudative. A bloody effusion before anticoagulation suggests infarction or an alternative diagnosis (tuberculosis, malignancy, trauma). Embolic effusions tend to appear early and unilaterally. More specific features, including segmental oligemia (Westermark's sign) and Hampton's hump (a wedge-shaped peripheral density resulting from pulmonary infarction), are unusual. Infiltrate may represent parenchymal hemorrhage (resolving rapidly without effusion) or infarction (resolving slowly, often accompanied by a bloody effusion). Fresh infarcts always are pleural based and cavitate frequently. Because the dual parenchymal blood supply usually protects against tissue ischemia, infarction occurs most commonly in patients with preexisting cardiopulmonary disease. When resolving, the infiltrate often rounds up to form a spheroid "nodule." Multiple, widely scattered, cavitating infiltrates that develop acutely suggest septic emboli.

SPECIALIZED DIAGNOSTIC TESTS

It is clear that clinical judgment plays an indispensable role in the diagnosis of pulmonary embolism. Special diagnostic studies should only be ordered for patients considered to have a "high likelihood" of having a pulmonary embolism based on clinical judgment. Because ventilation–perfusion (VQ) scans are noninvasive and essentially without risk, they are often ordered reflexly for patients with dyspnea or chest pain. (These studies are not inexpensive; however, sometimes costing more than $1000.) This practice frequently creates a dilemma when the result of a VQ scan is at odds with the clinical presentation. The situation most often encountered is one

in which a "low probability" or "indeterminate" scan is returned in a patient with a low clinical probability of having a pulmonary embolism. A consultant is then summoned to explain the results. Such patients are often unnecessarily subjected to angiography to demonstrate that a VQ scan abnormality is not the result of an embolism. The best strategy is not to perform a VQ scan unless (*a*) the clinical likelihood of PE is high and (*b*) if the VQ scan proves non-diagnostic there is a commitment to pursue the diagnosis with angiography or leg studies.

Ventilation–Perfusion Scans

A perfusion scan is performed by injecting radioactive macroaggregated albumin, a compound with a particle size exceeding the diameter of the alveolar capillary. The radioactive albumin then becomes trapped in perfused lung areas. Areas devoid of perfusion are suspect for pulmonary embolism but also can result from tumor, obstructive lung disease, or hypoxic vasoconstriction induced by airspace disease. Therefore, atelectasis, emphysema, and pneumonia all can induce perfusion defects. In an attempt to exclude airspace disease as a cause of a perfusion defect, a chest radiograph is performed routinely. Because infiltrates can change rapidly in hospitalized patients, the comparison chest radiograph should be obtained within hours of the scan. The diagnosis of PE is more likely when the perfusion scan defect occurs in an area without apparent disease on chest radiograph.

To further increase the specificity of the perfusion scan, a ventilation scan can be added to the diagnostic package. Because not all airspace disease is apparent on plain CXR, the ventilation scan is used to identify poorly ventilated areas that could cause regional reductions in perfusion. When a large perfusion defect occurs in a normal area on plain chest radiograph that also is normally ventilated on VQ scan, the diagnosis of PE is likely. The ventilation scan (xenon or diethylenetriamine penta-acetic acid) improves specificity for embolism; gross ventilation–perfusion (VQ) mismatching often allows a diagnosis to be made with confidence. However, matching VQ abnormalities sometimes occur in embolic disease due to bronchoconstriction, atelectasis, or secretion retention. Conversely, mismatching can occur when no embolus is present.

Criteria for "high probability" and "low probability" scans vary with the interpreter but generally depend on the size, number, and distribution of perfusion defects, as well as their relationship to chest radiograph and ventilation scan abnormalities. A perfusion defect much larger than a corresponding density on chest film suggests embolism; a perfusion defect equal to or smaller than the radiographic abnormality suggests that embolism is less likely. A similar rule applies even more strongly to areas of ventilation–perfusion mismatching. Experts often disagree among themselves in interpretation of VQ scans; consequently, the false–positive rate may be very high in some centers. In general, scans are interpreted as falling into one of four categories: (a) normal, (b) low probability, (c) intermediate probability, and (d) high probability. Probably a more practical scheme for interpreting VQ scans is to classify all scans as only normal, high probability, or indeterminate.

The most useful of all scans, a perfectly normal perfusion study effectively rules out a clinically significant embolism. The single rare exception to this rule may be submassive PE confined to the pulmonary outflow tract, producing symmetric reduction in flow as a result of central obstruction. (MRI or contrasted spiral CT scans can often detect such clots non-invasively.) The second most useful VQ result is the finding of multiple mismatched ventilation–perfusion defects of segmental or greater size. Such a result in the setting of a high clinical probability results in at least an 85% likelihood of a PE.

Unfortunately, most scans are interpreted as low or intermediate probability (i.e., indeterminate), which is the least helpful radiographic finding. A "low-probability" or indeterminate scan should not be confused with a normal scan. A substantial fraction (up to 15%) of patients with low probability scans (matched subsegmental defects) have angiographically demonstrable emboli. Similarly, up to 50% of patients with indeterminate scans (matched or mismatched segmental defects) have emboli. Therefore a "low-probability" or indeterminate scan almost always requires additional diagnostic testing if the clinical suspicion of PE is high.

The problem of a false–positive scan is common for the ICU patient in whom the prevalence of underlying cardiopulmonary disease is high. In general, perfusion scan defects in patients with proven pulmonary emboli are multiple and bilateral. Very rarely will PE result in complete absence of perfusion to an entire lung with the contralateral lung being normal. The diagnosis of PE is suspect when perfusion defects are single or unilateral. Complete unilateral absence of perfusion with a normal contralateral lung probably is more likely to be the result of a bronchial cyst, congenital pulmonary artery defect, mediastinal tumor, or central mucous plug than the result of PE.

Emboli isolated to the upper lobes are unusual in ambulatory patients whose blood flow, when upright, distributes preferentially to the bases—this rule is often violated in bedridden patients in the ICU.

Angiography

Angiography is the definitive test for PE and also is capable of yielding alternative diagnoses. In almost all cases, it is prudent to perform a VQ scan before an angiogram. If the VQ scan is normal, angiography is unnecessary; if it shows perfusion defects, it guides the angiographer to the site for safe selective injections. Measurement of intracardiac and pulmonary artery pressures and cardiac output should be obtained with each pulmonary arteriogram. Such measurements confirm alternate diagnoses (e.g., primary pulmonary hypertension, mitral stenosis) if the angiogram fails to show clot. With appropriate care, angiography can be performed safely in most hemodynamically stable patients. There is often undue concern about the potential for "false–negative" angiograms if obtained hours or days after the onset of symptoms—the angiogram usually remains positive long after the embolic event. Although best performed promptly, angiography still is worth undertaking as long as 1 week after the onset of symptoms. Criteria for an angiographic diagnosis must include an intraluminal filling defect or an abrupt convex "cutoff." (Oligemia and vessel tortuosity are nondiagnostic.) In the absence of overt lower extremity thrombosis, a negative angiogram, carefully performed within 48 hours of the onset of symptoms, indicates a negligible risk of clinically significant embolization for weeks afterward. Angiograms performed without "cut films," selective injections, multiple views, and magnification may miss a small embolus. The clinical significance of such small emboli, however, is unclear.

Risks of arteriography have been greatly overstated—the overall mortality rate is lower than 0.01%. Likewise, there is a low risk of allergic dye reaction and vascular damage (right ventricular or pulmonary artery perforation). Catheter-induced arrhythmias usually are self-limited or easily treated. The greatest risks are incurred during contrast injection in patients with severe pulmonary hypertension, but even then, patients can safely undergo selective angiography with nonionic contrast media. If subsequent thrombolytic therapy is contemplated, punctures of noncompressable vessels must be avoided; catheters are probably best introduced via peripheral cutdown to minimize bleeding complications.

Bedside arteriography using a balloon flotation catheter has been tried for critically ill patients who are unable to leave the ICU. Unfortunately, bedside injections are much less sensitive and specific than studies performed in the angiography suite. Therefore, this test is helpful if positive but

cannot confidently exclude emboli. Digital subtraction angiography does not seem to offer substantial advantages over standard techniques.

DIAGNOSTIC PLAN

Because of the complexity of making the diagnosis, no universally applicable diagnostic protocol can be recommended; however, one strategy is suggested in Figure 23.1. It is generally agreed that a negative angiogram rules out clinically significant embolic disease and documents a low risk of embolization in the near future. It also is clear that a normal perfusion scan rules out the need

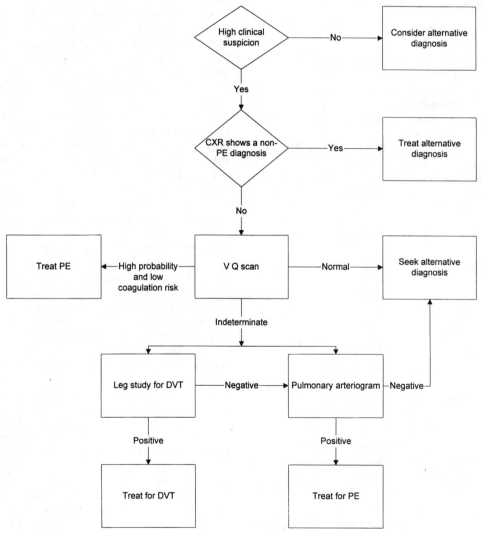

FIG. 23–1. Flow diagram of one strategy for evaluating patients with suspected pulmonary embolism. VQ, ventilation–perfusion lung scan; CXR, chest radiograph; DVT, deep venous thrombosis; PE, pulmonary embolism.

for pulmonary angiography. Between these limits, the decision to perform or withhold angiography is based, in large part, on the need for diagnostic certainty and the reliability of lung scan in detecting perfusion defects. Many clinicians use the perfusion lung scan only to exclude embolism or as a map for selective angiography. Others rely heavily on patterns of scan defects for guidance. Because the therapy of DVT and PE usually is identical, demonstrating a DVT obviates the need for a pulmonary arteriogram. Indeed, one-third or more patients with nondiagnostic ventilation–perfusion scans may avoid pulmonary arteriography by undertaking a diagnostic leg study for DVT. Based on currently available information, the following diagnostic strategy seems defensible.

Angiogram Almost Certainly Needed

1. High risk for anticoagulation (CNS trauma, active ulcer disease, etc.).
2. Thrombolytic therapy or vena caval interruption contemplated.
3. Lung parenchymal disease renders nuclear scans uninterpretable.
4. Paradoxical embolism suspected (to document right-to-left shunt or PE).
5. Low-probability VQ scan result with a high clinical suspicion. (Leg studies are a viable alternative.)

Angiogram Probably Not Needed

Clinical Likelihood of PE Low

1. Normal perfusion scan.
2. Perfusion defect much smaller than chest radiograph abnormality.
3. Ventilation defect much larger than perfusion defect.
4. Few matched subsegmental defects.

Clinical Likelihood of PE High

1. VQ scan shows more than one lobar or more than two segmental mismatched defects, with a chest radiograph showing no acute changes in involved areas.
2. VQ scan is indeterminate, but leg study reveals DVT.

With less convincing data, the decision to perform angiography should be based on the weight of clinical suspicion, the consequences of an undiagnosed embolic syndrome in patients with limited cardiopulmonary reserve, and the ability of the patient to safely undergo the procedure.

PROGNOSIS AND RATE OF RESOLUTION

A significant percentage of patients with massive PE die before the diagnosis is made, usually within the first hours of embolization. Adequately anticoagulated patients who survive for several hours have an excellent prognosis. If heparin anticoagulation is not begun, further clinically significant embolization occurs in at least one-third of cases. This risk falls to less than 10% with therapy. Whether or not embolism is treated, subclinical recurrence of PE (new lung scan defect) is very common. Both subclinical and clinically apparent recurrences usually occur within the first several days of initiating therapy. For well-anticoagulated patients, such early episodes represent embolization of preformed thrombus, not additional thrombus proliferation. Therefore, early reembolization does not necessarily imply ''anticoagulation failure.'' Because the thrombus is already formed, vena caval filtering may be the only therapy that might lower the incidence of pulmonary embolism, although this point remains to be proven.

Hemodynamic and gas exchange abnormalities usually reverse rapidly in patients who survive long enough for treatment to be started. Distal migration or fragmentation of clot certainly plays a role in this improvement, but it is likely that vasoactive mediators (e.g., thromboxane and prostacyclin) are also operative. Although the role of cyclooxygenase antagonists or inhibitors in PE remains uncertain, such drugs are very safe and preliminary data are sufficiently encouraging to foster further clinical study of severely ill patients. Angiographic findings can improve within 12 to 48 hours but usually require 2 to 3 weeks or longer for complete resolution. Likewise, perfusion scan defects may disappear quickly (over days), but most resolve over weeks to months. Most (approximately 85%) of all perfusion defects resolve within 3 months; defects persisting at that time are likely to be permanent. Repeat VQ scanning at 6 to 12 weeks can document resolution of clot. Chronic pulmonary hypertension and cor pulmonale due to multiple ''silent'' emboli rarely occurs; however, repetition of symptomatic embolic episodes can cause this problem. Furthermore, in a small percentage of cases, clot organizes within central vessels to produce a surgically treatable form of pulmonary hypertension.

MANAGEMENT

Anticoagulation

Acute Phase

Heparin is the drug of choice, given initially as a large bolus (approximately 10,000–20,000 units) to achieve immediate effect and then subsequently administered by continuous infusion of 1,000–2,000 units/hour). One schema for heparin dosing is presented in Table 23.1. Although not optimal, effective heparin therapy also can be given subcutaneously (approximately 7,500–10,000 units every 6 hours) if venous access is problematic. When given in this manner, dosage must be guided by PTT measurements.

In the acute period, it is probably better to err on the side of overanticoagulation than undertreatment. Therefore, it is important to ensure that therapeutic anticoagulation has been achieved within 4 to 6 hours of starting therapy by measuring the PTT. (Heparin should not be withheld pending the results of diagnostic studies unless the risk of anticoagulation outweighs the clinical suspicion of PE.) For the critically ill patient with thrombosis, heparin is a difficult drug to use—it is rarely possible to precisely target the PTT with initial dosing.

TABLE 23–1

HEPARIN DOSING STRATEGY

Initiation:
  Bolus: 10,000–20,000 units i.v. (70–150 units/kg)
  Initial infusion: 1,000–2,000 units/hour (15–40 units/ kg/hour)
  Obtain PTT in 4–6 hours

IF PTT < 1.5 times control:
  Repeat bolus: 5,000–10,000 units i.v.
  Increase infusion rate by 20–25%
  Recheck PTT in 4–6 hours

If PTT 1.5–3 times control:
  Recheck PTT in 4–6 hours
  If two consecutive PTTs in this range, change to daily checks of PTT

If PTT >3 times control:
  Patient not bleeding:
    Decrease heparin infusion rate by 20%
    Recheck PTT in 4–6 hours
  Patient bleeding:
    Interrupt heparin infusion and reconsider therapy:
      Should an IVC filter be inserted?
      Can heparin be restarted safely at a lower infusion rate?

Because heparin metabolism varies considerably among patients and over time in any given individual, the rate of heparin administration must be adjusted to maintain a target PTT of approximately 1.5 times normal. A PTT of more than 1.5 times control is not, however, a guarantee that preformed thrombus will not embolize. The PTT often oscillates around the target value, seemingly without regard to dosing. Instead of "chasing" the PTT with large changes in heparin, a reasonable strategy is to make modest changes in dosing and then reassess the effect. Whenever the PTT is below the target value, a bolus of heparin (5,000–10,000 units) and an increase in the infusion rate of approximately 20% usually brings the PTT into range. Dosing changes should be followed by a PTT in 4 to 6 hours. The half-life of heparin averages approximately 90 minutes in patients with active thrombosis. Therefore, unless the PTT exceeds 2.5 to 3.0 times the control value or the patient is bleeding, it is unwise to stop a heparin infusion; to do so results in a subtherapeutic PTT in approximately half the time. A better strategy is to reduce the infusion rate by 20 to 25% and recheck the PTT in 6 to 12 hours.

Rarely, "therapeutic" PTT values are difficult to achieve, even with high infusion rates of heparin. In such patients, preformed antiheparin or anticardiolipin antibodies and deficiencies of antithrombin III or proteins C or S should be suspected. Most "heparin failures" (reembolization) occur in patients who *consistently* have not been kept anticoagulated. Conversely, the risk of embolization because of an isolated subtherapeutic PTT is minuscule. Heparin should be continued for more than 5 days, which is sufficient time to allow fresh clot to dissolve or organize. Although bed rest often reduces swelling and discomfort in the legs of patients with DVT, the effectiveness of bed rest to prevent dislodging clots remains unproven. In practice, many physicians confine patients to bed for the first 24 to 48 hours of therapy as much to improve patient comfort as to reduce the risk of embolization. Once two consecutive therapeutic PTTs have been achieved, it is reasonable to reduce the frequency of PTT sampling to once daily. Measuring PCV and platelet count on a 1- to 3-day basis is a defensible strategy to detect asymptomatic anemia or thrombocytopenia.

Fixed dose subcutaneous LMWH is as effective as adjusted-dose continuous infusion of heparin for treating established DVT, and it is likely that similar results will be shown for PE.

Chronic Phase

After the completion of heparin therapy, antithrombotic prophylaxis usually is maintained with warfarin to prolong the PT to 1.2 to 1.5 times the control (INR 2.0–3.0). Because the prothrombin time should be "in range" 3 to 5 days before heparin is stopped, it makes sense to initiate warfarin simultaneously with heparin. Large "loading" doses of warfarin do not prolong the PT more rapidly than conventional doses and may paradoxically increase the thrombotic tendency by rapidly depleting vitamin-K-dependent anticlotting proteins. The duration of anticoagulation must reflect not only the risk for recurrence and its potential physiologic consequences but also the risk of the therapy. Because the rate of recurrence falls exponentially with time from discharge, an arbitrary period of anticoagulation of 3 to 6 months seems reasonable for patients recovering from trauma or surgery. Patients at continued high risk of recurrence, including those with genetic or acquired coagulopathies who have had two or more thrombotic episodes, should be anticoagulated indefinitely or until the risk abates. Although a bit more effective than fixed low doses of subcutaneous heparin, outpatient warfarin requires surveillance of the PT and is associated with a higher incidence of bleeding complications.

Thrombolytic Therapy

Unquestionably, streptokinase, urokinase, and tissue plasminogen activator accelerate the rate of angiographic clot resolution, sometimes dramatically. Unfortunately, these drugs have not been shown to decrease morbidity or mortality from PE, and the incidence of adverse effects is considerable. The many problems associated with thrombolytic agents are reviewed in Chapter 21 (Angina and Myocardial Infarction). Most problematic is the risk of hemorrhage, especially intracranial bleeding. Therefore, contraindications include any condition that predisposes to serious bleeding. Puncture of noncompressible venous sites (e.g., subclavian) must not be performed while thrombolytics are administered. The potential for devastating hemorrhage and absence of demonstrated mortality benefit makes many physicians question the role of thrombolytic agents in the treatment of PE. By weighing the risk:benefit ratio, it seems reasonable to reserve thrombolytic drugs for patients with (a) angiographically

proven massive PE and unstable hemodynamics and (b) those with profound leg swelling from DVT. When used, these drugs should be initiated as soon as possible after the thrombotic event has been confirmed. A loading dose and continuous infusion is given over a 12- to 72-hour period, depending on the condition treated and its clinical response. Ideally, the infusion rate is altered to keep thrombin time between 2 and 5 times the control value. (The PT and PTT also will be variably prolonged.) At the conclusion of thrombolytic therapy, heparin is begun as thrombin time and PTT fall to approximately 1.5 times normal. Aminocaproic acid can be used topically to stop local oozing or systemically to counteract thrombolysis if serious bleeding occurs. Reversal of the coagulation disorder also can be accomplished with fresh frozen plasma or cryoprecipitate.

SURGERY: CAVAL INTERRUPTION AND EMBOLECTOMY

Surgical interruption of the vena cava should be considered for patients who (a) sustain recurrent life-threatening emboli from the lower extremities or pelvis despite adequate anticoagulation, (b) cannot receive thrombolytic or anticoagulation safely, (c) suffer massive embolism or paradoxical systemic emboli, (d) develop septic embolism from the lower extremities, (e) clearly cannot withstand the hemodynamic effects of another embolism.

Recurrent emboli during the first few days of heparin infusion may be due to the original clot and do not necessarily indicate that heparin is ineffective. To be considered a heparin failure, embolism must recur after the PTT has been held continuously in the therapeutic range over several days. Options for interruption of the inferior vena cava (IVC) include ligation, narrowing the caval lumen by clipping, and percutaneous placement of an intravenacaval filter (mesh, "bird's nest," umbrella or Greenfield). Of these options, percutaneous filter placement is most frequent. The clipped or filtered vena cava clots off eventually in one-third or more of cases within the first 2 years. Ligation of the IVC forces the collateralizing process earlier and usually results in pedal edema (less of a problem with the other techniques). In experienced hands, the venacaval filter has a significant advantage over open procedures. Reported rates of clotting are lower and efficacy is greater than with alternative techniques. Rarely, such IVC filters perforate the cava or migrate to the heart or pulmonary outflow tract—potentially lethal events.

Mechanical methods reduce the risk of life-threatening embolism for at least several months if the source of embolism is the deep veins of the pelvis or thigh. Obviously, IVC filters have no effect on embolic risk if the source is in the upper extremities. Large collaterals eventually may develop, but most published surgical reports suggest that the risk of clinically important embolization through these vessels is low. Because venous return is impeded for a few days after caval ligation, the procedure itself can be dangerous in patients with impaired cardiac function. Caval clipping and filter insertion are better tolerated than ligation and are just as effective, except in treating septic embolism.

Emergent pulmonary embolectomy is rarely successful. Most patients surviving long enough for the diagnosis of PE to be made by angiography respond to thrombolytic or anticoagulant therapy alone. It is only in those patients who are gravely ill and deteriorating under treatment that this heroic form of therapy should be considered. On the other hand, a surgical approach to chronic persistent central emboli may offer the only chance of relieving disability and potentially lethal pulmonary hypertension in carefully selected individuals. For patients with suspected chronic thrombotic pulmonary hypertension, a VQ scan should demonstrate abnormalities that can then be confirmed by pulmonary angiography. Magnetic resonance imaging is often helpful diagnostically. Although less risky than an acute procedure, embolectomy for chronic thrombotic pulmonary artery disease remains hazardous.

KEY POINTS

1. Pulmonary emboli are difficult to diagnose. After developing a high clinical suspicion, the best diagnostic strategy is to review a chest radiograph and ABG for an alternative diagnosis. Then and only then, a VQ scan should be obtained.

2. Most VQ scans are nondiagnostic and require either a pulmonary arteriogram showing PE or leg study showing DVT for confirmation. A normal VQ scan or a high probability scan probably is sufficient for clinical decision making. A contrasted spiral CT scan can often reveal central emboli in those who cannot undergo angiography.

3. Full-dose anticoagulation with heparin should be started empirically for almost all patients suspected of having a PE or DVT, unless bleeding risk is prohibitive.

4. The risk of PE recurrence is a function of the duration of time spent with a PTT below 1.5 times control; therefore, early and aggressive anticoagulation is indicated. Doses of heparin should be adjusted every 4 to 6 hours until the PTT is in the therapeutic range; then, the frequency of monitoring can be greatly reduced.

5. There is a much less certain relationship between a high PTT and bleeding than there is between a low PTT and thrombosis.

6. Thrombolytic or surgical therapy is rarely needed for DVT or PE.

SUGGESTED READINGS

1. A Collaborative Study by the PIOPED Investigators. Value of the ventilation perfusion scan in acute pulmonary embolism: results of the prospective investigation of pulmonary embolism diagnosis (PIOPED). JAMA 1990;263: 2753–2759.
2. Ansell JE. Oral anticoagulant therapy 50 years later. Arch Intern Med 1993;153:586–596.
3. Bell WR, Simon TL, DeMets DL. The clinical features of submassive and massive pulmonary emboli. Am J Med 1977;62:355–360.
4. Hull RD, Hirsh J, Carter CJ, et al. Pulmonary angiography, ventilation lung scanning and venography for clinically suspected pulmonary embolism in the abnormal perfusion scan. Ann Intern Med 1983;98:891–899.
5. Hull RD, Hirsh J, Carter CJ, et al. Diagnostic efficacy of impedance plethysmography for clinically suspected deep-vein thrombosis. A randomized trial. Ann Intern Med 1985;102:21–28.
6. Koopman MMW, and the Tasman Study group. Treatment of venous thrombosis with intravenous unfractionated heparin administered in the hospital as compared with subcutaneous low-molecular weight heparin administered at home. N Engl J Med 1996;334:682–687.
7. Levine M, Gent M, Hirsh J. A comparison of low-molecular weight heparin administered primarily at home with unfractionated heparin administered in the hospital for proximal deep-vein thrombosis. N Engl J Med 1996;334: 677–681.
8. Litin SC. Current concepts in anti-coagulant therapy. Mayo Clin Proc 1995;70:266–272.

9. MacMillan JC, Milstein SH, Samson PC. Clinical spectrum of septic pulmonary embolism and infarction. J Thorac Cardiovasc Surg 1978;75:670–679.
10. Moser KM, Fedullo PF. Venous thromboembolism. Three simple decisions. Chest 1983;83:117–121, 256–260.
11. Sharma GV, Cella G, Parisi AF, Sasahara AA. Thrombolytic therapy. N Engl J Med 1982;306:1268–1276.
12. Schulman S, Rhedin AS. A comparison of 6 weeks with 6 months of oral anticoagulant therapy after a first episode of venous thromboembolism. N Engl J Med 1995;332:1661–1665.
13. Urokinase-streptokinase pulmonary embolism trial: a national cooperative study. JAMA 1984;229:1606–1613.
14. Warkentin TE. Heparin-induced thrombocytopenia in patients treated with low molecular weight heparin or unfractionated heparin. N Engl J Med 1995;332:1330–1335.
15. Wheeler AP, Jaquiss RDB, Newman JH. Physician practices in the treatment of pulmonary embolism and deep venous thrombosis. Arch Intern Med 1988;148:1321–1325.

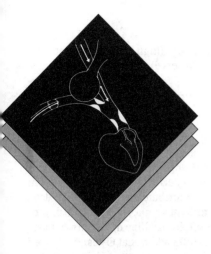

CHAPTER 24

Oxygenation Failure

OXYGENATION FAILURE—DEFINITIONS

Respiratory failure may be considered a problem in one or more of the steps necessary to sustain mitochondrial energy production. Dysfunction may occur in ventilation (the movement of gases between the environment and the lungs; see Chapter 25), in intrapulmonary gas exchange (the process in which mixed venous blood releases CO_2 and becomes oxygenated), in gas transport (the delivery of adequate quantities of oxygenated blood to the metabolizing tissue), or in tissue gas exchange (the extraction or use of O_2 and release of CO_2 by the peripheral tissues).

The latter two steps in this process may fail independently of the performance of the lung or ventilatory pump. Tissue O_2 delivery depends not only on the partial pressure of arterial oxygen (PaO_2) but also on nonpulmonary factors—cardiac output, hemoglobin (Hgb) concentration, and the ability of Hgb to take up and release O_2. Cardiogenic shock, anemia, and carbon monoxide poisoning provide clinical examples of O_2 transport failure (see Chapter 40). Laboratory abnormalities characteristic of such conditions are lactic acidosis and reduced O_2 content of mixed venous blood (even in the face of adequate arterial oxygen tension).

Failure of O_2 uptake refers to the inability of tissue to extract and use O_2 for aerobic metabolism. The clearest clinical examples of a derangement in this terminal phase of the oxygen transport chain are cyanide poisoning, in which cellular cytochromes (key enzymes in the electron transport process) are inhibited, and septic shock. During sepsis, there is failure of an often generous cardiac output to distribute appropriately and/or an inability of the tissues themselves to make use of the O_2 available. Unlike transport insufficiency, failure of tissue uptake is distinguished by normal or high values for mixed venous oxygen tension, saturation, and content. Therefore, some indices that are helpful in other forms of oxygenation failure, i.e., cardiac output, arterial O_2 tension, and mixed venous O_2 saturation (SvO_2), may not reflect impaired tissue O_2 uptake; lactic acidosis may be the sole laboratory indicator. Therapy directed at failure of the O_2 transport and uptake mechanisms is discussed in detail elsewhere (see Chapters 1 and 3). The following discussion focuses on the problems that bear on the performance of the lung in oxygenating the arterial blood and ventilatory failure.

MECHANISMS OF ARTERIAL HYPOXEMIA

Six mechanisms may contribute to arterial oxygen desaturation (Table 24.1):

1. Inhalation of a hypoxic gas mixture or severe reductions of barometric pressure
2. Hypoventilation
3. Impaired alveolar diffusion of oxygen
4. Ventilation–perfusion (VQ) mismatching
5. Shunting of systemic venous blood to the systemic arterial circuit
6. Abnormal desaturation of systemic venous blood

TABLE 24-1
MECHANISMS OF ARTERIAL HYPOXEMIA

Low inspired FiO_2
Hypoventilation
Impaired diffusion
VQ Mismatching
Shunt
Desaturated mixed venous blood*

* In the presence of other mechanisms for hypoxemia.

LOW INSPIRED OXYGEN FRACTION (FiO_2)

A decrease in the partial pressure of inhaled oxygen occurs in toxic fume inhalation, in fires that consume O_2 in combustion, and at high altitudes because of reduced barometric pressure.

HYPOVENTILATION

Hypoventilation causes the partial pressure of alveolar oxygen (PAO_2) to fall when alveolar oxygen is not replenished quickly enough in the face of its ongoing removal by the blood. Although PaO_2 may fall much faster than $PaCO_2$ rises during the initial phase of hypoventilation or apnea, the steady-state concentration of PaO_2 is predicted by the alveolar gas equation:

$$PAO_2 = PiO_2 - PaCO_2/R.$$

In this equation, PiO_2 is the partial pressure of inspired oxygen at the tracheal level (corrected for water vapor pressure at body temperature), and R is the respiratory exchange ratio, i.e., the ratio of CO_2 production to oxygen consumption at steady state. Transiently, R can fall to very low values as oxygen is taken up faster than CO_2 is delivered to the alveolus. Such a mechanism explains post-hyperventilation hypoxemia and some forms of hypoxemia that accompany hemodialysis.

IMPAIRED DIFFUSION

Impaired oxygen diffusion prevents complete equilibration of alveolar gas with pulmonary capillary blood. Although this mechanism has uncertain clinical importance, many factors that adversely influence diffusion are encountered clinically: increased distance between alveolus and erythrocyte, decreased O_2 gradient for diffusion, and shortened transit time of the red cell through the capillary (high cardiac output with limited capillary reserve).

VENTILATION-PERFUSION MISMATCHING

Ventilation-perfusion (VQ) mismatching is the most frequent contributor to clinically important O_2 desaturation. Lung units that are poorly ventilated in relation to perfusion cause desaturation; high VQ units contribute to physiologic dead space but not to hypoxemia. The relationship of O_2 content to PaO_2 is curvilinear. At normal barometric pressure, little additional O_2 can be loaded onto blood with already saturated Hgb, no matter how high the O_2 tension in the overventilated alveolus may rise. Because samples of blood exiting from different lung units mix gas contents (not partial pressures), overventilating some units in an attempt to compensate for others that are underventilated does not maintain PaO_2 at a normal level. Therefore, when equal volumes of blood from well-ventilated and poorly ventilated units mix, the blended sample will have an O_2 content halfway between them but a PaO_2 disproportionately weighted toward that of the lower VQ unit. Even though total V_E and Q may be absolutely normal, regional VQ mismatching will cause PaO_2 to fall.

Supplemental O_2 will impressively reverse hypoxemia when VQ mismatching, hypoventilation, or diffusion impairment is the cause. (The PAO_2 of even poorly ventilated units climbs high enough to achieve full saturation.) After breathing 100% O_2 for a sufficient period of time, only perfused units that are totally unventilated (shunt units) contribute to hypoxemia. However, when hypoxemia is caused by alveolar units with very low VQ ratios, relatively concentrated O_2 mixtures must be given before a substantial change in the PaO_2 is observed (see Fig. 5.2 in Chapter 5, Respiratory Monitoring).

SHUNTING

The term "shunt" refers to the percentage of the total systemic venous blood flow that bypasses the gas-exchanging membrane and transfers venous blood unaltered to the systemic arterial system. Changes in FiO_2—either upward or downward—have very little influence on PaO_2 when the true shunt fraction, as measured on pure oxy-

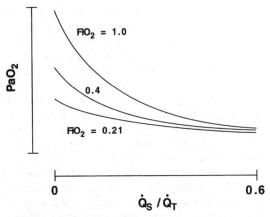

FIG. 24–1. Relationship of arterial oxygen tension (PaO_2) to true shunt fraction ($\dot{Q}_S/\dot{Q}_T$) for three values of inspired oxygen fraction (FiO_2). Variations of FiO_2 exert negligible effects on PaO_2 when true shunt exceeds 30%.

gen exceeds 30% (Fig 24.1). In contrast, venous admixture of similar magnitude is variably responsive, to the extent that low VQ units account for the hypoxemia. Shunt can be intracardiac, as in cyanotic right-to-left congenital heart disease, the opening of a patent foramen ovale due to right ventricular overload, or the result of passage of blood through abnormal vascular channels within the lung, e.g., pulmonary arteriovenous communications. However, by far the most common cause of shunting is pulmonary disease characterized by totally unventilated lung units that cannot respond to oxygen therapy. After an extended exposure to an FiO_2 of 1.0, all alveoli that remain open are filled with pure oxygen. Therefore, the shunt fraction ($\dot{Q}_S/\dot{Q}_T$) can be calculated from the following formula:

$$\dot{Q}_S/\dot{Q}_T = [(CcO_2 - CaO_2)/(CcO_2 - CvO_2)]$$

In this equation, C denotes content, and the lower case letters c, a, and v denote end-capillary, arterial, and mixed venous blood, respectively. In making such calculations, end-capillary and calculated alveolar oxygen tensions are assumed to be equivalent. For a patient breathing pure O_2, shunt percentages lower than 25% can be estimated rapidly by dividing the alveolar to arterial O_2 tension difference (approximately 670 − PaO_2) by 20, assuming also that the $PaCO_2$ and CvO_2 are normal. Note that some absorption atelectasis may occur in very low VQ areas when pure oxygen is breathed, adding to the measured shunt. In the clinical setting, however, the magnitude of this artifact usually is small.

At inspired oxygen fractions lower than 1.0, true shunt cannot be estimated reliably by an analysis of oxygen contents, but "venous admixture" or "physiologic shunt" can. (Note that many authors refer to venous admixture from any cause as "shunt.") Any degree of arterial O_2 desaturation can be considered as if it all originated from true shunt units. To calculate venous admixture, CcO_2 in the shunt formula is estimated from the ideal alveolar PO_2 at that particular fraction of inspired oxygen (FiO_2).

Many indices have been devised in an attempt to characterize the efficacy of oxygen exchange across the spectrum of FiO_2. Although no index is completely successful, the $PaO_2:P_{alv}O_2$ ratio and the alveolar to arterial oxygen tension difference $(A-a)$ O_2 are often used (see Chapter 5, Respiratory Monitoring). Both, however, are affected by changes in SvO_2, even when the lung tissue itself retains normal ability to transfer oxygen to the blood. Another imprecise but commonly used indicator of gas exchange is the $PaO_2:FiO_2$ ratio (the P:F ratio). In healthy adults, this ratio normally exceeds 400, whatever the FiO_2 may be. Hypoventilation and changes in the inspired O_2 concentration minimally alter these ratios in the absence of FiO_2-related absorption atelectasis or cardiovascular adjustments.

ABNORMAL DESATURATION OF SYSTEMIC VENOUS BLOOD

The admixture of abnormally desaturated venous blood is an important mechanism acting to lower PaO_2 in patients with impaired pulmonary gas exchange and reduced cardiac output. CvO_2, the product of Hgb concentration and SvO_2, is influenced by cardiac output ($\dot{Q}$), arterial oxygen saturation (SaO_2), and oxygen consumption (VO_2):

$$SvO_2 \approx SaO_2 - [\dot{V}O_2/(Hgb \times \dot{Q})].$$

It is clear from this equation that SvO_2 is directly influenced by any imbalance between $\dot{V}O_2$ and oxygen delivery. Thus, anemia uncompensated by an increase in cardiac output or a cardiac output too low for metabolic needs can cause both SvO_2 and PaO_2 to fall when the venous admixture percentage is abnormal.

Fluctuations in SvO_2 exert a more profound influence on PaO_2 when the shunt is fixed, as in regional lung diseases (e.g., atelectasis), than when the shunt varies with changing cardiac out-

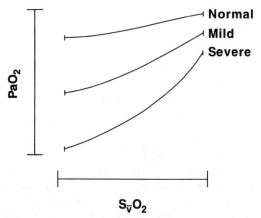

FIG. 24–2. Influence of mixed venous oxygen saturation ($S\bar{v}O_2$) on PaO_2 in patients with mild and severe lung disease. Variations in $S\bar{v}O_2$ related to an oxygen consumption/delivery imbalance have minimal effects on PaO_2 in normal subjects but may profoundly affect PaO_2 in patients with extensive lung disease.

put, as it tends to do in diffuse lung injury (acute respiratory distress syndrome [ARDS]) (Fig 24.2). Even when SvO_2 is abnormally low, PaO_2 will remain unaffected if all mixed venous blood gains access to well-oxygenated, well-ventilated alveoli. A marked decline in SvO_2 without arterial hypoxemia occurs routinely during heavy exercise in healthy subjects. Therefore, abnormal VQ matching or shunt is necessary for venous desaturation to be a contributing mechanism in hypoxemia.

COMMON CAUSES OF HYPOXEMIA

Oxygenation crises are categorized conveniently by their radiographic appearances, which give important clues to the appropriate management approach. Lung collapse (atelectasis), diffuse or patchy parenchymal infiltration, hydrostatic edema, localized or unilateral infiltration, and a clear chest radiograph are common patterns (Fig 24.3).

ATELECTASIS

Variants of Atelectasis

There are several morphologic types and mechanisms of atelectasis. Regional microatelectasis develops spontaneously in a healthy lung during shallow breathing when it is not periodically stretched beyond its usual tidal range. Plate-like atelectasis may be an exaggeration of this phenomenon due to regional hypodistention (e.g., pleural effusion or impaired diaphragmatic excursion). Both micro- and plate-like atelectasis occur most commonly in dependent regions. Lobar collapse usually results from gas absorption in an airway plugged by retained secretions, a misplaced endotracheal tube, or a central mass. External bronchial compression and regional hypoventilation are important in some patients. Micro- and plate-like atelectasis occur routinely in patients on prolonged uninterrupted bedrest and in postoperative patients who have undergone upper abdominal incisions.

Potential consequences of acute atelectasis are worsened gas exchange, pneumonitis, and increased work of breathing. PaO_2 drops precipitously to its nadir within minutes to hours of a sudden bronchial occlusion, but it then improves steadily over hours to days as hypoxic vasoconstriction and mechanical factors increase pulmonary vascular resistance through the local area. Whether an individual patient manifests hypoxemia depends heavily on the vigor of the hypoxic vasoconstrictive response, the abruptness of collapse, and the tissue volume involved. If small areas of atelectasis develop slowly, hypoxemia may never surface as a clinical problem.

Diffuse microatelectasis may be radiographically silent but detectable on physical examination by dependent (posterior or basilar) end-inspiratory rales, which improve after several sustained deep breaths ("sighs") or coughs. Plate atelectasis yields similar physical findings plus tubular breath sounds and egophony over the involved area. Lobar atelectasis gives a dull percussion note and diminished breath sounds if the bronchus is occluded by secretions but tubular breath sounds and egophony if the central airway is patent. (The latter findings correlate well with the presence of air bronchograms on chest radiograph.) Plate atelectasis develops most frequently at the lung base above a pleural effusion or above a raised, splinted, or immobile hemidiaphragm. Lobar atelectasis occurs most commonly in patients with copious airway secretions and limited power to expel them. Acute upper lobe collapse is less common and tends to resolve quickly because of comparatively good gravitational drainage. Collapse of the left lower lobe is more frequent than collapse of the right lower lobe, perhaps because of its retrocardiac position and its smaller caliber,

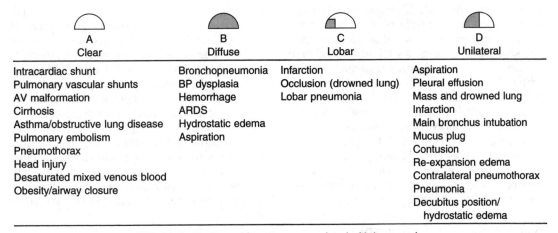

A	B	C	D
Clear	Diffuse	Lobar	Unilateral
Intracardiac shunt	Bronchopneumonia	Infarction	Aspiration
Pulmonary vascular shunts	BP dysplasia	Occlusion (drowned lung)	Pleural effusion
AV malformation	Hemorrhage	Lobar pneumonia	Mass and drowned lung
Cirrhosis	ARDS		Infarction
Asthma/obstructive lung disease	Hydrostatic edema		Main bronchus intubation
Pulmonary embolism	Aspiration		Mucus plug
Pneumothorax			Contusion
Head injury			Re-expansion edema
Desaturated mixed venous blood			Contralateral pneumothorax
Obesity/airway closure			Pneumonia
			Decubitus position/ hydrostatic edema

FIG. 24–3. Radiographic patterns associated with hypoxemia.

sharply angulated bronchus. Lobar atelectasis may be complete or partial, but in either case, it is radiographically recognized by opacification, displaced fissures, compensatory hyperinflation of surrounding tissue, and obliterated air/soft tissue boundaries (see Chapter 11). Small amounts of pleural fluid are a natural concomitant of lobar collapse and do not necessarily signify an additional pathologic process.

Management of Atelectasis

Prophylaxis

Effective prevention of atelectasis in high-risk patients counteracts shallow breathing and improves secretion clearance. Obesity, chronic bronchitis, secretion retention, neuromuscular weakness, pain, and advanced age are predisposing factors. Atelectasis is to be expected whenever the patient is prevented from taking a deep breath by pain, splinting, or weakness. Upper abdominal, thoracic, and lower abdominal incisions are associated with the highest incidence of postoperative atelectasis (in that order). Preoperatively, the airways should be maximally dilated and free of infection. Postoperatively, patients should be encouraged to breathe deeply, to sit upright, and to cough vigorously. Pain should be relieved, but alertness should be preserved. Frequent turning and early mobilization are among the most important prophylactic maneuvers. Continuous positive airway pressure (CPAP) may be helpful, especially for intubated patients. Respiratory therapy (RT) techniques such as airway suctioning, incentive spirometry, and chest physiotherapy are prophylactically (as well as therapeutically) effective in well-selected patients (see Chapter 18).

Treatment

Whenever possible, mobilization is the best treatment. Periodic deep breathing effectively reverses plate and microatelectasis. Sustained deep breaths are particularly effective. Whether a higher lung volume is achieved by positive airway pressure or by negative pleural pressure is immaterial, assuming that a similar extent and distribution of distention occurs in both cases. Although rational, the place of positive end-expiratory pressure in treatment of established collapse has not been clarified. Relief of chest wall pain helps reduce splinting and enables more effective coughing. Intercostal nerve blocks with anesthetic agents such as bupivacaine may be effective for 8 to 12 hours. Intrapleural instillation of lidocaine or bupivacaine (via catheter) can be effective occasionally, but pleural anesthesia may induce temporary ipsilateral diaphragmatic paralysis. Epidural narcotics also may be effective in certain settings. Retained secretions must be dislodged from the central airways. For the unintubated patient, effective bronchial hygiene is inconsistently accomplished with blind tracheal suctioning alone. Pharyngeal airways certainly help, but they are not well tolerated by patients who are awake and are not intended for extended care (see Chapter 6). Vigorous respiratory therapy initiated soon after the onset of lobar collapse can reverse most cases of atelectasis due to airway plugging within

24 to 48 hours. As a rule, fiberoptic bronchoscopy should be reserved for patients with symptomatic lobar collapse who lack central air bronchograms and who cannot undergo (or fail to respond to or tolerate) 48 hours of vigorous respiratory therapy (external chest physiotherapy, internal percussive ventilation at pulmonary resonant frequency, etc.). Even whole lung collapse usually merits at least one respiratory therapy treatment before bronchoscopy is performed. After reexpansion, a prophylactic respiratory therapy program should be initiated to prevent recurrence. Adjunctive measures (e.g., bronchodilators, hydration, and frequent turning) should not be ignored.

DIFFUSE PULMONARY INFILTRATION

When fluid or cellular infiltrates cause alveolar flooding or collapse, severe refractory hypoxemia may result. Fluid confined to the interstitial spaces may cause hypoxemia as a result of peribronchial edema, VQ mismatching, and microatelectasis; however, interstitial fluid itself does not interfere with oxygen exchange. Very few processes are confined exclusively to the air spaces or to the interstitium. Radiographic signs of alveolar filling include segmental distribution, coalescence, fluffy margins, air bronchograms, rosette patterns, and silhouetting of normal structures. A diffuse infiltrate is said to be largely ''interstitial'' if these signs are largely absent and the infiltrate parallels the vascular distribution. Any diffuse interstitial process will appear more radiodense at the bases than at the apices, in part because there is more tissue to penetrate and because vascular engorgement tends to be greater there. Alveoli also are less distended at the bases, so the ratio of aerated volume to total tissue volume declines.

The major categories of acute disease that produce diffuse pulmonary infiltration and hypoxemia are pneumonitis (infection and aspiration), cardiogenic pulmonary edema, intravascular volume overload, and the ARDS. From a radiographic viewpoint, these processes may be difficult to distinguish; however, a few characteristic features are helpful.

Hydrostatic Edema

Perihilar infiltrates (sparing the costophrenic angles), a prominent vascular pattern, and a widened vascular pedicle suggest volume overload or incipient cardiogenic edema (Fig. 24.4). A gravitational distribution of edema is highly consistent with well-established left ventricular failure (or longstanding, severe volume overload), especially when accompanied by cardiomegaly and a widened vascular pedicle. Patchy peripheral infiltrates that lack a gravitational predilection and show reluctance to change with position suggest ARDS. Interestingly, septal (Kerley) lines and distinct peribronchial cuffing are very seldom seen in classic ARDS (see below). On the other hand, prominent air bronchograms are quite unusual with hydrostatic etiologies but occur commonly in permeability edema (ARDS) and pneumonia.

Variants of Hydrostatic Edema

Hydrostatic pulmonary edema (HPE) may occur in multiple settings that have differing implications for prognosis and treatment. The most familiar form of HPE accompanies left ventricular failure. In this setting, signs of systemic hypoperfusion and inadequate cardiac output often accompany oxygenation failure. However, HPE can develop even with a normally well-compensated ventricle during transient heart dysfunction (ischemia, hypertensive crisis, arrhythmias). When the myocardium fails to fully relax during diastole (''diastolic dysfunction''), superimposed loading or temporary disturbances of left heart contractility (e.g., ischemia), mitral valve functioning, or heart rate or rhythm may cause rapid, transient alveolar flooding known as ''flash pulmonary edema.'' In this setting, an impressive radiographic appearance may both develop and resolve with impressive speed.

Acute Lung Injury and ARDS

The acute respiratory distress syndrome (ARDS) was originally called ''adult'' respiratory distress syndrome. In current parlance, acute lung injury is the general term that refers to all degrees of radiographically apparent, diffuse hypoxemic lung injury. ARDS is the most severe form of acute lung injury. ''Acute respiratory distress syndrome'' is an imprecise term that is often applied to any acute diffuse parenchymal infiltration associated with severe hypoxemia and not attributable to HPE. However, the ARDS designation is most useful when restricted to acute noncardiogenic pulmonary edema with certain characteristic features:

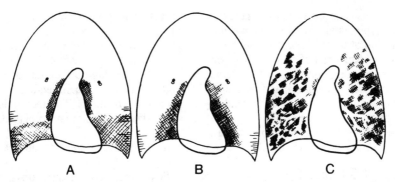

FIG. 24–4. Radiographic patterns in patients with impaired oxygenation due to congestive heart failure (left), vascular congestion due to volume overload (middle), and ARDS (right). Kerley lines, widened vascular pedicle, costophrenic angle sparing, blurred hilar structures, and paucity of air bronchograms help distinguish congestive heart failure from ARDS (Reprinted with permission from Milne et al. Am J Roentgen 1985;144:879–894).

1. Delay between the precipitating event and the onset of dyspnea
2. Impaired respiratory system compliance
3. Markedly reduced aerated lung volume
4. Refractory hypoxemia
5. Delayed resolution

The pathogenesis of permeability edema is almost certain to vary with the inciting event. Despite its many diverse causes, sepsis, aspiration, and multiple trauma account for most cases. The core pathophysiology of ARDS is sufficiently similar to warrant a common treatment approach. A prominent feature of all forms of ARDS is injury to the alveolar–capillary membrane from either the gas side (e.g., smoke inhalation, aspiration of gastric acid) or the blood side (e.g., sepsis, fat embolism). Increased membrane permeability allows seepage of protein-rich fluid into the interstitial and alveolar spaces. Such fluids inhibit surfactant, contributing to widespread atelectasis. Although wedge pressure usually remains normal, increased pulmonary vascular resistance and some degree of pulmonary hypertension are almost invariable in the latter stages of severe disease. Extreme pulmonary hypertension is a very poor prognostic sign. Diffuse pulmonary infiltration with a normal wedge pressure can be seen in other problems, such as flash pulmonary edema and partially treated heart failure. Apart from any difference in capillary pressure, permeability edema differs from hydrostatic edema in that it resists clearance by diuretic therapy and initiates a cellular inflammatory response that may require weeks to recede and even longer to heal.

Rapidly Resolving Noncardiogenic Edema

A few disorders that fall loosely under the heading of ARDS are worth noting because of their fundamentally different pathophysiology and clinical course. In certain settings, transient disruption in the barrier function of the pulmonary capillary can occur without overt endothelial damage. Neurogenic and heroin-induced pulmonary edema, for example, are two problems in which a transiently elevated pulmonary venous pressure is believed to open epithelial tight junctions, forcing extravasation of proteinaceous fluid. However, resealing and resolution of edema occur promptly without widespread endothelial damage or protracted inflammation. A similar process may be seen in settings such as severe metabolic acidosis and cardiopulmonary resuscitation. From the alveolar side, certain inhalational injuries (e.g., limited chlorine or ammonia gas exposure) can produce a dramatic initial picture, only to clear rapidly over a brief period.

HYPOXEMIA WITH A CLEAR CHEST RADIOGRAPH

It is not uncommon for patients to present with life-threatening hypoxemia without major radiographic evidence of infiltration. In such cases, occult shunting and severe VQ mismatching are the most likely mechanisms (Table 24.1). Intracardiac or intrapulmonary shunts, asthma and other forms of airway obstruction, low lung volume superimposed on a high closing capacity (e.g., bronchitis in a supine obese patient), pulmonary embolism, and occult microvascular communications (such as occur in patients with cirrhosis) are potential explanations. Hypoxemia is amplified by profound desaturation of mixed venous blood, by reversal of hypoxic vasoconstriction with therapeutic vasoactive agents (e.g., nitroprusside, calcium channel blockers, and dopamine), and by the severe VQ imbalance consequent to acute head injury. (Acute oxygenation crises following head trauma has been termed "nonedematous respiratory distress syndrome" or "NERDS.")

UNILATERAL LUNG DISEASE

Unilateral infiltration or marked asymmetry of radiographic density suggests a confined set of etiologic possibilities, most of which occur in highly characteristic clinical settings (Fig. 24.3). Marked asymmetry of radiographic involvement should prompt an especially careful search for an unaddressed and readily reversible cause of hypoxemia. In some cases, especially pneumonitis or airway plugging, precautions also should be taken against generalization of the process.

TECHNIQUES TO IMPROVE TISSUE OXYGENATION (TABLE 24.2)

BASIC THERAPEUTIC PRINCIPLES

Although atelectasis, fluid overload, and infection often yield to specific measures, the treatment

TABLE 24-2

TECHNIQUES TO IMPROVE TISSUE OXYGENATION

Increase FiO_2

Increase mean lung volume and alveolar pressure
  PEEP/auto-PEEP
  Extend inspiratory time fraction

Decubitus, upright, or prone positioning

Bronchodilation

Improve O_2 delivery/consumption ratio
  Reduce O_2 requirements
    Work of breathing
    Fever
    Agitation
  Increase cardiac output
  Increase hemoglobin

Remove pulmonary vasodilators (e.g., nitroprusside)

Consider adjunctive support
  Vibration
  Nitric oxide or inhaled prostacyclin

of diffuse lung injury remains largely supportive. The primary therapeutic aims are to maintain oxygen delivery, to relieve an excessive breathing workload, and to establish electrolyte balance while preventing further damage from oxygen toxicity, barotrauma, infection, and other iatrogenic complications. To these ends, the clinician should keep a few fundamental principles in mind.

Minimize the Risk: Benefit Ratio

Positive airway pressure, oxygen, and vasoactive drugs are potentially injurious. Therefore, there should be frequent reassessment of the need for current levels of positive end-expiratory pressure (PEEP), FiO_2, and the use and intensity of ventilator support. An oxygen saturation of 85% may be acceptable if the patient has adequate oxygen-carrying capacity and circulatory reserve without signs of oxygen privation (e.g., lactic acidosis). Similarly, allowing $PaCO_2$ to climb (buffering pH, if necessary, with $NaHCO_3$) may minimize the ventilatory requirement and reduce the risk of barotrauma (see Permissive Hypercapnia, below, and Chapter 8, Practical Problems and Complications of Mechanical Ventilation). Mean intrathoracic pressure can be reduced by allowing the patient to provide as much ventilatory power as possible, compatible with ventilatory capability and comfort.

Prevent Therapeutic Misadventures

Patients should be kept under direct observation at all times by well-trained personnel ready to intervene 24 hours per day. Paralyzed patients must be watched with special care, because ventilation is totally machine-dependent. Furthermore, the hands must be restrained in semiconscious, agitated, confused, or disoriented patients who receive mechanical ventilation; ventilator disconnections and extubations can abruptly produce lethal arrhythmias, hypoxemia, asphyxia, or aspiration. Special caution is warranted for orally intubated patients, who tend to self-extubate readily (see Chapter 6). In the setting of pulmonary edema, the interruption of PEEP for even brief periods (suctioning, tubing changes) may cause profound, slowly reversing desaturation as lung volume falls and the airways rapidly flood with edema fluid. The stomach should be decompressed in most recently intubated patients who demonstrate air swallowing vomiting or ileus. For mechanically ventilated patients, the clinician must stay alert to the possibility of tension pneumothorax, especially for patients with radiographic evidence of pneumomediastinum or subcutaneous emphysema (see Chapter 8). Because of the very high incidence of tissue rupture, prophylactic chest tubes may be indicated for patients who form tension cysts that evolve on serial films.

Consider ARDS to be a Multisystem Disease

Intravascular volume must be regulated carefully (see below). Although excessive administration of fluids clearly must be avoided to minimize lung water and improve oxygen exchange, severe fluid restriction may compromise perfusion of gut and kidney. Appropriate levels of nutritional support and prophylaxis for deep venous thrombosis, skin breakdown, and gastric stress ulceration should be considered for all mechanically ventilated or immobile patients (see Chapter 18, General Supportive Care).

The routine early use of corticosteroids is not justified; adverse changes in immunity, mental status, metabolism, and protein wastage tend to outweigh any potential therapeutic benefit in the first week of the course. ARDS caused by known vasculitis, fat embolism, or allergic reactions may be an exception to this rule. Corticosteroids may also be lifesaving in certain steroid-responsive diseases that mimic ARDS (e.g., bronchiolitis obliterans, pulmonary hemorrhage syndromes, *Pneumocystis carinii* pneumonia). Moreover, under such life-threatening circumstances, adrenal insufficiency occurs with surprising frequency; if the presentation is compatible, this problem should be pursued diagnostically and stress doses of hydrocortisone should be given (see Chapter 32, Endocrine Emergencies). Corticosteroids also may help resolution in the fibroproliferative stage of this illness, but there is no firm consensus on this point. Ibuprofen seems to hold promise in blocking some of the systemic manifestations of inflammation, but the indications and risks of this drug for this specific setting need better definition.

IMPROVING TISSUE OXYGEN DELIVERY

In the setting of acute lung injury, attention focuses on maintaining an adequate oxygen delivery:consumption ratio while reversing the underlying lung pathology. Oxygen delivery is the product of cardiac output and the O_2 content of each milliliter of arterial blood. Techniques for improving cardiac output are discussed in detail in Chapter 3 (Support of the Failing Circulation). The O_2 carrying capacity can be improved by increasing Hgb concentration and optimizing its dissociation characteristics. Both factors may be important. Increasing Hgb tends to increase mixed venous oxygen saturation as it reduces the need for any rise in cardiac output compensatory to anemia. Both of these actions (lower cardiac output and higher mixed venous O_2 saturation) tend to reduce venous admixture. Hgb performance is improved by reversing alkalemia to facilitate O_2 offloading. As Hgb concentration rises, blood viscosity increases, retarding passage of erythrocytes through capillary networks. Therefore, actual O_2 delivery can be impaired as hematocrit (Hct) rises higher than 50%. Although the optimal Hct in patients with an oxygenation crisis is unknown, it makes sense to restore Hct to 35 to 40%. More extensive supplementation increases the risks of transfusion without proven benefit (see Chapter 14, Transfusion and Blood Component Therapy).

A very high percentage of the oxygen contained in blood is bound to Hgb; the proportion of oxygen solubilized in plasma is very small (3%) at ambient pressure. However, in severe anemia, the Hgb-bound fraction is disproportionately small, so that total O_2-carrying capacity is boosted significantly when 100% O_2 is used. Breathing pure oxygen also helps dissociate carbon monoxide from Hgb. After carbon monoxide exposure, high partial pressures of O_2 (particularly those delivered under hyperbaric conditions) can deliver life-sustaining quantities of dissolved O_2 (see Chapter 40).

Because extravascular water accumulates readily in the setting of permeability edema, fluids should be used judiciously to keep the wedge pressure as low as feasible, consistent with adequate oxygen delivery. Liberal use of inotropes and other vasoactive drugs occasionally can be helpful, especially in certain postoperative or posttrauma settings. Driving the cardiac output to ''supraphysiologic'' levels, however, does not seem to be routinely helpful for medical patients with ARDS.

Oxygen Therapy

Increasing the FiO_2 improves PaO_2 in all instances in which shunt is not responsible for desaturation. The goal is to increase the saturation of Hgb to 85 to 90% or more without risking O_2 toxicity. Oxygen toxicity is both concentration-dependent and time-dependent. As a rule, very high inspired fractions of oxygen can be used safely for brief periods as efforts are made to reverse the underlying process. Sustained elevations in FiO_2 greater than 0.6 result in inflammatory changes and eventual fibrosis in experimental models; therefore, it seems logical that efforts are made to keep FiO_2 lower than 0.65 during the support phase of acute lung injury.

PEEP, Positioning, and Other Techniques for Raising Lung Volume

PEEP and other techniques (e.g., inverse ratio ventilation) for increasing mean alveolar pressure are often successful in maintaining lung volume recruitment (see Chapter 9, Positive End-Expiratory Pressure). Virtually all patients benefit from low levels of PEEP (3–5 cm H_2O), which help to compensate for the loss of volume that accompanies the supine posture and translaryngeal intubation. There is no evidence, however, that low to moderate levels of PEEP help in prophylaxis against the onset of ARDS. Although PEEP may be highly effective in the relaxed subject, its volume-recruiting effects can be negated by patient effort. Vigorous expiratory muscle action forces the chest to a lung volume lower than the equilibrium position. When this happens, relaxing or silencing the expiratory muscles by sedation (and/or paralysis, if needed) can prove very helpful. When infiltration is predominantly unilateral, PEEP may be ineffective or hazardous, because it causes already functional lung units to overdistend. In this setting, repositioning the patient (e.g., to a lateral decubitus posture) or the combination of selective intubation and independent lung ventilation may allow individual tailoring of the pattern of lung inflation, FiO_2, and PEEP, thereby improving oxygenation and reducing the risk of barotrauma.

The potential benefits of position changes often are overlooked. Alert patients should remain upright, if possible, and recumbent patients should be turned every few hours. (This is especially important during coma or paralysis.) Intermittent shifts from the supine to the prone position often help dramatically in reversing hypoxemia in the early stage of ARDS (see below). Alternating lateral decubitus positions puts different regions of the lung on maximal stretch and improves the secretion drainage of the uppermost lung. Indeed, the incidence of pulmonary infections may be reduced by such mechanisms. Several types of motorized beds perform this function continuously, although the patient generally is rotated through less extreme angles. When one lung is affected differentially, oxygenation occasionally improves dramatically with the good lung in the dependent position, but this is not observed reliably. Care should be taken to ensure that secretions from the infiltrated lung are not aspirated into the airway of the dependent viable lung during this process.

Recruiting Maneuvers

It must be remembered that PEEP itself does not recruit atelectatic lung units but only keeps recruited units from recollapsing. To accomplish maximal recruitment, sufficient pressure must be applied to exceed opening pressure, and sufficient total PEEP must be applied to exceed the closing pressure. It stands to reason, therefore, that periodic application of sustained high-pressure "recruiting" breaths (in a patient with a normal chest wall, 35 cm H_2O CPAP applied for at least 15 seconds) may be needed to achieve and sustain optimal arterial oxygenation when small tidal volumes are used for patients with acute oxygenation failure, as they often are in ARDS.

Secretion Management and Bronchodilation

Although ARDS often is regarded as a problem of parenchymal injury, airway edema, bronchospasm, and secretion retention often contribute to hypoxemia. Retained secretions pose an overlooked problem that increases endotracheal tube resistance, infection risk, the hazard of barotrauma, and maldistribution of ventilation. For some patients with diffuse lung injury, profound bradycardia develops during ventilator disconnections, discouraging airway suctioning. Although hypoxemia occasionally contributes, this bradycardia usually is reflex in nature and responds to prophylactic (parenteral) atropine or reapplication of positive airway pressure. Circuits that do not interrupt PEEP during suctioning may offer some advantage.

Reducing Oxygen Requirements

Reducing the tissue demand for O_2 can be as effective as improving oxygen delivery. Fever, agitation, overfeeding, vigorous respiratory activity, shivering, sepsis, and a host of other commonly observed clinical conditions can markedly increase VO_2. Fever reduction may have therapeutic value, but shivering must be prevented in the cooling process. Sedation and the use of antipyretics rather than cooling blankets make good therapeutic sense. (Although phenothiazines may prevent shivering, their use may inhibit the cutaneous vasodilation necessary for rapid heat loss.)

Paralysis is a valuable adjunct to reduce oxygen consumption and improve PaO_2 in patients who remain agitated or fight the ventilator despite more conservative measures. Although paralysis is helpful during the first hours of machine support, protracted paralysis must be avoided for several reasons. Paralysis places the entire responsibility of achieving adequate oxygenation and ventilation on the medical team. Furthermore, the patient is defenseless in the event of an unobserved ventilator disconnection. Paralysis also silences the coughing mechanism and creates a monotonous breathing pattern that encourages secretion retention in dependent regions. Finally, protracted and unmonitored paralysis may cause weakness or devastating neuromyopathy (see Chapter 17).

MECHANICAL VENTILATION OF ACUTE LUNG INJURY AND ARDS

Conventional Approach

The basic principles of managing acute lung injury (ALI) are well accepted. The primary objective is to accomplish effective gas exchange at the least inspired oxygen fraction (FiO_2) and pressure cost. The relative hazards of oxygen therapy, high pressure ventilatory patterns, and abnormal target values for arterial blood gases, pH, and cardiac output, are vigorously debated (Table 24.3).

Most traditional ventilatory strategies used in intensive care evolved directly from anesthetic and surgical postoperative practice. When the lungs are uninjured and their capacity to expand remains normal (as is common in the periopera-

tive period), large tidal volumes (V_T) of 10 to 15 mL/kg generate only modest end-inspiratory transalveolar pressure. In fact, large tidal volumes prevent the microatelectasis that accompanies monotonous shallow breathing and are needed by many spontaneously breathing patients to satisfy high ventilatory demands (e.g., metabolic acidosis). Postoperatively, the mandatory respiratory rate usually is adjusted to "normalize" pH and/or $PaCO_2$, and sufficient PEEP is used to achieve acceptable O_2 delivery at what is assumed to be a nontoxic FiO_2. (An FiO_2 less than 0.65 is commonly targeted.) Typically, airway pressures are monitored but not rigidly constrained.

With few modifications, this high tidal volume, normoxic, normocapnic ventilation paradigm was developed as the standard approach to supporting most critically ill patients as well. Consequently, tidal volumes that exceed 800 mL and end-tidal (plateau) alveolar pressures greater than 50 cm H_2O are still common in many intensive care units during the ventilation of ARDS. How best to select "optimal" PEEP remains controversial, but many practitioners advocate using the *least* PEEP consistent with accomplishing acceptable arterial oxygenation. Others rely on computations of systemic oxygen delivery or best tidal compliance to make their selections of PEEP and V_T. Unfortunately, the machine settings that achieve all important clinical objectives do not invariably coincide. A relatively small but growing number of practitioners are now shifting first priority from optimizing gas exchange, oxygen delivery, or respiratory system compliance to a strategy that minimizes the potentially injurious effects of mechanical ventilation.

Ventilator-Induced Lung Damage

Implications of Evolving Histology

Histologic findings evolve continuously (but heterogeneously) over the course of acute lung injury (Table 24.4). It is reasonable to assume that all lung regions sustain the initial insult more or less simultaneously and that, in the most severe cases, proliferation, organization, remodeling, and fibrosis sequentially follow an initial phase of edema and atelectasis. Although parenchymal damage is widespread, the nature, severity, pace of evolution, and perhaps even the stage of injury vary from site to site within the damaged lung. Early in the course of ARDS, gravitationally dependent areas are extensively consolidated and atelectatic, whereas nondependent regions tend to aerate better. Regional blood flows and vascular

TABLE 24–3

APPROACHES TO ARDS VENTILATION

Conventional	"Lung protective"
Large tidal volume	Small tidal volume
Minimum PEEP	"Sufficient" PEEP
Normalize $PaCO_2$	Permissive hypercapnia
Unrestrained Paw*	Pressure limitation

* Airway Pressure

TABLE 24–4

CHARACTERISTICS OF EARLY AND LATE-PHASE ARDS

	Early Phase (0–3 days)	Late Phase (>7 days)
Structural collagen	Strong	Degraded
Atelectasis	Prevalent	Less prevalent
Edema	Prevalent	Less prevalent
Mechanics	Heterogeneous	Less heterogeneous
Ventilator lung injury	Edema and hemorrhage	Pneumothorax Cystic barotrauma

pressures also vary (Fig. 24.5). Changes of body position alter lung (or chest wall) mechanics, influence the radiographic findings, and affect gas exchange. Although counter examples occasionally occur, perhaps 60 to 70% of patients respond to prone positioning by improving PaO_2 significantly during this early phase of ARDS (see below). The efficacy of PEEP in improving oxygen exchange relates directly to the reversal of atelectasis and the redistribution of lung water. It

is not surprising, therefore, that PEEP's effectiveness in improving oxygen exchange tends to decline as time passes.

The collagen framework of the normal lung remains relatively intact during the first days of injury but later weakens as inflammation gradually degrades structural protein and nonuniformly remodels the lung's architecture. Therefore, the same pressures that were withstood acceptably well initially may cause alveolar disruption after the disease is well established. This may explain the tendency for radiographically detectable barotrauma to occur late in the course of the disease—often well after gas exchange abnormalities have noticeably improved and ventilatory pressures have declined.

Dangers of Excessive and Insufficient Lung Volumes (see Chapter 8)

After acute injury, only a fraction of the injured lung is accessible to gas; in severe cases, no more than one-third of all alveoli remain patent. Considering that well-ventilated lung units may retain nearly normal elastance and fragility, the apparent

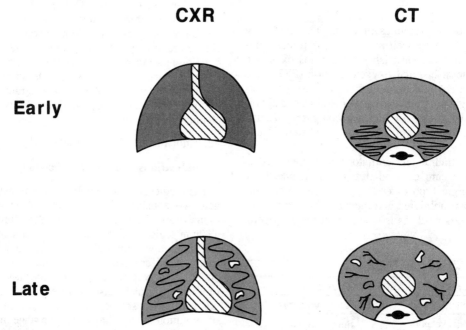

FIG. 24–5. Chest radiographic (CXR) and computed tomographic (CT) appearance of the chest in early and late phases of ARDS. The lung seems to be diffusely and uniformly affected in the early stage. However, CT demonstrates a preponderance of atelectasis in the dependent (dorsal) regions. Later, infiltrates are more widely distributed and cystic spaces often form. In this stage, atelectasis is less prevalent and infiltrates are more evenly distributed in the transverse plane of the CT.

"stiffness" of the lung in the early phase of ALI is better explained by fewer functioning alveoli than by a generalized increase in recoil tension. Increased tissue recoil contributes more significantly later on, when cellular infiltration is intense, edema has been reabsorbed or organized, atelectasis is less extensive, and fibrosis is under way. Because the lung's reduced functional compartment must accommodate the entire tidal volume, large (conventional) tidal volumes may cause overdistention, local hyperventilation, and inhibition or depletion of surfactant. Moreover, during rapid inflation to high transalveolar pressures, intense shearing forces may develop at the junctions of structures that are mobile (aerated lung units) with those that are immobile: collapsed or consolidated alveoli, distal conducting airways (see Chapter 8, Complications of Mechanical Ventilation).

Tidal pressures within the alveolus must neither rise too high at any time during the disease course nor fall too low during the first 3 to 5 days of treatment. Experimental damage resulting from overdistension of the alveolar–capillary membrane has been documented convincingly. The absolute value of peak inflation pressure is not the stretching pressure nor the true causative variable of barotrauma; instead, peak *transalveolar* pressure (roughly approximated by the difference between alveolar and pleural pressures) is the relevant variable. The plateau pressure is perhaps the best clinical correlate of peak alveolar (but not necessarily *trans*alveolar) pressure. The severity of "stretch injury" seems greatest when maximum transalveolar pressures exceed 25 to 30 cm H_2O and insufficient PEEP cannot keep dependent lung units fully recruited. Failure to maintain a certain *minimum* alveolar volume in the early phase of ALI may induce or accentuate lung damage. Unsupported by PEEP, certain collapsible alveoli may wink open and closed with every tidal cycle, generating shearing stresses within junctional tissues and tending to deplete surfactant. Increases in cycling frequency and duration of exposure to adverse ventilatory patterns accentuate any tendency for damage. The magnitude of blood flow in these stressed areas also may play an important role.

Bronchiolar dilatation, cystic changes, and/or microabscesses can be demonstrated in most patients with ALI ventilated for lengthy periods with peak airway pressures considered modest by traditional clinical standards. Such airway damage not only impairs gas exchange but also predisposes secretion retention and pulmonary infection.

Importance of Cycling Frequency

At levels of minute ventilation and tidal volume that are traditionally accepted, the ventilator may cycle in excess of 30,000 times per day (20 cycles per minute, 60 minutes/hour, 24 hours/day). Even if the tidal pressure profile is only slightly damaging, the cumulative effect might be severe. It is very important to reduce V_E requirements and cycling frequency whenever high cycling pressures are in use.

P_{flex} and the Choice of PEEP

A lower inflection (P_{flex}) region on the static pressure–volume curve of the passive respiratory system suggests the existence of a population of alveoli at risk for excessive tidal stresses (Fig. 24.6). Not all patients exhibit a lower P_{flex} region, but those who do are likely to experience extensive end-expiratory atelectasis at lower levels of PEEP. Indeed, arterial oxygenation often improves markedly as the end-expiratory pressure range just below P_{flex} is exceeded. Many investigators currently believe that tidal excursions into the lower inflexion range must be avoided and that persistent collapse of inflamed tissue is detrimental. Either provision of sufficient PEEP or the progression of disease over time obliterates the "P_{flex} zone" as well as narrows the hysteresis of the static pressure-volume curve. In contrast, in late-stage ARDS, high PEEP levels may simply add to the risk of lung rupture, or when peak pressure is capped, (out of a concern for barotrauma) increasing PEEP may reduce the safe operating tidal volume.

As a composite of the behaviors of all alveoli within the heterogeneous lung, the contours of the static pressure–volume curve obscure very important regional differences. Alveoli in dependent regions are most susceptible to collapse and those in nondependent regions are vulnerable to overdistention. This variability of opening pressures helps account for the *zones* (rather than *points*) of lower and upper inflection.

Implications of Pressure Limitation for Tidal Volume

The tidal volumes that correspond to the restricted range of safe ventilating pressures are ap-

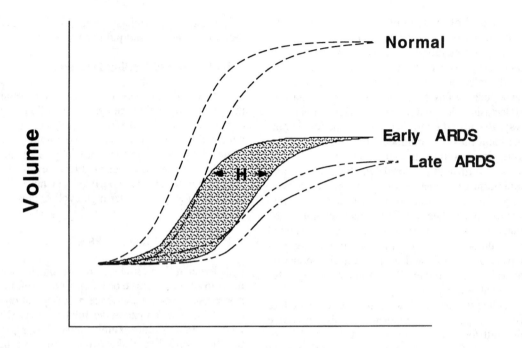

FIG. 24–6. Pressure–volume curves of the respiratory system in the earlier and late stages of ARDS. In the earlier stage of ARDS, distinct lower and upper inflection zones are evident, and the hysteresis (H) between inspiratory and expiratory limbs is prominent. Later, the inflection zones are less well demarcated and hysteresis is reduced.

proximately 4 to 8 mL/kg of lean weight or 300 to 600 mL for a 75-kg patient. However, because values for lung and chest wall compliance vary through wide ranges in different patients, unique values for tidal volume that are consistent with desirable pressure limits cannot be prespecified. Therefore, when using a flow-controlled, volume-cycled mode of ventilation, V_T should be adjusted with guidance by plateau pressure and the response of oxygen exchange to increments of tidal volume. The need to constrain tidal volume suggests the potential value of high-frequency ventilation.

Modes of Mechanical Ventilation in ARDS

Something of a mystique has developed around the topic of mode selection in ARDS. Although many would disagree, we believe that many choices are equivalent, as long as the practitioner ensures adequate O_2 delivery at a safe FiO_2, follows the same guidelines for lung protection, and remains alert to the potential shortcomings and complications of the mode in use. As a rule, spontaneous ventilation should be encouraged, except when oxygenation is marginal, heart function is seriously compromised, or ventilatory efforts are labored. It has been argued that newer techniques such as pressure control, pressure-regulated volume control, inverse ratio ventilation, and airway pressure release ventilation confer advantages over more traditional approaches, but none has yet been shown in a fair comparison to be consistently superior to its alternatives. The general concepts of ventilating the patient with ALI or ARDS are outlined elsewhere (see Chapter 7, Indications and Options for Mechanical Ventilation). The important difference in managing patients with ARDS is that the choices of maximum allowed tidal pressure and chosen level of PEEP may be crucial to safe ventilatory support.

Alternative Ventilatory Strategies

Permissive Hypercapnia

Carbon dioxide retention is often an inevitable consequence of a ''lung-protective'' strategy that tightly restricts applied pressure and maintains a certain minimum (end-expiratory) lung volume (see also Chapter 7). Maintaining normocapnia may not be appropriate if the cost is impaired lung healing and a heightened risk of extending tissue damage. "Permissive hypercapnia," a strategy that allows alveolar ventilation and peak ventilatory pressures to fall and $PaCO_2$ to rise, may reduce barotrauma and enhance survival in status asthmaticus and ALI, as several nonrandomized or retrospective studies without concurrent controls have suggested. The basis for any possible survival advantage has not yet been determined. However, the lung acutely damaged by stretch injury is susceptible to pneumonia and may be a source of inflammatory mediators transferred to the systemic circulation. Disruption of the lung's architecture also may promote bacteremia.

Physiologic Effects of Hypercarbia The physiologic effects of CO_2 retention are determined by the severity of hypercapnia and the rate of its buildup (Table 24.5). Except in the most severe cases or those complicated by extraordinary CO_2 production, the CO_2 retention that results from the pressure-targeted ventilation itself is generally modest ($PaCO_2 < 70$ mmHg). Chronic hypercapnia of this magnitude seems to have few notable side effects, other than the reduction in ventilatory drive attendant to compensatory metabolic alkalosis. Although gradual elevations of $PaCO_2$ (2.5 mmHg increase per hour) are often tolerated remarkably well, allowing hypercapnia may not be advisable for all patients with ALI

TABLE 24–5
CONSEQUENCES OF HYPERCAPNIA

System	Effect*
Respiratory	Reduced alveolar PO_2 Rightward shift of Oxy-Hgb curve Impaired diaphragm function Pulmonary vasoconstriction Worsened VQ mismatching
Renal	Enhanced bicarbonate reabsorption
CNS	Cerebral vasodilation Increased intracranial pressure Depressed consciousness Biochemical changes
Cardiovascular	Reduced cardiac contractility** Stimulation of sympatho-adrenal axis Lower systemic vascular resistance

* Most effects wane with time as cellular and extracellular pH readjust
** Only if not offset by adrenergic reflex compensation

TABLE 24–6
CONTRAINDICATIONS TO PERMISSIVE HYPERCAPNIA

Intracranial hypertension
  Head trauma
  Hemorrhage
  Severe systemic hypertension
  Space-occupying lesions
Cardiovascular instability
Cor pulmonale
β-blockade
Severe, uncorrected metabolic acidosis

(e.g., patients with coexisting head injury, recent cerebral vascular accident, or significant cardiovascular dysfunction [Table 24.6]). *Acute* elevations in $PaCO_2$ increase sympathetic activity, raise cardiac output, heighten pulmonary vascular resistance, alter bronchomotor tone, impair skeletal muscle function, dilate cerebral vessels, and impair central nervous system function. Carbon dioxide retention may be tolerated poorly by patients with autonomic insufficiency, β-blockade, or other conditions interfering with sympathetic tone and compensatory mechanisms.

Especially over the short-term, arterial pH may not closely reflect the pH of the intracellular environment. The magnitude of any intracellular acidosis resulting from permissive hypercapnia, however, is almost certain to be less than the profound intracellular pH changes produced by ischemia. Because CO_2 affects cardiac output and influences vascular and bronchomotor tone, it is uncertain if hypercapnia disturbs ventilation–perfusion matching or modulates the extent of lung injury and edema during the course of mechanical ventilatory support. Implementation of permissive hypercapnia often requires deep sedation and/or paralysis, a requirement that may be associated with serious side effects: impaired secretion clearance, fluid retention, and residual muscle weakness. Moreover, permissive hypercapnia may not be advisable (or even possible to implement safely) in the setting of coexisting metabolic acidosis or uncorrected hypoxemia.

Adjuncts to the Ventilatory Management of ARDS

Recently, there has been renewed interest in devising ways in which to accomplish effective arterial oxygenation without inflicting further damage on the injured lung. Some of these innovations modify the fundamental nature of ventilatory support (high frequency ventilation), whereas others provide gas exchange external to the lungs (extracorporeal or intravenacaval gas exchange), alter body position (prone positioning), or administer therapeutic agents designed to improve ventilation–perfusion matching (nitric oxide, aerosolized prostacyclin). One technique modifies the nature of the gas-carrying medium itself (partial liquid ventilation). Each of these adjuncts should be considered as promising techniques that currently are just beyond the perimeter of routine clinical practice.

High-Frequency Ventilation

When conducted at an appropriate lung volume and frequency, high-frequency ventilation (HFV) seems well aligned with current principles of lung protection and has a clear rationale. To this point, however, its superiority has been neither shown nor disproven.

Extrapulmonary Gas Exchange

Partial substitution for the lung's gas exchanging function reduces the requirement for ventilating pressure. Methods for assisting in the process of exchanging respiratory gases include extracorporeal membrane oxygenation (ECMO), extracorporeal CO_2 removal (ECCO$_2$R), and intravenacaval gas exchange (IVOX). All are costly, highly technical methods best undertaken by an experienced and dedicated team. Each has a good rationale, and laboratory experience and various clinical reports have been encouraging; however, for adult patients, none has been confirmed by well-controlled trials to add consistently to routine measures. Although initial experience with these exotic techniques has been frustrating, promise is held for well-selected patients.

Prone Positioning

Frequent changes of body posture are integral to normal activity, but positional variation is forgone for lengthy periods in the bedridden, critically ill patient. By tradition, the patient is cared for in the supine position, which allows more direct eye contact with the caregivers, family, and visitors, as well as better access to the vascular system and vital structures, thereby facilitating nursing care. Cardiopulmonary resuscitation must be conducted in the supine position. Despite these undeniable advantages, there is good reason to question our current practice of using only the supine orientation. A growing interest in therapeutic positioning has been stimulated by the observation that the prone position improves oxygen exchange in 50 to 70% of patients treated in the early phase of ARDS, allowing the physician to reduce both FiO$_2$ and PEEP. Recruitment of dorsal lung units with a more even distribution of pleural pressure and improved ventilation–perfusion matching seems best to explain this benefit. Airways serving the expansive dorsal regions generally are better drained in this position as well. Based on theoretical considerations and limited personal experience, prone positioning is less likely to benefit patients with large continuous pleural air leaks, especially if pneumothorax is radiographically evident and bilateral. When the lung is surrounded by gas, the normal pleural gradient of pressure is erased or altered substantially, making the effect of prone positioning unpredictable. Under such circumstances, prone positioning should be attempted with caution—if at all.

Practical Points in Prone Positioning (Table 24.7)   Although hemodynamic parameters tend to remain unchanged, hypotension, desaturation, and arrhythmias may occur during the process of turning from the supine to the prone position. These transient problems generally do not persist and can be minimized by using sedation, prior airway suctioning, and 100% oxygen during the maneuver. Continuous arterial pressure monitoring, electrocardiography, and pulse oximetry are strongly advised. Deep sedation and occasionally paralysis will be required to secure patient compliance. Attention also must be given to preserving the position and patency of intravascular lines and endotracheal tubes during the turning process.

TABLE 24–7

PRACTICAL POINTS FOR PRONE POSITIONING IN ARDS

Soft bed

Secure endotracheal tube and all lines before transition

Sedate and preoxygenate before turning

Monitor carefully during transitions

Support shoulders and hips

Adjust PEEP and tidal volume after positioning

Protect eyes, facial areas

Exercise special caution if bronchopleural fistula present

Flip one to three times daily

Use of a soft (air-cushioned) bed is all but mandatory for comfort. Pillows must be used to support the hips, pelvis, shoulders, and head. Patients with tracheostomies present a particular challenge. The compliance of the respiratory system generally changes little in shifting to the prone position. This is variable, however; tidal volume should be monitored (and adjusted if necessary) during pressure-controlled ventilation, which is influenced by any position-related changes in chest wall compliance. Furthermore, for the same plateau pressure, peak pressures may change if flow-controlled volume-cycled ventilation is used. For similar reasons, a given level of PEEP may be more or less effective in one position versus the other. Although the optimal frequency of supine–prone interconversions is not clear, in current practice, most experienced centers "flip" patients once or twice daily. Supine repositioning allows certain nursing procedures (washing, line dressing changes, etc.) to be delivered and helps resolve facial edema. It seems reasonable to assign the relative duration of each position in proportion to the gas exchange response. (For example, equal times would be assigned if only a minor important gas exchange difference is observed between positions.) Prone repositioning should be reevaluated often in the first 3 to 5 days of illness, after which time it tends to lose its oxygen-exchange effectiveness.

Partial Liquid Ventilation

Perfluorocarbons (PFCs) proposed for clinical purposes are environmentally innocuous liquids at room temperature that dissolve extraordinary volumes of oxygen and carbon dioxide, allowing effective gas exchange to take place. Biologically inert and immiscible in both aqueous and lipid media, they cause no known tissue reaction—even during extended use. Perfluoro-octyl bromide (Perflubron), a PFC currently undergoing clinical trials, has a desirably low vapor pressure (it clears itself by evaporating slowly), a high spreading coefficient (it distributes homogeneously), and a low surface tension. Although its viscosity is similar to water, perflubron has nearly twice the density; airway secretions and alveolar exudates float on it, allowing such debris to migrate centrally for airway suctioning. Infections may occur less commonly in a lung filled with inert, nonnutritive liquid hostile to bacterial growth, but this is unproven. Its radiodensity may interfere with conventional imaging. Perflubron has the potential to keep surfactant-deficient al-

veoli open by two distinct mechanisms: (a) reduction of interfacial surface tension; and (b) physical distention by noncompressible fluid ("liquid PEEP"). The former property may be especially important in the infant respiratory distress syndrome, whereas alveolar splinting may assume primacy in ARDS.

Sustained *partial* liquid ventilation (PLV) preserves the key benefits of liquid breathing while allowing gas ventilation to proceed with standard mechanical ventilators and connecting circuitry. Initial clinical experience has been promising. In stark contrast to total liquid ventilation, PLV is implemented rather simply. The liquid preferentially distends the dependent alveoli most in need of expansion during the initial phase of ARDS, providing the vertically graded "PEEP-like" effect required by the underlying pathoanatomy. Simultaneously, blood flow diverts toward nondependent regions, which receive a disproportionate share of the gaseous tidal volume. Reduced venous admixture, therefore, has at least two explanations—effective oxygen exchange directly across alveolar units reopened by liquid, and redirection of pulmonary arterial blood toward the better ventilated nondependent regions. The exciting potential of perfluorocarbons in ARDS has yet to be confirmed.

Tracheal Gas Insufflation

An alternative to allowing extreme or rapidly developing hypercapnia or to using extrapulmonary techniques for gas exchange in ARDS is to enhance the efficiency of CO_2 elimination at low V_T and cycling pressures by the tracheal insufflation of fresh gas (TGI). This minimally invasive approach reduces the effective series (anatomic) dead space by bypassing the airway proximal to the carina during inspiration, by washing out the PCO_2 of this same region during expiration, or both (Fig. 24.7). During TGI-aided ventilation, fresh gas delivery occurs either throughout the respiratory cycle (continuous catheter flow) or only during a segment of it (phasic catheter flow). In either mode, the crucial variable seems to be the volume of fresh gas injected per breath during expiration. During expiration, low-to-moderate continuous flows of fresh gas introduced near the carina dilute the proximal anatomic dead space (dead space flushing). At high catheter flow rates, turbulence generated at the catheter tip also can enhance gas mixing in regions beyond its orifice, thereby contributing to CO_2 elimination. Expiratory insufflation seems to be the safest and most

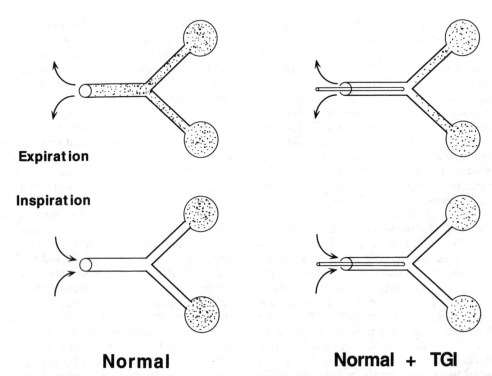

FIG. 24–7. Tracheal gas insufflation (TGI). CO_2-laden gas that fills the central airways at end-expiration is recycled to the alveolus with the subsequent inspiration. Expiratory flushing of CO_2 from the central airway by fresh gas helps improve CO_2 elimination and reduces dead space. The effectiveness of TGI is reduced when a high alveolar dead space lowers the end-expiratory tracheal CO_2 concentration but enhanced when hypercapnia raises the concentration of CO_2 in the central airways during expiration.

effective modality of implementing TGI, avoiding problems with overpressuring the airway, allowing manipulation of the inspiratory time fraction without influencing inspired tidal volume, and minimizing the volumes of fresh gas that must be injected to achieve a given level of CO_2 elimination.

Because much lower concentrations of CO_2 are delivered to the central airway, TGI loses its effectiveness when there is a large amount of alveolar (as opposed to anatomic and apparatus) dead space. ARDS, emphysema, and pneumonia are typical examples of such diseases. Conversely, permissive hypercapnia boosts the expiratory CO_2 concentration within the trachea, improving the effect of TGI.

Used improperly, TGI has the clear potential to cause mucosal damage, secretion retention, and interference with catheter suctioning. These effects should be mitigated by adequate humidification, using selective expiratory TGI, and the injection of fresh gas via channels imbedded within the walls of the endotracheal tube itself. Injection

of catheter gas retrograde to the exhalation stream tends to increase expiratory resistance and generate auto-PEEP; continuous gas injection allows the TGI injector to act as a constant flow generator during inspiration when the machine's valves are closed, risking overdistention. Excessive auto-PEEP and barotrauma are distinct possibilities when high gas flow rates are used—whatever the injection mode (selective expiratory or continuous). The experience of workers using transtracheal ventilation in outpatients with COPD, as well as other results with TGI in critically ill patients, indicate that once perfected, it may eventually prove helpful in a variety of acute and chronic settings. Because of its potential to moderate the rate and extent of CO_2 retention, TGI would appear particularly well suited to serve as an adjunct to a pressure-targeted, lung-protective ventilatory support for ARDS.

Inhaled Nitric Oxide and Prostacyclin

Nitric oxide (NO) is a key biologic mediator of smooth muscle relaxation. When inhaled, NO has the therapeutic potential to dilate the pulmonary vasculature in well-ventilated regions, tending to reduce pulmonary hypertension and improve the matching of ventilation and perfusion in an unevenly damaged lung. Inhaled nitric oxide is only active locally, as it is quenched immediately upon exposure to hemoglobin. Extremely low concentrations of NO achieve nearly full effect; biologic activity often is detectable at concentrations as low as 2 ppm, and beneficial effects are saturated fully at 20 to 40 ppm in most patients. The physiologic effects of NO in ARDS are highly variable—sometimes dramatic, but often quite modest. Although the onset and offset of the effects of NO are extremely rapid, gradual accommodation to its beneficial vasodilatory effects can result in rebound vasoconstriction when it is terminated abruptly. High concentrations of NO and minute quantities of its associated oxides, NO_2^{-1} and NO_3^{-2} are histotoxic and must be avoided. Although extremely appealing physiologically, the eventual place of NO in the management of ARDS has not yet been settled. At present, it seems most likely to benefit those cases in which hypoxemia is refractory to other measures or when hypoxic vasoconstriction accentuates symptomatic pulmonary hypertension.

Vasodilating aerosols (inhaled prostacyclin and lysosome-encapsulated prostaglandin E) operate by the same principle of selectively increasing perfusion to well-ventilated regions. Each may also inhibit inflammation and reduce pulmonary artery pressure. Although their physiologic effects can be dramatic, their routine clinical benefit has yet to be demonstrated.

A Pressure-Targeted Approach to Ventilating ALI and ARDS

Although definitive clinical data are needed to confirm the wisdom of adopting a pressure-targeted approach, a rational strategy for ventilating patients with ALI can be formulated based on firm theoretical and experimental grounds (Table 24.8). Such a strategy recognizes that several mechanically distinct alveolar populations coexist within the acutely injured lung, that a poorly chosen ventilatory pattern can be damaging, and that the underlying pathophysiology changes over time. This approach gives higher priority to controlling maximal and minimal transalveolar pressures than to achieving normocapnia.

Assuming that oxygen and ventilatory demands have been minimized, that FiO_2 is kept ≤0.65,

TABLE 24–8

A LUNG-PROTECTIVE STRATEGY FOR VENTILATING ARDS

Tailor ventilatory strategy to the phase of the disease (generous PEEP in early stage; withdraw PEEP later)

Minimize oxygen demands

Hold $FiO_2 < 0.65$

Minimize pulmonary vascular pressures

Control alveolar pressure, not $PaCO_2$

Maintain full recruitment of unstable alveoli in the early phase

Maintain total end-expiratory P_{alv} (PEEP + auto-PEEP) several cm H_2O above P_{flex}. In general, this will be more than 7 cm H_2O but less than 20 cm H_2O

Avoid large V_T and use least P_{alv} required to meet *unequivocal* therapeutic goals

Hold tidal transalveolar pressure <35 cm H_2O

Consider making necessary increases in mean P_{aw} by changing the inspiratory time fraction

Consider specialized adjunctive measures to improve gas exchange and O_2 Delivery*

---

* In addition to such standard measures as skillful management of pulmonary vascular pressure, repositioning, recruiting maneuvers, and use of cardiotonic agents, specialized adjunctive measures might include (where available) such experimental methods as $ECCO_2R$, inhaled nitric oxide or prostacyclin, partial liquid ventilation, and intravenous (IVOX) or intratracheal catheter-assisted gas exchange (TGI).

P_{alv}, alveolar pressure; P_{flex}, lower inflection zone of the static pressure volume relationship of the respiratory system.

and that fluid balance and cardiac function have been optimized, the essential strategic elements are as follows.

First, sufficient end-expiratory transalveolar pressure must be used to avert tissue damage resulting from surfactant depletion or stresses associated with repeated opening and closure of collapsible units during the tidal breathing cycle. The total PEEP applied (the sum of PEEP and auto-PEEP) should be sufficient to obliterate any lower inflection zone of the pressure–volume curve of the respiratory system, which at tidal volumes of 7 to 8 mL/kg generally occurs at a pressure of 10 to 15 cm H_2O in the early phase of ARDS. In truth, there is an inflection range rather than a single inflection point, as dependent alveoli in the lower regions of the lung require a greater end-expiratory alveolar pressure to maintain patency than those above them. Improved arterial oxygenation tends to parallel effective recruitment, and

CO_2 retention is a consequence of alveolar over-distension. Although actual construction of the pressure–volume curve (by any of a variety of static or dynamic methods) is theoretically appealing, for some patients, it is inadvisable to eliminate spontaneous breathing efforts. One simple way to select the best PEEP (with or without spontaneous efforts) is to first choose the operating tidal volume (4–7 mL/kg), initially setting PEEP at 8 to 10 cm H_2O. PEEP is then increased in small (2 cm H_2O) steps, looking for (a) an increase in peak static (plateau) pressure that exceeds the previous increment, signaling overdistention and (b) markedly improved oxygenation that corresponds to obliteration of the P_{flex} zone. (Under certain circumstances, a reasonable alternative to the empirical PEEP step approach is to gradually extend the inspiratory time fraction to create auto-PEEP.) Failure of oxygenation to improve significantly after two successive PEEP steps "and a recruiting manueuver" strongly suggests that nearly full recruitment had been achieved with that tidal volume at a lower PEEP value. PEEP should be lowered accordingly.

Second, because alveolar subpopulations with nearly normal elastic properties may coexist with flooded or infiltrated ones, the clinician must avoid applying transalveolar pressures greater than normal lung tissue is designed to sustain at its maximum capacity (30–35 cm H_2O). This pressure generally corresponds to end-inspiratory static airway pressures ("plateau" pressures) of 35 to 50 cm H_2O, depending on the stiffness of the chest wall. Pressures in this range generally are sufficient to reopen closed airways. Whatever the appropriate maximal pressure setting might be for an individual patient, it seems wise to avoid the upper inflexion range of the static pressure–volume curve whenever possible. Incursion into this zone is signaled by deterioration of tidal compliance and, for a passively inflated patient, by convexity of the inspiratory airway pressure curve to the horizontal (time) axis during constant flow ventilation.

Relatively small tidal volumes often result from imposing these upper and the lower bounds on ventilatory pressure. Therefore, periodic recruiting maneuvers (e.g., CPAP of 35 to 45 cm H_2O sustained for 10 to 30 seconds, according to re-sponse and hemodynamic tolerance) may be needed for some patients to maintain adequate lung volume and avoid hypoxemia. One interesting approach to making selections of PEEP and tidal volume when using pressure-controlled ventilation is to fix maximal airway pressure at approximately 30–40 cm H_2O, depending on chest wall stiffness, and to begin with PEEP of 8 cm H_2O. PEEP is then increased gradually while maintaining maximal airway pressure constant (allowing V_T to fall) until the point at which calculated tidal compliance begins to decline—one definition of the optimum PEEP value.

Third, under conditions of passive inflation (no spontaneous efforts), the practitioner should adjust mean airway opening pressure ($P_{\overline{aw}}$) to achieve acceptable pulmonary O_2 exchange by extending the inspiratory time fraction (T_I/T_T) or by raising PEEP. Cardiac output is supported as necessary to offset any detrimental effects of rising $P_{\overline{aw}}$. Extending improves the distribution of ventilation and may help to recruit or hold open otherwise collapsible lung units. Raising PEEP (and preserving a well-tolerated T_I/T_T) may be the preferred option, however, when the patient retains control of the breathing rhythm.

Fourth, when not contraindicated, hypercapnia should be accepted from the onset of therapy (buffered, when necessary, by judiciously infused sodium bicarbonate or other buffer) in preference to violating the guidelines of controlling alveolar pressure. Pharmacologic buffering also may be needed to allow hypercapnia when deep sedation and/or paralysis are not used. The strategy of permissive hypercapnia may be difficult to implement in the presence of metabolic acidosis, when other measures (e.g., dialysis) may be needed adjunctively.

Fifth, the prone position should be considered from the outset of management. Prone positioning generally offers its greatest oxygenation benefit early in the course of illness. When both available and necessary, consider the use of such adjunctive measures as nitric oxide, tracheal gas insufflation, or partial liquid ventilation.

Sixth, after the first 3 to 5 days of treatment, begin to reduce PEEP and the frequency of prone positioning as oxygenation allows, seeking to reduce maximum alveolar pressure and prevent alveolar rupture.

KEY POINTS

1. Six mechanisms may contribute to arterial oxygen desaturation: (*a*) inhalation of a hypoxic gas mixture, (*b*) alveolar hypoventilation, (*c*) impaired alveolar diffusion of oxygen, (*d*) ventilation–perfusion (VQ) mismatching, (*e*) shunting of systemic venous blood to the systemic arterial circuit, and (*f*) abnormal desaturation of systemic venous blood in the presence of a VQ abnormality.

2. Oxygenation crises are categorized conveniently by their radiographic appearance. Lung collapse (atelectasis), diffuse or patchy parenchymal infiltration, fluid overload, localized or unilateral infiltration, and a clear chest radiograph are distinct patterns that suggest specific etiologies and approaches to treatment.

3. Atelectasis is perhaps the most common cause of hypoxemia for the bedridden, critically ill, and postoperative patient. Potential consequences are worsened gas exchange, pneumonitis, and increased work of breathing. Mobilization, CPAP, and assiduous bronchial hygiene are keys to successful prevention and management.

4. ARDS is characterized by a delay between the precipitating event and the onset of dyspnea, impaired respiratory system compliance due primarily to the loss of functional lung units, a markedly reduced aerated lung volume, hypoxemia refractory to modest concentrations of inspired oxygen, pulmonary hypertension, and delayed resolution. The associated high protein edema resolves more slowly than hydrostatic edema.

5. Basic therapeutic principles in treating oxygenation crisis are to minimize the risk:benefit ratio, to prevent therapeutic misadventures, and to minimize tissue oxygen requirements (e.g., by sedation and antipyretics). ARDS should be considered as a potentially multisystem disease.

6. Shifts of body position alter the regional distributions of ventilation and perfusion and may be associated with changes in tidal and end-expiratory volumes. The regional distribution of any given lung volume clearly is altered by the prone position. In the early phase of ARDS, the prone position may dramatically improve the efficiency of arterial oxygenation for an unchanging ventilatory pattern and level of applied PEEP.

7. Manipulation of peak, mean, and end-expiratory alveolar pressures plays a crucial role in achieving adequate arterial oxygenation at an acceptable FiO_2. Moderately high pressures may be needed to increase lung volume enough for dependent airways to open. End-expiratory alveolar pressure (total PEEP, the sum of PEEP and auto-PEEP) helps maintain patency of alveolar units at risk for collapse. Mean airway pressure reflects average lung size and correlates with oxygenation efficiency.

8. High tidal volume/low PEEP strategies may extend alveolar injury or retard healing of already injured tissues. In the early phase of ARDS, avoiding excessive transpulmonary stretching pressures while maintaining sufficient end-expiratory transpulmonary pressure seems to be the least damaging ventilatory strategy. This approach often results in low tidal volumes (depending on lung compliance) and the need to accept CO_2 retention (permissive hypercapnia).

9. Many choices for ventilatory mode are equally defensible, as long as the practitioner ensures adequate oxygen delivery, follows similar guidelines for lung protection, and remains alert to the potential shortcomings and complications of the mode in use.

10. The essential elements of a pressure-targeted approach to ventilating ARDS are: (*a*) to minimize oxygen and ventilation demands; (*b*) to apply sufficient end-expiratory and end-inspiratory pressures to maintain nearly complete recruitment of functional alveoli; (*c*) to avoid overstretching the lung; (*d*) to accept hypercapnia unless there is a serious neurologic or cardiovascular contraindication; (*e*) to implement prone positioning whenever possible from the outset of treatment in the difficult to oxygenate patient; and (*f*) to consider the potential benefit of adjunctive ventilatory aides (such as NO and partial liquid ventilation).

SUGGESTED READINGS

1. Amato MB, Barbas CS, Mederios DM, et al. Beneficial effects of the "open lung approach" with low distending pressures in acute respiratory distress syndrome. Am J Respir Crit Care Med 1995;152:1835–1846.

2. Armstrong BW Jr, MacIntyre NR. Pressure-controlled, inverse ratio ventilation that avoids air trapping in the adult respiratory distress syndrome [Comments]. Crit Care Med 1995;23(2):279–285.

3. Brooks-Brunn J. Postoperative atelectasis and pneumonia. Heart Lung 1995;24(2):94–115.

4. Coggeshall JW, Marini JJ, Newman JH. Improved oxy-

genation after muscle relaxation in the adult respiratory distress syndrome. Arch Intern Med 1985;145: 1718–1720.

5. Cohen A, King T, Downey G. Rapidly progressive bronchiolitis obliterans with organizing pneumonia. Am J Respir Crit Care Med 1994;149(6):1670–1675.

6. Colice GL, Matthay MA, Bass E, et al. Neurogenic pulmonary edema. Am Rev Respir Dis 1984;130:941–948.

7. Demling R. Adult respiratory distress syndrome: current concepts. New Horizons 1993;1(3):388–401.

8. Elliott CG. Pulmonary sequelae in survivors of the adult respiratory distress syndrome. Clin Chest Med 1990; 11(4):789–800.

9. Gattinoni L, Pelosi P, Crotti S, Valenza F. Effects of positive end-expiratory pressure on regional distribution of tidal volume and recruitment in adult respiratory distress syndrome. Am J Respir Crit Care Med 1995;151: 1807–1814.

10. Gattinoni L, Pelosi P, Vitale G, et al. Body position changes redistribute lung computed tomographic density in patients with acute respiratory failure. Anesthesiology 1991;74:15–23.

11. Hickling K. Ventilatory management of ARDS: can it affect the outcome? Intensive Care Med 1990;16:219.

12. Hickling KG, Henderson SJ, Jackson R. Low mortality associated with permissive hypercapnia in severe adult respiratory distress syndrome. Intensive Care Med 1990; 16:372–377.

13. Lachmann B. Open up the lung and keep the lung open. Intensive Care Med 1992;18(6):319–321.

14. Leach CL, Greenspan JS, Rubenstein SD, et al. Partial liquid ventilation with perflubron in premature infants with severe respiratory distress syndrome. N Engl J Med 1996;335(11):761–767.

15. Levin D, Morriss FC, Toro LO, et al. Drowning and near-drowning. Pediatr Clin North Am 1993;40(2):321–336.

16. Marinelli W, Ingbar D. Diagnosis and management of acute lung injury. Clin Chest Med 1994;15(1):517–546.

17. Marini J. Evolving concepts in the ventilatory management of acute respiratory distress syndrome. Clin Chest Med 1996;17(3):555–575.

18. Marini JJ. New options for the ventilatory management of acute lung injury. New Horizons 1993;1(4):489–503.

19. Marini JJ. Postoperative atelectasis: pathophysiology, clinical importance, and principles of management. Respir Care 1984;29:516–528.

20. Marini JJ. Pressure-targeted, lung-protective ventilatory support in acute lung injury. Chest 1994;105(Suppl 3): 109S–115S.

21. Marini JJ, Kelsen SG. Re-targeting ventilatory objectives in adult respiratory distress syndrome: new treatment prospects—persistent questions. Am Rev Respir Dis 1992;146:2–3.

22. Meduri G. Late adult respiratory distress syndrome. New Horizons 1993;1(4):563–577.

23. Merritt T, Heldt G. Partial liquid ventilation—the future is now [Editorial]. N Engl J Med 1996;335(11):814–815.

24. Morris AH, Wallace CJ, Menlove RL, et al. Randomized clinical trial of pressure-controlled inverse ratio ventilation and extracorporeal CO_2 removal for adult respiratory distress syndrome. Am J Respir Crit Care Med 1994;149: 295–305.

25. Pappert D, Rossaint R, Slama K, et al. Influence of positioning on ventilation-perfusion relationships in severe adult respiratory distress syndrome. Chest 1994;106: 1511–1516.

26. Paulson T, Spear R, Peterson B. New concepts in the treatment of children with acute respiratory distress syndrome. J Pediatr 1995;127(2):163–175.

27. Pelosi P, D'Andrea L, Vitale G, et al. Vertical gradients of regional lung inflation in adult respiratory distress syndrome. Am J Respir Crit Care Med 1994;149:8–13.

28. Schuster DP. What is acute lung injury? What is ARDS? Chest 1995;107:1721–1726.

29. Stoller JK, Kacmarek RM. Ventilatory strategies in the management of the adult respiratory distress syndrome. Clin Chest Med 1990;11(4):755–772.

30. Tietjen P, Kaner R, Quinn C. Aspiration emergencies. Clin Chest Med 1994;15(1):117–135.

31. Weiss S, Hudson L. Outcome from respiratory failure. Crit Care Clin 1994;10(1):197–215.

32. Weiss S, Lakshminarayan S. Acute inhalation injury. Clin Chest Med 1994;15(1):103–116.

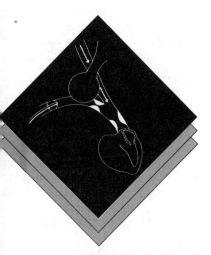

CHAPTER 25

Ventilatory Failure

PATHOGENESIS OF VENTILATORY FAILURE

DEFINITION

Ventilatory failure is the inability to sustain a sufficient rate of CO_2 elimination to maintain a stable pH without mechanical assistance, muscle fatigue, or intolerable dyspnea. Failure to maintain adequate alveolar ventilation usually is recognized by CO_2 retention and acidosis. Although a rise in $PaCO_2$ to a level higher than 50 mm Hg has been suggested as a hallmark, ventilatory failure can occur even when $PaCO_2$ falls to a value lower than its chronic level (which itself may exceed 50 mm Hg). For example, a modest metabolic acidosis may exhaust the limited ventilatory reserve of a patient with quadriplegia, severe airflow obstruction, or acute respiratory distress syndrome (ARDS). In similar fashion, hypocapnic alkalosis may deteriorate to ''normal'' values for pH and $PaCO_2$ as ventilatory failure develops in a fatiguing asthmatic patient. Conversely, many patients comfortably maintain $PaCO_2$ levels higher than 50 mm Hg on a chronic basis, without satisfying the aforementioned definitions.

MECHANISMS OF VENTILATORY FAILURE

Pulmonary venous blood delivers CO_2 to the lungs, where it normally diffuses into the alveolar space. Oxygen is replenished and CO_2 is eliminated by the pumping action of the chest muscles. Moving fresh air in and out of an unperfused lung unit fails to eliminate CO_2. Similarly, lung units that are meagerly perfused also contribute to wasted ventilation—the physiologic ''dead space'' (see Chapter 5, Respiratory Monitoring).

Normally, ventilatory drive adjusts the output of the muscular pump in proportion to metabolic activity to maintain pH within narrow limits. Inadequacy of the ventilatory pump in relation to the level needed to prevent acute CO_2 retention gives rise to clinical evidence of ventilatory failure. To maintain effective ventilation, an appropriate signal must first be sent from the brain to the ventilatory muscles. The muscles must then contract with adequate force and coordination to generate the fluctuating pleural pressure that drives airflow. Ventilatory work depends on the difficulty of gas movement and the minute ventilation requirement. Three major mechanisms cause or contribute to ventilatory failure: deficient central drive, ineffective muscular contraction, and excessive workload (Table 25.1). The primary physical signs of ventilatory overstress or fatigue are vigorous use of accessory ventilatory muscles, tachypnea, tachycardia, diaphoresis, and paradoxical motion of the chest or abdomen. In late-stage disease, the breathing pattern may become gasping or irregular.

GENERAL PRINCIPLES OF MANAGING VENTILATORY FAILURE

Ventilatory failure is managed by defining its cause, correcting reversible factors, and providing mechanical support when required. If the cause of ventilatory failure is not obvious, bedside measurements intended to define the mechanisms at

TABLE 25–1

CAUSES OF VENTILATORY FAILURE

Airflow obstruction	Ineffective musculature
Upper airway obstruction	Thoracic configuration
Extrathoracic	Chronic
Intrathoracic	Kyphoscoliosis
Functional (obstructive sleep apnea)	Thoracoplasty
Lower airway obstruction	Acute
Asthma	Pneumothorax
COPD	Pleural effusion
Bronchial stenosis (transplant,	Flail chest
trauma, tumor)	Hyperinflation
Muscular weakness	Inadequate ventilatory drive
Skeletal muscles	Intrinsic
Weakness	Congenital
Neuromuscular impairment	Chronic loading (obesity, severe airflow obstruction)
Quadriplegia	Advanced age
Myopathy	Endocrine disturbance
Diaphragm paralysis	Extrinsic
Functional	Drugs/sedatives
Hyperinflation	Sleep deprivation
Drugs, electrolytes	Metabolic alkalosis
	Nutritional insufficiency

work are especially important. Ventilatory workload is reflected in the V_E and in the machine pressures needed to deliver the tidal volume (see Chapter 5). Important factors contributing to the minute ventilation requirement include levels of alertness, agitation, pain or discomfort, body size and temperature, pathologic metabolic stress (sepsis, trauma, burns), ventilatory dead space fraction, nutritional status, and the work of breathing itself. The difficulty of chest inflation per liter of ventilation is best gauged by the peak dynamic and static (plateau) inflation pressures, as well as the estimated values for resistance, compliance, and auto-PEEP. Neuromuscular function is evaluated by observing the ventilatory pattern, the tidal volume and breathing frequency, the actions of the respiratory muscles, and by determining the maximal inspiratory pressure developed against an occluded airway. At the bedside, the appropriateness of ventilatory drive is often best assessed by examining the pH and $PaCO_2$ in relation to breathing effort. (For example, if $PaCO_2$ is high and pH is low, drive may be deficient, muscular reserve may be inadequate, or both; evidence of patient agitation, dyspnea, or distress argues for primacy of the latter.) The tidal mouth occlusion pressure ($P_{0.1}$) is just now coming into clinical use as a quantitative drive index, believed to be helpful when assessing the continuing need for machine support. As a strength-dependent index, the $P_{0.1}$ probably should be referenced to the maximal inspiratory pressure.

Correcting Reversible Factors

The investigation of the cause for ventilatory failure should be guided by a systematic evaluation of ventilatory drive, V_E, the work of breathing, and neuromuscular performance; therapy to reverse ventilatory failure should be guided by knowledge of the underlying defect (Table 25.2). For example, the V_E requirement may be diminished by reducing fever, agitation, and dead space. Impedance can be improved by relieving airway obstruction (bronchodilation, secretion clearance, placement of a larger endotracheal tube), increasing parenchymal compliance (reduction of atelectasis, edema, and inflammation), and improving chest wall distensibility (drainage of air or fluid from the pleural space, relief of abdominal distention, muscle relaxation, or analgesia). Neuromuscular efficiency should be optimized by ensuring alertness, maintaining the patient as upright as possible, relieving pain, and by correcting electrolyte disturbances, nutritional deficiencies, and endocrine disorders. Although Addison's disease is rare, adrenal insufficiency is surprisingly common among critically ill and chronically debilitated patients undergoing major physiologic stress. Measures that improve cardiac output or

TABLE 25–2

REVERSIBLE FACTORS IN VENTILATORY FAILURE

Excessive ventilation requirement	Impaired muscle strength and endurance
Metabolic acidosis	Nutritional deficiency
Increased CO_2 generation	Electrolyte disturbances
Fever	$PO_4{}^{-3}$, Mg^{+2}, K^+
Agitation	Endocrine disorders
Work of breathing	Inadequate cardiac output
Excessive calories	Myasthenia/Parkinson's disease
Increased dead space	Hyperinflation
Airway apparatus	Drugs (β-blockers, calcium channel blockers)
Hypovolemia	Impaired ventilatory drive
Vascular obstruction	Drugs (sedatives/analgesics)
Increased impedance to ventilation	Malnutrition
Secretions	Sleep deprivation
Bronchospasm	Metabolic alkalosis
Airway apparatus	Hypothyroidism
Pleural air or fluid	
Abdominal distention	
Auto-PEEP	
Pulmonary edema	

arterial oxygenation also will improve neuromuscular performance. Treatable neuromuscular disorders (e.g., myasthenia, myositis, Parkinson's disease) should not be overlooked. Some problems of decreased ventilatory drive are self-limited (e.g., sedative or opiate overdose); others improve with nutritional repletion, hormone replacement (hypothyroidism), or recovery of mental status. Few respond to nonspecific ventilatory stimulants such as progesterone. Unfortunately, many such problems are refractory to drug manipulation and must be treated by optimizing ventilatory mechanics with the goal of reducing the work of breathing sufficiently to restore compensation.

Mechanical Support

Willingness to institute mechanical ventilation should be directly proportional to the risk of deterioration without support and inversely proportional to the anticipated difficulty of eventual weaning. The general principles of intubation, mechanical ventilation with positive pressure, and weaning have been presented elsewhere (see Chapters 6, 7, 8, and 10). Noninvasive ventilation offers an attractive option for many patients with mild to moderate disease with rapidly reversible etiologies for ventilatory failure.

SPECIFIC PROBLEMS CAUSING VENTILATORY FAILURE

AIRFLOW OBSTRUCTION

Airflow may be limited at any level of the tracheobronchial tree. Even in the absence of underlying lung pathology, discrete lesions cause symptomatic airflow obstruction if located at the level of the larynx, trachea, or central bronchi (upper airway obstruction). Mediastinal compression due to fibrosis, granuloma, or neoplasia can narrow the trachea or major bronchi. Diffuse diseases of the airways (asthma, chronic bronchitis, emphysema) usually limit flow in peripheral air channels (<2 mm in diameter). For certain patients with asthma, however, the primary problem may center on the larynx and upper airway. Airflow obstruction also can occur with such chronic conditions as bronchiectasis, cystic fibrosis, sarcoidosis, eosinophilic granuloma, and certain occupational lung diseases (e.g., silicosis). Aspiration, reflux esophagitis, morbid obesity, retained airway secretions, and congestive heart failure routinely contribute to airflow obstruction.

Upper Airway Obstruction

Sedentary patients with low ventilation requirements and upper airway obstruction may remain relatively symptom-free until the airway lumen achieves a surprisingly small dimension. Dyspnea then progresses disproportionately to any further decrements in caliber. The complaints of upper airway obstruction may be impossible to distinguish from those of lower airway disease and may include cardiovascular as well as pulmonary symptoms.

Signs and Symptoms of Upper Airway Obstruction

The following signs and symptoms are particularly suggestive of upper airway obstruction (Table 25.3).

1. *Inspiratory limitation of airflow.*
2. *Stridor.* This shrill, inspiratory sound is particularly common with extrathoracic obstruction. In an adult, stridor at rest usually indicates a very narrow aperture (diameter < 5 mm). Frequently, stridor is mimicked by secretions pooled in the retropharynx.
3. *Difficulty clearing the central airway of secretions.*
4. *Cough of a "brassy" or "bovine" character.*
5. *Altered voice.* Hoarseness may be the only sign of laryngeal tumor or unilateral vocal cord paralysis. (Although not itself a cause of obstruction, unilateral cord paralysis frequently is associated with processes that do cause obstruction.) Cords paralyzed bilaterally do cause obstruction, but they usually meet near the midline, so that the voice may be "breathy" or soft but remains audible. Vocal cord paralysis impairs the ability to generate sound, so that the patient must increase airflow for each spoken word. Only short phrases can be spoken before the next breath, and the patient may sense dyspnea when conversing.
6. *Marked accentuation of dyspnea and signs of effort by exertion or hyperventilation.* The explanation of this nonspecific phenomenon is mechanical. During vigorous inspiratory efforts, negative intratracheal pressures and turbulent inspiratory airflow tend to narrow a variable extrathoracic aperture. Exertion is unusually stressful because obstruction worsens rather than improves during inspiration, as it does in asthma or chronic obstructive pulmonary disease (COPD).
7. *Change in breathing symptoms with position changes or neck movement.*
8. *Failure to respond to conventional bronchodilator therapy and/or steroids.*
9. *Unexpected ventilatory failure upon extubation or precipitous reversal of ventilatory failure by tracheal intubation alone, without ventilatory support.*
10. *Sudden pulmonary edema.*

During asphyxia and severe choking episodes, very forceful inspiratory efforts markedly lower intrathoracic pressure, increase cardiac output, and stimulate the release of catecholamines and other stress hormones. The increased loading conditions of the heart, in conjunction with augmented transcapillary filtration pressures, encourage the formation of pulmonary edema.

Diagnostic Tests

The diagnostic workup of upper airway obstruction may include routine films, computed tomography (CT) or magnetic resonance imaging (MRI) scans of the neck and trachea, and visualization by bronchoscopy or laryngoscopy (mirror, direct, or fiberoptic). Main bronchial obstruction caused by foreign body, tumor, or mediastinal fibrosis may give rise to strikingly asymmetric ventilation and perfusion scans. In cooperative patients, similar information may be available through a comparison of full inspiratory with full expiratory chest radiographs. In stable patients, pulmonary function tests should include inspiratory/expiratory flow–volume loops, maximal voluntary ventilation, and diffusing capacity, as well as routine unforced and forced expiratory spirometry (Table 25.4). Typically, upper airway obstruction (UAO) impairs inspiratory flow more

---

TABLE 25–3

SIGNS AND SYMPTOMS OF UPPER AIRWAY OBSTRUCTION*

Inspiratory limitation of airflow

Stridor

Impaired secretion clearance

Brassy or bovine cough

Breathy voice

Disproportionate exercise intolerance

Symptom variation with neck movement

Failure to respond to bronchodilators

Rapid reversal of dyspnea upon intubation

Fulminant episodic pulmonary edema

Frequent panic attacks

* Incidence of these signs will vary with nature, location, and severity of the obstruction.

TABLE 25–4

PULMONARY FUNCTION TESTS SUGGESTIVE OF UPPER AIRWAY OBSTRUCTION

Disproportionately reduced peak flow

Maximal midinspiratory flow < maximal midexpiratory flow

Vital capacity well preserved despite severely reduced FEV_1

Specific airway conductance low despite nearly normal FEV_1

$MVV^* < 30 \times FEV_1$

End-expiratory flows relatively well preserved

DLCO/VA** well preserved

* Maximum voluntary ventilation (L/minute)
** DLCO referenced to single breath lung volume (FRC)

than expiratory flow; impairs peak flow and airway resistance disproportionately to FEV_1; and responds extraordinarily well to a low-density gas (helium–oxygen) but not well to bronchodilators (unless there is simultaneous bronchospasm). Maximum voluntary ventilation typically is much less than the value predicted from spirometry, whereas vital capacity may be comparatively normal, relative to FEV_1.

Diffuse airway diseases such as asthma and COPD tend to produce a different pulmonary function test profile. However, asthma can have a significant upper airway component, and occasionally, stridor will be a prominent presenting sign. Often, these patients benefit from anxiolytics or psychotropic drugs, as well as bronchodilators and steroids. Unlike the diffuse obstructive diseases, which alter lung volume, distribution of airflow, and diffusing capacity, upper airway obstruction tends to leave the parenchyma unaffected. Diffusing capacity is relatively well preserved.

The flow–volume loop contour depends on (*a*) the fixed or variable nature of the obstruction and (*b*) the intrathoracic or extrathoracic location (Fig. 25.1). A fixed lesion inside or outside the thorax blunts maximal inspiration and maximal expiration to a similar degree, giving a "squared off" loop contour. A variable *extrathoracic* lesion, surrounded by atmospheric pressure, retracts inward when subjected to negative inspiratory airway pressure but dilates when exposed to positive airway pressure. Conversely, a variable *intrathoracic* lesion, surrounded by a pleural pressure more negative than airway pressure, dilates on in-

halation. On exhalation, the lesion is pushed inward to critically narrow the airway. Unilateral main bronchial obstruction may not give rise to such characteristic curves.

Management of Upper Airway Obstruction

The basic principles of managing upper airway obstruction can be summarized as follows: patients with symptoms at rest should be kept under continual surveillance and well monitored until the acute crisis resolves. Although certainly indicated, pulse oximetry may give a false sense of security, as O_2 saturation may remain within broad normal limits until the brink of total airway obstruction, physical exhaustion, or full respiratory arrest is reached. Postextubation glottic edema and laryngeal swelling resulting from thermal injury usually peak within 12 to 24 hours and then recede over the following 48 to 72 hours. Racemic epinephrine aerosols may help reduce glottic edema as they bronchodilate the lower airway to reduce the vigor of breathing efforts. For spontaneously breathing patients not already receiving ventilatory support, intubation and tracheostomy kits, as well as a 14-gauge needle (for cricothyroid puncture), should be at the bedside for emergent use. Oxygen can be insufflated via the needle until an airway is secured (see Chapter 6). Intravenous bronchodilators (e.g., metaproterenol or terbutaline) can be given if diffuse bronchospasm is unresponsive to inhaled agents. Release of bronchospasm is particularly important in the setting of an upper airway obstruction. Relief of lower (small) airway obstruction reduces the intrapleural pressure swings and the severity of upper airway (particularly extrathoracic) obstruction. If there is inflammatory obstruction, tactile stimulation of the involved region must be avoided and steroids may be helpful. Occasionally, the noninvasive application of continuous positive airway pressure (CPAP) or bilevel positive airway pressure (BiPAP) helps splint open the site of critical stricture. The patient should be kept calm but alert. If the patient does not struggle to breathe and maintains acceptable arterial blood gases, the following supportive measures may help temporarily while attention is directed toward reversal of the primary cause:

Head-up posture
Racemic epinephrine by aerosol
Corticosteroids (of uncertain benefit)
Helium–oxygen by mask

Flow Volume Loops in Airflow Obstruction

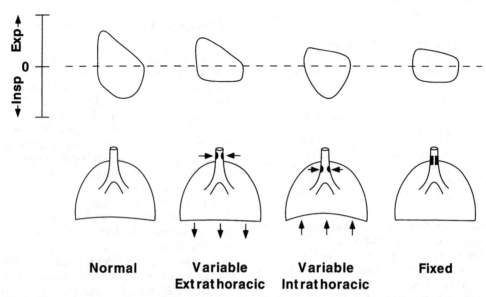

FIG. 25–1. Flow volume loops in upper airway obstruction. Maximal rate of inspiratory airflow is disproportionately curtailed as negative tracheal pressure accentuates resistance through a variable extrathoracic lesion. In similar fashion, the positive pleural pressures generated during forced exhalation selectively limit airflow across a variable intrathoracic lesion. A fixed lesion at either site limits the maximum flows in both phases.

Endotracheal intubation or tracheostomy may be needed if ventilatory failure ensues or secretions cannot be cleared. These procedures should be attempted only by experienced personnel.

Care of the Fresh Tracheostomy   Decannulation of a recent tracheostomy in a patient with upper airway obstruction may present a genuine emergency. As a prophylactic measure, many surgeons provide stay sutures to help locate and elevate the stoma. Others immobilize the tube by suturing it in place. If decannulation occurs, the first priority should be to maintain oxygenation as attempts are made to reestablish the airway. Oxygen should be provided by face mask or over the open stoma until the airway can be resecured. At least one brief attempt to reinsert the original tube usually is warranted, but this occasionally proves to be difficult. A tracheostomy of one size smaller should be kept at the bedside, as well as endotracheal tubes of one and two smaller sizes to serve as a temporary airway until the definitive tracheostomy can be reestablished by experienced personnel. Which-

ever airway is selected, proper location must be ensured quickly by the unopposed passage of a suction catheter and effortless manual insufflation and recovery of the tidal volume. If the trachea cannot be entered within the first few minutes, consideration must be given to immediate oral intubation, unless this is contraindicated by spinal injury, aberrant cervical anatomy, pharyngeal pathology, etc. (see Chapter 6).

Obstructive Sleep Apnea

Although usually considered an "outpatient" problem, obstructive apnea is observed quite often in the intensive care unit (ICU) environment. The typical patient is obese, middle aged, male or postmenopausal, or predisposed by pharyngocervical anatomy—but numerous exceptions to these stereotypes are encountered, especially under the provocation of physiologic stress, sedation, and fatigue. The well-monitored patient will demonstrate typical oscillations of the continuous oximeter and pulse tracings during sleep (Fig. 25.2),

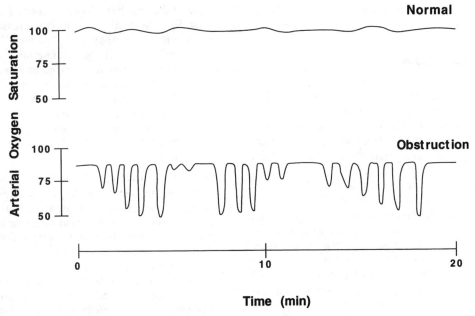

FIG. 25–2. Characteristic pulse oximetry tracings for patients with recurrent functional occlusion of the upper airway during sleep. When the upper airway obstructs repeatedly, the patient may spend a significant proportion of total sleep time under hypoxemic conditions.

and the heroic snoring efforts are hard to miss in these closely observed subjects. Most (but not all) patients will demonstrate evidence of CO_2 retention during wakefulness as well—a consequence of impaired drive to breathe coincident with or resulting from loaded breathing in a predisposed subject. A tentative diagnosis is made by extended sleep oximetry (with or without electrocardiogram [ECG] and blood pressure recording). As in the outpatient setting, nocturnal noninvasive ventilatory support (e.g., with CPAP or BiPAP, if necessary) is extremely helpful for patients who will tolerate this intervention.

Asthma

Causes

Asthma is an extraordinarily common disease characterized by airway inflammation, edema, and bronchospasm. The episodic airflow obstruction that results from these processes reverses partially or completely with medication. The trigger for inflammation and bronchospasm may be: (*a*) an inhaled or ingested allergen; (*b*) a bronchial irritant causing reflex bronchoconstriction (infection, endotracheal tube stimulation, smoke, fumes and odors, aspirated food, oral secretions, or excessively dry, humid, or cold air); (*c*) emotion; (*d*) exercise; (*e*) sinus drainage; (*f*) gastroesophageal reflux; or (*g*) pulmonary venous congestion or cardiac dysfunction. Obese patients often have a disproportionately reduced resting lung volume and correspondingly increased airway resistance. For such patients, relative small changes in airway caliber may cause wheezing and hypoxemia. Asthma may cause airway obstruction that never remits completely, but unlike emphysema, it does not routinely disrupt the parenchyma.

Herpes Simplex Tracheobronchitis It should be kept in mind that herpes simplex laryngotracheobronchitis can masquerade as refractory asthma, particularly in the intubated elderly patient with or without antecedent immune compromise. Infiltrates and fever are uncommon. Oropharyngeal signs of herpes often are absent or obscured. The diagnosis is supported by recovery of virus or viral antigen from sputum but must be confirmed by direct inspection. Bronchoscopic findings include an erythematous and friable mucosa that sometimes ulcerates. A fibrinous, pearly white membrane often lines the airway. The problem may prove refractory to corticosteroids and bronchodilators until treated definitively with intravenous acyclovir.

Physical Diagnosis

When admitted to the ICU, most patients relate a history of gradually worsening dyspnea. These patients usually require intensive therapy extending over several days before resolution. Other patients, typically in a young age category, develop life-threatening bronchospasm and ventilatory failure with frightening suddenness. Inspissated mucus and edema are less prevalent, whereas emotion, an identifiable provocative agent (e.g., aspirin) or allergen exposure, and asthmatic stridor often figure prominently in the presentation.

Patients may report few symptoms despite impressively abnormal examination findings and pulmonary function tests. Patients often report co-existing problems with nasal or sinus congestion and drainage. Dyspnea characteristically begins or worsens at night or in the early morning. Cough, rather than dyspnea, may be the major complaint. Hoarseness or gastroesophageal reflux suggests chronic nocturnal aspiration of small volumes of gastric contents. Substernal chest pain developing suddenly in a young patient with asthma suggests associated bronchitis or mediastinal emphysema due to alveolar rupture. A patient who is unable to converse in complete sentences has severe airflow obstruction or concomitant severe weakness. Because wheezing depends both on degree of obstruction and velocity of airflow, it appears in mild obstruction, reaches a loud intensity in moderate obstruction, and disappears in very severe obstruction. Wheezing may be audible only when the patient is supine. Wheezes do not necessarily imply asthma. The differential diagnosis includes left ventricular failure, pulmonary embolism, upper airway obstruction, and bronchitis (acute or chronic).

Specific Danger Signs

Deteriorating Mental Status Deteriorating mental status often is a harbinger of physical exhaustion and impending ventilatory arrest. Sleep deprivation, muscle fatigue, sustained high levels of catecholamine stimulation, and acute cerebral acidosis (occurring just before arrest) are likely contributing factors. When patients with asthma decompensate, they often do so suddenly. A low threshold should be maintained for intubating a disoriented, lethargic patient.

Arterial Pulsus Paradoxus Exceeding 15 to 20 mm Hg Normally, as arm cuff pressure is reduced, the discrepancy (the "paradox") between the point at which the first intermittent systolic Korotkoff sounds are detected and the arterial pressure at which all are heard is less than 8 mm Hg. The paradox increases as airflow obstruction worsens. This phenomenon is believed to result from the wide phasic swings of intrapleural pressure necessary for ventilation, which have several effects:

1. Inspiration effectively "afterloads" the left ventricle. Surrounded by very negative pleural pressure, the left ventricle must, nonetheless, raise intracavitary pressure to systemic levels. Systolic pressure falls during inspiration; reduced left ventricular afterload occurs during forced exhalation.
2. Although inflow to the right atrium increases during inspiration, preload to the left ventricle decreases simultaneously because a relatively small aliquot of blood returns to the left atrium, due to low right ventricular output during the preceding exhalation. Furthermore, the expanded right ventricle impairs left ventricular filling to a small degree during inspiration because the left and stretched right ventricles share myocardial fibers, the interventricular septum, and the pericardial space.

Severe Hyperinflation Hyperinflation abates as the severity of obstruction subsides. The increase in resting lung volume is produced by the combined effects of air trapping (the physical inability of narrowed airways to move sufficient air at lower lung volume to satisfy the minute ventilation requirement), and the need to hold airways open to minimize the work of breathing. Moreover, in very severe attacks of asthma, many air channels are plugged completely and do not communicate with the central airway at all. When such plugging is extensive, severe hyperinflation is evident on the chest radiograph, but auto-PEEP measured in the intubated patient may be misleadingly low, as it reflects only those pressures that correspond to alveoli that communicate with the airway (Fig. 25.3). There probably is considerable regional variation in the auto-PEEP values, whereas the end-inspiratory alveolar pressures may not differ greatly from site to site. In these cases, therefore, the end-inspiratory plateau pressure is a much better indicator of gas trapping when tidal volume and PEEP are fixed. Unless otherwise explained, a high plateau pressure despite a normal

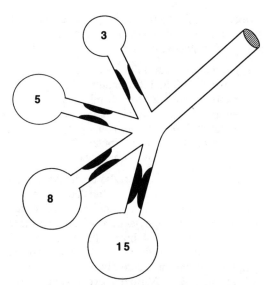

FIG. 25–3. Regional variation in auto-PEEP. The greatest tendency for airway closure and gas trapping tends to occur in dependent regions. Although end-expiratory airway occlusion reflects the average auto-PEEP among open alveolar units, the highest levels of auto-PEEP are encountered by alveoli cut off from the airway opening.

or low tidal volume indicates widespread gas trapping. A marked disparity between that high-plateau pressure and a low measurable auto-PEEP (and/or between the appearance of the hyperinflated chest radiograph and auto-PEEP) suggests extensive airway plugging as the basis for gas trapping.

CO_2 Retention/Acidosis/Cyanosis When the patient remains well compensated, an acute attack of asthma usually causes mild alveolar hyperventilation and mild-to-moderate hypoxemia. (Typically, pH is greater than 7.40, $PaCO_2$ is less than 40 mm Hg, and PaO_2 breathing air generally exceeds 60 mm Hg in a patient without underlying cardiopulmonary disease of another type.) Compensated asthma is unique among the obstructive diseases in promoting alveolar hyperventilation. Significant central cyanosis (implying marked arterial desaturation or cor pulmonale), elevated $PaCO_2$, and acidosis are important danger signs. However, if the patient does not seem fatigued and exhibits a normal mental status, these findings by themselves do not demand intubation and mechanical support; once appropriate therapy is under way, progressive deterioration in pH, $PaCO_2$, muscular strength, or mental status do require intubation and mechanical support.

Management

An attack of asthma may be brief, mild, and self-limited or may continue with such protracted severity as to require extraordinary measures. As a rule, the longer the attack persists, the more slowly it responds to treatment. Asthma must be managed aggressively, with prompt escalation of the therapeutic regimen if the attack does not "break" quickly.

In-Hospital Treatment Lethargy or disorientation, obvious fatigue, and deteriorating arterial blood gases are grounds for immediate admission to the ICU (Table 25.5). A single arterial specimen showing mild acidosis or $PaCO_2$ elevation should be interpreted cautiously. Most such patients will require admission to the ICU, but if the patient is alert and both the arterial blood gases and the patient show prompt and marked improvement with treatment, ICU admission is sometimes avoidable. Oxygen, corticosteroids, bronchodilators, and intravenous fluids are required for virtually all patients. For specific indications, antibiotics and ventilatory support are needed as well. During an established attack, the patient may not seem to improve for days, only to recover rapidly thereafter without a major change in therapy.

Oxygen Oxygen should be administered by nasal prongs or mask to all patients with less than full saturation of hemoglobin.

Inhaled Bronchodilators Although central to management, bronchospasm is by no means the entire (or sometimes even the primary) problem for patients with asthma who require intensive care. Termination of the inflammatory response, resolution of mucosal edema, and clearance of airway secretions are perhaps more important. In the setting of status asthmaticus, bronchodilating aerosols do not penetrate deeply into obstructed airways. (This is especially true for the intubated patient receiving mechanical ventilatory support).

TABLE 25–5

DANGER SIGNS IN ASTHMA

Deteriorating mental status

Arterial pulsus paradoxus > 15–20 mm Hg

Severe hyperinflation

Increasing CO_2 retention despite Rx

Cyanosis unresponsive to oxygen supplementation

Retained central airway secretions

Congestive heart failure

Unstable hemodynamics

Because a large fraction of a metered dose deposits ineffectively in the pharynx, the nonintubated patient using a metered-dose inhaler should be encouraged to use a spacer and/or to rinse the oral cavity with water and expectorate to avoid swallowing absorbable medications. It is generally acknowledged that more frequent dosing of β_2 agonists is required during an acute exacerbation of asthma. There is no convincing evidence, however, that continuous nebulization is preferable to the same total dose given intermittently. Moreover, intermittent administration encourages the frequent reassessment appropriate to this setting.

It must be remembered that a rapid response to bronchodilators is not to be expected in the patient with full-blown status asthmaticus who already has been admitted to the ICU and that there are important costs and hazards associated with frequent administration of high-dose β-agonists. Very frequent intermittent dosing may interfere with sleep and/or rest of an exhausted patient. Regardless of dosing method, β-agents induce agitation, tachycardia, arrhythmia, or hypokalemia. Such an intense treatment schedule may be counterproductive. These side effects and hazards are even more prevalent when nonaerosol (enteral or parenteral) β-agents are used.

In the hyperacute phase, albuterol can be given every 30 to 120 minutes unless there are limiting side effects. For most patients with asthma, the anticholinergic agents (e.g., ipratropium, atropine) are no more effective than the β_2 agonists (and less effective than they are in COPD). Because ipratropium is absorbed poorly from the airway mucosa, tachycardias, arrhythmias, and hypokalemia are decidedly less common than with the adrenergic agents; therefore, to reduce side effects, many clinicians elect to use them alternately with the β_2 bronchodilators. Ipratropium currently is not approved for use in asthma; efficacy should be documented individually and should not be administered more often than QID, for fear of drying secretions, blurring vision, or causing mental status changes. (These occur much less commonly than with atropine.) When so severely ill, many patients prefer a wet nebulizer to a metered-dose canister, even though some comparative studies fail to show a bronchodilating advantage. Wet nebulization of more than 10 to 15 mg of albuterol (or its equivalent) may be associated with undesirable cardiovascular stimulation, a fall in serum potassium concentration, or lactic acidosis. If inhaled bronchodilators are pre-scribed, careful attention should be directed to the duration of effective action, which varies with dosage. For standard doses:

isoproterenol: <60 minutes
isoetharine: 90 to 120 minutes
metaproterenol: 120 to 240 minutes
albuterol: 180 to 360 minutes
pirbuterol: 300 to 480 minutes
salmeterol: 480 to 720 minutes
ipratropium: 240 to 420 minutes

Rapidity of onset tends to be inversely proportional to duration of action. Inhaled corticosteroids, cromolyn, and necrodomil aerosols, which are intended for prophylactic use, have no place in the management of hospitalized patients. In fact, their irritant effects actually may worsen symptoms during the acute phase.

Corticosteroids Virtually every patient hospitalized for asthma should be given corticosteroids promptly and in high doses. Steroids reduce inflammation, help thin secretions, block components of the allergic response, and perhaps enhance responsiveness to β-adrenergic bronchodilators. Whether super-high doses of steroids (>125 mg of methylprednisolone every 6 hours) are preferable to moderately high doses (60–100 mg every 6 hours) is unknown. The question is not academic; apart from the financial cost, high-dose steroids often interfere with sleep, mood, cooperation, and thinking, as well as disturb glucose homeostasis. Although high-dose steroids are generally safe and well tolerated for short periods, profound neuromyopathy, manifest by elevated levels of creatine kinase and protracted weakness, is believed to result from the use of corticosteroids alone or in combination with extended neuromuscular blockade with nondepolarizing agents (see below and Chapter 17). Nevertheless, the danger of uncontrolled asthma clearly outweighs the danger of administering steroids for a brief period. The therapeutic effects of a single corticosteroid bolus are evident within 4 to 6 hours, peaking within 12 to 16 hours. There remains considerable disagreement regarding optimum delivery methods, doses, and schedules of administration. One rational recommendation is to administer an initial dose of 1.0 to 3.0 mg/kg of methylprednisolone (or equivalent) intravenously, followed by a similar dose every 6 to 12 hours until the attack is broken. (For many patients, the oral route is equally efficacious and dramatically more cost effective than parenteral dosing.) Once symptoms have improved considerably, the dosage can then be cut back to moderately high doses (0.5–1.0 mg/kg twice a day) for a few days before tapering gradually to the prehospital dose over 3 weeks. An inhaled steroid can be added at approximately 10 to 14 days, if indicated. Final tapering to the preattack dose should be performed by the outpatient physician.

Sedation, Paralytics, and Iatrogenic Neuromyopathy Many patients hospitalized with status asthmaticus are so exhausted that they sleep deeply and require little or no sedation during the first few hours of their intubation. Others, however, will require deep sedation and even muscle relaxants to reduce the ventilatory requirement to tolerable levels and to accept the permissive hypercapnia required to apply safe levels of airway and alveolar pressure (see Chapter 24, Oxygenation Failure, and discussion below). Neuromyopathy presents a serious risk in the controlled ventilation of the asthmatic patient. During the period of immobilization, myopathy manifests in the short term as elevation of muscle enzymes, and later as profound weakness requiring weeks to months for reversal. In all reported cases of asthma, high-dose corticosteroids were given. Most myopathic patients also received nondepolarizing paralytic agents uninterruptedly for longer than 48 to 72 hours, often without depth of relaxation monitoring. On the basis of current evidence, it seems advisable to limit the use of muscle relaxants to those who clearly need them and to use only the amounts necessary to accomplish partial paralysis for the shortest possible time. This need for paralysis is best established by attempting to withdraw the muscle relaxant entirely several times per day, thereby also allowing the physician to gauge the adequacy of sedation. "Train of four" monitoring, titrating to a two-twitch response, is also rational when continuous paralysis is targeted. This alternative, however, runs the risk of unnecessarily delaying withdrawal of the paralytic agent and may mask underlying alertness.

Theophylline Although clearly useful for some outpatients, theophylline derivatives must be used very cautiously (if at all) in status asthmaticus, with appropriate respect for their low therapeutic ratio. Failure of the left or right ventricle, hepatic disease, life-threatening illness, and certain drugs (notably ciprofloxacin and histamine-blocking drugs) slow its catabolism. Both efficacy and toxicity of theophylline roughly parallel its blood level; 10 to 20 μg/mL is a safe therapeutic range. As with most bronchodilators, greater ef-

fect can be achieved with higher doses, but response relates only logarithmically to dose, and the incidence of toxic effects accelerates at higher serum levels. Theophylline holds a very questionable place in the treatment of the patient with acute asthma who is receiving β-agonists and corticosteroids simultaneously. Some experienced practitioners believe that it improves diaphragmatic function, helps mobilize secretions, and improves cardiac contractility, but these potential benefits are controversial. The weight of current evidence suggests that theophylline seldom adds to the bronchodilating effect of an optimized β-aerosol regimen and it has little value as a stimulant to respiratory drive.

The warning signs of theophylline toxicity (nausea, abdominal discomfort) may not be sensed or reported by seriously ill patients; therefore, frequently obtained serum levels are mandatory. Cardiac arrhythmias predictably develop at levels greater than 25 μg/mL; in predisposed patients, it is likely that theophylline contributes to arrhythmogenesis at much lower levels. Central nervous symptoms (agitation, confusion, seizures) appear routinely at levels greater than 35 μg/mL but can be seen in a lower range. Theophylline seizures are problematic because of their resistance to standard anticonvulsants. An intravenous bolus of theophylline (aminophylline) can precipitate profound hypotension or sudden respiratory arrest. After a loading dose is given cautiously, aminophylline is best delivered by continuous pump infusion via a peripheral (not central) intravenous line.

Magnesium Sulfate Magnesium sulfate possesses some bronchodilating effects, believed to relate to modulation of calcium ion fluxes in smooth muscle. Studies conflict, however, regarding its value in refractory asthma. Although the toxicity of a 1.2-gm dose in patients with normal renal function seems limited to flushing and mild sedation, most patients given full doses of conventional bronchodilators experience little additional benefit.

Fluids The patient should be amply hydrated (2–3 L of fluid daily) to aid thinning of secretions, but excessive fluids are unnecessary and may cause volume overload. Although physiologic saline may help lubricate viscid secretions and facilitate airway suctioning in intubated patients, non-isotonic aerosols (mist therapy) may exacerbate obstruction due to bronchospasm or cause swelling in situ of retained secretions. Sodium bicarbonate is a hypertonic agent that may help lubricate or thin sticky mucus. Because of its irritating nature (see below), intratracheal sodium bicarbonate should be preceded immediately by an inhaled bronchodilator, if used at all.

Respiratory Therapy   Secretion retention is a very serious problem in asthma and is caused partly by the unusually tenacious nature of the sputum. Many airways are totally plugged, impeding dislodgment of the mucus. Unfortunately, chest percussion and postural drainage are relatively ineffective and poorly tolerated until a measure of bronchospasm has been relieved (usually the second or third day). Until that point, coaching to cough, bronchodilator inhalation, airway humidification, and oxygen therapy approach the limits of useful respiratory therapy services for the nonintubated patient. Noninvasive ventilation and CPAP are tolerated poorly by most patients with severe disease but are worth attempting in cooperative patients with more moderate illness (see Chapter 7, Indications and Options for Mechanical Ventilation). Iodinated glycerol compounds (e.g., potassium iodide) have little role in the treatment of acute airflow obstruction because their actions are delayed for days to weeks. Mucolytics (such as hypertonic $NaHCO_3$, acetylcysteine, and DNA splitting enzymes) may irritate the twitchy airways of the decompensated asthmatic and must be used concurrently with or immediately after an inhaled bronchodilator.

Mechanical Ventilation   Mental status or blood gas deterioration that occurs despite aggressive medical therapy is an important indication for ventilator support. Unlike many patients with COPD, patients with asthma tend to sustain adequate alveolar ventilation during attacks until sudden decompensation occurs. Mechanical support may afford the rest needed for recovery and should not be delayed once a firm indication appears. Although most patients with asthma can be disconnected from the ventilator within 3 to 5 days of intubation, others require much longer.

The basic principles of ventilator management during status asthmaticus do not differ greatly from those of other conditions. However, hemodynamic compromise and certain forms of barotrauma (pneumomediastinum, pneumothorax) are a greater risk due to gas trapping. Peak alveolar end-inspiratory (plateau) pressure should be monitored closely and kept lower than 30 cm H_2O. For most patients, this will mean the acceptance of hypercarbia and respiratory acidosis ("permissive hypercapnia"). Deep sedation and, in severe

cases, muscle relaxants, may be required to impose this gentler breathing pattern.

As a guideline, a tidal volume of 7 mL/kg, a backup frequency of 12 to 16 breaths/minute, and a decelerating flow waveform of 80 to 100 L/minute usually produces a satisfactory starting point. Failure to keep plateau pressure less than 30 cm H_2O prompts reductions of frequency or tidal volume. Administration of bicarbonate may be advisable if pH is less than 7.20, but this recommendation is also controversial. Some physicians allow pH to fall to 7.10 (or even lower) if the patient demonstrates physiologic tolerance, but this extreme approach cannot be advocated for general use. The degree of dynamic hyperinflation is determined by the severity of airflow obstruction, the size of the tidal volume, and the duration of expiration. The duration of expiration is most effectively extended by decreasing the breathing frequency (and minute ventilation). Using relatively rapid inspiratory flow rates and low compliance ventilator tubing during volume-cycled ventilation (to shorten the delivery time required for an effective tidal volume) will also help somewhat. For the same inspiratory time, a decelerating inspiratory flow waveform will help the distribution efficiency within the mechanically heterogeneous lung.

Positive End-Expiratory Pressure (PEEP) The place of PEEP in the management of asthma remains controversial. When resistance is volume-dependent, as it tends to be in this setting, PEEP helps even the distribution of ventilation and may possibly help improve bronchodilator penetration. In spontaneously breathing patients, PEEP may reduce the triggering threshold and the work of breathing. However, if expiration is not flow-limited, adding PEEP could simply raise both peak and mean alveolar pressures. As a rule, a low level of PEEP (<8–10 cm H_2O) can be added, as long as end-inspiratory plateau pressure does not rise.

Chronic Obstructive Pulmonary Disease

Characteristic Features

The obstructive pulmonary diseases associated with cigarette smoking (emphysema and chronic bronchitis) often coexist but are quite different processes. Emphysema destroys the alveolar surface membrane and blood vessels, reducing elastic recoil and diffusing capacity, leaving the airways collapsible but morphologically intact;

emphysematous obstruction of the airway is a functional, not anatomic, problem. Conversely, chronic bronchitis causes airway damage, bronchospasm, and sputum production but leaves the parenchyma unaffected.

Pure emphysema is clinically distinguishable from chronic bronchitis. On the chest radiograph, bullae, hyperlucency, diminished peripheral vascular markings, and increased lung volume are seen in emphysema. These findings differ from the increased bronchovascular markings and more normal lung volumes of chronic bronchitis. Patients with pure emphysema produce little or no sputum. Conversely, chronic bronchitis is defined as an airway disease in which there is habitual sputum production, especially in the morning. (That characteristic is shared by other airway diseases, such as sinusitis and bronchiectasis.)

Emphysemic patients tend to be breathless with minimal exertion but usually do not enter the hospital with exacerbations of their disease until they near the terminal phase. In contrast, patients with chronic bronchitis often seem relatively indifferent to their obstruction but decompensate more frequently.

The caricatures of patients with emphysema as "pink puffers" and patients with chronic bronchitis as "blue bloaters" are overdrawn. Many—if not most—have elements of both. Emphysema tends to destroy capillaries and alveolar septae in proportion to one another, preserving near-normal arterial blood gases at the cost of elevated minute ventilation. Diffusing capacity is routinely impaired. Bronchitis, on the other hand, produces extensive VQ mismatching and hypoxemia, without impairing the diffusing capacity adjusted for the volume of aerated tissue (see Chapter 24). Despite these general characteristics, many patients with advanced emphysema do not have vigorous ventilatory drives, whereas some with chronic bronchitis do. Thus, some patients with emphysema with moderate obstruction retain CO_2 and are not breathless, whereas many patients with chronic bronchitis are "blue puffers," especially as they near the terminal phase of illness.

Patients with emphysema tend to be more malnourished than those with chronic bronchitis. Pulmonary hypertension marks the end stage of both diseases, but for different reasons. In pure emphysema, pulmonary capillaries are destroyed, but normal oxygen saturation of arterial blood is the rule. In chronic bronchitis, pulmonary hypertension develops earlier, as a consequence of persistent alveolar hypoxia. Therefore, cor pulmonale

in a patient with bronchitis and hypoxemia may be partially reversed with supplemental oxygen. Cor pulmonale in emphysema is an ominous sign, responding poorly to therapy unless hypoxemia coexists. Even when relatively symptom free, both types of patients tend to experience tachycardia at rest.

Associated Problems

Hyperinflation helps speed expiratory airflow but increases the elastic work of breathing. More importantly, the inspiratory musculature is placed at a serious mechanical disadvantage (Fig. 25.4).

Poorly ventilated cystic spaces may fill when the surrounding parenchyma is infiltrated or flooded, simulating cavities or lung abscesses. However, distinction by chest film or CT usually can be made easily, and the prognosis for quick resolution is much better than for abscess.

Pneumonia and congestive heart failure (CHF) often complicate COPD but are often difficult to recognize because the parenchyma is hyperinflated and disordered and because the heart may appear small, despite enlargement.

Heart rhythm disturbances—typically atrial—are characteristic of decompensated COPD.

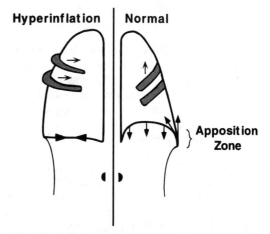

FIG. 25–4. Respiratory muscle compromise during acute hyperinflation. Normally, the curved hemidiaphragm is positioned optimally to splay the ribs outward by its bucket handle action and by the positive outward abdominal pressure exerted on the ribs in the zone of apposition. The hyperinflated patient may have a flattened diaphragm with no useful inspiratory force vector, lose the zone of apposition, and inspire against the inward recoil of the horizontal ribs. Simultaneously, the work of breathing is increased (see Chapter 10).

Management

Etiology of the Exacerbation The exact cause for many exacerbations of COPD remains unknown. Ischemic heart disease and diastolic dysfunction often coexist. Entry into a rapid atrial rhythm often precipitates dyspnea and altered gas exchange. Cor pulmonale is notoriously difficult to diagnose accurately, especially when a high-quality echocardiogram is unavailable. Numerous patients with severe disease blame climatic changes. However, treatable causes for deterioration (infection, pneumothorax, pleural effusion, congestive failure, embolism, etc.) must be sought (Table 25.2).

Oxygen Therapy Although it is true that high inspired fractions of oxygen may cause catastrophic blunting of ventilatory drive in susceptible individuals, judicious administration of the correct dose of oxygen can be lifesaving.

Reversal of hypoxemia may diminish hypoxic drive and work of breathing. In symptomatically hypoxic patients, oxygen improves alertness and muscular function and helps relieve cor pulmonale as well. (For this latter reason, oxygen often proves an effective diuretic.)

Although Venturi masks deliver a fixed FiO_2 and should be employed when control of the inspired O_2 fraction is crucial, nasal prongs are more comfortable for patients with dyspnea and allow expectoration without interrupting the flow of oxygen.

Any patient relieved of hypoxemia will retain slightly more CO_2 because hypercapneic drive and hypoxic drive are both reduced as supplemental oxygen is given. Two rules are useful: first, patients at risk to retain excessive CO_2 are those who already manifest some degree of hypercapnia before O_2 therapy is initiated. Second, in otherwise stable patients given "low-flow" oxygen, the rise in $PaCO_2$ generally is less than 10 mm Hg and usually occurs within the first hour of oxygen administration. Therefore, rather than withhold oxygen, the appropriate strategy is to raise PaO_2 to 55 to 60 mm Hg, watch the patient closely for signs of obtundation, obtain blood gases 20 to 30 minutes after the FiO_2 was increased, and adjust the oxygen flow rate accordingly. The proper primary endpoint is an acceptable PaO_2, documented by blood gas analysis.

Medication Regimen Bronchodilator therapy is similar to that already described for asthma. Anticholinergic aerosols, however, may be somewhat more effective in these "irritant" forms of bronchospasm. It is necessary to remember that the reversible bronchospasm component in COPD is usually small and that the patients are generally older and more fragile than those with asthma. Fluid/electrolyte balance, oxygen therapy, and respiratory therapy assume greater importance. Improving nutrition is helpful over the medium and long term.

Thick, green or deep yellow sputum with polys and Gram-stainable intracellular organisms should be treated with an appropriate antibiotic, whereas sputum eosinophilia suggests the probable utility of corticosteroids. (Both medications are given almost routinely, even in the absence of such data.) The choice of antibiotic should be guided by the sputum smear and by knowledge of the organisms to which these patients are vulnerable (i.e., *Haemophilus influenzae, Streptococcus pneumoniae, Neisseria, Branhamella,* etc.) (see Chapter 26, Common ICU Infections). If no organism is seen, a virus or mycoplasma are probable infectious causes of the exacerbation. In some regions of the country, *Legionella* is a prevalent community-acquired pathogen that is difficult to identify on Gram stain.

A patient who continues to do poorly despite appropriate initial measures probably should receive a trial of corticosteroids for at least 3 to 4 days. Massive doses of corticosteroids similar to those given in asthma should be avoided. Very high doses of steroids disrupt thinking, interfere with sleep, encourage protein wasting, elevate blood urea nitrogen (BUN) and white blood cell count, predispose to infection, and cause fluid retention. Metabolic alkalosis, hyperglycemia, and gut dysfunction or ulceration also are to be expected. When used, a reasonable schedule is to give 0.5 mg/kg of methylprednisolone or its equivalent every 6 hours during the first 24 to 48 hours of an acute crisis, with rapid tapering thereafter. Given steroids, some patients improve both baseline function and response to bronchodilators. Such persons have been termed "hidden asthmatics."

Management of fluids and diuretics is difficult, especially in the presence of cor pulmonale. Without solid evidence for intravascular volume depletion or overload, fluid loading or diuresis should be undertaken cautiously in a well-monitored setting.

Respiratory Therapy Respiratory therapy may assume a critical role in the management of hospitalized patients with chronic airflow obstruction. Most problems can be reversed by relieving hypoxemia, treating infection or fluid overload, and improving secretion clearance with the respiratory therapy techniques of coughing, deep breathing, and intensified bronchodilator therapy. The patient must be actively stimulated to cough, using endotracheal suctioning and/or vibropercussion of the chest wall or airway if necessary. Chest vibropercussion and postural drainage are quite effective when tolerated. However, no physiotherapy technique should be continued unless its efficacy can be documented.

Intubation and Mechanical Ventilation
Whenever possible, intubation and mechanical ventilation must be avoided for the following reasons:

1. Most patients without advanced cor pulmonale tolerate mild-to-moderate hypoxemia and mild acidosis quite well.
2. An effective cough clears the peripheral airways better than endotracheal intubation and suctioning.
3. Patients with COPD are at particular risk for the complications of mechanical ventilation (e.g., infection, hypotension, barotrauma) and can be exceptionally difficult to wean, due to the high work/cost of breathing, weakness, and muscular discoordination.
4. When intervention is early enough, some patients may respond well to noninvasive ventilation by nasal cannula or facial mask (see Chapter 7, Indications and Options for Mechanical Ventilation). Although extremely promising, additional development of noninvasive ventilation will be required before it can realize its full potential. Despite encouraging reports, many centers lack the highly trained and motivated nursing and respiratory care practitioners required to implement this technique safely, effectively, and expeditiously in this challenging setting. Early intervention, careful coaching of the patient, and a high degree of vigilance are essential to a successful outcome. In hypoxemic patients, great care should be taken to ensure delivery of the appropriate oxygen fraction at all times. Noninvasive ventilatory support is perhaps best delivered by a well-fitting mask attached to a full capability ICU ventilator.

Indications for Intubation Indications for intubation include deteriorating mental status, loss of effective cough (with retained secretions in central airways), progressive respiratory acidosis despite aggressive medical and respiratory therapy, and unstable hemodynamics.

If mechanical assistance is necessary, care should be taken not to overventilate with respect to the previous chronic state of CO_2 retention, a condition signaled by the sudden development of metabolic alkalosis when mechanical assistance is begun.

Throughout the course of ventilatory support, the staff must check periodically for evidence of dynamic hyperinflation (''auto-PEEP'') and its response to PEEP. Simultaneous airway pressure and flow tracings help greatly in this assessment (see Chapter 5). The auto-PEEP effect is associated not only with cardiovascular consequences but also with increased work of breathing. Increases in end-expiratory alveolar pressure secondary to air trapping and expiratory effort occur very commonly during spontaneous breathing as well. Weaning must be undertaken as soon as feasible but conducted cautiously to avoid cardiopulmonary decompensation or panic attacks (see Chapter 10, Weaning).

Treatment of Arrhythmias and Cardiac Dysfunction Atrial and ventricular arrhythmias of all types occur commonly, due to right atrial overdistension, catecholamine release, medication effects, pH and electrolyte disturbances, hyperinflation-related heart–lung interactions, and hypoxemia. The onset of atrial fibrillation can severely impair the efficiency of the ventricular pump and precipitate deterioration. Multifocal atrial tachycardia (chaotic but coordinated atrial contraction originating from at least three pacemaking foci; see Chapter 4, Arrhythmias, Pacing, and Cardioversion) is a characteristic rhythm that often responds only to the relief of metabolic derangement and respiratory failure. In certain cases, a calcium channel blocker such as verapamil or diltiazem can effectively slow the rate. Caution is indicated, however, because these agents may possibly worsen ventilation–perfusion (VQ) matching, impair myocardial performance or impede conduction (see Chapters 3, 4, and 22). In such patients, coexisting ischemic cardiac disease is common and may present with atypical signs or symptoms. The clinician should remain vigilant to the possibility of occult ischemia, congestive heart failure, and diastolic dysfunction—as well as cor pulmonale.

Nutrition The ability of the patient with COPD to cope with the respiratory workload depends on the strength and endurance of the ventilatory pump. Reversal of chronic malnutrition cannot be accomplished quickly, but maintaining adequate calorie intake is vital. Diaphragmatic bulk parallels body weight. Although it is possible to generate excessive CO_2 by overfeeding, this seldom presents a problem for hospitalized patients who are able to eat normally. Instead, attention should focus on providing adequate nutrition (2000 calories daily). Large meals or brisk enteral feedings may cause abdominal distention, discomfort, and breathing difficulty.

Neuromuscular Dysfunction

Functional Anatomy of the Respiratory Muscles

In healthy individuals, quiet tidal breathing is accomplished by active inhalation and passive deflation. The inspiratory muscle group is composed of the diaphragm (responsible for the major portion of ventilation at all but extreme work rates) and the accessory group, primarily the external and parasternal intercostal, scalene, and strap muscles of the neck. Expiratory muscle action is required for expulsive efforts (cough, sneeze, defecation), for high levels of ventilation (>20 L/minute), and for breathing against a significant resistive load (as during an exacerbation of asthma or COPD). An increased workload and impaired pump function often coexist. Because maintenance of alveolar ventilation requires a pressure gradient sufficient to overcome resistive and elastic forces, any condition that interferes with the ability to generate negative intrathoracic pressure (e.g., weakness, abnormal thoracic configuration, or muscular incoordination) will stress the system and may lead to ventilatory failure. Alternatively, conditions that increase the force requirement may lead to the same outcome, even without pump impairment.

Components of Pump Efficiency

Muscular Strength   Muscular strength depends on the bulk of the muscle, its contractility, the integrity of its innervation, and its loading conditions. Advanced age and poor nutrition are associated with reduced skeletal muscle mass. Contractility is influenced by the muscle's chemical environment. Derangements of Ca^{+2}, Mg^{+2}, PO_4^{-3}, K^+, CO_2, pH, and perhaps Fe^{+2} are particularly important to correct. The shorter the inspiratory muscle fiber and the greater its velocity of shortening, the less forceful will be the contrac-

tion for any specified level of neural stimulation. The greater the "afterload" faced by the muscle (due to resistive or elastic loading), the less effectively will muscle contraction perform useful external work. Achieving adequate intravascular volume ensuring optimal cardiac function and normalizing hemoglobin concentration help to maintain ample O_2 delivery to these metabolically active tissues.

Thoracic Configuration   However well individual muscle fibers contract, geometric alignment determines how effectively the force generated accomplishes ventilation. When totally flattened, for example, the diaphragm develops tension that tends to pull the ribs inward in an expiratory rather than inspiratory action (Fig. 25.4). Partially for this reason, acute hyperinflation represents an important impediment to effective ventilation.

Muscular Coordination   In generating negative intrathoracic pressure, the inspiratory muscles normally contract synchronously to either displace volume directly or to stabilize the rib cage or abdomen so that the inspiratory actions of complementary muscles work effectively together and are not offset by expiratory activity. Both a stable chest wall and coordinated muscular activity are essential to pump efficiency.

Common Pump Disorders

Chest Wall Configuration

Obesity and Ascites   Massive obesity and ascites are common disorders of chest wall configuration. The stiff chest wall and abdomen afterload the muscles of inspiration. However, although the diaphragm must push against the abdominal contents, impairing diaphragmatic descent, the abdomen can provide a fulcrum around which the diaphragm can flare the rib cage outward, expanding its volume. Thus, more extensive rib cage displacement may compensate for the reduced caudal displacement of the diaphragm, so that quiet breathing is little compromised. Under the stress of increased ventilation requirements, however, higher tidal volumes are needed, and the elastic work of breathing may increase dramatically. With the abdominal contents thrusting against the diaphragm, the equilibrium position of the chest wall is displaced to a lower volume, so that functional residual capacity (FRC) tends to fall. In comparison to patients without chest wall abnormality, higher levels of PEEP are needed to produce the physiologically effective changes in lung volume that influence oxygenation. This is especially true in the supine position, in which abdominal forces push the underside of the diaphragm cephalad. Airway calibers are reduced commensurately as FRC falls and resistance to breathing increases. Moreover, the tendencies for hypoxemia and positional desaturation are increased because the patient often tends to breathe below the "closing volume" of the lung. (This is particularly true in the setting of bronchitis or airway edema.) In managing the obese, pregnant, or ascitic patient, special attention must be paid to maintaining an upright position, which minimizes abdominal pressure, and to supplementing inspired O_2 when necessary.

Pleural Effusion and Pneumothorax Although massive pleural effusion and pneumothorax generally are not believed to be problems of chest wall configuration, in fact, both can cause dyspnea by this mechanism (see Chapter 8, Practical Problems and Complications of Mechanical Ventilation). For example, either may flatten or invert the ipsilateral diaphragm and drive the accessory inspiratory muscles to a hyperinflated position. In this configuration, the individual muscle fibers are foreshortened and the geometry does not permit efficient inspiratory motion. Thus, a major component of the relief of dyspnea after thoracentesis or chest tube placement relates to the recovery of an effective mechanical advantage for the diaphragm.

Flail Chest If large or painful, flail segments may dissipate a portion of the force developed by the intact ventilatory musculature or lead to "splinting", secretion retention, hypoxemia, and ineffective ventilation. Bronchial hygiene, analgesia, and ventilatory support form the cornerstones of treatment until the chest wall stabilizes and the pain recedes.

Kyphoscoliosis Kyphoscoliosis and ankylosing spondylitis seriously distort the other component of the thoracic shell, the rib cage. Both disorders seriously impair the inspiratory capacity, preventing the deep breaths needed for exertion or coughing. Functional residual capacity tends to be well preserved. Initially, the problem is purely one of configuration, but the inability to ventilate and clear secretions effectively from disadvantaged areas can lead to reduced lung compliance and hypoxemia later in the course. Difficulty increases in proportion to the bony deformity. In scoliosis, for example, serious respiratory problems attributable solely to its mechanical disadvantage are seldom evident until angulation ex-

ceeds 100°. Muscles that would ordinarily have an inspiratory action can be placed into a neutral or expiratory alignment by bony distortion. In addition, the chest cage becomes difficult to deform with tidal breathing efforts. Severe hypoxemia and cor pulmonale are frequent late complications. For such patients, maintaining the airway free of retained secretions and infection, treatment of hypoxemia, and ensuring appropriate electrolyte balance and nutrition are key to effective management.

Muscular Strength and Coordination Diaphragmatic paralysis and quadriplegia provide complementary opposing examples of regional muscular weakness. As such, both disorders present inherent problems of impaired muscular coordination as well as loss of effective muscle bulk and strength.

Diaphragm Certain events and acute problems observed in the ICU may result in diaphragmatic dysfunction: pneumonia, surgery, radiation, trauma, and anesthetic complications provide common examples. A paralyzed diaphragm tends to rise rather than fall during the inspiratory half-cycle. As a passive membrane, it moves in accordance with the transmural pressure gradient across it. As intra-abdominal pressure rises and intrathoracic pressure falls, the diaphragm tends to ascend into the chest. In the chronic setting, unilateral diaphragmatic paralysis only modestly impairs ventilatory capability, with vital capacity falling approximately 20 to 30% from its normal value. Quiet tidal breathing is little affected, and many such patients remain relatively asymptomatic throughout life. Symptoms only surface under periods of stress or in the presence of a comorbid problem. Although causes of permanent unilateral paralysis can sometimes be identified (e.g., tumor, infection, radiation, or surgery), the origin of most remains unknown.

By contrast, bilateral diaphragmatic paralysis is a devastating illness that usually is idiopathic. These patients must sustain the entire ventilatory burden using the accessory muscles. When upright, the expiratory muscles can contract to drive the diaphragm high into the chest at end exhalation. When expiratory tone is released, the falling abdominal pressure sucks the diaphragm caudally, thus aiding inspiration. In the supine position, this gravity-dependent mechanism cannot work, and the abdomen moves paradoxically inward during inspiration. Therefore, these patients experience extreme orthopnea and often present with sleep disturbances and headache related to nocturnal CO_2 accumulation. Vital capacity shows significant positional variation, falling by more than 30% in the transition from the upright to supine orientation. Many such patients can sustain ventilation for many hours when upright but need ventilatory support (invasively or noninvasively) for rest periods, especially during sleep. Although a positive-pressure ventilator is used most commonly for this purpose (with or without airway intubation), a negative-pressure body suit also can be employed, without the need for tracheostomy or facial mask. Poor regional ventilation in dependent areas, frequently combined with the need for tracheostomy, causes problems with atelectasis, pneumonitis, and bronchiectasis in basilar regions. Because diaphragmatic function seldom returns, treatment is supportive. Therapy centers on maintaining optimal secretion clearance, keeping the lungs free of infection, and optimizing nutrition.

Skeletal Muscle Weakness and Paralysis
The severity of ventilatory problems relating to spinal cord injury relates to the level of the lesion and, to some extent, to the time elapsed since the injury occurred. Ventilatory effectiveness can improve significantly in the weeks after the injury, as neural function improves, muscle tone alters the compliance of the chest wall, and any functional accessory muscles strengthen. In the usual forms of quadriplegia (levels at or below C_5), diaphragmatic function is well preserved. Unfortunately, some accessory inspiratory muscles may be compromised, and a variable fraction of expiratory power is routinely lost. Quadriplegic patients and those with acute myopathy often maintain excellent ventilation during quiet breathing but have little or no reserve. Expulsive activity may be severely impaired. For some patients, any pneumonia is potentially life threatening; secretions cannot be raised, and the ventilatory requirement is increased. Various techniques and devices are available to assist coughing, including manual compression, chest vibration, airway oscillation, and cough amplifiers that use a biphasic (positive–negative) pressure applied at the airway opening.

Paradoxically, some quadriplegic patients breathe more easily in the recumbent position than when upright. Presumably, the enhanced diaphragmatic curvature of the supine position, as well as the larger area of apposition of the diaphragm to the lower rib cage, improves mechanical efficiency. Like diaphragmatic paralysis, the focus should center on reducing the ventilatory requirement and on keeping the lungs free of infection. For patients who do not have an effective cough, secretion retention and mucus plugging is a continual risk. Vital measures are maintenance of optimal nutrition, prevention of aspiration, optimized bowel motility, prevention of abdominal distention, and prophylactic respiratory therapy, supplemented by assisted coughing (when feasible, indicated, and not contraindicated by abdominal distention, esophageal incompetence, severe thoracic deformity, spinal fracture, etc.). When some expiratory force can be generated (thoracic cord interruptions), abdominal compression may assist the coughing effort by splinting the abdomen and allowing intrathoracic pressure to build. Marginal patients often benefit from noninvasive nocturnal ventilatory support. Severely compromised patients who cannot effectively clear the airway with noninvasive aids or who have other airway, lung, or chest wall diseases will require tracheostomy and conventional ventilation.

KEY POINTS

1. Three major mechanisms cause or contribute to ventilatory failure: deficient central drive, ineffective muscular contraction, and excessive breathing workload. Important factors contributing to the minute ventilation requirement include levels of alertness, agitation, pain, body temperature, metabolic stress, ventilatory dead space fraction, nutritional status, and the work of breathing itself.

2. An investigation of the cause for ventilatory failure should include systematic evaluation of ventilatory drive, minute ventilation, the pressure required per liter of ventilation, and neuromuscular performance. Therapy to reverse ventilatory failure should be guided by knowledge of the underlying defect.

3. Signs and symptoms suggestive of upper airway obstruction include the following: inspiratory limitation of airflow; stridor; difficulty clearing airway secretions; altered voice or cough; marked accentuation of dyspnea by exertion or hyperventilation; and altered breathing symptoms with position changes or neck movements. Specialized pulmonary function testing (such as complete flow volume loops) help document upper airway obstruction.

4. The nonintubated patient with upper airway obstruction may benefit from maintaining the head-up position, breathing helium–oxygen mixtures, and receiving PEEP or CPAP. Glottic edema that occurs postextubation may respond to racemic epinephrine aerosols. Other key measures include decreasing pleural pressure swings by reducing minute ventilation requirements, relieving bronchospasm, and eliminating retained airway secretions.

5. An asthmatic attack may be triggered by a host of provocative stimuli that include the following: bronchial irritation, allergen inhalation, emotion, exercise, sinus drainage, gastroesophageal reflux, and pulmonary venous congestion.

6. Specific danger signs in asthma that warn of the need for urgent intubation include deteriorating mental status, a wide paradoxical pulse, severe hyperinflation, inability to talk in complete sentences, CO_2 retention, acidosis, and cyanosis.

7. Secretion plugging of the airways may be very widespread in status asthmaticus. Appropriate therapeutic interventions include β-adrenergic aerosols, corticosteroids, and mechanical ventilation. Magnesium sulfate, anticholinergic aerosols, theophylline derivatives, and vigorous respiratory therapy are of less certain benefit during the acute phase of support of asthma.

8. Many patients with COPD also have underlying heart disease that complicates their management. This may take the form of cor pulmonale or ischemic left ventricular disease. Atrial arrhythmias are unusually common and problematic for these patients. PEEP or CPAP often helps to offset auto-PEEP and improve triggering sensitivity, thereby decreasing the work of breathing. Respiratory therapy assumes a crucial role in the management of many such patients.

9. Only a minority of severely decompensated patients with COPD admitted to an ICU respond to noninvasive ventilation. Those that do are usually caught early. When ventilatory support is needed, care should be taken to avoid overventilating the patient and to maintain adequate nutrition.

10. For patients with neuromuscular diseases, derangements of calcium, magnesium, phosphate, potassium, and pH may impair respiratory muscle function. Other important causes are acute hyperinflation, derangements of thoracic configuration (obesity, pleural effusion or pneumothorax, kyphoscoliosis), and deficits in muscular strength and coordination (diaphragmatic weakness, quadriplegia).

11. Although isolated disorders of central ventilatory drive are quite uncommon causes of respiratory failure, they frequently serve as a background condition that leads to acute decompensation when the breathing workload increases or the muscular capability is impaired. Sedatives, sedating antidepressants, psychotropic agents, hypnotics, and opiates must be used very cautiously in elderly patients, patients with chronic sleep deprivation, and patients with subacute or chronic CO_2 retention.

SUGGESTED READINGS

1. Aboussouan L, Stoller J. Diagnosis and management of upper airway obstruction. Clin Chest Med 1994;15(1): 35–54.
2. Aubier M, Trippenbach T, Roussos C. Respiratory muscle fatigue during cardiogenic shock. J Appl Physiol 1981; 51:499–508.
3. Bach J. Respiratory muscle AIDS for the prevention of pulmonary morbidity and mortality. Semin Neurol 1995; 15(1):72–83.
4. Bach JR. Update and perspectives on noninvasive respiratory muscle AIDS. Part 1: the inspiratory AIDS. Chest 1994;105(4):1230–1240.
5. Bradley T, Phillipson E. Central sleep apnea. Clin Chest Med 1992;13(3):493–505.
6. Brochard L, Isabey D, Piquet J, et al. Reversal of acute exacerbations of chronic obstructive pulmonary disease by inspiratory assistance with a face mask. N Engl J Med 1990;323:1523–1530.
7. Brown L. Respiratory dysfunction in Parkinson's disease. Clin Chest Med 1994;15(4):715–728.
8. Cherniack N. The central nervous system and respiratory muscle coordination. Chest 1990;97(Suppl 3):52S–57S.
9. Corrado A, Gorini M, De Paola E. Alternative techniques for managing acute neuromuscular respiratory failure. Semin Neurol 1995;15(1):84–89.
10. Curtis J, Hudson L. Emergent assessment and management of acute respiratory failure in COPD. Clin Chest Med 1994;15(3):481–500.
11. Derenne J, Fleury B, Pariente R. Acute respiratory failure of chronic obstructive pulmonary disease. Am Rev Respir Dis 1988;138(4):1006–1033.
12. Epstein S. An overview of respiratory muscle function. Clin Chest Med 1994;15(4):619–640.
13. Goldstein R. Hypoventilation: neuromuscular and chest wall disorders. Clin Chest Med 1992;13(3):507–521.
14. Guilleminault C, Stoohs R, Quera-Salva MA. Sleep-related obstructive and nonobstructive apneas and neurologic disorders. Neurology 1992;42(7 Suppl 6):53–60.
15. Hotes L, Johnson J, Sicilian L. Long-term care, rehabilita-

tion, and legal and ethical considerations in the management of neuromuscular disease with respiratory dysfunction. Clin Chest Med 1994;15(4):783–795.

16. Hoyt J. Persistent paralysis in critically ill patients after the use of neuromuscular blocking agents. New Horizons 1994;2(1):48–55.

17. Kamp D. Physiologic evaluation of asthma. Chest 1992; 101(Suppl 6):396S–400S.

18. Kelly B, Luce J. The diagnosis and management of neuromuscular diseases causing respiratory failure. Chest 1991; 99(6):1485–1494.

19. Leatherman J. Life-threatening asthma. Clin Chest Med 1994;15(3):453–480.

20. Leatherman J. Mechanical ventilation in obstructive lung disease. Clin Chest Med 1996;17(3):577–590.

21. Leatherman J, Ravenscraft S. Low measured auto-positive end-expiratory pressure during mechanical ventilation of patients with severe asthma. Hidden auto-positive end-expiratory pressure. Crit Care Med 1996;24(3):541–546.

22. Lynn D, Woda R, Mendell J. Respiratory dysfunction in muscular dystrophy and other myopathies. Clin Chest Med 1994;15(4):661–674.

23. MacNee W. Pathophysiology of cor pulmonale in chronic obstructive pulmonary disease. Part 1. Am J Resp Crit Care Med 1994;150(3):833–852.

24. Marini JJ. Should PEEP be used in airflow obstruction? Am Rev Respir Dis 1989;140(1):1–3.

25. Marini JJ, Roussos C, eds. Ventilatory failure. Berlin: Springer-Verlag, 1991.

26. Martin RJ, ed. Clinics in chest medicine. Vol. 16. Philadelphia: WB Saunders, 1995.

27. Parsons P. Respiratory failure as a result of drugs, overdoses, and poisonings. Clin Chest Med 1994;15(1): 93–102.

28. Peruzzi W, Smith B. Bronchial hygiene therapy. Crit Care Clin 1995;11(1):79–96.

29. Polito A, Fessler H. Heliox in respiratory failure from obstructive lung disease. N Engl J Med 1995;332(3): 192–193.

30. Ranieri V, Giuliani R. Physiologic effects of positive end-expiratory pressure in patients with chronic obstructive pulmonary disease during acute ventilatory failure and controlled mechanical ventilation. Am Rev Respir Dis 1993;147(1):5–13.

31. Rochester D, Esau S. Assessment of ventilatory function in patients with neuromuscular disease. Clin Chest Med 1994;15(4):751–764.

32. Rossi A, Polese G, De Sandre G. Respiratory failure in chronic airflow obstruction: recent advances and therapeutic implications in the critically ill patient. Eur J Med 1992;1(6):349–357.

33. Rubini F, Rampulla C, Nava S. Acute effect of corticosteroids on respiratory mechanics in mechanically ventilated patients with chronic airflow obstruction and acute respiratory failure. Am J Resp Crit Care Med 1994;149(2 Pt 1):306–310.

34. Sassoon CS, Gruer SE. Characteristics of the ventilator pressure and flow-trigger variables. Intensive Care Med 1995;21(2):159–168.

35. Schmidt G, Hall J. Acute or chronic respiratory failure. Assessment and management of patients with COPD in the emergency setting. JAMA 1989;261(23):3444–3453.

36. Slack R, Shucart W. Respiratory dysfunction associated with traumatic injury to the central nervous system. Clin Chest Med 1994;15(4):739–750.

37. Strumpf DA, Millman RP, Hill NS. The management of chronic hypoventilation. Chest 1990;98(2):474–480.

38. Sugerman H. Pulmonary function in morbid obesity. Gastroenterol Clin North Am 1987;16(2):225–237.

39. Tobin MJ. Respiratory muscles in disease. Clin Chest Med 1988;9(2):263–286.

40. Tuxen DV, Williams TJ, Scheinkestel CD, et al. Use of a measurement of pulmonary hyperinflation to control the level of mechanical ventilation in patients with acute severe asthma. Am Rev Respir Dis 1992;146(5 Pt 1): 1136–1142.

41. Unterborn J, Hill N. Options for mechanical ventilation in neuromuscular diseases. Clin Chest Med 1994;15(4): 765–782.

42. Wiener C. Ventilatory management of respiratory failure in asthma. JAMA 1993;269(16):2128–2131.

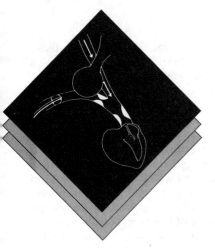

CHAPTER 26

Common ICU Infections

SUSPECTING INFECTION

Infection may be suspected on the basis of localizing signs (e.g., swelling, erythema, wound discharge) or localizing symptoms (e.g., pain, dyspnea, cough) but most commonly is questioned because of the presence of a generalized phenomenon, such as fever or leukocytosis. Fever afflicts at least half of all patients during their stay in the intensive care unit (ICU) and usually is an important clue to the presence of infection. The magnitude and pattern of fever, typically defined as a temperature exceeding 101 to 101.4°F, has been attributed undue significance; unfortunately, fever characteristics have little diagnostic significance. It is essential to recognize that not all fever is due to infection. Several diseases just as deadly as disseminated infection can induce fever, among them neuroleptic malignant syndrome, malignant hyperthermia, and the endocrine disorders of hyperthyroidism, adrenal insufficiency, and pheochromocytoma. Noninfectious causes of febrile syndromes are discussed in detail in Chapter 28 (Thermal Disorders).

For some patients, diagnosis of infection is more difficult because both localizing and generalized signs are unimpressive. Patients infected with human immunodeficiency virus (HIV) often have minimal tissue inflammation when infected. Elderly patients often have reduced fever responses compared to younger patients. Both neutropenia and immunosuppressive drug therapy tend to reduce the local response to infection, making erythema, pain, swelling, and pus formation less likely.

COMMON SCENARIOS

Three categories account for most infections seen in the ICU: primary bacterial infections that prompt admission (e.g., meningitis, pneumonia, urinary tract infection); nosocomial infections (e.g., catheter-related sepsis, nosocomial pneumonia); and infections of the immune-compromised host. The broad and important topic of infection cannot be addressed comprehensively herein; therefore, we have focused the discussion on the most common and serious infections occurring in the ICU. Perhaps more than with any other problem, therapy of infection must be individualized. Patient characteristics profoundly influence the likely site of infection and pathogens. The selection of antimicrobials must be tailored to individual patient allergies and organ dysfunctions. Furthermore, individual hospitals have vastly different spectra of bacteria causing a particular clinical syndrome and even within a hospital antibiotic susceptibility can vary widely by ICU. Therefore, practitioners must have a thorough knowledge of the patient being treated and the susceptibility pattern of the hospital in which they practice.

Antimicrobial use is constantly evolving and the staggeringly large number of antibiotic choices available can be intimidating. Because of the selection now available, there is almost always more than one potentially effective antimicrobial combination for any given infection, and few situations exist in which selections are dogmatic. Suggestions for antibiotic therapy made in the following section are based on the most common pathogens and their usual susceptibility patterns while considering the frequency and severity of side effects and ease and cost of administration. Currently, we have both the luxury and liability of many "broad-spectrum" antibiotic choices. The luxury of covering a large number of potential pathogens comes at a high price. Many practitioners have grown accustomed to one "set" of antibiotics and now lack the knowledge needed to cope with unique pathogens or patient characteristics. Indiscriminate use of broad-spectrum antibiotics is rapidly producing multidrug-resistant bacteria. Methicillin-resistant *Staphylococci* and penicillin-resistant *Pneumococci* were rare or unheard of when the first edition of this book was written but are now epidemic. New and menacing pathogens such as vancomycin-resistant *enterococci* have been recognized and, unless patterns of antibiotic use change, it is likely such infections will grow in importance. Caution must be used in the selection of antibiotics as these are the only class of drugs that, when misused, can injure not only the patient being treated but also may injure nearby patients and patients to be admitted to the ICU in the future. For example, the routine use of vancomycin to treat all cases of diarrhea in the ICU is one potential method of "selecting out" vancomycin-resistant organisms. These highly resistant organisms then reside in the ICU environment, ready to infect subsequent patients.

URINARY TRACT INFECTIONS

CAUSES

The urinary tract is the most common site of ICU infection, accounting for almost 40% of all documented infections. Although urinary tract infections (UTIs) usually are inconsequential, the mortality rate for a bacteremic urinary infection approaches 30%. Risk factors for bacterial UTI include presence of a urinary catheter, female gender, diabetes, and advanced age. Colonization of urinary catheters occurs at a rate of about 5 to 10% per day, and most ICU-acquired UTIs occur in such colonized patients. Presumably, the colonized catheter permits retrograde passage of pathogenic bacteria into the bladder, where bacteria adhere and proliferate. Urinary catheter composition (Teflon rather than rubber) may reduce the infective risk; however, there is no evidence that changing the catheter or external application of antibiotic ointment decreases risk. Critical factors

in preventing nosocomial UTI are sterile catheter insertion, early catheter removal, and use of a closed drainage system.

DIAGNOSIS

The diagnosis of UTI is all but certain when more than 10^5 bacteria/mL are isolated from culture of freshly collected urine. This level of bacteriuria correlates well with presence of more than one organism per high-power field of unspun urine. Unfortunately, fewer bacteria do not exclude the presence of infection, they only make it less likely. True infections have been documented with colony counts as low as 10^2/mL. *Escherichia coli,* the most common bacterial isolate, occurs in about 30% of UTIs. *Enterococci* and *Pseudomonas* are each recovered about 15% of the time in the ICU population. *Klebsiella* and *Proteus* species represent less common isolates. Contrary to previous teaching, in many cases, pure cultures of *Staphylococcus epidermidis* represent infection, not contamination. The clinical problem of *Candida* in urine is addressed separately (below). In the absence of frank pyuria or quantitative culture data, it is difficult to differentiate colonization from infection in critically ill patients with indwelling catheters. In the tenuous patient with bacteriuria, it is probably best to err on the side of brief, organism-directed antibiotic therapy. For more resilient patients in the ICU, treatment of asymptomatic bacteriuria may be deferred safely.

Pyocystis, an invasive infection of the bladder wall, may complicate oliguria or anuria, especially for patients requiring hemodialysis. In this setting, reduced urine flow allows bacteria to proliferate to massive numbers in the bladder. For oliguric patients with obscure fever, the bladder should be catheterized and the urine sediment should be examined. Murky, turbid, culture-positive urine establishes the diagnosis.

Recovery of *Candida* species in urine is a common event that often produces great consternation. The choice of therapy for isolated *Candiduria* should be based on a clinical judgment regarding whether the patient is "colonized" or "infected." Unfortunately, there are few reliable signs to distinguish these conditions. A clinical picture of sepsis, with recovery of *Candida* from blood cultures as well as urine is indicative of disseminated infection that should be treated with intravenous amphotericin B. Conversely, finding small numbers of yeast in an asymptomatic patient with an indwelling urinary catheter rarely requires treatment (except expedited removal of the catheter). The most difficult situation occurs when large numbers of yeast or clumps of hyphal forms are found in the urine of an asymptomatic patient or a patient with only modest fever. Although suggestive of invasive infection, such patients usually respond promptly to fluconazole (oral or intravenous), especially if the urinary catheter can be removed. In this setting, parenteral amphotericin B probably should be reserved for immunocompromised patients or those with limited physiologic reserves. Although widely used, bladder irrigation with an amphotericin B solution is time consuming, expensive, of uncertain benefit, and confounding to accurate assessment of urine output. Luckily, the availability of fluconazole has made bladder irrigation unnecessary.

TREATMENT

The aggressiveness of therapy should parallel the clinical severity of the acute syndrome and the underlying illness of the patient. As a rule, presumed UTIs should be treated aggressively because patients in the ICU often have impaired immunity (diabetes, HIV infection, immunosuppressive therapy); numerous indwelling devices (e.g., vascular catheters, prosthetic heart valves, pacemakers); and marginal physiologic reserves.

The treatment of UTI includes the promotion of urinary flow and drainage, removal of urinary catheters (when feasible), and antibiotic therapy. Not all patients with bacteriuria require prolonged courses of expensive, broad-spectrum, intravenous antibiotics. Otherwise stable, immunocompetent patients, capable of eating or tolerating enteral nutrition, can be treated successfully using enteral antibiotics (e.g., ampicillin, trimethoprim-sulfa, quinolones). Oral therapy is not appropriate for septic patients or patients with obstructive uropathy or a focal complication (e.g., renal abscess). In seriously ill patients, an intravenous aminoglycoside plus an antipseudomonal penicillin or third-generation cephalosporin should be administered. Cephalothin or vancomycin may be substituted in penicillin-allergic patients. If *Enterococci* or *Staphylococci* are deemed likely based on examination of the urine, vancomycin probably should be first-line therapy. Urine concentrations of renally excreted antibiotics often are dramatically higher than those used in *in vitro* (Kirby-Bauer) sensitivity testing; therefore, urinary infections often can be cured using an antibiotic to which the bacteria are found to be ''resis-

tant.'' Because drainage bags provide important reservoirs for urinary pathogens, manipulations of the closed drainage system should be undertaken, only when necessary and conducted with appropriate sterile precautions. Furthermore, drainage bags should not be raised above the level of the bladder. Doing so, even briefly, as often occurs during patient transport, produces urinary stasis and retrograde flow of potentially highly contaminated urine.

PNEUMONIA

PATHOGENESIS

Pneumonia-producing organisms usually enter the lower respiratory tract in aspirated upper airway secretions or through inhalation of infective aerosols. Hematogenous seeding is a less common mechanism. Unless the inoculum is very large, glottic closure, cough, and mucociliary clearance normally provide an effective mechanical defense (Table 26.1). Even when mechanical barriers fail, infection usually is averted by effective cellular (neutrophil and macrophage) and humoral immunity (antibody secretion). Unfortunately, both mechanical and immune defenses are jeopardized commonly in critically ill patients, even those without a recognizable immune deficiency. Common conditions that allow proliferation of organisms leading to pneumonia are listed in Table 26.2. The organism causing pneumonia in a given patient is highly dependent on where the infection was acquired and on individual patient characteristics.

DIAGNOSIS

In the community, a patient with acute onset of fever, dyspnea, and cough productive of purulent

TABLE 26–1

CONDITIONS PROMOTING LUNG INOCULATION

Aspiration
    Depressed consciousness
    Swallowing disorders
    Nasogastric and tracheal tubes

Hematogenous
    Bacteremia

Infected aerosol
    Contaminated ventilator tubing and humidifiers

TABLE 26–2

CONDITIONS ALLOWING PROLIFERATION OF MICROORGANISMS IN LUNG

Impaired immunity

Parenchymal necrosis

Malnutrition

Steroids/cytotoxic drugs

Alcohol

Diabetes

Secretion retention

Atelectasis

Smoking

Obstructive lung disease

Neuromuscular weakness

Cytotoxic drugs

Acute respiratory distress syndrome

Viral infections

---

sputum is likely to be suffering from bacterial pneumonia. Leukocytosis with a predominance of neutrophils and distinct (new) infiltrate(s) on chest radiograph are strong supporting data. The predominance of a single morphologic bacterial form on Gram's stain of sputum demonstrating an overwhelming predominance of neutrophils further bolsters the case. Finally, the diagnosis is established unequivocally by recovering the same organism from blood and sputum cultures. The presentation is seldom so classic, even with community-acquired pneumonia: fever may be mild, infiltrates may be subtle, and self-medication with antibiotics often obscures a bacteriologic diagnosis.

In the ICU, making a correct clinical diagnosis of pneumonia can be even more difficult. Diagnosis of nosocomial ICU pneumonia is difficult for several reasons. Fever and leukocytosis are nonspecific, and patients often have several potential nonpulmonary sites to explain these findings. In addition, the chest radiograph is rarely diagnostic, because infiltrates of pneumonia are mimicked by atelectasis, aspiration pneumonitis, pulmonary infarction, pleural effusion, and pulmonary edema. Finally, widespread use of antibiotics inhibits the ability to recover a single pathogenic organism and, even when sputum cultures are positive, small numbers of numerous colonizing bacteria usually are the yield.

Causative Organism

The causative organism of pneumonia differs dramatically when comparing pneumonia ac-

quired in the community to that acquired in the hospital. Common causes of community-acquired pneumonia and their clinical associations are shown in Table 26.3. In the community, *Streptococci*, especially *Pneumococci, Haemophilus influenzae, Mycoplasma*, and a variety of viruses are the most common pathogens in otherwise "healthy" adults. Many underlying conditions vary this spectrum, however. In addition to the organisms listed above, patients with alcoholism, diabetes, or heart failure are prone to infection with *Klebsiella, Legionella*, enteric gram-negative rods, and less commonly, *Staphylococci*. When aspiration is a potential etiologic factor (e.g., alcoholism, drug abuse, esophageal disorders), *Bacteroides* and other anaerobes become

TABLE 26–3

CLINICAL ASSOCIATIONS IN COMMUNITY-ACQUIRED PNEUMONIA

Patient Characteristics	Likely Organisms
Healthy young adult	*Streptococcus pneumoniae, Mycoplasma*, Viruses, Chlamydia
Healthy adult	*S. pneumoniae, Haemophilus influenzae, Mycoplasma*
Prone to aspiration Stroke Esophageal disease Alcoholism Seizures Alcohol abuse Recent dental work	*S. pneumoniae, Bacteroides*, oral anaerobes
Chronically ill Diabetes COPD Alcoholism Heart failure Low-dose corticosteroids	All organisms listed for healthy adult plus *Klebsiella* spp., enteric gram-negatives, Legionella, *Staphylococcus aureus, Branhamella* spp.
Postinfluenza	*Streptococcus pneumoniae, Staphylococcus aureus, H. influenzae*
Cystic fibrosis	*S. aureus, Pseudomonas* spp.
AIDS or HIV with CD4 < 200	*Pneumocystis carinii, S. pneumoniae, H. influenzae, Mycobacterium tuberculosis*, fungal infection (geographic predilection)
Neutropenia	All organisms listed for chronically ill plus *Aspergillus, Mucor*, and *Candida*.

more likely. *Staphylococcus aureus* frequently is recovered from patients with ''post-influenza'' pneumonia and *Pseudomonas* species, and *Staphylococci* are common etiologic organisms among patients with cystic fibrosis.

In the ICU, a different, hospital-specific spectrum predominates. Gram-negative rods (*Pseudomonas aeruginosa, Klebsiella* species, *Enterobacter* species, *Escherichia coli, Proteus,* and *Serratia*) cause approximately 50% of all ICU pneumonias. Which gram-negative organism predominates at a given hospital has a great deal to do with antibiotic pressure placed on the environment. *Staphylococcus aureus* causes another 10 to 15% of infections. The predominance of gram-negative rods and *Staphylococci* seen in the hospitalized patient is explained partially by the rapid rate at which the oropharynx of the critically ill patient is colonized. Almost all critically ill patients are colonized with nonnative gram-negative bacteria (many of which are antibiotic resistant) by the third hospital day.

All too often in the ICU, a specific pathogen cannot be identified, despite good sampling methods and symptomatology compatible with acute pneumonia. Mixed aerobic/anaerobic infection, *Mycoplasma, Chlamydia, Legionella,* and viral agents become more likely candidates under these conditions. Fungal pneumonia (*Candida, Aspergillus,* or *Mucor*) is common for the neutropenic patient (<500 neutrophils/mm^3) but is very unusual for the immunocompetent patient. When fungal pneumonia is diagnosed in the immunocompetent patient, it usually is the result of hematogenous seeding with candida.

Patients infected with HIV present a unique set of problems. When the CD4 T-cell counts are normal, patients infected with HIV are susceptible to the same organisms as any other adult in the risk categories outlined in Table 26.3. As the CD4 count declines, and especially as it falls below 200 cells/mm^3, the spectra of infecting organisms change somewhat. Although routine bacterial pathogens still predominate, *Pneumocystis carinii, Mycobacterium tuberculosis,* atypical mycobacteria, and fungal infections become more likely. There is a rough correlation between the CD4 count and the infecting organism, but the linkage is not sufficiently strong to forgo clinical evaluation for presumptive diagnosis. Potential pathogens also are influenced by the use of prophylactic therapy (e.g., oral trimethoprim-sulfa or aerosolized pentamidine).

Regardless of the patient substrate, the choice of initial therapy for a bacterial pneumonia is always accompanied by some uncertainty, even in the presence of a Gram's stain ''typical'' of a specific organism. Historical features can help immensely in sorting through the diagnostic possibilities of community-acquired pneumonia. For example, the sudden onset of chills, pleurisy, rigors, and high temperature are characteristic features for *pneumococcus* in a young adult. On the other hand, these findings may be inconspicuous in an older person, in whom confusion or stupor often predominate. A history of seizures, drug abuse, alcoholism, or swallowing disorder focuses attention on the possibility of aspiration. Recent travel history, occupational or recreational exposure, and concurrent family illnesses can help diagnose of an unusual organism (Table 26.4). A pulse rate that fails to rise in proportion to fever (pulse–temperature dissociation) suggests an ''intracellular pathogen'' such as *Legionella, Mycoplasma,* Q fever, psittacosis, or tularemia. *Mycoplasma* often causes pharyngitis, myringitis, or conjunctivitis. Contrary to popular teaching, extrapulmonary symptoms (diarrhea, central nervous system disease) are no more common in Legionnaires' disease than in other bacterial pneumonia.

Unlike community-acquired pneumonia, nosocomial pneumonia offers few historical clues to diagnosis. Occasionally, however, a skin rash, gingival disease, or purulent sinus drainage help narrow the possibilities. Numerous classic roent-

TABLE 26–4

CLUES TO UNUSUAL CAUSES OF PNEUMONIA

Diagnosis	Historical Clue
Histoplasmosis	Excavation, bird exposure, Ohio Valley Travel
Coccidiomycosis	Travel to southwestern United States
Tularemia	Tick bite or exposure to skinned animals
Brucellosis	Slaughterhouse work
Psittacosis	Exposure to pet birds
Q fever	Sheep contact
Varicella	Family exposure
Measles	Family exposure
Respiratory syncytial virus	Family exposure
Blastomycosis	Hunting, deep woods exposure
Erlichiosis	Tick bite

genographic features have been described, including lobar consolidation without air bronchograms (central obstruction), bulging fissures (*Klebsiella*), infiltrate with ipsilateral hilar adenopathy (*Histoplasmosis,* tularemia, tuberculosis), widespread cavitation (*Staphylococcus, Aspergillus*), and sequential progression to multilobar involvement (*Legionella*). These findings are not sufficiently consistent, however, to be of real value in confirming the diagnosis. For example, virtually any pneumonic infiltrate can imitate cavitation or pneumatocele formation in a patient with emphysematous bullae.

DIAGNOSIS

Although the history provides clues to the etiologic organism, laboratory studies are the cornerstone of the diagnostic workup. Leukopenia, an ominous prognostic sign, often results from overwhelming infections, particularly those due to *Staphylococcus, Pneumococcus,* or gram-negative organisms. A differential count that is not significantly left-shifted suggests the possibility of virus, *Mycoplasma,* or *Legionella.* Cultures of blood and pleural fluid (when present) must be obtained and, if positive, are the most convincing evidence of a causative organism. Unfortunately, such specimens are usually nondiagnostic, even in seriously ill patients, and sampling of pulmonary secretions becomes the primary diagnostic modality.

The aggressiveness of the diagnostic evaluation should parallel the severity of the illness. In an otherwise healthy young person with a lobar pneumonia and good oxygenation, empiric therapy or treatment based on Gram's stain alone is acceptable. For the septic, profoundly hypoxemic, or immunocompromised patient, however, a more systematic evaluation is often prudent. When performed correctly, stain and culture of pulmonary secretions remain the most likely techniques to yield a diagnosis. For patients with severe community acquired pneumonia, the best quality sputum often is obtained immediately after endotracheal intubation when forceful coughing and suctioning yields large quantities of lung secretions not yet contaminated by ICU colonization. Expectorated sputum is appropriate for analysis and culture only if there is a high ratio of inflammatory to epithelial cells. Apart from the Gram's stain, direct immunofluorescent antibody staining for *Legionella* and tuberculosis are other useful methods for processing the expectorated sample

that can yield an immediate, but presumptive, diagnosis. Inhalation of a nonisotonic aerosol, particularly if given via an ultrasonic nebulizer, can stimulate a productive cough in patients otherwise unable or unwilling to expectorate. When adequate sputum cannot be obtained, nasotracheal suctioning can be helpful. Transtracheal aspiration has been all but abandoned with wide availability of fiberoptic bronchoscopy.

Properly performed on selected patients, fiberoptic bronchoscopy is a valuable technique for evaluation of pneumonic infection. In general, bronchoscopic procedures should be reserved for those who are seriously ill, immunocompromised, or unresponsive to conventional therapy. When a decision is made to perform bronchoscopy, bronchoalveolar lavage and protected brush sampling are both reasonable and probably complementary procedures. When more than 10^3 to 10^4 organisms/mL are isolated, infection with the recovered organism is likely. Fewer bacteria are suggestive of a possible diagnosis of pneumonia, but also may be seen with a partially treated bacterial pneumonia. Performing transbronchial biopsies on mechanically ventilated patients is not done commonly because of the perceived risk of pneumothorax but is probably worth a try if the only diagnostic alternative is open or thoracoscopic lung biopsy. In this situation, the risks of developing a pneumothorax while on the mechanical ventilator must be balanced against the potential yield and the clinician's ability to promptly recognize and correct the pneumothorax. (Important: the incidence of pneumothorax is 100% after open lung biopsy.) In addition, there are situations in which a diagnosis can be made only by tissue biopsy. Transthoracic needle aspiration often yields an adequate specimen but exposes the patient to attendant risks of pneumothorax and bleeding. Open lung biopsy is rarely necessary for patients with intact host defenses.

The optimal diagnostic evaluation of a pneumonic process for patients infected with HIV is evolving and varies greatly by institution and practitioner. For patients with normal or minimally reduced CD4 counts, mild to moderate illness and a history and physical examination compatible with acute bacterial pneumonia, empiric antibacterial therapy after obtaining cultures is reasonable. For patients with reduced CD4 counts, progressive dyspnea, nonproductive cough, elevated lactic dehydrogenase (LDH), and a radiograph with a interstitial or ground glass pattern, empiric therapy for *Pneumocystis* and close observation may be reasonable. (This is especially true for patients not receiving *Pneumocystis* prophylaxis.) For patients with low CD4 counts, severe hypoxemia, uncharacteristic CXR infiltrates, or an unusual exposure history, early bronchoscopy is the most prudent option. When bronchoscopy is performed, bronchoalveolar lavage alone is often not sufficient; fungal infections, tuberculosis, and *Pneumocystis* are all missed at an unacceptable rate without transbronchial biopsy. Because of the wide variety of potential radiographic presentations of tuberculosis, it probably is wise for all patients with HIV and abnormal chest radiographs to be placed in respiratory isolation until a diagnosis of tuberculosis can be excluded reasonably.

TREATMENT

Nutrition, fluid, electrolyte, and oxygen support of the patient with bacterial pneumonia are noncontroversial and applied universally. The initial choice of antibiotic(s) must be guided not only by the nature of the suspected organism but also by the severity of the illness and underlying patient factors. Thus, although treatment should be directed as specifically as possible for patients who are only moderately ill, the initial therapy of a compromised patient with serious illness should include "broad-spectrum" coverage. There is little margin for error for critically ill patients with pneumonia; however, one can never cover all potential pathogens. Holes in coverage always exist, and there is almost always more than one acceptable combination of antibiotics. The selection of antibiotic therapy represents a calculated bet against the most likely organisms.

Recognizing the imprecision in the following descriptions, otherwise healthy patients with community-acquired pneumonia caused by an unknown organism who exhibit little systemic toxicity can be treated safely with ampicillin or erythromycin alone usually given orally. If the same patient seems toxic, reasonable initial treatments include any of the following combinations: ampicillin plus ofloxocin; a third-generation cephalosporin; or extended-spectrum penicillin plus erythromycin or doxycycline. The following caveats apply: if postinfluenza pneumonia is suspected or if the patient is from a geographic region with a high prevalence of penicillin-resistant *pneumococci,* the addition or substitution of vancomycin should be considered. For patients with a high likelihood of aspiration, clindamycin plus

an aminoglycoside represent a good initial choice. Community-acquired pneumonia in a patient with HIV is discussed above.

Because a second chance to institute the correct therapy cannot be guaranteed, broad empiric coverage is necessary for the toxic patient with nosocomial pneumonia. Coverage in this situation must include enteric gram-negative rods (including multiply resistant organisms), *Streptococci* (including penicillin-resistant organisms), *Staphylococci* (including MRSA). Regardless of the appearance of the Gram's stain, empiric therapy for critically ill patients should include an extended-spectrum penicillin plus an aminoglycoside or a third-generation cephalosporin plus an aminoglycoside. In addition, serious consideration should be given to the addition of vancomycin. (Vancomycin also can be used to cover essentially all forms of gram-positive aerobic infection in penicillin-allergic patients.) Erythromycin or doxycycline should be added if there is an "atypical" clinical or radiographic presentation or if fever persists despite usual therapy. Patients who are likely to contract *Staphylococcal* infection (e.g., recent influenza, neutropenia, or a suggestive sputum Gram's stain) should receive an anti-*Staphylococcal* penicillin or vancomycin. Recently, methicillin-resistant *Staphylococci* have surfaced as important pathogens in many institutions. In such hospitals, vancomycin represents first-line coverage.

Because highly resistant bacteria can be transferred between patients in the ICU, measures to decrease cross-contamination are essential. Careful hand washing between patient contacts dramatically decreases the risk of nosocomial infection. Use of latex gloves does not diminish the need for hand washing. Whenever suctioning intubated patients, gloves should be worn on both hands to prevent staff acquisition of herpetic infections and transfer of pathogenic bacteria. It is essential, however, that these gloves be removed before contacting another patient.

One pneumonic infection that deserves special discussion is pulmonary tuberculosis. Although patients may be admitted to the ICU with signs and symptoms typical of pulmonary tuberculosis (cavitary apical infiltrates, cachexia, fever), the presentation often is much more subtle. Tuberculosis in the ICU can take on almost any clinical or radiographic presentation. Cavitary lung disease is only marginally more common than the "miliary pattern" of punctate interstitial infiltrates, lobar pneumonia, "empyema," lung nodule, or diffuse bilateral infiltrate compatible with acute respiratory distress syndrome (ARDS). For every patient with respiratory failure due to infection who is admitted to the ICU, especially if infected with HIV, the diagnosis of tuberculosis should be considered. When the suspicion of tuberculosis is high, respiratory isolation should be instituted as quickly as possible and maintained until evidence suggests that the likelihood of contagion is low. (This is accomplished simply by examining two or more good-quality sputum smears for acid-fast organisms.) The implications of missing a case of tuberculosis are enormous: potential death or disability of the infected patient and transmission of infection to the staff and other nearby immunocompromised patients.

EMPYEMA AND PARAPNEUMONIC EFFUSIONS

DEFINITION

Small amounts of pleural fluid routinely accumulate adjacent to pneumonias and such collections are termed ''parapneumonic effusions.'' Most parapneumonic effusions are transudative in nature (protein < 3.5 gm/dL or 50% of the serum level; LDH < 200 U/dL or 60% of the serum level) and self-limited. The term ''complicated parapneumonic effusion'' has been applied to juxtapneumonic effusions, the characteristics of which fall somewhere between a transudate and an empyema. Usually exudative by protein and LDH criteria, leukocyte counts usually are less than 20,000/mm^3, and glucose levels fall between the serum value and 20 mg/dL. The pH of such effusions has received great attention and has been attributed undue significance. Although it is true that the lower the pH, the more likely a pleural effusion is to have characteristics of an empyema (see below), the pH alone neither makes the diagnosis of an empyema nor dictates therapy. Effusions with a pH less than 7.0 (with a normal arterial pH) are likely to be empyemas and likely to require tube thoracostomy, but such conclusions are not always true. An acidotic, thin, clear, or slightly cloudy sterile fluid does not necessarily require tube thoracostomy, whereas a thick, viscous, protein- and leukocyte-rich effusion would require thoracostomy, regardless of fluid pH.

Empyema is defined literally as ''pus'' in the pleural space, but unfortunately, physicians vary widely in their definition of ''pus.'' The diagnosis of empyema is not made by laboratory testing,

and there are no specific laboratory cutoffs for what constitutes an empyema. Not all empyemas grow bacteria in culture, and many do not even have visible microorganisms present on Gram's stain examination. If infected with bacteria, especially anaerobic bacteria, the odor of an empyema is memorable. Generally accepted characteristics of an empyema are grossly cloudy or opaque appearance and thick, viscous character due to high levels of protein and leukocytes. Certainly, not all infected pleural fluids are thick. Yet, it is the physical characteristics of the fluid that make empyema important to diagnose and treat appropriately. Unless grossly infected effusions that can be managed successfully with thoracentesis (thin, free-flowing fluid) and antibiotic therapy alone do not require chest tube drainage. Recent data suggest that intrapleural streptokinase can dramatically reduce the need for pleural decortication if used early in the clinical course. Amazingly, intrapleural streptokinase is associated with a low risk of either allergic reaction or coagulation disorder. The large number of leukocytes in empyema fluids suggests that DNAase might also be useful. Several types of pleural effusions can mimic an empyema: chylothorax, rheumatoid effusion, tuberculous effusion, and resolving hemothorax all can have the thick, turbid appearance characteristic of empyema.

The clinical presentation of empyema can be subtle. The diagnosis should be suspected in patients with unresolving or hectic fever and pleural effusions that do not improve with antibiotic therapy. Empyema becomes more likely if the suspect fluid collection is adjacent to a pneumonia. Because ICU chest films are often taken supine or semiupright, the classic ''layering'' of an effusion can be missed. Decubitus views, ultrasound, or CT enhance the likelihood of finding an empyema, especially a small or loculated one. For febrile or frankly septic patients, especially those with an underlying pneumonia, the search for an empyema is reasonable.

THERAPY

Four basic principles apply to treating empyema: early diagnosis, reversal of underlying problems, appropriate antibiotic therapy, and thorough drainage. Of these, drainage is most important. Because there are no radiographic or physical examination features to distinguish an empyema from a routine pleural effusion, thoracentesis is required. Early diagnosis reduces the early complications (sepsis and respiratory failure) and the late complication (fibrothorax). When turbid, viscous, pleural fluid (especially if foul smelling) is obtained at thoracentesis, cultures for aerobic and anaerobic bacteria, tuberculosis, and fungi should be sent. In addition to routine cell counts and chemistry analysis, it is prudent to obtain triglyceride and cholesterol levels to exclude a diagnosis of chylothorax, which can have an empyema-like appearance. (Effusions due to rheumatoid disease also can have a similar appearance.) The pleural fluid should be Gram's-stained to search for microbes and sputum and blood cultures should be obtained. Antibiotic coverage should be chosen initially on the basis of the Gram's stain and then fine-tuned by culture results. The usual etiologic suspects for pneumonia also cause empyema (*Streptococcus pneumoniae, Haemophilus influenzae,* anaerobic mouth flora, *Bacteroides*); however, *Staphylococci* also are frequent causes.

Prompt insertion of large-bore thoracostomy tubes sufficient to completely drain the pleural space usually is appropriate. Several tubes often are necessary because of the multiloculated nature of the effusions. Chest CT guidance can be invaluable in guiding placement of these tubes. Effusions that do not resolve with antibiotics and tube thoracostomy may require exploration and drainage at thoracotomy. Failure to resolve the acute process satisfactorily can require late pleural stripping or decortication.

INTRAVASCULAR CATHETER-RELATED INFECTIONS

INCIDENCE

Intravascular catheter-related infections remain one of the top three causes of nosocomial sepsis, in some series affecting as many as 20% of ICU occupants. Despite the use of antibiotics and a much greater understanding of the mechanisms of catheter-related infections, the case fatality rate for catheter-associated bacteremia remains between 10 and 20%.

MECHANISMS

Three basic mechanisms can produce catheter-related infections. (*a*) Most commonly, catheters are colonized at the skin–air interface, after which bacteria migrate toward the patient along the outer surface of the catheter. Subcutaneous and eventual intravascular migration results in local infec-tion, if bacterial growth is controlled by host defense or antibiotic therapy, or bacteremia, if bacterial growth is uncontrolled. (*b*) Catheters also can become colonized by exposure to circulating microorganisms introduced into the circulation at a distant site. As foreign bodies, catheters routinely incite surrounding thrombosis, forming a "fibrin sheath" around the catheter in the vessel lumen. This microenvironment is a stagnant, fertile environment for pathogen growth. Sources of bacteria or fungi far distant from the catheter (e.g., peritoneal or urinary tract infection) can seed these indwelling lines. (*c*) Much less commonly, catheter-related infections are due to the infusion of a contaminated intravenous fluid or drug. Although, in theory, such infusate contamination can occur with any drug, the problem has been reported most commonly with parenteral nutrition solutions and propofol, an intravenous sedative/anesthetic with a lipid vehicle.

RISK FACTORS

Risk factors for catheter-related infection can be divided roughly into two groups: patient factors that are often uncontrollable, and physician and environmental factors that can be altered. Recognized patient characteristics for those at particular risk for catheter-related infection include diabetes mellitus, immunosuppressive therapy (especially neutropenia) and immune deficiency diseases, skin diseases at the insertion site, and presence of sepsis from a distinct source.

Physician and environmental factors increasing the risk of intravascular catheter infection include: (*a*) catheter placement under emergency or nonsterile conditions; (*b*) insertion of large or multilumen catheters; (*c*) catheterization of a central vein; (*d*) prolonged catheterization at a single site; (*e*) placement by surgical cutdown; and (*f*) inexperience of the operator. Most catheter infections can be prevented by using sterile technique when inserting, dressing, changing, and reconnecting catheters and by minimizing the frequency of catheter entry. Although unproven to reduce the risk of infection, use of surgical gowns, caps, and masks is widely recommended, inexpensive, and therefore a reasonable practice for elective insertions. For unclear reasons, inexperience with catheter insertion is a powerful predictor of infection. It is not clear whether catheters become contaminated during insertion or if less experienced operators are prone to produce more tissue trauma during the insertion process. Multilumen catheters or catheters entered repeatedly (even for antibiotic administration) seem to have a higher infection rate. Neither antibiotic ointment applied at the catheter entry site nor systemic antibiotics convincingly decrease the risk of bacteremia. Data regarding the risk of infection in relation to the site of catheterization are confusing and contradictory. No clear data indicate that the internal jugular or femoral sites are at high risk for infection when the duration of catheterization is controlled. Although the risk of pneumothorax is averted, the femoral approach limits leg movement, predisposes deep venous thrombosis, and places the catheter in a region prone to contamination by urine and stool. In general, central venous catheters are more likely to become infected than peripheral catheters (possibly by virtue of the duration of catheterization). Pulmonary artery monitoring catheters and multilumen catheters (risk, 10–20%) are more likely to be infected than single-lumen catheters (risk, approximately 5%). Interestingly, venous catheters are more likely to be infected than arterial catheters. Whether this differential risk is related to the shorter duration of arterial catheterization, the greater flow of blood in the artery, or the site of placement (usually in the radial artery) is unclear. Hypertonic fluids (peripheral total parenteral nutrition [TPN]) or highly caustic drugs (e.g., amphotericin, diazepam, methicillin, erythromycin) may induce a chemical phlebitis, facilitating bacterial superinfection.

To minimize the risk of infection, intravenous sites should be monitored daily and connecting tubing should be changed every 24 to 48 hours. Blood withdrawal increases the risk of infection, as does the filling of tubing systems in advance of their use. Even minute quantities of blood or fat provide nutrients adequate to support the growth of most bacteria; therefore, changing tubing after infusing blood or lipids reduces infection risk. Continuous flush solutions and pressure-monitoring devices attached to arterial catheters pose special hazards. Reducing the number of catheter entries for blood sampling will reduce infection risk. Glucose-containing fluids promote bacterial growth in the transducer dome, tubing, and flush solutions. It is especially important to avoid contamination during calibration. Contamination of Swan-Ganz catheters may be reduced by minimizing the number of cardiac output determinations and by using sterile precautions during preparation and introduction of the injectate. Because of the escalating risk of infection, central venous, arterial, and Swan-Ganz catheters should be removed within 3 to 5 days of placement whenever possible. Obviously, there are situations in which all potential access sites have been exhausted or the risk of catheter reinsertion outweighs the risk of infection posed by leaving an existing catheter in place. Therefore, the need for and timing of catheter replacement must be individualized within the guidelines above. There are no credible data to support a practice of routine changing of catheters over a flexible guidewire and doing so in patients with established sepsis makes little sense unless all other sites and options for catheter insertion have been exhausted.

DIAGNOSIS

Although redness, pain, and swelling around the insertion site strongly suggest infection, these signs are often absent in patients with catheter-related phlebitis. Local (soft-tissue) catheter infections may be confirmed by Gram's staining and culturing the catheter and by "milking the wound" to provide material for Gram's stain. Because intravascular infections usually produce recurrent, sometimes continuous low-level bacteremia, collecting several sets of cultures obtained over hours to days is sensible. A positive blood culture withdrawn through a potentially contaminated intravenous line does not necessarily establish a diagnosis of catheter sepsis. Obtaining the same organism from a blood culture at a distant site is, however, strong evidence of catheter-related infection. In patients with suspected "line" sepsis, the catheter, tubing, and fluids should be replaced with fresh components. Before catheter removal, the skin should be cleansed with alcohol. The distal centimeter of the catheter tip should then be sent in a sterile container for culture and Gram's stain. Semiquantitative culturing is performed by rolling the tip of the catheter across a culture plate. If more than 15 colonies of a single organism are isolated, infection is more likely than colonization. The catheter tip should not be placed into any solution for transport—doing so renders quantitative culturing impossible. Routine catheter changes over a guidewire are not rational in patients with sepsis or inflamed entry sites and are not necessary for asymptomatic patients. Guidewire changes might make sense for patients in whom alternate sites for catheter insertion have been exhausted or who are deemed to be at high risk for insertion of a catheter at a fresh site (coagulopathy, tenuous respiratory status, bilateral femoral vein thrombosis).

COMMON ORGANISMS

Gram-negative rods, *Staphyloccus aureus, S. epidermidis,* and *Candida* cause most catheter-related infections, although enteric gram-negative rods also are recovered with some frequency. Although rare, blood cultures growing *Enterobacter agglomerans, Pseudomonas cepacia, Enterobacter cloacae, Serratia marcesens, Citrobacter freundi,* or *Corynebacterium* species should suggest a contaminated intravenous solution.

TREATMENT

Contaminated catheters should be removed and cultured as outlined above (this includes Portacath and Hickman devices). Blood cultures should be obtained from a site separate from the catheter insertion site. Considering the high incidence of methicillin-resistant *Staphylococci* in many ICUs, initial empiric antibiotic therapy for the patient with sepsis from a suspected intravenous line source should include vancomycin in doses adjusted for renal function. In units in which MRSA is rare, an anti-*Staphylococcal* penicillin is a reasonable initial choice (patients who are allergic to penicillin should receive vancomycin). In either case, additional coverage for gram-negative organisms should be initiated with an anti-*Pseudomonal* penicillin, a third-generation cephalosporin, and an aminoglycoside or imipenem. Recovery of *Candida* from the catheter tip and blood culture usually requires parenteral amphotericin B therapy.

PERSISTENT BACTEREMIA

For patients with persistent bacteremia or fungemia, line sepsis, and septic thrombophlebitis must be distinguished from bacterial endocarditis. The diagnosis of endocarditis usually obligates treatment with parenteral antibiotics for 4 to 6 weeks, whereas shorter courses of therapy are reasonable for line sepsis after the catheter is removed. The following factors all favor a diagnosis of endocarditis: (*a*) a new or changing (especially regurgitant) heart murmur; (*b*) valvular vegetations on echocardiogram; (*c*) physical stigmata of endocarditis; and (*d*) persistent bacteremia or fungemia after removal of the suspect intravenous catheter. Negative blood cultures should not dissuade the clinician from a diagnosis of endocarditis for patients with other stigmata: a small fraction of patients remain culture-negative off

antibiotics, and an even larger group are difficult to diagnose because antibiotics suppress bacterial recovery. The transesophageal echocardiogram has greatly enhanced the sensitivity of echocardiography to detect and stage heart valve lesions. For patients in the ICU, the presence of vegetations on the right-sided valves does not firmly make a diagnosis of bacterial endocarditis; central venous and pulmonary artery catheters crossing these valves can induce sterile vegetations.

It is difficult to make generalizations about endocarditis in critically ill patients because the condition may have been acquired in the community or may be a nosocomial problem, situations which have vastly different etiologic organisms, locations, and treatments. For patients with prosthetic valves who do not inject illicit substances, the left-sided heart valves (mitral and aortic) are most often affected by endocarditis and, in such cases, the disease is either a subacute or acute problem caused by *Streptococci* (40%), *Staphylococcus aureus* (20–30%), or *Enterococci* (10–20%). The *viridans* group of *Streptococci* are more common causes of the subacute form, whereas the acute variety is more commonly *Staphylococcal.* For patients with prosthetic valves who inject themselves with intravenous drugs and for hospitalized patients subject to nosocomial bacteremia, the disease differs. For such patients, endocarditis is much more likely to be acute in nature and is most commonly caused by *Staphylococcal* or *Streptococcal* species. For these groups, gram-negative rods and *Candida* also are recovered with a much greater frequency. Furthermore, infection developing while in an ICU or that associated with intravenous drug abuse is much more likely to occur on right-sided heart valves.

For patients with suspected endocarditis, several blood cultures should be obtained (preferably before initiating antibiotic therapy). A 12-lead electrocardiogram also should be obtained to look for evidence of conduction defects or arrhythmias, which can suggest the occurrence of valve ring abscess. When a clinical diagnosis of endocarditis is confirmed, at least a surface echocardiogram should be performed to look for vegetations, valve ring abscess, and rupture of valve leaflets. Each of these conditions is associated with increased morbidity (peripheral emboli), the need for surgical intervention, and mortality (possibly 50% higher than in the absence of these findings). The sensitivity of echocardiography has improved since the introduction of transesophageal techniques, which are now capable of detecting small

TABLE 26–5

CAUSES AND THERAPY OF ENDOCARDITIS

Patient Characteristic	Likely Organisms	Initial Therapy
"Normal" host, community-acquired infection	Streptococci (especially virdans) Staphylococcus aureus Enterococcus	Nafcillin or oxacillin plus penicillin and gentamicin. Substitute vancomycin in penicillin allergic patients or if resistant Staphylococci or Enterococcus recovered.
Prosthetic valve disease	Early postoperative S. epidermidis Gram-negative rods Diptheroids	Vancomycin plus aminoglycoside
	Late postoperative (As above for "normals")	As above for normals
Intravenous drug users	S. epidermidis S. aureus including MRSA, gram-negative rods	Vancomycin plus aminoglycoside.
	Candida	Amphotericin B, consider 5-flucytocisine and surgery
ICU acquired	Same organisms and therapy as for i.v. drug users.	

vegetations, and those in positions previously not visible by surface echocardiography.

Intravascular foreign bodies (venous and arterial catheters, pacing wires) should be removed to the extent possible. Empiric antibiotic therapy should be initiated against the most likely organisms based on history or clinical situation (Table 26.5). If valvular insufficiency, valve ring abscess, or fungal endocarditis is suspected or found, consultation with a cardiothoracic surgeon is indicated. Although most cases of subacute bacterial endocarditis on native valves can be managed successfully with antibiotics alone, gram-negative or fungal infections, valvular incompetence, valve ring abscess, and disease on a prosthetic valve often require surgical intervention.

Persistent unexplained bacteremia (or, more rarely fungemia), particularly when accompanied by pain, swelling, or redness at an intravenous site and recovery of a catheter-related organism, may signal suppurative thrombophlebitis, a condition that is often confused with endocarditis. A low threshold for surgical exploration should be maintained because this often subtle and highly lethal disease seldom will be cured unless the suppurated vessel is excised, despite the use of appropriate antibiotics.

INFECTIOUS DIARRHEA

Diarrhea is an extremely common problem for critically ill patients. Its etiology usually is multi-factorial but rarely is caused by bacteria commonly associated with outpatient infectious diarrhea (e.g., Salmonella, Shigella, Campylobacter, and Yersinia). When "infectious," a much more common condition is antibiotic associated or "pseudomembranous colitis." Hypoalbuminemia and drugs that promote bowel motility, destroy normal colonic flora, or have osmotic effects are common precipitants (see also Chapter 16, Nutritional Assessment and Support). Although it is entirely reasonable to perform stool cultures and examine the stool for ova and parities for patients admitted to the ICU with diarrhea, repeated culturing of patients with loose, frequent stools is expensive and of very low yield.

ANTIBIOTIC-ASSOCIATED AND PSEUDOMEMBRANOUS COLITIS

Pathophysiology

Pseudomembranous colitis is caused by a toxin produced by Clostridium difficile. This clostridial toxin directly attacks colonic cells, producing the areas of mucosal damage that form the characteristic "pseudomembrane." Although classically described after intravenous clindamycin therapy, C. difficile may overgrow the normal flora of patients receiving essentially any parenteral or oral antibiotic. Less commonly, colonic overgrowth of other microorganisms (e.g., Staphylococci, Candida) in response to antibiotic therapy can give rise to a similar picture.

Signs and Symptoms

Pseudomembranous colitis typically presents with watery diarrhea on the fourth to ninth day of antibiotic therapy. Although usually guaiac-positive, the stool is rarely bloody. However, bloody stools may result from one form of the disease localized to the hepatic flexure. Crampy periumbilical and hypogastric pain and low-grade fever are common, whereas an "acute abdomen" is rare (see Chapter 37).

Diagnosis

No routine laboratory test is diagnostic, but leukocytosis occurs in almost 80% of cases. As with other forms of inflammatory colitis, red blood cells and leukocytes usually are detectable in the stool specimen. Diagnosis is confirmed by culturing *Clostridium difficile* in profusion from the stool or by detecting bacterial toxin in a fecal specimen. The toxin assay is less sensitive but more specific than stool culture. (Some patients without pseudomembranous colitis have small numbers of *C. difficile* cultured from stool.) (If a diagnosis of *Staphylococcal* or *Candidal* antibiotic-associated diarrhea is being entertained, the microbiology laboratory should be notified when the stool specimen is submitted. Growth of *Staphylococci* or *Candida* may not be reported as pathogenic unless near-pure cultures result or unless the laboratory is alerted in advance.) Sigmoidoscopy usually visualizes the colonic pseudomembrane, but in a small fraction of patients (about 10%), only the right colon is involved. In such cases, full colonoscopy is required to find the characteristic lesions. Barium enema lacks sufficient resolution to be useful in diagnosis.

Treatment

The offending antibiotic should be discontinued and fluid and electrolyte support should be administered. Antidiarrheal agents should not be used, because they may prolong colonic dwell time, thereby increasing the severity of the colitis. There is no evidence that using corticosteroids or that giving lactobacilli to change the fecal flora is beneficial. Because the toxin as well as the organism may be transmitted nosocomially, all patients with this disease should be placed on enteric precautions. Because it is promptly effective, inexpensive, and not associated with the induction of bacterial resistance seen with vancomycin, metronidazole in doses of 500 mg orally every 8 hours for 10 days is the therapy of choice. Vancomycin (125–250 mg orally every 6 hours) for 10 days is the therapy of choice for documented failures of metronidazole. Intravenous metronidazole and vancomycin are ineffective. Bacitracin also has been used in doses of 25,000 units orally, four times daily, but is of uncertain benefit. Treatment may fail due to reinfection, emergence of a vancomycin-resistant strain, or bacterial transformation into a dormant spore phase. When therapy fails, relapses usually occur within 2 weeks of stopping treatment. Most episodes of recurrent or persistent diarrhea are not due to colitis associated with *Clostridium difficile* but with one of the more benign, noninfectious causes outlined above.

SINUSITIS

Although radiographic evidence of sinusitis can be demonstrated in most supine patients with nasogastric tubes, nasal packing, or nasotracheal tubes, sinusitis often is overlooked as a source of occult fever in critically ill patients. Nosocomial sinusitis usually is polymicrobial with gram-negative rods and *Staphylococci* predominating. *Pseudomonas* is not uncommon. Frequently, cryptic fever is the only clinical feature. Headache and facial pain may be impossible to detect in comatose or intubated patients. Nasal discharge usually is absent. The paucity of overt clinical signs may allow purulent sinusitis to advance to a life-threatening infection of the central nervous system. Its remote position and contiguity to vital structures renders sphenoid sinusitis an unusually insidious process. Because bedside sinus radiographs are worthless (particularly for visualizing the sphenoid sinus), CT of the head with attention directed to the sinuses is the preferred method of diagnosis.

The best treatment for nosocomial sinusitis is prevention. Whenever possible, insertion of ostia-obstructing tubes into the nose should be avoided. For orally intubated patients, a Salem® orogastric tube also can be placed easily for aspiration of the stomach or for feeding. An orogastic tube does not increase the level of patient discomfort and completely avoids the problems of ostial obstruction. When feeding tubes must be inserted through the nose, small-bore, flexible tubes should be used. Most cases of sinusitis respond to tube removal, decongestants, and antibiotics. Empiric antibiotic selection should include an anti-*Staphylococcal* penicillin and an aminoglycoside. More specific therapy can be guided by Gram's stain and culture of sinus cavity aspirates. For community-acquired sinusitis, *Haemophilus influenzae* is a common etiologic organism that often requires therapy with a β-lactamase-resistant drug, such as a third-generation cephalosporin. Surgical intervention may be necessary for patients with suppurative complications of sinusitis (e.g., retroorbital cellulitis, osteomyelitis, and brain abscess).

MENINGITIS

Bacterial meningitis should be suspected in all patients with mental status changes, fever, and signs of meningeal irritation. When neurologic symptoms begin, they often progress rapidly, but most patients with bacterial meningitis have been symptomatic for days before presentation. The presentation often is subtle in the ICU, where intubation, sedation, and/or paralysis limit communication. Fever and leukocytosis may be the only clues. When meningitis results from malignancy, tuberculosis, or fungal infection, the presentation is even more subtle and more likely to include focal neurologic deficits. Although focal deficits are possible with uncomplicated meningitis, the presence of focal lesions should raise the question of brain abscess, subdural empyema, or epidural abscess. Bacterial meningitis may be mimicked by several noninfectious conditions, including drug reactions to trimethoprim-sulfa and OKT3, carcinomatous meningitis, subarachnoid hemorrhage, systemic lupus, and sarcoidosis.

ORGANISMS

The microbiologic etiology varies with the site of acquisition (community versus hospital) and patient age. The *Pneumococcus* is the most common organism in community-acquired, adult meningitis. Sinusitis, otitis, pneumonia, and endocarditis coexist frequently. *Neisseria meningitides* is the second most frequent cause of sporadic meningitis. Nontypeable strains of *Haemophilus influenzae* represent the third. Although unusual in any setting, *Listeria* and enteric gram-negative rods are especially rare when meningitis is acquired outside the hospital. In hospital-acquired meningitis, *Staphylococcus aureus* or *S. epidermiditis* and enteric gram-negative rods are the leading etiologies, particularly in the postoperative setting.

DIAGNOSIS

Examination and culture of spinal fluid provide the only conclusive method of diagnosing meningitis. In the absence of papilledema or focal neurologic deficits suggestive of a mass lesion, lumbar puncture (LP) may be performed safely without CT scan. (Uncontrolled coagulopathy or significant thrombocytopenia constitute other relative contraindications to LP.) A lumbar puncture may be impossible technically because of poor patient cooperation or lumbar disease. In such patients, cisternal puncture or LP under fluoroscopy may secure a specimen of spinal fluid.

Spinal fluid pleocytosis with a granulocytic predominance usually is documented in infected patients. The spinal fluid glucose level usually is less than 50% of the peripheral blood glucose value and cerebrospinal fluid (CSF) protein concentration often exceeds 100 mg/dL. Gram's stain of spun spinal fluid demonstrates the organism in three of four cases of bacterial meningitis. It should be noted that seizures, tumors, trauma, and intracranial hemorrhage can mimic the CSF picture of meningitis. In particular, subarachnoid hemorrhage can present remarkably like bacterial meningitis. To differentiate these two conditions, it is useful to centrifuge a sample of freshly obtained spinal fluid and then examine the fluid for xanthochromia characteristic of subarachnoid hemorrhage.

Culture establishes a definitive diagnosis of meningitis. Although cultures of spinal fluid are positive in more than 90% of untreated cases of bacterial meningitis, the specimen may be rendered sterile by even a single dose of oral antibiotic. However, antibiotics rarely change the pattern of cells, glucose, or protein measurements in CSF for 12 to 24 hours. Leukocyte counts of 100/ mm^3, protein levels higher than 100 mg/dL, and glucose values lower than 30 mg/dL are typical in bacterial meningitis. If spinal fluid cultures are sterile, latex agglutination tests may reveal the etiology, especially when *Pneumococcus* or *Haemophilus influenzae* is causative. Because of wide cross-reactivity, these agglutination tests are least helpful in establishing or ruling out *Neisseria* infections. Blood cultures, positive in one-third of patients with bacterial meningitis, should be obtained before instituting antibiotics. After the diagnosis of bacterial meningitis has been established, the clinician should be careful to exclude underlying pneumonia, abscess, or endocarditis before deciding on the dosing and duration of treatment. Viral, neoplastic, fungal, and tuberculous organisms all cause meningitis but generally present less urgently than acute bacterial meningitis.

TREATMENT

Although not nearly as contagious as widely believed, patients with suspected bacterial meningitis probably should be isolated until the organism is identified and 24 to 48 hours of antibiotic therapy have been administered. Even if spinal fluid cannot be obtained because of technical problems or concern over safety of the procedure, antibiotics should be administered as rapidly as feasible. If lumbar puncture is contraindicated or technically impossible, empiric therapy should be initiated as efforts are undertaken to establish a delayed diagnosis by blood culture or latex agglutination testing. Antibiotic therapy and its route of administration (intravenous, intrathecal) should be guided by Gram's stain and culture of centrifuged spinal fluid. Although meningeal inflammation improves the penetration of most antibiotics into the CSF, certain drugs cross much more efficiently than others. For example, penicillin, chloramphenicol, and selected third-generation cephalosporins cross the blood–brain barrier easily, whereas aminoglycosides and other cephalosporins may fail to achieve effective concentrations. Penicillin has long been the drug of choice for community-acquired meningitis when lancet-shaped gram-positive cocci are present unequivocally. In regions of the country where the risk of penicillin-resistant *Pneumococci* is high, vancomycin should be included in initial coverage. Small gram-negative rods suggest *Haemophilus influenzae,* making a third-generation cephalosporin (e.g., cefotaxime, ceftriaxone) the drug of choice. If Gram's stain suggests an enteric (large) gram-negative rod or if there is evidence of a parameningeal focus (sinusitis, spinal osteomyelitis), an aminoglycoside should be added to a third-generation cephalosporin. (Aminoglycosides are never sufficient therapy alone, and even when clearly indicated for gram-negative infections, consideration should be given to intrathecal administration.) For cases in which spinal fluid cannot be obtained or is nondiagnostic, a third-generation cephalosporin with or without ampicillin or penicillin is the safest alternative. Because the spectrum of causative organisms in the hospitalized patient is so broad, initial therapy should include vancomycin, a third-generation cephalospo-

rin, and an aminoglycoside. Because acid-fast smears and cultures are negative in most patients with tuberculous meningitis, empiric antituberculous therapy should be considered for patients with chronic meningitis syndromes, especially if the CSF glucose concentration is low.

Patients with acquired immunodeficiency syndrome (AIDS) certainly can acquire any form of bacterial meningitis but a diagnosis of *Cryptococcus neoformans,* the most common cause of meningitis in AIDS, must be pursued. The CSF inflammatory response in patients with AIDS is often minimal; therefore, absence of an impressive pleocytosis should not dissuade one from the diagnosis of meningitis, especially if the glucose is low. Although an India ink examination of CSF reveals organisms in only 50% of cases, the CSF Cryptococcal antigen is positive in almost 90%. Combining these two tests promptly identifies the disease in most patients. The remainder are diagnosed when cultures return positive. Because Cryptococcal infection is so frequently a cause of meningitis in patients with AIDS, empiric amphotericin B probably is indicated unless CSF examination clearly indicates a bacterial cause. Tuberculous meningitis should also be considered when the patient infected with HIV presents with a syndrome of meningitis but has minimal CSF abnormalities. The higher frequency of brain abscess, toxoplasmosis, and central nervous system lymphoma in HIV-infected individuals necessitates a low threshold for head CT or MRI scanning, especially if focal defects are apparent on examination.

COMPLICATIONS OF MENINGITIS

Four important complications of acute bacterial meningitis are (*a*) cerebral edema, (*b*) inappropriate antidiuretic hormone (ADH) syndrome, (*c*) obstructive hydrocephalus, and (*d*) seizures. Because one in three adults with meningitis experiences seizures, prophylactic anticonvulsant therapy is rational. Signs of increased intracranial pressure (e.g., lethargy, papilledema, third nerve palsy, hemiparesis) should prompt emergent evaluation for cerebral edema or hydrocephalus by CT scanning. Hyponatremia should raise concern for syndrome of inappropriate antidiuretic hormone secretion (SIADH).

Craniotomy patients are at particular risk of meningitis caused by *Staphylococci* and gram-negative rods in the early postoperative period. Conversely, the *Pneumococcus* is responsible for more than 90% of late meningeal infections in patients with persistent posttraumatic CSF leakage. Septic cerebral embolism (e.g., from subacute bacterial endocarditis) or parameningeal infection (epidural abscess, brain abscess, sinusitis, and otitis media) are often confused with meningitis because they produce similar symptomatology and CSF pleocytosis. Paraspinal tenderness accompanied by radicular pain or weakness should be a clue to epidural abscess. *Staphylococcus aureus* is the causative organism in more than one-half of such cases. Brain abscess most often is a polymicrobial infection due to *Staphylococci, Streptococci,* and anaerobes. Abscess may develop by extension from the sinuses or ears or by hematogenous seeding (infected dialysis shunts, heart valves) or longstanding purulent lung disease (abscess, bronchiectasis). Brain abscess rarely is confused with uncomplicated bacterial meningitis because it usually presents with a less toxic picture and focal neurologic signs. Unless otherwise guided by results of culture, penicillin together with chloramphenicol or metronidazole should comprise the treatment. In selected cases, a third-generation cephalosporin or anti-*staphylococcal* agent may be indicated. Surgical intervention generally is reserved for lesions that compress vital structures, those unresponsive to medical management, and those for which malignancy is a strong alternative possibility.

SOFT TISSUE INFECTIONS

Most skin infections seen in the ICU are polymicrobial because they result from wounds incurred in surgical or accidental trauma, decubitus ulcers, therapeutic or illicit vascular punctures or because they occur in patients with compromised defenses and vascular insufficiency (especially diabetes). The most impressive of these are gas-producing infections, which usually develop in the setting of tissue ischemia or gross contamination. Risk factors for gas-forming infection include diabetes, penetrating foot lesions, peripheral vascular disease, and open trauma. Gas-producing infections may be classic gas gangrene with myonecrosis or a mixed organism (synergistic) necrotizing fasciitis. Both may spread with alarming speed. A mixture of aerobic and anaerobic organisms (gram-positive cocci and gram-negative rods) cause most gas-producing soft tissue infections. Classic clostridial gangrene is much less common. To achieve a successful outcome, a combined medical/surgical treatment approach must be executed rapidly.

Cultures of blood should be obtained, in conjunction with biopsy or aspiration culture of the affected tissue. Although the choice of antibiotics should be guided by Gram's stain and culture, empiric regimens usually include an anti-*staphylococcal* penicillin and penicillin G, with or without an aminoglycoside. Wide debridement or amputation frequently is required for control. If not up to date, tetanus immunization and toxoid should be administered.

Most soft tissue infections at intravenous sites are the result of *Streptococci* and *Staphylococci* present on the patients skin. In the colonized ICU patient, gram-negative rods may be causative. Removal of the catheter, application of warm compresses, and administration of analgesics and antibiotics usually resolve such infections rapidly. Treatment with a penicillinase-resistant penicillin usually will suffice. In less serious cases, oral therapy is acceptable. If methicillin-resistant *Staphylococci* are likely, vancomycin represents appropriate initial therapy.

Toxigenic *Staphylococcus aureus* presents a unique set of problems. Although toxic shock syndrome, an uncommon but lethal disease mediated by the *Staphylococcal* toxin TSST-1, was first reported in menstruating women using high-absorbency tampons, the syndrome clearly can occur in men. Traumatic or postoperative wound infections may serve as the source for the toxin, even when the surgical wound itself appears uninfected. Toxic shock syndrome should be suspected in any patient with the triad of fever, erythematous (eventually exfoliative) rash, and shock. Therefore, toxic shock can be confused with Rocky Mountain spotted fever, Stevens-Johnson syndrome, leptospirosis, measles, or a drug eruption. Because toxic shock syndrome is a toxin-mediated disease, local cultures are often positive for *Staphylococci* but blood cultures usually are negative. Therapy includes appropriate drainage (surgical drainage of wounds, removal of tampons), anti-*Staphylococcal* antibiotics (vancomycin is a good initial choice), and general supportive therapy with fluids, oxygen, and vasopressors.

INFECTION IN THE IMMUNE COMPROMISED HOST

GENERAL CONSIDERATIONS

Few clinical problems present a greater diagnostic challenge than fever in the immune compromised host. Because such patients often have impaired function of multiple organ systems and are undergoing treatment with toxic chemotherapeutic agents, possible etiologies span a wide range of noninfectious and infectious agents. Multiple causes frequently coexist. Patients in this category have primary deficits of T-lymphocyte (cell-mediated), B-cell (antibody), or granulocyte (phagocytic) function. Knowledge of the type of immune deficit can help narrow the differential diagnosis. For example, T-cell disorders predispose patients to viruses and fungi, whereas B-cell disorders and granulocytopenia predispose patients to bacterial pathogens. Although loss of humoral immunity and T-cell function predispose patients to infection, profound neutropenia (<1000 granulocytes/mm^3) is the defect that represents the greatest risk to life. Fever in such patients constitutes a true medical emergency. In this setting, the speed with which appropriate therapy is begun largely determines outcome. Unfortunately, establishing a specific diagnosis often proves difficult. Such patients frequently fail to produce suppuration or other localizing signs of inflammation. Regardless of the type of immune defect or site of inflammation, the etiologic organism usually is one that normally resides as a commensal in the host. Although any site may be the target of infection, a few problems are characteristic in the neutropenic patient. These include mucosal infections (e.g., mucositis, gingivitis), "primary bacteremia," soft tissue phlegmons (e.g., perirectal abscess), and atypical pulmonary infiltration.

PULMONARY INFILTRATES

The problem of diagnosing pulmonary infiltrates in the immunocompromised patient is complex, and only a few salient features can be covered here. For febrile neutropenic patients, infection must always be the leading diagnostic consideration; however, progression of the primary neoplastic process, hemorrhage, pulmonary edema, graft-versus-host disease, radiation, and drug reaction are frequent causes of pulmonary infiltrates. Although virtually any organism can cause pulmonary infiltration in the compromised host, the clinician often can integrate knowledge of the immune defect, epidemiology, and clinical and laboratory data to narrow the spectrum of likely possibilities and formulate a logical approach. As a first consideration, the underlying disease may give some clue to the nature of the

pathogen. For example, AIDS, a problem predominantly of helper T lymphocytes, so predisposes a patient to *Pneumocystis,* mycobacteria, fungal, and cytomegalovirus (CMV) infections that a presumptive diagnosis often is suggested by the radiographic and clinical pictures alone. Nonetheless, the spectrum of possibilities remains wide until the cause is confirmed by biopsy or fluid examination. Epidemiologic factors also are important to consider. The duration of hospitalization before the development of pneumonitis influences the microbiology. For example, *Pseudomonas, Candida,* and *Aspergillus* infections are most likely to develop after many days in the hospital, whereas the likelihood of routine (community prevalent) pathogens wanes after the first few days of hospital confinement. Renal transplant recipients are unusually prone to CMV, *Herpes simplex, Cryptococcus, Aspergillus,* and *Pneumocystis carinii* infections during the period of maximal T-cell suppression, 1 to 6 months after operation. Neutropenic patients are highly susceptible to gram-negative bacteria and fungal infections (*Aspergillus* and *Mucor* become common infecting organisms if neutropenia is sustained longer than 3 weeks). Concurrent infection with two or more organisms occurs commonly in patients with AIDS and in those undergoing renal or marrow transplantation. CMV, *Cryptococcus,* and *Nocardia* frequently are recovered in conjunction with other pathogens. (CMV and *Pneumocystis* are commonly associated.) Superinfections also occur frequently in immune-suppressed patients, particularly during sustained neutropenia and prolonged high-dose immunosuppressive therapy.

Certain clinical findings are especially noteworthy. *Legionella, Strongyloides,* and *Cryptosporidium* may cause diarrhea and pulmonary infiltration. Concurrent infiltration of lungs and skin may result from *Pseudomonas, Aspergillus, Candida,* and *Varicella-zoster.* Hepatic and pulmonary disease tend to coexist during infections with *CMV, Nocardia,* mycobacteria, and necrotizing bacteria (*Pseudomonas, Staphylococcus*).

Evaluation and Therapeutic Approach to Pulmonary Infiltrates

Unfortunately, these problems often defy easy diagnosis, and a tissue biopsy frequently is needed. The pace of the disease may be very rapid, so that the objective is to cover broadly while attempting to establish a specific etiologic diagnosis expediently and safely. Two important questions must be answered to deal effectively with a life-threatening pulmonary process in a compromised host. First, considering that the process seems to be infectious and that the course cannot be determined easily, does a precise diagnosis need to be established or is empirical therapy sufficient? Second, if a precise diagnosis is required, what is the most efficacious technique for a fragile, critically ill patient? These questions are not straightforward and remain the subject of intense controversy. In general, the approach should vary with the severity of illness, the pace of advancement, coagulation and ventilation status, the strength of ancillary information, and the experience of available personnel with specific invasive procedures. If a diffuse pattern on chest radiograph cannot be distinguished confidently from pulmonary edema, a brief trial of diuresis may be prudent before proceeding to invasive diagnostic measures. Even when pneumonitis is certain, the astute clinician considers the potential contributions of hypoproteinemia and hydrostatic forces to the density of the infiltrates. Unless contraindicated, "diuresis before biopsy" is a good rule of thumb. Sputum examination, when possible, is an obvious first step. Transtracheal aspiration and transthoracic needle biopsy are dangerous, low-yield procedures in this setting and probably should be withheld.

Ancillary Data

Both the characteristics of the chest radiograph at any single point in time and its rate of progression can provide helpful diagnostic clues. Localized infiltrates, either consolidated or nodular, are most consistent with bacterial or fungal infection, hemorrhage, or thromboembolic disease. Bilateral "interstitial" infiltrates, on the other hand, suggest volume overload, *Pneumocystis,* mycobacteria, or virus. However, serious lung infections may develop without causing pulmonary infiltrates, particularly in neutropenic patients. A fulminant evolution suggests a bacterial process or a noninfectious etiology (fluid overload, embolism, ARDS). Conversely, a process requiring 1 to 2 weeks for full expression calls to mind mycobacterial, parasitic, or systemic fungal diseases. The severity of hypoxemia is another key observation. Explosive life-threatening depressions of blood oxygen tension are typical for bacterial, viral, and *Pneumocystis* infections but are less common with more indolent fungal and mycobacterial processes. Examination of body fluids from extrapulmonary sources can suggest a presumptive diagnosis for the chest infiltrate. Spinal fluid may demonstrate *Cryptococcus* but does not prove that the roentgenographic infiltrates are related. Nonetheless, in the appropriate setting, pleural and joint fluids should be tapped, examined, and cultured and a stool specimen should be sent for parasite detection. Although blood cultures are unquestionably important, serologic testing rarely provides definitive information in an appropriate time frame.

Pulmonary Secretions and Tissue

Sputum is produced less frequently by the compromised host than by immune competent patients, especially when neutropenia is present. Nonetheless, when sputum can be obtained, its careful examination may reveal the responsible pathogen. In addition to the routine Gram's stain, a direct fluorescent antibody test for *Legionella,* a phase contrast or cytologic preparation for Blastomycosis, an acid-fast stain for mycobacteria and *Nocardia,* and a silver stain for *Pneumocystis* and fungal elements are highly worthwhile. Concentrated sputum specimens may reveal *Strongyloides.* In patients with AIDS, such a profusion of *Pneumocystis* organisms is harbored that expectorated specimens often reveal them. Unfortunately, cultures of many pathogens require days to weeks for growth and the nearly universal practice of early, multiple broad-spectrum antibiotic use routinely obscures the diagnosis.

The Need for Biopsy

If a specific diagnosis is not in hand after review of clinical data and laboratory results, the next step should be guided by the strength of clinical suspicion and the urgency of making the correct diagnosis. In most instances, bronchoscopy should be the first invasive procedure. Although coagulopathy and the need for mechanical ventilation are moderate contraindications to forceps biopsy, lavage, and gentle brushings can be obtained safely when care is taken to administer platelets and/or deficient clotting factors beforehand. Bronchoscopic yield varies greatly with the disease process and with the timing and method of conducting this procedure. For example, when all specimen-gathering techniques (biopsy, brushings, and lavage) are used, a specific diagnosis can be established about 50% of the time. In special instances, such as patients with AIDS, the yield is considerably higher.

Open lung biopsy often is delayed because of its perceived morbidity and expense. In fact, open biopsy, a 20- to 40-minute procedure, conducted early in the course of the illness is well tolerated, safe, and often helpful. It is the most reliable means of securing tissue for histologic diagnosis while establishing effective hemostasis in patients at high risk for bleeding. Video assisted thoracoscopy is another approach of merit in patients with good hemostasis. The expense of open biopsy should be considered along with the high cost of empiric multiantibiotic therapy. Not only are the four, five, or six drug combinations used expensive, some of the commonly used agents (trimethoprim/sulfa [TMP-SMX], aminoglycosides, and amphotericin) carry substantial risk of toxicity for kidneys and bone marrow. Whatever the value of open lung biopsy may be when undertaken early in the course of disease, it is clearly less valuable after broad-spectrum antibiotics have been given for a prolonged period. In such instances, it is unusual for open biopsy to add sufficient new information to warrant its attendant drawbacks. Failure to define a specific etiology should not mandate continuation of empiric antibiotics indefinitely. Not only can antibiotic management be streamlined when a specific diagnosis has been made, but also rational reductions in therapy can be made in the patient improving on multiple drugs. Usually, this takes the form of removing the next least likely beneficial or most toxic antibiotic from the combination every 1 to 2 days. The process of trimming antibiotic coverage often is delayed until patients are no longer granulocytopenic. Even while patients remain on multiple antibiotics, the clinician must remain alert to "superinfection" with a new or resistant organism. Furthermore, if a patient fails to improve with specific therapy directed against a known pathogen, a second organism commonly is present. For example, patients with AIDS and confirmed *Pneumocystis* pneumonia who fail to respond to TMP/SMX often have coexistent CMV infection. When no specific diagnosis has been made and the clinician is forced to choose a regimen, it should be remembered that *Legionella* and *Pneumocystis* are among the most lethal and common pathogens. For the immune compromised patient without a diagnosis, a third-generation cephalosporin and an aminoglycoside or quinilone, plus erythromycin or doxycycline and TMP-SMX, are often chosen as initial therapy. When methicillin-resistant *Staphylocci* are prevalent, vancomycin often is added or substituted. In centers in which fungi present a major problem, amphotericin often is begun very

early in the course. The use of ultra–broad-spectrum antibiotics (such as imipenem) may help to greatly simplify initial coverage, but such drugs present their own set of problems in terms of expense and the induction of multiply resistant bacteria.

Nonpulmonary Sites of Infection

Neutropenia most frequently is an iatrogenic complication of antineoplastic chemotherapy. These same drugs profoundly impair host ability to maintain the integrity of tissues having rapid cellular turnover (e.g., bowel wall and the mucosa of gingiva and rectum). Therefore, it is not surprising that diffuse necrotizing colitis, anorectal cellulitis, and typhlitis (a severe bacterial infection of the cecum mimicking appendicitis) are frequent sources of infection. Violation of the normally intact integument by intravenous catheters, surgical incisions, or decubitus ulcers also opens a portal for bacterial entry. Therefore, for febrile neutropenic patients, physical examination should routinely include catheter entry sites and the gingival and perirectal regions. Lack of tenderness with gentle palpation of the anal verge usually suffices to exclude this as a site of infection. All too often, no site is found for bacteremia or the sepsis syndrome.

GENERAL PRINCIPLES

Survival of neutropenic patients depends on early empiric therapy with more than one antibiotic effective against the infecting organism. The most common organisms include gram-negative rods (particularly *Pseudomonas*), *Staphylococci*, and fungi (e.g., *Aspergillus* and *Candida*). Patients with impaired cell-mediated immunity are more likely to be infected with *Pneumocystis* or *Candida*. When a site of infection is clearly definable, antibiotics should be chosen against the likely organisms. However, neutropenic patients frequently lack localizing signs of inflammation and no likely source is found in most cases (even with careful examination). In such cases, cultures of blood, urine, sputum, and skin lesions should be obtained. Even though pyuria may be absent, microscopic examination of the urine may reveal large numbers of organisms. Broad-spectrum antibiotics, including an extended-spectrum penicillin (e.g., ticarcillin) or third-generation cephalosporin plus an aminoglycoside, should be initiated. The empiric use of vancomycin is unwarranted unless the patient is allergic to penicillin or there is a reason to suspect a methicillin-resistant *Staphylo-*

coccal infection. In many centers, amphotericin is begun if the patient remains febrile for more than 72 hours after institution of broad-spectrum antibiotics.

POST-SPLENECTOMY INFECTIONS

Serious infections after splenectomy usually are due to encapsulated bacteria (e.g., *Pneumo-*

cocci, Salmonella, Haemophilus). Loss of the spleen's phagocytic function allows unchecked bacterial proliferation. Similarly, loss of hepatic phagocytic function in patients with cirrhosis makes them subject to overwhelming infection. *Salmonella* and *Vibrio* species are two unusual pathogens seen in such patients. Therefore, in patients without a spleen, the prevention of infections and the early institution of antibiotics are essential.

KEY POINTS

1. The speed with which an infectious diagnosis is pursued and the invasiveness of the techniques used generally should parallel the severity of illness of the patient. Stable patients with functioning immune systems and good physiologic reserves require less aggressive diagnostic approaches, whereas critically ill, fragile patients usually deserve rapid, definitive diagnosis.

2. For the unstable, infected, or septic patient, broad-spectrum empiric antibiotic therapy should be instituted after obtaining appropriate cultures. As a rule, for such patients, it is best initially to give too many rather than too few antibiotics—second chances to choose the appropriate therapy may not arise.

3. Antibiotics should be selected based on cul-

ture results, if available, and on microscopic examination of body fluid specimens if not. In the absence of diagnostic material, the clinical history and presumed site of infection should be the primary determinants of antibiotic selection.

4. When several equally effective alternatives exist to treat the same infection, choose the combination with the best side effect and cost profile. Oral therapy and parenteral dosing of a long-acting antibiotic on an infrequent schedule are the best methods of reducing antibiotic costs.

5. Antibiotic choices should be reassessed on a daily basis, keeping in mind that antibiotics rarely, if ever, reverse the effects of any infection in less than 48 to 72 hours. Antibiotic choices should be trimmed to the simplest effective combination as clinical response and culture data become available.

SUGGESTED READINGS

1. Armstrong D. Problems in management of opportunistic fungal diseases. Rev Infect Dis 1989;11(Suppl 7): S1591–S1599.
2. Bartlett JG. Anaerobic bacterial infections of the lung. Chest 1987;91:901–909.
3. Berger HA, Morganroth ML. Immediate drainage is not required for all patients with complicated parapneumonic effusions. Chest 1990;97:731–735.
4. Brewer NS, MacCarty CS, Wellman WE. Brain abscess: a review of recent experience. Ann Intern Med 1975;82: 571–576.
5. Caplan ES, Hoyt NJ. Nosocomial sinusitis. JAMA 1982; 247:639–641.
6. Cercanado E, Rodriguez M, Romero T, et al. Prevention and treatment of central venous catheter sepsis by exchange via guidewire. Arch Intern Med 1990;150: 1417–1420.
7. Chesney PJ. Clinical aspects and spectrum of toxic shock syndrome: overview. Rev Infect Dis 1989;11:S1–S7.
8. Corona ML, Peters SG, Narr BJ, et al. Infections related to central venous catheters. Mayo Clin Proc 1990;65: 979–986.
9. Faling JL. New advances in diagnosing nosocomial pneumonia in intubated patients. Part 1. Am Rev Respir Dis 1988;137:253–255.
10. Fang GD, Fine M, Orloff J, et al. New and emerging etiologies for community acquired pneumonias with implications for therapy. Medicine 1990;69:307–316.
11. Feingold SM. Anaerobic pleuropulmonary infections. Chest 1990;97:1–2.
12. Gallis HA. Amphotericin B: thirty years of clinical experience. Rev Infect Dis 1990;12:308–329.
13. Garibaldi RA, Burke JP, Dickman ML, et al. Factors predisposing to bacteriuria during indwelling urethral catheterization. N Engl J Med 1974;291:215–219.
14. Graybill JR, Marshall LW, Charache P, et al. Nosocomial pneumonia. Am Rev Respir Dis 1973;108:1130–1140.
15. Greenlee JE. Approach to diagnosis of meningitis: cerebrospinal fluid evaluation. Infect Dis Clin North Am 1990; 4:583–598.
16. Gross TJ, Chavis AD, Lynch JP. Noninfectious pulmonary diseases masquerading as community-acquired pneumonia. Clin Chest Med 1991;12:363–393.

17. Hampton AA, Sheretz RJ. Vascular access infections in hospitalized patients. Surg Clin North Am 1988;68: 57–71.

18. Kaufman BA, Tunkel AR, Pryor FC, et al. Meningitis in the neurosurgical patient. Infect Dis Clin North Am 1990; 4:667–701.

19. Krowka MJ, Rosenow EC, Hoagland HC. Pulmonary complications of bone marrow transplantation. Chest 1985;87:237–246.

20. Lambert RS, George RB. Diagnosing nosocomial pneumonia mechanically ventilated patients: which techniques offer the most reliability and the least risk? J Crit Illness 1987;2:57–62.

21. Maki DG, Weise CE, Sarafin HW. A semiquantitative culture method for identifying intravenous-catheter-related infection. N Engl J Med 1977;296:1304–1309.

22. Maki DG. Nosocomial bacteremia. Am J Med 1981;70: 719–732.

23. Maki DG. Risk factors for nosocomial infection in the intensive care unit. Arch Intern Med 1989;149:30–35.

24. Marcy TW, Reynolds HY. Pulmonary consequences of congenital and acquired immunodeficiency states. Clin Chest Med 1989;10:503–519.

25. Meunier-Carpentier F, Kiehn TE, Armstrong D, et al. Fungemia in the immunocompromised host: changing patterns, antigenemia, high mortality. Am J Med 1981;71: 363–370.

26. Nishijima H, Weil MH, Shubin H, et al. Hemodynamic and metabolic studies on shock associated with gram-negative bacteremia. Medicine 1973;52:287–294.

27. Norwood S, Ruby A, Civetta J. Catheter related infections and associated septicemia. Chest 1991;99:968–975.

28. O'Brien JT, Geiser EA. Infective endocarditis and echocardiography. Am Heart J 1984;108:386–394.

29. Orringer MB. Thoracic empyema—back to the basics. Chest 1988;93:901–902.

30. Penn RL. Choosing initial antibiotic therapy in the pneumonia patient. J Crit Illness 1986;1:57–67.

31. Platt R, Polk BF, Murdock B, Rosnen B. Mortality associated with nosocomial urinary tract infections. N Engl J Med 1982;307:637–642.

32. Robbins MJ, Eisenberg ES, Frishman WH. Infective endocarditis: a pathophysiologic approach to therapy. Cardiol Clin 1987;5:545–562.

33. Robbins MJ, Soeiro R, Frishman WH. Right sided valvular endocarditis: etiology, diagnosis, and an approach to therapy. Am Heart J 1986;111:128–135.

34. Rosenow EC, Wilson WR, Cockerill FR. Pulmonary disease in the immunocompromised host (Parts 1 and 2). Mayo Clin Proc 1985;60:473–487, 610–631.

35. Schaeffer AJ. Catheter associated bacteremia. Urol Clin North Am 1986;13:737–747.

36. Stone HH, Martin JD. Synergistic necrotizing cellulitis. Ann Surg 1972;175:702–711.

37. Stover DE. Diagnosis of pulmonary disease in the immunocompromised host. Semin Respir Med 1989;10: 89–100.

38. Warren JW. Catheter associated urinary tract infections. Infect Dis Clin North Am 1987;1:823–854.

39. Wilson WR, Giuliani ER, Danielson GK. General considerations in the diagnosis and treatment of infective endocarditis. Mayo Clin Proc 1982;57:81–85.

40. Wispelwey B, Tunkel AR, Scheld WM. Bacterial meningitis in adults. Infect Dis Clin North Am 1990;4:645–659.

41. Varkey B, Rose HD, Kutty CP, Politis J. Empyema during a ten year period. Arch Intern Med 1981;141:1771–1776.

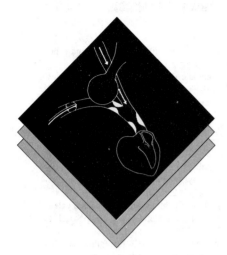

Sepsis Syndrome

TERMINOLOGY

Because the word "sepsis" means different things to different people, a meaningful discussion of the clinical problem is often difficult. Well-accepted, standardized, but arguably imprecise definitions of the clinical syndrome and its variations now exist. The constellation of fever or hypothermia, tachycardia, and tachypnea define the vital sign abnormalities of the "systemic inflammatory response syndrome" (SIRS). SIRS represents an organismic level response to inflammation that may or may not be due to infection. When a major organ system failure results from this inflammatory process, the syndrome is termed "severe SIRS." Common limits for vital sign abnormalities of SIRS are a temperature lower than 96°F or higher than 100.4°F, a pulse greater than 90 to 100 beats per minute in the absence of intrinsic heart disease or pharmacotherapy limiting heart rate response; and tachypnea with a respiratory rate higher than 20 breaths per minute. In mechanically ventilated patients, a minute volume criteria of 10 L/minute is customarily applied. Abnormalities in the circulating leukocyte (WBC) count are frequent enough in SIRS to constitute a diagnostic hallmark. Interestingly, elevations in WBC count higher than 10,000/mm³ or declines to levels lower than 4,000/mm³ can be seen.

When SIRS is caused by infection, the condition is termed "sepsis." Correspondingly, when an acute organ system failure occurs in a patient with infection-induced SIRS, the resulting syndrome is termed "severe sepsis." Patients who develop hypotensive cardiovascular system failure are said to have "septic shock." The multiple organ failure (MOF) syndrome is progressive cumulative failure of organ systems, most commonly the result of unresolved infection, and often culminates in death. Although strict criteria are lacking, MOF is best defined as a state of generalized progressive inflammation. The rather complex relationship of infection, SIRS, severe SIRS, sepsis, and severe sepsis are illustrated in Figure 27.1. The operational definition of sepsis is outlined in Table 27.1. The remainder of this discussion will focus on the features of the most important of these disorders, the clinical syndromes of severe sepsis and multiple organ failure.

EPIDEMIOLOGY

The roughly 500,000 cases of severe sepsis that occur each year represent a huge medical and economic problem. The average age of patients with sepsis is approximately 55 years, and for unclear reasons, there is a slight male predominance. Despite these observations, sepsis has no age or gender boundaries. Although sepsis certainly can develop de novo in previously healthy patients outside the hospital, it more commonly begins in hospitalized patients, most often in those with a recent medical or surgical intervention. In fact, most patients have been hospitalized for 5 to 10 days before the onset of the condition. Victims of trauma or complicated surgical procedures, immunosuppressed patients, and patients with chronic debilitating medical conditions are most

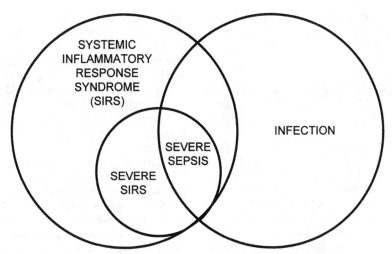

FIG. 27–1. Systemic inflammatory response syndrome (SIRS) is defined by a specific pattern of vital sign abnormalities. Infection is the presence of a microbe within the host at a normally sterile site. When infection causes SIRS, the resulting syndrome is called sepsis (central overlap). If an organ failure results from sepsis, the syndrome is called severe sepsis.

TABLE 27–1

SEPSIS SYNDROME CRITERIA

I. Clinical evidence of infection (required)

II. Major criteria (two of four required)
   Fever or hypothermia (temperature > 100.4°F or <96°F)
   Tachypnea or high minute ventilation (respiratory rate >20 or minute ventilation >10 L)
   Tachycardia (pulse >90 in absence of intrinsic heart disease or drug therapy inhibiting tachycardia)
   Leukocytosis or leukopenia (WBC >10,000/mm³ or <4,000/mm³) or >10% band forms on differential.

III. Acute impairment of organ system function (one required)
   Altered mental status (reduction in Glasgow coma score >2 points)
   Hypotension (SBP <90 mm Hg or fall in BP >40 mm Hg refractory to fluid challenge)
   Impaired gas exchange or acute respiratory distress syndrome (PaO_2/FiO_2 ratio <300)
   Metabolic acidosis/lactic acidosis
   Oliguria or renal failure (urine output <0.5 mL/kg/hour)
   Hyperbilirubinemia
   Coagulopathy (platelet count <100,000/mm³; INR > 2.0; PTT > 1.5 × control or elevated fibrin degradation products)

at risk. Over all, approximately 40% of patients with sepsis die, many from underlying diseases or disorders; but perhaps half of the deaths are attributable to the septic process itself. Although mortality averages 40%, certain subgroups such as hypothermic patients and extremely old patients seem to have a substantially worse prognosis. Curiously, even with the development of intensive care units, highly effective antibiotics, and sophisticated support technologies such as dialysis, parenteral nutrition, mechanical ventilation, and cardiovascular support drugs and devices, the mortality rate of sepsis appears not to have declined significantly during the last century. The reasons for the stable death rate are speculative. Perhaps the advancing age of the population, the increasing violence of trauma, the aggressive use of immunosuppressive therapy in cancer and transplantation, and the expanding population of patients infected with human immunodeficiency virus (HIV) are all partly responsible. Regardless, the current morbidity and mortality are unacceptably high and billions of dollars are spent caring for this desperately ill group of patients. The good news about sepsis is that survivors usually are returned to their premorbid level of function; that is, sepsis rarely results in a chronic debilitating illness.

After onset of the syndrome, the average survivor requires 7 to 14 days of intensive care support. For most patients, much of this time is spent on a mechanical ventilator. After weaning and ICU discharge, another 10- to 14-day hospital stay is typical. Thus, the time from hospital admission to discharge averages 3 to 5 weeks for most survivors. Because of its lengthy and technologically complex therapy, sepsis poses a substantial economic burden on society.

RELATIONSHIP OF INFECTION TO SEPSIS

Recovery of a pure growth of a pathogenic organism from a normally sterile site (e.g., blood, synovial fluid, or cerebrospinal fluid) diagnoses infection; however, most infected patients do not develop sepsis. This fact suggests that it is not infection per se that results in sepsis but rather the combination of infection and host response. Interestingly, a clear microbiologic explanation for sepsis is absent in many patients. Over all, cultures obtained from patients meeting clinical criteria for severe sepsis grow some organism 60 to 80% of the time, but many of these positive cultures represent colonization or contamination. Common examples of a ''positive'' but clinically insignificant culture result include growth of skin flora in one of several blood culture bottles, the recovery of a light growth of *Staphylococcus aureus* in the suctioned sputum of a chronically ventilated patient, or demonstration of a few colonies of *Candida albicans* in the urine of a patient with an indwelling urinary catheter. Perhaps the most convincing evidence of infection in the septic patient comes when several blood cultures return growth of an identical pathogenic organism consistent with the patient's clinical situation. For example, recovery of *Escherichia coli* in multiple blood cultures taken from an elderly man with pyuria and bladder outlet obstruction is credible and significant. Unfortunately, blood culture confirmation occurs in no more than 20 to 30% of patients.

Amazingly, the severity of the inflammatory response does not depend on the presence of infection. In fact, noninfected patients with severe SIRS due to pancreatitis, trauma, or burns have identical physiology, clinical presentation, and outcome as infected patients meeting criteria for ''severe sepsis.'' Again, this observation suggests that infection is not integral to the SIRS/sepsis syndrome but that microbiologic stimulation acts merely as one trigger for the disease.

The relative frequency of sites of infection causing sepsis are illustrated in Figure 27.2. In almost all studies, the lung is the most common site of infection resulting in sepsis, accounting for almost half of the cases in most series. Urinary tract infections, intra-abdominal infections, and all other sites comprise the remainder, each with roughly equal frequency. Obviously, the probable site of infection will vary widely, depending on the patient population studied.

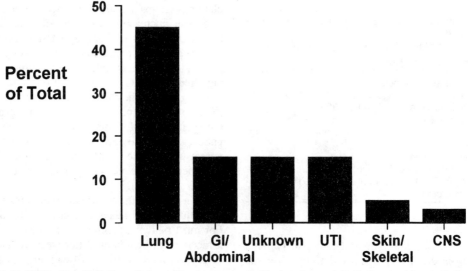

FIG. 27–2. Distribution of infections that result in severe sepsis. The lung is consistently the most frequent site causing sepsis.

CLINICAL MICROBIOLOGY

Bacteria, fungi, parasites, and viruses all can incite severe sepsis. Probably because of the relatively high frequency of bacterial infection and relative ease in their recovery, bacteria are commonly implicated. Because of the shear difficulty in culturing the organisms, viruses are least commonly identified. Approximately 70 to 80% of all "septic" patients have a bacteriologic isolate recovered, but it is not always certain that the bacteria recovered is the cause of the syndrome. In approximately 20 to 30% of patients exhibiting a septic picture, a bacterial pathogen can be recovered from the bloodstream. The frequency of gram-positive versus gram-negative bacteria in reported series varies widely, but currently the split is roughly 50–50. Theoretical discussions of the frequency of gram-positive or gram-negative infections as a cause of sepsis syndrome are of little use: the frequency of each type of bacteria varies with time, often "cycling" under the pressure of antibiotic use. Furthermore, knowledge of the overall rates of each type of bacteria are not helpful in designing therapy for the individual patient. Under most circumstances, the critically ill septic patient requires empiric antimicrobial therapy for both groups of bacteria until a more certain diagnosis can be made.

PATHOPHYSIOLOGY

The severity of the sepsis syndrome most often is dictated not by the inciting organism but rather by the specificity and ferocity of the host response to that triggering event. The same inflammatory mechanisms that are detrimental when unchecked in the septic patient probably are beneficial on the average day. Certainly, inflammation is beneficial when it limits spread of local infection or injury. It is only when rogue, diffuse unbridled inflammation occurs that it becomes detrimental.

The cellular and biochemical understanding of sepsis syndrome is rapidly evolving; new mediators are being discovered daily. At the risk of becoming rapidly dated, it makes sense to simplistically outline a paradigm of our understanding of the sequence of inflammatory events in sepsis (Fig. 27.3). Currently, it is believed that a multistage "cascade" occurs in which an initial trigger causes the production of a limited number of "early" mediators, followed over a period of hours by a larger number of secondary mediators

TABLE 27–2

COMMON MEDIATORS OF SEPSIS AND THEIR ACTIONS

Agent	Action
Cellular elements	
Monocytes and macrophages	Production of TNF and IL-1
Neutrophils	Tissue destruction via oxidant and protease mechanisms
Eicosanoids	
Prostaglandins	
Prostacyclin	Vasodilation, inhibition of platelet aggregation
Thromboxane	Vasoconstriction, platelet aggregation
E series prostaglandins	Renal vasodilation, inhibition of cytokine generation
Leukotrienes	
Cytokines	
Tumor Necrosis factor	Activates neutrophils, causes IL-1, IL-6, and IL-8 production, promotes leukocyte/vessel wall adhesion
Interleukin-1	
Interleukin-6	
Interleukin-8	Neutrophil chemoattractant
Oxidants	
H_2O_2, $HOCl^{-2}$, O_2^{-}	Direct injury of lipids, nucleotides, and proteins
Proteases	Destruction of vital cellular proteins, including antioxidants

(Table 27.2). Much of the structure of this cascade is inferred from in vitro and animal experiments, but data from clinical trials also support the schema. For most patients, it is believed that an initial "toxic trigger" stimulates cellular production of inflammatory mediators. The trigger is often a protein, lipid, or carbohydrate compound shed or released from a microbe but may be an activated complement, a component of the clotting cascade, or remnants of dead host tissue. Possibly most notorious of these inciting toxins is endotoxin, the integral cell wall lipopolysaccharide component of gram-negative bacteria. Endotoxin is far from being the only important microbiologic toxin; however, staphylococcal toxic shock syndrome toxin (TSST-1) and group B streptococcal (GBS) toxin are other well-recognized triggers. The septic trigger usually is only present transiently in the circulation and commonly es-

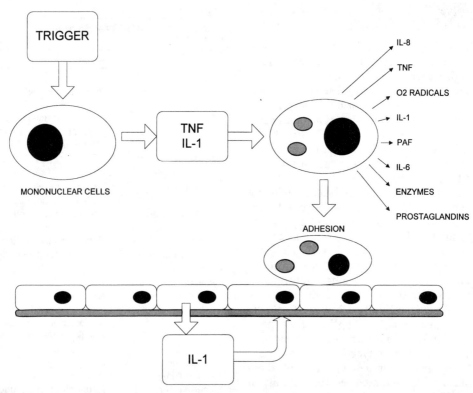

FIG. 27–3. Simplified representation of the early chemical events in sepsis syndrome. In most cases, an inflammatory stimulus (upper left) activates tissue based and circulating mononuclear cells. The resulting production of tumor necrosis factor (TNF) and interleukin 1 (IL-1) can subsequently activate every nucleated cell. In response to TNF, other cells, especially neutrophils (upper right), release additional interleukins, more TNF, oxidant radicals, prostaglandins, leukotrienes, and proteases. TNF and IL-1 also activate adhesion molecules on neutrophils and vascular endothelium, resulting in cellular binding and vessel injury (bottom).

capes detection, even when sophisticated monitoring is performed. For example, even with state-of-the-art methodology, fewer than one-half of patients exhibiting septic shock ever have detectable endotoxin in plasma. It should be noted that the development of sepsis does not require bacteremia or endovascular infection: toxic products may be released into the bloodstream from localized sites (e.g., abscesses) or directly from the colon (gut translocation), even when viable organisms do not circulate.

Two of the earliest inflammatory mediators triggered are members of a group of proteins known collectively as "cytokines." These cytokines, tumor necrosis factor (TNF), and interleukin 1 (IL-1) have received the most attention as experimental targets for modifying the inflammatory response because they are produced rapidly, are potent inflammatory agents, and are identified in the tissues and circulation of many septic patients. Furthermore, there is a rough correlation between the levels of TNF in plasma, the duration of cytokine presence, and outcome. Simply stated, the higher the serum TNF level and the longer the level remains elevated, the worse the prognosis. Substantial controversy exists regarding the significance of finding cytokines in the circulation and the relative importance of TNF and IL-1. That controversy not withstanding, probably the most important compound is TNF, because it serves as the major intermediate for other compounds, including IL-1, IL-6, IL-8, numerous enzymes, prostaglandins and leukotrienes, oxidant radicals, platelet-activating factor, and nitric oxide. Evidence suggests that TNF and IL-1 are synergistic and that TNF production is required for maximal expression of other cytokines downstream. Within minutes of a stimulus, TNF can be detected in the circulation of many sepsis victims and is followed temporally by IL-1, IL-6, and IL-

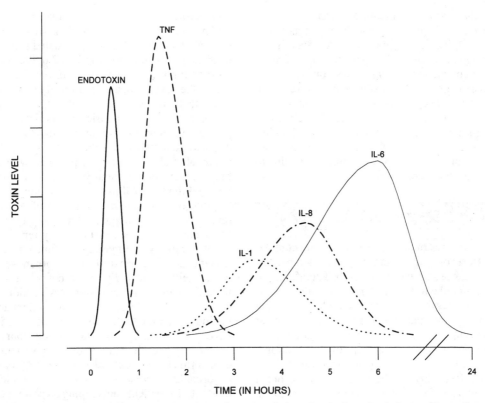

FIG. 27–4. Idealized illustration of cytokine release after presentation of a single toxic challenge. The toxin typically is present for a short period of time. Within minutes of stimulation, tumor necrosis factor is released into the circulation, peaking in concentration within 1 to 2 hours. After TNF, the pattern of release of interleukin 1, 6, and 8 is more variable. Il-6 usually is detectable in the circulation for the longest period of time.

8 (Fig. 27.4). TNF and IL-1 are not stored but are produced rapidly after a triggering event. Experimentally, TNF and IL-1 antagonists can alter the effects of a septic challenge in animals, but clinical trials have yet to confirm these findings. Fascinating new data suggest that one TNF Fab antibody fragment can eliminate TNF from the circulation, alter the production of interleukins, and change the clinical manifestations of some sepsis-like diseases.

CLINICAL DIAGNOSIS

Sepsis has many classic presentations: group B streptococcal sepsis observed in newborns, meningococcemia seen in young children, and staphylococcal toxic shock syndrome of adults. Such classic presentations, which include recovery of a specific microorganism, are the exception, however, and not the rule. Sepsis is a clinical diagnosis,

not one made by noting a single specific laboratory value or positive culture. Although fever is almost universally present (>90% of diagnosed cases), it may be minimal or absent in elderly patients, patients with chronic renal failure, or patients receiving steroids or other anti-inflammatory drugs. Hypothermia occurs in approximately 10% of cases of sepsis and is a particularly poor prognostic sign with mortality rates ranging as high as 80%. This high mortality rate probably is not due to the temperature itself but due to the close linkage of hypothermia with chronic underlying disease, shock, and gram-negative bacteremia. Data suggest that the ferocity of the biochemical response may be greater in hypothermic patients as compared to febrile patients.

Respiratory rate is a second key vital sign, because tachypnea is one of the early harbingers of sepsis. Although possible, the diagnosis of sepsis should be questioned in patients without tachypnea or abnormalities of gas exchange, because more than 90% of patients develop hypoxemia sufficient to require oxygen therapy (usually a PaO_2/FiO_2 ratio below 300). Tachycardia is a cardinal sign of sepsis. Unless patients have intrinsic cardiac conduction system disease or are receiving medications to block tachycardia (e.g., β-blockers), tachycardia is nearly universal. Abnormalities in circulating leukocyte (WBC) count also are frequent enough to be considered an initial diagnostic criteria. Typically, WBC can elevate to more than 10,000 cells/mm³ or decline to less than 4,000 cells/mm³.

ORGAN SYSTEM FAILURES

In fatal cases of severe sepsis, it is the cumulative effects of multiple organ system failures that usually cause patients to succumb. Therefore, understanding the usual onset, duration, and resolution of organ system failure and methods of organ support assume paramount importance. A clear relationship between the number of organ failures due to sepsis and the mortality of the syndrome exists. Each new organ system failure adds roughly 15 to 20% to the baseline risk of death of 10 to 15% for all ICU occupants (Fig. 27.5).

Patients average slightly more than two failing organ systems at the time of diagnosis. The frequency of various organ failures noted at the time of diagnosis is shown in Figure 27.6. Perhaps the most common constellation of serious organ failures is the development of pulmonary dysfunction and shock. (Most patients meeting criteria for shock also will be oliguric at least transiently.) Despite the multiplicity of causes, the pattern organ system failures seen in severe sepsis shows remarkable similarly among patients, with most failures developing rapidly (usually within 72 hours). Figure 27.7 illustrates the interesting relationship between the average time of onset and reversal of the organ system failures with respect to the onset of sepsis. Most organ system failures develop rapidly; pulmonary dysfunction, hypotension, and oliguria reflect the organ systems most likely to fail early in the course of sepsis, whereas central nervous system dysfunction tends to develop later. Because chest radiograph abnormalities take time to develop, meeting criteria for ARDS also tends to occur later in the course.

Not only does the number of organ system failures correlate with outcome, the severity of each abnormality also is important. For example, the mortality for patients developing a creatinine ele-

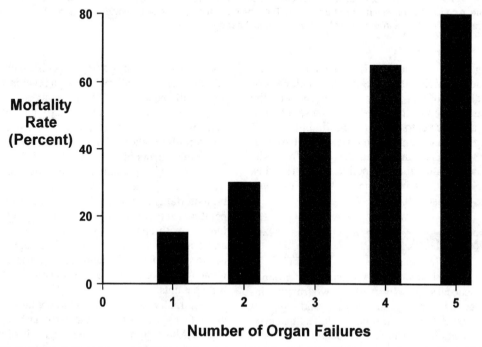

FIG. 27–5. Relationship between mortality and the number of organ systems failing because of sepsis. Each additional failing organ system raises the overall mortality rate by 15 to 20%.

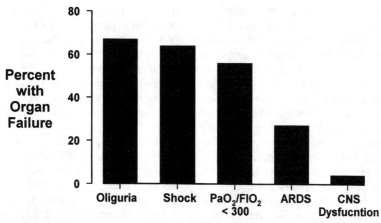

FIG. 27–6. Prevalence of organ system failures at the time of diagnosis of severe sepsis.

vation higher than 3.5 mg/dL as the result of sepsis may reach 80%, whereas a creatinine level of of 2 to 3.5 carries a mortality risk of near 50%. A level lower than 2.0 mg/dl predicts approximately a 30% risk of death.

SPECIFIC ORGAN SYSTEM FAILURES

PULMONARY

Pulmonary (oxygenation) failure rarely is absent and usually is the first dysfunction to be rec-ognized. Perhaps oxygenation failure is common because the lung is the only organ to receive the entire cardiac output; therefore, any inflammatory mediator contained in blood thoroughly bathes the lung. The lung's large vascular surface area and delicate endothelial–epithelial capillary structure also may play a role in its sensitivity to injury. Or perhaps it is much more simple, in that patients complain of dyspnea when they become hypox-emic or when lung compliance declines, and tech-niques for detecting pulmonary dysfunction (ox-imetry, arterial blood gases, and chest radiography) are applied promptly to patients who appear ill in any fashion.

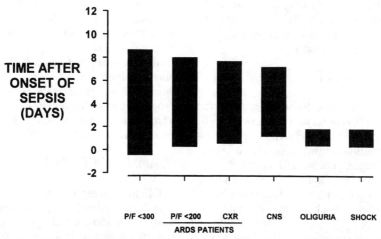

FIG. 27–7. Pattern of onset and reversal of organ failures in severe sepsis. The average time of onset of each organ dysfunction relative to the onset of sepsis is illustrated by the bottom limit of each bar. The top of each bar represents the average time of reversal after the onset of sepsis. As can be seen, most organ failures occur rapidly after the onset of sepsis. Shock has a short average duration, whereas lung dysfunction is prolonged. The development of central nervous system dysfunction tends to be delayed.

Sepsis puts many demands on the respiratory system, requiring an increased minute ventilation to maintain oxygenation and compensate for metabolic (lactic) acidosis. In the septic patient, frequently airflow resistance is increased and lung compliance is reduced, resulting in an overall increase in the work of breathing. These increased demands occur at a time when ventilatory power is compromised by diaphragmatic dysfunction and reduced perfusion of the muscles of respiration. The imbalance of respiratory muscle oxygen supply and demand often leads to combined hypoxic and hypercapnic respiratory failure.

Most patients with severe sepsis require intubation and mechanical ventilation. The average duration of mechanical ventilation for survivors is 7 to 10 days. Fortunately, fewer than 5% of patients require chronic mechanical ventilation and less than 1 in 10 patients requires oxygen 30 days after onset of the disease. Of all patients with severe sepsis, 35 to 45% eventually develop full-blown acute respiratory distress syndrome (ARDS), defined as a PaO_2/FiO_2 ratio less than 200 with diffuse bilateral infiltrates resembling pulmonary edema on chest radiograph (not as a result of heart failure). If ARDS develops, it happens rapidly, with most afflicted patients manifesting the syndrome within 48 hours of onset. Interestingly, in ARDS, there is only a rough correlation of PaO_2/FiO_2 ratio (P/F ratio) with mortality until the ratio falls below 150, when the P/F ratio becomes a powerful predictor of death. Paradoxically, the chest radiograph adds little prognostic information after the P/F ratio and lung compliance are considered. The good news about pulmonary dysfunction is that in essentially all survivors, lung injury reverses within 30 days.

CIRCULATORY FAILURE

Hypotension sufficient to meet criteria for shock (systolic blood pressure [BP] less than 90, or a fall in BP of more than 40 mm Hg unresponsive to fluid administration) is present in about one-half of all septic patients at the time of diagnosis and develops in one-half of the remainder within the first 5 days of illness. Understandably, of all organ failures, shock has the shortest duration, averaging only 24 hours. "Chronic" shock is rare: patients not reversing the shock state usually die quickly. Surprisingly, mean arterial pressure alone is a poor indicator of prognosis—pharmacologic elevation of blood pressure usually is achieved easily; therefore, mean arterial pressure

of treated patients with "shock" does not differ from that of patients without shock. Clinicians can be lulled into a false sense of security if vasopressor therapy is not taken into consideration. A mean arterial pressure of 60 mm Hg in a patient receiving norepinephrine is indicative of a vastly different prognosis than that of a patient with an identical pressure who is not on vasopressor support.

For most hypotensive patients with sepsis, invasive monitoring will initially reveal a low pulmonary capillary wedge pressure (PCWP) and a normal or modestly elevated cardiac output with a low systemic vascular resistance (SVR). Cardiac filling pressures usually are low because of some combination of reduced intake (e.g., vomiting or diarrhea), increased insensible losses (sweating and tachypnea), and increased vascular permeability. Therefore, initial fluid requirements for resuscitation often are substantial. It is not uncommon to require 4 to 6 L of crystalloid to raise the wedge pressure into a range producing optimal cardiac performance (commonly 14–18 mm Hg). If, however, underlying myocardial disease is present or if aggressive fluid resuscitation has been undertaken, the PCWP can be normal or even elevated.

The septic process can also blunt myocardial performance sufficiently to reduce baseline cardiac output. Therefore, it is easy to see how septic shock with an elevated wedge pressure and a low or low normal cardiac output may be mistakenly labeled "cardiogenic shock." The key to proper diagnosis is calculation of the SVR, which usually is reduced in sepsis. When volume-challenged, most patients who eventually survive sepsis exhibit a rise in cardiac output, but the slope of the cardiac performance curve is flatter than that of normal subjects. Failure to raise the cardiac output when the wedge pressure is boosted is a poor prognostic sign that may reflect impaired cardiovascular reserve or presence of a myocardial depressant factor such as TNF.

RENAL FAILURE

Oliguria (urine output < 0.5 mL/kg/hour) is very common early in sepsis and tracks closely with shock. Reversal of hypotension usually corrects the defect in urine production. As might be expected, patients with both shock and oliguria have a worse prognosis than those with either condition alone or those without either organ failure. As many as 80% of patients with sepsis syndrome develop at least transient oliguria, but it rarely persists beyond 5 days. (Approximately 10 to 15% of patients have oliguria of longer duration.) Although the creatinine level often rises modestly in patients with sepsis (range, 2.0 to 3.0 mg/dL), it is distinctly uncommon to develop frank renal failure from sepsis. Overall, fewer than 5% of patients with sepsis syndrome require hemodialysis, and in essentially all of these cases, support is temporary. It is rare to develop permanent dialysis-dependent renal insufficiency from sepsis.

METABOLIC ACIDOSIS

Metabolic (lactic) acidosis develops somewhat later in the course of sepsis than shock, lung injury, or oliguria. The reason for development of lactic acidosis is controversial. Clearly, in some patients with low oxygen delivery (DO_2) resulting from hypoxemia, anemia, or low cardiac output, impaired DO_2 alone could produce anaerobic metabolism. Over all, however, this group is relatively small. It is much more common that lactic acidosis results from maldistribution of cardiac output in which some organs are ''ischemic'' whereas others are luxuriantly perfused. Lactate also could accumulate because of a basic intracellular malfunction induced by sepsis—probably at the mitochondrial level. In a sense, the mitochondrial failure can be viewed as an ''organelle'' failure much like other organ failures described. Although a great deal of attention has been given to boosting DO_2 as a method to prevent or reverse anaerobic tissue metabolism and lactic acidosis, it is not at all clear that increasing DO_2 reduces anaerobic metabolism in all patients.

COAGULATION DISORDERS

The cause of coagulation disorders in patients with sepsis is multifactorial in most cases. Although direct activation of the clotting system may occur, probably the most important mechanisms are endothelial cell activation and damage. The incidence of coagulation disorders varies among patients with sepsis, depending on the defining criteria. Whereas mild to modest thrombocytopenia (platelet counts, 75–100,000/mm^3), minimal reductions in fibrinogen level, and trivial prolongations of the prothrombin and partial thromboplastin times are very common; full-blown, disseminated intravascular coagulation is distinctly rare. Although uncommon, when disseminated intravascular coagulation does occur, it carries an extremely poor prognosis.

CENTRAL NERVOUS SYSTEM FAILURE

A slight decline in central nervous system (CNS) function, usually measured as a deterioration in the Glasgow coma score of 2 or more points, is a later manifestation of sepsis. Surprisingly, even this minor decline in cerebral function portends a dismal prognosis. It is interesting that any clinical scale of CNS function that relies so heavily on volitional actions can predict outcome, considering the frequency of use of sedative and paralytic agents.

GASTROINTESTINAL FAILURE

The gut is an early victim of the septic response, in that perfusion is diverted to more ''essential'' organ systems. Therefore, in sepsis, especially that associated with shock, the peristaltic function of the gut temporarily ceases, producing ileus. Shortly after BP and oxygenation are stabilized, gut function tends to return to normal. Thus, enteral feeding usually is feasible 1 to 2 days after the onset of sepsis. In fact, it makes little sense to attempt full enteral nutrition until hemodynamic stability is achieved. Gut ischemia also is at least partly responsible for the higher incidence of gastrointestinal (GI) bleeding seen in septic patients. Upper GI bleeding occurs with substantial frequency unless pharmacologic prophylaxis is undertaken or early feeding can be accomplished. Nearly routine use of histamine blockers, antacids, or sucralfate probably is indicated until enteral nutrition can be reestablished. Although controversial, the hypoperfusion of the enteral mucosa also has been associated with leakage or ''translocation'' of bacteria and their toxins to the lymphatic and portal circulations.

Profound hypotension, especially when prolonged, also can lead to hepatocellular injury—the so-called ''shock liver'' syndrome. Shock liver is characterized by significant increases in hepatic transaminases and bilirubin, whereas alkaline phosphatase tends to remain in the normal range or rise minimally.

SEPSIS THERAPY

Because no specific treatment exists for sepsis syndrome, the therapy for all patients has similar core elements: supportive care for failing organ systems, drainage of closed space infection, and institution of appropriate antibiotic therapy.

ANTIMICROBIAL THERAPY

Initially, a low threshold for obtaining cultures of blood, urine, and sputum should be held. Appropriate cultures of wound discharge, ascitic fluid, pleural fluid, and cerebrospinal fluid should be performed based on the history and clinical examination. The likelihood of making a culture diagnosis is maximized by obtaining specimens before antibiotics are initiated, but in some circumstances, this is not practical. For example, for a septic patient with suspected meningitis and a focal neurologic defect, it may be prudent to obtain a head CT before lumbar puncture; however, it probably is not wise to delay antibiotic therapy while awaiting a scan. In this situation, it is better to begin empiric therapy, even if it may delay or obscure a specific bacteriologic diagnosis. Although it makes sense to initiate antibiotics in a timely fashion, beginning antibiotic therapy in most other situations *not* an "emergency." In fact, little data exist to suggest that antibiotics alter the morbidity or mortality of sepsis syndrome occurring in the first few days of illness. Ultimately, however, establishing appropriate antibiotic coverage is important: patients with sepsis who do not have the offending organisms properly treated have a 10 to 20% higher mortality rate than those receiving adequate microbiologic coverage. Failure to respond to seemingly appropriate antimicrobial therapy may be the result of undrained closed space infection (e.g., empyema, intra-abdominal abscess), presence of a resistant organism(s), insufficient drug levels, or simply insufficient time for response after starting therapy. Obviously, drainage of closed-space infections is crucial for cure.

Antibiotics should be chosen based on individual patient factors (e.g., immunosuppression, allergies, and underlying chronic illnesses), the presumptive site of infection, pattern of local antibiotic resistance, and examination of body fluids/specimens. Unless the etiologic agent is known with a very high degree of certainty, broad-spectrum antibiotic coverage is indicated until culture and sensitivity data return. Unfortunately, changes in resistance patterns induced by indiscriminate past use of antibiotics now frequently necessitate three or sometimes even four antibiotics to provide empiric coverage.

When no clear site of infection can be found, therapy with a third-generation cephalosporin and aminoglycoside probably is reasonable. In many cases, vancomycin also should be added to this primary coverage if penicillin-resistant *Pneumococci* or *Staphylococci* (especially methicillin-resistant) are prevalent regional pathogens. Similarly, if the suspicion of an "atypical" organism causing pneumonia is high, addition of doxycycline or erythromycin is reasonable. Finally, high suspicion of an anaerobic infection should often prompt addition of metronidazole or clindamycin. Within reason, it is best to begin therapy in the critically ill patients with too broad a spectrum and then narrow coverage as more clinical data become available. With that caveat, antibiotic coverage should be reassessed on a daily basis and unnecessary drugs should be stopped promptly. Contrary to popular wisdom, antibiotic therapy is not benign. Use of excessive or unnecessary antibiotic therapy is costly, predisposes patients to allergic reactions and drug toxicity, and perhaps most importantly, breeds the emergence of highly resistant bacteria.

In the absence of diagnostic clinical specimens, the presumed site of infection probably is the most helpful information upon which to select antibiotics. An in-depth discussion of appropriate empiric coverage based on the presumptive site of infection is covered in Chapter 26 (Common ICU Infections). Antibiotic coverage must be tailored to the individual patient history. The lung is, by far, the most common site of infection identified in approximately 50 to 60% of septic patients. In most clinical series, this is followed by an intra-abdominal or pelvic source in 25 to 30% of patients and an unknown site in a similar percentage. The urinary tract, skin, and central nervous system are somewhat less frequent sites. Obviously, even when appropriate initial antibiotic choices are made, the doses of antibiotics also must be customized to the ever-changing levels of renal and hepatic function.

RESPIRATORY SUPPORT

Because of the high frequency of hypoxemic respiratory failure, airway intubation, supplemental oxygen, and mechanical ventilation usually are necessary for the septic patient. The specifics of airway control and the principles and problems of mechanical ventilation are presented in detail in Chapters 6 through 9; however, some unique features of sepsis-induced lung injury deserve mention. More than 80% of sepsis victims eventually develop respiratory failure sufficient to require mechanical ventilation, and nearly all require supplemental oxygen. Therefore, for patients with sepsis, tachypnea (respiratory rate higher than 30), and marginal oxygenation, it is prudent to plan for elective intubation. It is counterproductive to pretend that rapidly evolving tachypnea and desaturation will resolve spontaneously. Doing so often results in emergent intubation of an apneic patient and only rarely can patients sustain a respiratory rate greater than 30 breaths per minute.

There is no clear best mode of ventilation for the septic patient; however, it makes sense to provide full support (assist control or an intermittent mandatory ventilation [IMV] rate sufficient to provide more than 75% of the minute ventilation requirement) during the period of initial instability. Full support, especially for patients in shock, provides mechanical assistance that permits redistribution of cardiac output from the respiratory muscles to other parts of the body. The effect of ventilatory support can be substantial, in many cases amounting to an effective 20% boost in systemic oxygen delivery relative to demand.

Occasionally, the drive to breathe is so high that sedation must be administered to match the respiratory efforts of man and machine. Fortunately, paralysis is rarely necessary if appropriate sedation is provided and the ventilator is adjusted carefully. To maximize patient matching and comfort, special consideration should be given to altering the gas flow delivery pattern, flow rate, and tidal volume.

Although a single precise predictor of ventilator-associated barotrauma does not exist, there is a strong association of barotrauma with transalveolar pressures higher than 30 to 35 cm H_2O. Practically, maximum tidal alveolar pressure is best gauged clinically by the plateau pressure unless the chest wall is very stiff. Sufficient data now exist to recommend limiting plateau pressure to 35 cm H_2O to reduce the risk of overexpansion of the lung and barotrauma. This pressure guideline often requires reduction of the tidal volume to 5 to 6 mL/kg, usually resulting in some degree of hypercapnia.

Supplemental oxygen should be administered to maintain an acceptable saturation (in most cases, SaO_2 higher than 88%). The real and immediate risk of hypoxemia should not be traded for the potential future risk of oxygen toxicity. Lower saturation limits are acceptable for young, otherwise healthy patients, whereas higher targets may

be appropriate for patients with critical organ perfusion deficits (e.g., myocardial ischemia or recent stroke). Many uncertainties surround the potential for oxygen toxicity; however, common practice is to attempt to reduce the FiO_2 to a level of 0.6 or less provided saturation is acceptable. If higher FiO_2 levels are required, sequential upward titration of PEEP usually is undertaken. It is probably still true that the "best PEEP" is the lowest PEEP which keeps the lung fully recruited and provides acceptable O_2 delivery with an FiO_2 below 0.6. Some minimal level of PEEP is probably beneficial for all mechanically ventilated patients, to raise functional residual capacity and minimize injury induced by the repeated phasic opening and closing of alveoli. In most cases, 5–10 cm H_2O PEEP is sufficient to achieve the former goal. However, the optimal PEEP to prevent repetitive alveolar opening and closing is unknown. (Recent data hint that levels higher than 5 cm H_2O may provide better protection for patients with ARDS [see Chapters 8 and 9]). Despite the emotion surrounding the selection of an ideal combination of PEEP and FiO_2, practically most patients with ARDS end up receiving an FiO_2 between 40 and 60% and PEEP of 7 to 15 cm H_2O pressure.

CARDIOVASCULAR SUPPORT

In the setting of severe sepsis, circulatory shock usually is defined as a systolic BP lower than 90 mm Hg or a decrease in normal systolic BP of more than 40 mm Hg unresponsive to fluid administration. At the onset of the syndrome, most patients with sepsis-induced shock have substantial volume depletion with variable degrees of systemic vascular dilation and myocardial dysfunction. Left ventricular filling pressures are usually low because patients with sepsis have been deprived of oral intake, have increased fluid losses (from sweating, panting, vomiting, or diarrhea), and have dilated capacitance vessels and increased endothelial permeability. The average septic patient requires 4 to 6 L of crystalloid fluid replacement or a comparable volume expanding amount of colloid to optimize left ventricular filling. There is no demonstrated difference in efficacy of crystalloid and colloid in achieving successful resuscitation. Obviously, a smaller volume of colloid will be required to achieve any given increase in wedge pressure; however, neither colloid nor crystalloid is confined entirely to the vascular compartment in sepsis. Although less colloid is required, volume expansion is achieved at substantial cost—colloid risks allergic reactions and its price is often 20 to 100 times that of an equivalent dose of crystalloid. Fluid is often initially given empirically, but when infused volumes exceed 2 to 3 L, invasive pulmonary artery monitoring catheters commonly are inserted. The only way to be certain of adequate left ventricular preload is to directly measure wedge pressure. (A less desirable alternative is to give fluid until pulmonary edema develops.) Because myocardial compliance and transmural pressure are highly variable, the optimal left ventricular filling pressure for each patient must be derived empirically and should be reevaluated frequently. Typically, this is accomplished by measuring hemodynamics in response to serial fluid challenges several times daily.

A detailed discussion of cardiovascular support is provided in Chapter 3 (Support of Failing Circulation); however, a few points deserve highlighting here. As a rule, vasopressor or cardiostimulatory agents should be reserved for patients in whom the circulating volume has been restored. Vasopressors often are ineffective in volume-depleted patients and can be detrimental if employed in doses that compromise perfusion to vital tissues. As a practical matter, most physicians initiate pharmacologic circulatory support with dopamine, in a low dose (<5 μg/kg/minute), and then titrate the infusion upward to achieve the desired clinical result. This makes sense based on the pharmacology of dopamine. "Low-range" doses are likely to have β-adrenergic stimulating effects, boosting cardiac output. In addition, dopamine will have some degree of dopaminergic effect, possibly improving renal blood flow. As doses are increased, dopaminergic effects persist; the strength of β-stimulation increases, and eventually α-adrenergic effects become clinically significant. Therefore, dopamine may counteract the myocardial depression of sepsis and increase an abnormally low systemic vascular resistance. Although entirely empiric, some clinicians substitute or add dobutamine to an existing pressor regimen if cardiac output appears inappropriately low. When profound reductions in systemic vascular resistance are responsible for hypotension and shock, it is also a common practice to add an α-adrenergic stimulant (Neosynephrine or norepinephrine) to the pharmacologic regimen. One widely held misconception is that the use of potent α-adrenergic agents "guarantees" a poor outcome. To the contrary, sometimes it is only after norepinephrine is begun that systemic vascular re-

sistance (SVR) increases, in turn raising mean arterial pressure and organ perfusion. In certain settings (e.g., cor pulmonale) failure to raise systemic blood pressure will deprive the heart of the perfusion gradient it needs to pump effectively.

Physicians and nurses often become anxious when the required dose of any vasoactive drug is higher than that in their past experience. However, it should be kept in mind that individual patient responsiveness to vasopressors can vary widely (perhaps a log variation). Therefore, there are no absolute limitations for vasopressor doses in shock. When very high doses of vasoactive agents are required, however, consideration should be given to several specific causes of refractory hypotension, including intravascular volume depletion, adrenal insufficiency, profound acidosis, pericardial constriction or tamponade, and tension pneumothorax. The systemic blood pressure to target should take into consideration the patient's chronic blood pressure, specific organ requirements, and clinical indicators of response.

A normally functioning brain, adequate (>0.5 mL/kg/hour) urine output, evidence of adequate peripheral skin and digit perfusion, and a reasonable level of oxygenation are the appropriate goals of shock therapy, not a specific value of oxygen delivery, wedge pressure, blood pressure or cardiac output. These clinical perfusion goals usually are met when cardiac output is in the 7- to 10-L range, arterial lactate concentrations are declining, and oxygen delivery measurements are slightly above those for a resting healthy patient.

Because hemodilution accompanies resuscitation with colloid or crystalloid, administration of packed red blood cells is often required to maintain hemoglobin concentrations in the range of 10 to 12 gm/dL.

THERAPY OF METABOLIC ACIDOSIS

Lactic acidosis is a common finding in septic patients. Fortunately, it is usually a mild and self-limited problem that resolves when intravascular volume deficits are corrected. When lactic acidosis results from low cardiac output and hypotension, it is likely to be improved by increasing arterial pressure. Conversely, when cardiac output and arterial pressure are normal or high, no data convincingly demonstrate a benefit of further increasing output. Survival correlates best with lactate levels and not serum pH; therefore, one might expect that direct buffering of an abnormal pH would not be expected to improve outcome, unless the underlying reason for lactate generation is corrected simultaneously. This suspicion has been borne out in clinical trials showing that pH correction with sodium bicarbonate or dichloroacetate does not benefit victims of lactic acidosis. Even though experimental data do not support the practice, as a practical matter, many physicians feel compelled to intervene when pH measurements decline below approximately 7.10.

SUPPORT OF THE KIDNEY

The kidney commonly experiences transient dysfunction early in the septic process; more than 80% of patients develop transient oliguria. Oliguria usually is reversed by simple fluid administration to correct underlying volume depletion. For patients with shock, a combination of volume repletion and vasoactive drug administration may be required to raise cardiac output or SVR sufficiently to perfuse the kidney. Because the kidneys also may serve as a source of sepsis, it is important to exclude urinary tract infection—especially that associated with obstruction. There is no credible clinical evidence indicating that the use of dopamine (in any dose range) serves to protect the kidney from injury or improve a patient's outcome. Likewise, diuretic therapy has not been shown to improve outcome in oliguric patients,

despite the observation that nonoliguric patients with acute renal failure have a lower mortality rate than do oliguric patients. Perhaps the most important intervention to protect the kidneys of patients with sepsis is to avoid potentially nephrotoxic medications whenever possible. As renal function declines early in the septic process, any number of toxic drugs may accumulate to the point that they cause systemic toxicity or accentuate the injury to the kidney. Probably the most important class of compounds in this regard are antibiotics. The potential nephrotoxic effects of antibiotic therapy again emphasize the importance of rationally directed antibiotic therapy.

NUTRITIONAL SUPPORT

A thorough discussion of nutritional assessment and support is provided in Chapter 16. As with all other critically ill patients, there are two basic "truths" about nutrition. First, prolonged starvation (weeks to months) is fatal, and second, any patient can tolerate several (3 to 5 days) without feeding. Almost every other aspect of nutritional support is arguable. Even with the disagreements about nutrition, there are some common practices among physicians. Nutritional support usually is withheld until hemodynamic and respiratory stability is achieved. (Typically, this requires 1 to 2 days.) Most practitioners now favor the enteral route of support because it provides a

TABLE 27–3

EXPERIMENTAL THERAPIES FOR SEPSIS

Category	Proposed Action	Result
Corticosteroids	Nonspecific anti-inflammatory	Failed multiple human trials, possibly increases infection risk
Naloxone	Opioid receptor antagonist	May transiently raise blood pressure, no effect on survival
Cyclooxygenase inhibitors	Reduce thromboxane and prostacyclin	Biochemically effective, improved vital signs, no demonstrated improvement in survival, overall very safe
Anti-endotoxins	Inactivate Gram-negative toxins	Failed in several trials, harm suspected from one agent
IL-1 receptor antagonist	Block IL-1 action	No improvement in physiology or survival
TNF antibodies	Inactivate TNF	No certain benefit. No evidence of harm. Trials ongoing
TNF receptor antagonists	Block TNF action	Dose-dependent increase in mortality
Antioxidants	Prevent oxidant-mediated cellular injury	Trials ongoing

more complete or balanced form of nutrition and it affords the theoretical benefits of preserving gut mucosa. In addition, enteral nutrition is substantially less expensive than intravenous supplementation and avoids the complications associated with the central venous catheters required for effective parenteral nutrition. At this time, there is no compelling evidence to suggest that any particular enteral feeding formula or particular balance of components is superior to another for the patient with sepsis.

Simply stated, the current level of knowledge supports giving a mixture of carbohydrate, protein, and lipid (based on the patient's estimated needs) via an enteral route after hemodynamic stability is achieved. For patients with prolonged

($>$5 days) gut dysfunction, parenteral nutrition may be indicated.

EXPERIMENTAL THERAPIES

To date, there is no specific therapy for sepsis despite numerous experimental investigations. In some cases, the study drug has been shown definitively to be ineffective and, in other cases, insufficient data exist to make conclusions about the efficacy of therapy. A detailed discussion of the problems associated with the experimental therapy of sepsis is well beyond the scope of this text. An overview of the experimental approaches by category and a simplistic summary of human experimental results are presented in Table 27.3.

KEY POINTS

1. Severe sepsis is a syndrome caused by infection and defined by the presence of vital sign abnormalities and new organ system failure caused by the ensuing inflammation. It differs from SIRS only by the fact that infection is present. Both SIRS and sepsis are the result of a poorly directed, uncontrolled, or excessively exuberant host response to the initiating stimulus.

2. Sepsis is common and carries approximately a 40% risk of death. Outcome is influenced strongly by the number and severity of organ system failures that occur. Average mortality risk increases approximately 15 to 20% for each organ system failure.

3. Most survivors of sepsis recover to their

baseline level of function within 30 days. Hemodialysis, mechanical ventilation, or vasopressor support are rarely needed beyond 2 to 3 weeks.

4. The lung and circulatory system are the two most commonly injured organ systems. Both manifest dysfunction early in the septic process. Circulatory failure usually reverses rapidly or is fatal, whereas respiratory failure often requires 7 to 14 days of ventilatory support. Transient oliguria is very common, but frank renal failure requiring dialysis is rare.

5. No specific sepsis therapy exists: drainage of closed-space pus, appropriate antimicrobial therapy, organ system support, and meticulous attention to avoid nosocomial infections constitute the best plan for success.

SUGGESTED READINGS

1. Balk RA, Bone RC., eds. Septic shock. Crit Care Clin 1989;5:1–194.
2. Bernard GR, Reines HD, Metz CA, et al. Effects of a short course of ibuprofen in patients with severe sepsis. Am Rev Respir Dis 1988;137:1543.
3. Bone RC, Fisher CJ, Clemmer TP, Slotman GJ, Metz CA, Balk RA. Sepsis syndrome: a valid clinical entity. Crit Care Med 1989;17:389–393.
4. Bone RC, Fisher CJ, Clemmer TP, et al. A controlled clinical trial of high-dose methyl-prednisolone in the treatment of severe sepsis and septic shock. N Engl J Med 1987;317:653–658.
5. Bone RC, Fisher CJ, Clemmer TP, et al. Early methylprednisolone treatment for septic syndrome and adult respiratory distress syndrome. Chest 1987;932:1032–1036.
6. Christman JW, Wheeler AP, Bernard GR. Cytokines and sepsis: what are the therapeutic implications? J Intensive Care 1991;6:172–182.
7. Dorinsky PM., eds. The sepsis syndrome. Clin Chest Med 1996;volume 17.
8. Lefer AM. Induction of tissue injury and altered cardiovascular performance by platelet activating factor: relevance to multiple systems organ failure. Crit Care Clin 1989;5:331–352.
9. Luce JM, Montgomery AB, Marks JD, et al. Ineffectiveness of high dose methylprednisolone in preventing parenchymal lung injury and improving mortality in patients with septic shock. Am Rev Respir Dis 1988;138:62–68.
10. Horbar JD, Soll RF, Sutherland JM, et al. A multicenter randomized, placebo-controlled trial of surfactant therapy for respiratory distress syndrome. N Engl J Med 1989;320:959–965.

11. Spragg RC, Richman P, Gilliard N, Merritt TA, et al. The use of exogenous surfactant to treat patients with acute high-permeability lung edema. Prog Clin Biol Res 1989; 308:791–796.

12. Veterans Administration Systemic Sepsis Cooperative Study Group. Effect of high dose glucocorticoid therapy on mortality in patients with signs of systemic sepsis. N Engl J Med 1987;317:659–665.

13. Wheeler AP, Bernard GR. Applications of molecular biology and biotechnology: antibody therapy of sepsis. J Crit Care 1996;11:77–94.

14. Wheeler AP. Immunological therapy of endotoxemia. In: Brigham KL, ed. Endotoxin and the lungs. New York: Marcel Dekker, 1994; 351–392.

15. Wheeler AP, Brigham KL. Cytokine antibodies and antagonists in the treatment of sepsis. In: Landon J, Chard T, eds. Therapeutic antibodies. London: Churchill Livingstone, 1994; 199–224.

16. Wheeler AP, Bernard GR. Immunological therapy of endotoxemia: anti-endotoxin antibodies. In: Landon J, Chard T, eds. Therapeutic antibodies. London: Churchill Livingstone, 1994; 177–198.

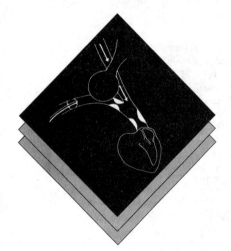

CHAPTER 28

Thermal Disorders

NORMAL TEMPERATURE REGULATION

Body temperature is normally tightly regulated between 36° and 37.5°C. The net temperature is the result of the balance between heat generated and heat lost. Heat dissipation occurs primarily by radiation and evaporation at the skin surface, with a lesser contribution from exhaled gas. When heat production rises (e.g., exercise) or heat loss declines (e.g., environmental exposure), sweating, cutaneous vasodilation, and hyperventilation return temperature toward normal. Behavioral responses (shedding clothing, drinking cool liquids, cessation of exercise) also act to lower temperature. If mechanisms for heat loss fail to keep pace with heat generation, body temperature rises. Significant reductions in body temperature usually are the result of exposure to low ambient temperatures. Vasoconstriction and behavioral responses (donning extra clothing, seeking a warm environment) counteract excessive heat loss, but exercise and shivering are the only effective methods of raising heat production. In general, the body is much better adapted to losing excess heat than it is to rapid heat production. (Options for heat generation are much less effective.)

TEMPERATURE MEASUREMENT

TYPES OF MEASURING DEVICES

The technique used to measure temperature is critical in detecting fever or hypothermia. Mer-

cury thermometers usually are unable to detect temperatures lower than 94°F or higher than 105°F and fail to record values below the initial "shaken" level. Mercury thermometers respond rather slowly to temperature changes; use of an electronic device or thermocouple (e.g., on a pulmonary artery catheter) is preferable when recording temperature extremes and rapid fluctuations. Infrared sensing ear canal probes capable of accurate estimation of core temperature within seconds currently are available. Plastic strip thermometers have limited accuracy and recording range.

SITES OF MEASUREMENT

Recorded oral temperatures are routinely reduced below true core values when respiratory rates exceed 18 breaths per minute. Rectal temperatures avoid the artifacts seen with oral recordings due to varying respiratory rates, poor thermometer–patient contact, and temperature aberrations caused by smoking or oral consumption of hot or cold liquids. Although usually accurate, rectal temperatures may spuriously indicate hypothermia in patients with colonic impaction or intense mucosal vasoconstriction. Axillary temperatures often underestimate core temperature due to poor thermometer–skin contact and wide differences between skin and core temperature. Esophageal temperature measurement is an effective "noninvasive" way to measure core temperature, but it requires specialized equipment. Infrared sensing of external ear canal temperature very closely parallels core temperature and is not subject to influence by eating, drinking, or smoking, as is oral temperature. The temperature of pulmonary artery blood may be monitored continuously using the thermistor-tipped pulmonary artery catheter. Freshly voided urine also provides a source for on-line measurement of central temperature by specialized collection systems.

HYPOTHERMIA

DEFINITION AND PROBLEMS IN DETECTION

Patients with uremia, hypothyroidism, malnutrition, and congestive heart failure often have mildly reduced (1–3°F) basal temperatures. For these patients, a "normal" or slightly increased temperature may represent fever. Clinical hypothermia, a core temperature below 35°C (95°F), frequently escapes detection because symptoms are nonspecific and because most thermometers fail to record in the appropriate range.

ETIOLOGY

Most hypothermia is multifactorial in origin. (Environmental exposure subsequent to intoxication or a primary neurologic event is a common sequence of events.) Hypothermia also may be caused by medications that (*a*) alter the perception of cold; (*b*) increase heat loss through vasodilation; or (*c*) inhibit heat generation. (Phenothiazines and barbiturates are frequent offenders.) Common contributing metabolic conditions include adrenal insufficiency, hypoglycemia, and myxedema. Hypothyroidism decreases heat production, blunts the shivering response, and impairs temperature perception. Consequently, myxedema is an etiologic factor in up to 10% of cases of hypothermia. Hypopituitarism, sepsis, diabetic ketoacidosis, malnutrition, and mass lesions of the central nervous system also may induce hypothermia. (The topic of hypothermic sepsis is discussed in detail in Chapter 27.) An intact skin covering and the ability to vasoconstrict are essential to the regulation of core temperature. Therefore, burns and spinal cord injuries both impair the ability to conserve heat. Hypothermia is observed commonly during and immediately after general anesthesia because of exposure to the body to low ambient temperatures and the use of drugs that blunt the vasoconstrictor response (e.g., neuromuscular blockers).

CLINICAL MANIFESTATIONS

Vasoconstriction to conserve heat and shivering to generate heat are important initial compensatory mechanisms to prevent hypothermia. Unfortunately, both responses are blunted by a variety of underlying diseases or drugs and by profound hypothermia. Progressive hypothermia depresses metabolism of essentially all organ systems. The key physiologic events occurring during hypothermia are illustrated in Figure 28.1.

Cardiovascular

Hypothermia decreases cardiac conduction and slows repolarization, prolonging all measured electrocardiographic (ECG) intervals and eventually causing atrioventricular (AV) nodal blockade. Characteristic deformations of the J-point (Osbourn waves) may be seen on the ECG, but are neither sensitive nor specific indicators of core temperature. Myocardial irritability is increased at temperatures lower than 86°F. Conversely, asystole may supervene at temperatures lower than 60°F. Disproportionate reductions of cardiac output and blood pressure often result in metabolic acidosis.

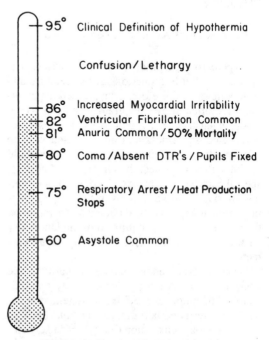

FIG. 28–1. Benchmarks in hypothermia.

Neurologic

Cerebral oxygen consumption is roughly halved for each 10°C (18°F) decline in temperature, making the central nervous system (CNS) more tolerant of reduced perfusion during hypothermia. Initial CNS responses to hypothermia include decreased respiratory drive, lethargy, and fatigue. Coma usually develops when core temperatures fall below 80°F. Concurrent with the loss of consciousness, deep tendon reflexes disappear and the pupils become fixed. Asymmetric cranial nerve dysfunction rarely results from hypothermia, unless an independent CNS event (trauma or stroke) has occurred. Complete neurologic recovery is possible after an hour or more of asystolic cardiac resuscitation of patients with hypothermia.

Renal

Early in hypothermia, tubular dysfunction produces a "cold diuresis" of large volumes of dilute urine (often with an osmolarity <60 mOsm/L). Late in the course of hypothermia, volume contraction and arterial vasoconstriction profoundly decrease renal blood flow. At temperatures lower than 81°F, most patients become anuric.

Respiratory

Correction of Arterial Blood Gas Values

Hypercarbic respiratory drive generally decreases parallel to reductions in temperature and metabolic rate. Therefore, a suppressed hypercarbic drive often allows respiratory acidosis to develop, even though hypoxic drive is preserved. Altered consciousness and an increased volume of respiratory secretions warrant a low threshold for intubation to protect the airway. Furthermore, special caution must be exercised when interpreting arterial blood gas values in this setting. It is important always to record patient temperature on the requisition and to inquire from the laboratory whether the reported values are temperature corrected.

When analyzed under standard conditions, the uncorrected pH is falsely depressed by approximately 0.01 units per 1°F fall in core temperature, whereas arterial carbon dioxide tension ($PaCO_2$) and arterial oxygen tension (PaO_2) are falsely elevated by 2 to 4% per 1°F. Artifactual increases in

gas tensions occur because higher partial pressures are required to keep CO_2 and O_2 in solution as cold blood is warmed to 37°C during analysis. Furthermore, oxygen binds less avidly to warmed hemoglobin, releasing more into solution. If unaccounted for, these artifacts may prompt poor clinical decisions: (a) the use of sodium bicarbonate to treat an artifactual acidosis; (b) overventilation in response to artifactual hypercarbia; (c) withholding supplemental oxygen because reported PaO_2 values seem adequate.

Hematologic

Hypothermia-induced diuresis decreases plasma volume, causing hemoconcentration and increased serum viscosity. The resulting sluggish blood predisposes patients to deep venous thrombosis. The oxyhemoglobin dissociation curve shifts to the left in hypothermia, further decreasing tissue oxygen delivery. Total leukocyte counts usually are normal or slightly increased, but isolated granulocytopenia may be seen. Thrombocytopenia, a common finding, is believed to result from platelet sequestration.

Other Complications

Counter-regulatory hormones, including cortisol, epinephrine, glucagon, and growth hormone, are increased in hypothermia, frequently causing hyperglycemia. Skeletal and cardiac muscle enzymes may increase in response to membrane dysfunction or rhabdomyolysis. Pancreatitis, ileus, and deep venous thrombosis are common. Although deep venous thrombosis often complicates hypothermia, subcutaneous heparin is absorbed poorly and full anticoagulation is risky. Coexisting or precipitating infections (particularly pneumonia and meningitis) complicate as many as 40% of hypothermia cases. Cold-induced stiffness of the abdominal wall or neck often confounds clinical interpretation by simulating acute abdomen or meningitis.

TREATMENT

General Principles

Many hypothermia deaths are iatrogenic. Overly aggressive treatment, including excessive use of adreneogic agents and prophylactic pacemakers, should be avoided; rewarming, close observation, and gentle patient handling are key factors in successful therapy. Fluids should be replaced cautiously to maintain blood pressure and vital organ perfusion. Central venous catheters are preferred for fluid and drug administration because peripheral intravenous lines are difficult to place (due to vasoconstriction) and allow only sluggish infusion. Delivery of vasoactive drugs to the central circulation may be delayed significantly if administered peripherally. Central venous catheters should not be advanced into the right atrium or ventricle, where they may stimulate life-threatening arrhythmias. Serum amylase should be routinely determined as pancreatitis is a common complication of hypothermia. A gently inserted nasogastric tube is useful in management, not only to counter gut hypomotility but also to enable gastric lavage for rewarming. Because many medications have prolonged actions in hypothermia, all drugs must be given cautiously, particularly those that are degraded hepatically.

Rewarming

The aggressiveness with which hypothermia is reversed depends not only on the depth of temperature depression but also on its physiologic manifestations. Caution must be exercised in reversing well-tolerated hypothermia. Passive external rewarming with ordinary blankets usually is adequate if the temperature is higher than 91°F. Active external rewarming may shunt blood away from deep vital tissues to the body surface, producing visceral hypoperfusion and hypotension. Because active external rewarming has been associated with higher mortality rates than passive external or active internal rewarming, it is not recommended.

Internal rewarming may be performed by several methods. Cardiopulmonary bypass and mediastinal lavage are the most rapid methods, but for logistical and safety reasons, are not the techniques of choice. Peritoneal lavage with warmed fluid is an attractive option because it may raise core temperature as quickly as 4°C per hour and can be instituted rapidly. Warmed, fully humidified oxygen (via an endotracheal tube at temperatures up to 46°C) delivers heat more slowly, raising core temperature approximately 1°C per hour. Warm gastric lavage is an adjunctive technique but is not particularly effective when used alone and increases the risk of aspiration in the nonintubated patient. Although insufficient by itself, infu-

sion of warmed intravenous fluids also augments other rewarming methods.

Patients with Cardiovascular Instability

The primary therapeutic goal for patients with life-threatening arrhythmias should be rewarming the core quickly to temperatures higher than 85°F, a threshold below which defibrillation and antiarrhythmic therapy are often ineffective. Bretylium has been reported to be more helpful than lidocaine or procainamide for suppressing ventricular arrhythmias in hypothermia, but no controlled trials have been performed. Digitalis preparations should be avoided. Pacemakers increase myocardial irritability and the risk of ventricular fibrillation. Therefore, they should not be used in the absence of a clear indication.

DIAGNOSIS OF DEATH

Prolonged resuscitative efforts (hours) can prove successful in hypothermia. Therefore, patients with hypothermia must be rewarmed to temperatures exceeding 85°F before death is declared.

HYPERTHERMIA

CAUSES OF TEMPERATURE ELEVATION

In the intensive care unit (ICU), sudden temperature elevations usually signal infection, making it prudent to perform a directed physical examination and, if indicated, obtain appropriate cultures and institute empiric antibiotics. Although infection is the most common explanation, several life-threatening noninfectious causes of fever frequently are overlooked (Table 28.1). Interestingly, conditions producing elevated temperatures in patients in the ICU rarely respond well to acetaminophen. Nonsteroidal anti-inflammatory drugs (e.g., ibuprofen) seem to be much better antipyretic agents than acetaminophen for these patients.

SYNDROMES OF EXTREME HYPERTHERMIA

Even brief episodes of extreme hyperthermia (core temperature higher than 105°F) may perma-

TABLE 28–1

NONINFECTIOUS CAUSES OF FEVER

Heatstroke	Drug allergy
Neuroleptic malignant syndrome	Hyperthyroidism
	Pheochromocytoma
Malignant hyperthermia	Status epilepticus
Allergic drug or transfusion reaction	Vasculitis
	Crystalline arthritis (gout and pseudogout)
Autonomic insufficiency	α-agonist drugs
Malignancy	
Stroke or CNS hemorrhage	Anticholinergic drugs
Alcohol withdrawal/delirium tremens	Salicylate intoxication

nently injure the CNS and must be reduced to safer levels as quickly as possible. In addition to thyroid storm (see Chapter 32, Endocrine Emergencies), four noninfectious conditions producing high fever include: (*a*) classic or nonexertional heatstroke; (*b*) exertional heatstroke; (*c*) neuroleptic malignant syndrome; and (*d*) malignant hyperthermia. All of these conditions are associated with dramatic elevations in core temperature and demand immediate recognition and therapy. Clinical features, etiology, and treatment of these diseases are presented in Table 28.2.

NONEXERTIONAL (CLASSIC) HEATSTROKE

Causes and Mechanisms

Classic heatstroke is a potentially lethal disorder that should be suspected in all patients exposed to high ambient temperatures who develop

altered mental status. Heatstroke is defined by a triad of: (*a*) fever (temperature higher than 105°F), (*b*) hot dry skin, and (*c*) CNS dysfunction. Other organ systems (renal, hematologic) frequently are affected, but their involvement is not necessary for diagnosis. Evaporation of moisture from the skin surface is normally the primary mechanism of heat dissipation, but high humidity and poor air circulation impair the efficiency of this process. Nonexertional heatstroke occurs most commonly among elderly individuals because of an impaired ability to dissipate heat due to decreased sweat production, decreased skin blood flow, impaired hypothalamic regulation, and the use of drugs impairing heat loss. Individuals who are poor, elderly, or inner-city residents are at highest risk. Impaired heat loss also may be seen with extensive burns or skin diseases (e.g., scleroderma) and with the use of occlusive dressings or ointments that cover large skin areas. Low cardiac output, dehydration, and use of β-blockers, diuretics, or peripheral vasoconstrictors reduce cutaneous perfusion and may contribute to heatstroke by this mechanism. CNS tumors, stroke, and certain drugs (e.g., cocaine, lysergic acid diethylamide [LSD], amphetamines) may disrupt hypothalamic heat regulation. Other drugs may produce heatstroke through increased heat production (e.g., cocaine, tricyclics, lithium, or alcohol withdrawal), by impairing heat loss (e.g., anticholinergics, phenothiazines, diuretics, and tricyclics), or by a combination of these two mechanisms.

Laboratory studies commonly are abnormal in nonexertional heatstroke. Arterial blood gases should be corrected for temperature. The most

TABLE 28–2

FEATURES OF HEATSTROKE, NEUROLEPTIC MALIGNANT SYNDROME, AND MALIGNANT HYPERTHERMIA

Feature	Malignant Hyperthermia	Neuroleptic Malignant Syndrome	Classic Heat Stroke	Exertional Heat Stroke
Usual age	<30	<30	>60	Any age
Common precipitants	Succinylcholine, halogenated anesthetics	Neuroleptics	Diuretics, tricyclics, anticholinergics	Hot environment Confining garments
Mechanism	Increased heat production ? Impaired Ca^{++} reuptake	Increased heat production ? Dopamine receptor blockade	Impaired heat loss	Impaired heat loss
Therapy	Remove offending agent, dantrolene	Dantrolene, bromocriptine	External cooling	External cooling

?, questionable mechanism.

common acid–base pattern is respiratory alkalosis, but metabolic acidosis commonly is superimposed. Outcome correlates poorly with the degree of acidosis. Rhabdomyolysis often is responsible for the hypocalcemia, hypokalemia, and elevations in creatinine phosphokinase (CPK) and serum glutamic oxaloacetic transaminase (SGOT) that commonly accompany heatstroke, although rhabdomyolysis is more common in exertional heatstroke. Abnormal coagulation studies are seen in about 10% of patients, and hyponatremia occurs in about half of all cases.

Complications and Prognosis

Renal damage from heatstroke is the result of dehydration, hyperuricemia, and rhabdomyolysis and is much more common in exertional heatstroke than classic heatstroke. This difference is based on the higher incidence of volume depletion and rhabdomyolysis. Heatstroke also may result in "high output" heart failure. Prolonged fever, exceedingly high temperature, and elevated serum lactate values portend CNS damage and death.

Treatment

With the exception of therapy to rapidly lower temperature, the treatment of heatstroke is supportive. Core temperature should be lowered to <103°F as quickly as possible. The most effective method of cooling is through the use of convection and evaporation, not conduction. Spraying unclothed heatstroke victims with tepid water and using a fan to encourage evaporation cools most patients to lower than 103°F within 60 minutes. Ice packing or ice water immersion produces conductive heat loss rapidly but has major limitations in addition to the difficulty of implementation. Immersion causes intense peripheral vasoconstriction, encouraging maintenance of the core temperature. Furthermore, rebound elevations of temperature may be more common after ending treatment. Fluid deficits in heatstroke average approximately 1.5 L, but the extent of dehydration is highly variable. α-agonists and atropine in support of the circulation should be avoided whenever possible, because drug-induced peripheral vasoconstriction further impairs heat loss.

EXERTIONAL HEATSTROKE

Causes

Exertional heatstroke usually is the result of vigorous physical exercise by an otherwise healthy young person in a hot, humid environment. (Occult sickle cell trait and sickle cell C disease occasionally have been discovered in apparently healthy, black military recruits suffering heatstroke.) Victims of exertional heatstroke commonly are involved in activities they continue long after perceiving the sensation of extreme heat (e.g., military training, firefighting, law enforcement, athletic activity). Furthermore, these patients often are wearing heavy or restrictive equipment that impairs heat loss. In addition to environmental stress, predisposing factors include dehydration and lack of training and acclimatization.

Clinical Features

Clinical features include temperature higher than 105°F, altered mental status, hypotension, tachycardia, and tachypnea. Laboratory data often suggest a diagnosis of rhabdomyolysis with elevated SGOT, CPK, and myoglobinuria. Renal function tests often are abnormal as a result of dehydration and rhabdomyolysis. Hemoconcentration can be profound and tends to be more frequent and severe in exertional than classic heatstroke because of the greater fluid losses.

Treatment

Therapy includes discontinuing activity, moving the patient to a cooler environment, rehydration, and external cooling. Removal of clothing and spraying the patient with cool water seem to be the best method to rapidly lower temperature. Blowing a fan across the disrobed victim may accelerate evaporative heat loss. Even with rapid lowering of body temperature, mortality rates as high as 10% have been reported.

MALIGNANT HYPERTHERMIA

Causes

Malignant hyperthermia is a rare but dramatic disorder caused by excessive heat generation in muscle, probably a result of altered calcium kinetics. Malignant hyperthermia is most commonly a disease of young people in which the temperature may rise as fast as 2°C (3.6°F) per minute within minutes of drug exposure. Although usually rapid in onset, hyperthermia can be delayed up to 12 hours after drug exposure and, therefore, should be considered in the differential diagnosis of early, severe postoperative fever (post-anesthesia). Predisposition to malignant hyperthermia is an autosomal dominant trait usually expressed after exposure to anesthetic drugs. Halothane and succinylcholine precipitate more than 80% of all cases of malignant hyperthermia, although other halogenated anesthetics, neuromuscular blockers, ketamine, and phencyclidine (PCP) can be responsible. Muscle biopsy and provocative testing can help make the diagnosis before the onset of the syndrome in most patients at risk.

Diagnosis

The diagnosis must be a clinical one recognized by the occurrence of (*a*) muscular rigidity, (*b*) high and rapidly developing fever (often 41–45°C); and (*c*) tachycardia. Extreme muscle activity causes increased oxygen consumption and CO_2 production. Malignant hyperthermia produces hypoxia, hypercarbia, and metabolic acidosis, which may cause arrhythmias and skin mottling. The differential diagnosis of malignant hyperthermia includes thyroid storm and pheochromocytoma. Neither lumbar puncture nor electroencephalogram (EEG) is helpful in explaining the altered mental status. Phosphate, uric acid, and muscle enzymes (CPK, lactic dehydrogenase, lactate dehydrogenase [LDH], aldolase) are elevated routinely as a result of rhabdomyolysis.

Complications

Massive increases in metabolic rate cause hypercapnia, hypoxemia, and hypoglycemia in a large percentage of cases. When not treated promptly, malignant hyperthermia can produce severe muscle damage with necrosis and soft tissue calcification. Circulating myoglobin may produce renal failure. In such cases, renal damage may be averted by alkalinizing the urine and by maintaining blood pressure and tubular flow. High cardiac output with low systemic vascular resistance may result in hypotension, but dopamine or α-agonists should be used cautiously because vasoconstriction may retard heat loss. Tissue hypoxia is more intense in malignant hyperthermia than in heatstroke or neuroleptic malignant syndrome, accounting for a higher incidence of cardiac arrhythmias and muscular damage.

Direct thermal toxicity may cause neuronal death. The hippocampus and the Purkinje cell layer of the cerebellum are particularly vulnerable, accounting for a high incidence of movement disorders after recovery. Prophylactic anticonvulsants may prevent the seizures that occur almost universally in malignant hyperthermia. Prophylactic use of histamine blockers or antacids is indicated to counteract the tendency for gastrointestinal hemorrhage. Hepatic necrosis and cholestasis are seen infrequently. Late hematologic effects include increased leukocyte and platelet counts, coagulopathy resulting from impaired liver function, and direct thermal activation of platelets and clotting factors.

Treatment

Malignant hyperthermia is a true emergency; mortality relates directly to the magnitude and duration of peak temperature. Even brief delays in therapy may prove fatal. Anesthesia must be terminated immediately and breathing circuit elements must be changed out. Direct external cooling and specific treatment with dantrolene (2–10 mg/kg) should be initiated as soon as possible. Dantrolene may uncouple excitation–contraction mechanisms and inhibit calcium release to stop heat generation, but response to dantrolene is not diagnostic (heatstroke and neuroleptic malignant syndrome also may respond). Corticosteroids do not improve outcome and should not be used. Drugs believed safe in malignant hyperthermia include nitrous oxide, barbiturates, diazepam, pancuronium, and opiates. Patients with malignant hyperthermia usually have normal circulating volume, unlike patients with exertional heatstroke who are typically dehydrated.

NEUROLEPTIC MALIGNANT SYNDROME

Definition

Like malignant hyperthermia, neuroleptic malignant syndrome is a rare drug-induced hyperthermic syndrome characterized by fever, muscle rigidity, altered mentation, and frequently accompanied by pulmonary dysfunction and autonomic instability. It differs, however, regarding precipitating factors, underlying mechanism, time course, prognosis, and patient substrate. Laboratory abnormalities all are nonspecific and include elevated CPK, leukocytosis, and elevated liver function tests. Lumbar puncture and head computed tomography (CT) are not diagnostically helpful. Other diseases in the differential diagnosis of neuroleptic malignant syndrome include heatstroke, pheochromocytoma, anticholinergic toxicity, and monoamine oxidase (MAO) inhibitor crisis.

Causes

Neuroleptic malignant syndrome occurs in fewer than 1% of all patients receiving neuroleptic drugs. Phenothiazines, butyrophenones, and thioxanthines all have been associated with the syndrome, but haloperidol is the single most frequently recognized association. Interestingly, neuroleptic malignant syndrome has been reported only rarely in patients in the ICU who receive intravenous haloperidol for agitation. Most patients develop symptoms within 4 weeks of initiating therapy or increasing drug dosage; however, the syndrome may occur after a single dose or at any time during therapy. Neuroleptic malignant syndrome also has been reported when anti-Parkinsonian (dopaminergic) drugs are discontinued abruptly. Regardless of etiology, symptoms develop over 24 to 72 hours and usually last about 10 to 14 days. (A longer duration may accompany longer-acting neuroleptics.) The cause of neuroleptic malignant syndrome is uncertain but probably is due to blockade of dopaminergic receptors in the corpus striatum. Acetylcholine receptor blockade is proposed as a second potential mechanism. Dehydration and muscular exhaustion predispose patients to neuroleptic malignant syndrome.

Clinical Features

Rapid onset of significant fever, muscle rigidity, altered sensorium, autonomic instability, and extrapyramidal movement disorders characterize the syndrome. As is evident, clinical features alone may not distinguish this syndrome from malignant hyperthermia (especially for the immediately postoperative patient treated with haloperidol for agitation).

Laboratory

Laboratory abnormalities all are nonspecific and include elevated CPK, elevated creatinine, leukocytosis, and elevated liver function tests. Lumbar puncture and head CT are not helpful.

Complications

Even with appropriate treatment, neuroleptic malignant syndrome is fatal in 20 to 30% of cases and frequently is complicated by rhabdomyolysis, acute myocardial infarction, and persistent movement disorders. Not all patients with neuroleptic malignant syndrome relapse when rechallenged with similar neuroleptic drugs. Although the degree of crossover between malignant hyperthermia and neuroleptic malignant syndrome is unknown, some patients who have had malignant hyperthermia undergo uneventful therapy with neuroleptic drugs, suggesting that malignant hyperthermia and neuroleptic malignant syndrome have different etiologies, despite a similar clinical appearance.

Treatment

As with malignant hyperthermia, the treatment of neuroleptic malignant syndrome requires stopping the offending drug and administering dantrolene in intravenous doses up to 10 mg/kg. Although not proven to be effective, external cooling measures seem reasonable. Bromocryptine, amantadine, and neuromuscular paralysis with pancuronium also may be useful in controlling the muscular rigidity.

KEY POINTS

1. Body temperature is the result of the net balance between heat generated and heat lost. In general, loss of heat is a much more efficient process than heat generation when environmental stresses act to displace body temperature from normal.

2. The method of temperature measurement is important in recognizing fever or hypothermia. Many thermometers cannot detect temperatures below 94°F or above 105°F. In the ICU, a thermocouple on a pulmonary artery monitoring catheter sampling central blood (core temperature) is the most accurate but obviously invasive method. Oral and axillary temperatures are much less accurate because of problems of tachypnea and poor thermometer–body contact, respectively. The most practical reliable temperature monitoring site in the ICU patient is the rectum.

3. Hypothermia usually is multifactorial in origin, involving exposure to low ambient temperatures in a patient with infection, hypothyroidism, or drug or alcohol use. Reduced temperatures alter the function of every major body system.

Although controversial, passive external rewarming probably is the best method for most patients with initial temperatures at or above 91°F. Passive rewarming can be supplemented by warmed gastric lavage, heated humidified ventilator gas, and warmed intravenous fluids. Peritoneal lavage or cardiopulmonary bypass are rarely necessary.

4. Exertional and nonexertional heatstroke, although due primarily to environmental stress, often are complicated by underlying cardiovascular diseases and medication and illicit drug use. Lowering ambient air temperature and spraying the patient with a windblown mist of water are the most efficient methods to achieve rapid cooling. Fluid replacement is adjunctive; deficits are much more prominent in patients with exertional heatstroke than classic heatstroke.

5. Malignant hyperthermia, a potentially lethal syndrome, precipitated by use of inhalational anesthesia and neuromuscular blockade, must be considered as a cause of fever in the operative and perioperative periods. When the characteristic muscle rigidity and high fever are recognized, precipitating drug exposure must be terminated and a combination of external cooling and dantrolene must be initiated.

6. Neuroleptic malignant syndrome, another chemical-induced hyperthermic disease, can be caused by neuroleptic drug use or withdrawal of dopaminergic agents. Onset may occur any time neuroleptic drugs are used but is more common with the initiation of therapy or with a change in drug dose. Termination of the offending drug and dantrolene therapy are indicated.

SUGGESTED READINGS

1. Biancolini CA, Del Bosco CG, Jorge MA, et al. Active core rewarming in neurologic, hypothermic patients: effects on oxygen-related variables. Crit Care Med 1993; 21:1164–1168.
2. Caroff SN, Mann SC. Neuroleptic malignant syndrome. Med Clin North Am 1993;77:185–202.
3. Costrini A. Emergency treatment of exertional heatstroke and comparison of whole body cooling techniques. Med Sci Sports Exerc 1990;22:15–18.
4. Danzl DF, Hedges JR, Pozos RS. Hypothermia outcome score: development and implications. Crit Care Med 1989; 17:227–231.
5. Gallant EM, Ahern CP. Malignant hyperthermia: responses of skeletal muscles to general anesthetics. Mayo Clin Proc 1983;58:758–763.
6. Graham BS, Lichtenstein MJ, Hinson JM, et al. Non-exertional heatstroke: physiologic management and cooling in 14 patients. Arch Intern Med 1986;146:87–91.
7. Guze BH, Baxter LR. Neuroleptic malignant syndrome. N Engl J Med 1985;313:163–166.
8. Hudson LD, Conn RD. Accidental hypothermia. JAMA 1974;227:37–40.
9. Kelman GR. Nomograms for correction of blood PO_2, PCO_2, pH and base excess for time and temperature. J Appl Physiol 1966;21:1484–1487.
10. Knochel JP. Heat stroke and related heat stress disorders. Dis Mon 1989;35:301–377.
11. Kurlan R, Hamill R, Shoulson I. Neuroleptic malignant syndrome. Clin Neuropharmacol 1984;7:109–120.
12. Nelson TE, Flewellen EH. The malignant hyperthermia syndrome. N Engl J Med 1983;309:416–418.
13. Otto RJ, Metzler MH. Rewarming from experimental hypothermia: comparison of heated aerosol inhalation, peritoneal lavage and pleural lavage. Crit Care Med 1988;16: 869–875.
14. Reuler JB. Hypothermia: pathophysiology, clinical settings, and management. Ann Intern Med 1978;89: 519–527.
15. Rohrer MJ, Natale AM. Effect of hypothermia on the coagulation cascade. Crit Care Med 1992;20:1402–1405.
16. Sakkas P, Davis JM, Janicak PG, Wang ZY. Drug treatment of the neuroleptic malignant syndrome. Psychopharmacology Bulletin 1991;27(3):1–4.
17. Simon HB, Daniel, GH. Hormonal hyperthermia: endocrinologic causes of fever. Am J Med 1979;66:257–263.
18. Simon HB. Hyperthermia. N Engl J Med 1993;329: 483–487.
19. Welton DE, Mattox KL, Miller RR, et al. Treatment of profound hypothermia. JAMA 1978;240:2291–2292.
20. Weyman AE, Greenbaum DM, Grace WJ. Accidental hypothermia in an alcoholic population. Am J Med 1974; 56:13–20.
21. Wong KC. Physiology and pharmacology of hypothermia. West J Med 1983;138:227–232.

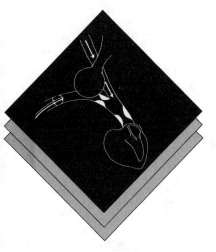

CHAPTER 29

Acute Renal Failure and Dialysis

Because the kidney's excretory function can be taken over by dialysis and its metabolic functions can be compensated for pharmacologically or by the actions of the lung and liver, the kidney represents the only organ whose total failure is not necessarily fatal. Since the first edition of this book, a greater appreciation of the importance of maintaining adequate perfusion and avoiding nephrotoxic compounds may have reduced the incidence and severity of acute renal failure. Furthermore, when acute injury renders the kidney nonfunctional, dialysis and other support technologies have improved markedly.

INDICES OF RENAL FUNCTION

Because the kidney is the primary excreter of nitrogenous waste, concentrations of blood urea nitrogen (BUN) and creatinine track renal function. The extreme variation of urea load and the ability of the tubule to absorb filtered urea renders BUN less reliable than creatinine for this purpose. As general guidelines, the BUN increases 10 to 15 mg/dL/day and creatinine increases 1 to 2.5 mg/dL/day after abrupt renal shutdown. The serum potassium usually rises less than 0.5 mEq/L/day, and HCO_3^- falls by approximately 1 mEq/L/day. Under the catabolic stress of burns, trauma, rhabdomyolysis, steroids, sepsis, or starvation, the rates of change of these parameters may be doubled. In contrast to BUN, daily creatinine production is relatively constant. A rising creatinine indicates that the rate of production exceeds its clearance by glomerular filtration. Therefore, a stable elevation of creatinine implies that a new steady state has been achieved at a decreased glomerular filtration rate (GFR). Until creatinine stabilizes, the severity of acute renal dysfunction and creatinine clearance cannot be assessed reliably. Because serum creatinine lags behind the deterioration in GFR, drug doses usually are overestimated during the development of acute renal failure. If shutdown continues, creatinine usually levels out at approximately 12 to 15 mg/dL, depending on catabolic state. (Rhabdomyolysis can cause creatinine to transiently exceed this value.) Ketones, dobutamine, flucytosine, and cefoxitin can cause artifactual elevations in measured serum creatinine.

Urine volume usually reflects kidney perfusion, whereas urine-specific gravity parallels concentrating ability (tubular function). Therefore, renal blood flow probably is adequate in nonoliguric patients. Furthermore, patients producing concentrated urine are unlikely to have significant tubular damage. Certain calculated indices may be helpful in separating problems of perfusion from those of tubular dysfunction (Table 29.1).

ETIOLOGY OF ACUTE RENAL FAILURE

Approximately 20% of critically ill patients develop acute renal failure—an incidence five times that of the general hospital population. As is the case with pneumonia, the etiology of renal failure differs drastically depending on whether the condition develops in the community or in the hospital and the chronicity of the process. For example,

TABLE 29–1

LABORATORY INDICES IN ACUTE RENAL FAILURE

	Prerenal	Intrarenal
BUN/Creatinine	>10:1	≈ 10:1
Urinary Na^+ concentration	<20 mEq/L	>40 mEq/L
Urine osmolality	>500 mOsm/L	<300–400 mOsm/L
Urine creatinine/plasma creatinine	>40	<20
Urine Na^+/creatinine clearance	<1	>2
Na^+ clearance/creatinine clearance (FeNa)	<1	>1
Urine sediment	Normal	Active

poorly controlled hypertension and diabetes mellitus are the most common etiologies of chronic or slowly developing renal failure outside the hospital. When acute renal failure develops outside the hospital, glomerulonephritis, vasculitis, and obstructive uropathy are the most common causes. In contrast, acute renal failure developing in the hospital is much more likely to be the result of hypoperfusion or drug toxicity.

Acute renal failure may be classified as oliguric (<15 mL/hour) or nonoliguric. The mortality of oliguric renal failure (approximately 50%) is at least two-fold greater than nonoliguric failure, a difference that probably stems from the high incidence of shock and sepsis, leading to the oliguric form. Because 25 to 50% of acute renal failure is induced by volume depletion or nephrotoxic drug use, prevention is key. Acute renal failure may result from a variety of causes acting through one of three common mechanisms: (*a*) hypoperfusion (prerenal); (*b*) outlet obstruction (postrenal); or (*c*) parenchymal disease (intrarenal) (Fig. 29.1).

PRERENAL FAILURE

Hypoperfusion accounts for half of all cases of acute renal failure; therefore, prevention of hypotension or rapid reversal is probably the single most effective therapy. Although prolonged renal ischemia alone may lead to acute renal failure, in most cases, the etiology is multifactorial (i.e., sepsis, drugs, and hypotension). In general, mean arterial pressures below 60 to 70 mm Hg for longer than 30 minutes risk renal injury. Renal hypoperfusion results from circulatory failure, hypotension, vascular obstruction (e.g., renal artery stenosis, vasculitis, or bland clot or cholesterol embolization), or maldistribution of cardiac output (as in sepsis). Marked increases in intra-abdominal pressure, usually exceeding 40 mm Hg,

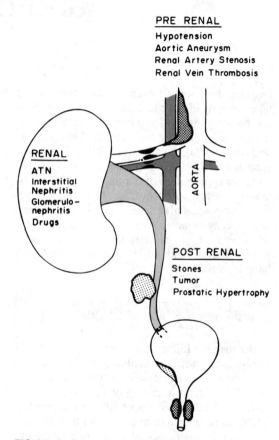

FIG. 29–1. Common causes of acute renal failure in the intensive care unit.

resulting from the accumulation of ascitic fluid, blood, or post-surgical edema in a closed abdomen also can effect pre-renal physiology. The hepatorenal syndrome and the renal response to positive end-expiratory pressure (PEEP) mimic prerenal physiology by redistributing blood flow away from the filtering glomerulus.

Indicators of Intravascular Volume Status

Orthostatic blood pressure is a helpful clinical measure of intravascular volume status in healthy persons. However, few critically ill patients can be tested in this fashion, and autonomic insufficiency may render such changes less reliable for patients who are diabetic, elderly, or bedridden. Dry mucous membranes, skin laxity, and absence of axillary moisture also may be clues to hypovolemia. Unfortunately, these signs also prove unreliable in patients with hyperpnea or advanced age.

Because noninvasive methods to assess fluid status (chest radiograph and echocardiogram) are not sensitive tests of intravascular volume depletion, invasive monitoring is often undertaken (see Chapter 2, Hemodynamic Monitoring). The need for invasive monitoring is controversial, however, because no particular values for wedge pressure, cardiac output, or systemic vascular resistance guarantee sufficient or inadequate renal blood flow. That is, the pressure and flow at the level of the glomerulus are gauged poorly by hemodynamic indices obtained from a pulmonary artery monitoring catheter.

In prerenal failure, the urinalysis is normal or minimally abnormal with hyaline casts and other nonspecific sediment. A prerenal state prompts the tubule to reabsorb sodium and water, yielding a concentrated urine with low sodium. Typically, the urine sodium is less than 20 mEq/L, the urine osmolality exceeds 500 mOsm/L, and the urine specific gravity is above 1.015. The fractional excretion of sodium (FeNa) is another commonly used index to identify prerenal conditions. FeNa is calculated as the ratio of the product of the urine sodium concentration times the plasma creatinine concentration to the product of the plasma sodium concentration times the urine creatinine concentration.

FeNa =

$$100 \times [([\text{Urine sodium}] \times [\text{Plasma creatinine}])/$$

$$([\text{Plasma sodium}] \times [\text{Urine creatinine}])]$$

FeNa values less than 1% generally are indicative of prerenal disease, whereas values greater than 3% usually reflect acute tubular disorders such as acute tubular necrosis. For urine sodium or FeNa measurements to be valid, the underlying sodium reabsorbing capacity of the renal tubule must be intact. For this reason, chronic renal failure, hypoaldosteronism, and metabolic alkalosis may all render tests of urine sodium invalid. Likewise, diuretic therapy invalidates urine sodium determinations for at least 24 hours after administration. Osmotic agents (glucose, mannitol, radiographic contrast material) also may confuse interpretation of urine chemistry values by producing dilute urine.

Although the BUN may be disproportionately high because of increased urea production resulting from tetracycline, corticosteroids, or gastrointestinal (GI) bleeding, an elevated BUN:creatinine ratio more commonly results from reduced tubular urine flow and increased tubular reabsorption of urea nitrogen. Therefore, in prerenal states, the BUN:creatinine ratio usually is elevated (>10:1). Because the renal tubules cannot absorb creatinine, reduced tubular flow rates have no effect on the creatinine concentration if GFR is preserved. Comparing urea clearance to creatinine clearance will determine whether increased urea production or decreased urea excretion is the cause of an elevated BUN. If the urea:creatinine clearance ratio is >1, increased production is the likely etiology. The most common clinical task is to differentiate prerenal disease from acute tubular necrosis. Table 29.1 compares the more common renal function indices in these two conditions. Imaging studies of the kidneys also may provide clues to the cause of acute renal failure (Table 29.2). In pure prerenal azotemia, the kidneys should be of normal size when imaged with ultrasound, CT, or nuclear medicine techniques. Small kidneys suggest a more chronic process.

POSTRENAL FAILURE

After prerenal causes have been excluded, obstructive or postrenal causes (e.g., urinary calculi, tumor, prostatic hypertrophy, blood clot, retroperitoneal hemorrhage) should be considered. Even though obstructive disease accounts for only 1 to 10% of cases of acute renal failure, this reversible problem should not be overlooked. The pattern of decline in urine flow can provide a valuable clue to the presence of obstructive disease. In both prerenal and intrarenal failure, the development of oliguria or anuria usually is gradual over a period of hours to days, whereas an abrupt cessation of urine flow often occurs with obstructive uropathy. (Clearly, urethral obstruction by prostatic enlargement, trauma, or blood clot is the most common cause of anuria.) Upper tract obstruction produces anuria only if it is bilateral or if it occurs in a patient with a single kidney or drainage pathway.

Urethral obstruction may be excluded immediately or confirmed by the attempt to place a uri-

TABLE 29–2

KIDNEY SIZE AS A CLUE TO THE ETIOLOGY OF RENAL FAILURE

Normal	Enlarged	Small
Acute glomerulonephritis	Amyloidosis	Chronic renal failure
Acute tubular necrosis	Acute glomerulonephritis	Chronic hypertension
Acute cortical necrosis	Acute interstitial nephritis	
Acute interstitial nephritis	Obstructive uropathy	
Hepatorenal syndrome	Renal vein thrombosis	
Malignant hypertension	Acute transplant rejection	
Renal artery obstruction		
Scleroderma		

nary catheter into the bladder. Because of the high incidence of urinary collecting system abnormalities, however, urinary bladder catheterization alone never excludes the possibility of more proximal obstructive uropathy. In patients with indwelling catheters, the possibility of clogged catheter should not be overlooked as a potential cause of sudden anuria. Renal ultrasonography or CT scans can detect hydronephrosis and urinary obstruction within or proximal to the bladder, and nuclear renal scans assess flow or tubular function. The intravenous pyelogram (IVP) is not likely to be useful in obstructive uropathy unless stones or trauma are suspected. Furthermore, IVP contrast is potentially nephrotoxic.

In obstructive uropathy, the urinalysis is usually normal, at least initially, and urine chemistries are seldom helpful. A notable exception would be discovery of hematuria, suggesting papillary necrosis, or obstruction by renal stone or clot.

INTRARENAL FAILURE

The urinalysis and urinary chemistry profile provide vital clues to distinguish prerenal from intrarenal causes for acute renal failure (Tables 29.1 and 29.3). However, no single index of renal function yields a specific diagnosis in acute renal failure. For example, although the fractional excretion of sodium (FeNa) usually is higher than 1 when "intrarenal" failure occurs, diuretic use, glycosuria, mannitol, and prolonged urinary obstruction can produce identical findings. Similarly, the urinalysis can be very informative if it reveals red cell casts, eosinophils, or crystals but rarely is unequivocal. The size of the kidneys also may provide a useful clue to the etiology of renal failure. The kidneys usually are small when renal failure is chronic. In contrast, normal size or large

kidneys are much more common in acute renal failure. Renal enlargement is indicative of a limited number of acute etiologies, including obstruction, renal vein thrombosis, and transplant rejection (Table 29.2).

There are three major categories of acute intrarenal failure: (a) tubular disorders, (b) interstitial nephritis; and (c) glomerulonephritis or small-vessel vasculitis.

Tubular Disorders

After prerenal azotemia, nephrotoxic drugs are the most common cause of acute renal failure. Patients who are elderly, dehydrated, hypertensive, diabetic and/or have mild underlying renal dysfunction and myeloma are at particular risk of drug-induced renal insufficiency. Aminoglycosides, contrast agents, cyclosporine, platinum-

TABLE 29–3

URINE SEDIMENT IN ACUTE RENAL FAILURE

Urine Sediment	Associated Etiology
Red cell casts	Glomerulonephritis, vasculitis, trauma
Heme pigmented casts	Hemoglobinuria, myoglobinuria
Leukocyte casts	Pyelonephritis, papillary necrosis
Renal tubular casts	Acute tubular necrosis
"Muddy" granular casts	Acute tubular necrosis
Leukocytes	Urinary tract infection, interstitial nephiritis
Eosinophils	Interstitial nephritis
Crystals	Urate, oxalate (ethylene glycol)

based chemotherapeutic agents, angiotensin-converting enzyme (ACE) inhibitors, and nonsteroidal anti-inflammatory drugs (NSAIDs) are the most commonly implicated causes.

Aminoglycosides cause renal insufficiency in 10 to 20% of all individuals who receive them by binding and damaging cellular proteins in the proximal tubule. The resulting acute tubular necrosis is most likely when elevated trough levels of drug are sustained. (Aminoglycoside peak levels correlate with antibacterial efficiency, whereas trough levels predict toxicity.) Toxicity is potentiated by preexisting renal disease, volume depletion, and concomitant use of other nephrotoxins. The risk of developing acute renal failure differs only modestly among the most commonly used aminoglycosides. Because it is prolonged exposure of the renal tubule to drug and not peak levels that seem to be the critical determinant of renal damage, dosing aminoglycosides once daily (commonly 5 mg/kg) lowers the risk of nephrotoxicity. Such a dosing schedule also is more convenient and less costly. Because the duration of exposure is the most substantial risk factor for toxicity, limiting the duration of therapy and dosing less frequently reduces risk. Frequent mistakes when using aminoglycosides are to administer multiple doses each day and to empirically treat patients at high risk of toxicity for prolonged periods without a clear indication. This tendency is not restricted to aminoglycosides; however, many physicians underestimate the toxicity and overestimate the benefits of antibiotics, even when infection is unproven. Although aminoglycoside loading doses need no modification, maintenance doses should be reduced in proportion to GFR. (For example, a patient with 50% of predicted GFR should receive approximately 50% of the standard maintenance dose). Serum peak and trough levels should be determined after approximately five half-lives (when steady-state concentrations are achieved). Fortunately, almost all patients with aminoglycoside-induced renal failure recover sufficient renal function to obviate long-term dialysis.

Radiographic contrast agents rarely cause renal insufficiency in patients with normal baseline renal function but frequently produce acute renal failure in patients with underlying renal disease, diabetes mellitus, or paraproteinemia. Risk is proportional to the number of exposures and volume of contrast (highest when doses exceed 2 mL/kg). The toxicity of radiographic contrast may be reduced by prophylactic fluid loading; however, the protective effects of loop diuretics and mannitol are less certain.

NSAIDs may impair renal function in patients with prerenal azotemia, shock, heart failure, cirrhosis, and nephrotic syndrome, but their risk to the average patient in the intensive care unit (ICU) probably has been exaggerated. Prostaglandin E_2 (PGE_2), an endogenous vasodilator, is pivotal in maintaining renal blood flow in patients with high renin/angiotensin states. In such patients, NSAIDs can block PGE_2 formation, decreasing renal blood flow. Furthermore, NSAIDs encourage sodium, potassium, and fluid retention and inhibit diuretic action. If NSAIDs are used, aspirin and sulindac are perhaps the best options. (Recent data reveal that ibuprofen may be used safely in patients with sepsis for several days without significant risk.)

ACE inhibitors reduce renal perfusion and may precipitate renal failure when perfusion is marginal, especially among patients with bilateral renal artery stenosis or a single kidney. Luckily, prompt discontinuation of the ACE inhibitor usually results in rapid return of renal function to baseline. The combination of ACE inhibitors and NSAIDs is especially detrimental to renal function because of synergistic effects on perfusion.

The cellular pigments myoglobin and hemoglobin may induce acute renal failure when released into serum during hemolysis or rhabdomyolysis. Both myoglobin and hemoglobin precipitate in the renal tubules, obstructing them and causing formation of heme-pigmented tubular casts. Contrary to popular belief, rhabdomyolysis does not always result from trauma and may be relatively asymptomatic. Sepsis, seizures, drugs, and prolonged immobilization all can be etiologic, and half of all patients have no complaints of muscle pain, tenderness, or weakness. Clues to rhabdomyolysis include rapidly increasing creatinine with disproportionate rises in potassium, phosphate, and uric acid. Volume loading, osmotic diuretics, and alkalinizing agents may help keep these compounds in solution, thus encouraging their elimination and preventing renal failure.

Interstitial Nephritis

Acute interstitial nephritis is a common but frequently unrecognized allergic event in the renal interstitium, usually in response to a specific drug. Penicillin, sulfonamides, thiazides, ciprofloxacin, rifampin, furosemide, ACE inhibitors, and cimetidine are reported causes. Interstitial nephritis may present with fever, eosinophilia, and rash; however, oliguria and a rising creatinine level are often the only indications. Laboratory clues to di-

TABLE 29–4

COMPLICATIONS OF ACUTE RENAL FAILURE

Metabolic	Cardiovascular	Neurologic
Hyponatremia	Fluid overload	Neuropathy
Hyperkalemia	Hypertension	Dementia
Hypocalcemia	Arrhythmias	Seizures
Hyperphosphatemia	Pericarditis	Hyperuricemia
Hematologic	**Gastrointestinal**	**Infectious**
Anemia	Nausea and vomiting	Urinary tract
Coagulopathy	Gastrointestinal bleeding	Sepsis
		Intravenous catheter
		Pneumonia

agnosis include eosinophilia and eosinophiluria. Hansel's stain is necessary to document urinary eosinophilia. (Wright's stain is pH dependent and often fails to demonstrate eosinophils in the urine.) Removal of the offending drug and high-dose corticosteroids are accepted treatments.

Glomerulonephritis and Vasculitis

Although glomerulonephritis and vasculitis represent a relatively common etiology for acute renal failure developing outside the hospital, they are uncommon causes of abrupt renal failure in the ICU. The diverse spectrum of these disorders includes post-streptococcal glomerulonephritis, rickettsial infection, subacute bacterial endocarditis, systemic lupus erythematous (SLE), malignant hypertension, and drug-related vasculitis. Urinalysis reveals an active sediment containing leukocytes, protein, and the hallmark of glomerulonephritis, red blood cell (RBC) casts. Specific diagnosis may be aided by measurement of serum complement, antinuclear antibody (ANA), rheumatoid factor latex agglutination, hepatitis B surface antigen, and blood culture. Therapy is directed at the underlying condition (e.g., antibiotics for endocarditis, steroids for SLE, and cytotoxic therapy for polyarteritis).

COMPLICATIONS AND TREATMENT OF ACUTE RENAL FAILURE

For established renal failure, treatment is supportive: maintaining acid–base status and electrolyte balance near normal limits and filtering the blood of toxic substances while the kidney recovers function. Because the only therapy after renal failure is established is supportive, it is clear that the best treatment is primary prevention.

Avoiding circulatory crises and recognizing urinary obstruction can prevent most cases of acute renal failure. Careful use of nephrotoxic drugs in appropriate doses is the next most important preventative measure. Volume expansion is effective prophylaxis against acute renal failure induced by contrast agents, rhabdomyolysis, cisplatinum, methotrexate, or cyclophosphamide.

The initial approach to ongoing acute renal failure should be to eliminate prerenal factors, exclude obstructive uropathy when possible, and reverse oliguria. After prerenal and postrenal causes have been excluded, careful review of the history, physical examination, and laboratory and medication records may give clues to the cause. Unfortunately, acute renal failure often occurs in the setting of multiorgan failure, in which potential etiologies are numerous. In this situation, combined renal and respiratory insufficiency is particularly ominous; mortality exceeded 90% in several published series. Interestingly, even with appropriate dialysis, morbidity and mortality remain high as a result of nonuremic causes (Table 29.4). For patients with acute renal failure, supportive care must be meticulous to maximize chances for survival. It is most important to avoid such iatrogenic complications as infection related to monitoring devices, fluid and electrolyte imbalances, drug toxicity, and inappropriate nutritional support.

FLUID MANAGEMENT

Nonoliguric acute renal failure is associated with lower mortality than the oliguric variety. Unfortunately, clinical studies reporting this differential mortality rate often are misinterpreted. A response to measures designed to restore urine flow is not necessarily an indication of improved renal function but simply may serve as an indicator of a patient's overall physiologic condition. Perhaps responders have better baseline renal function or more substantial cardiovascular reserves than nonresponders. Although it has not been proven that restoring urine flow reduces mortality, attempting to convert oliguric to nonoliguric renal failure probably is worthwhile because it vastly simplifies fluid management. Unless there are obvious signs of intravascular congestion, a fluid challenge should be performed first when attempting to reverse oliguria. Volume loading then should be followed by a large dose of loop diuretic (e.g., furosemide, 1 mg/kg). Although single doses of osmotic agents (mannitol, 25–50 gm) also may be effective, these risk volume overload and hyperosmolarity. Measures to reverse the oliguric state are most likely to be successful when undertaken shortly after the reduction in urine flow. When 8 hours or more have elapsed, efforts to restore urine flow by volume loading routinely fail. Invasive monitoring should be considered for patients with tenuous cardiovascular or pulmonary status, but the limitations of the pulmonary artery monitoring catheter in the oliguric patient must be recognized. No unique combination of wedge pressure, cardiac output, and systemic vascular resistance measurements guarantee adequate glomerular blood flow. Dopamine may be a useful adjunct in the treatment of acute renal failure due to hypoperfusion or maldistribution of blood flow. At doses less than 5 μg/kg/minute, dopamine has predominantly renal vasodilating (dopaminergic) and natriuretic (aldosterone antagonist) effects that complement the action of loop diuretics. The vasoactive dose of dopamine varies widely, and if low-dose therapy is ineffective in promoting urine flow, doses higher than 5 μg/kg/minute are worth trying, especially in patients with marginal blood pressure. Contrary to popular belief, the dopaminergic stimulatory properties of this agent are *not* lost (but may be overwhelmed) at higher doses.

ELECTROLYTE DISORDERS

Hyperkalemia, hyponatremia, hypermagnesemia, and hyperphosphatemia are the major electrolyte disturbances of acute renal failure. The primary approach to each disorder is to modify input and/or enhance removal of solute or fluid, as detailed in Chapter 13 (Fluid and Electrolyte Disorders). It is worth noting here that oral phosphate binders (aluminum-containing antacids) usually are capable of suppressing the serum phosphate sufficiently to prevent hypocalcemia. Because

magnesium excretion is impaired in patients with acute renal failure, products containing magnesium (antacids and cathartics) should be avoided.

Water, sodium, and potassium intake should be adjusted to match measured urinary output and normalize serum values. In the resolution phase of acute tubular necrosis, patients frequently undergo a polyuric phase 3 to 4 weeks after onset. Fluid losses may be life-threatening unless appropriately replaced to maintain circulating volume. The cause of the polyuric phase is not known with certainty but probably results from tubular dysfunction in the face of recovering GFR and excess total body water.

INFECTION

Infection-induced multiple organ failure is arguably the most common cause of death in acute renal failure. With the possible exception of pyocystis, a pus-filled nondraining bladder, the infections acquired by patients with renal failure do not differ from those of other patients in the ICU. Nosocomial pneumonia and intravenous-catheter-related infections are most frequent. Among patients dying with renal failure, however, there may be a disproportionate occurrence of intra-abdominal sepsis. The clues to suspect infection and the techniques to diagnose and treat various infections are outlined in Chapter 26 (Common ICU Infections).

BLEEDING DISORDERS

Hemorrhage (primarily GI) accounts for many of the deaths among patients with renal failure. Bleeding is common in acute renal failure due to the inhibitory actions of uremic toxins on platelets and factor VIII. The key to reversing coagulation disorders is to improve the environment in which the platelets and clotting factors function. Most commonly, this is accomplished by treating a reversible cause of renal failure or by dialysis. Replacement of factor VIII with cryoprecipitate or fresh frozen plasma (FFP) may transiently help to correct bleeding defects (see Chapter 14, Transfusion and Blood Component Therapy). Likewise, arginine vasopressin (DDAVP) will improve bleeding time temporarily in uremic patients by increasing levels of factor VIII complex. Platelet transfusions also may briefly improve hemostasis before invasive procedures.

NUTRITION

The production of uremic toxins can be reduced by minimizing catabolism and providing sufficient

TABLE 29–5

CHARACTERISTICS OF BLOOD PURIFICATION METHODS

	Efficiency of Solute Removal		Disequilibrium Syndrome	Cardiovascular Instability	Cause of Hypoxemia	Protein Losses
	Small	Large				
Peritoneal dialysis	Low	Medium	Rare	Rare	High volume	Present
Hemodialysis	Very high	Low	Frequent	Frequent	Acetate/cellophane membrane	Absent
Intermittent hemofiltration	High	High	Frequent	Rare	None	Absent
Continuous hemofiltration	Low	Very high	None	None	None	Absent

calories to prevent protein wasting. Except in interstitial nephritis and some forms of renal vasculitis, corticosteroids should be avoided because of their catabolic effects and suppression of immune function. For most patients with acute renal failure, caloric requirements generally range from 2500 to 3000 calories per day. Sufficient carbohydrate (>100 gm/day) and fat calories should be provided to prevent the catabolism of body protein for energy production. For patients who do not undergo dialysis, protein intake should be limited to 40 to 50 gm/day, most of which should be of high biologic value. In dialyzed patients, protein intake may be liberalized (80–100 gm/day); however, it should be recognized that higher protein intake may necessitate more frequent dialysis. Folate and pyridoxine must be supplemented because they are lost through hemodialysis.

Although controversial, total parenteral nutrition (TPN) using hypertonic glucose, and l-amino acids may reduce the mortality of acute renal failure and hasten recovery of renal function. If TPN is used, a formulation low in Na^+, Mg^{+2}, PO_4^{-3}, and K^+ is mandatory. Insufficient data exist to accurately compare the efficacy of enteral to parenteral nutritional support.

DRUG THERAPY

The need for all drugs should be questioned in acute renal failure. Any drug that may impair renal function should be discontinued or its dosage should be modified appropriately. Renally metabolized or excreted drugs usually require reductions in dosage. As a general guideline, the dosage needs revision in proportion to its percentage of elimination by the kidney and the degree of renal impairment. Dosing of each drug susceptible to renal excretion should be guided by published nomograms. Even when dosage is calculated precisely, serum levels of drugs with a low therapeutic index must be followed.

DIALYSIS

Three basic methods of fluid and solute removal can be used to treat the manifestations of renal failure: ultrafiltration, a process in which fluid and the solute it contains is removed from blood by convection; hemodialysis, a continuous-flow, high-efficiency system combining diffusion and convection to remove fluid and solute from blood; and peritoneal dialysis, a method that uses intermittent exchanges of hypertonic dialysate to draw fluid and solutes across the peritoneal surface. A summary of the characteristics of each of the blood purification methods is provided in Table 29.5.

Ultrafiltration is appropriate when removal of intravascular volume (salt and water) is a primary objective. For example, ultrafiltration has been used successfully to treat metabolic acidosis, replacing filtered fluid with $NaHCO_3$. Unfortunately, uremic toxins (small and mid-molecular-weight molecules) are removed inefficiently. Therefore, ultrafiltration is sometimes used in conjunction with intermittent dialysis. Ultrafiltration can be accomplished using a dialysis machine to power the flow of venous blood across a dialysis membrane or by using the patient's arteriovenous pressure gradient to drive flow through a hollow fiber cartridge. When performed using a dialysis machine, short periods of venovenous filtration can remove large amounts of fluid. When driven by arterial pressure alone, the process is less efficient but inefficiency is counterbalanced by continuous application. Typically, filtration becomes ineffective when mean arterial pressure falls below 60 mm Hg. The rate of filtration may be increased by restricting venous outflow (raising venous pressure), by increasing the arterial pressure, or by increasing the transmembrane filtration pressure (applying suction to the shell surrounding the permeable fibers or by lowering the collection bag if suction is not applied) (Fig. 29.2).

HEMOFILTRATION

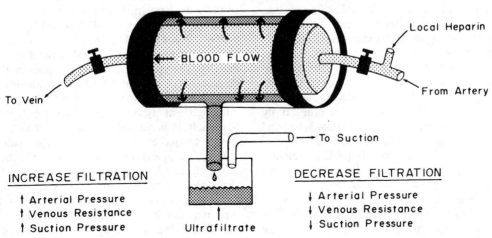

FIG. 29–2. Mechanism of continuous arteriovenous hemofiltration and regulation of ultrafiltrate production.

However, applying suction risks rupture of the filter's fibers. Filtration rate may be decreased by restricting the arterial inflow (by clamping the arterial line). Local anticoagulation (usually with heparin) is required and, unfortunately, the anticoagulant effect often becomes systemic. Clotting of the cartridge used for continuous arteriovenous hemofiltration is common despite anticoagulation. Without careful monitoring of output, patients are prone to volume depletion even though the rates of fluid removal are low.

Hemodialysis provides high blood flow rates across a large, very selective permeable membrane. Consequently, hemodialysis represents the only practical method of removing large quantities of fluid and uremic toxins rapidly. Furthermore, by altering the dialysate present on the opposite side of the permeable membrane, acid–base status and electrolyte concentrations can be manipulated quickly. In the setting of acute renal failure, the indications for dialysis are: (a) fluid overload; (b) refractory hyperkalemia or hypermagnesemia; (c) life-threatening acidosis; (d) symptomatic uremia (e.g., pericarditis, seizures, coma, bleeding, nausea, and vomiting); (e) presence of a dialyzable toxin (salicylate, methanol, ethylene glycol). Dialysis is almost always instituted when the serum creatinine exceeds 8 mg/dL or the BUN approaches 100 mg/dL. In catabolic patients, early dialysis (to maintain creatinine levels lower than 4 mg/dL and BUN lower than 50 mg/dL) may improve outcome.

Acutely, access to the circulation for hemodialysis is achieved by inserting a multilumen central venous catheter. Because of their rigid construction, such catheters are prone to perforate vascular structures during insertion and to erode through vessel walls over time. Particular care should be used in catheter insertion to ensure that the catheter advances easily over the guidewire. Once in place, a radiograph should be obtained to confirm that the catheter tip is aligned with the luminal axis and does not terminate in the heart.

Although more efficient than the peritoneal approach, hemodialysis requires cardiovascular stability; rapid shifts of fluid between intracellular and extracellular compartments are not well tolerated by hemodynamically unstable patients. Hypotension during dialysis is perhaps the most common significant problem. Fluid and electrolyte shifts, reactions to the dialysis membrane or dialysate, and impaired cardiac performance all have been implicated. Many hypotensive episodes result from excessively rapid reduction in preload and respond quickly to crystalloid and low-dose vasopressor support. If transfusion is planned, administration of blood during dialysis helps minimize hypotension. The residual effects of antihypertensive agents used for blood pressure control before institution of dialysis also may contribute to cardiovascular instability. If hypotension recurs with each dialysis session or occurs after only small volumes of fluid have been removed, a reaction to the dialysis membrane or to acetate in the dialysis bath should be suspected.

During hemodialysis, intraneuronal tonicity may not track the abrupt shifts in fluid/solute composition that occur in the extracellular compartment, producing the "dialysis disequilibrium" syndrome. Nausea, vomiting, confusion, seizures, and coma all may be manifestations of the syndrome which occurs most commonly in patients with high BUN concentrations undergoing initial dialysis. Disequilibrium can be minimized by using brief dialysis sessions, low flow rates, and a small surface area dialyzer. Administration of osmotically active compounds (NaCl, mannitol, or dextrose) also can reduce the frequency and severity of the syndrome.

Depending on the choice of dialyzing membrane and dialysate, hypoxemia during hemodialysis may result from leukostasis within the pulmonary capillaries (cuprophane membrane) or from hypoventilation (acetate buffer). Hypoventilation occurs as CO_2 diffuses into the dialysate, reducing the stimulation of ventilatory chemoreceptors.

Peritoneal dialysis can be undertaken in most patients who have a freely communicating and uninflamed peritoneal cavity but is considerably less efficient than hemodialysis in removing toxins or correcting electrolyte imbalances. The major advantages of peritoneal dialysis are the absence of significant hemodynamic effects and the lack of need for vascular access. The process requires insertion of a peritoneal dialysis catheter, which incurs minimal risk. After catheter insertion, 1 to 3 L of dialysis solution is slowly introduced into the peritoneal cavity and allowed to "dwell" for 30 to 40 minutes before drainage. This 1-hour dialysis cycle can be repeated continuously or can be automated using a "cycler." An osmotic gradient for fluid removal is created by using hyperosmolar (350–490 mOsm/L) glucose concentrations (1.5–4.25 gm/dL) in the dialysate. Standard concentrations of sodium and chloride are slightly hypotonic compared to plasma. Concentrations of other electrolytes (potassium and calcium) can be varied from patient to patient. Although hemodynamically well tolerated, peritoneal dialysis is not always feasible or risk-free. The technique cannot be performed on patients with recent laparatomy or active intra-abdominal infection. In addition, abdominal distention during high-volume peritoneal dialysis may drive the diaphragm cephalad, causing atelectasis, hypoxemia, and increased work of breathing. Instilled dialysate also may leak into the chest, resulting in pleural effusion, further impairing lung function. Electrolyte imbalance, significant hyperglycemia, and peritonitis are encountered commonly.

PROGNOSIS

The prognosis of patients with acute renal failure is determined more by the underlying conditions precipitating renal failure than by renal dysfunction itself. Patients do not die from renal failure if dialysis is instituted. Recent data indicate that among patients who do not succumb to their underlying illness, recovery of renal function is the rule rather than the exception.

KEY POINTS

1. The development of acute renal failure is associated with a significant increase in mortality in critically ill patients despite the existence of dialytic support capable of replacing the filtering function of the kidney. Because no specific therapy exists for treating acute renal failure, prevention is critical.

2. Prerenal azotemia and obstructive uropathy are rapidly reversible causes of acute renal failure that should be sought in every case of acute renal failure.

3. Acute renal failure not caused by prerenal or postrenal causes commonly is the result of hypoperfusion and drug-induced disease.

4. Drug therapy must be selected carefully and adjusted for the degree of renal insufficiency.

5. For most patients with uremic symptoms, temporary hemodialysis represents the best option for managing fluid status, uremia, and electrolyte and acid–base disorders. If fluid overload is the sole problem, hemofiltration represents a reasonable alternative.

6. When acute renal failure occurs in the setting of sepsis and multiple organ failure, renal function can be expected to return to near-baseline levels, provided the patient survives the critical phase of illness.

SUGGESTED READINGS

1. Appel BB. Aminoglycoside nephrotoxicity. Am J Med 1990;159:427–443.
2. Better OS, Stein JH. Early management of shock and prophylaxis of acute renal failure in traumatic rhabdomyolysis. N Engl J Med 1990;322:825–829.
3. Bryan CS, Stone WJ. Antimicrobial dosage in renal failure: a unifying nomogram (updated version). Clin Nephrol 1977;7:81.
4. Cameron JS. Acute renal failure: the continuing challenge. Q J Med 1986;228:337–343.
5. Cerra FB, Anthore S. Colloid osmotic pressure fluctuations and the disequilibrium syndrome during hemodialysis. Nephron 1974;13:245–249.
6. Cullen D, Coyle J, Teplick R, et al. Cardiovascular, pulmonary and renal effects of massively increased intra-abdominal pressure in critically ill patients. Crit Care Med 1989;17:118–121.
7. Dixon BS, Anderson RJ. Nonoliguric acute renal failure. Am J Kidney Dis 1985;6(2):71–80.
8. Graziani G, Cantaluppi A, Casati S, et al. Dopamine and furosemide in oliguric acute renal failure. Nephron 1984; 37:39–42.
9. Kaplan AA, Longnecker RE, Folkert VW. Continuous arteriovenous hemofiltration. Ann Intern Med 1984;100: 358–367.
10. Lazarus JM. Complications in hemodialysis: an overview. Kidney Int 1980;18:S77.
11. Macguire WC, Anderson RJ. Continuous arteriovenous hemofiltration in the intensive care unit. J Crit Care 1986; 1:54–56.
12. Miller TR, Anderson RJ, Linas SL, et al. Urinary diagnostic indices in acute renal failure. Ann Intern Med 1978; 89:47–50.
13. Misson RT, Cutler RE. Radiocontrast-induced renal failure. West J Med 1985;142:657–664.
14. Paller MS. Drug induced nephropathies. Med Clin North Am 1990;74:909–917.
15. Ronco C, Feriani M, Chiaramonte S, et al. Pathophysiology of ultrafiltration in peritoneal dialysis. Perit Dial Int 1990;2:119–126.
16. Speigel DM, Ullian ME, Zerbe GO, Berle T. Determinants of survival and recovery in acute renal failure patients dialyzed in intensive care units. Am J Nephrol 1991;11: 44–47.
17. Velez RL, Woodward TD, Heinrich WL. Acetate and bicarbonate hemodialysis in patients with and without autonomic dysfunction. Kidney Int 1984;26:59.
18. Voerman HJ, Strack von Schijndel RJ, Thijs LG. Continuous arterial-venous hemodiafiltration in critically ill patients. Crit Care Med 1990;18:911–914.

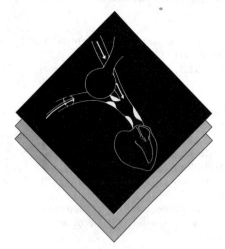

CHAPTER **30**

Clotting and Bleeding Disorders and Anticoagulation Therapy

In the intensive care unit (ICU), bleeding disorders are diagnosed substantially more commonly than clotting disorders. The disparity in diagnostic rates occurs in part because bleeding disorders often display visible signs, whereas thrombotic disorders usually have more protean manifestations. This variation also is explained partly by the fact that routine in vitro laboratory tests detect defective clotting, not an excessive thrombotic tendency; Less is known about disorders producing excessive thrombotic activity. Furthermore, although no single routine laboratory test is indicative of thrombosis, the prothrombin time (PT) alone is a good screening test for most bleeding disorders. In fact, nearly all clinically significant bleeding disorders can be screened for by the addition of a partial thromboplastin time (PTT) and platelet count to the PT. Unfortunately, no abnormal in vitro clotting test value guarantees that bleeding will occur and normal values do not exclude a risk of bleeding with certainty.

BLEEDING DISORDERS

Vascular endothelium, clotting proteins, and platelets comprise the key components of the hemostasis mechanism. Only when two or more of these hemostatic components are defective is spontaneous or uncontrollable hemorrhage likely; impairment of any single factor seldom provokes clinical bleeding. However, because many patients require the ICU by virtue of conditions that violate vascular endothelial integrity (e.g., surgery, trauma, sepsis), it only requires the addition

of a platelet or soluble factor disorder to induce bleeding.

APPROACH TO THE BLEEDING PATIENT

History

The history provides important clues to the etiology of bleeding. With few exceptions, the rarer hereditary disorders produce deficiency or dysfunction of a single clotting factor, whereas the much more common acquired disorders usually cause multiple factor abnormalities. All congenital bleeding disorders are autosomal, except for the sex-linked recessive hemophilias and the very rare Wiskott-Aldrich syndrome. The hemophilias are the most common congenital bleeding disorders. Deficiencies of factors VIII (hemophilia A) and IX (hemophilia B) account for 85% and 12% of congenital bleeding diatheses, respectively. The X-linked recessive inheritance pattern of these diseases dictates an almost exclusively male occurrence. The next most common inherited disorder is von Willebrand's disease, an autosomal dominant disorder producing platelet and/or vessel wall dysfunction. All other inherited factor deficiencies are very rare autosomal recessive conditions; therefore, a negative family history virtually excludes a diagnosis of hereditary coagulopathy.

The coagulation history must include more than just a report of "easy bleeding" or "bruising." Specific answers to the following questions should be sought

1. Has there been prior life-threatening hemorrhage?

2. Has bleeding required transfusion or reoperation?
3. If surgery has been performed (especially oral
surgery), was there excessive bleeding?

The answers to these first three questions can be
very telling; an adult who has never experienced
significant bleeding spontaneously or after surgery or trauma is extremely unlikely to have a
congenital clotting disorder.

4. When did hemorrhage occur in relation to
trauma or surgery? (Immediate intraoperative
bleeding suggests a platelet disorder, whereas
delayed bleeding is more indicative of a soluble factor problem.)
5. What drugs are currently taken? Particular attention should be paid to drugs affecting platelet function (e.g., aspirin, alcohol, and nonsteroidal anti-inflammatory agents) or those
impairing synthesis of vitamin-K-dependent
clotting proteins (warfarin and antibiotics).

Physical Examination

The examiner should search for evidence of pe-
techiae (especially in dependent, high-venous-
pressure areas), purpura, and persistent oozing
from skin punctures or mucosal sites. Such findings are most characteristic of platelet disorders.
Palpable purpura is a sign of small artery occlusion usually associated with vasculitis due to col-
lagen-vascular disease (polyarteritis, systemic
lupus erythematosus [SLE]), endocarditis, or sepsis (especially that resulting from gram-negative
rods or meningococcus). Larger vessel occlusions
from disseminated intravascular coagulation
(DIC) may cause the extensive ecchymoses of
purpura fulminans. In contrast, factor deficiencies
(especially the hemophilias) usually cause deep
muscle and joint bleeding that results in ecchymoses, hematomas, and hemarthroses.

Laboratory Tests

Basic screening clotting tests are indicated for
patients undergoing surgery or invasive procedures and for those with a history that suggests a
bleeding disorder. Clotting tests also are useful
for patients undergoing massive transfusion, anticoagulation, or thrombolytic therapy. When evaluation of clotting status is indicated, a platelet
count, PT, and PTT usually suffice to exclude
clinically important bleeding disorders, but a

bleeding time should be added when platelet dysfunction is suspected. (A PT and PTT will not
detect factor XIII deficiency, a rare cause of hemorrhage.) Not all prolongations of the PT and/or
PTT signify an increased risk of hemorrhage. Deficiencies of factor XII, high-molecular-weight
kininogen or prekallikrein or the presence of anticardiolipin antibody, also known as lupus anticoagulant, may prolong in vitro clotting tests
without increasing bleeding risk. To limit interlaboratory variability in PT testing, most hospitals
now report the standardized international normalized ratio (INR) as well as the PT in relation to the
patient's own baseline or the laboratory's control.

It has long been routine to measure PT, PTT,
and platelet count at the time of admission in almost all hospitalized patients. However, in the absence of a history suggesting hemophilia, von
Willebrand's disease, or heparin use, routine determination of the PTT is extremely unlikely to
yield a true positive abnormality and thus is
wasteful. Likewise, the common practice of measuring both the PT and PTT for all patients receiving warfarin or heparin anticoagulation is also ill
considered; PTT determinations are unnecessary
during warfarin therapy alone and repeated PT
determinations rarely add to the care of patients
receiving only heparin.

INTERPRETATION OF ABNORMAL CLOTTING TESTS

In general, the singular observation of a PT prolonged by 1 or 2 seconds or a PTT prolonged by
as much as 5 seconds should not raise concern in
the absence of active bleeding. In fact, abnormalities of such magnitude in the PTT usually do not
warrant further investigation. Limiting evaluation
of minor PTT abnormalities is an acceptable practice because very few disorders occurring in the
ICU cause an isolated progressive prolongation
of the PTT (e.g., heparin therapy) and the history
will dictate further evaluation for hemophilia or
von Willebrand's disease. On the other hand, it is
often prudent to recheck an isolated prolongation
of the PT of even a few seconds, because many
diseases or interventions undertaken in the ICU
can progressively prolong the PT (e.g., antibiotic
therapy, starvation, progressive hepatic failure).
In the absence of ongoing bleeding, most clinicians do not exhibit undue concern over isolated
reductions in platelet count until levels approach
$100,000/mm^3$. As platelet counts fall below this

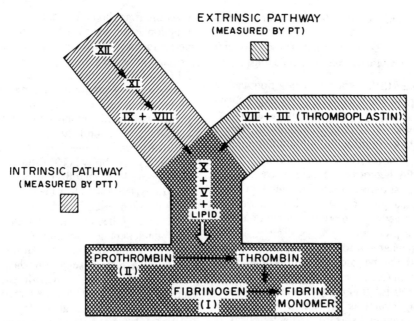

FIG. 30–1. Relationship of PT and PTT to the clotting cascade. Deficiencies of factors in the doubly cross-hatched region (the intersection of intrinsic and extrinsic pathways) produce abnormalities of both tests. The thrombin time tests only the final conversion of fibrinogen to fibrin monomer. Factor XIII (not shown) stabilizes the linkup of fibrin monomers into organized clot.

threshold, bleeding risk increases progressively, and even more strikingly if functional platelet abnormalities exist. As with the PT, many diseases and therapies present in the ICU population can progressively alter the platelet count, and a search for the cause of thrombocytopenia and periodic rechecking of platelet counts is prudent when they decline to the 100,000/mm³ range.

The PT and PTT may be prolonged individually or together. Each potential combination of abnormalities suggests a limited specific set of diagnostic possibilities and a reasonable plan for evaluation.

PROTHROMBIN TIME

The PT is a test of the extrinsic clotting pathway in which factors II, V, VII, and X are activated by adding tissue thromboplastin and calcium to the sample. Because the endpoint of the prothrombin test is clot formation, deficiencies of factor VII (or any factor below factor X in the clotting cascade) can prolong the PT (Fig. 30.1). A normal PT requires each factor in the sequence to have more than 30% of normal activity. Common causes of a prolonged PT are listed in Table 30.1.

The uncommon combination of a normal PTT

TABLE 30–1

COMMON CAUSES OF A PROLONGED PROTHROMBIN TIME

Liver disease

Disseminated intravascular coagulation

Vitamin K deficiency

Warfarin

Excessive heparin

Salicylate poisoning

Circulating anticoagulants

Dilutional coagulopathy

with a prolonged PT is explained by selective deficiency of factor VII. This rarely occurs as a chronic condition, but because factor VII has the shortest half-life of all vitamin-K-dependent clotting proteins (approximately 6 hours), isolated prolongation of PT can occur in early vitamin K deficiency, hepatic failure, or warfarin therapy.

ACTIVATED PARTIAL THROMBOPLASTIN TIME

The PTT tests the intrinsic pathway by adding phospholipid and kaolin, silica, or other particu-

TABLE 30–2

COMMON CAUSES OF A PROLONGED PARTIAL THROMBOPLASTIN TIME

Spurious results (underfilled tube)
Delay in performing assay
Circulating anticoagulants
Heparin
Hemophilia
Von Willebrand's disease

late to activate coagulation. The PTT tests all clotting proteins except factor VII simultaneously, making it the most sensitive test of clotting factor abnormalities but less specific than the PT for the same reason (Fig. 30.1). The combination of a normal PT and a prolonged PTT usually indicates an inherited deficiency or dysfunction of factors VIII, IX, XI, or XII. When both PT and PTT are abnormal, an acquired bleeding disorder almost always is responsible. Common causes of a prolonged activated PTT are listed in Table 30.2. An accurate PTT determination is highly dependent on the presence of a standardized ratio of citrate anticoagulant to blood. Therefore, underfilled blood collection tubes often result in apparent PTT prolongations and may serve as the most common cause of an isolated PTT increase.

COMBINED ABNORMALITIES

Because the extrinsic and intrinsic pathways share common factors, diseases or therapies altering one pathway often affect the other. An overview of the diseases and defects in which isolated or combined abnormalities of the PT and PTT are seen is presented in Table 30.3.

THROMBIN TIME

The thrombin time is a test of the final step in the coagulation cascade that is performed by adding thrombin to an anticoagulated sample, thereby converting fibrinogen to fibrin (see Fig. 30.1). Because only the terminal step in a complex clotting array is surveyed by this test, it detects only a limited number of clotting abnormalities. Fibrinogen levels lower than 100 mg/dL, most commonly from DIC, thrombolytic therapy, or dysfunctional fibrinogen, may prolong the thrombin time. Heparin, fibrin degradation products, and abnormal immunoglobulins also prolong the thrombin time by interfering with thrombin-induced fibrinogen conversion.

BLEEDING TIME

The bleeding time is primarily a test of platelet function but also can be influenced by platelet number and tissue fragility. The bleeding time often will be prolonged if platelets number less than $80,000/mm^3$ and will almost always be prolonged if counts fall below $50,000/mm^3$. As a rule, bleeding times are unreliable when platelet counts fall below $100,000/mm^3$. Unfortunately, a normal or high platelet count does not ensure a normal bleeding time because platelet function may be selectively impaired. Together, a platelet count and bleeding time effectively screen for platelet problems by testing platelet number, adhesion, and aggregation. The bleeding time often is abnormal in patients with uremia and in those receiving drugs that impair platelet function (e.g., aspirin and other nonsteroidal anti-inflammatory drugs). The bleeding time is also prolonged by rare inher-

TABLE 30–3

| Activated PTT | Prothrombin Time | |
	Normal	Prolonged
Normal	Defect: factor XIII Frequency: very rare Dx test: urea solubility assay	Defect: isolated to extrinsic pathway (e.g., early: starvation, warfarin, liver disease, or dilution) Frequency: relatively common but transient Dx test: factor VII assay
Prolonged	Defect: intrinsic pathway (e.g., heparin, hemophilia A and B) Frequency: uncommon Dx test (exclude heparin) then: If bleeding check: VIII, IX, XI levels No bleeding check: prekallikrein, XII, high-molecular-weight kininogen	Defect: combined intrinsic/extrinsic defect (e.g., DIC, liver failure, warfarin, starvation, thrombolytic Rx) Frequency: most common Dx test: DIC panel; fibrinogen; factors II, V, and X; liver function assessment

ited platelet disorders (Bernard-Soulier and Wiskott-Aldrich syndromes), by von Willebrand's disease, and by severe hypofibrinogenemia. Although abnormal platelet function will be detected by a bleeding time, the degree of prolongation correlates poorly with the tendency to bleed.

INHIBITOR TESTING

Only approximately 30% activity of each clotting factor is needed to result in normal clotting assays; therefore, combining equal portions of normal plasma and plasma from a patient with a factor deficiency will yield normal PT and PTT results, unless a factor inhibitor (e.g., anticardiolipin antibody, factor VIII inhibitor, heparin) is present.

FIBRINOGEN AND FIBRIN DEGRADATION PRODUCTS

Fibrinogen levels may be reduced as a result of impaired production or increased consumption. Because fibrinogen is an acute phase reactant released from the liver, it may be elevated in hepatitis or other conditions that cause liver inflammation. Therefore, even if consumption is increased, fibrinogen levels may remain in the normal range.

Fibrin degradation products (FDPs), fibrin monomers, d-dimers, and fibrinopeptide A are all products resulting from the lysis of fibrinogen. Although the fibrin monomer and d-dimer tests are the most sensitive and specific, FDP measurements are most widely available. Recently, clinical investigations have claimed a high predictive value of a negative d-dimer assay in excluding thromboembolic disease (deep venous thrombosis and pulmonary embolism). At present, however, it is premature to use d-dimer levels as definitive evidence against the presence of thromboembolic disease (also see Chapter 23, Venous Thrombosis and Pulmonary Embolism).

PLATELET DISORDERS

CAUSES OF PLATELET-RELATED BLEEDING

Bleeding can occur when either platelet number or function is inadequate. If platelet counts are normal but the bleeding time is prolonged, the next step is to determine whether the problem is

TABLE 30–4

DRUGS INHIBITING PLATELET FUNCTION

Aspirin

Nonsteroidal anti-inflammatory agents

Alcohol

High-dose penicillin or ticarcillin

Moxalactam

Heparin

the platelet itself or caused by the circulating plasma. Platelet defects are assayed by aggregation studies. Plasma of such patients should be evaluated for factor VIII activity. (Humoral factors impairing platelet function include severe hypofibrinogenemia or von Willebrand's disease.)

PROBLEMS OF PLATELET FUNCTION

Drug effects, uremia, DIC, leukemia, von Willebrand's disease, or paraproteinemia can explain a prolonged bleeding time with normal platelet count. The most common drugs to impair platelet function are listed in Table 30.4.

Significant drug-induced abnormalities of platelet aggregation may not be reflected by the bleeding time. Platelet function may be impaired by drug combinations even when any single drug acting alone would be well tolerated. (The most common combination causing platelet dysfunction is aspirin and alcohol.) Platelet function requires at least 24 hours to recover after discontinuing the responsible medication. Some drugs (like aspirin) injure platelet function irreversibly, so that hemostasis is restored only by transfusion or formation of new platelets over a period of days. (Platelets can be generated at a rate sufficient to restore levels by 10 to 30% each day.) Aspirin should be avoided in patients with bleeding disorders, and in patients with unexplained bleeding, it is important to ask specifically about salicylate-containing over-the-counter medicines. Alcohol inhibits platelet production and action in several ways. Heavy alcohol use predisposes patients to trauma, encourages nutritional deficiencies, and directly injures the marrow. Given in high doses, most penicillins bind to the platelet surface, preventing interaction with von Willebrand's factor (VWF). (This does not occur with methicillin or cephalosporins.) Uremic toxins diminish factor VIII/VWF activity and, like paraproteinemia, interfere with interaction between the platelet and the vessel wall.

THERAPY OF PLATELET DYSFUNCTION

Bleeding rarely occurs in patients with isolated platelet dysfunction. Unless sequestered or destroyed, transfused platelets quickly restore coagulation competency. Platelet transfusions effectively correct dysfunction induced by aspirin or the cardiac bypass pump. Platelet transfusion also is transiently useful when the platelet environment is abnormal, as in uremia, paraproteinemia, or after treatment with high-dose penicillin or dextran. However, it is better to correct the underlying defect, using dialysis, plasmapheresis, or by discontinuing the offending drug. Defects caused by uremia and von Willebrand's disease may, at least temporarily, be corrected with fresh frozen plasma, vasopressin analog desmopressin (DDAVP), or cryoprecipitate. Corticosteroids often improve the bleeding time when antiplatelet antibodies cause thrombocytopenia.

PROBLEMS OF PLATELET NUMBER—THROMBOCYTOPENIA

The bleeding time is potentially prolonged when the count of normal platelets falls below $100,000/mm^3$ (<10 platelets per high-power field on peripheral blood smear). Although counts higher than $50,000/mm^3$ are acceptable for most types of operations, levels higher than $100,000/mm^3$ are preferred for cardiac procedures or neurosurgery. Spontaneous bleeding is rare with a count of more than 20,000 to $50,000/mm^3$ normally functioning platelets, but at this level, bleeding may occur even with minor trauma. When counts fall below $20,000/mm^3$, spontaneous bleeding is possible. Normally, approximately 10% of platelets appear "large" on the peripheral smear, reflecting recent production. These large, young platelets produced by an active marrow are more hemostatically effective. Therefore, at any given count, bleeding is more likely to occur if thrombocytopenia results from impaired platelet production (rather than increased destruction).

Mechanistically, thrombocytopenias usually are classified as disorders of production and destruction. Common causes of thrombocytopenia are outlined in Table 30.5. Idiopathic thrombocytopenia (ITP), acute leukemia, and aplastic crisis are the most likely causes of severe thrombocytopenia (<$10,000/mm^3$).

TABLE 30–5
CAUSES OF THROMBOCYTOPENIA

Production defects	Consumption defects
Impaired production	Immune-mediated destruction
Drugs	ITP
Infection (hepatitis, CMV, TB)	Drugs (heparin, rifampin, penicillin, sulfonamide, phenytoin)
Myelodysplasia	Lymphoma
Radiation	Systemic lupus
Ineffective production	Non–immune-mediated destruction
B12/folate deficiency	DIC
Myeloproliferative disease	Dilutional coagulopathy
	Postbypass pump
	Splenomegaly
	Prosthetic cardiac valves
	Thrombotic thrombocytopenic purpura
	Hemolytic uremic syndrome

Impaired Production

In the ICU, isolated production defects are rare; when inadequate production accounts for thrombocytopenia, anemia and leukopenia usually coexist (i.e., complete marrow failure). In such cases, platelets are small and bone marrow examination shows a decreased number of megakaryocytes. Marrow failure may result from alcohol or radiation, a deficiency of vitamin B_{12} or folate, infection with hepatitis B or cytomegalovirus, high-dose chemotherapy, or marrow infiltration with tumor, fibrosis, or granuloma. Selective failure of platelet production may occur with the use of gold, sulfas, and thiazides.

Increased Consumption

Excessive platelet consumption may be due to immunologic or nonimmunologic mechanisms. Nonimmunologic platelet consumption occurs in DIC, sepsis, microangiopathic hemolysis, thrombotic thrombocytopenic purpura (TTP), hemolytic uremic syndrome (HUS), after cardiopulmonary bypass and with splenic sequestration. Anemia, leukopenia, and a normal or hyperplastic marrow usually accompany thrombocytopenia due to hypersplenism. Laboratory clues to excessive platelet consumption include disproportionate numbers of large (young) platelets on peripheral smear and an increased number of marrow megakaryocytes.

Immunologic-mediated destruction may result from drugs, systemic vasculopathies, idiopathic thrombocytopenic purpura, posttransfusion purpura, or lymphoma. Antiplatelet antibodies stimulated by drugs (e.g., quinidine, sulfa, digoxin, methyldopa, heparin, and morphine) can cause complement-mediated platelet destruction. Removal of the offending drug elevates platelet counts substantially within 5 days, but full recovery may take 3 to 4 weeks. Platelet transfusions and steroids may help restore platelet counts rapidly after the offending drug is removed.

In acute ITP, immunologic platelet destruction usually follows a childhood viral illness. Steroids frequently are helpful if thrombocytopenia persists more than several weeks. In adults, ITP usually presents as a chronic disease, with counts ranging from 20,000 to 80,000. The spleen is the major site of platelet destruction of the IgG-coated platelets. Splenectomy is indicated for the 10 to 20% of patients who fail to respond to steroids, immune globulin, and vincristine. Vincristine and other chemotherapeutic agents have been replaced largely by use of intravenous immune globulin. Anemia in ITP is secondary to blood loss, not immune hemolysis. Interestingly, despite sometimes profound reductions in platelet count, life-threatening bleeding is rare.

Heparin also can induce the formation of IgG antibodies that may cross-react with platelet Fc receptors, causing thrombocytopenia. Onset usually is approximately 1 week after initiation of heparin but may occur as rapidly as 24 hours in sensitized patients. Although the syndrome is most common among patients receiving high-dose heparin, even the modest amounts used for subcutaneous deep venous thrombosis, prophylaxis or intravenous catheter flushing can cause disease. An estimated 1 to 5% of heparin recipients will develop thrombocytopenia (typically platelets decline to between 40,000 and 60,000/mm^3); however, only a minority will exhibit bleeding or clotting as a consequence. Clotting is more common than hemorrhage, but thrombosis is seen in only 10% of patients with the syndrome. Withdrawal of heparin is the treatment of choice. Alternative anticoagulants such as ancrod may be used. Platelet transfusions should be avoided if possible.

SPECIFIC CLOTTING DISORDERS

HEMOPHILIA

The hemophilias are sex-linked recessive diseases producing clinical bleeding in affected males. Spontaneous hemorrhage in hemophilia A (factor VIII deficiency) or hemophilia B (factor IX deficiency) usually occurs only when factor levels dip below 5% of normal (most commonly less than 1%). Therefore, female carriers possessing 50% of normal factor VIII or IX levels are spared bleeding complications. Despite these guidelines, a less than ideal correlation exists between factor levels and bleeding tendency.

Laboratory examination in both diseases most commonly reveals a prolonged PTT, with normal PT, platelet count, bleeding time, and thrombin time. Specific levels of factors VIII and IX are required to distinguish hemophilia A from B.

The urgency of therapy must be guided by the amount and location of bleeding; massive hemorrhage or bleeding into the brain or upper airway are most urgent. Surgery and invasive procedures in hemophiliacs require maintenance of factor levels higher than 50% for 14 days after the procedure. In critical operative sites (e.g., brain, spinal cord), activities approaching 100% are desirable. Topical aminocaproic acid (Amicar) may be effective at controlling localized mucosal or venipuncture bleeding.

Although factor VIII is present in fresh frozen plasma (FFP) and cryoprecipitate, specific factor VIII concentrate usually is the most practical replacement vehicle because of cost and fluid volume considerations. The 8- to 12-hour half-life of transfused factor VIII dictates twice daily dosing. In factor IX deficiency (hemophilia B), replacement of the deficient factor can be accomplished with FFP or factor IX concentrates. Care must be exercised in administration of factor IX concentrates, which may induce venous thrombosis and DIC if given in excessive amounts. The biologic half-life of factor IX is longer than factor VIII, permitting once daily dosing for most patients. (For recommendations on the replacement of factors VIII and IX, see Chapter 14, Transfusion and Blood Component Therapy.)

LIVER DISEASE

In addition to its role in clearing FDPs, the liver produces albumin and all clotting factors except the factor VIII/VWF complex. Therefore, a low serum albumin concentration supports hepatic insufficiency as the etiology of the coagulation disorder. When the liver is responsible for a coagulopathy, laboratory examination typically reveals decreased fibrinogen, increased circulating levels of FDPs, prolonged PT and PTT, and an increased thrombin time (due to FDPs). Such a laboratory pattern is identical to that seen with DIC; however, detecting d-dimers and fibrin monomers favors a diagnosis of DIC.

Liver disease and vitamin K deficiency decrease levels of factor VII, the vitamin-K-dependent factor with the shortest half-life. This reduction leads to early increases in the PT. Because multiple factors (II, VII, IX, and X) are deficient in liver disease, FFP is the replacement product of choice if immediate correction is necessary. In less urgent situations, vitamin K usually will suffice. Vitamin K also should be given empirically to virtually all patients with liver-related coagulopathy because it is difficult to distinguish liver disease from pure vitamin K deficiency. Unless correction is urgent, vitamin K usually should be injected subcutaneously. Intravenous administration carries the risk of anaphylaxis, and intramuscular injections can cause hematoma formation. Platelet counts usually are normal in liver disease unless there is coexisting hypersplenism or DIC. When platelet counts are significantly decreased ($<50,000/mm^3$), platelet concentrates may be administered but, unfortunately, are often ineffective.

VITAMIN K DEFICIENCY

Vitamin K deficiency may develop in any patient deprived of a balanced diet for 7 to 14 days. Because broad-spectrum antibiotic therapy may eliminate the enteric bacteria required for the production of vitamin K when intake is insufficient, malnourished patients and those receiving broad-spectrum antibiotic therapy are at particular risk. Fat-soluble vitamin K is incompatible with many total parenteral nutrition (TPN) preparations and, if omitted, must be given separately. Warfarin compounds can produce vitamin K deficiency by preventing carboxylation to the active form. Malabsorption (from pancreatic insufficiency) and bile salt deficiency (from ductal obstruction) also may prevent vitamin K absorption.

Vitamin K is required for the formation of factors II, VII, IX, and X. Although depletion of vitamin K eventually extends both the PT and PTT, prolongation of the PT is more marked and occurs earlier because factor VII (extrinsic pathway) has the shortest half-life of all clotting proteins. (Vitamin K deficiency also may reduce production of the anticlotting proteins C and S and antithrombin III, a problem that may cause seemingly paradoxical thrombosis.) FFP corrects the clotting disorder of vitamin K deficiency very rapidly (two to three bags usually suffice). Parenteral vitamin K usu-

ally corrects the deficiency within 24 to 48 hours if liver function is normal.

DISSEMINATED INTRAVASCULAR COAGULATION

DIC should be considered strongly for any patient with the combination of diffuse bleeding or clotting, elevations in PT and PTT, and a decreased platelet count. DIC is not self-perpetuating but requires continuous activation of the clotting mechanism. Such stimulation most frequently results from vascular damage or sepsis. In DIC, thrombin activation stimulates plasmin-mediated thrombolysis. Fibrin split products are formed in this process. With concurrent clotting and fibrinolysis, factors V and VII, fibrinogen, and platelets are consumed rapidly. Bleeding results if consumption outstrips production. The causes of DIC are numerous but usually relate to tissue inflammation from infection, tumor, or release of the products of conception into the circulation. Cytotoxic drugs, heatstroke, and shock, as well as vascular disruption (e.g., aortic aneurysm) also may cause DIC.

Diagnosis of DIC usually is straightforward. Early in the course, the PTT may be shortened as thromboplastin is released into the circulation. Later, the PT and PTT are prolonged due to depletion of fibrinogen, factors V and VII, and the anticoagulant action of FDPs. The platelet count usually is less than $150,000/mm^3$ and the fibrinogen level usually is less than 150 mg/dL. (Fibrinogen concentration may be in the normal range if levels were elevated initially, as with hepatitis or in pregnant patients.) The hallmark of DIC is an increase in the levels of fibrin degradation products (FDPs) or fibrin monomers to titers higher than 1:40. Large platelets usually are seen on peripheral smear along with fragmented red blood cells (RBCs), suggestive of microangiopathic hemolysis. A laboratory picture similar to DIC may be seen in dilutional coagulopathy or in hepatic failure if complicated by thrombocytopenia from splenic sequestration or platelet destruction.

The treatment of DIC is to reverse the underlying cause and to supplement consumed clotting factors. FFP may be used to replace factors V and VII. Platelets should be administered for severe thrombocytopenia. Cryoprecipitate may be used to replace fibrinogen if levels are markedly depressed. There is no clear evidence that heparin is beneficial, possibly except when DIC is due to acute promyelocytic leukemia. Trials using antithrombin III replacement in DIC are ongoing.

DILUTIONAL COAGULOPATHY

Dilutional coagulopathy occurs during massive hemorrhage, when replacement of a substantial fraction of the circulating volume leads to wash-out of platelets and clotting factors. After 10 units of packed red blood cells are transfused, it is generally recommended to give 2 units of FFP and 6 units of platelets for every additional 4 to 6 units of packed RBCs. The major diagnostic dilemma is to separate dilutional coagulopathy (increased PT and PTT, decreased platelet count) from DIC, a distinction that is made most reliably by FDP or fibrin monomer assay. While awaiting laboratory confirmation, the best strategy is to administer 2 units of FFP; if the clotting disorder is dilutional, FFP will correct the defect.

CIRCULATING ANTICOAGULANTS

Circulating anticoagulants are immunoglobulins that inhibit the action of clotting proteins. These circulating inhibitors are seen most commonly in patients with hemophilia, acquired immunodeficiency syndrome (AIDS), advanced age, and with certain drugs (e.g., penicillin and chlorpromazine). The most notable circulating anticoagulant occurs in systemic lupus, in which the action of factors II, V, IX, and X are impaired. Although termed the "lupus anticoagulant," also known as antiphospholipid antibody, such proteins are much more commonly associated with thrombosis than hemorrhage. Screening for a circulating anticoagulant is done by performing a PT and PTT on a mixture of equal parts of normal and patient plasma. If a simple factor deficiency is the cause of abnormal clotting, the addition of normal plasma will provide 50% activity and will normalize clotting tests. However, if an inhibitor is present, clotting tests tend to remain abnormal. Circulating anticoagulants often increase only the PTT, mimicking the laboratory findings of hemophilia. (Antiphospholipid antibodies are also commonly associated with mild thrombocytopenia.) In urgent circumstances, therapy may include massive replacement of the affected factors or the use of activated factor X.

VON WILLEBRAND'S DISEASE

Von Willebrand's disease (VWD), an autosomal dominant trait, decreases the activity of the factor VIII/VWF complex, thereby reducing the adherence of platelets to sites of vascular injury. VWD usually presents with hemorrhage after trauma, mucosal bleeding, or menorrhagia. Laboratory findings include an increased bleeding time with a normal platelet count and a prolonged PTT. Because factor VIII/VWF is an acute-phase reactant, the physiologic stress of illness or even hemorrhage may increase plasma factor levels, thereby obscuring the diagnosis. Several subtypes of VWD exist, each of which requires a slightly different diagnostic approach and treatment. Because of the complexities of diagnosing and treating VWD, hematologic consultation is valuable. Cryoprecipitate may be used to replace VWF, but as a pooled blood product, cryoprecipitate risks viral contamination avoided by use of specific factor VIII concentrates. Target VWF levels in bleeding patients or those undergoing surgery are 80 to 100 U/dL in the immediate perioperative period. DDAVP may be used to transiently increase the endogenous release of factor VIII, thereby avoiding transfusion in patients requiring only temporary normalization of hemostasis (e.g., patients undergoing brief invasive procedures). Although tachyphylaxis to desmopressin has been described, mild cases of VWD can be managed successfully with doses administered every 12 to 24 hours.

PARAPROTEINEMIA

When present in large amounts, serum proteins of the IgG, IgM, and IgA classes may impair clotting. Such problems usually occur in patients with myeloma or Waldenstrom's macroglobulinemia. Plasmapheresis reduces the serum protein level and reverses the coagulopathy.

BLEEDING DURING THROMBOLYTIC THERAPY

Almost any clotting test will confirm the presence of a "lytic state" during the administration of thrombolytic agents (e.g., streptokinase, urokinase, or tissue plasminogen activator). The thrombin time, however, most directly monitors the effect of thrombolytic drugs by examining the final step in the clotting cascade (the conversion of fibrinogen to fibrin). As an index of the effectiveness of thrombolytic activity, the thrombin time should be maintained at two to five times the baseline value when assessed 4 hours after the initiation of therapy. If bleeding occurs during thrombolytic therapy, cryoprecipitate and FFP can rapidly correct the clotting abnormalities. Because hemorrhage during thrombolytic therapy usually is a consequence of poor patient selection (e.g., elderly, traumatized) or the result of invasive procedures during the lytic period, most bleeding episodes can be avoided. Although there is no clearly demonstrated therapeutic superiority of one thrombolytic agent over another in most situations, side effects may differ. For example, central nervous system hemorrhage events are more common when tissue plasminogen activator (TPA) is used to treat myocardial infarction.

ANTICOAGULANT THERAPY

Bleeding during anticoagulation usually indicates a coexisting disturbance of vascular integrity or platelet function. Gastrointestinal or genitourinary tract hemorrhage occurring at therapeutic levels of anticoagulation usually indicates an underlying structural lesion. Risk factors for anticoagulant-induced bleeding include advanced age, alcohol and aspirin use, and female gender.

Heparin is a poorly understood complex drug with a half-life of approximately 90 minutes. Used subcutaneously in prophylactic doses (5000–8000 units every 8–12 hours), the PTT usually remains unaffected and bleeding is very rare unless heparin-induced thrombocytopenia (HIT) occurs. The goal of full dose ''therapeutic'' anticoagulation with heparin is to prolong the PTT to 1.5 to 2 times a control value. (Either the patient's baseline PTT or the midpoint of the laboratory normal range may be used to determine individual patient targets.)

There is little evidence to suggest anything more than a weak correlation of PTT values between 1.5 and 3 times control and bleeding tendency during heparin therapy. Because heparin inhibits the action of thrombin and factor Xa, it can and does often prolong the PT as well as the PTT. However, if the PT or PTT are ''infinitely'' prolonged (>100 seconds), the tendency for unprovoked bleeding may be increased. The therapy of heparin overdose includes discontinuation of the drug and the administration of protamine (1 mg per estimated unit of circulating heparin).

Much more common than heparin excess is the underdosing of heparin in thrombotic conditions. For patients with active thrombosis, larger doses of heparin than those commonly used may be required to interrupt thrombosis. Unfortunately, there is no way to standardize the ''clot burden'' to guide therapy. The most common error in heparin dosing is not to administer a bolus of heparin

and increase the rate of heparin infusion for patients with subtherapeutic PTTs. When a subtherapeutic PTT is encountered, failure to bolus and increase the heparin infusion rate results in a PTT in the therapeutic range in only 50 to 60% of cases. When a ''high'' PTT is encountered, physicians often interrupt heparin infusions for prolonged periods of time, the result being a subtherapeutic level of anticoagulation when next measured. In most cases, prolongation of the PTT to more than 2 times control does not require interruption of heparin therapy, but merely reduction in the infusion rate of 20 to 25%. (An obvious exception would be in the patient suffering hemorrhage while anticoagulated.) Interruption of a continuous infusion of heparin for more than 2 to 3 hours almost always results in a subtherapeutic PTT, except in the setting of massive overdosage.

Heparin-induced thrombocytopenia (HIT) develops in 5 to 10% of hospitalized patients given heparin. HIT seems to be induced by the formation of antibodies to heparin that cross-react with platelet surface antigens. (Bovine heparin is more likely than porcine heparin to induce the syndrome.) HIT usually is manifest within the first 7 days of heparin therapy and is most common in patients receiving larger doses of heparin. However, the syndrome may occur at any time during heparin therapy and has been reported in patients only receiving subcutaneous heparin or the tiny amounts infused in the maintenance of continuously flushing vascular access catheters. Early reports of a very low incidence of HIT when using low-molecular-weight heparin probably are not true. The most serious complication of HIT is not bleeding but thrombosis. Although only approximately 10% of patients developing HIT experience thrombosis, the ''white clot syndrome'' of diffuse venous and arterial thrombosis induced by platelet aggregation may carry a mortality rate as high as 25%. Treatment of HIT should include an alternate method of anticoagulation (e.g., warfarin, ancrod, or hirulog). Platelet transfusions should be avoided. Insertion of a venacaval filter and surgical removal of arterial clot may be beneficial in selected cases. Among patients developing HIT, future heparin exposure should be avoided if at all possible; however, short-term exposure (several hours) often is well tolerated.

Low-molecular-weight heparins (LMWHs) (e.g., enoxiparin) are depolymerized antithrombin III activators fractionated from standard heparin. Little endothelial uptake and low serum protein binding provide high bioavailability and slow clearance. The result is that intermittent subcutaneous dosing of LMWH is sufficient to provide DVT prophylaxis, and recent data suggest that it may be sufficient therapy for established DVT. Among patients undergoing lower extremity surgery (e.g., hip or knee replacement), LMWH possibly is superior to warfarin and standard heparin therapy for DVT prophylaxis. Minor interactions of LMWH with VWF produces fewer platelet inhibitory actions than standard heparin and may account for the lower incidence of hemorrhage observed in several clinical trials of DVT prophylaxis and therapy. There are little data to suggest that LMWH differs from standard heparin in the incidence of thrombocytopenia. Studies have clearly shown the efficacy of LMWH for treatment of DVT, and similar trials will likely prove LMWH efficacious for pulmonary embolism. Such trials may allow many patients with DVT and PE to be treated safely in the outpatient setting, reducing hospital length of stay and cost.

Warfarin (coumarin) inhibits production of vitamin-K-dependent proteins (II, VII, IX, X) prolonging the PT to a greater degree than the PTT. The intensity of warfarin anticoagulation should be guided by the severity of the thrombotic consequences. Because of interlaboratory variation in testing procedures, most hospitals now report the PT in relation to an "international normalized ratio" (INR) in addition to the ratio of the observed PT to the patient's baseline or laboratory control. INR reporting standardizes the intensity of anticoagulation among hospitals. The goal of warfarin therapy in deep venous thrombosis or pulmonary embolism traditionally has been to maintain PT at 1.5-2.5 times the patient's baseline or laboratory control (INR 3–4.5). More intense anticoagulation has been advocated for patients with mural cardiac thrombi and mechanical prosthetic heart valves. However, recent evidence suggests that PT values 1.25 to 1.5 times control (INR 2–3) are adequate for most conditions and such less-intense anticoagulation lowers hemorrhagic risk.

Changes in previously stable levels of anticoagulation often are due to fluctuations in warfarin metabolism or protein binding induced by the addition or discontinuation of other drugs (e.g., erythromycin, phenobarbital, phenytoin). The intensity of anticoagulation also is increased by drugs that compete with warfarin for albumin binding (sulfas, sulfonureas, indomethacin, and phenylbutazone). For patients with warfarin-induced bleeding and firm indications for chronic anticoagulation (prosthetic heart valves, recurrent embolism), interruption of warfarin for 2 to 4 days usually is uneventful. If more precise control of anticoagulation is needed, heparin may be substituted temporarily. Vitamin K usually is sufficient to reverse the anticoagulant effect of warfarin for patients with an excessively prolonged PT without bleeding. However, vitamin K does not provide ideal reversal because its effect may be delayed for 6 to 24 hours and reanticoagulation may be difficult if greater than 1 mg of vitamin K is given. In more urgent cases, FFP will promptly (but temporarily) reverse anticoagulation.

Warfarin-induced skin necrosis is a rare complication of warfarin anticoagulation traditionally associated with rapid anticoagulation using "loading doses" of warfarin. Pathologically, the mechanism of necrosis is the formation of microvascular thrombosis, leading to the hypothesis that necrosis is the result of inhibiting production of the anticlotting vitamin-K-dependent proteins C and S. It has been postulated that warfarin-induced necrosis is most likely to occur in protein-C-deficient patients; however, at this time, a clear relationship is uncertain.

HYPERCOAGULABLE DISORDERS

Knowledge regarding hypercoagulable or thrombotic disorders is much less complete than that for bleeding disorders. Currently available laboratory tests cannot reliably predict a thrombotic tendency and the assays possibly useful to predict thrombotic tendency are not routinely available in all hospitals. Most episodes of arterial and venous thrombosis cannot be linked to any well-defined inherited or acquired prothrombotic blood disorder. That is, a hypercoagulable state classically described in Virchow's triad usually cannot be identified. Most patients with a thrombotic event do, however, have the risk factors of stasis and vascular intimal damage or inflammation. Until recently, it was believed that fewer than 5% of unselected patients with a thrombotic event had an identifiable prothrombotic condition. The discovery of factor V abnormalities (activated protein C resistance), however, now suggests that as many as 20% of patients with thrombotic episodes may have a genetic cause. The most common causes of an identifiable hypercoagulable disorder are outlined in Table 30.6. Useful clinical clues to raise suspicion of an inherited or acquired thrombotic tendency are outlined in Table 30.7.

TABLE 30-6

MOST COMMON IDENTIFIED ABNORMALITIES OF THE HYPERCOAGULABLE STATE

Activated protein C resistance
Protein C deficiency
Protein S deficiency
Antithrombin III deficiency
Anticardiolipin antibody
Dysfibrinogenemias

TABLE 30-7

CLINICAL CLUES TO HYPERCOAGULABLE DISORDERS

Family history of thrombotic events (usually venous)
Thrombotic event at an early age
Thrombosis without identifiable risk factor
Recurrent clotting episodes
Thrombosis at unusual site (upper extremity)
Recurrent spontaneous abortions

INHERITED THROMBOTIC DISORDERS

Deficient quantities or activity of three specific plasma proteins, antithrombin III (ATIII) and proteins C and S, have been linked to a thrombotic tendency. Unfortunately, there are no clinical features to distinguish patients with these disorders, and levels of all three of these proteins can be reduced by liver disease, DIC, pregnancy, or the occurrence of a thrombotic event not precipitated by the protein deficiency. It is likely that most affected individuals do not experience significant thrombotic episodes unless additional thrombotic risk factors occur. When clotting does occur, deep venous thrombosis of the leg seems to be the most likely event. Arterial thrombosis or visceral, cerebral, or upper extremity thromboses occur rarely. Protein and functional assays now exist for all three proteins; however, numerous difficulties still exist in performing and interpreting results of such tests. Therefore, the involvement of a hematologist in the evaluation of a patient with a prothrombotic disorder is prudent. As a first step in the evaluation of patients with a suspected clotting disorder and activated protein C assay, a functional assay for ATIII (heparin cofactor assay), and functional assays for protein C and an immunologic assay for protein S are reasonable.

Antithrombin III

Antithrombin III (ATIII) is a naturally occurring serine protease plasma anticoagulant that acts to inhibit the action of activated factors IX, X, and XI and thrombin. The predominant activity of ATIII is to irreversibly inactivate thrombin. The rate at which ATIII inactivates thrombin can be increased dramatically (up to 10,000-fold) by the addition of heparin. ATIII deficiency usually is inherited as an autosomal dominant trait and it is estimated that somewhere between 1 in 2000 and 1 in 5000 adults is heterozygous for the protein. Spontaneous mutations (acquired disease) have been described rarely, and pregnancy, liver disease, DIC, nephrotic syndrome, and acute thromboses have been reported to reduce ATIII levels in genetically normal persons. Protein-deficient heterozygotes are at a particularly increased risk for thrombotic events. Deficient homozygotes have not been identified, suggesting that such a severe deficiency is lethal in fetal life or childhood. Two general types of ATIII deficiency have been identified: reductions in plasma protein level or activity. The most common form of the disorder is a combined reduction in plasma protein level and functional activity. Normal ATIII levels but decreased functional activity represents the next most common form of the disorder. Immunologic assays can measure the protein level, but functional assays usually are required to quantitate protein anticoagulant activity in the absence of heparin (progressive assay) or in the presence of heparin (heparin cofactor assay). An antithrombin III concentrate is now available for treatment of deficient patients; however, the mainstay of therapy remains lifelong anticoagulation for patients with demonstrated thrombotic events and ATIII deficiency.

Protein C Deficiency

The clinical presentation of protein C, a thrombin-activated vitamin-K-dependent serine protease deficiency is similar to that of ATIII deficiency. Activated protein C (APC) inhibits the activity of activated factors VIII and V and increases fibrinolytic activity. Heterozygotes for the autosomally dominant inherited protein exhibit partial deficiency. As many as one in 200 persons in the general population may be heterozygous for protein C. Protein C levels also can be reduced by liver disease, DIC, use of chemotherapy, or the occurrence of an acute thrombotic event. Because warfarin reduces both protein C and S levels, laboratory determinations of protein levels during warfarin therapy are unreliable. Submaximal function of the enzyme also may result, even when levels are normal. The importance of protein C deficiency is less certain than that for ATIII; many patients with reduced protein C levels are asymptomatic. Therapy for protein C deficiency includes warfarin. Purified protein C and activated protein C infusions represent experimental options. Warfarin-induced skin necrosis has been associated with the institution of oral anticoagulation, especially when loading doses of warfarin are used. However, warfarin-induced necrosis is a rare event, even for patients with protein C deficiency.

Protein S Deficiency

Protein S, another vitamin-K-dependent protein, complexes with activated protein C, potentiating its anticoagulant effect. Protein S also is associated with carrier protein C4b. Although protein assays for protein S exist, the free-protein fraction is difficult to measure reliably. The most common form of protein S deficiency is a decrease in total level, although disorders in which the functional activity is decreased with normal total activity also have been described. Therapy for protein S deficiency is warfarin anticoagulation.

Activated Protein C (APC) Resistance

In vitro clotting assays of blood of some patients with thrombotic diseases exhibit a resistance to the anticoagulant effect of activated protein C. A mutation in the amino acid sequence of factor V is the most common cause of APC resistance. In preliminary studies, 20 to 40% of patients with thrombotic episodes exhibit APC re-

sistance, and APC resistance may be the most common genetic risk factor for deep venous thrombosis. The presence of activated protein C resistance can be screened for using a modified activated PTT test. It should be noted that some functional assays for protein S are sensitive to APC resistance and can yield a false diagnosis of protein S deficiency. Protein and functional assays must be performed when patients are not receiving anticoagulant therapy. Fortunately, genetic assays are now available that can directly detect the factor V defect. A major advantage is the ability to diagnose the defect in patients receiving anticoagulant therapy. The genetic assay provides superior accuracy to functional assays but will miss APC resistance caused by any other defect except the arginine–glycine substitution in factor V.

LUPUS ANTICOAGULANT/ ANTIPHOSPHOLIPID (ANTICARDIOLIPIN) ANTIBODY

Antiphospholipid antibody (APLA) is an IgG antibody directed against cardiolipin-phospholipid, which constitutes a substantial risk for thrombosis. The antibody also produces abnormalities of in vitro clotting studies and has been associated with the occurrence of spontaneous abortions. Antibody titer correlates best with the risk for thrombosis. APLA should be suspected in an appropriate clinical setting when the baseline PTT is prolonged, especially if the platelet count is low. APLA can be confirmed using a factor Xa clotting time, a kaolin-activated PTT, a dilute Russell viper venom time, or a dilute one-stage prothrombin time. Alternatively, direct measurement of antibody titer can be performed. Therapy for patients with APLA syndrome includes intense warfarin anticoagulation.

KEY POINTS

1. Most bleeding disorders seen in the ICU are the result of acquired deficiencies of multiple clotting factors, whereas most hereditary disorders stem from a single soluble factor deficiency. Hemophilia A (factor VIII deficiency) and hemophilia B (Factor IX) deficiency constitute 90% or more of hereditary bleeding disorders. Because these two conditions can be detected by a PTT and are rarely the result of a spontaneous mutation, they can be excluded easily from consideration by family history and a PTT.

rhage and often are treated with platelet transfusions. Platelet counts do not provide information about platelet function.

5. Liver disease, vitamin K deficiency, dilutional coagulopathy, and DIC are the most common soluble factor problems encountered in the ICU. All can have elevations of the PT and PTT. The presence of high levels of fibrin degradation products and a lower platelet count favors DIC. Vitamin K deficiency and liver disease often can be distinguished by searching for additional historical or chemical evidence of a liver disease,

2. A PT, PTT, and platelet count performed after a careful, detailed history, which includes a review of current medications, can detect essentially all significant acquired bleeding disorders seen in the ICU.

3. Coagulation tests often are performed indiscriminately. The PTT is rarely necessary unless a patient is receiving heparin, and the PT is of essentially no use to monitor heparin's effects. Similarly, patients receiving warfarin need not have PTT determinations.

4. Platelet numbers correlate roughly with the tendency to bleed. At platelet counts higher than $50,000/mm^3$, the risk of spontaneous bleeding is low, platelet transfusions are rarely necessary, and most procedures can be performed safely if platelets function normally. In contrast, platelets counts lower than $20,000/mm^3$ are associated with spontaneous hemor-

especially a problem of synthetic function. Although dilution and DIC can appear similar, dilutional coagulopathy is less likely to exhibit fibrin degradation products.

6. When using standard heparin for thromboembolic disease, a loading dose followed by a continuous infusion is almost always necessary to achieve the usual target level of anticoagulation of a PTT 1.5 to 2 times the baseline. Lower PTTs usually require an additional bolus and increases in infusion rate of 20 to 25% to promptly achieve anticoagulation.

7. Identifying a specific cause for thrombosis is uncommon. Clues that should trigger a laboratory search for a thrombotic condition are unprovoked clotting, clotting at an early age, repeated episodes of thrombosis, a positive family history of clotting, and a history of repeated spontaneous abortions.

SUGGESTED READINGS

1. Alpern JB. Coagulopathy caused by vitamin K deficiency in critically ill, hospitalized patients. JAMA 1987;258:1916–1919.
2. Ansell JE. Oral anticoagulant therapy—50 years later. Arch Intern Med 1993;153:586–596.
3. Bachmann F. Diagnostic approaches to mild bleeding disorders. Semin Hematol 1980;17(4):292–305.
4. Bick RL, Baker WF. Disseminated intravascular coagulation syndromes. Hematol Pathol 1992;6:1–24.
5. Bone RC. Modulators of coagulation. A critical appraisal of their role in sepsis. Arch Intern Med 1992;152:1381–1389.
6. Bowie ESW, Owen CA Jr. Hemostatic failure in clinical medicine. Semin Hematol 1977;14(3):341–364.
7. Brown RB, Klar J, Teres D, et al. Prospective study of clinical bleeding in intensive care unit patients. Crit Care Med 1988;16:1171–1176.
8. Corrigan JJ, Ray WL, May N. Changes in the blood coagulation system associated with septicemia. N Engl J Med 1968;279:851–856.
9. Counts RB, Haisch C, Simon TL, et al. Hemostasis in massively transfused trauma patients. Ann Surg 1979;190(1):91–99.
10. Deykin D. The clinical challenge of disseminated intravascular coagulation. N Engl J Med 1970;283:636–644.
11. Feinstein DI. Diagnosis and management of disseminated intravascular coagulation: the role of heparin therapy. Blood 1982;60:284–287.
12. George JN, Shattil SJ. The clinical importance of acquired abnormalities of platelet function. N Engl J Med 1991;324:27–39.
13. Hull RD, Raskob GE, Rosenbloom D, et al. Optimal therapeutic level of heparin therapy in patients with venous thrombosis. Arch Intern Med 1992;152:1589–1595.
14. King DJ, Kelton JG. Heparin-associated thrombocytopenia. Ann Intern Med 1984;100:535–540.
15. Kitchens CS. Approach to the bleeding patient. Hematol Oncol Clin North Am 1992;6:983–989.
16. Kottke-Marchant K. Laboratory diagnosis of hemorrhagic and thrombotic disorders. Hematol Oncol Clin North Am 1994;4:809–853.
17. Malpass TW, Harker LA. Acquired disorders of platelet function. Semin Hematol 1980;17:242–258.
18. Menache D, Grossman BJ, Jackson CM. Antithrombin III. Physiology, deficiency, and replacement therapy. Transfusion 1992;32:580–588.
19. Penner JA. Managing the hemorrhagic complications of heparin administration. Hematol Oncol Clin North Am 1993;7:1281–1289.
20. Rosenberg RD. Role of antithrombin III in coagulation disorders. State of the art review. Am J Med 1989;87(Suppl 3B):1S–67S.
21. Schafer AI. The hypercoagulable states. Ann Intern Med 1985;102:814–828.
22. Simonneau G, Charbonnier B, Decousus H, et al. Subcutaneous low molecular weight heparin compared with continuous intravenous unfractionated heparin in the treatment of proximal deep venous thrombosis. Arch Intern Med 1993;153:1541–1546.
23. Woodman RC, Harker LA. Bleeding complications associated with cardiopulmonary bypass. Blood 1990;76:1680–1697.

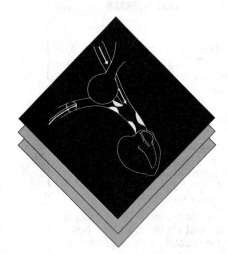

Hepatic Failure

CLASSIFICATION OF ACUTE HEPATIC FAILURE

Acute hepatic failure can arise as a primary process in a previously healthy person (e.g., acetaminophen overdose, acute viral hepatitis), as an exacerbation of a chronic liver disease (e.g., cirrhosis, chronic active hepatitis), or as part of the multiorgan failure syndrome of critical illness. Whatever the cause, certain key manifestations are shared as one or more of the five major functions of the liver are disrupted: (*a*) maintenance of acid–base balance through the metabolism of lactate; (*b*) drug and toxin metabolism; (*c*) glucose and lipid metabolism; (*d*) protein synthesis (including immunoglobulins, clotting factors, and albumin); and (*e*) phagocytic clearance of organisms and circulating debris.

ACUTE HEPATIC FAILURE AS A PRIMARY PROCESS

When fulminant hepatic failure develops as a primary process, the manifestations evolve over a period of less than 4 weeks in a previously healthy person. The most advanced form of this syndrome, fulminant hepatic necrosis, is produced by a wide variety of noxious insults and proves fatal in 75 to 90% of cases. Common etiologies of acute hepatic failure are listed in Table 31.1. Consistently, viral hepatitis is the most common cause of fulminant hepatic failure, followed closely by drug (particularly acetaminophen) toxicity.

Viral Hepatitis

The risk of developing hepatic failure from hepatitis is minor (<1%), but because viral hepatitis is the most frequent cause of hepatic failure, a review of infectious hepatitis is warranted. At least six viruses are known to cause severe hepatitis: A; B; non-A non-B (or C); δ agent; Epstein-Barr virus; and cytomegalovirus. Hepatitis B and C account for more than 90% of cases of viral hepatitis; hepatitis A accounts for about 5% of cases. Hepatitis B and C are transmitted predominantly through the exchange of body fluids. Accidental or intentional needle sticks and sexual intercourse are the most common modes of transmission. Although blood transmission probably represents the highest relative risk, saliva and semen also transmit the virus. Testing the blood supply for hepatitis B and monitoring the liver function tests of donors has dramatically reduced the risk of transfusion-induced disease. After exposure to the DNA containing hepatitis B virus, a 2- to 3-month incubation period passes as the virus proliferates. During this time, viral surface antigen (HbsAg) can be detected in the serum of infected patients. Nonspecific, gastrointestinal (GI), systemic, and rheumatologic symptoms precede the onset of overt jaundice. Jaundice is accompanied by elevations in liver transaminase (SGOT, SGPT) and, in most patients, by the disappearance of surface antigen. In a small minority of patients, the surface antigen persists in the circulation and signifies the presence of chronic hepatitis B (and potential infectivity). Antibodies to the virus core antigen appear in the serum during

TABLE 31–1

ETIOLOGIES OF FULMINANT HEPATIC NECROSIS

Viral	Chemical hepatotoxins
Hepatitis A, B, C, δ	Carbon tetrachloride
Adenovirus	Benzene
Varicella-Zoster	Ethylene glycol
Cytomegalovirus	Ethanol
Ebstein-Barr	Phosphorus
Drug ingestions	**Miscellaneous**
Halogenated anesthetics	Reye's syndrome
Acetaminophen	Fatty liver of pregnancy
Tetracycline	Toxic mushrooms—
Isoniazid	*Amanita phalloides*
Rifampin	Wilson's disease
Phenytoin	Sickle-cell disease
Methyldopa	Budd-Chiari syndrome
Valproic acid	Autoimmune hepatitis
Anabolic steroids	
Sulfonamides	

the incubation period and are typically present for several months after the illness resolves. Antibodies to the surface antigen develop during the period of clinical convalescence and may persist for years. The δ agent is an incomplete viral particle that can reinfect patients previously infected with hepatitis B or can coinfect with hepatitis B. Patients infected with hepatitis B and the δ agent have a poor prognosis, frequently developing acute hepatic failure. An effective vaccine to hepatitis B exists, and for workers in the intensive care unit (ICU) who do not have protective levels of naturally occurring antibodies, vaccination makes sense because of the high level of occupational exposure.

In contrast to hepatitis B, hepatitis C is an RNA virus, is difficult to detect, and is more likely to be clinically subtle in its initial stages. Jaundice is rare with the acute illness, and when it does occur, it is mild. Despite this ''mild'' initial illness, hepatitis C is a major cause of chronic hepatitis and cirrhosis.

Hepatitis A is the third most frequent cause of viral hepatitis but differs in many respects from hepatitis B, C, or the δ agent. Hepatitis A is acquired by the fecal–oral route and often produces an asymptomatic infection in children. After ingestion, an average incubation period of a month precedes the onset of nonspecific constitutional and GI symptoms. In some patients, an icteric phase then follows, which is associated with abnormalities of liver transaminase and coincides with the appearance of IgM antibodies to the virus in serum. Adults often have more severe cases of

the disease than children. Fortunately, hepatitis A rarely is associated with either fulminant hepatic failure or chronic hepatitis. Cytomegalovirus and Epstein-Barr virus are much less common causes of clinically important hepatitis and only rarely are associated with fulminant liver failure.

ACUTE HEPATIC FAILURE AS A SECONDARY PROCESS

Although fulminant liver failure occurs only rarely as a primary process, life-threatening hepatic dysfunction often develops in patients with limited reserves, when another even relatively minor insult tips the balance. This injury can occur when nutritive flow is compromised by congestive heart failure or shock or when hepatocytes are damaged by circulating mediators of inflammation, as in sepsis syndrome.

DIAGNOSIS OF ACUTE HEPATIC FAILURE

The clinical diagnosis of acute hepatic failure cannot be made until biochemical signs of liver and central nervous system (CNS) dysfunction are present. Irritability, confusion, and vomiting are all early signs of CNS involvement. Fever is common early in the course, whereas hypothermia is more frequent later. Ascites and peripheral edema reflect portal hypertension and hypoalbuminemia but are not necessary for diagnosis. The patient with acute hepatic failure is typically tremulous and hyperventilating; a liver ''flap'' and sustained clonus can be often elicited. Hypoxemia is present in most patients, and the acute respiratory distress syndrome (ARDS) complicates about one-third of all cases.

LABORATORY FEATURES

Leukocytosis with neutrophilia and hepatic transaminase elevations usually are present. Marked hyperbilirubinemia commonly precedes a fall in serum albumin and prolongation of the prothrombin time, both of which are late signs of hepatic failure. Extensive hepatic destruction may impair gluconeogenesis, giving rise to hypoglycemia. Low-grade disseminated intravascular coagulation (DIC) commonly results from decreased synthesis of clotting factors, together with failure of the liver to clear fibrin degradation products. Deficient hepatic production of antithrombins also may predispose patients to thrombosis. In acute hepatic failure with encephalopathy, arterial ammonia concentrations usually are elevated; a normal ammonia level in a patient with altered mental status may help to exclude the diagnosis of hepatic encephalopathy. (Ammonia levels may be elevated spuriously by venous rather than arterial sampling or by improper specimen handling. Conversely, ammonia levels may be artifactually low in patients with severe protein malnutrition.)

THERAPY

There is no specific therapy for acute hepatic injury, except that caused by acetaminophen (see Chapter 33, Drug Overdose and Poisoning). Because there is no specific therapy, the prognosis of acute hepatic failure is dismal once profound coma develops, with survival rates averaging less than 20%. Patients with fulminant hepatic failure should be cared for in an ICU because of their numerous unstable physiologic problems. On admission, a toxicologic survey should be obtained which includes acetaminophen levels. Basic laboratory studies including blood counts, liver hepatic transaminases, platelets electrolytes, creatinine levels, an arterial blood gas analysis, and tests of hepatic synthetic function: albumin and prothrombin times.

As a minimum, a peripheral intravenous catheter, nasogastric tube, and urinary catheter are necessary for most patients. Patients should be positioned with the head of the bed elevated to decrease the risks of aspiration and formation of cerebral edema. Neurologic status should be monitored frequently. Prophylactic therapy for gastric ulceration should be undertaken. Supportive care includes maintenance of adequate nutrition and hemodynamic support as well as monitoring for the most frequent complications: (a) hepatic encephalopathy; (b) cerebral edema; (c) bacterial infection; (d) GI bleeding; (e) coagulopathy; and (f) renal failure.

Some centers have begun to offer liver transplantation as a therapeutic option for acute hepatic failure. Because short-term survival rates of 50 to 75% have been achieved with transplantation, appropriate patients who deteriorate despite maximal medical therapy should at least be considered for transplant. Unfortunately, the procedure is still plagued with problems and as many as one-half of all good candidates will die while waiting for a liver. It should be noted that transplantation is best reserved for the patient with isolated liver failure—for example, it clearly cannot not benefit patients who have sustained irreversible brain damage from hypoxia, intracranial bleeding or intracranial hypertension.

COMPLICATIONS

HEPATIC ENCEPHALOPATHY

Hepatic encephalopathy, also known as portosystemic encephalopathy, is the most frequent fatal complication of acute hepatic failure. Although hepatic encephalopathy is the most common cause of mental status alterations, it is important to exclude other more readily reversible causes of altered consciousness, including (a) hypoglycemia, (b) infection, (c) electrolyte imbalance, (d) drug overdosage (particularly sedatives), (e) hypoxemia, (f) profound sleep deprivation, and (g) vitamin deficiency. Hypoglycemia is particularly important because it develops in as many as 40% of all patients and the condition is easily reversible.

Encephalopathy arises when severe liver disease causes shunting of toxin-laden portal blood around the liver directly into the systemic circulation. Ammonia, fatty acids, mercaptans, and other false neurotransmitters have been implicated as causative, but there is no clear consensus. Encephalopathy may produce focal neurologic deficits as well as alterations in consciousness, intellectual performance, and personality. In salvageable patients, mental status changes usually respond to appropriate therapy within several days.

Regardless of the specific biochemical cause, a number of precipitating factors are known to worsen the encephalopathy of liver failure. Gastrointestinal hemorrhage increases the gut protein load and ammonia production. Intravascular volume depletion from bleeding or diuretic use worsens mental status by reducing hepatic and renal perfusion and predisposing patients to contraction alkalosis. In turn, alkalosis and hypokalemia increase ammonia production and impair its excretion, further worsening mental status. Excessive withdrawal of ascitic fluid may translocate fluid from the vascular space to the peritoneal cavity, further decreasing hepatic perfusion. Because of the complications associated with volume depletion, weight lost through the use of diuretics or fluid restriction must not exceed 1 to 2 pounds per day. Failing renal function accentuates the accumulation of ammonia and other toxins. Almost any systemic infection may alter mental status, but the most common infection precipitating encephalopathy is spontaneous bacterial peritonitis.

All drugs (but particularly sedatives and narcotics) must be used with extreme caution when hepatic metabolism is impaired. Histamine blockers also should be used cautiously because of the likelihood of impaired mentation in patients with liver disease. The diagnosis of hepatic encephalopathy is made on clinical grounds and supported by elevated blood ammonia levels, specific electroencephalogram (EEG) findings, or increases in spinal fluid glutamine. Hyperpnea and hyperventilation are common. Although computed tomographic (CT) scanning of the brain can only reveal nonspecific cerebral edema in hepatic encephalopathy, an EEG occasionally demonstrates characteristic abnormalities (high-amplitude δ and triphasic waves). Unfortunately, the EEG usually demonstrates only nonspecific, diffuse slowing. Evoked potential testing has been advocated as a specific and sensitive marker of encephalopathy, but whether it offers an advantage over the EEG is not yet clear.

For patients with subtle encephalopathy or for cases in which the diagnosis is in doubt, a therapeutic trial should be undertaken after other causes of reversible encephalopathy are excluded. Response to therapy for hepatic encephalopathy usually occurs within 3 to 4 days if the diagnosis is correct. Correction of precipitating causes (bleeding, drugs, infection, alkalosis, hypovolemia) are key to improvement. However, after hepatic encephalopathy is established, restricting protein intake and preventing GI bleeding reduce the substrate available for the production of cerebral toxins. Aromatic amino acids (e.g., phenylalanine, tyrosine) have been implicated in the encephalopathy of liver failure; therefore, branched-chain amino acids (e.g., valine, leucine, and isoleucine) have been advocated as a potentially useful therapy.

Laxatives and enemas decrease fecal generation of nitrogenous toxins, but profuse or protracted diarrhea sufficient to cause fluid depletion and electrolyte abnormalities must be avoided. Lactulose, a synthetic nonabsorbable and poorly digestible disaccharide, usually is used to reduce the intestinal burden of toxins. Lactulose is broken down by colonic bacteria to lactic and acetic acids, compounds that promote bowel transit. Although effective in encephalopathy associated with chronic hepatic failure, it is controversial whether lactulose reduces the encephalopathy of fulminant hepatic failure. When used, lactulose is initially administered hourly until a laxative effect is produced. It is then continued in doses sufficient to produce one to two soft stools per day. As with other laxatives, excessive lactulose-induced diarrhea may deplete intravascular volume-worsening hepatic encephalopathy, and sometimes precipitating the hepatorenal syndrome. Neomycin is a poorly absorbed broad-spectrum antibiotic that is sometimes used as an alternative to lactulose. When given in 2- to 4-gm oral doses or administered as an enema once or twice daily, neomycin reduces the number of intestinal bacteria forming these toxic compounds. Because as much as 5% of the drug may be absorbed systemically, renal insufficiency may occur when large doses are given to patients with pre-existing renal dysfunction. Rarely, neomycin causes reversible diarrhea, nephrotoxicity, and ototoxicity. Occasionally, patients respond to neomycin but not to lactulose or vice versa. Experimental therapy of hepatic encephalopathy with L-dopa or bromocryptine is of unknown effectiveness.

SPONTANEOUS BACTERIAL PERITONITIS

Spontaneous bacterial peritonitis (SBP) is a common complication of acute hepatic failure in which bacteria seed the peritoneal cavity. In most cases, bacteria are believed to cross directly into the ascitic fluid through the bowel wall. Hypoperfusion often precipitates SBP, presumably by impairing bowel wall integrity. In patients with ascites, sudden deterioration of renal function or mental status, rapid weight gain, or ascites that becomes resistant to diuretic therapy all should prompt consideration of SBP. Untreated SBP is fatal in 60 to 90% of cases; even with early antibiotic treatment, the fatality rate remains near 40%. The observed high mortality rate despite treatment may be due to delayed diagnosis and institution of therapy or may reflect the high incidence of debilitation and multiple organ failure in this population. Classically, SBP may be recognized by the triad of fever, abdominal pain, and encephalopathy. However, SBP differs from peritonitis of other causes in that fever, abdominal pain, and tenderness are often subtle. Approximately 25% of all patients with SBP have only extra-abdominal symptoms, and 5% of patients are entirely asymptomatic.

Nothing short of obtaining peritoneal fluid can

exclude the diagnosis of SBP. A peritoneal fluid pH less than 7.31, a gradient in pH between the serum and acidic fluid of more than 0.1 unit, or an ascitic fluid lactic acid level higher than 32 mg/dL are suggestive. Diagnosis is confirmed when bacteria are seen on Gram's stain or grow in culture. An absolute leukocyte count in the ascitic fluid that is higher than 500/mm^3 should prompt empiric therapy, particularly if polymorphonuclear leukocytes predominate.

Enteric gram-negative rods are the most common organisms, but 15% of patients with SBP have polymicrobial infections and 5% grow anaerobes. The single most likely organism is *Escherichia coli,* but pneumococcal infections also are prevalent. Because bacteremia occurs in approximately 50% of cases, blood cultures should be obtained. An aminoglycoside given with ampicillin or an extended-spectrum penicillin (ticarcillin/clavulinate, ampicillin/sulbactam) is appropriate initial coverage for most patients.

CEREBRAL EDEMA

The intracranial hypertension induced by cerebral edema is another cause of altered mental status in acute hepatic failure. The physical examination is rarely helpful in detecting cerebral edema, and the head CT scan is insensitive to this diagnosis. (The CT can be very helpful, however, to rule out other causes of decreased mental status.) Unfortunately, even when diagnosed accurately, the elevated intracranial pressure caused by hepatic failure generally fails to respond to treatment that is effective in other forms of cerebral edema (see Chapter 35, Head and Spine Trauma). Surgical decompression and dexamethasone seem to be of little or no benefit. Hyperventilation is only transiently beneficial, and although mannitol (25–50 gm) may temporarily reduce edema, there is no evidence that survival rates are increased. Furthermore, there is no evidence that mortality is improved through direct monitoring of CSF pressure. Death due to cerebral herniation may be sudden and unexpected and is observed in 80% of fatal cases of acute hepatic failure coming to autopsy.

INFECTION

By decreasing opsonins, complement levels, and phagocytosis, hepatic failure predisposes patients to infection. As many as 80% of patients with acute hepatic failure develop serious infections, 25% of which are bacteremic. Ten to 20% of patients with acute hepatic failure die of bacterial infection. Fever and leukocytosis are not commonly seen (occurring in only 30% of cases). *Staphylococci* and *streptococci* followed by gram-negative rods are the predominant organisms of bacteremia. Prophylactic antibiotics offer no benefit. Pneumonia, SBP, and catheter-related sepsis are especially common infections and are largely preventable with good supportive care.

GI BLEEDING

Because GI bleeding frequently produces shock, hepatic encephalopathy, or hypoperfusion that initiates acute renal failure, it is often the proximate cause of death in patients with hepatic failure. Coagulopathy frequently accentuates the tendency for GI blood loss. Although antacids, sucralfate, and histamine (H$_2$) blockers are all effective in preventing stress ulceration, H$_2$ blockers are difficult to use safely in acute hepatic failure because of impaired drug metabolism and CNS side effects.

COAGULATION DISORDERS

Because of the liver's central role in maintaining hemostasis, it is not surprising that bleeding accounts for the death of one-third of all patients with fulminant hepatic failure. The frequency of bleeding and clotting disorders is understandable because all clotting factors are produced by the liver, with the exception of factor VIII/von Willebrand's factor (see Chapter 30, Clotting and Bleeding Disorders and Anticoagulation Therapy). In addition, Kupffer cells also play a key role in the clearing activated clotting proteins from the circulation. Furthermore, the liver is responsible for production of the major anticlotting proteins (antithrombin III and proteins C and S). Thrombocytopenia is common, usually related to DIC. Vitamin K safely augments production of certain several factors (II, VII, IX, X). Because renal (as well as liver function) is often impaired, volume overload is a common complication when fresh frozen plasma is used to reverse clotting factor deficiencies.

RENAL FAILURE

Renal insufficiency develops in up to one-half of all patients with acute hepatic failure and is most common in the setting of acetaminophen toxicity. Two types of renal insufficiency may accompany acute hepatic failure: acute tubular necrosis (ATN) and the hepatorenal syndrome (HRS). Blood urea nitrogen (BUN) levels are not a reliable indicator of renal function in acute hepatic failure because the liver's production of urea nitrogen is impaired. The diagnosis and therapy of ATN is outlined elsewhere (see Chapter 29, Acute Renal Failure and Dialysis).

HRS is a unique form of oliguric renal failure seen in patients with severe liver failure characterized by increasing serum creatinine, oliguria, and failure to respond to fluids or diuretics. Urinary sodium values are typically very low (<10 mEq/L). Because of its high fatality rate and failure to respond to treatment, HRS must be prevented. It is especially important to avoid nephrotoxic drugs and the intravascular volume depletion that results from untreated GI hemorrhage, overzealous paracentesis, or excessive diuretic usage. The role of low-dose dopamine and other experimental agents such as atrial natriuretic factor have not yet been defined.

NUTRITION

Adequate nutrition is important to the survival of patients with acute hepatic failure. Although sufficient calories and protein of high biologic value must be provided, high-protein loads should be avoided. Vitamin K, thiamine, and folate are required by most patients. Sufficient glucose should be given to provide protein-sparing effects (see Chapter 16, Nutritional Assessment and Support). It may be advantageous to use branched-chain (rather than aromatic) amino acids in total parenteral nutrition (TPN) preparations to minimize encephalopathy. Restoring a positive nitrogen balance is a major goal of nutritional repletion and may be assessed by standard tests of urine urea nitrogen. Lipid infusions are of limited usefulness because the failing liver cannot process fats readily.

PULMONARY COMPLICATIONS

Aspiration, pneumonia, atelectasis, and abnormal ventilation–perfusion (VQ) matching all contribute to the frequent development of hypoxemia in patients with acute hepatic failure. Acute VQ mismatching probably is due to failure of the damaged liver to clear vasodilating humoral substances. A reduced level of consciousness, abdominal distention from ascites, and splinting from pain caused by a swollen liver all can produce hypoxemia by causing atelectasis. Pulmonary edema due to fluid overload, hypoalbuminemia, impaired cardiac contractility, and increased vascular permeability all may occur.

MISCELLANEOUS COMPLICATIONS

Many hepatically metabolized drugs are potentially lethal in acute hepatic failure. Because narcotics, sedatives, and anesthetics severely depress mental status and glottic reflexes in these sensitive patients, indiscriminate use may have a fatal outcome; careful dosing and patient monitoring are mandatory. Long-acting sedatives given frequently or in large doses should be avoided because of cumulative drug effects. If sedation is necessary, small doses of short-acting drugs without active metabolites (e.g., oxazepam) should be used. If neuromuscular paralytic agents are used, those not requiring hepatic metabolism are favored (e.g., succinylcholine, pancuronium, and atracurium).

Ascites frequently is present in acute hepatic failure and, on occasion, a pleuroperitoneal communication may allow ascitic fluid to enter the chest, producing a symptomatic pleural effusion. The development of ascites with or without pleural fluid may impair ventilation and increase the work of breathing. Usually, sodium and water restriction and diuretic therapy are sufficient to limit ascites to manageable levels. Spironolactone, a potassium-sparing diuretic, alone or in combination with a loop diuretic, usually is effective. When diuretics fail, large-volume paracentesis may temporarily improve gas exchange and patient comfort. Rarely, ascites can become so tense that venous return is impaired and urine flow is impeded, in essence, "abdominal tamponade." The reductions in urine flow can result from compression of the ureter, renal vein, or artery. Removal of large volumes of ascites can, on occasion, precipitate hypotension, which responds to intravenous volume replacement. Controversy persists about the relative benefits of colloid and crystalloid in this situation.

PROGNOSIS

Outcome is determined largely by patient characteristics, the cause of hepatic failure, and severity of hepatic failure. Outcome is best for young patients between the ages of 10 and 40 years. Fulminant hepatic failure caused by non-A non-B hepatitis or drugs (exclusive of acetaminophen) is associated with poor prognosis. Similarly, development of coma, a bilirubin level higher than 18 mg/dL, an arterial pH lower than 7.30, a prothrombin INR higher than 3.5, or less than 10% activity of any specific clotting factor are poor prognostic indicators. The occurrence of any other associated organ failure (e.g., ARDS or acute renal failure) also dramatically reduces the chances for survival.

EXPERIMENTAL TREATMENT

All published studies using corticosteroids in acute hepatic failure demonstrate increased protein catabolism, and a higher incidence of infection without hepatic improvement. There is no evidence that prostaglandin infusions, plasmapheresis, exchange transfusion, hyperimmune globulin, or cross-species circulation improves survival. In survivors of fulminant acute hepatic failure, combined therapy with insulin and glucagon may cause the remaining liver to regenerate at a faster rate, but no benefit on survival has been demonstrated. As outlined earlier, some centers are aggressively pursuing liver transplantation for acute hepatic failure.

KEY POINTS

1. Only hepatic failure caused by acetaminophen has a specific therapy; therefore, supportive care is the basis for treating most patients with hepatic failure.

2. Loss of the liver's drug-detoxifying capacity radically alters the pharmacokinetics of most medications used in the ICU. Drugs, doses, and schedules must be reconsidered carefully and drugs metabolized extensively by the liver should be avoided.

3. Intravascular volume is often normal or depleted despite total body fluid overload in patients with acute hepatic failure. Therefore, hemodynamic and renal status is very tenuous in these patients.

4. Altered mental status in patients with hepatic failure frequently has a second treatable cause that is not hepatic encephalopathy (e.g., hypoglycemia, sepsis, increased intracranial pressure, drug intoxication).

5. Loss of hepatic function impairs immunocompetence to such a degree that infection is a major killer. Primary bacteremias and spontaneous bacterial peritonitis are common and should be considered constantly.

6. Because of the central role of the liver in maintaining hemostasis, acute hepatic failure often is complicated by bleeding complications, commonly from the gastrointestinal tract.

SUGGESTED READINGS

1. Alexander WF, Spindel E, Harty RF, et al. The usefulness of branched chain amino acids in patients with acute or chronic hepatic encephalopathy. Am J Gastroenterol 1989;84:91.
2. Ash SR. Treatment of acute hepatic failure with encephalopathy: a review. Int J Artif Organs 1991;14:191.
3. Bernuau J, Rueff B, Benhamou JP. Fulminant and subfulminant liver failure: definitions and causes. Semin Liver Dis 1986;6:97.
4. Behari DJ, Gimson AES, Williams R. Cardiovascular, pulmonary and renal complications of fulminant hepatic failure. Semin Liver Dis 1986;6:119.
5. Boks AL, Brommer EJP, Schalm SW, et al. Hemostasis and fibrinolysis in severe liver failure and their relation to hemorrhage. Hepatology 1986;6:79.
6. Brems JJ, Hiatt JR, Ramming KP, et al. Fulminant hepatic failure: the role of liver transplantation as primary therapy. Am J Surg 1987;154:137.
7. Chapman RW, Forman D, Peto R, et al. Liver transplantation for acute hepatic failure? Lancet 1990;335:32.
8. Clark R, Rake MO, Flute PT, et al. Coagulation abnormalities in acute liver failure: pathogenetic and therapeutic implications. Scand J Gastroenterol 1973;8(Suppl 19):63L.
9. Conn HO, Fessel JM. Spontaneous bacterial peritonitis in cirrhosis: variations on a theme. Medicine 1971;50:161–197.
10. Dunn GD, Hayes P, Breen KJ, et al. The liver in congestive heart failure: a review. Am J Med Sci 1973;265:174–189.
11. Dymock IW, Ticker JS, Woolf IL, et al. Coagulation studies as a prognostic index in acute liver failure. Br J Haematol 1975;29:385.
12. Ede RJ, Williams R. Hepatic encephalopathy and cerebral edema. Semin Liver Dis 1986;6:107.

13. Fagan ES, Williams R. Fulminant viral hepatitis. Br Med Bull 1990;46:462.
14. Gammal SH, Jones AE. Hepatic encephalopathy. Med Clin North Am 1989;73:793.
15. Gelman S. Hemodynamic support in patients with liver disease. Transplant Proc 1991;23:1899.
16. Guarner F, Hughes RD, Gimson AES, et al. Renal function in fulminant hepatic failure: hemodynamics and renal prostaglandins. Gut 1987;28:1643.
17. Harrison PM, Wendon JA, Gimson AES, et al. Improvement by acetylcysteine of hemodynamics and oxygen transport in fulminant hepatic failure. N Engl J Med 1991; 324:1852.
18. Hoyumpa AM, Desmond PV, Arant GR, et al. Hepatic encephalopathy. Gastroenterology 1979;76:189–195.
19. Iwatsuki S, Steibner A, Marsh JW, et al. Liver transplantation for fulminant hepatic failure. Transplant Proc 1989; 21:2431.
20. Karvountzis GG, Redeker AG, Peters RL. Long term follow up studies of patients surviving fulminant viral hepatitis. Gastroenterology 1974;67:870.
21. Krowka MJ, Cortese DA. Pulmonary aspects of liver disease and liver transplantation. Clin Chest Med 1989;10: 593.
22. Lidofsky SD, Bass NM, Prager MC, et al. Intracranial pressure monitoring in patients with fulminant hepatic failure. Hepatology 1992;16:1.
23. MacDougall BRD, Williams R. H₂-receptor antagonists and antacids in the prevention of acute gastrointestinal hemorrhage in fulminant hepatic failure. Two controlled trials. Lancet 1977;1:617.
24. MacDougall BRD, Williams R. H2 receptor antagonists in the prevention of acute upper gastrointestinal hemorrhage in fulminant hepatic failure. Gastroenterology 1978; 74:464.
25. Munoz SJ, Robinson M, Northrup B, et al. Elevated intracranial pressure and computed tomography of the brain in fulminant hepatocellular failure. Hepatology 1991;13: 209.
26. Nora LM, Bleck TP. Increased intracranial pressure complicating hepatic failure. J Crit Illness 1989;4:87.
27. O'Grady JG, Alexander GJM, Hayllar KM, et al. Early indicators of prognosis in fulminant hepatic failure. Gastroenterology 1989;97:439.
28. Rakela J, Mosely JW, Edwards VM, et al. A double-blinded, randomized trial of hydrocortisone in acute hepatic failure. Dig Dis Sci 1991;36:1223.
29. Ring-Larsen H, Palazzo V. Renal failure in fulminant hepatic failure and terminal cirrhosis: a comparison between incidence, types and prognosis. Gut 1981;22:585.
30. Rizzetto M, Verme G. Delta hepatitis-present status. J Hepatol 1985;1:187–193.
31. Roberts HR, Cederbaum AL. The liver and blood coagulation: physiology and pathology. Gastroenterology 1972; 63:287.
32. Rolando N, Harvey F, Brahm J, et al. Prospective study of bacterial infection in acute liver failure: an analysis of fifty patients. Hepatology 1990;11:49.
33. Sherlock S, Parbhoo SP. The management of acute hepatic failure. Postgrad Med J 1971;47:493.
34. Trewby PN, Warren R, Conti S, et al. Incidence and pathophysiology of pulmonary edema in fulminant hepatic failure. Gastroenterology 1978;74:859.
35. Tygstrup N, Ranek L. Assessment of prognosis in fulminant hepatic failure. Semin Liver Dis 1986;6:129.
36. Tygstrup N, Ranek L. Fulminant hepatic failure. Clin Gastroenterol 1981;10:191.
37. Williams R. Fulminant hepatic failure. Postgrad Med J 1983;4(Suppl 59):33–41.
38. Williams R, Gimson A. Management of acute liver failure. Clin Gastroenterol 1985;14:93–104.
39. Wyke RJ, Rajkovic IA, Eddleston ALW, et al. Defective opsonization and complement deficiency in serum from patients with fulminant hepatic failure. Gut 1980;21:643.

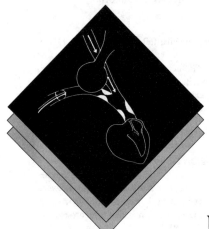

CHAPTER 32

Endocrine Emergencies

THYROID DISEASE

The most common "thyroid disorder" seen in the intensive care unit (ICU) is the sic euthyroid syndrome, which is not a thyroid disorder at all but rather a peripheral alteration in the binding and metabolism of thyroid hormone caused by critical illness. Although significant hyperthyroidism or hypothyroidism are substantially less common, profound excess or deficiency of thyroid hormone is life threatening, can be confused with many other nonendocrine conditions, and generally is amenable to simple therapy.

SEVERE HYPERTHYROIDISM AND THYROID STORM

Definitions

No absolute signs differentiate thyroid storm from severe hyperthyroidism. In addition to accentuated signs and symptoms of hyperthyroidism, thyroid storm is more likely to exhibit fever (often exceeding 100°F) and tachycardia (pulse greater than 100 per minute). Ancillary features include a goiter, congestive heart failure, arrhythmias, tremor, diaphoresis, diarrhea, elevated liver function tests, and psychosis.

Etiology

Historically, surgery performed on large goiters with poor preoperative preparation was the most common cause of thyroid storm, but currently, thyroid storm usually results from an acute infec-

tion, withdrawal of antithyroid drugs, or nonthyroid surgery. Recognizable Graves' disease is present in most patients with severe hyperthyroidism. Although iodine ingestion initially increases thyroxine (T4) production, it then temporarily suppresses T4 release. However, after 10 to 14 days, serum iodine levels decline, allowing discharge of large amounts of newly formed T4 into the circulation. For this reason, radioactive iodine, cardiac catheterization dye, intravenous pyelogram (IVP) contrast, and oral iodinated contrast may precipitate delayed thyroid storm in predisposed individuals. Accidental or intentional overdose with exogenous T4 rarely leads to thyroid storm, except in massive ingestions.

Laboratory Tests

For the critically ill patient with thyroid storm, the diagnosis must be a clinical one, because the results of thyroid function tests often are delayed and because comparable elevations in total T4, free T4, and T3 are seen in both mild and severe hyperthyroidism. (Free T4 levels tend to be higher in patients with thyroid storm.) Among patients with Graves' disease, occasionally only T3 concentrations are elevated (T3 thyrotoxicosis). TSH levels will be low to undetectable in all cases of hyperthyroidism. Elevated hepatic transaminases often indicate life-threatening disease. Rarely, hypercalcemia may be present. In thyroid storm, the leukocyte count usually is normal or slightly elevated, but relative lymphocytosis is common, a feature that may aid in differentiating thyroid disease from infectious causes of fever.

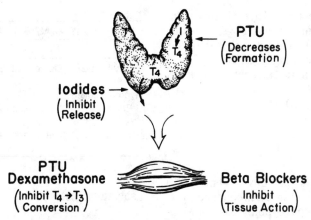

FIG. 32–1. Sites of action of antithyroid medications.

Treatment

The treatment of thyroid storm is fourfold: (*a*) block T4 formation, (*b*) prevent T4 release, (*c*) prevent peripheral conversion of T4 to T3, and (*d*) inhibit the tissue effects of T4 (Fig. 32.1). Propylthiouracil (PTU) and methimazole both block T4 synthesis, an action that develops its full clinical effect over days. Of the two choices, PTU is preferred because of its additional ability to block the conversion of T4 to its biologic active form (T3) in peripheral tissues. (Inhibition of T4 to T3 conversion also may be accomplished by dexamethasone and to a minor degree by propranolol.) Although PTU is preferred over methimazole, allergic reactions may occur with its use, and late, dose-dependent agranulocytosis is a real risk. Low doses of PTU represent a particularly good choice of therapy for the pregnant patient because the drug crosses the placental barrier poorly. One advantage of methimazole is its ability to be administered by rectal suppository in patients who are unable to take oral medicines.

Release of preformed T4 into the circulation is blocked rapidly by a supersaturated oral solution of iodine (5 drops of SSKI solution three times a day) or by dexamethasone (2 mg intravenously every 6 hours). Unfortunately, even complete blockade of T4 release does not terminate hyperthyroid crisis because circulating T4 has a very long half-life. PTU and iodine are only available as oral preparations, therefore, administration may prove difficult in the critically ill patient. Because iodine inhibits thyroid uptake of PTU and methimazole, these drugs must be administered at least 2 hours before iodine therapy. β-blockers

blunt the tissue actions of thyroid hormone, but the need for adrenergic blockade is questionable if other appropriate therapy is initiated. If a β-blocker is used, it makes some sense initially to select a short-acting agent such as esmolol to gauge the patient's response to β-blockade. If adverse consequences develop from β-blockade, the drug can be terminated rapidly. In cases of deliberate overdose of thyroid hormone, oral administration of bile-acid-sequestering drugs can prevent absorption of the thyroid hormone. In extreme cases of overdose, plasmapheresis or peritoneal dialysis may be used to remove thyroid hormone from the circulation.

Complications

Clinical heart failure occurs in half of patients with thyroid storm. Although classically described as a "high output" state, many patients have normal or even low cardiac outputs and elevated wedge pressures and may be harmed by the use of β-blockers. In contrast, hypertension and tachycardia seen in thyroid storm may respond well to β-blockade. Tachyarrhythmias associated with thyroid storm may be controlled with a combination of digoxin, β-blockers, and verapamil. (The ultra–short-acting β-blocker, esmolol may be particularly useful.) Fever from increased metabolic rate may be controlled by direct external cooling, but salicylates should be avoided because of their tendency to displace T4 from serum proteins, worsening thyroid storm. Therapy of thyroid storm must include nutritional support because of increased caloric requirements. (Folate and B vitamins are also consumed rapidly and should be supplemented.) Thyroid storm increases the metabolism of many drugs, including some of those useful in its treatment (β-blockers and dexamethasone), making larger doses of these drugs necessary on a more frequent schedule.

SEVERE HYPOTHYROIDISM (MYXEDEMA COMA)

Definition

Hypothermia, central nervous system (CNS) dysfunction, and hypotension differentiate myxedema coma from simple hypothyroidism. Myxedema is a rare but reversible cause of several common syndromes precipitating ICU admission, including (a) severe ileus suggestive of bowel obstruction, (b) respiratory failure (including failure to wean), (c) heart failure, (d) hypothermia, and (e) coma.

Etiology

Hypothyroidism usually (in more than 90% of cases) results from primary failure of the thyroid gland and not pituitary insufficiency. Interestingly, severe myxedema usually does not become manifest until some intercurrent illness complicates preexisting hypothyroidism (e.g., infection, surgery, hypothermia, trauma, and drugs, particularly sedatives). For unclear reasons, hypothyroidism is much more likely to occur in women and during the winter months of the year. Most patients hospitalized with severe hypothyroidism have had the condition for some time; admission to the hospital is often precipitated by discontinuing thyroid replacement therapy.

Diagnosis

The diagnosis of myxedema coma must be a clinical one, because thyroid function tests rarely are available in a timely fashion and therapy must be initiated promptly to achieve optimal outcome. The common physical signs of hypothyroidism include (a) obesity, (b) dry puffy skin, (c) characteristic facies, (d) sinus bradycardia, (e) decreased relaxation phase of deep tendon reflexes, and (f) nonpitting edema. Pleural and pericardial effusions and ascites also are often detected. Less commonly, hoarseness, macroglossia, and hair loss are noted. Paradoxically, hypertension is a more common presentation than hypotension.

TABLE 32–1

LABORATORY ANALYSIS OF HYPOTHYROIDISM

	Total T4	Free T4	TSH
Sic euthyroid	Decreased	Normal or decreased	Normal
Hypothyroidism			
Primary	Decreased	Greatly decreased	Increased
Secondary	Decreased	Decreased	Decreased or zero

Laboratory Tests

Anemia, hyponatremia, hypoglycemia, hypercapnia, and hypoxemia are common in hypothyroidism but are not diagnostic. Marked elevations in cholesterol also are noted frequently. The hyponatremia seen in hypothyroidism is often multifactorial, reflecting inappropriate antidiuretic hormone (ADH) secretion and combined treatment with diuretics and hypotonic fluids.

The laboratory hallmark of primary hypothyroidism is an elevated serum concentration of thyroid-stimulating hormone (TSH) accompanied by low total and free T4 levels (Table 32.1). (The much less common secondary or ''pituitary'' form of the disease is characterized by a low T4 and low TSH.) Many nonthyroidal illnesses decrease the T3 and total T4 levels without impairing thyroid function, the so-called ''sic euthyroid'' state. In this syndrome, decreased T4 binding protein and altered T4 metabolism lead to a decreased total T4 with normal or slightly depressed free T4, a reduced T3, and normal or minimally elevated TSH. The sic euthyroid condition does not require thyroid hormone replacement therapy. Rarely, chronic dopamine infusion may inhibit pituitary release of TSH, inducing a false laboratory pattern suggesting a sic euthyroid state in a truly hypothyroid patient.

Treatment

Because orally administered drugs are poorly absorbed in myxedema, T4 initially should be administered intravenously. No controlled studies have been conducted to guide dosing, but reasonable starting daily doses of thyroxine in myxedema range from 0.2 to 0.5 mg intravenously. (There does not seem to be benefit from larger initial doses.) Commonly, 0.5 mg of T4 is given in the first 24 hours, followed by 0.05 to 0.1 mg each day thereafter. Some clinical response usually is seen within 6 to 12 hours. T4 doses should be somewhat reduced in patients with known ischemic heart disease or angina because abrupt elevation of thyroxine may precipitate cardiac ischemia. In normotensive, euthermic patients, the initial dose may be as low as 0.1 mg. Current knowledge does not support the practice of administering T3.

When hypothyroidism is suspected, adrenal function also must be tested because an adrenal crisis may be precipitated if T4 is administered to patients with concurrent adrenal insufficiency. To avoid missing a diagnosis of adrenal insufficiency, the most practical approach is to perform a cortisol stimulation test when thyroid function tests are obtained and begin empiric stress doses of corticosteroids while awaiting the results (see Adrenal Insufficiency, below). Hypoglycemia occurs frequently enough to warrant urgent evaluation in acutely ill patients with altered mental status and suspected hypothyroidism. Arterial blood gases should be analyzed in most patients because suppressed ventilatory drive leading to hypercapnic respiratory failure is common. Hyponatremia is treated effectively by temporary water restriction. Hypotension and hypoperfusion should be treated with thyroxine and corticosteroids as well as the fluids and vasopressors dictated by usual hemodynamic indicators. Many patients will have concomitant hypothermia requiring treatment (see Chapter 28, Thermal Disorders).

Complications

Aspiration pneumonitis is a very common complication for patients with reduced mental status secondary to hypothyroidism and often precipitates acute lung injury. The obesity and immobility of the profoundly hypothyroid patient predispose patients to the formation of atelectasis, decubitus ulcers, and deep venous thrombi. Prevention of these common complications is covered in detail in Chapter 18 (General Supportive Care).

ADRENAL DISEASES

ADRENAL INSUFFICIENCY

Etiology

The physiologic effects of adrenal insufficiency result from deficiencies of cortisol and/or aldoste-

rone. Primary adrenal insufficiency results from direct adrenal gland destruction. Tuberculosis, fungal disease, surgery, infarction, metastatic malignancy, autoimmune disease, and hemorrhage are the most frequent causes. Hemorrhagic adrenal insufficiency is seen most commonly in septic patients and in anticoagulated patients, especially after cardiopulmonary bypass. Critically ill patients with the acquired immunodeficiency syndrome (AIDS) also have an increased frequency of adrenal insufficiency. For patients with AIDS, cytomegalovirus, metastatic neoplasm, or ketoconazole therapy are the most common culprits; however, in many patients, the etiology remains obscure.

In the more common, secondary form of adrenal insufficiency, pituitary secretion of adrenocorticotrophic hormone (ACTH) is insufficient to maintain adequate levels of cortisol, but aldosterone secretion remains normal because it is not regulated by ACTH. Secondary adrenal insufficiency results from direct trauma, tumor growth (especially pituitary adenoma), or infarction of the pituitary gland. Pituitary infarction may occur when hemorrhage occurs in a preexisting pituitary adenoma, when primary hemorrhage occurs in the anticoagulated patient, when trauma disrupts a feeding artery, or when the postpartum patient suffers spontaneous infarction. The abrupt withdrawal of exogenous steroids mimics secondary adrenal insufficiency because ACTH secretion remains depressed as the exogenous corticosteroid is rapidly cleared from the circulation. Because aldosterone levels remain normal or near normal, secondary adrenal insufficiency seldom results in dehydration or hyperkalemia. Conversely, primary adrenal insufficiency frequently demonstrates these features. In most patients, adrenal crisis is precipitated by an intercurrent illness that causes volume depletion (vomiting/diarrhea) or vasodilation (sepsis). Surgery increases the risk of adrenal crisis through both of these mechanisms and by increasing cortisol clearance.

A rare, tertiary form of adrenal insufficiency also exists in which granulomatous disease or neoplasm destroys the hypothalamic pathways necessary for signaling the pituitary release of ACTH. Diagnosis and replacement therapy for this condition parallels that for secondary adrenal insufficiency.

The drugs ketoconazole, etomidate, and aminoglutethimide all interfere with normal steroidogenesis and may precipitate adrenal insufficiency. In addition, drugs that accelerate hepatic metabolism of exogenously administered corticosteroids (e.g., rifampin, phenytoin, and barbiturates) can also precipitate adrenal insufficiency.

Signs and Symptoms

Weakness, fatigue, anorexia, fever (as high as 40°C), and nausea are the most common presenting signs of adrenal insufficiency, regardless of etiology. Shock may be the initial presentation in adrenal failure complicated by infection or dehydration. In anticoagulated patients, flank pain and a fall in hematocrit may be the presenting signs of adrenal hemorrhage. Mild to moderate diffuse abdominal pain also has been reported. Occasionally, the pain is sufficiently severe to prompt exploratory laparotomy, a potentially lethal intervention for the patient with adrenal insufficiency. Cutaneous hyperpigmentation is seen only in primary adrenal insufficiency. (A functioning pituitary gland is necessary to produce the ACTH-like melanocyte-stimulating hormone responsible for hyperpigmentation.) Loss of body hair may be seen in women with primary adrenal insufficiency as a result of a loss of adrenal androgen production but is not a feature in men because of the unaffected testicular production of androgens.

Laboratory Examination

Urinary sodium wasting (resulting in hyponatremia) and renal potassium retention (causing hyperkalemia) are seen predominantly in primary adrenal insufficiency in which aldosterone is lacking. Conversely, the isolated cortisol deficiency of secondary adrenal insufficiency impairs free water excretion but rarely causes hyperkalemia. Hypercalcemia may be seen in either form of adrenal insufficiency because cortisol is required to regulate gastrointestinal absorption and renal excretion of calcium. Although the total leukocyte count usually is normal, the percentage of eosinophils and lymphocytes often is increased. Mild normochromic normocytic anemia is very common. Hypoglycemia may be the presenting manifestation of either primary or secondary adrenal insufficiency. Volume depletion seen with all forms of adrenal insufficiency elevates the blood urea nitrogen (BUN).

Tests of Adrenal Function

Because adrenal insufficiency is life threatening, it is important to institute cortisol replacement before laboratory confirmation of the diagnosis. The following protocol may be used to simultaneously diagnose and treat adrenal failure.

1. Draw baseline blood cortisol and ACTH levels.
2. Administer an ACTH analog (intravenous Cortrosyn, 250 μg).
3. Obtain cortisol levels 30 and 60 minutes after ACTH injection.
4. Begin empiric glucocorticoid therapy. (Dexamethasone represents a good therapeutic choice because it is potent and will not significantly interfere with initial serum cortisol assays.)

If such testing reveals a baseline cortisol value exceeding 25 μg/dL or a brisk (approximately twofold) rise after stimulation, a diagnosis of adrenal insufficiency is very unlikely. A high baseline cortisol that fails to stimulate adrenal reserve that may require supplementation during severe stress. For patients who fail to respond to single-dose ACTH stimulation, a 3-day ACTH (Cortrosyn) infusion may be required to distinguish between primary and secondary forms of the disease. (The primary form of the disease will not respond to even prolonged ACTH analog infusion because the adrenal gland is destroyed or unresponsive.) The usual responses to a brief ACTH stimulation test in various clinical scenarios are illustrated in Table 32.2.

Treatment

Glucocorticoids and salt-containing fluid are the essence of therapy. If adequate amounts of salt-containing crystalloid are infused, mineralocorticoid hormones are not immediately necessary in either form of adrenal insufficiency. In persons with normally functioning pituitary–adrenal axes, cortisol levels may rise 10-fold above baseline levels under periods of maximal stress to a daily equivalent of 300 to 400 mg of hydrocortisone. Therefore, patients with acute adrenal insufficiency require relatively large doses of corticosteroids. Although hydrocortisone (100 mg every 6 to 8 hours) often is given intravenously because of its mineralocorticoid effects, dexamethasone (2–5 mg every 8 hours) is a useful alternative because it does not interfere with serum cortisol assays. Table 32.3 provides several equivalent doses of corticosteroids for replacement therapy. Although not required in every case, intravenous steroid administration avoids potential problems of delayed or incomplete absorption in the unstable patient.

TABLE 32–2

USUAL RESPONSE TO ACTH STIMULATION

| Pituitary Adrenal Axis Status | ACTH Level | Cortisol Level | |
		Baseline	Post-ACTH Stimulation
Normal	Normal	Normal	Increased
Primary adrenal failure	Marked increase	Low	Low
Secondary adrenal failure	Low or normal	Low	Increased
Post-steroid withdrawal	Low	Low or normal	Mild increase*

* Requires 24-hour ACTH infusion for confirmation.

TABLE 32–3

STRESS REPLACEMENT DOSES OF CORTICOSTEROIDS

Dexamethasone	7.5–30 mg/day
Hydrocortisone	200–300 mg/day
Methylprednisolone	40–80 mg/day
Prednisone	50–100 mg/day

Although mild hyperkalemia is seen commonly, potassium concentrations seldom rise to dangerous levels in adrenal insufficiency. Hyperkalemia usually is corrected rapidly with volume expansion and glucocorticoids alone. (Potassium binding resin or dialysis is rarely necessary.) Because adrenal insufficiency impairs gluconeogenesis, intravenous fluids should include adequate glucose.

WITHDRAWAL OF EXOGENOUS STEROIDS

A cushingoid appearance always should be a clue to the use of exogenous corticosteroids and the potential for pituitary–adrenal axis suppression. Adrenal insufficiency as a result of exogenous steroid therapy is a surprisingly rare event considering the frequency with which corticosteroids are used. The likelihood of developing adrenal insufficiency after withdrawal of steroids is related directly to the daily dose of corticosteroid and the duration of therapy. Partial or complete adrenal suppression from exogenous corticosteroids may occur with as little as 7 days of low-dose prednisone (20–30 mg). Prolonged steroid use may impair adrenal responsiveness for as long as 1 year after withdrawal of exogenous steroids (Fig. 32.2). After discontinuing exogenous corticosteroids, the ACTH response returns first (usually within 90 days); however, several months

often pass before normal cortisol response to ACTH is restored. Patients who demonstrate a normal cortisol response to ACTH stimulation are unlikely to have subnormal adrenal response to stress. If the adrenal responsiveness of a critically ill patient is questionable, adrenal function should be tested and cortisol replacement should be given empirically. For patients of questionable adrenal status who require immediate surgery, administration of 100 mg of intravenous hydrocortisone before and after surgery will provide sufficient perioperative coverage.

EXCESSIVE CORTICOSTEROID ADMINISTRATION

High doses of corticosteroids predispose patients to infection and produce protein wasting, poor wound healing, mental status alterations, sleep disruption, and glucose intolerance. Long-term exposure also may cause intracranial hypertension, bone loss, aseptic necrosis, glaucoma, pancreatitis, and cataract formation. Adverse steroid effects are minimized by (a) using the lowest effective dose, (b) using a short-acting steroid preparation such as hydrocortisone, (c) administering the full daily requirement in a single morning dose, and (d) using alternate day therapy where possible.

DISORDERS OF GLUCOSE METABOLISM

GENERAL CARE OF THE CRITICALLY ILL DIABETIC PATIENT

Several important principles apply to treatment of glucose abnormalities in the ICU.

1. Critical illness induces a state of relative insulin resistance due to release of stress hormones (glucagon, epinephrine, cortisol).

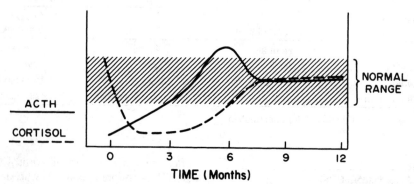

FIG. 32–2. ACTH and cortisol levels following abrupt termination of prolonged glucocorticoid therapy at time 0.

2. Starvation, sepsis, and drug therapy complicate diabetes management by unpredictably altering the effectiveness of insulin. Although "tight" control of blood glucose has been shown to reduce long-term morbidity of diabetes, similar data do not exist to justify intensive glucose control in the ICU. Rapid changes in glucose metabolism and a high propensity to develop hypoglycemia makes tight control risky.

The following suggestions comprise a rational approach to managing the critically ill, nonketotic diabetic patient.

1. Avoid interruption of feedings.
2. Eliminate or significantly reduce the proportion of long-acting insulin. (Instead, monitor blood glucose values frequently and treat with small doses of regular insulin.)
3. Withhold oral hypoglycemic agents: their hypoglycemic effects may persist much longer than desired.
4. Do not substitute urine tests for serum tests of glucose. (At best, urine tests are time-delayed measures of serum levels and are less precise.)
5. Use bedside glucose determinations liberally.

HYPOGLYCEMIA

Hypoglycemia is a relative term used to describe a blood glucose level that is insufficient to meet current metabolic demands. Although many patients are symptomatic at glucose concentrations less than 50 mg/dL, a large number of young, otherwise healthy patients may have plasma glucose levels of 40 mg/dL or less without symptoms. The early symptoms of hypoglycemia are generally those of adrenergic excess (e.g., sweating, tachycardia, and hypertension) and depend not only on the absolute blood glucose value but also on the rate of its decline. Blood glucose should be determined rapidly in patients with altered mental status to rule out hypoglycemia, even if focal neurologic deficits are present. Seizures also may be the presenting symptom but are a more common manifestation in children than in adults. If glucose concentrations cannot be measured readily in a patient with suspected hypoglycemia, administration of 50 to 100 mL of dextrose with an appropriate amount of thiamine is indicated.

Insulin Reactions

Hypoglycemia episodes induced by insulin ("insulin reactions") are the most common cause of hypoglycemia in patients younger than 30 years of age. When combined with alcohol ingestion, insulin reactions represent the most common causes of hypoglycemia in all patients. Insulin reactions are particularly common in the ICU because renal insufficiency impairs insulin clearance and because hospitalized diabetics frequently do not receive regular feedings. (Long-acting insulins and oral hypoglycemics amplify this risk.) Insulin-induced hypoglycemia also may occur when insulin injected into suboptimally perfused tissue is later absorbed as perfusion is reestablished. High insulin levels and low C-peptide levels in the hypoglycemic patient suggest intentional or inadvertent insulin overdosage. Patients with little or no functional pancreatic tissue are at particular risk for hypoglycemia because of their inability to produce and release the counter-regulatory hormone glucagon. In addition, drugs that block the adrenergic response (especially β-blocking drugs) can blunt the counter-regulatory effects of epinephrine released during a hypoglycemic crisis.

Oral Hypoglycemic Agents

Oral hypoglycemic agents are a poor choice for glucose control in the hospitalized diabetic because of their long half-life and frequent interactions with other drugs. Patients with hypoglycemia due to these agents should be observed closely because of the potential for prolonged or recurrent symptoms. Hypoglycemia due to oral agents is often refractory to glucose alone and may require combined therapy with hydrocortisone, glucagon, and diazoxide. Advanced age and renal failure prolong the half-life of these drugs and their attendant toxicity. Hypoglycemic action also is potentiated by butazolidin, sulfonamides, probenecid, and salicylates. Furthermore, oral hypoglycemics interact with such commonly used medications as phenytoin, phenothiazines, rifampin, and thiazides.

Other Causes of Hypoglycemia

Overwhelming infection may produce hypoglycemia by multiple mechanisms, including hepatic hypoperfusion or failure, renal insufficiency, depletion of muscle glycogen, and starvation. Alcohol suppresses gluconeogenesis, restricts nutrient intake, and induces a low insulin state that favors free fatty acid release and ketone production. Consequently, alcoholic patients may present with hypoglycemia and a mixed ketoacidosis and lactic acidosis. By the time such patients seek medical attention, the ingested alcohol often has been completely metabolized; therefore, blood alcohol levels are often zero. Glucose, thiamine, and fluids comprise the key elements in the treatment of alcoholic acidosis with hypoglycemia. Although ketoacids are present, insulin does not speed resolution of the acidosis and may precipitate or exacerbate hypoglycemia. Sodium bicarbonate rarely is necessary, possibly only to maintain the pH above 7.10.

Other causes of hypoglycemia include hepatic failure (due to cirrhosis, tumor infiltration, or massive hepatic necrosis), renal failure, salicylate poisoning, and insulin-secreting tumors. Surgery and other states of physiologic stress blunt the effect of insulin while stimulating the release of counter-regulatory hormones. Imbalance of these effects may cause circulating glucose to rise or decline unpredictably to dangerous levels. To prevent hypoglycemia in the surgical patient, it is prudent to monitor glucose closely and to decrease (but not discontinue) preoperative insulin. A useful strategy is to administer one-half of the regular insulin dosage before surgery, despite the fasting state. The key to preventing hypoglycemia is frequent intraoperative and postoperative glucose testing.

Artifactual hypoglycemia may occur when glucose is metabolized in blood samples with extremely high leukocyte counts. Leukocyte-induced hypoglycemia occurs most commonly when glucose measurement is delayed for hours. Inactivating leukocyte metabolism using oxalate-fluoride-containing blood collection tubes can prevent this problem.

Treatment of Hypoglycemia

Unless otherwise contraindicated, intravenous glucose should be administered empirically to all patients with abruptly altered, undiagnosed changes in mental status or neurologic function, even when focal. Two ampules of D50W (100 gm glucose) are always sufficient to acutely raise the serum glucose levels above 100 mg/dL. Larger doses simply increase serum osmolarity. When hypoglycemic patients of unknown or questionable nutritional status are treated with glucose, thiamine (1 mg/kg) should be given concurrently to prevent Wernicke's encephalopathy. For all cases of hypoglycemia, it is prudent to closely monitor the patient and recheck the serum glucose frequently. On rare occasion, hypoglycemia is refractory to bolus glucose administration alone. In such cases, constant infusion of D10W, with hydrocortisone (100 mg intravenously) and/or glucagon (1 mg intravenously per liter of D10W), will augment the blood glucose.

DIABETIC KETOACIDOSIS

Precipitating Factors

Diabetic ketoacidosis (DKA) is a common, serious condition, the mortality of which remains at 5 to 15% despite aggressive therapy. DKA is the result of a deficiency of insulin, usually with a relative excess of counter-regulatory hormones. Most commonly, DKA is precipitated by noncompliance with diet or medications, although infection frequently contributes. Stroke, myocardial infarction, trauma, pregnancy, pancreatitis, and hyperthyroidism also are potential precipitants.

Physical Features

The most prominent physical features of DKA (hypotension, hypoperfusion, and tachypnea) are the result of the two major metabolic derangements—volume depletion and metabolic acidosis. Deep and rapid "Kussmaul" respirations are an attempt to compensate for metabolic acidosis. Recognition of DKA is not difficult, but some "classic" features are seldom seen. For example, although obtundation is frequent, frank coma is rare (<10% of cases). Fever is not a part of DKA in the absence of infection. In fact, slight reductions in temperature are much more frequent. (This is particularly true if the temperature is measured orally in a hyperventilating patient.) Vomiting is very common and often is the result of ileus induced by ketonemia, dehydration, and electrolyte imbalance. Unexplained features of DKA include pleurisy and abdominal pain. The fact that abdominal pain almost always resolves rapidly with correction of the acidosis can help distinguish DKA from more serious causes of abdominal pain. Therefore, patients with undiagnosed acute abdominal pain should have glucose and ketone determinations before undergoing other diagnostic or "therapeutic" procedures.

Laboratory Features

Metabolic acidosis, ketosis, and hyperglycemia are the laboratory hallmarks of DKA. Ketone measurements should be made initially in patients with hyperglycemia to confirm the diagnosis, but there is little value in serial measurements of ketones. Plasma ketoacid levels will be reflected in the anion gap, and as the total quantity of ketoacids decline, the anion gap narrows. In patients with DKA, three ketones are present in chemical equilibrium (acetoacetate, acetone, and β-hydroxy butyrate), but only acetoacetate is measured by the nitroprusside reaction most commonly used to detect ketones. Normally, β-hydroxy butyrate exceeds acetoacetate by a 3:1 ratio, but in severe acidosis, β-hydroxybutyrate may be present in concentrations 12-fold greater than acetoacetate. As the acidosis improves, the dynamic equilib-

rium shifts in favor of acetoacetate, and ketone concentrations may seem to worsen (another potential reason not to get serial ketone determinations).

Glucose levels typically range between 400 and 800 mg/dL, but they may be lower in young, well-hydrated patients whose preserved glomerular filtration facilitates glucose clearance. Leukocytosis ($>20,000/mm^3$) with a predominance of granulocytes may occur, even in the absence of infection. Loss of free water due to osmotic diuresis may lead to hyperosmolarity and hemoconcentration; therefore, even mild reductions of measured packed-cell volume in patients with DKA suggest underlying anemia or active bleeding.

The osmotic effects of glucose translocate water from the intracellular to the extracellular space, producing hyponatremia. Sodium concentration declines approximately 1.6 mEq/L for each increase of 100 mg/dL of glucose. Because serum glucose seldom exceeds 1000 mg/dL, it is unlikely for the serum sodium to fall below 120 mEq/L on an osmotic basis alone. Artifactual depressions of sodium concentration may be seen in DKA when triglycerides contribute substantially to plasma volume. Because acidosis shifts potassium from the intracellular to the extracellular compartment, most patients with DKA have normal or elevated potassium values despite sizable (200–700 mEq) total body deficits. With appropriate volume expansion, insulin therapy, and correction of the acidosis, potassium values can plummet. Therefore, even a normal serum potassium value noted at admission should be tracked closely. Total body depletion of magnesium and phosphorus are extremely common. After urine flow is reestablished, it is reasonable to offer oral replacement therapy of both ions, although no certain benefit has been demonstrated.

Serum creatinine is elevated commonly by dehydration-induced decreases in glomerular filtration rate (GFR). (With colorimetric assays, ketones may cause artifactual elevations in creatinine.) For obscure reasons, the serum amylase (particularly the salivary isoenzyme) also may be elevated in DKA.

Treatment

The most important aspects of DKA therapy are adequate fluid replacement and careful record keeping. The single best indicator of successful therapy is narrowing of the anion gap; a single measurement reflecting correction of both lactic acidosis and ketoacidosis. Total body deficits of fluid range between 5 and 10 L, with sodium deficits averaging 300 to 500 mEq. Adequate circulating volume should be replenished rapidly with normal saline in patients with evidence of hypoperfusion. After immediate stabilization, the aim should be to restore 50 to 75% of the deficit within 24 hours. Isotonic saline, Ringer's solution, or half-normal saline all are reasonable alternatives for fluid replacement after initial resuscitation. Physical examination, urine output, and frequent electrolyte measurements should guide subsequent fluid and electrolyte administration.

For patients with DKA and hypotension refractory to repletion of volume and pH correction, one should consider the following: (*a*) bleeding (particularly gastrointestinal or retroperitoneal); (*b*) septic shock, especially from urinary tract infection (UTI) or pneumonia; (*c*) adrenal insufficiency; (*d*) pancreatitis; and (*e*) myocardial infarction.

An initial insulin bolus of 0.1 to 0.5 units/kg followed by an infusion of 0.1 units/kg/hour should suffice for most patients. Insulin infusions should be titrated by infusion pump for accurate delivery. The initial goal should be to reduce plasma glucose by 75 to 100 mg/dL each hour. Initially, glucose measurements at 1- to 2-hour intervals should guide the rate of insulin and fluid administration. Failure of glucose to decline significantly within 2 to 3 hours indicates insulin resistance and should prompt doubling the insulin dosage. Insulin infusions should be continued until serum ketones are cleared and the anion gap is normalized, even if supplemental glucose must be used to prevent hypoglycemia. (Practically, this usually requires 12 to 24 hours, at which time the patient usually is able to eat.) Premature termination of insulin infusions is the most common cause of "relapsing DKA."

Sodium bicarbonate rarely is necessary in DKA and may be indicated only if the pH is below 7.10 or the patient demonstrates refractory hypotension or respiratory failure. (pH correction can help reduce the ventilatory requirement and improve diaphragmatic function in patients with respiratory fatigue or limited ventilatory capacity.) When insulin is provided to the patient with adequate hepatic perfusion, the liver regenerates bicarbonate from ketones and lactate. Loss of ketones in the urine of well-hydrated patients with normal renal function can result in a loss of "HCO_3 equivalents." When normal saline is used for resuscitation, a self-limited and mild hyperchloremic aci-

dosis often results. Sodium bicarbonate therapy is not without risk: because ketones normally regenerate bicarbonate, patients receiving exogenous base frequently develop a "rebound" alkalosis. Furthermore, the osmolality of a 50-mL ampule of $NaHCO_3$ is nearly fivefold greater than normal saline; therefore, aggressive bicarbonate therapy may exacerbate hyperosmolarity. In addition, rapid reversal of acidemia shifts the oxyhemoglobin curve leftward, exacerbates hypokalemia, and may cause paradoxical CNS acidosis.

Spontaneous or iatrogenic arrhythmias induced by acid–base and electrolyte disturbances are a major preventable cause of cardiovascular morbidity in DKA. For example, insulin and bicarbonate can rapidly drive potassium across the cell membranes, dramatically decreasing the serum K^+. Therefore, after adequate urine flow is reestablished, potassium should be administered to most DKA patients. Usually, 10 to 20 mEq per hour is required to maintain normal potassium levels, but on occasion, up to 60 mEq per hour may be necessary. Magnesium and phosphate also should be monitored. Hypophosphatemia may decrease 2,3-diphosphoglyceric acid (2,3-DPG) levels and muscle strength, but phosphate administration has yet to be shown to improve outcome. Risks of phosphate therapy include acute hypocalcemia and tissue deposition of calcium-phosphate complexes, occasionally inducing acute renal failure. Hypoglycemia, a common complication of aggressive DKA therapy, may be prevented through vigilant monitoring.

HYPEROSMOLAR NONKETOTIC COMA

Hyperosmolar nonketotic coma (HNKC) is a disorder of glucose metabolism in which plasma osmolality is elevated dramatically (often >350 mOsm/L) and plasma glucose concentrations are increased profoundly (often >1000 mEq/L). Contrary to its name, coma is neither a requisite nor common feature. Insulin levels in HNKC are sufficient to prevent ketone formation but insufficient to prevent hyperglycemia. Patients with HNKC also generate fewer ketones than patients with DKA because they tend to have lower levels of lipolytic hormones (i.e., growth hormone and cortisol). Glycosuria, a compensatory mechanism limiting increases in serum glucose, is tightly linked to GFR; therefore, HNKC is more common in elderly patients and in those underlying renal dysfunction. Patients with impaired perception of thirst (e.g., elderly patients) and/or deprived of

TABLE 32–4

FEATURES OF DKA AND HYPEROSMOLAR COMA

Characteristic	DKA	Hyperosmolar Coma
Insulin levels	Very low to absent	Low
Lipolytic hormone levels	High	Lower
Typical glucose	400–800	≈1000
Acidosis	Severe	Minimal
Ketones	High	Low or absent
Dehydration	Moderate	Severe

access to free water also are predisposed. HNKC often is precipitated by an intercurrent illness that produces volume depletion or promotes hyperglycemia (e.g., sepsis, stroke, diarrhea, vomiting, or corticosteroid or diuretic use). Unlike DKA, in which the accumulating ketoacids stimulate ventilation and produce dyspnea, patients with HNKC are often minimally symptomatic and maintain near-normal acid–base status for long periods of time. It is not until profound volume depletion limits organ function that these patients seek medical attention. The chemical and clinical features of DKA and HNKC are contrasted in Table 32.4.

Laboratory features of HNKC are similar to those of DKA, except that ketoacidosis is absent or minimal, whereas glucose values often are extremely elevated (>1000 mg/dL). Marked hyperglycemia produces the hyperosmolarity that characterizes this disorder (see Chapter 13, Fluid and Electrolyte Disorders). Total body water is severely is severely depleted in HNKC, largely due to a prolonged osmotic diuresis. Nonetheless, the osmotic effects of high glucose levels help maintain intravascular volume. Although *intravascular* volume usually is better preserved in HNKC than in DKA, it is at the expense of the intracellular compartment. This effect is responsible for the primary clinical expression of HNKC-life-threatening depression of neurologic function. Because the osmotic effect of glucose is required to maintain intravascular volume, insulin administration before restoring circulating volume with isotonic fluids can cause sudden and profound hypotension by producing a rapid shift of glucose and water into cells. As with DKA, hypokalemia and hypophosphatemia are common.

Correction of HNKC must be cautious, because abrupt reversal of serum hyperosmolarity may produce intracellular water intoxication mani-

fested by dysphoria and seizures. Despite differences in pathophysiology, the cornerstone of treatment of HNKC is similar to that of DKA: initial restoration of circulating volume with normal saline. (For such patients, normal saline represents a relatively hypotonic fluid.) Initial fluid replacement using D5W or half-normal saline can precipitate rapid cellular swelling (especially in the brain) as fluid enters the dehydrated, hypertonic cells. In general, complete fluid replacement should be targeted to occur over 24 to 48 hours. Low-dose insulin therapy should be initiated only after circulating volume has been repleted as evidenced by stable blood pressure and adequate urine output. Subsequent insulin administration and free water repletion should be guided by serial electrolyte and glucose determinations.

DIABETES INSIPIDUS

Diabetes insipidus (DI) is a life-threatening illness that results from a failure of the pituitary–hypothalamic axis to release sufficient antidiuretic hormone (ADH) or from a failure of the kidney to respond to the released hormone. Pituitary or hypothalamic trauma, surgery, or infarction are the most common causes of "central" DI; however, involvement of the pituitary gland with granulomatous disease or metastatic carcinoma also are seen. Transient DI lasting 3 to 7 days may follow closely on the heels of head trauma, meningitis, or pituitary injury. In 25 to 30% of patients, no cause for DI can be determined.

The kidneys' inability to respond to ADH is referred to as "nephrogenic DI." Hypokalemia, hypocalcemia, chronic pyelonephritis, polycystic kidney disease, sarcoidosis, amyloidosis, sickle cell disease, and chronic use of medications such as loop diuretics, lithium carbonate, and demeclocycline can all impair renal responsiveness to ADH.

Loss of the action of ADH results in a dilute urine (osmolality < 200 mOsm/L) even though the plasma is hyperosmolar. Clinical signs include polyuria and polydipsia; however, if oral intake is inadequate, the clinical presentation may be one of hypovolemic shock. The diagnosis of DI is confirmed by demonstrating a rise in urine osmolality within 2 hours of administration of 5 units of aqueous vasopressin subcutaneously or 1 μg of des-amino-arginine vasopressin (DDAVP). Increases in urine osmolality of 50% suggest central DI, whereas lesser rises suggest nephrogenic DI.

In central DI, computed tomography (CT) or magnetic resonance imaging (MRI) of the head may demonstrate pathology in the region of the hypothalamus or pituitary. Adrenal failure (ACTH deficiency) accompanies DI in approximately one-third of trauma-induced cases and therefore should be sought in accident victims with DI.

Treatment of DI consists of aggressive free water replacement guided by electrolyte and osmolarity determinations. Aqueous vasopressin (5–10 units intramuscularly or subcutaneously every 4–6 hours or 2 μg of DDAVP every 12 hours) is adequate hormone replacement therapy. Hormone replacement therapy usually is dramatic; urine volume responds within hours. Chlorpromazine, clofibrate, and carbamazepine are poor choices for control of DI and should be avoided.

KEY POINTS

1. Endocrine disorders often have subtle presentations in the ICU. Altered mental status (DKA, hypothyroidism, and hyperthyroidism), failure to wean from mechanical ventilation (adrenal insufficiency and hypothyroidism), and refractory hypotension (adrenal insufficiency, diabetes insipidus) are the most common clinical presentations in which endocrinologic causes are overlooked.

2. Severe hypothyroidism and hyperthyroidism must be suspected and treated on clinical grounds; laboratory tests often are too delayed to be useful. Because gastrointestinal absorption of medications in patients with thyroid disease is not predictable, initial dosing is often best accomplished intravenously.

3. To avoid hypoglycemia in the ICU: make every effort not to interrupt regular feedings; avoid oral hypoglycemic and long-acting insulin; and check bedside blood glucose values frequently in patients with diabetes.

4. Fluid administration and low-dose insulin are mainstays in the care of diabetic ketoacidosis. Reduction in the anion gap is the single most informative laboratory test that can be monitored.

5. Because hypertonic glucose is responsible for maintaining the circulating volume in patients with hyperosmolar nonketotic coma, adequate volume resuscitation is essential before beginning insulin therapy.

6. Maintain a high suspicion of adrenal insufficiency. When suspected, diagnostic investigation (Cortrosyn stimulation test) and institution of therapy (isotonic saline and corticosteroids) should be undertaken simultaneously.

7. Suspect diabetes insipidus when large volumes of dilute urine are accompanied by hyperosmolar hypernatremia. In such patients, it is probably most prudent to confirm the diagnosis by supplementing ADH rather than performing a water deprivation test, which can prove fatal for the critically ill patient.

SUGGESTED READINGS

1. Arem R. Hypoglycemia associated with renal failure. Clin Endocrinol Metabol 1989;18:103–121.
2. Arky RA. Hypoglycemia associated with liver disease and ethanol. Clin Endocrinol Metabol 1989;18:75–86.
3. Artega E, Lopez JM, Rodriguez JA, et al. Effect of the combinations of dexamethasone and sodium ipodate on serum thyroid hormones in graves disease. Clin Endocrinol 1983;19:619.
4. Baruh S, Sherman L, Markowitz S. Diabetic ketoacidosis and coma. Med Clin North Am 1981;65:117–132.
5. Beigelman PM. Potassium in severe diabetic ketoacidosis. Am J Med 1973;54:419–420.
6. Bitton RN, Wexler C. Free triiodothyronine toxicosis: a distinct entity. Am J Med 1990;88:53.
7. Brooks MH, Waldenstein SS. Free thyroxine concentrations on thyroid storm. Ann Intern Med 1980;93:694.
8. Byyny RL. Withdrawal from glucocorticoid therapy. N Engl J Med 1976;295:30–35.
9. Chanson P, Jedynal CP, Czernichow P. Management of early postoperative diabetes insipidus with parenteral desmopressin. Acta Endocrinol 1988;117:513.
10. Chapmin J, Wright AD, Nattrass M, et al. Recurrent diabetic ketoacidosis. Am J Med 1985;78:54–60.
11. Cobb WE, Spare S, Reichlin S. Neurogenic diabetes insipidus: management with DDAVP (1 desamino-8-D-arginine vasopressin). Arch Intern Med 1978;88:183.
12. Cooper DS. Which antithyroid drug? Am J Med 1986;80:1165.
13. Cooper DS, Ridgeway EC. Clinical management of patients with hyperthyroidism. Med Clin North Am 1985;69:953.
14. Domm BM, Vassallo CL. Myxedema coma with respiratory failure. Am Rev Respir Dis 1973;107:843.
15. Dorin RI, Crapo LM. Hypokalemic respiratory arrest in diabetic ketoacidosis. JAMA 1987;257:1517.

16. Ericksson MA, Rubenfeld S, Garder AJ, et al. Propranolol does not prevent thyroid storm. N Engl J Med 1977;296: 263–267.

17. Field JB. Hypoglycemia, definition, clinical presentations, classification and laboratory tests. Clin Endocrinol Metabol 1989;18:27.

18. Fischer KF, Lees JA, Newman JH. Hypoglycemia in hospitalized patients: causes and outcomes. N Engl J Med 1986;315(20):1245–1250.

19. Forfar JC, Muir AL, Sawers SA, et al. Abnormal left ventricular function in hyperthyroidism. N Engl J Med 1982; 307:1165.

20. Forfar JC, Caldwell GC. Hyperthyroid heart disease. Clin Endocrinol Metab 1985;14:491.

21. Fradkin JE, Wolff J. Iodine induced thyrotoxicosis. Medicine 1983;62:1.

22. Fulop M, Tawnebaum H, Dyer N. Ketotic hyperosmolar coma. Lancet 1973;2:635–639.

23. Ginsberg HN. Investigation of insulin resistance during diabetic ketoacidosis: role of counter-regulatory substances and effect of insulin therapy. Metabolism 1977; 26:1135–1146.

24. Gordon EE, Kabadi UM. The hyperglycemic hyper osmolar syndrome. Am J Med Sci 1976;271:265–268.

25. Graber AL, Ney RL, Nicholson WE, et al. Natural history of pituitary-adrenal recovery following long term suppression with corticosteroids. J Clin Endocrinol Metab 1965; 25:11–16.

26. Hale PJ, Crase J, Nattrass M. Metabolic effect of bicarbonate in the treatment of diabetic ketoacidosis. Br J Med 1984;289:1035–1038.

27. Hartzband PI, Van Herle AJ, Sorger L, et al. Assessment of hypothalamic-pituitary (HPA) axis dysfunction: comparison of ACTH stimulation, insulin-hypoglycemia and metyrapone. J Endocrinol Invest 1988;11:769.

28. Holvey DN, Goodner CJ, Nicoloff JT, et al. Treatment of myxedema coma with intravenous thyroxine. Arch Intern Med 1964;113:139.

29. Jurney TH, Cockrell JL, Lindberg JS, et al. Spectrum of serum cortisol response to ACTH in ICU patients. Correlation with degree of illness and mortality. Chest 1987; 92:292.

30. Kitabchi AE. Low dose insulin therapy in diabetic ketoacidosis: fact or fiction? Diabetes Metab Rev 1989;5: 337–363.

31. Lever E, Jaspan JB. Sodium bicarbonate therapy in sever diabetic ketoacidosis. Am J Med 1983;75:263–268.

32. Levy GS. The heart and hyperthyroidism: use of beta-adrenergic blocking drugs. Med Clin North Am 1975;59: 1193–1201.

33. Malouf R, Brust JCM. Hypoglycemia: causes, neurological manifestations, and outcome. Ann Neurol 1985;17: 421.

34. Mazzaferri EL. Adult hypothyroidism: causes, laboratory diagnosis and treatment. Postgrad Med 1986;79:75.

35. McCulloch W, Price P, Hinds CJ, et al. Effects of low-dose oral triiodothyronine in myxedema coma. Intensive Care Med 1985;111:259.

36. Membreno L, Irony I, Dere W, et al. Adrenocortical function in acquired immunodeficiency syndrome. J Clin Endocrinol Metab 1987;65:482.

37. Morris LR, Murphy MB, Kitbchi AE. Bicarbonate therapy in severe diabetic ketoacidosis. Ann Intern Med 1986;105: 836–840.

38. Moses AM. Clinical and laboratory observations in the adult with diabetes insipidus and related syndromes. Front Hormone Res 1985;13:156.

39. Nicoloff JT. Thyroid storm and myxedema coma. Med Clin North Am 1985;69:1005–1017.

40. Rao RH, Vagnucci AH, Amico JAL. Bilateral massive adrenal hemorrhage. Early recognition and treatment. Ann Intern Med 1989;110:227.

41. Refetoff S. Thyroid hormone therapy. Med Clin North Am 1975;59:1147–1162.

42. Robertson GL. Diagnosis of diabetes insipidus. Front Hormone Res 1985;13:176.

43. Robinson AG. DDAVP and the treatment of central diabetes insipidus. N Engl J Med 1976;294:507.

44. Robinson AG. Disorders of antidiuretic hormone secretion. Clin Endocrinol Metab 1985;14:55.

45. Roti E, Robuschi G, Gardini E, et al. Comparison of methimazole, methimazole, and sodium ipodate, and methimazole and saturate solution of potassium iodide in the early treatment of Graves' disease. Clin Endocrinol Metab 1988;28:305.

46. Roti E, Montermini M, Roti S, et al. The effect of diltiazem, a calcium channel blocking drug on cardiac rate and rhythm in hyperthyroid patients. Arch Intern Med 1988; 148:1919.

47. Sanson TH, Levine SN. Management of diabetic ketoacidosis. Drugs 1989;38:289–300.

48. Scarlett JA, Mako ME, Rubenstein AH, et al. Diagnosis of factitious hypoglycemia. N Engl J Med 1977;297:1029.

49. Schein RMH, Sprung CL, Marcial E, et al. Plasma cortisol levels in patients with septic shock. Crit Care Med 1990; 18:259.

50. Seltzer HS. Drug induced hypoglycemia. A review of 1418 cases. Clin Endocrinol Metab 1989;18:163.

51. Shenfeild GM. Influence of thyroid dysfunction on drug pharmacokinetics. Clin Pharmacol 1981;6:275.

52. Streck WF, Lockwood DH. Pituitary adrenal recovery following short-term suppression with corticosteroids. Am J Med 1979;66:910.

53. Sullivan JN. Saturday conference: steroid withdrawal syndromes. South Med J 1982;75:726–733.

54. Turlapaty P, Laddu A, Shrinivas V, et al. Esmolol: a titratable short-acting intravenous beta-blocker for acute critical care settings. Clin Pharm 1987;114:866.

55. Verbalis JG, Robinson AG, Moses AM. Postoperative and post-traumatic diabetes insipidus. Front Horm Res 1985; 13:247.

56. Wallis WE, Donaldson I, Scott RS, et al. Hypoglycemia masquerading as cerebrovascular disease. Ann Neurol 1985;18:510.

57. Wilson HK, Keuer SP, Lea AS, et al. Phosphate therapy in diabetic ketoacidosis. Arch Intern Med 1982;142: 517–520.

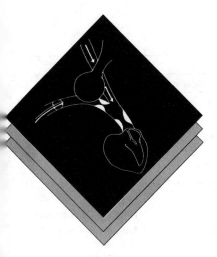

CHAPTER 33

Drug Overdose and Poisoning

Overdose and poisoning account for approximately 15% of all intensive care unit (ICU) admissions. Despite a myriad of potential toxins, only a few drugs account for more than 90% of all overdose cases. In adults, overdose is usually a deliberate ingestion of multiple drugs. In children, poisoning usually is an accidental ingestion of a single agent. Most poisonings occur in otherwise healthy patients younger than 35 years of age, which partially explains the low in-hospital mortality ($\approx$1%). (Most fatalities occur from arrhythmia or hypoventilation-induced anoxic brain damage before patients reach the hospital.)

DIAGNOSIS OF DRUG OVERDOSE

CLINICAL HISTORY

Although often erroneous, detailed historical information is important. Many patients overestimate the dose ingested; others have taken a drug that they do not report. Suicidal patients may attempt to conceal the nature of the ingested poisons, and patients ingesting illicit drugs often lack accurate knowledge of these substances or fail to provide information, fearing prosecution. Because patients may switch the contents of labeled prescription bottles and accidental overdose may result from pharmacy dispensing errors, it is always wise to examine the contents of prescription bottles to ensure that their contents match the label. In the drug history, it is important to seek the following information: (*a*) type of drug or toxin; (*b*) quantity consumed; (*c*) time elapsed since ingestion; (*d*) initial symptoms, including a history of vomiting or diarrhea; and (*e*) underlying diseases or other drugs taken.

PHYSICAL EXAMINATION

The physical examination is extremely valuable for the patient with a suspected overdose of unknown cause, because it may allow rapid classification of patients into classic ''toxic syndromes,'' which may guide initial therapy. The cardinal manifestations of these syndromes and their common causes are illustrated in Table 33.1 and discussed in detail below.

The first steps in treating a patient with poisoning are to assess the vital signs, secure the airway, and ensure adequate perfusion. The airway of the overdosed patient may be obstructed, particularly if narcotics or sedative drugs have been ingested. Intubation and artificial ventilation are required when the central drive to breathe is severely depressed. Hypoventilation is a clue to narcotic, sedative, or clonidine overdose. A patient sedate enough to allow unresisted endotracheal intubation almost certainly requires the airway protection and ventilatory support that intubation provides. Hyperventilation resulting from central nervous system (CNS) stimulation or induced metabolic acidosis should suggest salicylate, theophylline, amphetamine, cocaine, or methanol toxicity. Tissue hypoxia caused by cyanide or carbon monoxide also induces hyperventilation (see Chapter 40, Burns and Inhalational Injury).

511

TABLE 33–1

TOXIC SYNDROMES

Signs and Symptoms	Anticholinergic	Sympathomimetic	Narcotic/Sedative	Cholinergic
Mental status	Delirium	Delirium	Coma/lethargy	Confusion
Skin	Dry skin	Sweating	Normal	Sweating
Temperature	Fever	Fever	Hypothermic/normal	Normal
Pulse	Rapid	Rapid	Slow	Normal/slow
Respiration	Normal	Rapid	Slow/shallow	Normal
Blood pressure	Normal/elevated	Elevated	Normal/reduced	Normal or low
Pupils	Mydriasis	Mydriasis	Miosis	Normal
GI tract function	Decreased	Increased	Decreased	Diarrhea and vomiting
Other	Seizures	Seizures	Hyporeflexia	Muscle weakness Salivation Urinary incontinence

Blood pressure and perfusion should be assessed and corrected rapidly if inadequate. Anticholinergic, tricyclic, or sympathomimetic (e.g., cocaine, amphetamine) poisoning should be suspected in patients with marked tachycardia. Sinus bradycardia or conduction system block may result from overdoses of digitalis, clonidine, β-blockers, calcium channel blockers, or cholinergic drugs.

Although hypertension is a relatively nonspecific sign, *marked* hypertension should suggest amphetamine, cocaine, thyroid hormone, and catecholamine toxicities. Core temperature may give valuable clues as well. Hyperthermia suggests anticholinergic, amphetamine, or tricyclic poisoning or may be indicative of alcohol withdrawal, whereas hypothermia frequently accompanies alcohol or sedative–hypnotic overdose.

In the assessment of the poisoned patient, it is important not to overlook concurrent trauma or serious medical illness. For example, nearly one-half of all head injured motor vehicle accident victims also are intoxicated with alcohol or other substances. When trauma cannot be excluded in patients with altered mental status, it often is prudent to perform a head computed tomography (CT) scan and evaluate the cervical spine for injury while the evaluation and therapy of the overdose is ongoing. Similarly, drug or alcohol ingestion does not preclude a coexisting life-threatening medical illness such as meningitis or hypoglycemia.

The head should receive particularly close examination, both to exclude other causes of coma (e.g., head trauma, subarachnoid hemorrhage) and to provide data relevant to overdose. Inspection of the oral cavity may yield unswal-

TABLE 33–2

CHARACTERISTIC BREATH ODORS OF VICTIMS OF POISONING

Odor	Poison
Sweet/fruity	Ketones/alcohols
Almond	Cyanide
"Gasoline"	Hydrocarbons
Garlic	Organophosphates/arsenic
Wintergreen	Methyl salicylate
Pear	Chloral hydrate

lowed tablets or evidence of caustic injury. Breath odor may suggest a particular toxin (Table 33.2). For example, ketones give a sweet odor, whereas cyanide presents an almond scent. The characteristic smell of hydrocarbons is distinguished easily, as is the "garlic" odor of organophosphate ingestion.

Narcotics, organophosphates, and phenothiazines commonly produce miosis, whereas drugs with anticholinergic properties cause mydriasis. Nystagmus is often seen with phencyclidine (PCP) or phenytoin ingestion. Pupils that appear fixed and dilated can result from profound sedative overdose but are characteristic of glutethimide or mushroom poisoning. Pupils that are dilated but reactive suggest anticholinergic or sympathomimetic poisoning. Because any response to light (even if barely detectable) has prognostic implication, the pupillary response should be tested with a bright light in a darkened room. An ophthalmoscope focused on the plane of the iris serves the twin function of magnification and illumination.

LABORATORY TESTING

The electrocardiogram (ECG) can provide valuable clues in drug overdose and should be reviewed at the earliest appropriate time. Ectopy is common in sympathomimetic and tricyclic poisoning. High-grade atrioventricular (AV) block may be due to digoxin, β-blockers, calcium channel blockers, cyanide, phenytoin, or cholinergic substances. A wide QRS complex or prolonged QT interval suggests quinidine, procainamide, or tricyclic antidepressant overdose.

Arterial blood gases are necessary to assess acid–base status and gas exchange and may yield a specific clue to salicylate intoxication if they reveal a mixed respiratory alkalosis and metabolic acidosis. Severe metabolic acidosis with hyperventilation is common with cyanide or carbon monoxide poisoning (see also Chapter 40, Burns and Inhalational Injury).

Six relatively common poisonings elevate the anion gap: (*a*) salicylates; (*b*) methanol; (*c*) ethanol; (*d*) ethylene glycol; (*e*) paraldehyde; and (*f*) carbon monoxide. In the presence of a coexisting osmolar gap (the difference between calculated and measured serum osmolarity), ethanol and ethylene glycol become the most likely offenders. Ketoacidosis suggests ethanol, paraldehyde, or diabetes as potential culprits. If ketones are present without systemic acidosis, isopropyl alcohol is the probable etiology.

In addition to routine arterial blood gases, measurement of hemoglobin saturation and oxygen content may be helpful. Both methemoglobin and carboxyhemoglobin lead to a disparity between the measured oxygen content or hemoglobin saturation and that predicted from the arterial oxygen tension (PaO_2). Carboxyhemoglobin is elevated in carbon monoxide poisoning, and a number of ingested drugs can oxidize hemoglobin to methemoglobin. Profound methemoglobinemia may be recognized at the bedside by the chocolate brown color it imparts to blood.

Hypocalcemia is produced by the ingestion of ethylene glycol, oxalate, fluoride compounds, and by certain metals: manganese, phosphorus, and barium. Chest and abdominal radiographs may help identify radiopaque tablets of iron, phenothiazines, tricyclic agents, or chloral hydrate. When these drugs are involved, the abdominal radiograph may help to ensure that the gut has been emptied after emesis or gastric lavage. With hydrocarbon poisoning upright abdominal radiography may show a three-layered fluid/fluid/air level in the stomach (see Fig. 33.1).

USE OF THE DRUG SCREEN

Most qualitative drug screens assay blood or urine using thin-layer chromatography. Urine and gastric juice are the most reliable samples for toxin assay because many drugs rapidly cleared from the serum may be detected as unabsorbed drug or excreted metabolites. Unfortunately, the drug screen has limited usefulness because significant delays invariably occur before the results are available, many toxins are not identified on the

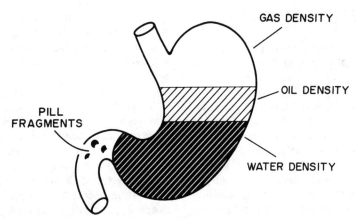

FIG. 33–1. Composite diagram of radiographic features seen on an upright film of the stomach region after ingestion of radiopaque tablets and/or selected liquid hydrocarbons.

TABLE 33–3	
DRUGS FOR WHICH QUANTITATIVE ASSAY IS HELPFUL	
Acetaminophen	Digitalis glycosides
Ethanol	Methanol
Theophylline	Salicylates
Ethylene glycol	Carbon monoxide
Iron	Lithium

TABLE 33–4	
POISONS NOT ABSORBED BY ACTIVATED CHARCOAL	
Lithium	Acids
Iron	Organophosphates
Alcohols	Hydrocarbons
Ethylene glycol	Heavy metals
Alkalis	Cyanide

screen, and the results seldom change empirical therapy. Many common drugs (e.g., aspirin, acet- aminophen, ethanol) are omitted from "routine" screens, and assays of each must be requested specifically. If a particular toxin is suspected, specific assay techniques may provide more rapid and quantitative results. A negative drug screen alone does not exclude overdose because of problems with sensitivity and timing of the test in relation to ingestion. Whenever there is doubt regarding drug screen results, clinical judgment should prevail. Specific therapy is available for certain toxins for which quantitative levels should be obtained to guide management (see Table 33.3).

TREATMENT OF DRUG OVERDOSE

Physiologic support is key to all overdose management. Three basic precepts help minimize the toxic effects of drug ingestion: (a) prevent toxin absorption; (b) enhance drug excretion; and (c) prevent formation of toxic metabolites. Depending on the drug ingested, appropriate therapy also may include antidote administration or toxin removal.

PREVENTION OF TOXIN ABSORPTION

After cardiopulmonary stabilization, the first step in the treatment of poisoning is to stop absorption. Although currently controversial, this is probably best accomplished by emptying the stomach using gastric lavage followed by instillation of activated charcoal. Induction of emesis with ipecac is rarely, if ever, indicated for the hospitalized patient. Commonly, long delays between ingestion and hospital presentation limit emesis effectiveness and, for patients with altered mental status or suppressed gag reflex, vomiting is dangerous. (Ipecac-induced emesis still may be useful in the prehospital setting for highly selected patients.) Emesis is not appropriate in ingestion

of corrosive chemicals or petroleum distillates nor should it be used for pregnant women or children younger than 6 months of age. Although equally effective as an emetic, apomorphine frequently produces significant respiratory depression and probably should not be used.

For patients with altered consciousness, the airway should be protected with a cuffed endotracheal tube before attempting gastric evacuation and lavage. Lavage should be performed in the left lateral decubitus position using a large orogastric (Ewald) tube. (Smaller nasogastric tubes fail to adequately remove pill fragments.) Vomitus or aspirated gastric contents should be sent for toxicologic analysis. Gastric lavage is more effective than emesis at eliminating unabsorbed drug, removing most toxins from the stomach if performed within 4 hours of ingestion. Some poisons may be recovered even after 12 hours, particularly if they form concretions or impair gastric emptying (e.g., drugs with anticholinergic properties, salicylates, meprobamate).

Activated charcoal may be given after emesis or lavage to absorb orally ingested drugs. Although the risks are small, activated charcoal frequently causes vomiting and may produce pneumonitis when aspirated. One gram of charcoal has enormous absorptive area (>1000 m^2) and achieves absorption of many toxins within minutes of administration; however, activated charcoal is not effective in reducing the toxic effects of a number of common poisons (Table 33.4). Although activated charcoal tends to constipate, cathartics may deplete fluids and electrolytes and repeated doses are not routinely needed unless large volumes or multiple doses of activated charcoal are given. "Charcoal briquette bowel" can result from retention of charcoal in the colon. If necessary, sorbitol is the preferred cathartic because it works faster than magnesium citrate and avoids the magnesium toxicity that can result if renal function is impaired. The only relative contraindication to the use of charcoal is acetaminophen overdose, in which activated charcoal may interfere with the absorption of N-acetylcysteine—an effect that is probably of little consequence. Other absorbents such as bile acid sequestrants (e.g., cholestyramine) also can be used to reduce absorption of specific agents such as thyroid hormone. For cutaneously absorbed toxins (e.g., organophosphates), washing the skin and removing contaminated clothing is particularly important.

ENHANCEMENT OF DRUG REMOVAL

Four therapeutic techniques enhance removal of circulating toxins: (a) "gut dialysis;" (b) ion trapping; (c) hemodialysis; and (d) hemoperfusion. Drugs undergoing enterohepatic circulation, such as theophylline, digoxin, phenobarbital, phenylbutazone, and carbamazepine, may be eliminated by "gut dialysis," a process using repeated doses of oral charcoal to bind drug excreted into the bile.

Charged molecules do not cross lipid membranes easily; therefore, ionized drugs are not absorbed readily from the stomach and fail to cross the blood–brain barrier. Furthermore, when inside the renal tubule, such molecules have a limited tendency to back-diffuse into the circulation. Altering the pH of body fluids to "ion-trap" drugs in the desired compartment (serum, gut, urine, etc.) is effective for only a small number of compounds. Alkalinization of the serum and urine, although often difficult to achieve, can impede transfer of weak acids (e.g., salicylates, tricyclics, phenobarbital, and isoniazid) across the blood–brain barrier and promotes their excretion. Conversely, acidification using ammonium chloride may accelerate excretion of weak bases such as amphetamine, strychnine, PCP, and quinidine. Urinary acidification is questionably effective and potentially dangerous for patients with renal or hepatic dysfunction.

Hemodialysis effectively clears low-molecular-weight, water-soluble molecules having a small volume of distribution (e.g., methanol and ethylene glycol). Salicylates and lithium also are dialyzed effectively. Charcoal hemoperfusion removes theophylline and other lipid-soluble drugs from the blood but may provoke hypocalcemia, initiate complement activation or coagulopathy, and result in air embolism.

INHIBITION OF TOXIC METABOLITE FORMATION

Some drugs, most notably acetaminophen, methanol, and ethylene glycol, are relatively inert when ingested but form highly toxic compounds during metabolism. Inhibition of toxin formation will be discussed below under specific therapy for these poisons.

SPECIFIC POISONS

ACETAMINOPHEN

Acetaminophen is safe when taken in recommended doses, but ingestion of as little as 6 gm may be fatal. (Usually, a fatal dose exceeds 140 mg/kg.) Acetaminophen is absorbed rapidly, especially when taken in the liquid form. The usual serum half-life is approximately $2\frac{1}{2}$ hours but lengthens with declining liver function. Normally, the drug is metabolized hepatically to nontoxic compounds by linkage with sulfates and glucuronide. The hepatic cytochrome P-450 system converts less than 5% of an ingested dose to reactive metabolites, which are then detoxified by conjugation with glutathione. However, during massive overdose, toxic metabolites overwhelm the glutathione supply and accumulate to cause liver damage. Conditions that induce the hepatic cytochrome P-450 system, including chronic use of ethanol, oral contraceptives, or phenobarbital, predispose patients to acetaminophen toxicity.

Most episodes of acetaminophen overdose are not life threatening and do not require specific therapy. Even in serious acetaminophen overdose, symptoms are minimal for the first 24 hours after ingestion, with the exception of nausea and vomiting. One to 2 days after ingestion, deteriorating liver function tests, right upper quadrant pain, and oliguria (due to the antidiuretic hormone [ADH]-like effects of acetaminophen) become evident. At this time, hepatic transaminase concentrations may peak in the tens of thousands of units. Hepatic necrosis and failure evolve within 3 to 5 days. (This toxicity is often manifest by a rising bilirubin level and prothrombin time and declining transaminases.)

As for all other drug ingestions, initial treatment should include evacuation of the stomach, in addition to hemodynamic and respiratory support. A specific antidote, N-acetylcysteine (NAC; Mucomyst®) is the drug of choice. Although concomitant charcoal administration may modestly reduce NAC absorption, a negative clinical effect is unlikely. Not all patients require therapy with NAC; the likelihood of hepatic toxicity may be predicted from the serum level using standard nomograms. Patients with pre-existing liver disease may develop symptoms at concentrations much lower than the nomogram predicts. NAC probably has a twofold action: directly binding the toxic metabolites of acetaminophen and repleting intracellular glutathione. To be effective, NAC should be given as early as possible—certainly within 16 hours of ingestion. An oral loading dose of 140 mg/kg is followed by 17 additional doses of 70 mg/kg at 4-hour intervals. (Shorter courses of therapy may predispose patients to recurrent toxicity.) Of note, liver injury induced by acetaminophen commonly predisposes patients to hypoglycemia, which should be closely monitored and treated. When massive hepatic necrosis develops, liver transplantation may be considered if irreparable brain injury has not occurred from hepatic-failure-induced cerebral edema.

SALICYLATES

Most salicylate overdose occurring in adults results from therapeutic misadventure, not intentional ingestion. In high doses, salicylates inhibit cellular enzymes and uncouple oxidative phosphorylation. The clinical presentation of salicylate overdose includes altered mental status, tinnitus, acidosis, hypoxemia, and (more rarely) hyperosmolarity, hyperthermia, and seizures. Initially, direct CNS stimulation causes a respiratory alkalosis and compensatory renal wasting of bicarbonate. Later, superimposed metabolic acidosis may produce a complex acid–base disturbance. Tachypnea may be absent if the patient has ingested a sedative or hypnotic concurrently. Large doses of aspirin may induce pulmonary edema, causing acute respiratory distress syndrome (ARDS).

Salicylate intoxication always should be considered in the differential diagnosis of an anion gap acidosis. The anion gap elevation results primarily from lactate and pyruvate generated during anaerobic glycolysis. (Ketones also are formed in response to decreased glucose and accelerated lipolysis.) However, very high serum levels of salicylate (>80 mg/dL) may directly contribute to the anion gap. In addition, large insensible fluid losses deplete intravascular volume, thereby stimulating aldosterone secretion, which depletes bicarbonate and potassium. Salicylate levels higher than 50 mg/dL commonly induce nausea and vomiting and may produce a metabolic alkalosis, leading to a "triple" acid–base disorder.

Salicylates inhibit the formation of prothrombin, impair platelet function, and irritate the gastric mucosa—all of which contribute to the risk of hemorrhage. Patients with salicylate-induced coagulopathy or bleeding should receive vitamin K and, if immediate reversal is necessary, fresh frozen plasma and platelets.

If therapy is to prevent morbidity, salicylate intoxication must be suspected on clinical grounds. In chronic salicylate toxicity, serum levels correlate poorly with toxicity but in acute intoxication, adverse effects are uncommon with serum levels below 30 mg/dL. Moderate toxicity often is seen with acute ingestions of 150 to 300 mg/kg. Another salicylate preparation, oil of wintergreen, represents a significantly greater risk; 1 teaspoon of the compound provides the amount of salicylate in almost 20 aspirin tablets. In acute salicylate poisoning, initial levels higher than 120 mg/dL, 6-hour levels higher than 100 mg/dL, or any levels higher than 500 mg/dL are associated with a high risk of death. Declining salicylate levels should not necessarily be reassuring but merely indicating transit of the salicylate from the plasma to tissue compartments. If salicylate levels are not immediately available, "Phenistix" test strips can demonstrate a purple color when serum levels exceed 70 mg/dL. Although purely qualitative, the ferric chloride urine test is helpful to rule out salicylate ingestion.

Gastric lavage followed by charcoal and cathartics can increase stool excretion. Salicylates normally are absorbed rapidly, but in massive overdoses, serum levels may continue to rise for up to 24 hours after ingestion due to delayed gastric absorption. As weak acids, salicylates remain nonionized at low serum pH and readily cross cell membranes; therefore, "ion trapping" may be used to lower toxicity and promote excretion. In addition to decreasing urinary excretion, an acidic pH favors movement of salicylates into cells and across the blood–brain barrier. Therefore, serum and urine pH should be monitored and kept alkaline with bicarbonate titration or dialysis. Hemodialysis is indicated for severe intoxications.

STIMULANTS

Patients experiencing stimulant (amphetamines, cocaine, and phencyclidine [PCP]) overdose characteristically present with agitation, hypertension, tachycardia, mydriasis, and warm moist skin. Occasionally, seizures occur. Nystagmus is a common feature in PCP intoxication. Cardiac ischemia induced by the vasoconstrictive and chronotropic effects of cocaine may cause acute myocardial infarction, even in young patients and those without coronary artery disease. Therefore, in cocaine intoxications, an electrocardiogram (ECG) should be obtained, and if suspicious, myocardial ischemia or injury should be confirmed or excluded by serial ECGs and cardiac enzyme determinations.

For most stimulant overdoses, specific treatment is lacking; however, maintenance of the airway, oxygenation, and control of blood pressure are universally indicated. Providing adequate hydration to maintain urine flow is important because many compounds in this class may precipitate rhabdomyolysis.

ALCOHOLS

Ethanol

Many suicide attempts involve ethanol, either alone or in combination with other drugs. Physiologic effects do not relate closely to serum concentrations, but blood levels higher than 150 mg/dL are inebriating. Coma usually requires levels higher than 300 mg/dL and death often supervenes when concentrations exceed 600 mg/dL. The therapy of acute alcohol intoxication is largely supportive. Ethanol may be removed by hemodialysis but is rarely necessary. One in five ethanol-intoxicated patients will transiently awaken in response to large doses of naloxone. There is no role for direct CNS stimulants in the treatment of ethanol intoxication.

Ethanol Withdrawal Syndrome

The ICU deprives the habituated patient of access to ethanol. Deprivation may precipitate withdrawal, a condition that is significantly more dangerous than intoxication. Symptoms of withdrawal usually start within 36 hours of the last drink (but may be delayed for 5 to 7 days). Measurable serum levels of ethanol do not exclude the diagnosis of withdrawal. Patients experiencing severe withdrawal (hallucinosis, delirium tremens ["DTs"]) are unpredictable, both in behavior and disease course. Delirium tremens is the most extreme form of ethanol withdrawal, profoundly altering mental status and initiating life-threatening autonomic instability. Therefore,

most patients with DTs should be managed in an ICU to avert such fatal complications as seizures, aspiration, arrhythmias, and suicide attempts. Symptoms of withdrawal (specifically DTs) often mimic infection or primary neurologic processes. It is important to emphasize, however, that 50% of febrile patients with DTs also have a concomitant infection, most frequently pneumonia or meningitis. The agitated withdrawal patient should be restrained in a lateral or prone position (not supine because of the risk of aspiration). Patients should be given nothing by mouth (NPO); all fluids, electrolytes, and vitamins (B_{12}, thiamine, folate) should be administered intravenously. Withdrawal may be prevented or aborted in its early stages through the use of oral benzodiazepines, but if fully manifest, intravenous diazepam or lorazepam becomes the sedative of choice. Benzodiazepines reduce hyperactivity and the risk of seizures. In this situation, intravenous benzodiazepines should be given frequently, in small doses, until the patient is calm but not obtunded. Haloperidol may be a very useful adjunct. After initial control with intravenous dosing is achieved, oral maintenance therapy should be instituted. Lorazepam has become a popular choice because it is a long-acting drug available in both oral and intravenous forms, it does not require hepatic metabolism, and it has no active metabolites (a particularly useful property in patients with liver disease). Although very effective in achieving controlled sedation, propofol has not be widely used for the indication. Phenothiazines probably should be avoided because they lower the seizure threshold. Titratable β-blockers may also be helpful in well selected hypermetabolic, tachycardic patients.

Methanol and Ethylene Glycol Toxicity

A tabular overview of the clinical and laboratory features of the most common alcohol poisonings is presented in Table 33.5. The toxicity of methanol and ethylene glycol results from the formation of organic acids from the parent compounds. Toxic metabolites of ethylene glycol include oxalic, glycolic, and glyoxylic acids. Formic acid and formaldehyde are responsible for methanol toxicity. In their early phase, the clinical picture of methanol or ethylene glycol ingestion resembles ethanol-related intoxication. However, as symptoms progress, almost any global CNS finding may be seen—coma, hyporeflexia, nystagmus, or seizures. Whereas the presentations

TABLE 33–5

FEATURES OF VARIOUS ALCOHOL
INTOXICATIONS

	Ethanol	Methanol	Ethylene Glycol	Isopro- panol
Osmolar gap	+	+	+	+
Ketones	+	−	−	+
Acidosis	+	+	+	−
Visual changes	−	+	−	−
Ca^{+2} oxalate crystals	−	−	+	−

of ethylene glycol and methanol are often indistinguishable, cardiovascular symptomatology (tachycardia, hypertension, pulmonary edema, and renal failure resulting from oxalate crystalluria) more frequently complement ethylene glycol. On the other hand, optic neuritis and blindness are hallmarks of methanol poisoning. Methanol or ethylene glycol ingestion should be suspected in any patient with acidosis and coexistent anion and osmolar gaps. It should be noted, however, that lethal levels of ethylene glycol (>20 mg/dL) may be present with minimal elevations in the osmolar gap.

The treatment of methanol or ethylene glycol poisoning is fourfold:

1. Remove any drug remaining in the stomach.
2. Prevent the formation of toxic metabolites.
3. Remove the parent drug from the circulation.
4. Treat metabolic acidosis.

Emergent dialysis should be performed in all patients with toxic serum levels. Formation of toxins is attenuated by using ethanol to compete with ethylene glycol or methanol for metabolism by alcohol dehydrogenase. To effectively inhibit toxic metabolite formation, an ethanol level higher than 100 mg/dL should be sustained by giving a loading dose of 600 mg/kg intravenously or orally (equivalent to about 4 ounces of whiskey), followed by a maintenance regimen (about 100 mL of 10% ethanol intravenously per hour or 25 mL of 40% alcohol orally at the same rate). Because hemodialysis enhances ethanol clearance, doses must be increased during the filtration procedure. Calcium replacement may be required for patients with ethylene glycol poisoning and symptomatic hypocalcemia.

SEDATIVE–HYPNOTIC DRUGS

Six major drugs or drug groups comprise this category: barbiturates, benzodiazepines, mepro-

bamate, methaqualone, chloral hydrate, and glutethimide. Although barbiturates historically were popular drugs with which to overdose, now perhaps benzodiazepines are seen with higher frequency. All sedative drugs depress consciousness and, in large doses, act as negative inotropes—occasionally causing cardiovascular collapse. The benzodiazepines, however, have a wide therapeutic range, and when taken alone, doses of 50 to 100 times the usual therapeutic dose may still be well tolerated. Unfortunately, ethanol is a common cofactor in benzodiazepine overdoses, substantially enhancing toxicity. In very large doses, benzodiazepines can produce neuromuscular blockade.

Flumazenil is a competitive receptor antagonist that reverses the respiratory and central depressant effects of benzodiazepines in approximately 80% of patients. High doses of benzodiazepines, long duration of therapy, and concomitant narcotic use lower the rate of reversal. Flumazenil has no beneficial effect on ethanol, barbiturate, narcotic, or tricyclic antidepressant-induced CNS depression. Because flumazenil is cleared rapidly by the liver, its duration of action is substantially shorter than that of most benzodiazepines. Akin to the naloxone–opioid story, as many as 10% of patients given flumazenil relapse into a sedated state, making careful observation essential. Intermittent doses of 0.2 mg at 1-minute intervals (up to 1 mg total) usually are effective. Flumazenil should be used cautiously because it may precipitate withdrawal symptoms (agitation, vomiting, and seizures), especially in chronic tricyclic antidepressant or benzodiazepine users. Flumazenil is expensive, rarely needed in the ICU, and should be regarded as no more than an adjunct to airway protection and ventilation in the management of benzodiazepine overdose. Supportive therapy remains the cornerstone of management in benzodiazepine overdose.

The treatment of barbiturate overdose is generally supportive; however, delayed gastric emptying induced by barbiturates makes evacuation of the stomach a key therapeutic maneuver. The airway must be protected before lavage. Barbiturates are metabolized hepatically before excretion; therefore, patients with underlying liver disease are most prone to toxicity. Even though barbiturates are weak acids, forced alkaline diuresis has little effect on total drug excretion and is potentially dangerous. After all drug has been cleared, patients chronically habituated to barbiturates (and selected other sedatives) may enter a withdrawal phase. Tremor and convulsions may require temporary reinstitution of phenobarbital in therapeutic doses with gradual tapering.

The anticholinergic effects of glutethimide also delay gastric emptying and may warrant stomach lavage long after ingestion of the drug. Instillation of activated charcoal may bind unabsorbed drug or drug metabolites undergoing enterohepatic circulation.

ORGANOPHOSPHATES AND CARBAMATES

Organophosphates and the related carbamate insecticides inhibit the action of acetylcholinesterase, thereby causing accumulation of acetylcholine at neuromuscular junctions. Early specific treatment is important, because binding of the toxin to acetylcholinesterase may become irreversible after 24 hours. Organophosphates initially stimulate but later block acetylcholine receptors. Organophosphates penetrate the CNS, but carbamates do not. Toxic manifestations usually appear within 5 minutes but may be delayed for 24 hours after exposure. (Toxicity evolves rapidly after inhalation but more slowly during cutaneous absorption.)

The clinical presentation may be remembered by the mnemonic "S.T.U.M.B.L.E.D.": Salivation, Tremor, Urination, Miosis, Bradycardia, Lacrimation, Emesis, Diarrhea—all expressions of cholinergic-muscarinic excess. In some patients, nicotinic effects (fasciculation, skeletal cramping, hypertension, and tachycardia) predominate. A garlic odor on the patient's breath also is suggestive of the diagnosis. Laboratory confirmation requires measurement of plasma pseudocholinesterase or erythrocyte cholinesterase. Acute reductions of enzyme activity by more than 90% correlate with severe toxicity. (With chronic exposures, enzyme levels may be reduced dramatically with few symptoms.) Alternatively, the diagnosis can be established by direct analysis of organophosphates in serum, gastric, or urinary samples. Laboratory findings also may include hemolytic anemia (seen with carbamates) and an anion gap metabolic acidosis. Bradycardia and heart block frequently result from cholinergic stimulation.

Skin decontamination is an essential component of initial treatment. High doses of anticholinergics may block muscarinic CNS effects but do not reverse nicotinic manifestations. (Atropine, 2 to 4 mg, usually is given intravenously until muscarinic symptoms are reversed.) Therapy should continue for at least 24 hours after exposure. Prali-

doxime (2-PAM) reverses the nicotinic (muscular) effects of organophosphates by uncoupling bound organophosphates from the esterases. However, treatment retains efficacy for only approximately 24 hours; therefore, it should be given as soon as possible in a dose of 1 gm, repeated once if necessary. 2-PAM is ineffective in carbamate poisoning.

THEOPHYLLINE TOXICITY

Impaired theophylline clearance occurs commonly in patients with obstructive lung disease and heart or liver failure. The potential for impaired clearance due to drug interaction is overlooked frequently, particularly for patients who have had ciprofloxacin, erythromycin, zileuton, or cimetidine added to chronic theophylline therapy. Smoking modestly improves the clearance of theophylline in patients without liver disease.

Toxic symptoms (tremors, arrhythmias, gastrointestinal [GI] upset) may occur at serum levels well within the therapeutic range (10–20 μg/mL), particularly in patients predisposed by advanced age or underlying CNS or cardiac disease (Table 33.6). A minority of hospitalized patients experience GI warning symptoms before having refractory seizures—the most life-threatening toxic manifestation. (The mortality of theophylline-induced seizures exceeds 40%, and a large percentage of survivors have persistent neurologic deficits.) Leukocytosis may result from catecholamine-induced demargination of leukocytes. Cardiac arrhythmias of all varieties occur, but serious arrhythmias generally do not emerge at therapeutic drug concentrations. Hyperglycemia can be treated effectively with β-blockers.

The treatment of theophylline intoxication initially includes correction of hypoxemia, acidosis, and electrolyte abnormalities. Oral charcoal should be administered after gastric lavage if ingestion is recent. When given in doses of 30 to 50 gm every 2 to 4 hours (up to a total dose of 120 gm), charcoal may double theophylline clearance.

TABLE 33–6

SIDE EFFECTS AND THEOPHYLLINE LEVELS

Theophylline Level	Side Effects
>20 mg/L	Nausea, vomiting, confusion
20–40 mg/L	Cardiac arrhythmias
>40 mg/L	Refractory seizures

Lidocaine is the drug of choice for theophylline-induced ventricular arrhythmias, whereas phenobarbital is the preferred anticonvulsant. Charcoal hemoperfusion probably is indicated for theophylline levels higher than 60 mg/L and for refractory arrhythmias or seizures.

DIGITALIS COMPOUNDS

All of the symptoms of digitalis glycoside poisoning are nonspecific (fatigue, weakness, nausea, visual complaints) and are common in the elderly population with cardiac disease. Therefore, a low threshold of suspicion must be maintained for digitalis toxicity. Renal insufficiency, hypothyroidism, heart failure, and electrolyte abnormalities (e.g., hypokalemia and hypomagnesemia) predispose patients to digitalis toxicity. Initiation of calcium channel blockers, type Ia antiarrhythmics, or amiodarone also can precipitate digitalis toxicity. The major toxicity of digitalis compounds is hyperkalemia and associated arrhythmia (AV nodal block, and increased automaticity) resulting from poisoning of the cellular sodium–potassium pump.

Treatment consists of activated charcoal to decrease drug absorption and normalization of serum magnesium and potassium levels. Atropine and pacing are indicated for severe bradycardia. Lidocaine and phenytoin are the drugs of choice for ventricular tachyarrhythmias. It is best to avoid quinidine, β-blockers, and calcium channel blockers. Specific therapy using Digibind®, a highly purified, ovine IgG Fab antibody fragment is indicated for digoxin levels greater than 6 mg/dL; when potassium exceeds 5 mEq/L; or when refractory tachycardia or bradycardia occur. The usual adult dose of 10 vials produces a response within 30 minutes. Digibind® is very safe—its only recognized toxicities are due to the reversal of digitalis effects (i.e., hypokalemia, congestive heart failure, and rapid ventricular response to atrial fibrillation). Because the Digibind®–digitalis complex is detected by digoxin assays, digoxin levels are not valid. With normal renal function, Digibind is cleared rapidly (48–72 hours) but clearance is reduced dramatically by renal insufficiency.

TRICYCLIC ANTIDEPRESSANTS

It is not surprising that tricyclic antidepressants (TCA) are the single most common cause of fatal drug overdose because they are used widely for depressed patients, have a long half-life, and accumulate in tissue. Despite the frequency of TCA overdose, in-hospital mortality remains below 1%. (Most deaths occur in the prehospital phase of illness.) Signs and symptoms of TCA overdose are predominantly anticholinergic. The phrase "hot as a hare, blind as a bat, dry as a bone, red as a beet, mad as a hatter" accurately describes severely intoxicated patients, who often demonstrate hyperthermia, fixed and dilated pupils, dry red skin, and CNS hyperactivity (hallucinations and psychosis). The differential diagnosis of TCA overdose includes other compounds having anticholinergic effects (e.g., atropine, phenothiazines, scolopamine, anti-Parkinson drugs, jimson weed, and mushroom poisoning).

Because of their tendency to produce ileus, TCAs may remain in the gut long after ingestion; therefore, gastric evacuation is a key therapeutic maneuver. Oral charcoal effectively binds TCAs during their enterohepatic circulation and should be administered as rapidly as possible. The role of repeated doses of charcoal in TCA overdose is controversial. Because TCAs are highly tissue bound, toxicity correlates poorly with ingested dose or serum level. That notwithstanding, plasma levels in excess of 1000 ng/mL often result in life-threatening toxicity. The ECG warns of cardiac (and CNS) toxicity when the QRS complex widens to more than 0.12 seconds. Widening of the QRS complex can provide a valuable clue to TCA overdose in the unconscious patient who has ingested an unknown drug.

Both supraventricular and ventricular arrhythmias complicate TCA overdose. Sinus tachycardia, conduction disturbances, and ventricular arrhythmias may persist long after serum levels normalize, because of avid tissue binding. Return of the QRS width to baseline is the best indication that the risk of significant arrhythmias has passed. Arrhythmias frequently respond to systemic alkalinization (pH > 7.50), which reduces the serum concentration of unbound drug. Lidocaine and phenytoin are the most helpful antiarrhythmics, but tricyclic antidepressant-induced arrhythmias may be refractory to all standard therapy. Type Ia drugs (quinidine and procainamide) should be avoided because of their tendency to further impede conduction. TCA-related hypotension usually is due to volume depletion. If fluid administration fails to restore blood pressure, α-agonists (e.g., norepinephrine) are the most effective vasopressors. Mixed-adrenergic agonists (e.g., dopamine, epinephrine) may paradoxically worsen the hypotension by increasing β-stimulation (increased heart rate and systemic vasodilation).

Interestingly, the tendency for seizures also may be predicted by a QRS complex width exceeding 0.12 seconds. Seizures, although undesirable in and of themselves, also induce systemic acidosis, which translocates TCA from plasma to tissue, potentially worsening the CNS and cardiac toxicity. Diazepam, phenytoin, and phenobarbital should be considered first-line anticonvulsants. In seizing patients with unstable hemodynamic or respiratory status, it may be necessary to use paralytic agents to establish an airway and effective circulation before the cerebral discharges are controlled. If used, extreme caution must be exercised with paralytic agents because they do not interrupt cerebral discharges even though they stop muscular convulsive activity. In such settings, continuous EEG monitoring is probably required.

Physostigmine, a rapidly acting anticholinesterase inhibitor that penetrates the blood–brain barrier, has been used in refractory seizures or ventricular arrhythmias, but its use is controversial. There is no evidence that physostigmine decreases mortality, and its own impressive spectrum of toxicity includes AV block, asystole, seizures, bronchospasm, and hypotension. If used, its short half-life necessitates hourly administration. Neither hemodialysis nor hemoperfusion are effective at TCA removal. Experimental therapy for TCA poisoning under development includes the use of widely cross-reactive antibodies in a strategy similar to that provided by Digibind®.

KEY POINTS

1. Victims of overdose rarely give a complete and accurate description of the quantity or type of medications ingested. In most adult cases, multiple substances are involved.

2. Basic treatment principles include limiting the amount of toxin absorbed, enhancing elimination of absorbed toxin, and preventing conversion of nontoxic compounds to toxic metabolites.

3. A tentative diagnosis in most overdose and poisoning cases can be made by physical examination and simple laboratory tests (electrolyte profile, creatinine, serum osmolarity, urinalysis).

4. With little intervention, the outcome for most victims of poisoning is excellent. Supportive care, with particular attention to maintaining an airway, oxygenation, and perfusion are the mainstay of the treatment. Becoming prematurely fixated on the details of specific antidotal therapy can lead to disastrous consequences if basic support of oxygenation and perfusion are ignored.

5. Drugs or poisons for which specific antidotes or therapies exist (especially acetaminophen, salicylates, methanol, ethylene glycol, digitalis) should be aggressively sought (including specific quantitative levels) and treated after initial stabilization.

SUGGESTED READINGS

1. Boehnert MT, Lovejoy FH. Value of the QRS duration versus the serum drug level in predicting seizures and ventricular arrhythmias after an acute overdose of tricyclic antidepressants. N Engl J Med 1985;313:474–479.

2. Caravati EM, Bossart PJ. Demographic and electrocardiographic factors associated with severe tricyclic antidepressant toxicity. Clin Toxicol 1991;29:31–43.

3. Chapman BJ, Proudfoot AT. Adult salicylate intoxication: Death and outcome in patients with high plasma salicylate concentrations. Quart J Med 1989;72:699–707.

4. Dugandzic RM, Tierny MG, Dickinson GE, et al. Evaluation of the validity of the Done nomogram in the management of acute salicylate intoxication. Ann Emerg Med 1989;18:1186–1190.

5. Frommer DA, Kulig KW, Marx JA, Rumack B. Tricyclic antidepressant overdose: a review. JAMA 1987;257:521–526.

6. Jay JS, Johanson WG, Pierce AK. Respiratory complications of overdose with sedative drugs. Am Rev Respir Dis 1975;112:591–598.

7. Kellerman AL, Fihn SD, Logerfro JP, et al. Impact of drug screening in suspected overdose. Ann Emerg Med 1987;16:1206–1216.

8. Litovitz TL, Schmitz BF, Bailey KM. 1989 Annual Report of the American Association of Poison Control Centers National Data Collection System. Am J Emerg Med 1990;8:394–442.

9. Marshall JB, Forker AD. Cardiovascular effects of tricyclic antidepressant drugs: therapeutic usage, overdose and management of complications. Am Heart J 1982;103:401–414.

10. Milne MD, Scribner BH, Crawford MA. Non-ionic diffusion and the excretion of weak acids and bases. Am J Med 1958;24:709–729.

11. Namba T, Nolte CT, Jackrel J, et al. Poisoning due to organophosphate insecticides. Am J Med 1971;50: 475–492.
12. Osterloh JD. Utility and reliability of emergency toxicologic testing. Emerg Med Clin North Am 1990;8: 693–723.
13. Rumack B, Peterson R, Koch G, et al. Acetaminophen overdose: 662 cases with evaluation of oral acetylcysteine treatment. Arch Intern Med 1981;141:380–385.
14. Smilkstein MJ, Knapp GL, Kulig KW, Rumack BH. Efficacy of oral N-acetylcysteine in the treatment of acetaminophen overdose. N Engl J Med 1988;319:1557–1562.
15. Smith TW, Butler VP, Haber E, et al. Treatment of life-threatening digitalis intoxication with digoxin-specific Fab antibody fragments: experience in 26 cases. N Engl J Med 1982;307:1357–1362.
16. Steinhart CM, Pearson-Shaver AL. Poisoning. Crit Care Clin 1988;4(4):845–872.

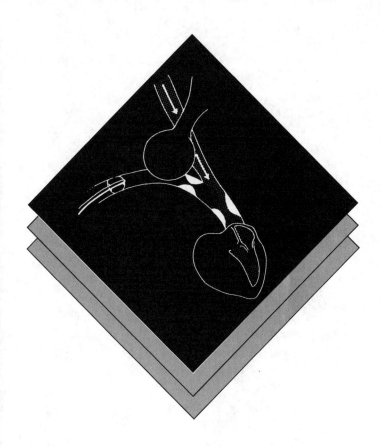

SECTION 3

Surgical Crises

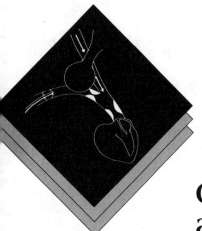

Coma, Stroke, Seizures, and Brain Death

ALTERED MENTAL STATUS

Altered mental status is an extremely common problem in the intensive care unit (ICU) but usually falls short of meeting the strict definition for coma. However, even these milder alterations in consciousness are associated with high mortality rates, unless they result from deliberate sedative administration. Although the frequency of conditions altering mental status varies with the specific patient population of each ICU, for the nontrauma patient, metabolic encephalopathy and seizures clearly are the most common causes. Prospective evaluation of the causes of metabolic encephalopathy in a medical ICU generally reveals that sepsis, hepatic failure, and renal failure are the most common antecedents (Fig. 34.1).

COMA

DEFINITIONS

Coma is a sleep-like state of unconsciousness from which the patient cannot be awakened. Although reflex movements (spinal reflexes and decorticate or decerebrate posturing) may occur, there is no speech or purposeful eye or limb movement. Less profound stages of suppressed consciousness are termed obtundation, stupor, and lethargy. Imprecise terms such as "semicoma" or "light coma" may confuse subsequent examiners and should be abandoned in favor of a less ambiguous description of the highest level of neurologic function.

PATHOPHYSIOLOGY

Consciousness has two components: arousal and awareness. Failure of arousal results from reticular activating system or diffuse bilateral hemispheric dysfunction. Continuous stimulation by the brainstem's reticular activating system is required for the appearance of wakefulness. Conversely, awareness, a cognitive function, requires coordinated function of both cerebral cortices. Arousal may occur without awareness, but the converse does not occur. From its origin in the midpons, the reticular activating system radiates diffusely outward to the cerebral cortex. It is this wide distribution that prevents coma, unless a diffuse process impairs both cerebral cortices or the reticular activating system is interrupted near its pontine origin. Although this simple schema generally explains arousal and awareness, data suggest that the dominant cortical hemisphere plays a disproportionate role in maintaining consciousness and selective damage to both frontal lobes can result in coma.

Coma may arise from a wide variety of diffuse or focal conditions affecting the central nervous system (CNS); however, all coma results from only four basic pathophysiologic mechanisms: (*a*) metabolic or toxic encephalopathy; (*b*) generalized seizures; (*c*) compression of the pons or cerebral cortices by structural lesions or increased intracranial pressure (ICP); and (*d*) inadequate cerebral perfusion. Regardless of cause, the extent of neurologic impairment of any potential cause of coma is modified by the patient's age and underlying cerebral and cardiovascular status. Sim-

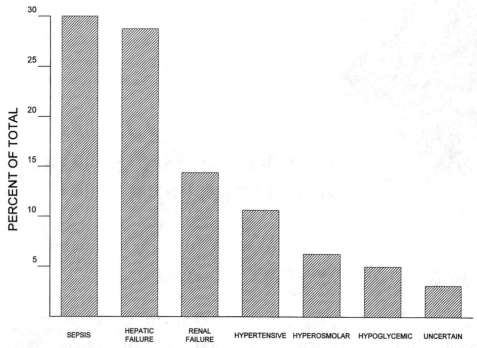

FIG. 34–1. Relative frequency of causes of mental status alterations in nontrauma patients in the ICU. Sepsis, hepatic failure, and renal failure rank as the most common causes.

ply stated, a metabolic insult that might not produce coma in a healthy young person could result in profound coma in an elderly patient with chronically impaired circulatory performance.

ETIOLOGY

Metabolic Disorders

Outside the neurosurgical setting (e.g., head trauma, subarachnoid hemorrhage, brain tumors), metabolic encephalopathy is the most common cause of coma. A comparison of the usual clinical features of structural and metabolic coma is presented in Table 34.1. Because metabolic encephalopathy affects the cortex and brainstem diffusely, abrupt focal defects and progressive rostrocaudal dysfunction seen with supratentorial mass lesions usually do not occur. Instead, patients exhibit slowly evolving symmetric deficits, often preceded by progressive somnolence or confusion. A variety of common disorders, including hypoxia, hypotension, dehydration, sepsis, hepatic encephalopathy, and uremia, all can contribute to impaired consciousness, but no absolute guidelines can be given regarding the magnitude of an isolated abnormality that is necessary to cause coma, especially because multiple derangements often coexist. Furthermore, the age of the patient, the

TABLE 34–1

CLINICAL CHARACTERISTICS OF CAUSES OF COMA

Characteristics	Cause of Coma	
	Traumatic or Vascular	Toxic or Metabolic
History	Injury	Toxin, drug exposure
Onset	Abrupt	Gradual
Rate of progression	Rapid (minutes) deterioration	Slower (hours) progression common
Pattern of progression	May be stuttering or gradual Rostrocaudal loss of function	Global impairment from the start No rostrocaudal pattern
Focality	Focal lesions common	Focal lesions rare

presence of underlying diseases, and the rapidity with which such disorders develop also determine their affect.

It is difficult to state with certainty threshold values for critical metabolites. However, as a rule, it is uncommon for a glucose level higher than 50 or less than 500 mg/dL, Na^+ higher than 120 or less than 150 mEq/L, Ca^{+2} less than 12 mg/dL, or Mg^{+2} less than 10 mg/dL to produce coma without other cause. Only rarely do disorders of other electrolytes produce unconsciousness. The precise cause of unconsciousness in patients with renal failure is unknown; however, uremia rarely causes coma until the blood urea nitrogen (BUN) exceeds 100 mg/dL. (Renal insufficiency probably alters consciousness through multiple mechanisms, including metabolic acidosis, electrolyte abnormalities, metabolic toxin accumulation, and increased permeability of the blood–brain barrier.) Likewise, the exact cause of coma in patients with liver failure is unknown, but accumulation of toxins (e.g., drug metabolites, ammonia) and cerebral edema both play some role in the process. Although there is a rough correlation between serum ammonia levels and mental status, no rules can be offered regarding the level of ammonia necessary to produce coma.

More firm guidelines can be offered with respect to the affect of hypoxemia and hypercapnia on consciousness. Tolerance for hypoxemia depends not only on the extent of desaturation but also on compensatory mechanisms available and the inherent sensitivity of the patient. The major mechanisms of acute compensation are increased cardiac output, increased O_2 extraction, increased anaerobic metabolism, and improved unloading of O_2 resulting from tissue acidosis. Most individuals without cardiac limitation or anemia remain asymptomatic until PaO_2 falls to less than 50 to 60 mm Hg. At that level, malaise, lightheadedness, mild nausea, vertigo, impaired judgment, and incoordination are noted. Confusion develops as PaO_2 falls into the range of 35 to 50 mm Hg. As PaO_2 declines below 35 mm Hg, urine output slows, bradycardia and conduction system blockade develop, lactic acidosis appears, and the patient becomes lethargic or obtunded. At levels near 25 mm Hg, the normal unadapted individual loses consciousness, and minute ventilation falls due to respiratory center depression.

Like all other metabolic toxins, the effects of carbon dioxide accumulation depend not only on the absolute level of CO_2 but also on its rate of accumulation. A CO_2 below 60 mm Hg is often asymptomatic, but as levels rise above this soft threshold, headache and lethargy commonly are observed. Asterixis and myoclonus occur as levels mount even higher but surprisingly massive elevations in CO_2 (often double normal values) usually are necessary to render a patient unconscious.

Generally, the cerebral perfusion pressure (mean arterial pressure [MAP] − intracranial pressure [ICP]) must exceed 50 mm Hg to perfuse the brain adequately; however, otherwise healthy patients may maintain consciousness despite severe reductions in MAP. In contrast, patients with cerebrovascular disease or elevated ICP may be underperfused at much higher pressures.

Sepsis frequently alters consciousness; however, changes in mental status usually fall short of true coma. The mechanisms are multifactorial. Obviously, direct infection of the CNS can render a patient unconscious. In addition, sepsis usually is associated with some degree of hypoxemia and almost two-thirds of septic patients will develop symptomatic hypotension; both factors contribute to changes in mental status. Possibly most interesting, however, is the finding that by stimulating formation of inflammatory proteins called cytokines (e.g., tumor necrosis factor and interleukin-1), sepsis may directly impair consciousness in the absence of hypotension, hypoxemia, or cerebral infection.

Sepsis-induced coma is particularly common in elderly febrile patients, in whom altered mental status presents a difficult management decision. The diagnostic possibilities commonly debated are meningitis, sepsis alone, and an intracranial structural lesion such as a brain abscess or hemorrhage. Obviously, early antibiotic therapy is desirable in all infectious situations, but confirming the diagnosis and nailing down a specific organism to guide antimicrobial therapy requires a lumbar puncture (LP). Unfortunately, LP incurs some small but real risk in the presence of coagulopathy or intracranial mass lesion; therefore, deciding the order in which to perform a head computed tomography (CT) scan, perform an LP, or administer empiric antibiotic therapy is often difficult and must be individualized. For a febrile patient without evidence of a focal neurologic defect, papilledema, or history of trauma, an LP is almost certainly safe and can be performed before or without a head CT scan. (Not too many years ago, the decision to perform an LP always was made by history and clinical examination alone.) If head trauma, papilledema, or focal neurologic deficit complicates the evaluation of a potentially in-

TABLE 34–2

COMMON REVERSIBLE CAUSES OF COMA

Hypoperfusion	Poisoning (see Chapter 33)
Hypoxemia	Carbon monoxide
Hypercapnia	Hypercalcemia
Hypoglycemia	Wernicke's encephalopathy
Status epilepticus	Temperature disorders
Myxedema	CNS infections (e.g., brain abscess, meningitis, encephalitis)
Hypertension	CNS hemorrhage

fected patient, probably the best course is to administer empiric antibiotic coverage and proceed to the CT scanner before lumbar puncture. In any case, if logistical limitations preclude prompt CT scanning and intracranial infection is a real consideration, it is best to begin treatment with appropriate antibiotics, even if doing so eventually impedes a definitive microbiologic diagnosis. Although it seems rational to administer antibiotics as quickly as practical in patients with suspected meningitis, there are little if any data to support the often quoted need to dose antibiotics within 1 hour of suspecting the diagnosis.

Drug ingestion or toxin exposure is perhaps the most frequent cause of nontraumatic coma. Opiates, benzodiazepines, ethanol, and tricyclic antidepressants are the most common classes of drugs implicated. Unconsciousness produced by toxic ingestion often is multifactorial: commonly, several consciousness-depressing drugs are ingested simultaneously and the drugs or toxins often lead to independent changes in oxygenation or perfusion that can cause coma in and of themselves. For example, tricyclic antidepressant overdose often is combined with alcohol ingestion. Although direct effects of either of these drugs alone can cause coma, each can also result in coma producing hypoventilation or hypotension sufficient to alter consciousness. A complete discussion of the problem of toxin ingestion is included in Chapter 33 (Drug Overdose and Poisoning). The common reversible causes of coma are summarized in Table 34.2.

Seizures

Generalized seizures may induce unconsciousness during the ictal phase or as a postictal phenomenon. Distinguishing a seizure from other metabolic or structural causes of coma is seldom difficult because (*a*) convulsive activity usually can be observed and (*b*) consciousness usually returns rapidly after the termination of a brief seizure in an otherwise healthy patient. Patients with underlying cerebral infarctions, metabolic encephalopathy, or prolonged seizures (status epilepticus) may sustain a prolonged postictal period. In turn, status epilepticus often has an underlying structural or metabolic cause. Thus, delayed return of consciousness after a seizure should suggest a structural lesion (e.g., tumors, stroke, subarachnoid hemorrhage, subdural hematoma) or an underlying metabolic disorder (e.g., hypoglycemia, toxin ingestion, or electrolyte disturbance). As with metabolic encephalopathy, seizures that cause loss of unconsciousness generally tend to produce symmetric neurologic defects unless there is an underlying structural abnormality. In contrast to metabolic encephalopathy, however, the loss of consciousness associated with seizures usually is instantaneous rather than gradual.

Structural Lesions

Although supratentorial mass lesions generally are confined to one hemisphere, they cause coma by increasing ICP or by impairing reticular activating system function through pressure on the brainstem. Unless located exactly in the midline, supratentorial mass lesions usually produce hemispheric (unilateral) findings that precede loss of consciousness. Because cerebral function is affected progressively in a rostrocaudal manner, there is a relatively predictable progression of signs. Supratentorial mass lesions, if unchecked, often cause uncal herniation across the cerebellar tentorium, manifest by a fixed dilated pupil, third cranial nerve palsy, and hemiplegia. In contrast, when infratentorial (brainstem) lesions cause coma, rapid or immediate loss of consciousness may be the initial manifestation. Such lesions (e.g., brainstem strokes, cerebellar hemorrhage) often are not associated with rostrocaudal progression and may be rapidly fatal.

INITIAL APPROACH TO THE COMATOSE PATIENT

History

Because pathophysiology and treatment differ radically, a metabolic or structural origin of coma must be distinguished as quickly as possible. The history is helpful in making this separation if it reveals trauma or documents drug or toxin ingestion. Sudden onset of coma suggests a seizure or a vascular event (e.g., subarachnoid hemorrhage, brainstem stroke). The onset of coma after minutes to hours of a focal deficit suggest supratentorial intracerebral hemorrhage with progressively increasing intracranial pressure. A history of a slowly evolving focal deficit occurring over days to weeks before loss of consciousness suggests abscess, tumor, or subdural hematoma, whereas a gradual progression to coma over minutes to hours without a focal deficit favors a metabolic cause. The specific setting in which coma develops may suggest trauma, hyperthermia, hypothermia, or a toxic exposure (e.g., organophosphates, carbon monoxide). Medications or poisons found near the comatose patient are particularly helpful. For example, not only may the offending toxin or drug(s) be discovered, but medication containers usually bear the name of the patient's physician, allowing additional history to be obtained. At the very least, knowledge of a patient's medications provides a sketchy picture of the overall health and underlying diseases. In patients with alcoholism, intoxication with alcohol, ethylene glycol, methanol, or isopropyl alcohol should be suspected. In patients with diabetes, hypoglycemia and diabetic ketoacidosis are equally common causes for coma. Underlying medical problems such as hypothyroidism, renal failure, cirrhosis, or psychiatric illness also suggest a greater likelihood of a metabolic etiology, whereas a clear history of falling, previous stroke, brain tumor, or chronic atrial fibrillation favors a structural or vascular problem. Patients with malignant tumors are subject to both structural lesions (metastases and hemorrhage) and metabolic causes (hyponatremia, hypercalcemia) of coma. Similarly, uncontrolled hypertension can induce metabolic (e.g., hypertensive encephalopathy) or structural (e.g., intracerebral hemorrhage) coma.

Physical Examination

The physical examination is most helpful in differentiating structural from metabolic causes of coma when it reveals evidence of focal, lateralizing signs. In such patients, a metabolic etiology is uncommon. (The most frequent exceptions to this rule occur in patients with hepatic failure, hypoglycemia, and those recovering from seizures.) Comatose patients always should be fully disrobed and examined for evidence of occult trauma. Although physical evidence of head trauma suggests primarily a structural cause, as many as 50% of patients with trauma also suffer from intoxication—often sufficient to produce coma. Boggy areas of the skull suggest depressed skull fracture, whereas Battle's sign (postauricular hematoma), "raccoon eyes," and bloody nasal or aural discharge suggest basilar skull fracture. For traumatized patients, it is critical to exclude cervical spine instability before the neck is manipulated because serious spinal injuries commonly accompany cranial lesions severe enough to cause coma. Diffuse mucosal bleeding may implicate coagulopathy as the cause of intracranial bleeding. Tongue lacerations or incontinence of stool or urine strongly suggest a recent seizure. Atrial fibrillation, a large heart, and recent myocardial infarction are associated with cerebral embolic disease. (In general, embolic disease is an uncommon cause of coma because of the limited area of cerebral infarction caused by small emboli.) Cardiac murmurs should raise suspicion of endocarditis-induced septic embolism or brain abscess. Arrhythmias only result in coma when they cause hypotension or cerebral emboli. Isolated carotid bruits are of little significance because vaso-occlusive carotid disease is a rare cause of coma. Nuchal rigidity suggests meningitis or subarachnoid hemorrhage.

Vital signs provide additional clues to diagnosis. Although hypertension may accompany any cause of increased intracranial pressure, severe hypertension suggests intracerebral or subarachnoid hemorrhage, particularly if accompanied by nuchal rigidity and focal neurologic signs. Hypertensive encephalopathy alone may produce coma and usually is characterized by a nonfocal examination and systolic blood pressures higher than 240 mm Hg or diastolic blood pressures higher than 130 mm Hg. Stimulant intoxication with amphetamines, cocaine, or phenylpropanolamine should at least be considered in patients with altered mental status and elevated blood pressures. Although young patients without underlying vascular or cerebral disease may remain awake with very low (40–50 mm Hg) mean arterial pressures, elderly patients, patients with chronic hypertension, and those with concurrent metabolic encephalopathy or structural lesions tolerate hypotension less well.

Heatstroke, neuroleptic malignant syndrome, malignant hyperthermia, stimulant intoxication, and any number of infections may cause fever sufficient to impair consciousness. Patients with hyperthermia or hypothermia frequently have an infection accompanying the primary temperature disorder that may itself disturb consciousness (e.g., pneumonia, brain abscess, or meningitis). Although aberrations of body temperature can directly cause coma, they rarely do so until core temperatures exceed 105°F or fall below 80°F (see Chapter 28, Thermal Disorders). Bradypnea and hypoventilation most often result from the sedative effects of drugs or alcohol, endogenous toxins, hypothyroidism, or far advanced brainstem compression. Tachypnea is a nonspecific finding but usually arises from one of four basic causes: (a) inappropriate ventilatory control; (b) hypoxemia; (c) compensation for metabolic acidosis; or (d) reduced lung or chest wall compliance. Contrary to popular teaching, specific "pathognomonic" respiratory patterns have little localizing or prognostic value, with one notable exception—discoordinated, irregular (ataxic) respirations usually indicate severe medullary impairment and impending respiratory collapse.

DETAILED NEUROLOGIC EXAMINATION

After the vital signs are obtained, ventilation and perfusion are stabilized, and initial history and physical are performed, neurologic function should be examined in a stepwise fashion. The five key features of the initial neurologic examination may be remembered by the mnemonic "SPERM:" (a) State of consciousness; (b) Pupillary response; (c) Eye movements; (d) Respiratory rate and pattern; and (e) Motor function.

State of Consciousness

Only four terms should be used to describe the level of consciousness: (a) alert; (b) lethargic (aroused with simple commands); (c) stuporous (aroused only with vigorous stimulation—usually pain); and (d) comatose (unarousable).

Pupillary Response

Pupil size, congruency, and response to light and accommodation should be described. Pupillary function is controlled by the midbrain. Therefore, if the pupils function normally, the cause of coma either is a structural lesion located above the midbrain or is metabolic. Small "pinpoint" pupils usually result from pontine hemorrhage or from ingestion of narcotics or organophosphates. (Meperidine frequently fails to produce the miotic pupils typical of other narcotics.) Pupillary re-

sponses almost always remain intact in metabolic causes of coma. (Exceptions to this rule include atropine and atropine-like substances and glutethimide intoxication in which "fixed and dilated" pupils may occur.)

Eye Movements

Normal movement of the eyes requires an intact pontomedullary-midbrain connection. The resting position of the gaze, the presence of nystagmus (horizontal, vertical, or rotatory), and the response to head movements (oculocephalic testing) or to cold tympanic membrane stimulation ("calorics") should be recorded. Cervical spine stability must be ensured before oculocephalic maneuvers are performed. Likewise, tympanic membrane integrity should be confirmed before caloric testing to prevent introduction of water into the cerebrospinal fluid through a basilar skull fracture. Although endogenous toxins accumulated from hepatic or renal failure usually do not impair coordinated eye movements, exogenous toxins (drugs) frequently impair eye movements. In pontine disorders, the medial longitudinal fasciculus is often dysfunctional, but sixth cranial nerve function is preserved. Therefore, ipsilateral abduction is intact, but contralateral adduction is impaired. Quite simply, if rotation of the head (oculocephalic) and vestibular stimulation (calorics) produce no change in eye position, the pons is nonfunctional. If only the eye ipsilateral to the stimulus abducts, a lesion of the medial longitudinal fasciculus (encapsulated by the pons) should be suspected.

Respiratory Rate and Pattern

Description of the respiratory pattern is less helpful than has been suggested previously; however, ataxic breathing is a marker of severe brainstem dysfunction. Despite the nonspecificity of most breathing patterns, the respiratory rate can provide valuable clues to the etiology of coma (see Physical Examination, above).

Motor Function

The highest observed level of motor function should be noted (e.g., "spontaneously moves all extremities," "withdraws right arm and leg from noxious stimulus," "no response to pain"). Motor function in pontine compression often is limited to extensor (decerebrate) posturing, whereas lesions above the pons can produce flexor (decorticate) posturing. If a structural lesion compresses the centers for respiration and heart rate control on the dorsal medullary surface, the patient will be flaccid, without eye movements, and will have midposition, unreactive pupils.

LOCALIZING THE LEVEL OF DYSFUNCTION

If history or examination reveals a sequential, rostrocaudal loss of function, either a supratentorial mass lesion or increased intracranial pressure is the most likely etiology of coma. A funduscopic examination that demonstrates papilledema is virtually diagnostic of increased intracranial pressure or hypertensive encephalopathy.

Although the thalamus–diencephalon cannot be examined directly, injury to this area usually causes lethargy but spares motor function. (Because pupillary and ocular movements are controlled by the midbrain and pons, respectively, they remain unaffected.) The respiratory pattern in thalamic dysfunction is unpredictable. Injury extending lower to the midbrain level usually results in loss of motor function and decorticate, or flexor, posturing. Although pupillary diameter usually is midposition (approximately 3 mm), midbrain injury tends to spare pupil reactivity and eye movements. When damage extends further to the pontine level, pupillary function is impaired routinely. Motor responses are often limited to extensor or decerebrate posturing. If compression progresses to involve the medulla, all motor function usually is absent, as are pupillary responses and eye movements. It is only at this medullary level that respiratory rhythm is predictably affected, becoming ataxic.

LABORATORY EVALUATION

Appropriate body fluid samples should be collected to evaluate the patient for metabolic and toxic coma. Such testing is indicated, even for patients with obvious head trauma, because of the possibility that a metabolic cause may coexist or may have precipitated the trauma (e.g., alcohol, carbon monoxide). Laboratory determinations should include indices of renal and hepatic function, serum glucose and electrolyte determinations, hematocrit and arterial blood gases, and when appropriate, carboxyhemoglobin determinations. The use of a screening toxicologic examination is discussed in detail in Chapter 33 (Drug Overdose and Poisoning).

TREATMENT

The major diagnostic differential is to separate neurosurgical causes of coma from metabolic causes, but initially in all cases, similar supportive treatment should be undertaken. An airway should be secured, perfusion should be stabilized, and oxygen should be administered. Immediately after obtaining appropriate laboratory specimens, an intravenous line should be established for the administration of fluids and medications. At a minimum, laboratory studies should include an arterial blood gas, hematocrit, and measurement of sodium, calcium, magnesium, creatinine, and liver function tests. During initial phlebotomy, it is also prudent to obtain a sample for future toxicologic analysis, should it become necessary. Because of its time-sensitive importance, glucose levels should be screened at the bedside. If testing is not available immediately or if the measured glucose value is low, 50% dextrose in water (D50W) and thiamine (1 mg/kg) should be given.

Naloxone, a narcotic antagonist, and flumazenil, a benzodiazepine antagonist, can temporarily reverse narcotic and benzodiazepine-induced coma, respectively, and thus serve as useful diagnostic tools. The duration of action of both antagonists is less than that of their agonist counterparts; therefore, neither compound is a reliable substitute for intubation and mechanical ventilation for patients with sedative-induced respiratory failure. Relapse into coma often follows a single dose of either reversing agent in patients who are not monitored closely.

After initial stabilization and primary evaluation, an in-depth neurologic examination and specific diagnostic testing can be undertaken. If the history, physical examination, or initial laboratory testing is suggestive of a drug overdose or poisoning, a toxicology profile, and, where indicated, specific levels of compounds not included in a typical toxicology screen (e.g., aspirin, acetaminophen, ethylene glycol, methanol) should be obtained. For most febrile comatose patients, immediate lumbar puncture, blood cultures, and institution of antibiotics are indicated. However, if lateralizing neurologic signs are present or there is a history of trauma, a head CT scan usually should precede lumbar puncture but not antibiotic administration.

STROKE

Cerebrovascular accident (CVA) or stroke is one of the world's leading causes of death and is a frequent precipitant of ICU admission. The common factor in all stroke syndromes is neuronal ischemia due to interruption of cerebral blood flow. The term "stroke," derived from the biblical reference to being "struck down" by the hand of God, implies an acute dramatic neurologic event. Although sudden profound neurologic events do occur, in the ICU population, the presentation usually is much more subtle and often atypical. Common occurrences such as altered mental status, speech disorders, a decreased level of consciousness, agitation, or the new onset of seizures may be the only manifestation. Not only are the presenting signs in ICU patients different, so is the etiology: whereas most strokes occurring in the community are due to vascular occlusive disease, in hospitalized patients, many more strokes are the result of cerebral emboli, often after an invasive medical procedure.

PATHOPHYSIOLOGY

Three pathophysiologic mechanisms account for all strokes: thrombosis, embolism, or hemorrhage. Five basic types of strokes result: thrombotic, embolic, lacunar, and hemorrhagic (intracerebral and subarachnoid), each with its own predisposing factors, typical clinical presentation, and specific treatment summarized in Table 34.3.

THROMBOTIC STROKE

Thrombotic strokes, the most common variety, result from the progressive occlusion of larger arteries (usually proximal branches of the carotid). Therefore, the risk of thrombotic stroke is related directly to age as the chronic risk factors of diabetes, hypertension, smoking, and hypercholesterolemia take their toll on vessel patency. Although large vessels usually are the target, thrombotic strokes can occur in small, perforating vessels, resulting in a specific pattern known as a lacune (see below). Acute stroke also may occur in patients with less than critical vascular narrowing when hypotension, hypoxemia, or coagulopathy tips the balance of cerebral oxygen supply and demand unfavorably.

The slow, progressive vascular narrowing results in premonitory ischemic episodes, transient ischemic attacks (TIAs), in as many as 40% of patients who ultimately sustain a thrombotic stroke. Much akin to unstable angina, TIA serves as a marker of a transition period during which stroke is likely. The risk of stroke correlates with the severity of the TIA—when temporary monocular vision loss (amaurosis fugax) is the only symptom, the risk of stroke is substantially lower

TABLE 34–3
CHARACTERISTICS OF STROKE SYNDROMES

Characteristic	Embolic	Thrombotic	Hemorrhagic
Time course	Abrupt, maximal defect at onset	Stuttering progression	Abrupt, rapid progression
Common locations	Cortical infarcts	Cortical infarcts	Internal capsule, basal ganglia
Predisposing factors	Atrial fibrillation Arterial catheter flushing Left ventricular aneurism or dilation Mitral stenosis Central venous catheter insertion DVT—Pulmonary embolism Atrial septal defect Endocarditis (especially fungal)	Heart failure Hypercholesterolemia Hypertension Smoking Diabetes	Hypertension Prodromal headache Cardiac catheterization Vascular malformation
Antecedent history	Recent myocardial infarction	TIA common Amaurosis fugax Central retinal artery occlusion	Recent thrombolytic therapy "Herald bleed possible"
Therapy	Antithrombotic	Antithrombotic Elective endarterectomy	Correction of coagulopathy Surgical evacuation of selected lesions

than when large transient hemispheric defects occur. A TIA is a powerful warning sign that must not be ignored, because at this stage, antithrombotic therapy or surgical intervention can abort disabling stroke in many patients. Unfortunately, other than TIAs, there are few if any reliable physical signs identifying patients at risk. A diminished carotid pulse or a carotid bruit are perhaps the best indicators of large-vessel occlusive disease.

Because thrombotic strokes usually infarct the cerebral cortex, in which sensory and motor functions are juxtaposed anatomically, equal losses of sensory and motor function to a given anatomic region occur. This is in contrast to small-vessel strokes (lacunes) occurring deeper in the brain, in which, by virtue of the neuronal pathway arrangement, widespread deficits of isolated sensory or motor function are possible. For thrombotic strokes, the supply distribution of the occluded vessel determines the pattern of neurologic deficit, which differs for the anterior, middle, and posterior cerebral artery circulations. Typically, thrombotic strokes present in a progressive "stuttering" fashion, presumably as in situ thrombosis progressively diminishes flow. When middle cerebral artery (MCA) flow is interrupted, the resulting sensory and motor deficits are greatest on the contralateral side of the face, with lesser deficits in the arm and leg. MCA occlusions of the dominant cortex also may produce an expressive or receptive aphasia when infarcting the anterior or posterior speech centers, respectively. A corresponding lesion of the nondominant hemisphere may produce only an acute agitated or confused state. Homonymous hemianopsia and conjugate eye deviation toward the side of the lesion are less common but characteristic features of MCA occlusion. (Although certainly possible from thrombosis, MCA occlusions are more likely to be the result of embolism.) Occlusion of the anterior cerebral artery produces the greatest neurologic deficits in the contralateral leg, followed in severity by the arm and then the face. A homonymous hemianopsia or loss of vision ipsilateral to the stroke also is possible. In such patients, frontal lobe signs of incontinence, grasp and suck reflexes, and perseveration also are seen commonly. Posterior cerebral artery occlusion generally does not affect the major centers for speech or motion; deficits are limited to homonymous hemianopsia, impaired recent memory, and prominent sensory loss.

The diagnosis of thrombotic stroke is a clinical one. The CT scan usually is normal in the acute period but occasionally may show low-density areas. A relatively low percentage (approximately 25%) of bland thrombotic strokes undergo hemorrhagic transformation within 48 hours. This conversion often is associated with some worsening of the neurologic deficit and can be confirmed by repeating a CT scan 48 to 72 hours after onset. Large strokes (>30% of a hemisphere), especially in elderly patients, present the greatest risk for this complication.

The supportive treatment common to all stroke victims is outlined below. Unfortunately, at this time, there is no convincing evidence that outcome of a completed thrombotic stroke is altered with anticoagulation, thrombolytic therapy, or surgery. Clinical trials using thrombolytic agents for thrombotic stroke in progress have failed to show consistent or dramatic benefit and results of these trials are sometimes contradictory. Recombinant tissue plasminogen activator (rTPA) given to patients within 3 hours of the onset of stroke does not improve early measures of neurologic function but may improve late (3-month) survival and function. In contrast, streptokinase, as tested in recent clinical trials, offers no such benefits. It is not clear whether there are intrinsic differences in efficacy between TPA and streptokinase or if the differences observed in these trials are related only to patient selection. (Patients in the streptokinase trials were entered up to 6 hours after the onset of stroke.) Both agents, however, are associated with significant risks of intracranial and extracranial bleeding and thus should be used only by experienced physicians in a hospital with neurosurgical backup.

Carotid endarterectomy is not indicated for treatment of acute thrombotic stroke, but for patients with chronic or recurrent symptoms of cerebral ischemia, endarterectomy may be beneficial. For symptomatic patients with a greater than 70% carotid stenosis, endarterectomy is of proven benefit if performed by an experienced surgeon in patients with a low (<6%) operative risk. When the stenosis is in the range of 50 to 70%, benefit is unproven but endarterectomy still is probably acceptable if the combined operative risk remains less than 6%. The morbidity and mortality rate must, however, be significantly lower (below 3%) to favor surgical intervention in the asymptomatic patient. Because of the rapid evolution of diagnostic techniques, an enduring discussion of the merits of diagnostic tests to evaluate the cerebral circulation is not possible. Currently, the cerebral arteriogram remains the gold standard.

Aspirin clearly reduces the incidence of thrombotic strokes when given prophylactically, particularly to patients with premonitory transient ischemia and can reduce the incidence of recurrent stroke. Unfortunately, aspirin does not abort stroke in progress or reverse established neurologic deficits.

EMBOLIC STROKES

Embolic strokes, overall the second most common variety, result from the sudden impaction of a plug in a small cerebral artery branch, usually giving rise to isolated cortical defects. Because complete small-vessel occlusion occurs nearly instantaneously, maximal neurologic deficits are typically observed at the time of embolization, but it is common for deficits to partially improve within 1 to 2 days. Although embolic strokes are considered to be second in frequency to thrombosis in the general population, patients in the ICU are at substantially higher risk of emboli because they are commonly subjected to procedures that predispose patients to arterial injury or thrombosis and cholesterol or air embolism (e.g., central venous catheterization, left heart catheterization, aortic balloon pump insertion, and invasive blood pressure monitoring). During such procedures, air, clot, or atherogenic material can be released or dislodged.

Cerebral embolism can result from foreign bodies, septic material, bland clot, air, or cholesterol fragments. Bland clot formed either in a sluggishly flowing carotid vascular system or in the heart of patients with mural thrombi, myocardial infarction, mitral valve disease, or atrial fibrillation is most common. Rarely, deep leg vein thrombi causes stroke as they cross a right-to-left intracardiac shunt to enter the cerebral circulation. In most cases, the intracardiac defect is a patent foramen ovale or atrial septal defect. Left-sided endocarditis is another potential source of embolism in the critically ill patient. Bacteria, fungi, and amorphous material sloughed by structurally abnormal or infected heart valves all can cause cerebral vascular plugging. It is often forgotten that arterial pressures generated when ''flushing'' a peripheral arterial line can exceed systolic blood pressure, thereby propelling catheter tip clot or system-contaminating air retrograde into the cerebral circulation. Foreign materials, either illicitly injected into the arterial system by the patient or resulting from fracture of arterial catheters, occasionally produce a cerebral embolism. Cerebral air emboli can result from disruption of the pulmonary veins by penetrating trauma or high ventilator inflation pressures, therapeutic misadventures during cardiac catheterization, rapid ascent from underwater diving, or from unusual sexual practices (predominantly in pregnant women).

As a rule the diagnosis of embolic stroke is not difficult to make. History usually reveals one or more predisposing conditions. In addition, the neurologic deficit typically is described as unexpected, immediate, and maximal in severity at onset. Because the heart is the most common embolic source, clinical examination often provides evidence of cardiac disease (e.g., arrhythmia, murmur, or cardiomegaly). Neurologic evaluation typically reveals a cortically based deficit with both sensory and motor loss to the same body region.

Because the volume of tissue infarcted normally is small and the infarcts rarely are hemorrhagic, the CT scan often is unremarkable. For patients with a history suggestive of embolic stroke without an obvious source, the combination of blood cultures to exclude endocarditis, cardiac monitoring to exclude arrhythmias, and an echocardiogram to diagnose mural thrombi and valvular lesions and to evaluate myocardial performance constitute a good initial diagnostic battery. Because of the superior sensitivity of transesophageal echocardiography in finding subtle valvular lesions, it should be considered for patients with a history suggestive of embolism who have a nondiagnostic surface echocardiogram.

The therapy of embolic stroke should be dictated by the embolic material and size of the stoke. Obviously, antimicrobial therapy is indicated for patients with emboli secondary to infective endocarditis. Valve replacement should be considered when large vegetations are present or when recurrent embolism occurs despite appropriate therapy. Myxomas should be excised, when feasible to do so. For patients with nonhemorrhagic embolic stroke from a cardiac source, heparin followed by warfarin with a target INR of 2 to 3 is indicated. Anticoagulation possibly should be delayed for 48 hours after the event to document absence of hemorrhage by CT scan. (Waiting 1–2 weeks to begin anticoagulation is prudent for patients at high risk for hemorrhagic transformation.) For patients with nonrheumatic atrial fibrillation, long-term warfarin has been demonstrated to reduce the risk of stroke by as much as 65% in patients older than 65 years of age. There is no evidence that thrombolytic therapy or anticoagulation is effective for ''stroke in evolution'' or completed embolic stroke.

LACUNAR STROKES

Lacunes are ischemic occlusive events of deep, tiny vessels within the brain, usually occurring in hypertensive individuals. Lacunar syndromes can result from bland infarction or hemorrhage. Most often, these events occur in the region of the internal capsule producing a large functional deficit, even though only a small area of brain is injured. Because neurons controlling distant body regions are grouped closely together, deficits of the face, arm, and leg are typically equal in severity. Similarly, because of the anatomic arrangement of neurons in this region, selective deficits of sensory or motor function can occur. This pattern of deficits is in distinct contrast to cortical infarcts, in which sensory and motor losses tend to occur in parallel, and the limbs and face usually are affected to varying degrees.

The CT scan may be normal or may show only a small lucency or density in patients with lacunes because of the typically small size of the infarct. With the exception of appropriate supportive care and blood pressure control, there is no specific therapy for a lacunar infarct.

HEMORRHAGIC STROKES

Hemorrhagic strokes usually occur in the basal ganglia (i.e., putamen, thalamus, caudate nucleus), pons, and cerebellum when small vessels rupture as the result of chronic hypertension or vessel wall defects. Bleeding into the hemispheric parenchyma is less frequent and more commonly the result of an arteriovenous malformation or venous hemangioma. The site, relative frequency, and clinical characteristics of hemorrhagic stroke are presented in Table 34.4. A rapidly progressive deficit is characteristic.

In addition to vascular defects, nonvascular risk factors also may contribute to the development of hemorrhagic stroke. These extracranial risk factors include drug (prescription or illicit) use and systemic vasculitic conditions. Warfarin and heparin account for approximately 10% of all cases of intracranial bleeding, and an approximate 1% risk of intracranial hemorrhage is associated with use of thrombolytic therapy for acute myocardial infarction. "Crack" cocaine, amphetamines, and phenylpropanolamine all can induce a hemorrhagic syndrome by boosting blood pressure or by inducing vasculitis.

There are three classical clinical presentations of hemorrhagic stroke: (a) hemiplegia, sometimes with hemisensory impairment, when the thalamus or basal ganglia are involved; (b) sudden-onset quadraparesis, pinpoint pupils, midposition eyes, and coma occur when the pons is the site of the injury; and (c) headache, ataxia, nausea, and vomiting when bleeding occurs in the cerebellum. The deficit of intracerebral hemorrhage usually is rapidly progressive, but late deterioration can be seen days after the initial bleed as the osmotic effects of extravasated blood worsen localized swelling. If hemorrhage ruptures into the ventricular system, obstructive hydrocephalus can occur with a slow progressive downhill course. Seizures are more common with hemorrhagic strokes than with bland ischemic lesions. Virtually all hemorrhagic strokes are recognized easily on CT scan by the presence of "bright white" extravasated blood in the region of the stroke.

As one of the few surgically amenable neurologic problems, cerebellar hemorrhage should be recognized quickly, confirmed radiographically, and corrected by evacuation. Serial CT scan evaluation is the best monitoring technique to select

TABLE 34-4

SITES AND CHARACTERISTICS OF INTRACEREBRAL HEMORRHAGE

Site	Frequency	Clinical Characteristics
Putamen	35%	Contralateral hemiparesis, hemisensory loss, dysphagia, or neglect
Thalamus	10%	Similar to putamen bleed plus forced downward gaze, upgaze palsy, unreactive pupils
Caudate nucleus	5%	Confusion, memory loss, hemiparesis, gaze paresis, intraventricular blood, and hydrocephalus common
Hemispheric cortical bleed	30%	Variable findings, depending on location
Cerebellum	15%	Headache, vomiting, gaze ataxia, nystagmus, cranial nerve palsies
Pons	5%	Quadriplegia, pinpoint pupils, gaze palsies, ataxia, sensorimotor loss

candidates who might benefit from clot evacuation. Evacuation generally is reserved for patients with posterior fossa hemorrhage more than 3 cm in diameter and those with rupture of blood into the third ventricle.

Finally, subarachnoid hemorrhage is a stroke syndrome in which headache, confusion, or coma are typical but paralysis rarely is seen. Although the headache very well may not be described as "the worst of my life," patients often identify the headache of subarachnoid hemorrhage as a unique event. Rupture of a Berry aneurysm or arteriovenous malformation allows escape of blood directly into the cerebral spinal fluid, where CT scanning and lumbar puncture offer rapid and reliable confirmation of the diagnosis. Initial mortality rates from subarachnoid hemorrhage approach 50%, with as many as one in four patients experiencing recurrent bleeding without surgical repair. Although treatment of subarachnoid hemorrhage is still evolving, initial stabilization usually is followed by arteriography and elective surgical repair.

When brain perfusion is impaired globally (e.g., shock, cardiopulmonary arrest), those regions at the border between two vascular distributions suffer the greatest. Ischemia of these so-called "watershed zones" results in three major clinical syndromes, including (a) bilateral upper extremity paralysis; (b) cortical blindness; and (c) memory impairment.

STROKE TREATMENT

The therapy of a specific stroke syndrome depends on its etiology and structural manifestations; however, the therapy of most strokes remains supportive. Notable exceptions include cerebellar hemorrhage and TIAs, for which surgery may be beneficial. The roles of anticoagulation and thrombolytic therapy in thrombotic stroke in evolution are still in flux. Because of the frequency of serious complications in stroke victims, simple prophylactic measures to prevent skin breakdown, gastric ulceration, and deep venous thrombosis make good sense (see Complications below).

Regardless of etiology, oxygenation and perfusion should be evaluated in all stroke patients. If the arterial blood is hypoxemic, supplemental oxygen should be administered; however, there is no evidence that supplemental oxygen assists normoxemic patients. Symptomatic arrhythmias, particularly those resulting in hypotension, should

be corrected immediately. Anemia should be corrected to a hemoglobin level of 10 gm/dL or greater.

The appropriate blood pressure target for stroke victims is controversial; however, transient, mild-to-moderate hypertension is very common in all forms of stroke. One point is clear: "normalizing" blood pressure in the chronically hypertensive stroke victim is likely to do more harm than good. A reasonable low-end target for mean arterial pressure in the adult is 110 to 120 mm Hg. For most stroke victims with systolic blood pressures lower than 180 mm Hg and diastolic blood pressure lower than 105 mm Hg, acute antihypertensive therapy probably is not indicated. With sustained diastolic blood pressures in the range of 105 to 120 mm Hg or systolic pressures in the range of 180 to 230 mm Hg, gradual reductions in blood pressure over several hours should be undertaken. Often, these can be accomplished using oral therapy. Persistent diastolic pressures higher than 120 mm Hg or systolic pressures greater than 230 mm Hg almost always warrant urgent (parenteral therapy). If pharmacotherapy is required, drugs without CNS depressant effects should be the primary agents. A complete discussion of blood pressure control is presented in Chapter 22 (Hypertensive Emergencies).

If there is clear evidence of symptomatic intracranial hypertension, immediate measures should be undertaken to lower intracranial pressure, including optimal patient positioning, seizure control, endotracheal intubation, hyperventilation, diuretics, and mannitol. In specific cases of intracranial hemorrhage noted above, surgical evacuation of clot should be considered. A complete discussion of increased intracranial pressure and its therapy is presented in Chapter 35 (Head and Spine Trauma).

An immediate head CT scan is indicated for essentially all stroke patients after initial stabilization to evaluate the magnitude and type of stroke. Thrombotic and embolic strokes eventually show hypodense areas in the distribution of the involved artery, but often early in the course of stroke, the CT is normal. In contrast, the CT shows a high-density (white) area in patients with hemorrhagic lesions. In addition to providing anatomic definition, the CT provides important prognostic information—strokes involving more than 30% of a hemisphere are at high risk for hemorrhagic transformation even if the infarct is bland initially. A repeat scan at 48 hours will identify most patients who will develop bleeding. Furthermore, hemispheric bleeds that rupture into the ventricular system have a worse prognosis. In specific settings, such as brainstem stroke, the MRI may add information to CT scan data; however, indications for an MRI are well beyond the scope of this text.

Unfortunately, recent well-performed trials have failed to resolve the question of acute thrombolytic therapy in bland infarction. Administration of streptokinase within 6 hours of the onset of stroke does not improve late death rates or stroke morbidity. In fact, thrombolytic treatment is associated with a higher 10-day mortality rate mainly because of the transformation of bland thrombotic strokes to the hemorrhagic variety. Because of these increased complications, streptokinase should not be used for acute therapy of bland infarction. In contrast, recombinant TPA given earlier in the course of stroke (less than 3 hours) is associated with long-term neurologic improvement compared to controls. When either compound is used, substantial risk of intracranial and extracranial hemorrhage exist and it is clear that thrombolytic therapy should be reserved for use by experienced personnel in medical centers prepared to deal with its potential complications.

The role of anticoagulation in stroke also remains controversial. Many of the analyses suggesting lack of efficacy or harm from anticoagulation are derived from small or otherwise flawed clinical studies, many of which were performed before CT scanning was a routine practice. Currently, CT scanning allows a much more precise classification of stroke type and the risks and benefits of varying intensities of anticoagulation are better appreciated. Although it is uncertain precisely which patients should be anticoagulated, it is clear that patients with hemorrhagic strokes, especially elderly patients, should not. Furthermore, patients with "large" strokes (involving more than one-third of a cerebral hemisphere) on CT scan should not be anticoagulated before a 48-hour period has passed. Failure to observe hemorrhage on a follow-up scan performed at 2 days is a relatively good predictor that hemorrhage will not occur. Because patients with poorly controlled hypertension also are probably at higher risk for anticoagulation, therapy should be withheld. If any stroke patient is to be helped by anticoagulation, nonhemorrhagic infarcts, especially those believed to be from a cardioembolic source, are perhaps the best candidates. Victims of cardioembolic strokes are at high risk of recurrent stroke within days to weeks of the initial event, thus preventing a second stroke may prove as important

TABLE 34–5

PHARMACOLOGIC THERAPY OF ACUTE STROKE SYNDROMES

Transient ischemic attacks
  Aspirin 325 mg/day (Ticlodipine 500 mg/day, an alternative for aspirin-sensitive patients
Complete ischemic stroke
  Aspirin 325 mg day to prevent recurrence
Progressive ischemic stroke
  Aspirin 325 mg/day OR heparin to PTT 1.5 times control for 3–5 days (especially for posterior circulation stroke)
  EXCEPTIONS: hemorrhagic infarcts, infarcts >30% of a hemisphere.
Cardioembolic stroke
  If hemorrhage absent on CT scan at 48 hours, begin heparin to PTT of 1.5 times control, THEN: warfarin targeted to INR of 2.0–3.0
  EXCEPTIONS: CVA involving >30% of cerebral hemisphere (high risk for hemorrhagic extension). Warfarin can be started without heparin for prophylaxis in atrial fibrillation.

as therapy for the first. When used, anticoagulation with heparin followed by long-term warfarin is indicated. Possibly more than with other thrombotic conditions, excessive anticoagulation should be avoided. In summary, current data suggest that heparin is best used to prevent future strokes, especially those due to cardioembolic phenomena, not to treat established strokes.

For patients with hemorrhagic strokes at the time of presentation, coagulation status should be evaluated using prothrombin and partial thromboplastin times and a platelet count. Anticoagulants and thrombolytic drugs should be stopped and an appropriate reversing agent should be used to correct the coagulation defect: vitamin K and/or fresh frozen plasma for warfarin; cryoprecipitate or amino caproic acid for thrombolytic complications; and nothing or protamine sulfate for heparin intoxication. A summary of standard pharmacologic approaches to stroke syndromes is presented in Table 34.5.

Hemodilution, calcium channel blockade, corticosteroids, and emergent carotid endarterectomy do not seem to have a beneficial effect in the therapy of acute stroke. The importance of strict control of glucose is debatable. Older studies show an association of hyperglycemia with poor neurologic outcome; however, it is very possible that hyperglycemia serves as only a marker of severity of brain injury rather than a cause of damage. Be-

UNPROVEN OR HARMFUL STROKE THERAPIES

Calcium channel blockers
N-methyl-d-aspartamate (NMDA) antagonists
Antioxidant compounds
Pit viper venom
Aminophylline
Hemodilution
Streptokinase
Corticosteroids

cause no cause-and-effect relationship between hyperglycemia and brain injury has been shown in humans, aggressive glucose control cannot be advocated. As a general principle, any degree of even transient hypoglycemia is likely to be more harmful than sustained mild hyperglycemia. Numerous other ineffective or harmful therapies have been used in stroke and are presented in Table 34.6.

COMPLICATIONS

In victims of stroke, deep venous thrombosis, decubitus ulcer formation, and gastric ulceration all are common. In fact, the largest gains in survival of stroke victims is achieved by preventing death from deep venous thrombosis and pulmonary embolism. By one estimate, more than one-third of stroke victims develop deep venous thrombosis in the absence of effective prophylaxis. Therefore, early institution of low-dose subcutaneous heparin prophylaxis (in patients at low risk for heparin-related complications) or venous compression devices may be one of the most efficacious treatments that can be employed in the stroke victim. Likewise, because gastric stress ulceration is common in stroke patients, either early enteral feeding, histamine blocker therapy, or sucralfate is prudent. Careful use of positioning, padding, turning, and therapeutic beds can prevent the devastating complication of skin breakdown. These seemingly mundane but critical issues of supportive care are covered in detail in Chapter 18 (General Supportive Care).

Seizures are a frequent complication of stroke; most seizures occur during the first 48 hours after the onset of symptoms. Often, a seizure is the presenting symptom. Despite the frequency of seizure activity, the role of prophylactic anticonvulsants remains controversial. If prophylactic anticonvulsants are used, it is reasonable to limit their use to the first few days after the onset of stroke, for patients with large infarcts and those who might be at particularly high risk from a seizure (e.g., patients with increased intracranial pressure).

Hydrocephalus is an uncommon complication of most forms of stroke but is far from rare in patients sustaining hemorrhagic infarction of the caudate or posterior fossa. Bleeds into the caudate nucleus rupture into the ventricular system with some frequency, sometimes resulting in a waning level of consciousness and hydrocephalus on CT scanning.

Respiratory complications of stroke, including aspiration pneumonitis and bacterial pneumonia, are extremely common and are responsible for most episodes of post-stroke fever.

SEIZURES

PATHOPHYSIOLOGY

A seizure results from paroxysmal neuronal discharge that causes generalized or focal neurologic signs. Most generalized seizures begin as a focal cortical discharge and proceed to a loss of consciousness with violent muscular spasms. Continuous partial (non-generalized) seizures may not result in coma and therefore often present a diagnostic challenge. Although seizure disorders have been classified in many different ways, it is probably most useful to think of them in terms of their duration (brief versus continuous) and scope (generalized versus focal). Duration is important because prolonged seizures irreversibly injure neuronal tissue. The most dangerous form of seizure activity is that known as status epilepticus, in which continuous seizures of more than 30 minutes duration occur or in which the patient experiences two or more seizures without return of consciousness. Focality is also noteworthy because focal seizures suggest a discrete structural abnormality. Although seizures usually present as localized or generalized phasic muscle spasms, in the ICU, seizures occasionally masquerade as unexplained coma or puzzling sensory or psychiatric disturbances. Because prolonged or persistent seizures are most important in terms of causing death or long-term impairment, the bulk of this discussion will be focused on status epilepticus—prolonged or uninterrupted seizures.

ETIOLOGY

Seizures are most prone to occur in patients at the extremes of age. In children and in elderly patients, the causes of seizures differ. Children most commonly have seizures as the result of fever, infection, or a change in anticonvulsant medications. In contrast, adults are much more likely to seize as a result of stroke, trauma, and drugs and alcohol. One of five basic pathophysiologic mechanisms is responsible for convulsions in most cases. Seizures arise from intrinsic electrical instability (epilepsy), toxic or metabolic disturbances (e.g., electrolyte imbalances, alcohol, drug effect), structural lesions (e.g., trauma or tumor), infectious causes (meningitis, cerebritis, brain abscess), or abnormalities of brain perfusion (global hypoxia). In general, these precipitating factors segregate into two prognostic groups. Patients with idiopathic epilepsy, subtherapeutic drug levels, and alcohol-related seizures tend to have an excellent prognosis. In contrast, victims of stroke, trauma, tumor, encephalitis, global hypoxia, or direct CNS poisons tend to have a poor prognosis.

High fever (especially in children), drug withdrawal (particularly anticonvulsant, alcohol, or sedatives), and iatrogenic overdoses of isoniazid, penicillin, tricyclic antidepressants, theophylline, or lidocaine are common metabolic causes. Many electrolyte disturbances responsible for coma also may induce seizures, especially when such changes occur abruptly (e.g., acute hyponatremia, disequilibrium after dialysis).

Although most seizure disorders that occur in outpatients are idiopathic, this is true less often in the ICU, where such treatable conditions as drug or alcohol withdrawal, metabolic imbalances, and acute structural lesions are more common and must be excluded. Most important among the metabolic precipitants are uremia, hypoglycemia, hypocalcemia, hypomagnesemia, and hyponatremia. CNS infections (meningitis, encephalitis, and brain abscess) are frequent causes of ictus; approximately one-third of adults with bacterial meningitis will experience a seizure. Human immunodeficiency virus (HIV) represents a particular hazard for CNS infections, including toxoplasmosis and viral encephalitis.

DIAGNOSIS

The diagnosis of seizures usually is made from the history and from the observation of an attack. Occasionally, historical features and/or the clinical appearance are so atypical as to require confirmatory testing by electroencephalography. In such cases, an intra-ictal electroencephalogram (EEG) recording may be diagnostic. Rarely, an EEG recording may reveal unsuspected seizure activity in a patient with unexplained coma. EEG localization of seizure discharge to the base of the temporal lobes (or intense uptake of radioisotope in the temporal lobes) suggests herpes encephalitis. A head CT or MRI scan is indicated in all patients with new-onset seizures, in those accompanied by a preceding or persistent focal neurological deficit, and in those refractory to simple medical therapy. In such patients, imaging often reveals a structural cause (e.g., vascular malformation, subdural or subarachnoid hemorrhage, primary or metastatic tumor, or hemispheric bleed). For patients with a known seizure disorder, a CT scan is not necessary to reevaluate each seizure; however, it should be remembered that even patients with epilepsy can develop strokes, tumors, and infectious intracranial process. Therefore, each episode of seizures should be evaluated by history and physical examinations to develop individual treatment plans.

SYSTEMIC EFFECTS OF SEIZURES

Brief ictal episodes are of little consequence if they do not occur while the patient is involved in a dangerous activity, if oxygenation and ventilation are maintained, and if the episode does not cause musculoskeletal injury. However, continuous electrical firing during prolonged seizures depletes cellular reserves of oxygen and adenosine triphosphate (ATP) and allows intracellular accumulation of calcium—processes that culminate in neuronal death. In humans, status epilepticus of 2 hours duration reliably results in permanent brain damage, but injury may begin as early as 30 to 60 minutes after the onset of seizures. Therefore, the long-lasting adverse effects of seizures usually are associated with status epilepticus, a condition in which uninterrupted seizure activity occurs or the patient fails to regain consciousness between intermittent but closely spaced ictal episodes. Seizure-induced neuronal damage does not require loss of consciousness nor convulsive muscular contraction.

Early and massive catecholamine release associated with prolonged seizures may induce arterial and intracranial hypertension and hyperglycemia. Alterations in arterial and pulmonary vascular pressures may give rise to post-ictal pulmonary edema. Fever resulting from both central thermostatic reset and sustained muscular activity may rise to dangerous levels (>105°F). Furthermore, thermoregulation may be disturbed for days, even after cessation of seizure activity. Temperature elevations related to seizures tend to respond poorly to antipyretics or paralytic agents. Because fever and leukemoid reactions (peripheral leukocyte counts often exceed 20,000 mm³) are common, infection often is suspected in seizure patients. Differentiating infection from seizure is confused further by the common finding of cerebrospinal fluid (CSF) pleocytosis. Leukocyte counts may reach 80 cells/mm³ and a predominance of neutrophils.

Profound and rapid-onset acidosis often accompanies seizure activity. One-half of patients with post-ictal acidemia exhibit lactic acidosis alone, whereas the other half exhibit a mixed respiratory and metabolic (lactic) acidosis. Although the seizure-associated acidosis may be severe (pH < 6.5), no evidence links pH with outcome and most patients resolve their acidosis within 1 hour. Increased free water losses from sweating and hyperventilation may increase serum osmolarity and sodium concentration. Hypotension and (rarely) seizure-induced cardiovascular collapse can further aggravate neurologic damage, but unlike the setting of ischemic brain injury, cerebral blood flow typically is increased in patients with seizures. The summation of direct cerebral damage and metabolic pandemonium induced by seizures can result in a mortality rates as high as 30 to 35% for patients with status epilepticus.

TREATMENT

The most important factors in determining the outcome of an episode of status epilepticus are the etiology of the episode and the time from onset to termination of the seizures. The longer that time, the more difficult it is to control the seizure and the worse the ultimate neurologic outcome. Protection of the airway and maintenance of perfusion are primary considerations. Aspiration must be guarded against by prompt termination of the seizure, by proper patient positioning (lateral decubitus), and endotracheal intubation in which clinical judgment dictates. (Without neuromuscular paralysis, it is sometimes dangerous and often impossible to perform endotracheal intubation on patients with seizures.) As with all causes of altered consciousness, electrolytes and glucose should be tested and normalized. When hypoglycemia is noted and treated, thiamine should be administered concurrently.

For patients who experience a solitary seizure or a small number of brief seizures with known

TABLE 34–7

THERAPY OF STATUS EPILEPTICUS

Step 1 (ABCDs)
  Establish an airway, administer oxygen
  Ensure circulation with adequate blood pressure
  Establish intravenous access
  Collect blood for routine laboratory studies and possibly toxicologic analysis
  Administer D50W (1 mg/kg) and thiamine (1 mg/kg), unless patient known to be normoglycemic or hyperglycemic
Step 2 (Rapidly achieve seizure control)
  Diazepam 5–10 mg i.v.
    or
  Lorazepam (0.05–0.2 mg/kg) 2–4 mg i.v. (initial doses of either may be repeated if necessary)
Step 3 (Achieve and maintain lasting seizure control)
  Phenytoin 15–18 mg/kg by slow i.v. infusion
Step 4 (Salvage therapy for resistant status epilepticus)
  Phenobarbital 150–400 mg slow i.v. infusion (<100 mg/minute)
Step 5 (Advanced treatment for refractory disease)
  General anesthesia (pentobarbital), paraldehyde, sodium valproate
  Pentobarbital (12 mg/kg) at 0.2–2.0 mg/kg/hour
Step 6 (Diagnostic evaluation)
  Evaluate electrolytes, oxygenation, acid–base status
  Consider CT, MRI, lumbar puncture, toxicologic evaluation

precipitant, long-term anticonvulsants are not always necessary; however, there is no disagreement that status epilepticus should be terminated pharmacologically as rapidly as possible. One strategy for acute anticonvulsant administration is given in Table 34.7. There is clearly no single ideal drug regimen for terminating seizures; however, benzodiazepines may represent the initial anticonvulsant of choice because of their rapid action, high effectiveness, and wide therapeutic margin. Benzodiazepines cannot be expected to provide long-term seizure control by themselves but can "break" seizures long enough to accomplish intubation if necessary and to initiate therapy with phenytoin, fosphenytoin, or another longer-acting drug. Initial intravenous doses of diazepam (0.1–0.2 mg/kg) or lorazepam (0.05–0.1 mg/kg) are equally effective in terminating seizure activity. The relatively short duration of action of benzodiazepines limits their effectiveness as long-term anticonvulsants and explains the rather high rate of seizure recurrence when these drugs are used alone. Hypotension and apnea are complications of benzodiazepine use but occur rarely

($<5\%$) unless other anticonvulsants (especially phenobarbital) have been administered.

Phenytoin is the preferred second drug to achieve long-term seizure control in patients with status epilepticus. Although phenytoin has received "bad press" because of its potential for adverse cardiovascular effects (arrhythmias, hypotension, conduction disturbances) when infused rapidly, it is a safe and effective drug in status epilepticus when given with appropriate caution. (No anticonvulsant is entirely free of side effects.) Because of its long half-life, seizure recurrence is rare after convulsive activity is terminated using phenytoin. Initial loading doses should not exceed 1 gm (15–18 mg/kg), with a maximum infusion rate of 50 mg per minute. (Additional carefully titrated doses, to a total of 30 mg/kg, may be necessary.) Therefore, a full adult dose of phenytoin usually requires 20 to 30 minutes for infusion. Phenytoin must be administered only in saline; it is not compatible with glucose-containing solutions. Although the adult daily maintenance dose averages 300 mg intravenously or orally, therapy should be guided by serum drug levels. Phenytoin toxicity may produce diplopia, horizontal and vertical nystagmus, slurred speech, ataxia, clumsiness, and somnolence. Paradoxically, phenytoin may even increase the frequency of seizures. Fosphenytoin, a potentially less toxic phenytoin precursor is now available. It is not yet clear if it has the superior efficacy needed to justify its substantial cost.

Fosphenytoin, a potentially less toxic phenytoin precursor, is now available. It is not yet clear if it has the superior efficacy needed to justify its substantial cost. Phenobarbital (150–400 mg) administered by slow intravenous infusion also may be used to terminate seizures, but its cardiorespiratory depressant action and interaction with other drugs often makes its use problematic. Because it is a weak acid, phenobarbital exists in the ionized state in the plasma of patients with seizures and acidemia. Ionization of phenobarbital may result in up to a 50% reduction in drug delivery to the brain in acidosis. Once administered, phenobarbital may have a prolonged (1- to 3-day) sedative effect, which may later complicate neurologic evaluation. Paraldehyde and sodium valproate have limited application in status epilepticus because these two preparations are no longer available in parenteral formulation.

Seizures refractory to combinations of benzodiazepines, barbiturates, and phenytoin may require "general anesthesia," consisting of intubation and administration of a volatile anesthetic (e.g., isoflurane) or a continuous infusion of a short-acting barbiturate (typically pentobarbital, 5–15 mg/kg load, followed by 1–2 mg/kg/hour or thiopental, 3–7 mg/kg load, followed by 50–100 mg/minute intravenously). Such a regimen is nearly always effective but may be required for 12 to 36 hours or longer to prevent seizure recurrence. Furthermore, use of vasopressor support is nearly always required and emergence from protracted coma induced by pentobarbital may require weeks. Propofol also has been suggested as a potential therapy for refractory status epilepticus, but data regarding its efficacy in this setting are limited. Additionally, the propensity to cause hypotension, a weak proepileptic effect, and substantial cost are other factors potentially limiting propofol use as an anticonvulsant. If general anesthesia is used for seizure control, continuous availability of EEG monitoring and expert neurologic consultation are indicated.

Status epilepticus occasionally is resistant to the initial step of pharmacologic control with benzodiazepines and phenytoin. Reasons for failure of this regimen include inadequate drug dosing, cerebral mass lesion (tumor or hemorrhage), or profound metabolic abnormality (hypoxemia, hyponatremia, or hypocalcemia).

BRAIN DEATH

Because the brain is the most sensitive organ to deprivation of oxygen and perfusion, its function may be irretrievably lost despite preservation of other bodily functions. Firm criteria for diagnosing brain death are important to establish to prevent wasting valuable medical resources and conversely to avoid premature abandonment of hope for potentially salvageable patients. Even with full support, patients meeting brain death criteria rarely survive beyond a few days. To diagnose brain death, the etiology of coma must be known with reasonable certainty. Hypothermia, drug overdose, neuromuscular blockade, and shock must be excluded. No sedative, narcotic, or anesthetic drugs may remain in the circulation. Furthermore, the patient must be observed over a prolonged period (approximately 24 hours) to document the stability of the clinical picture. Seizure activity and decerebrate or decorticate posturing are inconsistent with the diagnosis; however, reflexes of purely spinal cord origin are compatible. To confirm brain death, cerebral function must be absent at hemispheric, midbrain, pontine, and medullary levels. Lack of cortical function is evidenced by a totally unreceptive and unresponsive state. Patients in a persistently vegetative state lack awareness and responsiveness but appear awake because reticular activating system arousal pathways remain intact. Such patients do not meet brain death criteria. Patients with destructive lesions of the base of the pons that give rise to the "locked in" syndrome also appear unresponsive. Detailed testing, however, reveals that these patients are aware but unable to respond, except for eye opening and vertical eye movements. Brainstem death is confirmed by demonstrating the absence of pupillary, corneal, oculocephalic, oculovestibular, gag, and respiratory reflexes. Absent pupillary activity indicates loss of midbrain function. Inability to evoke eye movements confirms lost pontine function. Medullary dysfunction is ensured by demonstrating apnea when the patient is challenged by a profound hypercarbic stimulus. Apnea testing is performed by interrupting positive pressure ventilation while continuing oxygenation. After preoxygenation with an FiO_2 of 1.0, an O_2 catheter is introduced into the endotracheal tube. The patient is then observed for respiratory effort over a prolonged period of time. Such precautions ensure that the patient remains adequately oxygenated although unventilated. A $PaCO_2$ level higher than 60 mm Hg must be attained to ensure adequate ventilatory stimulation. For patients with apnea and functioning circulation, the $PaCO_2$ level normally rises 3 to 5 mm Hg per minute. Therefore, knowledge of the baseline $PaCO_2$ can be used to predict the apneic time necessary to ensure a $PaCO_2$ higher than 60 mm Hg. (In general, 4–6 minutes of apnea are required if the baseline $PaCO_2$ is normal.) For strictly legal reasons, some localities require confirmatory EEGs, brain perfusion scans, or other tests to document absence of cerebral activity or perfusion, but such tests are not necessary to establish a medical diagnosis of brain death. Furthermore, such tests are not foolproof. Isoelectric EEGs have been recorded as long as 4 days after the initial presentation of patients with drug-induced coma. Isoelectric tracings also may occur in patients who have lost cortical function but who retain brainstem activity (neocortical death). Such patients usually demonstrate a vegetative state in which arousal is intact but awareness is lacking. Brain death also may be confirmed by using contrast or radioisotope angiography to demonstrate absence of cerebral flow.

KEY POINTS

1. With the exception of patients with head trauma, metabolic encephalopathy is the most common cause of alterations in mental status seen in the ICU. For medical patients, sepsis, hepatic failure, and renal failure are the leading causes of mental status changes, apart from drugs.

2. An airway should be established and ventilation and perfusion should be restored in comatose patients so that the brain receives adequate quantities of glucose-replete, oxygenated blood. Only after this initial stabilization should further evaluation be undertaken.

3. The best therapy of stroke remains prevention—therapy for established or evolving stroke is controversial and minimally effective. Anticoagulation remains of unproven benefit in most patients with stroke and is likely to be dangerous in elderly patients and in patients with hemorrhagic or large strokes.

4. Among patients sustaining an acute CVA, a CT scan should be used to guide therapy after initial stabilization. Hemorrhagic strokes or those anatomically involving more than one-third of a cerebral hemisphere probably should not receive acute anticoagulation regardless of etiology.

5. Therapy of status epilepticus should be directed to terminate seizure activity as quickly as possible. This goal is best accomplished by ensuring oxygenation and perfusion and then administering an intravenous benzodiazepine followed by phenytoin while simultaneously assessing potential structural or metabolic precipitants of the seizure.

6. Brain death is a state of irreversible absence of function at all levels of the brain (cortex, midbrain, and brainstem). Clinically, this is manifest as an absence of arousal or response, absence of midbrain reflexes (predominantly cranial nerve signs), and absence of spontaneous ventilation, despite significant hypercarbia. The diagnosis generally cannot be made in the presence of ongoing hypothermia or drug intoxication.

7. Although the diagnosis can reliably be made clinically, local legal definitions or requirements for determining brain death preclude a universally valid plan for establishing brain death.

SUGGESTED READINGS

1. Aminoff MJ, Simon RP. Status epilepticus. Causes, clinical features and consequences in 98 patients. Am J Med 1980;69:657–666.
2. Bleck TP, Smith MC, Pierre-Louis SJ, et al. Neurologic complications of critical medical illness. Crit Care Med 1993;21:98–103.
3. Brown RD, Evans BA, Wiebers DO, Petty GW. Transient ischemic attack and minor stroke: an algorithm for evaluation and treatment. Mayo Clin Proc 1994;69:1027–1039.
4. Cascino GD. Generalized convulsive status epilepticus. Mayo Clin Proc 1996;71:787–792.
5. Cloyd JC, Gumnit RJ, McLain W. Status epilepticus. The role of intravenous phenytoin. JAMA 1980;244(13):1479–1481.
6. Diringer MN. Intracerebral hemorrhage: pathophysiology and management. Crit Care Med 1993;21:1591–1603.
7. Duffy FH, Lombroso C. Treatment of status epilepticus. Clin Neuropharmacol 1978;3:41–56.
8. Engel J, Troupin AS, Crandall PH, et al. Recent developments in the diagnosis and therapy of epilepsy. Ann Intern Med 1982;97:584–598.
9. Fisher CM. The neurological examination of the comatose patient. Acta Neurol Scand 1969;45(Suppl 36):4–56.
10. Fisher CM. Acute brain herniation: a revised concept. Semin Neurol 1984;44:417–421.
11. Gorelick PB. Stroke prevention. Arch Neurol 1995;52:347–355.
12. Guidelines for the determination of death: report of the medical consultants on the diagnosis of death to the President's Commission for the study of ethical problems in medicine and biomedical and behavioral research. Neurology 1982;32:395–399.
13. Leppik IE. Double blind study of lorazepam and diazepam in status epilepticus. JAMA 1983;249:1452–1454.
14. Levine SR. Acute cerebral ischemia in a critical care unit: review of diagnosis and management. Arch Intern Med 1989;149:90–98.
15. Levy DE, Coronna JJ, Singer BH, et al. Predicting outcome from hypoxic-ischemic coma. JAMA 1985;253:1420–1426.
16. Lowenstein DH, Alldredge BK. Status epilepticus in an urban public hospital in the 1980's. Neurology 1993;42:483–488.
17. Lowenstein DH, Aminoff M. Clinical and EEG features of status epilepticus in comatose patients. Neurology 1992;42:100–104.
18. Meldrum BS, Vigouroux RA, Brierley J. Systemic factors and epileptic brain damage. Arch Neurol 1973;29:82–87.
19. Orringer CE, Eustace JC, Wunsch CD, Gardner L. Natural history of lactic acidosis after grand-mal seizures. N Engl J Med 1977;297:311–316.
20. Patterson JR, Grabois M. Locked in syndrome: a review of 139 cases. Stroke 1986;17:758–764.
21. Penry JK, Newmark ME. The use of antiepileptic drugs. Ann Intern Med 1979;90:207–218.
22. Plum F, Posner JB. The diagnosis of stupor and coma, 3rd ed. Philadelphia: FA Davis, 1980.
23. Ropper AH, Kennedy SK, Russel L. Apnea testing in the diagnosis of brain death. J Neurosurg 1981;55:942–946.
24. Ropper AH. Lateral displacement of the brain and level of consciousness in patients with an acute hemisphereal mass. N Engl J Med 1986;314:953–958.
25. Rowan AJ, Scott D. Major status epilepticus. Acta Neurol Scand 1970;46:573–584.
26. Schmidley JR, Simon RP. Postictal pleocytosis. Ann Neurol 1981;9:81–84.
27. Shaner DM, McCurdy SA, Herring MO, Gabor A. Treatment of status epilepticus: a prospective comparison of diazepam and phenytoin versus phenobarbital and optional phenytoin. Neurology 1988;38:202–207.
28. Sherman DG, Dyken ML, Fisher M, et al. Antithrombotic therapy for cerebrovascular disorders. Chest 1992;102:529S–537S.
29. Simon RP. Physiological consequences of status epilepticus. Epilepsia 1985;26(Suppl 1):S58–S66.
30. Tassinari CA. Benzodiazepines: efficacy in status epilepticus. Lancet 1983;2:1145–1147.
31. Teasdale G, Jennett B. Assessment of coma and impaired consciousness Lancet 1974;2:81–83.
32. Wityk RJ, Stern BJ. Ischemic stroke: today and tomorrow. Crit Care Med 1994;22:1278–1293.

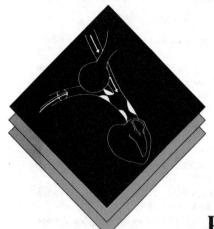

CHAPTER 35

Head and Spine Trauma

SPINAL CORD TRAUMA

MECHANISMS

Spinal cord injuries occur most frequently in the region subject to the greatest motion: the cervical area. Other life-threatening (intracranial, intrathoracic, or intra-abdominal) wounds should be sought in patients with spinal injury because they frequently accompany spinal trauma. Because spinal cord injury so often occurs in conjunction with head injury, all patients with head trauma should be treated initially as if they have sustained cord injury.

The spinal cord can be injured by three basic mechanisms: flexion–rotation, compression, or hyperextension. Cord contusion is the feature common to all three. A minority of cord injuries result from primary vascular disruption. Spinal cord injury should be suspected in every patient with trauma and back or neck pain and sensory or motor deficits.

Flexion–rotation injury of the neck usually occurs when the neck is hyperflexed onto the trunk out of the midline axis, disrupting the posterior spinal ligament. Motor vehicle accidents are the most common cause. At a minimum, patients with flexion–rotation injury require closed reduction and traction. If radiographs demonstrate displacement of a vertebral body by more than half of its width, instability and bilateral facet dislocation are likely. Displacement of less than one-half the width of the vertebral body suggests unilateral dislocation, which is a less serious problem. Such injuries are potentially unstable after reduction, but fewer than 10% require surgery for fixation. If facets in the lumbar region become "locked," surgery usually is necessary.

Compression injuries most commonly result from diving accidents. In this setting, bone fragments or expanding hematoma may lead to neural damage by protruding into the spinal cord. However, these injuries are inherently stable because spinal ligaments remain intact. The usual treatment is bed rest with skeletal traction.

Hyperextension ("whiplash") injuries in the cervical region usually are stable. These injuries occur in older patients with cervical arthritis and frequently are associated with bleeding into the spinal gray matter, producing a "central cord" syndrome.

INITIAL MANAGEMENT

All passive and active motion of the spine should be prevented in patients with suspected cord injury. Adequate ventilation and circulation should be ensured and oxygen should be administered if indicated. Autonomic instability often occurs in the early phase, so that mild hypotension is common. Judicious filling of the intravascular compartment is indicated, but because of disordered vasoregulation, it is important not to administer excessive volumes. Other measures key to the resuscitation of the trauma victim, such as central venous catheter and chest tube insertion, should be performed immediately.

Physical Examination

After spinal immobilization and stabilization of the airway and circulation, a detailed neurologic examination should be conducted. Complete spinal cord disruption produces loss of all sensory and motor function below the level of the injury, initially resulting in flaccid paralysis and loss of deep tendon reflexes that lasts for 2 to 7 days—the "spinal shock" phase. Incomplete cord injuries carry a better prognosis because some function is retained distal to the level of the injury. In a cooperative patient, many clinically important injuries may be diagnosed at the bedside. If the patient is able to take a spontaneous deep breath, cervical roots C2 through C5 probably are intact and diaphragm function is preserved. If the patient can raise and extend the arms, C5 through C7 are intact. The ability to open and close the hand ensures function of C7 through T1, whereas the ability to elevate the legs confirms the integrity of L2 through L4. Wiggling the toes indicates that L5 through S1 roots are functional. Normal anal sphincter function implies preserved function of roots S3 through S5.

RADIOGRAPHIC EVALUATION

After initial examination and stabilization, radiographs of the spine should be obtained. More than two-thirds of all spinal injuries may be seen on a single lateral view of the spine if proper technique is used. Even in cases in which bone injury does not occur, ligamentous injury may cause an expanding hematoma that results in cord compression. Thoracic and lumbar radiographs should be obtained if there is any suspicion of injury in those locations based on patient complaints or examination. It is important to visualize all seven cervical vertebrae because C7 is the vertebra most commonly injured but least commonly seen on portable radiographs. A "swimmer's view" or traction on the patient's arms may aid visualization of C7 and T1.

The alignment of the anterior and posterior aspects of each vertebral body, the alignment of the spinolaminal lines, and the contour of the spinous processes and vertebral bodies should be reviewed. The prevertebral space should be examined for evidence of widening due to hemorrhage. Open-mouth views should be obtained to look for odontoid fractures. Radiographs should visualize the entire spine if a fracture is found. (Up to 20% of patients have multiple levels of injury.) Computed tomography (CT) or myelography probably should be reserved for cases in which the extent of injury is unclear after clinical evaluation and plain radiographs or cases in which injury or limitation of motion precludes adequate visualization.

Therapeutic Interventions

Short-course, high-dose methylprednisolone (30 mg/kg bolus then 5.4 mg/kg/hour for the first day) improves neurologic outcome in most cord-injured patients but does not benefit patients with anterior spinal artery disruption (loss of motor function with preserved sensory function). Use of corticosteroids for longer than 24 hours predisposes patients to infection and possibly gastrointestinal ulceration and therefore is contraindicated.

Neurosurgical consultation should be sought at the earliest possible time. Although the indications for immediate surgery in spinal cord trauma are controversial, commonly accepted criteria include the following: (a) progressive loss of neurologic function due to suspected epidural or subdural bleeding; (b) a foreign body in the spinal canal; (c) cerebrospinal fluid (CSF) leak; and (d) bony instability requiring immobilization.

COMPLICATIONS

Progressive neurologic impairment is only one of the many complications of spinal cord injury. The most significant of these are iatrogenically induced by spinal manipulation or inappropriate administration of fluids or vasopressors to alter blood pressure. During the first 48 hours after spinal cord injury, the level of neurologic impairment often ascends by one to two vertebral levels.

Cardiovascular

Cord lesions above the T6 level interrupt sympathetic outflow, resulting in vasodilation, bradycardia, and hypothermia. Even in young, healthy persons, the loss of sympathetic tone usually produces a stable supine blood pressure in the range of 100/60 mm Hg. Hypovolemia, infection, or placement in the upright position often precipitates profound hypotension. The blood pressure is acceptable if urine output remains good and cerebration is clear. However, if mean arterial pressure (MAP) falls below 70 mm Hg, a fluid challenge may be indicated; invasive monitoring helps dictate proper therapy. Measures to reduce venous capacitance, including abdominal binding, Trendelenburg positioning, and compression stockings may help avoid postural hypotension.

Bradycardia often accompanies hypotension due to cord injury and does not require treatment unless symptomatic. Accommodation of the sympathetic and parasympathetic responses usually produces normal heart rates within 3 to 5 days after injury. However, unopposed vagal stimulation from pain, hollow viscus distention, hypoxemia, or endotracheal suctioning may produce profound bradycardia. If symptomatic bradycardia not caused by hypoxemia occurs, atropine, isoproterenol, or temporary pacing is useful. It is the loss of compensatory tachycardia early in the course of spinal cord injury that makes iatrogenic pulmonary edema common after even modest fluid administration. If unequivocal tachycardia is present in a hypotensive patient with spinal cord injury, suspect another condition such as sepsis, internal hemorrhage, or hypovolemia. Because autonomic paresis eliminates crucial vasoconstrictive reflexes, these patients have very limited stress reserves.

Respiratory

Respiratory impairment, the most common complication of spinal cord injury, results from respiratory muscle weakness, rib fractures, hemopneumothorax, lung contusion, and aspiration. Cervical roots 3, 4, and 5 innervate the diaphragm. Therefore, interruption of the cord above this level in an unsupported patient rapidly leads to apnea and death. Cervical spine injuries also cause problems when expiratory muscle weakness impairs cough and secretion clearance. The forced vital capacity (FVC) should be monitored several times daily in the acute phase of spinal cord injury. As a rule, such problems are unusual if FVC exceeds 1.5 to 2.0 L. If the FVC is less than this value in patients with injuries below the C5 level, direct injury to the phrenic nerve(s) should be suspected.

Because quadriplegic patients have little ventilatory reserve, any condition that further impairs ventilation or mandates an increased minute ventilation may lead rapidly to fatigue and ventilatory failure. Lesions above T10 most commonly cause respiratory difficulty by impairing cough, altering ventilation–perfusion distribution (causing hypoxemia), or decreasing inspiratory capacity. Low lung volumes and atelectasis occur not only because of intrinsic muscle weakness but also because abdominal distention (often from ileus) limits inspiration. Ventilation may be compromised further by unopposed parasympathetic responses that cause bronchorrhea and bronchoconstriction and increase the risk of vomiting and aspiration. Patients with spinal cord injury are particularly sensitive to the effects of neuromuscular paralytic agents.

Although seemingly paradoxical, quadriplegic patients often ventilate best in the supine position. Their only potential muscle of respiration (the diaphragm) is "cocked" into optimal position by such a posture through the upward pressure of the abdominal contents. Conversely, patients with isolated diaphragmatic paralysis ventilate best when fully erect. Upright positioning minimizes the cephalad pressure of the abdominal contents against the flaccid diaphragm. This action increases lung volume and helps stabilize the diaphragm during contraction of the accessory muscles of inspiration. Limitations of vital capacity and forcefulness of cough predispose patients with spinal cord injuries to pneumonia.

Genitourinary

Urinary tract complications (urosepsis, renal failure) are the most common cause of late death in patients with spinal cord injuries. Continuous Foley catheterization probably is indicated early in the hospital course to monitor urine output. Later, intermittent catheterization is preferred because of its reduced risk of infection. Micturition may be impaired for months after spinal cord injury. Regular surveillance cultures of urine help detect infection at an early stage. Prophylactic antibiotics may prevent bacteremia but are unlikely to maintain sterile urine in patients with indwelling catheters.

Gastrointestinal

Immediately after spinal cord injury, ileus that typically lasts 3 to 4 days may occur. Ileus is likely to be protracted if spinal cord injury is accompanied by retroperitoneal hemorrhage. For most patients, a nasogastric tube should be inserted until bowel sounds return. Daily measurements of abdominal girth also may help assess gastrointestinal (GI) motility and the possibility of colonic impaction. For patients with spinal cord injuries, the combination of tachycardia, hypotension, and absent bowel sounds should prompt consideration of an acute abdomen. (Because of sensory neurologic deficits, pain may be absent or atypical.)

Often, there is no certain way to rule out intra-abdominal catastrophe without laparotomy or paracentesis, although abdominal imaging procedures can provide some guidance. Pain referred to the shoulder or scapula is a particularly valuable sign of abdominal inflammation in patients with spinal cord injuries.

Nutrition may be withheld safely for approximately 5 days before caloric supplementation is begun. When ileus resolves, enteral feedings are preferred, if feasible, because of improved gut function, reduced cost, and avoidance of catheter-related infections. Peptic ulcer disease is common after spinal cord injury, and enteral feeding, antacids, and/or histamine blockers are useful preventative measures. As soon as bowel sounds return and enteral feeding begins, a program of bowel care with regular evacuation and stool softeners should be started to prevent constipation and impaction. The level of the spinal cord lesion will dictate whether evacuation is spontaneous, reflex, or manually induced.

Cutaneous

Skin breakdown is a costly and potentially lethal complication of spinal cord injury that presents a central focus for nursing care. When the skin is disrupted, numerous microorganisms infect the wound, causing local infections and making sepsis possible. Padding, frequent repositioning, physical therapy, and the use of rotating or air-cushioned beds are helpful in prevention. (The problem of skin breakdown is discussed in detail in Chapter 18, General Supportive Care.) Patients with spinal cord injuries (particularly quadriplegic patients) should not be placed in the prone position because of the possibility of hypoventilation, hypoxemia, and bradycardia, which occasionally are fatal.

Miscellaneous

After the return of spinal reflexes, patients with lesions above the T6 level may develop episodes characterized by hypertension, diaphoresis, piloerection, and flushing. This syndrome, autonomic hyperreflexia, must be recognized because it can prove fatal unless reversed rapidly by a simple expedient decompression of an overdistended viscus (usually bowel or bladder). For patients with excessive sympathetic activity, a vagally mediated compensatory bradycardia often occurs.

Thromboembolism is extremely common in the first 90 days after cord injury. The hemodynamic affect of embolism is accentuated by altered autonomic reflexes. Prophylactic heparin may be ef-

fective, but there are substantial risks of provoking hemorrhage in the early phase. Elastic and pneumatic compression stockings may be useful if anticoagulants are contraindicated.

HEAD TRAUMA

MECHANISMS—PATHOPHYSIOLOGY

High-speed motor vehicle accidents and falls account for most serious head and neck injuries. Head trauma from these incidents injures neural tissue by primary (direct brain tissue injury) or secondary mechanisms (vascular disruption and increased intracranial pressure [ICP]). The concussive forces produced by a blow to the head usually are greatest at the point of application and diametrically across the skull from the site of the blow (contrecoup injury). Bony prominences on the base of the skull also commonly cause injury, particularly to the inferior surfaces of the frontal and temporal lobes. Primary diffuse brain injury is characterized by immediate loss of consciousness. Unfortunately, prevention is all that can be offered to alter the course of the immediate primary brain injury. It is the secondary mechanisms of brain injury that can be influenced by skillful medical care.

Secondary brain injury, characterized predominantly by increased ICP, results from tissue edema, hydrocephalus, or mass lesions (fluid/blood accumulations, epidural or subdural hematomas, intracerebral hemorrhage, abscess, or empyema). Secondary brain injury is responsible for approximately one-half of the deaths occurring after head trauma. Therefore, optimal management of the secondary consequences of head trauma theoretically could reduce mortality by as much as 50%. Global ischemia and hypoxia and vascular disruption also increase the severity of cerebral injury. The clinical hallmark of secondary injury is a progressive decline in the level of consciousness after the initial injury.

Rarely, hemorrhage from scalp wounds may be substantial—even life threatening—in children, but almost always is controlled easily by direct pressure.

INITIAL MANAGEMENT

Nearly one-half of all patients with head injury have other accompanying life-threatening medi-

TABLE 35-1

THE GLASGOW COMA SCALE

Eyes	Open	Spontaneously	4
		To verbal command	3
		To pain	2
		No response	1
Best motor response	To verbal command	Obeys	6
	To painful stimulus	Localizes pain	5
		Flexion—withdrawal	4
		Flexion—decorticate	3
		Extension—decerebrate	2
		No response	1
Best verbal response		Oriented converses	5
		Disoriented converses	4
		Inappropriate words	3
		Incomprehensible sounds	2
		No response	1
Total			**3-15**

cal problems (hypotension, hypoventilation, hypoxemia, or hypercarbia) upon arrival to the hospital. Potentially lethal thoracic or abdominal injuries must be sought and corrected simultaneously by a multidisciplinary team. An unstable airway, ineffective ventilation, and reduced oxygen delivery, resulting from hypovolemia or anemia, must be corrected promptly.

The airway must be ensured. If intubation is required, "in-line" traction should be used to stabilize the spine. Hyperextension of the neck should be avoided. Often, fiberoptic-guided intubation or nasotracheal intubation can be useful to avoid manipulation of the potentially unstable spine. The route of intubation must be tailored to the individual. Basilar skull fractures or facial fractures usually contraindicate nasotracheal intubation. Awake or rapid-sequence intubation is preferred for most patients with head trauma because they often have full stomachs, predisposing to aspiration. Supplemental oxygen and mechanical ventilation should be used to counter respiratory acidosis and hypoxemia. Positive end-expiratory pressure (PEEP) should be used judiciously to reverse refractory hypoxemia, recognizing that PEEP may raise the outflow pressure of the central circulation, potentially increasing the formation of cerebral edema. Unless hypotensive, positioning the patient with head elevation of 15 to 20° will help limit the formation of cerebral edema. Care should be taken to prevent flexion of the neck, which can obstruct jugular venous outflow. After initial stabilization, a complete physical and neurologic examination should be performed while measures are instituted to manage increased ICP.

Physical Examination

After assessing the adequacy of the airway and blood pressure, neurologic examination should be conducted, including assessment using the Glasgow Coma Scale (GCS) (Table 35.1). The GCS is potentially useful as a prognostic tool and to help gauge the need for invasive ICP monitoring. Unfortunately, the neurologic examination of such patients is often difficult because it is complicated by the ingestion of ethanol or other intoxicants. In addition to a careful neurologic evaluation, the physical examination of patients sustaining head trauma should look for evidence of penetrating wounds, spinal cord damage, and depressed or basilar skull fractures (evidenced by blood behind the tympanic membrane, CSF rhinorrhea, "raccoon eyes," or discoloration behind the ears [Battle's sign]). Papilledema is a particularly useful finding in patients with head trauma, indicating an elevated ICP.

Radiographic Evaluation

It is difficult to give specific guidelines regarding which patients should undergo CT of the brain. Practically speaking, almost all patients with a history of high-speed collision, fall, loss of consciousness, or strong blow to the head will undergo CT scanning. It also is generally agreed that immediate CT scanning is indicated for patients with (*a*) GCS scores of 8 or lower; (*b*) GCS scores of 9 to 13 who have skull fractures; (*c*) a deteriorating level of consciousness; and/or (*d*) planned immediate surgery. Additionally, patients who are unconscious or who have a history of loss of consciousness after trauma will be scanned. Any patients suspected of significant head injury probably should undergo precautions for spinal injury and have radiographs of the spine obtained.

CRANIAL DISRUPTION

Linear skull fractures are of particular significance when they traverse the normal course of the middle meningeal artery, suggesting the possibility of epidural hematoma. Depressed skull fractures or penetrating injuries produce damage as the inner table of the skull is driven inward, injuring the brain surface. Such injuries usually result from the impact of small, high-velocity objects and carry a high risk of bacterial infection. Injuries causing skull fractures often are associated with intracranial bleeding. (The risk of intracranial hematoma is 10 times greater in patients with fractures).

Basilar skull fractures have unique associated injuries but also serve as markers for the severity of the overall head impact. Basilar fractures are seldom seen on plain radiographs and can be missed even by CT. CSF leakage into the sinuses is common when the floor of the middle cranial fossa is fractured. CSF leak into the external auditory canals seldom occurs immediately after trauma. Nasal bleeding occurs commonly when the floor of the anterior fossa is damaged. In such cases, transnasal tubes must not be inserted because of the possibility of passage through the base of the skull into the brain. Nasal packing should not be used in patients with CSF leakage because of the increased risk of meningitis. Febrile patients with basilar skull fractures must be treated as if meningitis is present, with a lumbar puncture and the early institution of antibiotics. Although recurrent meningitis is a feared complication of basilar skull fracture, CSF leaks seldom need surgical closure (fewer than 1% of all cases).

INJURY TO BRAIN TISSUE

Cerebral contusion due to rapid deceleration is the most common mechanism of brain injury. Subsequent cerebral edema and increased ICP may exacerbate damage. One form of this injury, the brainstem contusion syndrome, is character-

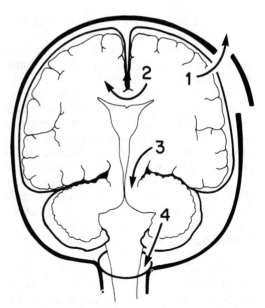

FIG. 35–1. Potential sites of brain herniation: (1) transcranial; (2) subfalcial; (3) transtentorial; (4) foraminal.

ized by intermittent agitation, disordered autonomic regulation, and episodic hyperthermia.

Mass lesions and the effects of cerebral edema produce secondary brain injury by displacing cerebral contents across anatomic boundaries or by globally decreasing perfusion (Fig. 35.1). Translocation may occur through bony defects or by subfalcial, transtentorial, or foraminal herniation.

Intracranial Hemorrhage

The risk of the three types of intracranial hemorrhage (epidural hematoma, subdural hematoma, and intracerebral hematoma) can be approximated by physical examination and knowledge of the presence of a skull fracture. Presence of a skull fracture and a low GCS score predict a high risk of intracranial hemorrhage. For example, patients with a normal GCS score (e.g., 15) and no skull fracture have less than a 1% risk of intracranial hemorrhage, whereas patients with GCS score less than 8 with a skull fracture have a 40% risk of intracranial hemorrhage. It is vital to diagnose and surgically correct intracranial hematomas as rapidly as possible. Data indicate that delaying repair for as little as 4 hours can triple the mortality rate (30–90%) of patients with these injuries.

Epidural hematoma occurs in approximately 20% of patients with severe closed head injury and usually presents as a rapidly expanding mass (blood) in a patient with a linear skull fracture. Vascular disruption usually occurs when the fracture crosses the course of the middle meningeal artery, the dural sinuses, or the foramen magnum. Most epidural hematomas occur over the temporal lobes, where the skull is thin and highly vascular. An enlarging epidural hematoma results most commonly in medial compression of the temporal lobe. Clinically, this process presents as loss of consciousness, contralateral hemiparesis, and a third nerve palsy with ipsilateral pupillary dilation. Only one-third of patients have a classic "lucid interval." When severe death eventually occurs, the midbrain is compressed against the tentorium. Because epidural hematoma has an associated mortality approaching 50%, it usually requires urgent neurosurgical intervention. Therefore, any patient with trauma who demonstrates a linear skull fracture or who loses consciousness (even transiently) probably should be admitted to the hospital for observation.

Acute subdural hematoma is an expanding mass that results from cortical contusion and laceration of a meningeal vessel. Like epidural hematoma, it is seen in about 20% of patients with serious closed head injury, is associated with high mortality, and usually requires immediate surgical intervention. In contrast to epidural hematoma, which usually requires substantial force, subacute or chronic subdural hematoma due to laceration of enlarged dural venous sinuses may occur as the result of a seemingly trivial injury. Subdural hematoma occurs most frequently in elderly patients because cortical atrophy stretches the subdural veins, predisposing them to injury. A typical presentation of a subacute or chronic subdural hematoma is slowly progressive confusion, somnolence, and headache leading eventually to hemiplegia. Anticoagulants greatly increase the risk of post-traumatic hematoma formation.

Intracerebral hematoma develops in approximately 40% of all cases of severe brain injury. The clinical presentation of intracerebral hematoma is dependent on the location of the bleeding. The CT scan is useful in delineating this mass, which appears initially as a dense, intraparenchymal collection of blood. If an intracerebral hematoma produces mass effect, it should be evacuated surgically.

INTRACRANIAL HYPERTENSION

Only three tissues occupy the intracranial cavity: brain substance, cerebrospinal fluid, and blood. None are readily compressible. Therefore, after head trauma, swelling of the brain substance, or blockage of the normal circulation or absorption of CSF leads to increased ICP, a process that may be mitigated by the movement of one of the "liquid" components (blood or CSF) out of the cranium.

Bleeding into the cranial vault is especially problematic. Not only does the bleeding increase ICP by mass effect, but also clotting of intraventricular blood may obstruct the circulation of CSF, producing obstructive hydrocephalus. Blood products within the CSF can elevate the ICP by two other mechanisms: clogging CSF absorption at the subarachnoid villi and increasing CSF osmotic pressure during red-cell lysis. Increased ICP reflects the severity of brain injury and is deleterious when it reduces tissue perfusion or encourages herniation of brain tissue. The swelling of injured tissue peaks within 72 hours of injury. ICP, however, can remain elevated for weeks if there has been significant intracerebral or intraventricular bleeding.

Cerebral Hemodynamics

ICP is normally quite low (<5 mm Hg) but often reaches critically high levels (20–40 mm Hg) in patients with head injuries. ICP should be kept low enough to maintain cerebral perfusion and prevent cerebral herniation (usually <20 mm Hg). The pressure perfusing the brain (the cerebral perfusion pressure [CPP]) is the difference between MAP and either the ICP or the pressure within the cerebral veins (whichever is higher). CPP normally exceeds 60 mm Hg, the lowest acceptable level is approximately 40 mm Hg. Neural dysfunction occurs when CPP is less than 40 mm Hg, and neuronal death occurs at CPP less than 20 mm Hg.

In healthy individuals, cerebral autoregulatory mechanisms sensitive to arterial oxygen tension (PaO_2), arterial carbon dioxide tension ($PaCO_2$), and blood pressure continuously adjust cerebral vascular resistance to maintain perfusion in proportion to metabolic need and changing perfusion pressure. Arterial blood gases, cerebral metabolism, and the components of perfusion pressure (blood pressure, ICP) must be watched cautiously in patients with head injuries because the autoregulatory mechanisms of injured tissue are impaired. In this setting, perfusion of these tissues directly parallels CPP and perfusion adequacy is influenced directly by cerebral metabolism.

COMPLICATIONS OF HEAD TRAUMA

Direct neuronal injury causes seizures with sufficient frequency that prophylactic use of an anticonvulsant (e.g., phenytoin) is prudent. Not only the brain suffers from head injury; almost every other organ system of the body can be adversely affected.

Direct injury to the hypothalamus or pituitary or increased ICP may disrupt the normal secretion of hypophyseal hormones. Loss of antidiuretic hormone (ADH) may cause acute diabetes insipidus (DI). DI usually indicates a poor prognosis, because it is usually the result of prolonged increases in ICP. Such patients can produce massive volumes (>1 L/hour) of dilute urine despite increasing serum osmolality. Typically, the serum sodium concentration exceeds 145 mEq/L when urine-specific gravity is below 1.003. Life-threatening hypovolemia and hyperosmolarity may result unless prompt treatment with hypotonic fluids and ADH are instituted. An empiric trial of aqueous vasopressin (5 units subcutaneously) is often diagnostic (see also Chapter 32, Endocrine Emergencies). In the absence of diabetes insipidus, hypotension in the head injured patient always should be assumed to signify blood loss at an extracranial site. With the exception of ACTH deficiency, which may result in adrenal insufficiency, loss of other pituitary hormones (e.g., growth hormone, thyroid-stimulating hormone) usually presents a nonurgent problem.

Disruption of the dura by penetrating trauma or boney fracture (e.g., basilar skull fracture) may provide a pathway for the entry of microorganisms into the CSF, resulting in recurrent posttraumatic meningitis. Nosocomial sinusitis resulting from obstruction of the sinus ostia by nasal tubes and impaired drainage in the supine position affects 10 to 15% of all patients with head injuries.

Serious head injury also may disrupt or cause blockage of normal channels of communication of CSF. Such disruptions may cause obstructive hydrocephalus with subsequent elevations in ICP.

Erosive (stress) gastritis occurs with great frequency, suggesting that the use of H_2 blockers, proton pump inhibitors, sucralfate, or antacids is wise. Because head injury induces a hypermetabolic state, caloric requirements are elevated and nutritional supplementation is often indicated (see Chapter 16, Nutritional Assessment and Support). After a brief period of post-traumatic ileus, enteral tube feeding usually is well tolerated until the patient can eat normally again. For patients with severe persistent neurologic deficits, consideration should be given to placement of a feeding gastrostomy tube. Insertion of a gastrostomy tube often is accomplished most efficiently at the same time a permanent tracheostomy is created.

Although full-blown acute respiratory distress syndrome (ARDS) may result from some combination of aspiration, chest trauma, shock, and massive transfusion, milder acute lung injury often follows head injury alone. Many hypoxemic patients with head injuries have normal chest radiographs. The mechanism of hypoxemia in these patients probably is related to autonomic alterations directly induced by the head trauma. Neurogenic pulmonary edema may result from head trauma, presumably because of catecholamine-induced, profound, transient pulmonary venoconstriction. Therapy consists of supportive care using oxygen and intubation, mechanical ventilation, and PEEP when indicated. The more mundane, but frequent pulmonary complications of aspiration pneumonitis and atelectasis usually respond to standard therapy. Aspiration risk can be minimized by preventing massive gastric residuals, elevating the head of the bed to 30 to 45°, and avoiding premature attempts at resuming eating. Atelectasis and "retained secretions" are best prevented and treated by maximizing activity, providing effective suctioning, and encouraging deep breathing and coughing. These standard measures can be problematic for patients with increased ICP, because each tends to further raise the pressure. For the tenuous patient with intracranial hypertension, deep sedation and intratracheal lidocaine can be used to block increases in ICP induced by suctioning. As expected, bronchoscopy offers little advantage for secretion clearance for these patients because it, too, is a potent stimulus to raise ICP.

Severe head trauma causes the systemic activation of the clotting cascade, probably through the release of brain thromboplastin. As many as one-fourth of all patients with head injuries will have laboratory features of disseminated intravascular coagulation. Specific therapy is rarely required as the defect is self-limited.

Deep venous thrombosis (DVT) occurs frequently after head and spinal cord injury. Prophylaxis is indicated clearly; however, substantial controversy exists concerning the best method. Because of the risk of heparin-induced or aggravated intracranial bleeding, a combination of graded compression stockings and intermittent pneumatic compression devices usually is preferred (see Chapter 23, Venous Thrombosis and Pulmonary Embolism).

Decubitus ulcers also are a common problem for patients with head and spine injuries. The best course of therapy is to prevent decubitus formation through padding, frequent repositioning, and maximizing activity. Especially high risk patients may be treated with specialized therapeutic beds. The topic of decubitus ulcer prevention and treatment is discussed in detail in Chapter 18 (General Supportive Care).

MONITORING PATIENTS WITH BRAIN INJURIES

Careful monitoring of the neurologic examination and use of the GCS is helpful, especially in mild to moderate injury. Although no specific electroencephalogram (EEG) pattern defines etiology or prognosis in head trauma, the EEG is useful to monitor for seizures and document the suppression of brain activity in barbiturate-induced coma. Unfortunately, the ICU is an electrically hostile environment in which EEG signal fidelity is often suboptimal. Serial CT scans give invaluable information regarding the nature and evolution of the injury process. However, the only way to accurately assess ICP in the seriously injured, comatose patient is to monitor it directly.

INTRACRANIAL PRESSURE MONITORING

There are three primary reasons to measure ICP: (a) to monitor patients at risk of life-threatening intracranial hypertension, (b) to monitor for evidence of infection, and (c) to assess the effects of therapy aimed at reducing ICP.

Mean ICP of a supine patient is normally approximately 10 to 15 mmHg, and the ICP waveform normally undulates gently in time with the cardiac cycle. Extreme fluctuations of the ICP waveform (>10 mm Hg) suggest a position near the critical inflexion point of the cranial pressure–volume curve, particularly when the contour shows a high "second peak" corresponding to the arterial pulse. Elevations in ICP to 15 to 20 mm Hg compress capillary beds and compromise the microcirculation. At ICP levels of 30 to 35 mm Hg, venous drainage is impeded and edema develops in uninjured tissue. ICP elevations of this degree produce a vicious cycle in which impeded venous drainage leads to accumulating edema and elevated ICP. Even when autoregulatory mechanisms are intact, cerebral perfusion

cannot be maintained if ICP rises to within 40 to 50 mm Hg of the MAP. When the ICP approximates MAP, perfusion stops and the brain dies. The urgency of reducing ICP may be assessed by following intracranial compliance, i.e., the response of ICP to a 0.1-mL challenge of sterile fluid injected through a ventricular catheter. This procedure is not risk free, however, and must be undertaken with extreme caution. Herniation can be precipitated unless the challenge is performed carefully.

In addition to sustained elevations of ICP, two specific transients have been described by Lundberg. "A waves," pressure elevations of 20 to 100 mm Hg for periods of 2 to 15 minutes, are always pathologic. A waves usually are associated with abnormal eye movements, posturing, and abnormal neurologic reflexes—physiologic responses resulting from inadequate cerebral perfusion during periods of extreme pressure elevation. Lundberg A waves indicate the likelihood of sudden deterioration and poor neurologic outcome. Lundberg "B waves" are lower in amplitude, shorter in duration, and usually occur in relation to respiratory variation. B waves have no associated physical findings at the time of occurrence and, unlike their A-wave counterparts, are not well correlated with neurologic outcome.

Of the three fluid components contained within the fixed cranial volume, only the volumes of CSF and blood may be changed (unless brain tissue is removed or made less edematous). Starting from normal levels, ICP shows little response to volume change until a critical inflexion point is reached. Thereafter, small increases in intracranial volume dramatically boost ICP, risking sudden neurologic deterioration (Fig. 35.2). Direct ICP monitoring is important, because changes in other clinical indices—reflexes, blood pressure, and heart rate—usually occur too late to avert disaster. Bradycardia, a preterminal sign, is the least reliable of all clinical indicators of increased ICP. (Tachycardia is seen more frequently.)

Specific Indications for Monitoring ICP

Closed Head Injury

It is not practical or necessary to monitor ICP in all patients with head trauma, but two groups of patients with head trauma seem to derive benefit: (a) patients with an abnormal CT scan at admission, and (b) patients with normal CT scans at admission but who present with hypotension,

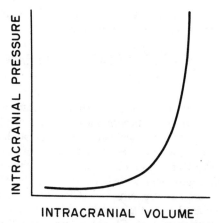
FIG. 35–2. Relationship of ICP to intracranial volume. ICP remains low until a critical volume is attained.

posturing, or age above 40 years. A normal CT scan of the head accurately predicts normal ICP in more than 80% of cases, whereas ICP is elevated in approximately 50% of patients when any specific lesion is observed on head CT. Midline shift of more than 7 mm or blood in the lateral ventricles is especially worrisome. Patients with head trauma and GCS scores lower than 7 frequently have an increased ICP, as do patients with decorticate/decerebrate posturing or abnormal evoked potential testing. Abnormal eye or pupil movements are unreliable guides to increased ICP. Repeat head CT is advisable at approximately 24 hours after injury to assess the progress of injury and to evaluate the degree of intracranial hypertension.

Reye's Syndrome

Increased ICP is a major cause of death in Reye's syndrome. Mortality approaches 100% without prompt diagnosis and treatment. Therapeutic reductions in ICP may reduce mortality to 20% or less, with survivors experiencing few sequelae. Therefore, ICP monitoring is indicated for patients with Reye's syndrome and GCS scores lower than 7.

Encephalopathy

As opposed to Reye's syndrome, the mechanism of increased ICP in acute hepatic failure of other etiologies and in other metabolic encephalopathies is largely unknown. At present, there

is little evidence to suggest that monitoring ICP reduces mortality in these disorders.

Brain Tumors

ICP monitoring rarely is necessary for patients with chronic supratentorial lesions. However, ventriculostomy may be useful preoperatively to allow reduction in the CSF volume of patients with large infratentorial lesions. For patients with large brain tumors or extensive edema on CT scanning, ICP monitoring may help guide therapy.

Contraindications to Monitoring

Coagulopathy (platelet count less than 100,000/mm^3) and prothrombin time (PT) or partial thromboplastin time (PTT) greater than two times control are strong contraindications to the placement of an ICP monitor. Isolated elevations of fibrin degradation products (FDPs) should not contraindicate catheter placement; FDP levels may be increased by brain trauma alone. Immunosuppressive therapy (particularly steroids) is a relative contraindication to ICP monitoring. If required, a subarachnoid bolt is preferred for such patients because of the lower risk of nosocomial infection.

Hardware and Devices

Ventricular Catheters

Ventricular catheters provide continuous, reliable data, enable compliance measurements to be performed, and allow therapeutic removal of CSF. Ventricular catheters may be inserted under local anesthesia at the bedside, through a burr hole in the skull.

Unfortunately, ventriculostomy presents several problems. Difficulty may be encountered in placing the catheter into a lateral ventricle compressed by extensive edema or mass lesion. To limit brain damage, no more than three passes should be attempted. After insertion, the CSF invariably shows evidence of catheter irritation (mild elevations of protein and leukocyte count). Infection is not uncommon (approximately 15%) after ventriculostomy and relates to duration of monitoring and to sterility of catheter placement and maintenance. (To avoid adding to the infection risk, cranial compliance testing must be undertaken with close attention to sterility of technique.) Prophylactic antibiotics have shown no benefit in reducing infection rates, but tunneling the catheter through the skin may be helpful. Because bleeding commonly accompanies insertion of ventricular catheters, coagulopathy strongly contraindicates placement.

Epidural Transducers

Although epidural transducers present a lower risk of infection than ventricular catheters, they are technically more difficult to insert. For accuracy, the transducer membrane must be precisely juxtaposed to the dura. Once placed, these devices are difficult to keep calibrated. Another drawback to the use of epidural transducers is the inability to remove CSF.

Subarachnoid Screws/Bolts

The subarachnoid screw is an open bolt inserted into the subarachnoid space through a burr hole (usually bored in the frontoparietal suture). During placement, the dura is opened and the screw is inserted onto the brain surface. Problems with the subarachnoid screw include infection and the potential for seriously underestimating ICP if not placed on the side of an existing mass lesion. Brain herniation into the device is the most common cause for device failure. Problems with damping and clotting are sufficiently frequent that regular flushing is mandatory. Such flushing, however, exposes patients to an increased risk of herniation and infection. Finally, these devices frequently are dislodged, even with meticulous care.

Problems with Intracranial Pressure Monitoring

Metallic monitoring devices preclude magnetic resonance imaging (MRI) scans and produce artifacts on CT scans that can obscure important information. Infection occurs in 2 to 5% of patients who undergo ICP monitoring and is most common if the devices remain for more than 5 days or if open drainage systems are used. *Staphylococcus epidermidis* is the most common infecting organism. Volume–pressure testing of cranial compliance adds to the infection risk. Prophylactic antibiotics have not been demonstrated to be effective.

As with any monitoring technique, poor quality data may lead to inappropriate therapy. The intraventricular catheter gives the most consistent data;

although the subarachnoid screw is less reliable, it carries the lowest risk of infection.

TREATMENT OF PATIENTS WITH BRAIN INJURIES

The viability of the injured brain depends on the critical balance of nutritional supply and demand. Because injured tissue cannot autoregulate blood flow to metabolic need, a key component of the treatment strategy focuses on reducing the metabolic requirement while boosting CPP. Therefore, mean arterial pressure and ICP must be maintained as close to their normal values as possible. (High elevations of ICP not only reduce CPP but also risk herniation.) Prophylactic anticonvulsant (phenytoin) therapy is indicated for most patients. Caution should be used when performing endotracheal suctioning as the process can acutely raise ICP to high levels. Because of the association of poor neurologic recovery with hyperglycemia, many practitioners favor resuscitation of patients with head injuries using non–glucose-containing solutions (normal saline); however, the importance of this practice is unclear.

THERAPY TO REDUCE INTRACRANIAL PRESSURE

Lowering Jugular Venous Pressure

The goal of reducing ICP is to maintain cerebral blood flow by keeping cerebral perfusion pressure at or above 60 mm Hg. Patient positioning can be important; neck flexion, head turning, and tracheostomy ties impede venous drainage and may rapidly elevate ICP. Therefore, the head should be elevated to 15° to 30° and maintained in a midline position. Tracheostomy ties and bandages should be applied loosely. Increases in intrathoracic pressure related to straining, suctioning, and coughing should be minimized. Seizures should be prevented. Special caution should be taken during ventilation with PEEP. High levels of PEEP have the potential to reduce MAP and raise ICP simultaneously. However, judicious use of PEEP is not strictly contraindicated, especially because the ICP of patients with trauma often exceeds the PEEP-affected pressure within the superior sagittal sinus. The very agitated patient may acutely raise central venous pressure, thereby raising ICP. In such cases, deep sedation and paralysis can reduce ICP.

Diuretics

Loop diuretics (furosemide and ethacrynic acid) have a twin therapeutic action—decreasing CSF production and producing a diuresis that reduces intravascular volume.

Osmotic Agents

When combined with loop diuretics, osmotic agents may produce marked but transient reductions in ICP. Diuretics help oppose the volume-expanding effect of osmotic agents. Glycerol and mannitol establish an osmotic pressure gradient between the CSF and blood, promoting fluid transfer from brain cells to the circulation. Increasing the blood osmolality by 10 mOsm/L has a net effect of acutely removing approximately 100 mL of intracellular water from brain cells. In doses that produce a serum osmolarity greater than 320 mOsm/dL, osmotic agents slowly penetrate the blood–brain barrier, gradually counterbalancing their own therapeutic effect. Furthermore, when given rapidly, large doses of osmotic agents may paradoxically expand the circulating volume, elevate ICP, and produce hemodilution. However, in the long term, excessive diuresis depletes intravascular and/or intracellular volume, delaying return to normal consciousness. Rebound intracranial hypertension is a significant problem that may be seen after discontinuation of any osmotic agent. High osmolarity (>340 mOsm/dL) should be avoided because it may depress consciousness or impair renal tubular function.

Hyperventilation

Hyperventilation is the most rapid method of temporarily lowering ICP. Acute reduction of $PaCO_2$ raises tissue pH, causing cerebral vasoconstriction in normally responsive cerebral vessels (Fig. 35.3). Within wide limits, reduced flow through normal brain tissue is well tolerated. As flow and vascular volume fall, ICP declines, thereby boosting CPP. Flow to injured, poorly autoregulated brain actually improves because flow through injured brain is dependent on CPP (Fig. 35.4).

Although moderate hyperventilation tends to reduce ICP, improve CPP, and improve nutrient flow to damaged tissue, extreme hyperventilation ($PaCO_2 < 25$ mm Hg) offsets this beneficial action by causing excessive vasoconstriction and

global reduction of perfusion. (Assuming a normal starting value, reducing $PaCO_2$ remains effective for approximately 48 hours; after that time, renal compensation restores acid–base status and eventually negates its effects.) Hyperventilation should be terminated gradually (over 24–48 hours) to avoid causing a rebound increase in ICP. Although the therapeutic benefits of deliberate hyperventilation are uncertain, it is clear that hypoventilation should be avoided; increased blood flow and vascular volume can drive ICP quickly to life-threatening levels. Associated hypoxemia accentuates the risk, because like hypercapnia, hypoxemia is a cerebral vasodilator of autoregulated brain tissue. Within the first 72 hours of injury, special caution should be exercised not to interrupt hyperventilation for more than brief periods. (For example, prolonged disconnections to determine whether the patient has spontaneous respirations may be ill advised during this period.)

Corticosteroids

Experimentally, corticosteroids seem to reduce CSF production and exert direct anti-edema effects in head trauma. However, there is no clear evidence that steroids benefit patients with head trauma, and it is clear that they increase the risk of nosocomial infection. In contrast to patients with head injuries, corticosteroids do reduce cerebral edema associated with tumors.

Ventriculostomy Drainage

The removal of CSF may acutely lower ICP, especially when the system is poised on the steep portion of the ICP–volume curve. Because CSF production is a continuous process, the effects of intermittent CSF removal are usually transient (<2 hours). Systems for continuously venting the CSF to maintain ICP at or below a given hydrostatic level are effective in reducing ICP but increase the risk of infection. Nonetheless, CSF drainage makes consummate sense in the setting of aqueductal blockage (by clotted blood in the fourth ventricle, for example). Here, venting the CSF output until clot lysis occurs (approximately 5–7 days) may prove to be lifesaving. Withdrawal of spinal fluid from the lumbar region may precipitate brain herniation by increasing the pressure gradient across the tentorium.

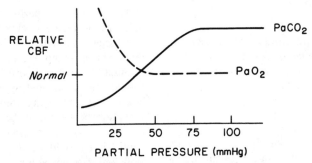

FIG. 35–3. Effect of arterial blood gas tensions on cerebral blood flow (CBF) in normal brain tissue (autoregulation intact). Whereas reductions of $PaCO_2$ lower CBF (and cerebral volume) in more or less linear fashion over the physiologic range, reductions in PaO_2 have an opposite effect that manifests only when the O_2 content of hemoglobin falls ($PaO_2 < 60$ mm Hg). Injured tissue may lose this ability to autoregulate flow in response to blood gas (or blood pressure) changes (see Fig. 35.4).

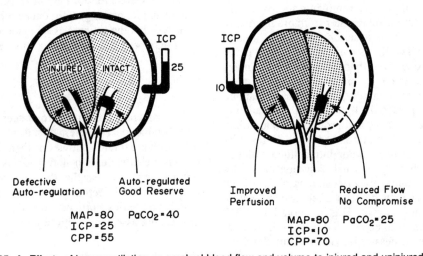

FIG. 35–4. Effects of hyperventilation on cerebral blood flow and volume to injured and uninjured brain.

Surgery

A direct attack on the cause of increased ICP may be indicated in such conditions as obstructive hydrocephalus (improved by shunting), tumor, or large but focal hemorrhage (particularly into the cerebellum). Prompt evacuation of a large subdural hematoma may be lifesaving and, if necessary, can be performed at the bedside. Removal of a cranial flap may be an effective (if short-lived) temporizing maneuver.

THERAPY TO MINIMIZE CEREBRAL METABOLISM

Fever and agitation greatly increase cerebral metabolic requirements and should be prevented. However, it may be a serious mistake to use methods of temperature control (e.g., cooling blankets) that induce shivering. Semiconscious patients are made more uncomfortable, thereby increasing cerebral metabolism and raising intrathoracic and intracerebral pressure. Antipyretics are preferable. High-dose barbiturates decrease cerebral metabolism and blood flow and, therefore, have been hypothesized to have a protective effect on injured brain. The role of barbiturates in head injury is controversial, and the decision to undertake such therapy should be considered carefully. These drugs depress cardiovascular function and attenuate both the EEG signals and the clinical parameters used for neurologic assessment. Barbiturate therapy for head injury probably mandates ICP monitoring. As an alternative to barbiturates, benzodiazepines can be used to reduce cerebral oxygen consumption.

THE RECOVERY PHASE

Recovery from reduced consciousness after cerebral trauma may be a prolonged process, much more so than after nontraumatic coma. It is not uncommon for patients with head trauma to require 1 year or longer to maximize their level of function. Patients with head trauma are fragile, even long after the injury. After the acute insult subsides, vigilance must be maintained to ensure that reversible factors do not impede the return to normal function. All too often, metabolic derangements (spontaneous or iatrogenic) are responsible for persistently depressed consciousness. Hyperosmolarity, hypovolemia, hyperglycemia, and hyponatremia frequently are induced by the therapies applied in the treatment of these disorders: diuretics, steroids, fluid restriction, osmotic agents, etc.

KEY POINTS

1. For victims of trauma with potential head or spine injury, airway patency, ventilation, oxygenation, and effective circulation are primary considerations. While achieving these goals, special attention should be afforded immobilization of the cervical spine.

2. After initial stabilization, a thorough neurologic examination and plain radiographs of the spine should be obtained. In many (if not most) cases of significant head or spine trauma, a head CT scan also is indicated to evaluate patients for the possibility of a surgically correctable lesion.

3. Patients with head and spine trauma should, whenever possible, be managed in a specialized neurologic care ICU with expert neurosurgical consultation.

4. After stabilization, mundane medical problems, including ileus, gastric stress ulceration, urinary tract infection, aspiration, atelectasis, deep venous thrombosis, and decubitus ulcers, present the largest challenges. Appropriate prophylactic measures should be instituted for each of these conditions as soon as possible.

5. Elevated ICP is a common secondary mechanism producing late, or secondary, brain injury. Unfortunately, measures to lower ICP, such as hyperventilation, corticosteroids, diuretics, and other osmotic agents, are not particularly effective for trauma-induced edema, and all methods have potential complications.

SUGGESTED READINGS

1. Becker DP, Miller JD, Ward JD, et al. The outcome from severe head injury with early diagnosis and intensive management. J Neurosurg 1977;47:491–502.
2. Bleck TP. Vegetative state after closed head injury. Neurol Chronicle 1992;1:10–11.
3. Borel C, Hanley D, Diringer MN, et al. Intensive management of severe head injury. Chest 1990;98:180–189.
4. Bracken MB, Shepard MJ, Collins WF, et al. A randomized, controlled trial of methylprednisolone or naloxone in the treatment of acute spinal cord injury: results of the second National Acute Spinal Cord Injury Study. N Engl J Med 1990;322:1405–1411.
5. Bruce DA, Gennarelli TA, Langfitt TW. Resuscitation from coma due to head injury. Crit Care Med 1978;6(4):254–269.
6. Cooper PR, Moody S, Clark WK, et al. Dexamethasone and severe head injury. J Neurosurg 1979;51:307–316.
7. Cooper KR, Boswell PA, Choi SC. Safe use of PEEP in patients with severe head injury. J Neurosurg 1985;63:552–555.
8. D'Amelio LF, Hammond JS, Spain DA, et al. Tracheostomy and percutaneous endoscopic gastrostomy in the management of the head injured patient. Am Surg 1994;60:180–185.
9. Duffy K, Becker D. State of the art management of closed head injury. J Crit Care Med 1988;3:291–302.
10. Eisenberg HM, Frankowski RF, Contant CF, et al. High dose barbiturate control of elevated intracranial pressure in patient with head injury. J Neurosurg 1988;69:15–23.
11. Feldman Z, Kanter MJ, Robertson CS, et al. Effect of head elevation on intracranial pressure, cerebral perfusion pressure and cerebral blood flow in head-injured patients. J Neurosurg 1992;76:207–211.
12. Frank JI. Management of intracranial hypertension. Med Clin North Am 1992;77:61–75.
13. Frost EAM. Effects of positive end expiratory pressure on intracranial pressure and compliance in brain injured patients. J Neurosurg 1977;47:195–200.
14. Grossman RG, Gildenberg PL, eds. Head injury. New York: Raven Press, 1981.
15. Gudeman SK, Miller JD, Becker DP. Failure of high-dose steroid therapy to influence intracranial pressure in patients with severe head injury. J Neurosurg 1979;51:301–306.

16. Heffner J, Sahn S. Controlled hyperventilation in patients with intracranial hypertension. Arch Intern Med 1983; 143:765–769.

17. Hooshmand H, Dove J, Houff S, et al. Effects of diuretics and steroids on CSF pressure. Arch Neurol 1969;21: 499–509.

18. Jennett B, Teasdale G. Management of head injury. Philadelphia: FA Davis, 1981.

19. Jennett B, McMillan R. Epidemiology of head injury. Br Med J 1981;282:101–104.

20. Lam AM, Winn HR, Cullen BF, et al. Hyperglycemia and neurological outcome in patients with head injury. J Neurosurg 1991;75:545–551.

21. Marsh ML, Marshall LF, Shapiro HM. Neurosurgical intensive care. Anesthesiology 1977;47:149–163.

22. Marshall LF, Smith RW, Shapiro HM. The outcome with aggressive treatment in severe head injuries. J Neurosurg 1979;50:20–25.

23. Mendelow AD, Teasdale G, Jennett B, et al. Risks of intracranial hematoma in head injured adults. Br Med J 1983;2187:1172–1176.

24. Miller JD. Significance and management of intracranial hypertension after head injury. In: Vincent JL, ed. Update in intensive care and emergency medicine. 1989;8: 496–501.

25. Miller JD, Butterworth JF, Gudeman SK. Further experience in the management of severe head injury. J Neurosurg 1981;54:289–299.

26. Miller JD, Becker DP, Ward JD, et al. Significance of intracranial hypertension in severe head injury. J Neurosurg 1977;47:503–516.

27. Moraine J, Brimioulle S, Kahn RJ. Effects of respiratory therapy on intracranial pressure. J Crit Care 1991;6: 197–201.

28. Muizelaar JP, Marmarou A, Ward JD, et al. Adverse effect of prolonged hyperventilation in patients with severe head injury. J Neurosurg 1991;75:731–739.

29. Robertson CS, Clifton GL, Taylor AA, et al. Treatment of hypertension associated with head injury. J Neurosurg 1983;59:455–460.

30. Ropper AH, Kennedy SK, Zervas NT. Neurological and neurosurgical intensive care. Baltimore: University Park Press, 1983.

31. Rosner MJ, Daughton S. Cerebral perfusion pressure management in head injury. J Trauma 1990;3:933–940.

32. Seelig JM, Becker DP, Miller JD, et al. Traumatic acute subdural hematoma: major mortality reduction in comatose patients treated within four hours. N Engl J Med 1981; 304:1511–1517.

33. Shapiro HM, Marshall LF. Intracranial pressure responses to PEEP in head-injured patients. J Trauma 1978;18: 254–256.

34. Sivakuman V, Rajshekhar V, Chardy MJ, et al. Management of neurosurgical patients with hyponatremia and naturiesis. Neurosurgery 1994;34:269–274.

35. Skull x-ray examinations after head trauma (recommendations by multi-disciplinary panel and validation study). N Engl J Med 1987;316:84–91.

36. Suggestions from a group of neurosurgeons. Guidelines for initial management after head injury in adults. Br Med J 1984;288:983–985.

37. White RJ, Likavec MJ. The diagnosis and initial management of head injury. N Engl J Med 1992;327:1507–1511.

38. Wilkinson HA. Intracranial pressure monitoring. In: Cooper PR, ed. Head Injury. Baltimore: Williams & Wilkins, 1982; 147–184.

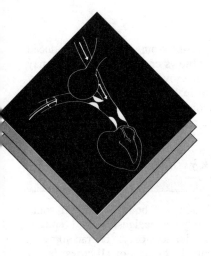

CHAPTER 36

Thoracic Trauma

EPIDEMIOLOGY

Almost 500,000 Americans suffer chest trauma each year. In most cases, the injuries are nonpenetrating and result from a misadventure involving a motor vehicle. When a motor vehicle accident proves fatal, more than one-half of the fatalities are directly due to serious thoracic trauma. Fortunately, most patients who survive long enough to be transported to a hospital will survive. Most deaths occur at the scene of the accident as a result of a catastrophic, unsalvageable injury such as aortic transection.

MECHANISMS OF CHEST TRAUMA

Blunt chest trauma may produce pneumothorax, neurologic dysfunction, respiratory failure, or cardiovascular instability. Our approach to such problems, which are common to a wide spectrum of critical illness, is detailed elsewhere (see Chapters 8, 35, 24, and 4, respectively). The current discussion focuses on those mechanical problems unique to blunt (nonpenetrating) chest injury. Rib fractures, increased intracavitary pressures, and shear forces are the major mechanisms producing intrathoracic injury in blunt chest trauma.

RIB AND STERNAL FRACTURES

During chest trauma, older, less elastic patients frequently sustain bony fractures that injure the lung perimeter. In contrast, the increased chest wall flexibility of younger patients tends to allow direct energy transfer to the intrathoracic organs, without rib breakage. In young patients, disarticulation of ribs is more common than rib fractures but results in identical physiologic alterations.

Rib fractures, the most common form of thoracic injury, usually occur in the midchest (ribs 5–9) along the posterior axillary line (the point of maximal stress). The uppermost ribs are damaged less frequently because of their intrinsic strength and protection by the shoulder girdle and clavicle. Therefore, fractures of the upper ribs imply a very forceful blow and should raise concern regarding injury of the major airways or great vessels. On the other hand, the flexibility of the lowermost ribs makes them less prone to injury. Therefore, fracture of the lower ribs (9–11) suggests an unusually powerful regional impact and the possibility of concurrent splenic, hepatic, or renal injury. The number of rib fractures roughly correlates with the force of impact and the risk of serious internal injury and death. The history and clinical examination should raise the suspicion of rib fractures, but even when present, fractures may not be confirmed by conventional radiographic views. (Initial plain chest radiographs fail to reveal as many as one-half of all rib fractures.) Aligned fractures of multiple ribs, ''curbstone fractures,'' usually result from striking a sharp edge. ''Cough fractures'' most frequently involve ribs 6 through 9 in the posterior axillary line. Although cough fractures produce significant pain, they are nondisplaced and difficult to detect. A bone scan occasionally is required for diagnosis.

Rib fractures often injure adjacent tissues as displaced rib ends or fragments cause lung laceration or contusion, pneumothorax, and hemothorax. Because the intercostal and internal mammary arteries are perfused under systemic pressure, large hemothoraces can occur when these vessels are disrupted by fractures. Pain associated with rib fractures frequently causes splinting, hypoventilation, secretion retention, and atelectasis—complications are minimized by adequate narcotic analgesia or intercostal nerve blocks. Fractures of multiple ribs at two or more sites may produce a free-floating, unstable section of the chest wall known as a flail segment. Forceful displacement also may disrupt chondral attachments, producing a flail sternum. Discovery of a flail sternum should raise concern for underlying blunt cardiac injury.

Sternal fractures usually occur in high-speed motor vehicle accidents when an unrestrained driver strikes the steering wheel or when automobile shoulder harnesses are used without lap belts. Complaints of pain and tenderness to palpation are signs indicating that a lateral chest radiograph should be obtained. Occasionally, the diagnosis can be made by palpating a "step" where two sternal segments are askew. Although sternal fractures may precipitate respiratory failure and delay weaning by causing pain and altering chest wall mechanics, their greatest significance lies as a marker of potential cardiac and bronchial injuries.

INCREASED INTRACAVITARY PRESSURES

Abrupt elevation of intracavitary pressures may rupture any air-filled or fluid-filled structure unbraced for the impact. Leak of orogastric secretions after esophageal rupture may result in mediastinitis or empyema. Alveolar rupture may cause pneumothorax, pneumomediastinum, or pulmonary hemorrhage. Sudden increases of intra-abdominal pressure can rupture the diaphragm, herniating the abdominal contents into the chest. Unprotected by the liver, the left hemidiaphragm is at greatest risk. By a similar mechanism, a distended stomach or urinary bladder also may rupture when the chest is struck forcefully.

SHEAR FORCES

To varying degrees, all intrathoracic structures are tethered to adjacent tissues. Consequently, shear forces produced by differential organ motion may cause visceral or vascular tears. Aortic rupture is the most serious injury produced by this mechanism; however, tracheobronchial disrup-

tion also may result from deceleration-induced shearing. Direct blows or rapid deceleration may tear pulmonary microvessels, causing pulmonary contusion. If the leak from these vessels is sufficient to form a discrete fluid collection, a pulmonary hematoma may form.

INITIAL MANAGEMENT OF CHEST TRAUMA

Most chest trauma can be managed with some combination of oxygen, analgesics, fluid replacement, and tube thoracostomy. Thoracotomy is necessary in only 15 to 20% of all cases. Initial therapy should consist of ensuring the ABCs: airway, breathing, and circulation. When patency of the airway or stability of respiratory drive are uncertain, intubation is indicated. Positive-pressure ventilation is initiated for reduced respiratory drive, or hypoxemia, or when pain or profoundly deranged chest wall mechanics prevent adequate spontaneous ventilation. After auscultation of the chest to ensure adequate symmetric airflow, a portable chest radiograph should be obtained to search for pneumothorax and intrathoracic vascular injury.

Hypotension in thoracic injury usually is the result of hypovolemia; therefore, the early insertion of two large-bore peripheral intravenous catheters is required. At the time of catheter insertion, blood should be obtained for determinations of electrolytes, creatinine, hematocrit, coagulation parameters, toxicologic screening, and blood cross-matching. When surface veins can be cannulated, the need for central venous catheterization is controversial; equivalent or greater volumes of fluid can be infused through large peripheral catheters and there is real risk of iatrogenic complications in the busy setting of the trauma room. Hypovolemia can result from injury to low-pressure (pulmonary or systemic veins) or from high-pressure systemic vessels. Bleeding from veins often will subside spontaneously, whereas arterial bleeding usually requires surgical intervention. Hypotension is not always the result of hypovolemia; pneumothorax and cardiac tamponade cause hypotension, partly by impeding the return of venous blood to the heart. Hence, constant vigilance for the development of neck vein distension or a quiet hemithorax must be maintained.

Because patients with chest trauma often have severe extrathoracic injuries, careful examination should be performed of the head, spine, and abdomen, looking for associated trauma.

SPECIFIC CONDITIONS

The problems of pneumothorax and barotrauma are covered in detail in Chapter 8.

BRONCHIAL AND TRACHEAL DISRUPTIONS

Fracture of the first two ribs, sternum, and clavicle are the most common bony injuries associated with airway disruption. Hemoptysis, atelectasis, subcutaneous emphysema, pneumomediastinum, or pneumothorax that fails to improve with tube thoracostomy are potential signs of major airway disruption. (The occurrence of bilateral pneumothoraces after blunt trauma strongly suggests this possibility.) Most (>80%) airway disruptions occur within 2 cm of the carina in the form of a spiral tear of the main bronchi or a longitudinal tear in the posterior membranous portion of the trachea (Fig. 36.1). If disruption of a major bronchus is complete, the amputated lung can fall away from its normal hilar position to rest on the diaphragm and posterior chest wall.

Immediate recognition of airway disruption is important to avert the atelectasis, infection, and bronchial stenosis associated with delayed repair. Fiberoptic bronchoscopy allows its detection and facilitates selective intubation with a dual-lumen tube. On the affected side, an attempt is made to position the inflatable cuff distal to the site of disruption. Partial disruption often is not detected until bronchial stenosis and atelectasis occur several weeks later. Because complete disruption generally is recognized earlier than partial disruption, it is associated with fewer long-term complications.

HEMOTHORAX

Hemothorax is diagnosed when the hematocrit of pleural fluid exceeds 5%. For hemodynamically stable patients, thoracentesis should confirm the diagnosis before chest tube placement. If a hemopneumothorax is present, immediate tube thoracostomy is indicated. Indications for tube drainage include the presence of more than 500 mL of blood in the chest or brisk ongoing hemorrhage into the pleural space.

Aortic tears or avulsion of intercostal or internal mammary vessels may produce massive bleeding. Rib fractures, esophageal tears, and avulsion of periesophageal vessels frequently accompany large hemothoraces. Tube thoracostomy drainage is satisfactory in most cases, but the natural course of an undrained hemothorax is highly variable. Exploratory thoracotomy should be strongly considered. If more than 1000 mL of blood is evacuated initially from the chest or if

SITES OF TRACHEO-BRONCHIAL DISRUPTION

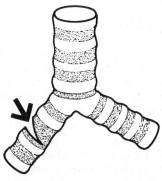 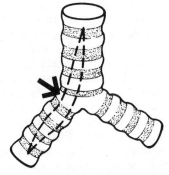

FIG. 36–1. Sites of tracheobronchial disruption. Bronchial tears usually occur posteriorly, within an inch of the carina, and most often in the right side.

there is continued bleeding of more than 100 mL per hour. Large effusions are less likely to reabsorb spontaneously and therefore require drainage. However, the late complications of hemothorax (fibrothorax, empyema, and trapped lung) are not prevented for certain by early evacuation of pleural blood.

PERICARDIAL TAMPONADE

Traumatic tamponade may be the result of aortic root disruption, coronary artery laceration, or rupture of the free ventricular wall. When cardiac rupture occurs, it usually is of the right atrium or ventricle and is rapidly fatal. The diagnosis of tamponade should be suspected when muffled heart sounds, hypotension, tachycardia, and elevated jugular pressure are noted. These findings assume particular significance when a fractured sternum is discovered. (Note that in hypovolemic patients, signs of elevated central venous pressure may be absent.) Echocardiography may support the diagnosis by showing pericardial fluid and/or diastolic collapse of the right atrium or ventricle. QRS alternans is rare but highly suggestive. Right heart catheterization can confirm the diagnosis by demonstrating diastolic equalization of pressures throughout the cardiac chambers, but diagnostic testing must not delay definitive therapy in the unstable patient. Although needle aspiration of pericardial fluid is a worthwhile initial approach, trauma-induced tamponade usually requires prompt surgical decompression ("drainage window") or pericardiectomy.

CARDIAC INJURY

Cardiac contusion should be considered whenever a displaced or fractured sternum, multiple rib fractures, or a convincing history indicates a significant blow to the chest (e.g., high-speed steering wheel or shoulder harness injury). Common consequences of cardiac contusion include arrhythmias (most common), myocardial ischemia, and conduction system defects (particularly heart block). Contusion may transiently produce "stunned myocardium", impairing cardiac output. Elevated cardiac isoenzymes of creatine phosphokinase (CPK) help confirm the diagnosis. Although the electrocardiogram (ECG) may demonstrate ST segment elevations that simulate myocardial infarction, reciprocal changes and Q waves are characteristically absent. Ventricular and atrial extra-systoles are very common. Tech-

netium pyrophosphate infarct scanning may reveal "hot" areas of myocardium in the contused region. The echocardiogram may be useful for diagnosis by revealing a focal area of hypokinetic myocardium. The supportive treatment of cardiac contusion is the same as that for acute myocardial infarction and includes close monitoring for arrhythmias, pump failure, and pericardial disease.

Any valve may be damaged by a blow to the heart. Disruption of the tricuspid valve may be apparent by physical examination demonstrating large jugular v waves and a systolic murmur that varies with respiration. Because of the elevated jugular venous pressure waves, tricuspid disruption can be confused with evolving pericardial tamponade. Rupture of the chordae or papillary muscles also can result in mitral valve insufficiency. Classically, evidence of reduced forward cardiac output is combined with a systolic murmur and overt pulmonary edema in this injury. Distinguishing tamponade, valvular disruption and cardiac rupture can be accomplished using surface echocardiography, transesophageal echocardiography, or diagnostic cardiac catheterization (see Chapter 2, Hemodynamic Monitoring).

AORTIC DISRUPTION AND DISSECTION

The aorta can withstand massive uniform elevations in transmural pressure (up to 2000 mm Hg) but tolerates the shear forces of impact injuries much less well. Most aortic ruptures occur just distal to the ligamentum arteriosum. (In a minority of cases, disruption occurs at the aortic root just above the aortic valve, in which case tamponade is common.) When rupture of the ascending aorta occurs, damage to the aortic valve or coronary arteries also is possible. Clues suggesting a high likelihood of vascular injury include a fatality in the same vehicle, fracture of the steering wheel by a driver, need for prolonged extrication from wreckage, being an "ejected" passenger, or a fall from a height greater than 30 feet.

Aortic disruption, a result of abrupt deceleration, usually is fatal at the accident scene. Older patients are more likely to suffer aortic avulsion. Amazingly, no evidence of external trauma is present in many patients with fatal aortic rupture; clearly, neither rib or sternal fractures are required for diagnosis. Clues to aortic disruption are similar to those for aortic aneurysm and include acute valvular insufficiency, hoarseness, dysphagia, carotid pulse differential, and an arm-to-leg blood pressure differential. Typically, when present,

RADIOGRAPHIC SIGNS OF LEAKING AORTIC ANEURYSM

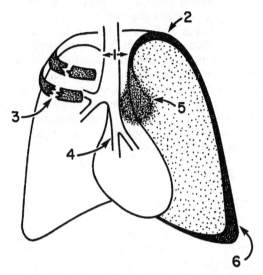

FIG. 36–2. Radiographic clues to aortic disruption include the following: (1) mediastinal widening (best detected on upright films); (2) apical pleural capping; (3) fractures of the first two ribs or sternum; (4) depression of the left main bronchus; (5) indistinct aortic knob; and (6) pleural effusion (shown here for a supine exposure with "ground glass" appearance of left lung field).

chest pain penetrates to the intrascapular region. Aortic disruption may present as a stroke syndrome if the carotid circulation is compromised. Occasionally, disruption of the aorta produces acute paraplegia as the anterior spinal artery take-off is damaged. Some radiographic clues to aortic aneurysm or disruption are illustrated in Figure 36.2. Angiography is currently more sensitive and specific than computed tomography (CT) scanning with contrast but non-invasive imaging is steadily improving. Although possible, tears and disruptions of the pulmonary artery rarely occur without penetrating injury.

DIAPHRAGM INJURIES

Blunt trauma may rupture the diaphragm, herniating the abdominal contents into the chest. Almost all such ruptures are left-sided, because the liver shields the right hemidiaphragm from direct injury. Disruption of the right hemidiaphragm suggests massive injury force. Major clues to diaphragmatic injury include a left-sided infiltrate or atelectasis, combined with signs and symptoms of bowel obstruction. Hearing bowel sounds above the diaphragm on physical examination or seeing air–fluid levels above the diaphragm on radiograph also are suggestive. CT scanning or plain radiographs taken after placement of contrast in the bowel may be confirmatory.

FLAIL CHEST

Flail chest results from multiple contiguous fractures of bony ribs or cartilaginous attachments that dislodge a free-floating section of rib cage or sternum. Restrained by negative intrapleural forces, the floating segment lags during inspiration, producing an apparent "paradoxical motion" during forceful breathing. This instability often goes unnoticed until vigorous efforts cause major swings in intrapleural pressure (as during weaning). Flail chest should be suspected in every patient with blunt chest trauma, particularly if rib fractures are evident. Whenever possible, a brief period of spontaneous breathing (5–10 breaths) should be observed to bring any flail segment to clinical attention.

A flail segment impairs normal coordinated action of the respiratory muscles and produces regional hypoventilation due to splinting and pain. Oxygen exchange is further impaired by underlying lung contusion and retained secretions. Although the work of breathing may be only modestly affected at low levels of ventilation, it rises dramatically during hyperpnea as breathing efficiency worsens. Because the sternum retains a relatively fixed position and is not located in a strategic position in relation to the ventilatory function of the rib cage, flail sternum usually is better tolerated than flail segments elsewhere.

For patients with extensive injury and ventilatory compromise, a high level of mechanical ventilatory assistance may help to reduce fluctuations of intrapleural pressure for the 7 to 14 days needed to stabilize the chest wall. More than in most patients, it is important to minimize the minute ventilation requirement and ensure excellent bronchial hygiene to reduce the breathing workload before weaning is attempted. Taping, sandbagging, or other attempts at external chest wall stabilization do not significantly lessen pain or improve ventilatory mechanics and may encourage atelectasis. Intercostal nerve blocks may reduce pain without impairing consciousness or ventilatory drive and thereby facilitate the weaning process.

PULMONARY CONTUSIONS

A forceful blow to the chest may contuse the lung at the site of impact or cause a contrecoup injury. This condition is nothing more than localized tissue bleeding and edema, which causes the consequent ventilation–perfusion mismatching leading to hypoxemia—often severe. Hemoptysis is common. Pulmonary contusion should be considered in all patients with ill-defined chest radiograph infiltrates and hypoxemia developing shortly after chest trauma, particularly when the radiographic abnormality is aligned with the known path of a forceful blow. Within 6 hours of trauma, pulmonary contusions are radiographically visible as localized, nonsegmental infiltrates. Resolution begins within 24 to 48 hours of injury and usually is complete within 3 to 10 days. Pulmonary contusions tend to be less severe in obese patients because of decreased energy transfer to the lung afforded by the thickened chest wall.

Occasionally, pulmonary contusions coalesce to form a pulmonary hematoma that typically appears as a spherical 1- to 6-cm density. A pulmonary hematoma is a large pocket of blood located deep within the pulmonary parenchyma. Hematomas arise from significant vascular disruption and may require weeks or months to clear. Resolution is often incomplete, leaving a permanent scar.

ESOPHAGEAL RUPTURE (BOERHAAVE'S SYNDROME)

Esophageal rupture should be suspected in patients with a history of major chest trauma and a pleural effusion, especially if it is left-sided or accompanied by pneumothorax. Empyema following blunt chest trauma should suggest the possibility of esophageal or diaphragmatic rupture with subsequent bacterial contamination of the pleural space. Although interscapular, substernal, or epigastric pains are common, fever, hypotension, a rapidly accumulating pneumothorax, or a pleural effusion may be the only manifestation. Thoracentesis is highly suggestive if it reveals an acidic exudative fluid. A marked elevation of pleural fluid amylase is often present, a result of leakage of salivary amylase into the pleural space. The diagnosis may be confirmed by observing macroscopic or microscopic evidence of food particles in fluid aspirated from the pleural space.

Esophageal rupture is a highly lethal condition with mortality approaching 2% per hour. Mediastinitis is the most frequent cause of death, fatal in almost one-half of patients within the first day. Chest radiographs demonstrate mediastinal widening and gas in the mediastinum or pleural space. Extravasation of swallowed contrast material into the mediastinum or pleural space confirms the diagnosis. Surprisingly, endoscopy is frequently unrevealing, and CT scan may only suggest the problem by demonstrating fluid with or without gas in the pleural space and mediastinum. Immediate surgical repair and drainage are indicated.

FAT EMBOLISM

The fat embolism syndrome may occur 1 hour to 3 days after trauma. Although fat embolism usually is associated with multiple long bone or pelvic fractures, diabetes, fatty liver, pancreatitis, joint surgery, and sickle cell anemia are other reported causes. It is theorized that lung injury is produced when lipases hydrolyze neutral triglycerides to liberate unsaturated fatty acids toxic to the pulmonary parenchyma. Fat confined to the pulmonary circulation may precipitate diffuse coagulopathy and clinical disseminated intravascular coagulation (DIC). Fat microglobules may even pass through the pulmonary capillary bed to enter the systemic circuit and produce characteristic retinal, central nervous system, and skin lesions.

A triad of confusion, pulmonary dysfunction, and skin abnormalities characterize this disorder. Frequent symptoms include cough, dyspnea, and pleuritic chest pain. These complaints often are accompanied by physical findings of fever, rales, tachypnea, and disorientation. Although a petechial rash over the upper torso may be present in the full-blown syndrome, it is unusual in less obvious cases. Serum and urine lipase levels may be elevated, and fat globules sometimes can be found in the urine, sputum, or bronchial lavage fluid. Retinal fat emboli also may be seen. Initially, the chest radiograph is normal in a large percentage of patients, despite severely impaired gas exchange. Decreased lung compliance, impaired diffusing capacity, hypoxemia, and respiratory alkalosis are common respiratory manifestations. In cases of fat-embolism-induced acute respiratory distress syndrome (ARDS), infiltrates may require 1 to 4 weeks to resolve. Early use of corticosteroids may be helpful, but this practice remains controversial.

LUNG TORSION

Lung torsion is an uncommon result of severe chest trauma that forces the lung to rotate on its hilar axis. A radiographic clue is reversal of the normal pattern of bronchovascular markings, with the major pulmonary vessels coursing cephalad rather than caudad. "Ground glass" opacification of the affected hemithorax may accompany this pattern, due to vascular congestion, edema, and atelectasis in the affected lung. Torsion must be reversed surgically to avoid infarction or gangrene.

KEY POINTS

1. Victims of chest trauma who survive to hospital admission have a generally good prognosis and uncommonly require thoracotomy: rib and sternal fractures and pulmonary contusions are the most common injuries.

2. Ensuring that the airway is patent and respiratory drive is adequate are critical first steps. Securing adequate venous access and draining pneumothoraces or hemothoraces are secondary priorities.

3. In the setting of thoracic trauma, hypotension is explained by relatively few possibilities. If the neck veins are flat, hemorrhage is most likely; if the neck veins are distended, cardiac tamponade, tricuspid valve disruption, and tension pneumothorax are leading candidates. Myocardial dysfunction secondary to blunt cardiac injury or infarction should always be considered.

4. Hemothorax, widening of the mediastinum, an arm/leg pulse or blood pressure deficit, thoracic inlet hematoma, and multiple rib or sternal fractures serve as clues to major vascular injury. Patients with these signs should be managed in a setting in which invasive diagnostic evaluation and immediate thoracotomy are possible.

5. Tracheobronchial injury should be suspected when hemoptysis or a large bronchopleural fistula is present or when a "drooping" lung is noted on chest radiograph. Early evaluation by bronchoscopy is indicated.

SUGGESTED READINGS

1. Kirsh MM, Sloan H. Blunt chest trauma: general principles of management. Boston: Little, Brown & Co., 1977.
2. Majeski JA. Management of flail chest after blunt trauma. South Med J 1981;74(7):848–849.
3. Rothstein RJ. Myocardial contusion. JAMA 1983; 250(16):2189–2191.
4. Bancewicz J, Yates D. Blunt injury to the heart. Br Med J 1983;286:497.
5. Berg GA, Kirk AJB, Reece IJ. Management of penetrating chest wounds. Hospital Update 1987;November: 949–961.
6. Bryan AJ, Angeleini GD. Traumatic rupture of the thoracic aorta. Br J Hosp Med 1989;41:320–326.
7. Buckman R, Trooszkin SZ, Flancbaum L, Chandler CD. The significance of stable patients with sternal fracture. Surg Gynecol Obstet 1987;164:261–265.
8. Mattox KL, Allen MK. Systematic approach to pneumothorax, hemothorax, pneumomediastinum and subcutaneous emphysema. Injury 1986;17:309–312.
9. Poole GV. Fractures to the upper ribs and injury to the great vessels. Surg Gynecol Obst 1989;169:275–282.
10. Taggart DP, Reece IJ. Penetrating cardiac injuries [editorial]. Br Med J 1987;294:1630–1631.

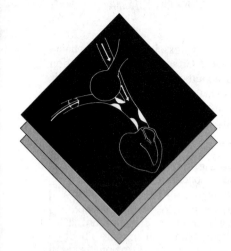

CHAPTER 37

Acute Abdomen

The specific problems of pancreatitis and gastrointestinal bleeding are discussed separately in Chapters 38 and 39, respectively. Diseases causing acute abdominal pain rarely present in a typical fashion in patients in the intensive care unit (ICU). Such seemingly trivial findings as a modest reduction in the intensity of bowel sounds, intolerance of tube feeding, or loose stools can be the first signal of serious abdominal pathology. Moreover, the single most important part of the diagnostic evaluation, the history, often is difficult or impossible to obtain from patients in the ICU. Patients with spinal cord injuries, those in coma, and those receiving corticosteroids or neuromuscular paralytic drugs may experience an abdominal catastrophe with few signs or symptoms. Therefore, ICU patients should undergo frequent abdominal evaluations, and a low threshold of suspicion for serious problems must be maintained.

Several principles should be kept in mind when evaluating critically ill patients with acute abdominal pain:

1. Carefully exclude emergent nonabdominal processes such as myocardial infarction and ruptured thoracic aortic aneurysm.
2. Until a firm diagnosis is established, consider the problem to be urgent and life threatening.
3. Make repeated observations—a changing examination provides valuable clues in diagnosing abdominal disorders.
4. Involve a surgeon and/or gynecologist early in the evaluation. (All consultants should follow the evolving course of the illness; furthermore, this strategy avoids unnecessary repetition of painful pelvic and rectal examinations.)
5. Avoid excessive use of analgesics or sedatives for patients with undiagnosed acute abdominal pain.
6. Withhold enteral feedings and medications as a precaution in the event that laparotomy becomes necessary.

HISTORY

An accurate history is key to the workup. Description of the onset and character of the pain as well as exacerbating or relieving factors is helpful in diagnosis. All conscious patients should be asked to localize the pain to a discrete site with one finger. Acute abdominal pain awakening patients from sleep or persisting longer than 6 hours frequently represents a surgical problem. Acute abdominal pain generally arises from one of three mechanisms: (*a*) visceral ischemia; (*b*) serosal inflammation; or (*c*) distention of hollow viscus. Pain of sudden onset suggests a vascular catastrophe or perforation of a hollow viscus. Pain of gradual onset that builds to a crescendo is more typical of hollow viscus overdistention, as is intermittent pain in a "colicky" pattern. Steady pain suggests serosal inflammation, especially when it is exacerbated markedly by changes in position or local pressure (rebound tenderness). A pleuritic component raises the possibility that an "intra-abdominal process" either abuts the inferior surface of the diaphragm or actually extends into the chest. (Conversely, lower lobe pneumonia and pericarditis may be diagnosed mistakenly as an acute abdominal process.)

New symptoms associated with pain, such as nausea or vomiting, change in bowel habits, or urinary symptoms, are extremely helpful. For obvious reasons, a history of hematemesis, hematochezia, or rectal bleeding is informative. A detailed gynecologic history is essential for all female patients. Special attention should be given to a history of previous gynecologic problems or a change in menstrual pattern.

PHYSICAL EXAMINATION

The specific site of the pain may be helpful in diagnosis. The abdomen should be examined visually first, then auscultated, and finally palpated. Palpating the abdomen as the first part of the examination is likely to produce voluntary guarding or induce bowel sounds, even in patients with severe ileus. The most painful area of the abdomen should be examined last. The abdominal examination must answer the following specific questions:

1. Is there rebound tenderness?
2. Are bowel sounds absent?
3. Are there palpable masses?
4. Is there evidence of free air or fluid in the abdomen?

A positive response to any of these questions strongly indicates that surgical intervention will be necessary. Peritoneal signs are the most reliable in predicting the need for urgent laparotomy. The development of shock in a patient with an acute abdomen also indicates a need for surgery.

ROUTINE LABORATORY TESTS

Routine laboratory tests rarely are diagnostic during acute abdominal pain. Leukocyte counts and white cell differentials may be normal, even with severe intra-abdominal disease, and a reduced packed cell volume (PCV) is indicative of either slow chronic blood loss or acute severe hemorrhage with volume replacement. The serum amylase can be helpful if pancreatitis is suspected, but both false–negative and false–positive results occur (see Chapter 38, Pancreatitis). Similarly,

elevations in hepatic transaminase, bilirubin, or alkaline phosphatase levels suggest liver disease but are nonspecific. The combination of acutely elevated bilirubin and alkaline phosphatase levels is probably most helpful, suggesting obstructive biliary tract disease. A triad of hyperkalemia, hyperphosphatemia, and metabolic acidosis (in the absence of renal failure) suggests well-advanced bowel infarction.

Because ectopic pregnancy represents a potentially fatal cause of abdominal and pelvic pain, and an intrauterine pregnancy dictates some diagnostic and management choices, a rapid, sensitive pregnancy test should be obtained in the evaluation of any potentially pregnant woman. The abdominal radiograph may give important clues to the etiology and urgency of acute abdominal pain and is discussed elsewhere in this text (see Chapter 11, Radiology in the Intensive Care Unit).

PLAIN FILMS OF THE ABDOMEN

For patients with acute abdominal pain, supine and upright films of the abdomen often are helpful but rarely diagnostic. For example, even when the film reveals "free air," such a finding does not guarantee gut perforation and furthermore does not localize the site of perforation. (Free air may be the result of pulmonary barotrauma with intra-abdominal dissection of air.) Similarly, finding multiple air–fluid levels in small bowel does not precisely identify the site or cause of bowel obstruction. Radiographic signs that should be sought include the following: (a) calcification, (b) mass effect, (c) extraluminal gas, (d) obliteration of normal soft tissue planes, (e) localized ileus, (f) thumbprinting of bowel, (g) evidence of gas in the biliary tree. Because it is difficult if not impossible to obtain upright films in critically ill patients, lateral decubitus views usually must be substituted. An upright chest radiograph also should be reviewed for all patients with acute abdominal pain to look for subdiaphragmatic air or a lower lobe pneumonia. For a more extensive discussion of plain films in abdominal disorders, see Chapter 11 (Radiology in the Intensive Care Unit).

ULTRASOUND

Ultrasonographic examination uses high-frequency sound energy to define anatomic structure and, when combined with Doppler technology, characterizes blood flow. Because wound dressings, adipose tissue, and air–tissue interfaces deflect ultrasonic energy, ultrasound (US) is a poor imaging mode for obese patients or patients with prominent bowel distention or abdominal surgical dressings. Ultrasound also suffers from the problem that the views it generates are difficult to interpret by the nonradiologist (unlike computed tomographic [CT] images). Ultrasound has the desirable features of being portable, rapidly accomplished, relatively inexpensive, and devoid of ionizing radiation.

Ultrasound is an excellent method for detecting pelvic processes (e.g., ectopic or intrauterine pregnancy, ovarian cysts, or pelvic tumors) in female patients. Likewise, because a bowel gas interface usually does not need to be crossed by the ultrasound beam in the right upper quadrant, ultrasound is excellent for viewing the liver and gallbladder. Therefore, ultrasound is an excellent method to detect cholelithiasis, biliary tract dilation, and pericholecystic fluid or edema. Clear images of the kidneys and ureters also can be obtained routinely because they can be imaged from the rear, avoiding overlying bowel gas. The presence or absence of bowel gas makes visualization of the pancreas inconsistent.

COMPUTED TOMOGRAPHIC SCANNING

The CT scan requires transport of the patient to the radiology suite, but in contrast to magnetic resonance (MR) scanning offers more rapid images and is not precluded by the presence of metallic devices. CT images are rather easy to interpret, even for the nonradiologist, and they offer high-resolution views of essentially every intra-abdominal structure. The CT scan does have some disadvantages, however; it requires ionizing radiation, usually requires contrast administration, and only offers ideal images in patients with sufficient body fat to adequately delineate tissue planes.

BILIARY SCANS

The performance of biliary tract scans relies on use of a radioactive analog of iminodiacetic acid, which, after administration, is taken up by the liver and secreted into the bile. There it outlines the major intrahepatic ducts, gallbladder, and common bile duct. Radionuclide scans (''-IDA'' scans) are sensitive but lack specificity for biliary tract inflammation, particularly in the absence of

gallstones. The high sensitivity of these tests renders them useful for excluding the diagnosis of cholecystitis if an adequate study is obtained. Failure to visualize the gallbladder may result from obstructive biliary tract disease, starvation, total parenteral nutrition use, or severe parenchymal liver failure—often the very problems necessitating ICU admission.

GALLIUM AND INDIUM SCANS

The question of abdominal abscess arises frequently and is difficult to resolve noninvasively. Whole-body or localized gallium and indium scans may be useful in the search for localized inflammation. Unfortunately, there are many problems in using these studies. Indium-labeled white blood cells (WBCs) are difficult to produce because the isotope is very expensive, short-lived, and cyclotron-generated. Indium scanning is likely not to work if WBCs are dysfunctional, as in patients with acquired immune deficiency syndrome (AIDS), malnutrition, or a need for dialysis. False–positive abdominal scans may result in pneumonia, sinusitis, gastrointestinal (GI) bleeding, or tumors of the bowel. Indium may be used to localize acute infections, but chronic infections may not have sufficiently numerous or active WBCs to enable visualization. Gallium[67] concentrates in any site of inflammation (not just areas of infection) and may visualize tumors, hematomas, fractures, infections, sarcoidosis, or acute respiratory distress syndrome (ARDS). Gallium is normally excreted into the colon and kidney, producing ''physiologic hot spots.'' Resolution is characteristically poor, and precise localization is difficult. In most cases the CT scan and US are more useful in diagnosing intra-abdominal conditions. Each has its own specific advantages and limitations, as outlined in Tables 37.1 and 37.2.

MAGNETIC RESONANCE IMAGING

Magnetic resonance imaging (MRI) has significant limitations in the ICU patient population because of the requirement for transport to the scanner, the long scanning times, and the prohibition against metallic support devices.

SPECIFIC CONDITIONS PRODUCING THE ACUTE ABDOMEN

Although age alone never makes nor excludes a specific diagnosis, a patient's age does give

TABLE 37-1

MERITS OF RADIOLOGIC DIAGNOSTIC METHODS FOR ACUTE ABDOMINAL PAIN

Characteristic	CT and Ultrasound (US)	Radionuclide Scans (Ga and In)
Operator dependence	Require directed study of a suspected area by skilled operator	Whole body scan
Specificity for inflammation	Failure to determine whether fluid collections contain leukocytes	More specific for the presence of WBCs
Rapidity	Rapidly accomplished	Usually requires 24–48 hours
Portability	Only US portable	Not portable
Body habitus	US best in thin patients; CT requires body fat to define tissue planes	Not as effective in obese patients

CT = computed tomography; Ga = Gallium; In = Indium

TABLE 37-2

CHARACTERISTICS OF CT, MR, AND US EXAMINATIONS

Computed Tomography	Magnetic Resonance Imaging	Ultrasound (US)
Not portable	Not portable	Portable
Expensive	Expensive	Less expensive
Can evaluate through wounds and bandages	Can evaluate through wounds and bandages	Requires skin contact
Better in fat patients	Body habitus not critical	Better in thin patients
Cross-sectional views best	Infinite number of views	Wide range of sectional views
Metal causes artifacts	Impossible with metal implants	Air causes artifact
Static images	Static images	Dynamic images possible
Uniform resolution across field	Uniform resolution across field	Limited area of high resolution
Not operator-dependent	Not operator-dependent	Highly operator-dependent
Requires contrast to distinguish vessels	Exquisite detail of flowing blood and soft tissues	Cystic and dilated structures provide best contrast; air interferes

TABLE 37-3

ASSOCIATION OF SPECIFIC DISEASES WITH PATIENT AGE

Condition	Age Predilection
Ruptured aortic aneurysm	Older
Ectopic pregnancy	Younger
Pelvic inflammatory disease	Younger
Ovarian tumor	Older
Mesenteric ischemia	Older
Cholecystitis	(Any age)
Pancreatitis	(Any age)
Small bowel obstruction	(Any age)
Colonic obstruction/perforation	Older
Diverticulitis	Older
Ulcer perforation	Younger

valuable clues to diagnosis (see Table 37.3). Similarly, the etiology of abdominal pain varies depending on whether the pain precipitated ICU admission or developed while the patient was in the ICU. Although ruptured ectopic pregnancy, aortic rupture, and pancreatitis do not commonly develop in the ICU, cholecystitis, appendicitis, and ulcer perforations commonly do.

The most rapidly lethal condition compatible with the presentation should be considered first, particularly for patients with overt abdominal signs and hypotension. The fulminant development of shock associated with acute abdominal pain usually is attributable to vascular disruption and intra-abdominal hemorrhage. Two conditions of this type in most urgent need of surgical intervention are ruptured abdominal aortic aneurysm and ruptured ectopic pregnancy.

RUPTURED ANEURYSM

Immediate diagnosis and surgical correction are needed to salvage patients with a ruptured abdominal aortic aneurysm. A ruptured or leaking aneurysm typically presents with back and abdominal pain and shock in a middle-aged or elderly patient with known arterial vascular disease. An expanding abdomen or pulsatile abdominal mass with the loss of one or both femoral pulses completes the classic presentation. The retroperitoneal irritation produced by a leaking abdominal aneurysm can mimic nerve compression or a ureteral stone by causing "sciatica" or groin pain. Rarely, rupture of an aortic aneurysm into the duodenum causes the massive hematemesis of an aortoenteric fistula. Unfortunately, hypotension often impedes comparison of pulse volumes, and examination of the abdomen and pulses may be difficult in obese patients. Because such patients are losing "whole blood," the hematocrit often remains stable until volume replacement is substantial or the patient nears exsanguination.

When clear signs and symptoms of a ruptured abdominal aneurysm are present, the patient should be taken directly to the operating room while initiating fluid and blood resuscitation. If the patient is hemodynamically stable, multiple large-bore intravenous lines should be inserted and blood cross-matched before diagnostic testing. A contrasted CT scan or aortic arteriogram are the best tests to confirm and delineate the aneurysm in the stable patient. Ultrasonography is a quick, noninvasive bedside test to confirm the presence of an aneurysm, but clear visualization may be obscured by the presence of bowel gas.

PELVIC DISEASE IN FEMALES

Ruptured ectopic pregnancy typically presents as acute abdominal pain, hypotension, vaginal bleeding, and a mass in the cul-de-sac. (Acute abdominal pain occurs in almost all patients; approximately three-fourths have vaginal bleeding, and approximately one-half have a pelvic mass; fever is rare.) A reported history of a recent menstrual period is unreliable and cannot be used to exclude pregnancy. Therefore, a serum β-human chorionic gonadotropin (HCG) should be performed on every fertile female with acute abdominal pain. Urinary HCG testing, although possibly more readily available, is less sensitive. Hematocrit determinations usually are not helpful because of the acute nature of any associated bleeding.

Ectopic pregnancy is especially likely in patients with a history of salpingitis, tubal ligation, prior ectopic pregnancy, and in patients using intrauterine devices for birth control. Young women with unexplained acute abdominal pain and shock should undergo immediate laparotomy for a presumed ruptured ectopic pregnancy. For patients with acute abdominal pain, stable blood pressure, and no evidence of peritoneal signs, elective serum pregnancy testing and ultrasonographic evaluation should be performed before surgery.

The transabdominal and transvaginal US examinations are complementary in evaluation of painful pelvic disease: lesions located "high" in pelvis (e.g., ovarian masses) are often best seen by transabdominal screening (if bowel gas does not obscure the view). Conversely, transvaginal scanning often is better at detecting early intrauterine pregnancy and ectopic pregnancies. Use of transabdominal scanning can detect pregnancy within 4 weeks of gestation—transvaginal scanning can detect the same gestational sac 1 week earlier. The only certain ultrasonographic sign of ectopic pregnancy is visualizing a gestational sac outside the uterus, although finding a viable intrauterine pregnancy is strong evidence against a concurrent ectopic pregnancy.

Ovarian tumors or cysts also may produce pelvic pain if they undergo torsion or ischemia. Rupture of a normal ovarian follicle into the peritoneum may produce worrisome but otherwise benign peritoneal signs.

Pelvic inflammatory disease (PID), the most common cause of pelvic pain in young women, is often difficult to differentiate from appendicitis or a ruptured ectopic pregnancy. PID usually starts within 7 days of the menstrual period, a helpful point in the differential with ectopic pregnancy. The pain of PID is gradual in onset and usually is bilateral, whereas the pain of appendicitis tends to be of sudden onset and unilateral when fully developed. Diffuse bilateral tenderness elicited by moving the cervix during pelvic examination is key to detecting PID. The US and CT features of PID are subtle and nonspecific unless a frank abscess forms. Untreated, PID can progress to the formation of a pus-filled Fallopian tube, a tubo-ovarian abscess (TOA). TOA is an especially common problem among women with repeated or prolonged episodes of PID. TOA is characterized by pelvic pain, fever and chills, and vaginal discharge. Examination reveals lower abdominal and adnexal tenderness (usually asymmetric). Leukocytosis occurs in approximately two-thirds of patients. Both US and pelvic CT scanning are excellent for imaging the lesion.

Most tubal abscesses are polymicrobial infections that include enteric aerobic gram-negative rods, *Hemophilus,* anaerobes, and *Streptococci.* Pelvic US is invaluable, demonstrating an adnexal mass in more than 90% of patients. Initial therapy should include appropriate cultures, hemodynamic stabilization, and administration of antibiotics. A second-generation cephalosporin plus doxycycline or clindamycin and gentamicin are rational combinations.

MESENTERIC ISCHEMIA

Mesenteric ischemia afflicts elderly patients, particularly those with underlying heart and vascular disease. The mortality of bowel infarction approaches 70%, primarily because of delayed diagnosis, but also because victims tend to be older and have other underlying diseases. The differential diagnosis includes bowel obstruction, diverticulitis, and inflammatory bowel disease.

Bowel ischemia may result from arterial or venous occlusion of the superior or inferior mesenteric vessels. Approximately 50% of patients with acute bowel ischemia have superior mesenteric artery disease. Superior mesenteric artery (SMA) occlusion usually presents as the sudden onset of acute abdominal pain and a striking leukocytosis. Conversely, inferior mesenteric artery occlusion (accounting for approximately 25% of bowel ischemia) usually has a more subtle, chronic pattern. Bowel infarction most often is the result of thrombotic occlusion near the aortic origin of mesenteric vessels in patients with extensive atherosclerotic vascular disease. In patients with slowly progressive occlusion, a history of "intestinal angina" may be elicited. Embolism, the second major mechanism producing bowel obstruction, is a more likely etiology in patients with chronic atrial fibrillation or recent myocardial infarction complicated by mural thrombosis. Vasculitis from lupus, radiation, or polyarteritis is rarely responsible. It has been recognized recently that many critically ill patients have nonocclusive bowel infarction due to generalized hypotension and use of vasopressor drugs. Initially, ischemia produces mucosal and submucosal injury and edema. Later, mucosal sloughing occurs. Unless corrected within 2 to 4 days, bowel necrosis and perforation occur, resulting in generalized peritonitis and death.

The signs and symptoms of mesenteric ischemia are often minimal and poorly localized. (A benign abdominal examination in a patient complaining of severe abdominal pain should be a tipoff to mesenteric ischemia.) The most common symptom of mesenteric occlusion is constant, nondiscrete back and abdominal pain. More than one-half of all patients have either occult blood in the stool or bloody diarrhea. Bowel sounds increase early in this process but decrease later. Shock may be the presenting symptom if perforation or infarction already has occurred. Atrial fibrillation or congestive heart failure are present in as many as one-half of all patients with bowel infarction.

Laboratory tests are seldom sufficiently specific or timely to aid in diagnosis. Although loss of circulating volume may cause hemoconcentration, more typically, the hematocrit remains normal as the leukocyte count rises. Refractory metabolic (lactic) acidosis in conjunction with increased levels of potassium and phosphate is typical of infarction. Unfortunately, these abnormalities often are recognized too late to affect favorably on crucial therapeutic decisions.

Plain abdominal radiographic findings (seen in a minority of cases) include an ileus localized to the area of bowel ischemia with dilation of large and small bowel loops and loss of haustral markings. Occasionally, gas may be seen in the portal venous system, in the bowel wall, or free in the peritoneal cavity. Hemorrhage and bowel wall edema may result in a classic "thumbprinting" pattern on the plain radiograph. CT of the abdomen can demonstrate the suggestive findings of bowel wall thickening, ascites, air in the portal vein, or focal bowel dilation with a high degree of sensitivity (approximately 85%). Occasionally, CT may demonstrate mesenteric vein thrombosis directly, which is diagnostic.

Angiography, the procedure of choice for diagnosis, also may aid in the therapy but must be performed without delay. Angiography distinguishes thrombosis, embolism, and vasoconstriction and allows the local infusion of a vasodilator, e.g., papaverine or nitroglycerin. (Angiography may fail to show occlusive disease in cases in which ischemia is caused by intense vasoconstriction or low cardiac output states.) Barium studies should not be performed if ischemic bowel is suspected, because barium prevents effective angiography and CT scanning, and extraluminal barium may cause peritonitis.

After initial stabilization with fluid and correction of electrolyte abnormalities, early angiographic diagnosis and surgical correction are crucial for a good outcome. In selected cases, infusion of papaverine or nitroglycerin may improve the perfusion of the ischemic gut, delaying or averting surgery. Thrombolytic agents are not of proven benefit. For patients with peritoneal signs, immediate surgery should follow confirmation of the diagnosis. At the time of surgery, nonviable segments of bowel should be removed. A "second look" operation 24 to 36 hours after revascularization has gained popularity to allow dying tissue time to demarcate. Prognosis is best when revascularization is performed on a "nonsurgical" abdomen. Unfortunately, the diagnosis of ischemic bowel disease often is overlooked or delayed until the clinical condition is too poor to permit salvage.

APPENDICITIS

In cases of appendicitis, early diagnosis is critical to prevent the major complications of perforation and abscess formation. Unfortunately, the pace and intensity of this surgical problem are highly variable. The classic features of acute appendicitis—midepigastric pain migrating to the right lower quadrant accompanied by nausea and vomiting—are seen in fewer than one-half of all ambulatory patients and in probably even fewer critically ill patients. The site of pain is not predictable because of the variable location of the cecum and appendix. Appendicitis often is overlooked in the absence of fever, leukocytosis, a localizing physical examination, or a "classic" history. Physical examination usually reveals a mildly elevated temperature with moderate acute abdominal pain. Generalized peritoneal signs are absent until perforation has occurred. Pelvic and rectal examinations are particularly helpful in localizing the pain to the right lower quadrant. Laboratory examination reveals an elevated WBC count in most patients, but leukocyte counts may be normal in older patients or in those receiving steroids or cancer chemotherapy. Even when perforation is demonstrated surgically, free intra-abdominal air is seen radiographically in only one-half of all patients. Standard CT scanning rarely shows the normal appendix; however, discovery of a mass in the cecal region, mesenteric edema, or thickening of the appendiceal wall are all suggestive of appendicitis. If the diagnosis is missed, the delayed suppurative complications are easily diagnosed by CT.

CHOLECYSTITIS AND CHOLANGITIS

In most cases originating outside the hospital (>90%), cholecystitis results from obstruction of the cystic duct by gallstones. For cases developing in the ICU, however, acalculous cholecystitis probably is more common. A low threshold for surgical intervention must be maintained to prevent mortality in patients with the common problems of cholecystitis and cholangitis. Many patients with these disorders in the ICU have coexisting problems. The increased mortality in elderly patients with biliary infection relates to delays in diagnosis and institution of therapy.

Bacterial infection plays a minor role in the development of cholecystitis. In contrast, cholangitis is a problem that arises primarily in elderly patients and occurs when bacteria reflux into a partially obstructed biliary duct, producing infection. Life-threatening bacteremia may result as infected bile, under pressure, seeds the bloodstream. Chronic or recurrent cholangitis may result in abscess or stricture formation.

Cholangitis and cholecystitis are most common among patients with gallstones, previous biliary surgery, pancreatic or biliary tumors, or other obstructions to bile flow. Instrumentation of the biliary tract, including endoscopic retrograde cholangiopancreatography (ERCP), surgery, or T-tube cholangiography, is a major risk factor. When cholecystitis occurs among ambulatory patients, gallstones are found 85 to 95% of the time; however, acalculous cholecystitis occurs commonly in hospitalized patients. Cholestasis may be key to the development of acalculous cholecystitis. Thus, acalculous cholecystitis tends to occur in patients deprived of the oral alimentation that produces the normal pattern of phasic gallbladder emptying.

Emphysematous cholecystitis (gas in the wall of the gallbladder) is an infectious complication of cholecystitis often seen in diabetic and immunocompromised patients. Gangrene and gallbladder perforation are very common in this condition and emergent cholecystectomy with common bile duct exploration is usually indicated.

The signs and symptoms of acute biliary inflammation are referred to as either a "classic" triad or pentad. The complete triad of cholecystitis (fever, chills, and right upper quadrant pain) occurs in about 70% of patients. The addition of mental status changes and shock completes the pentad of cholangitis in another 10% of patients. Either diagnosis is unlikely in the absence of fever. Nausea and vomiting are common but non-specific signs. Physical examination reveals right upper quadrant tenderness and guarding. A mass is palpated in the right upper quadrant in approximately 20% of patients. Physical findings of generalized peritonitis are rare and should suggest a complication (e.g., ruptured gallbladder) or another diagnosis (e.g., perforated ulcer).

The leukocyte count is elevated (12,000–15,000 cells/mm^3) in approximately two-thirds of patients with cholecystitis. Even when the total WBC count is normal, granulocytes usually predominate. Higher leukocyte counts should suggest cholangitis. The bilirubin level is elevated in 80% of cases of acute cholecystitis, but in most cases, it remains lower than 6 mg/dL. (A bilirubin level higher than 4 mg/dL is suggestive of a common bile duct stone.) Only 25% of patients are overtly jaundiced. The alkaline phosphatase usually is modestly elevated (less than two to three times normal) unless obstruction is severe or prolonged. Serum levels of liver transaminases usually are only modestly elevated. A low-grade coagulopathy is common, manifest as a decreased platelet count and prolonged prothrombin time. The serum amylase may be modestly elevated, even in the absence of pancreatitis.

Although plain radiographs visualize only 15 to 20% of gallstones, gas demonstrated in the biliary tract is virtually diagnostic of cholangitis. The oral cholecystogram has no role in diagnosis of acute cholecystitis. US will visualize gallstones and dilated biliary ducts reliably if obesity and bowel gas are minimal and sufficient time has elapsed for ductal distention to occur. US cannot reliably make the diagnosis of simple acute cholecystitis in the absence of ductal dilation, although gallbladder enlargement, wall thickening, and edema are suggestive. US also can occasionally find edematous changes within the pancreas that are suggestive of cholecystitis-induced pancreatitis. Patients with acalculous cholecystitis do not have evidence of gallstones, but "sludge" may be detected. In summary, ultrasound is sensitive and specific for gallstones but rarely can be more than suggestive for cholecystitis.

CT scanning may be a superior method of demonstrating dilated intrahepatic channels and processes in the region of the common bile duct, but lacks portability. Occasionally, thin-cut (2–4 mm) CT scanning will detect biliary tract stones missed by US because of its high resolution and superior ability to detect calcification. On CT, acute cholecystitis is indicated by gallbladder enlargement

(>5 cm) and wall thickening (>3 mm). The unusual occurrence of emphysematous cholecystitis also is seen easily.

Percutaneous cholangiography is a feasible and helpful diagnostic method if the biliary ducts are dilated but otherwise has a low yield. Unfortunately, percutaneous cholangiography fails to outline the pancreatic duct and may result in liver laceration, bile leak, and sepsis. A postoperative T tube in the biliary tract may provide a convenient channel for cholangiography.

Nuclear biliary scans also may be used to evaluate the function of the liver and biliary tract. A radioactive analog of iminodiacetic acid is administered, taken up by the liver and secreted into the bile, where it outlines the major intrahepatic ducts, gallbladder, and common bile duct. The gallbladder should demonstrate uptake within 30 to 60 minutes if normal. Delayed imaging at 4 hours that fails to visualize the gallbladder is highly suggestive of acute cholecystitis. Nonvisualization of the gallbladder is common in patients with cystic or common duct obstruction, but nonvisualization also may occur with starvation, pancreatitis, perforated peptic ulcer, use of total parenteral nutrition, and severe hepatic dysfunction. The specificity of biliary scans is high (>90%) if gallstones are present, but in acalculous cholecystitis, the specificity falls to approximately 40%.

ERCP requires a skilled operator and transport of a relatively stable patient to the radiology suite. This technique, however, allows direct visualization of the ampulla and radiographic visualization of the intrahepatic and pancreatic ducts—information that is helpful when malignancy is suspected. ERCP also offers the option of stone extraction, dilation of a stenotic ampulla, or stent placement.

For most patients with cholecystitis, frank cholangitis is not seen until more than 48 hours after ductal obstruction. Intraoperative bile cultures are positive in 85% of patients; two or more organisms grow more than 50% of the time. Although the most common organisms are *Escherichia coli, Klebsiella,* and *Streptococcus faecalis,* anaerobes (i.e., *Bacteroides fragilis* and *Clostridium perfringens*) are isolated in approximately 40% of infected patients.

Patients with cholangitis or cholecystitis should be stabilized hemodynamically, cultured, and given analgesics. Although antibiotic use is controversial, as a practical matter, most physicians use them. Antibiotics, however, are not an alternative to appropriate biliary drainage. Drugs normally excreted into bile are unlikely to achieve effective concentrations in unrelieved biliary obstruction. If antibiotics are used for cholecystitis, coverage should include broad coverage directed against gram-negative rods (aminoglycosides) and enterococci (e.g., ampicillin, vancomycin) as well as anaerobes (e.g., clindamycin, chloramphenicol, metronidazole, or cefoxitin). Although achieving adequate serum concentrations is important, the renal toxicity of aminoglycosides increases with biliary obstruction; therefore, special care must be exercised in their use. Doses should be adjusted by serum levels to an appropriate therapeutic index. Ampicillin is effective against most biliary pathogens and provides coverage of enterococcus (*Streptococcus faecalis*) not obtained by using cephalosporins. (For patients who are allergic to penicillin, vancomycin may be substituted for ampicillin.) Anaerobic coverage is particularly important in emphysematous cholecystitis; clostridial infections are demonstrated in nearly one-half of all such patients.

Most patients with cholecystitis should undergo semi-elective (within 72 hours) drainage of the biliary tract after hemodynamic stabilization. Surgical cholecystectomy remains the procedure of choice for acute cholecystitis. Mortality rates for cholecystectomy in this setting are less than 1% but may rise as high as 5 to 10% for patients older than 60 years of age. Urgent surgery is indicated for patients with empyema or perforation of the gallbladder and for those who deteriorate while receiving antibiotic and fluid support. Laparoscopic cholecystectomy, although safe and effective for elective cholecystectomy, has not yet been used widely in the emergent setting. (Early data suggest that it is likely to be safe and effective for most patients and, when technically not feasible, incisions can be extended for an open procedure.)

Early surgical intervention reduces the risk of suppurative complications, shortening hospital stay and mortality. Severity of illness in biliary tract obstruction should not preclude surgery because drainage offers the only chance for recovery. In the critically ill patient, it is generally best to perform the simplest effective procedure and to reoperate at a later time, if necessary. T-tube drainage of the biliary tract (with or without cholecystectomy) is effective, but the reliability of cholecystostomy alone is uncertain. Nonoperative options include percutaneous catheter drainage, a useful technique for the high-risk patient in the ICU or in terminally ill patients. Unfortunately, bile peritonitis, a potentially lethal problem, may complicate this procedure. ERCP is another option that may be performed without general anesthesia. ERCP is most helpful for stones impacted in the ampullary region, but cannulation can be difficult because of ampullary edema and obstruction.

SMALL BOWEL OBSTRUCTION

The triad of nausea, vomiting, and acute abdominal pain should suggest small bowel obstruction (SBO). SBO can be classified as (*a*) simple, (*b*) strangulated (in which vascular compromise is the predominant manifestation), or (*c*) closed loop (in which vascular compromise and complete bowel obstruction rapidly escalate intraluminal pressure). About three-fourths of cases are due to adhesions; incarcerated hernias and malignancy comprise most of the remainder. Inflammatory bowel disease, intussusception, and gallstones account for a small minority of cases.

On examination, occult blood in the stool signifies compromised bowel wall integrity. Incarcerated hernias or abdominal scars are suggestive physical findings. Bowel sounds usually are rushing and high pitched early in SBO, but later they become hypoactive. Flat abdominal radiographs are normal, but those taken with the patient in the upright position demonstrate small bowel dilation (>3 cm) and multiple air–fluid levels with distal evacuation of the colon and rectum. For patients who are unable to stand, a left lateral decubitus film can be diagnostic.

Treatment of SBO usually is less urgent than treatment of colonic obstruction. Strangulated bowel with perforation, a potentially disastrous problem, is often misdiagnosed as simple SBO. Unfortunately, there is no clinical way to distinguish between simple SBO and strangulated bowel. Good candidates for conservative management with nasogastric suction include patients who are hemodynamically stable, those with a partial SBO, those with recurrent obstruction after radiation therapy, and those with SBO occurring within 30 days of abdominal surgery. Failure to symptomatically improve with nasogastric suction suggests that operative intervention is required.

COLONIC OBSTRUCTION

Colonic obstruction, a disease predominantly of the elderly, presents with acute abdominal pain, obstipation (50%), and vomiting (50%). The most common causes of obstruction include colon cancer, diverticular disease, and volvulus. Impaction may imitate this picture. Approximately 20% of patients with colon cancer will have both perforation and obstruction, demonstrating free air on abdominal radiographs. Preoperatively, the etiology of colonic obstruction is often unknown, although the plain radiograph may be quite helpful. Plain radiographs are diagnostic of volvulus in more than 50% of patients. When radiographs show an acute increase of cecal diameter to more than 9 cm, perforation of the colon may be imminent.

Rarely, "pseudo-obstruction" (Ogilvie's syndrome) may occur in which signs and symptoms of bowel obstruction are present without a mechanical cause. Colonic pseudo-obstruction may be due to electrolyte imbalances (magnesium or potassium), anticholinergic drugs, myxedema, or ganglionic blockers. Pseudo-obstruction usually results from ileus of the right colon and is treatable by correction of the underlying disorder.

DIVERTICULITIS

Diverticulitis, the result of an inflamed pseudo-diverticulum, accounts for up to 10% of all abdominal pain in elderly patients. Even though diverticulitis has been referred to as "left-sided appendicitis," the pain has no typical pattern. Nausea, fever, and constipation are common, but vomiting is quite unusual.

Physical examination frequently demonstrates a palpable mass in the lower abdomen or pelvis. The stool, although often guaiac positive, rarely is bloody. Colonoscopy often is necessary to rule out neoplasm, because the extrinsic compression of the bowel caused by diverticulitis mimics colon carcinoma. The abdominal CT scan also can be useful, demonstrating bowel wall inflammation, pericolic edema, and fistula and abscess formation. (Steroid therapy may impair the "walling off" process and predispose to free perforation into the peritoneum.)

Medical therapy is successful in 80 to 90% of cases. Withholding food and providing mild analgesia, nasogastric suction, and intravenous fluids are standard. Broad-spectrum antibiotics (e.g., ampicillin plus clindamycin and an aminoglycoside) should be administered. Indications for operation in diverticulitis include perforation, obstruction, abscess formation, fistula tract formation, malignancy, and failure to respond to several days of conservative management.

RETROPERITONEAL HEMORRHAGE

Retroperitoneal hemorrhage rarely occurs spontaneously, usually resulting from trauma, surgery or invasive procedures (e.g., vena caval filter placement), thrombolysis, or anticoagulation. Most patients present with nonspecific flank or abdominal pain—a minority have shock or an acute abdomen. Although typically the PCV does not decline rapidly, the retroperitoneum is one of the few anatomic compartments capable of containing a massive hemorrhage without evidence of external blood loss. US may be suggestive but rarely is diagnostic. CT scan is the diagnostic procedure of choice to clearly demonstrate the extent of the bleeding, although it rarely identifies the precise source. Patients with adrenal hemorrhage as the result of infection or anticoagulation can have an identical presentation with nonspecific flank pain. The diagnosis is confirmed by a CT that demonstrates adrenal hemorrhage and by biochemical testing that often shows primary adrenal insufficiency (see Chapter 32, Endocrine Emergencies).

PERFORATED VISCUS

Free air detected under the diaphragm can be the result of a supradiaphragmatic or subdiaphragmatic process. Pulmonary barotrauma can result in dissection of air into the peritoneal cavity, making a certain diagnosis of a perforated viscus difficult in mechanically ventilated patients. When free air is detected below the diaphragm as a result of perforation of an intra-abdominal organ, the proximal GI tract is the most likely source. Because perforation of the stomach or duodenum is much more common than colonic perforation, an investigation of the upper GI tract should precede laparotomy for presumed colonic perforation in most cases.

Ulcer Disease

The perforated gastric or duodenal ulcer often is misdiagnosed as pancreatitis because of similar symptomatology (midabdominal pain radiating to the back, nausea, vomiting, and elevated serum amylase). Perforation more commonly complicates duodenal (5–10%) than gastric ulcers (<1%). Anterior ulcer perforation produces chemical peritonitis with diffuse acute abdominal pain and ileus. Approximately 80% of all ulcer perforations release free air into the peritoneal cavity. To demonstrate free abdominal gas, it may be necessary to position the patient upright or in the left lateral decubitus posture for 5 to 10 minutes before film exposure. Patients with perforated ulcers usually appear very ill, with diffuse acute abdominal pain, tenderness, and decreased bowel sounds. A minority of such patients have the abrupt onset of acute abdominal pain or a rigid abdomen. Perforations of the GI tract may be confirmed by demonstrating extravasation of Gastrografin® (not barium) into the peritoneum. Surgical intervention is indicated in ulcer disease for (a) intractable pain, (b) uncontrollable bleeding, (c) bowel obstruction, and (d) uncontained perforation. If the ulcer is located in the duodenum and the patient is stable, a definitive resection (vagotomy and drainage) should be performed. For unstable patients, however, the ulcer should be oversewn and the operation should be terminated quickly. Whenever possible, gastric ulcers should be resected because of the high potential for carcinoma.

Colonic Perforations

Perforation of the colon frequently is associated with colonic obstruction due to malignancy or diverticular disease. Diverticular perforation frequently is responsible for free intraperitoneal gas in elderly patients, but many (possibly most) perforated diverticuli do not liberate intraperitoneal gas.

UNUSUAL CAUSES OF ACUTE ABDOMINAL PAIN

Carcinoma is found in 5 to 10% of elderly patients with acute abdominal pain. Although no one knows the cause, patients with diabetic ketoacidosis often present with acute abdominal pain. (Diabetic ketoacidosis should be excluded in all patients before laparotomy.) Sickle cell disease may produce abdominal pain by causing ischemia or infarction of the bowel or spleen. Inferior myocardial infarction and pneumonia in the basilar segments of the lung may both present predominantly with abdominal discomfort. In these patients, nausea and vomiting also are common, mimicking acute cholecystitis. Typhlitis, bacterial invasion of the bowel wall in immunosuppressed patients, may be confused with ischemic colitis, diverticulitis, or appendicitis. Several forms of chemotherapy may produce nausea, vomiting, and GI bleeding (particularly cytosine arabinoside). As many as one-fourth of all leukemic patients have neoplastic infiltration of the bowel wall that may cause perforation, either in the natural history of the disease or shortly after the initiation of chemotherapy.

KEY POINTS

1. Patients in the ICU rarely have typical presentations of acute abdominal conditions—low-grade fever, mild agitation, or tube-feeding intolerance may be the only clues.

2. Extra-abdominal processes, especially thoracic diseases producing diaphragmatic distention, often mimic abdominal disasters.

3. A patient's age and underlying illnesses provide valuable clues to specific diagnosis, even in the absence of a detailed history.

4. When caring for patients with suspected abdominal disasters: (a) assume that the most life-threatening condition is causative; (b) avoid obscuring symptoms with excessive sedation or analgesics; (c) reexamine the patient regularly; (d) involve surgical and/or gynecologic consultants early in the evaluation; and (e) carefully select diagnostic tests likely to give an expeditious and definitive answer.

5. US is an excellent first imaging method for suspected lesions in the pelvis, right upper quadrant, or kidneys. CT scanning is better at imaging the entire abdomen but suffers from lack of portability.

SUGGESTED READINGS

1. Field S. Plain films: the acute abdomen. Clin Gastroenterol 1984;13(1):3–40.
2. Jordan GL Jr. The acute abdomen. Adv Surg 1980;14: 259–315.
3. Laing FC. Diagnostic evaluation of patients with suspected acute cholecystitis. Radiol Clin North Am 1983;21(3): 477–493.
4. Sallarides T, Hopkins W, Doolas A. Abdominal emergencies. Med Clin North Am 1986;70:1093.
5. Silen W, ed. Cope's early diagnosis of the acute abdomen. 16th ed. New York: Oxford University Press, 1983.

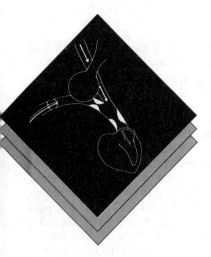

CHAPTER 38

Pancreatitis

PATHOPHYSIOLOGY

Some combination of direct cytotoxic injury, ductal obstruction, and bile and duodenal reflux is the stimulus initiating pancreatic injury. Regardless of the inciting stimulus, all pancreatitis results from organ damage caused by autodigesting enzymes. Trypsin and chymotrypsin, lipase, and elastase are responsible for damage to proteins, lipids, and elastin, respectively. Trypsin is not only destructive to proteins but is a potent activator of other proenzymes. Trypsin-induced activation of phospholipase A and the kinin–kallikrein system probably is responsible for many of the hemodynamic and permeability changes associated with pancreatitis. Enzyme-induced inflammation disrupts pancreatic ducts, breaks down vessel walls, causes fat necrosis, and kills both exocrine and endocrine pancreatic cells. The most severe cases of necrotizing pancreatitis are accompanied by hemorrhage. With the exception of alcohol-induced pancreatitis, most cases (more than 80%) are self-limited, leaving little residual pancreatic damage. Only rarely does acute pancreatitis progress to a chronic form.

ETIOLOGY

Cytotoxic effects of alcohol- and gallstone-induced reflux of bile into the pancreatic duct account for 80% of all cases of acute pancreatitis. Ethanol is a more likely etiology in men, whereas gallstones are a more frequent cause of pancreatitis in women. Other causes include trauma, tumors, medications, electrolyte disturbances, toxins, infections, and surgery (Table 38.1).

Gallstones causing acute pancreatitis usually affect the ampulla of Vater. Approximately one-half of all patients with gallstone pancreatitis have concurrent biliary tract infection (cholangitis), a complication that raises mortality dramatically. Two-thirds of patients with gallstone pancreatitis who do not undergo stone removal experience a recurrence of symptoms. Tumors of the pancreas and common bile duct or ampullary stenosis after biliary tract surgery also may induce pancreatitis by obstructing the free flow of bile.

Visualization of the pancreatic duct by endoscopic retrograde cholangiopancreatography (ERCP) reveals structural abnormalities, tiny stones, or thick biliary sludge in many cases of recurrent pancreatitis of obscure etiology. The ERCP procedure may elevate serum amylase in as many as 60% of patients; however, most of these cases are asymptomatic.

Ethanol leads the list of toxins and medications that commonly cause acute pancreatitis. Other direct pancreatic toxins include methanol, carbon tetrachloride, and organophosphate insecticides. Numerous medications have been implicated in causing acute pancreatitis (Table 38.2).

In lipid-induced acute pancreatitis, triglyceride levels usually exceed 1000 mg/dL. The diagnosis often is difficult to make because triglycerides interfere with assays of serum amylase and frequently are elevated, even when acute pancreatitis has another cause. Hypercalcemia-induced acute pancreatitis usually occurs in association with untreated hyperparathyroidism. After arteriographic

TABLE 38–1

CAUSES OF ACUTE PANCREATITIS

Common causes (~80%)
  Ethanol
  Gallstones

Less common causes (~15)
  Idiopathic
  Drug-induced
  Abdominal trauma

Rare causes (~5%)
  Hypertriglyceridemia
  Hypercalcemia/hyperparathyroidism
  End-stage renal failure
  Penetrating duodenal ulcer
  Organ transplant associated
  Pancreas divisum
  Ampullary stenosis or spasm
  Hereditary
  Pancreatic carcinoma
  Viral infections (CMV; mumps; hepatitis A, B, and C;
    EBV)
  AIDS-associated
  Pregnancy

TABLE 38–2

DRUGS IMPLICATED IN CAUSING PANCREATITIS

Acetaminophen	Angiotensin-converting enzyme
Asparaginase	inhibitors
Cimetadine	Azathioprine
Cytarabine	Corticosteroids
Diphenoxylate	Danazol
Estrogens	Ergotamine
Furosemide	Ethacrynic acid
Interleukin-2	Gold compounds
Mercaptopurine	Isoretinoin
Metronidazole	Methyldopa
Pentamidine	Nitrofurantoin
Procainamide	Piroxicam
Sulfonamides	Ranitidine
Tetracycline	Sulindac
Valproic acid	Thiazides

procedures, cholesterol emboli may incite acute pancreatitis; for unclear reasons, this complication is particularly likely in the anticoagulated patient. Pancreatitis also is common in patients undergoing solid organ transplantation, possibly due to use of cyclosporine.

DIAGNOSIS

SYMPTOMATOLOGY

Patients with pancreatitis usually present with severe, constant "boring" abdominal and/or back pain made worse by lying supine. Nausea, vomiting, and low-grade fever also are common. However, less than typical acute presentations (chest pain, shock, respiratory distress) often are encountered. Occasionally, the presenting signs of pancreatitis in patients in the intensive care unit (ICU) can be extremely subtle. Tube-feeding intolerance, hypocalcemia, or an unexplained fever or decline in hematocrit may be the only manifestations, especially in patients with impaired mental status. Acute pancreatitis can be difficult to distinguish from cholecystitis, mesenteric ischemia, ulcer disease (especially posterior duodenal ulcers), and colonic diverticular inflammation.

PHYSICAL EXAMINATION

Tachycardia is nearly universal because of pain and intravascular volume depletion. Volume depletion often produces hypotension. Epigastric tenderness with or without signs of peritoneal irritation is the most common finding on physical examination. (Rebound tenderness is not common because of the retroperitoneal location of the gland.) Pain often is worse when the patient is supine. Chest examination rarely reveals rales characteristic of atelectasis or acute lung injury. Bluish discoloration of the flanks (Grey-Turner sign) or periumbilical region (Cullen sign) are rare manifestations of retroperitoneal hemorrhage. Red subcutaneous nodules of fat necrosis and hypocalcemic tetanus are extremely rare.

LABORATORY FINDINGS

Leukocyte counts commonly range from 10,000 to 25,000 cells/mm^3. Early volume depletion frequently causes hemoconcentration and elevation of the blood urea nitrogen; later, anemia is the rule. Increased levels of stress hormones (glucagon, cortisol, and epinephrine) often produce hyperglycemia. Increased capillary permeability and chronic illness (especially alcoholism) commonly cause hypoalbuminemia. Transient hypertriglyceridemia and mild elevations in hepatic transaminase also are seen frequently.

CHEMICAL MARKERS OF PANCREATIC INFLAMMATION

Amylase and lipase are the two plasma enzymes most frequently assayed to diagnose pancreatitis. Unfortunately, many conditions unassociated with symptomatic acute pancreatitis elevate the amylase level, making this test much less specific than is perceived commonly (Table 38.3). For example, as many as one-third of all patients undergoing laparotomy and nearly one-fourth of those having major extra-abdominal surgery have elevated amylase levels without pancreatic manipulation or clinical evidence of acute pancreatitis. The specificity of amylase for diagnosing acute pancreatitis can be improved by using a cutoff of two to five times the laboratory upper limit of normal; however, the degree of serum amylase elevation has no prognostic value. Amylase determinations also lack sensitivity. Because peak amylase elevations usually occur within 24 hours of disease onset and then decline gradually, as many as one-third of patients with clinical and radiographic features of acute pancreatitis do not have elevated serum amylase values. High rates of false positive and false negative results limit the clinical utility of amylase clearance tests. (For example, renal failure is one of many conditions that increase the ratio of amylase clearance to creatinine clearance.)

Lipase is more specific than amylase as an indicator of pancreatitis. Lipase peaks later and clears more slowly than amylase, remaining elevated for up to 14 days. Therefore, it can help in making a diagnosis in a patient who presents later in the course of disease. Unfortunately, timely lipase determinations are not widely available, limiting their usefulness. Unlike amylase, lipase rarely is elevated in patients with burns, diabetic ketoacidosis, pelvic infection, salivary gland dysfunction, or macroamylasemia but, like amylase, may be elevated in renal failure. Assays of trypsinogen, methemalbumin, elastase, and phospholipase A are nonspecific tests used to support the diagnosis of pancreatitis but none of these has demonstrated any practical advantage over amylase or lipase determinations.

RADIOGRAPHIC STUDIES

The chest radiograph commonly demonstrates bibasilar atelectasis, diaphragmatic elevation, or pleural effusion. For patients with altered consciousness, diaphragmatic elevation or pleural effusion may be the initial indication of underlying subdiaphragmatic inflammation. Diffuse infiltrates suggest acute respiratory distress syndrome (ARDS). Abdominal films are never diagnostic but may reveal the suggestive signs of localized ileus, such as "the colon cutoff sign" or the "sentinel loop." Free air may enter the abdomen in cases of pancreatitis resulting from ulcer perforation. A "soap bubble" appearance of the pancreatic bed, calcifications suggestive of chronic pancreatitis, ascites, and widening of the duodenal sweep on upper gastrointestinal (GI) series offer other clues. Retroperitoneal inflammation may obscure the psoas margins.

Abdominal ultrasound is a useful bedside screening test for many patients with abdominal pain, but suboptimal visualization of the pancreas occurs in 40% of patients because of obesity or bowel gas. Ultrasound is good at detecting gallstones and biliary duct dilation and for observing the course of pancreatic pseudocysts but is inferior to computed tomography (CT) for detecting or staging pancreatitis and most of its complications.

CT scanning is the single best test to visualize the pancreas because it is unaffected by patient size or the presence of bowel gas. Although CT scanning demonstrates some radiographic abnormality in two-thirds of all patients with pancreatitis (pancreatic edema or necrosis or peripancreatic fluid collections) and is abnormal in all patients with severe disease, it provides an etiologic diagnosis in fewer than 25% of cases. Not all patients with pancreatitis must undergo CT scanning; the diagnosis and etiology of pancreatitis is apparent in most patients after history, physical examination, and measurement of serum amylase.

In addition to confirming the diagnosis, a reliable CT-scan-based scoring system has been devel-

TABLE 38–3

NONPANCREATIC CAUSES OF AMYLASE ELEVATION

Alcoholism	Abdominal trauma
Macroamylasemia	Perforated duodenal ulcer
Mesenteric ischemia	Small bowel obstruction
Morphine administration	Ectopic pregnancy
	Gallbladder disease
Lung cancer	Hepatic failure
Surgery	Ovarian tumors
Renal failure	Hydroxy ethyl starch administration
Diabetic ketoacidosis	
Endoscopic retrograde cholangiopancreatography	

TABLE 38–4

CT SCAN ASSESSMENT OF SEVERITY

Grade of acute pancreatitis	
Normal pancreas	0
Pancreatic enlargement	1
Inflammation of the pancreas and peripancreatic fat	2
One fluid collection or phlegmon	3
Two or more fluid collections	4
Degree of pancreatic necrosis	
No necrosis	0
Necrosis of one-third of pancreas	2
Necrosis of one-half of pancreas	4
Necrosis of more than one-half of pancreas	6
Total score	0–10

oped for assessing the severity of pancreatitis (Table 38.4). In this system, the presence of pancreatic enlargement, surrounding inflammation, peripancreatic fluid collections, and pancreatic necrosis correlate inversely with prognosis. Using this score, mortality may be less than 5% with scores of 0 to 3 but rises to 15 to 20% with scores of 7 to 10. Late complications are almost certain in patients with scores higher than 7.

CT scanning is prognostically useful but has its greatest value in documenting the late complications of peripancreatic fluid accumulation, pseudocyst formation, necrosis, and abscess development and drainage. Although diagnostic CT-directed aspiration is useful to establish infection, the role of therapeutic CT-directed drainage is controversial. Percutaneous aspiration fails when the fluid is extremely viscous or cannot be approached safely because of its location. In patients who are too ill to undergo a standard surgical approach, CT-directed drainage may be attempted as a temporizing option. Unfortunately, CT scanning technique is relatively expensive, inconvenient, and requires transport of the patient from the ICU. Magnetic resonance imaging (MRI) is time consuming, not universally available, and at present, seems to add little in the diagnosis or therapy of pancreatitis.

Because ERCP can exacerbate acute inflammation and cause infection, it probably should be reserved for trauma-induced pancreatitis or acute gallstone-induced pancreatitis in which stone extraction is anticipated. In traumatic cases, ERCP visualizes the damaged pancreatic duct, helping plan the repair. In moderate to severe cases of gallstone-induced pancreatitis, ERCP permits stone extraction (with or without sphincterotomy)

and reduces hospital stay, complications, and mortality. Extraction must occur within 24 to 48 hours of the onset of symptoms to abort a full-blown attack. ERCP also is useful in the first episodes of pancreatitis for patients older than 40 years of age, in whom ampullary tumors and pancreas divisum are more common findings.

PROGNOSTIC FEATURES

As with other critically ill patients, prognosis is determined largely by the number and severity of organ system failures (see Chapter 27, Sepsis Syndrome). Prognostication in pancreatitis has been studied extensively, and certain specific clinical features have been integrated to form the predictive Ranson and Glasgow scales (Table 38.5). These two clinical scales are used in addition to the CT-based scoring systems outlined above. Patients with fewer than three of the Ranson criteria fare well. Conversely, patients rarely survive if more than six of these criteria are present. A simplified Glasgow score has been developed along similar lines. Of all clinical features, pancreatic hemorrhage (usually caused by a nonalcoholic precipitant) carries the worst prognosis.

Death from alcohol-induced pancreatitis usually occurs early in the hospital course, often as a result of hypovolemia, whereas death from gallstone-induced pancreatitis usually occurs later, as

TABLE 38–5

ADVERSE PROGNOSTIC FEATURES OF ACUTE PANCREATITIS

Ranson Criteria	Simplified Glasgow Score
Age >55 years	Age >55 years
Calcium <8 mg/dL	Calcium <8 mg/dL
Glucose >200 mg/dL	Glucose >180 mg/dL
ARDS	PaO_2 <60 mm Hg
WBC >16,000/mm³	WBC >15,000/mm³
Rise in BUN >5 mg/dL	BUN >45 mg/dL
SGOT or LDH >350 units/dL	LDH >600 U/L
Falling hematocrit	Albumin <3.2 g/dL
Base deficit >4 mEq/L	
Repletion volume >6 L	

WBC, white blood cells; SGOT, serum glutamic oxaloacetic transaminase; LDH, lactic dehydrogenase; BUN, blood urea nitrogen; ARDS, acute respiratory distress syndrome.

a result of sepsis originating in devitalized hemorrhagic pancreatic tissue. Because peritoneal lavage has risks and does not provide superior prognostication to the use of abdominal CT or clinical scoring criteria, its use should be reserved for cases of diagnostic uncertainty.

MEDICAL THERAPY

A wide variety of experimental treatments (e.g., corticosteroids, anticholinergics, histamine blockers) have been tried in acute pancreatitis (Table 38.6), but there are little data to support their use. Therefore, the treatment of acute pancreatitis remains supportive.

Because marked reductions in circulating volume are common, adequate fluid resuscitation remains key to the initial management. Common causes of hypovolemia include extravascular ("third space") losses into the pancreas and retroperitoneum, intraluminal gut sequestration (due to ileus), and vomiting.

Withholding oral feeding makes sense to attempt to reduce pancreatic enzyme synthesis and release. Unfortunately, there is little evidence that this speeds resolution of inflammation. Continuous nasogastric suction has been used to decrease acid delivery to the duodenum and thereby decrease pancreatic stimulation but does not speed resolution. Nonetheless, nasogastric suction may help relieve ileus-related discomfort or intractable vomiting. Similarly, inhibition of gastric acid secretion using histamine blockers reduces the incidence of stress ulceration and upper GI bleeding but does not influence the course of acute pancreatitis. By hormonally suppressing pancreatic secretion, somatostatin may offer benefit if administered early in the course of severe disease.

Total parenteral nutrition (TPN) should be considered for symptomatic patients from whom food is withheld for longer than 3 to 5 days. Although

TABLE 38–6

UNPROVED THERAPIES FOR ACUTE PANCREATITIS

Anticholinergic drugs	Antiprotesases (aprontinin/gabexate)
Cimetidine	
Glucagon	Fresh frozen plasma
Nasogastric suction	Indomethacin
Prophylactic antibiotics	Peritoneal lavage
Total parenteral nutrition	Somatostatin

TPN does not exert therapeutic benefit in resolving pancreatitis, it provides some degree of nutritional support. Intravenous amino acids in TPN stimulate gastric acid production, but there is no evidence that amino acid or lipid preparations aggravate acute pancreatitis.

If narcotics are used to relieve pain, meperidine is preferred by many over morphine, which may evoke ampullary spasm; however, the superiority of one narcotic over another is unproven.

Prophylactic antibiotics are not indicated in all cases of pancreatitis but, because of the high incidence of biliary tract infection in gallstone-induced pancreatitis, antibiotics directed against enteric gram-negative rods, anaerobes, and enterococci are reasonable.

SURGICAL THERAPY

Although peritoneal lavage may be diagnostically useful to separate perforated viscus or trauma from acute pancreatitis, there is no evidence that peritoneal lavage reduces mortality or morbidity of acute pancreatitis. It remains possible, however, that a small subgroup of patients with severe or hemorrhagic disease may benefit.

Operative approaches do not benefit all patients with acute pancreatitis and should be reserved for patients who are likely to have gallstone-induced pancreatitis indicated by biochemical and ultrasonographic determinations and for patients with trauma-induced pancreatic duct disruption. There are four major indications for laparotomy in critically ill patients with acute pancreatitis—"the four Ds:" (a) **D**ecompression of biliary obstruction; (b) **D**iagnostic uncertainty; (c) **D**rainage of infected necrotic pancreatic tissue; and (d) **D**eterioration in the face of conservative therapy.

The clearest indication for early intervention is obstructive choledocholithiasis. The mortality rate from untreated gallstone-induced pancreatitis approaches 50% but is dramatically improved by early intervention. If extraction can be accomplished within 48 hours, endoscopic stone removal seems to be as successful as surgery in aborting pancreatitis, improving survival, and reducing infectious complications in patients with moderate to severe disease. Even though most cases of gallstone-induced pancreatitis will resolve spontaneously, removal of residual stones dramatically reduces the risk of recurrence.

Early surgery also is indicated for diagnostic uncertainty in which operative repair of an alter-

TABLE 38-7

BACTERIA RECOVERED IN PANCREATIC INFECTION

Escherichia coli

Pseudomonas species

Mixed anaerobic infections

Staphylococci

Klebsiella species

Proteus species

Streptococci

Enterobacter species

native diagnosis (e.g., perforated viscus, leaking aneurysm, mesenteric ischemia) would be vital. Late complications including nonresolving pseudocyst, infected pancreatic necrosis, fistula formation, and pancreatitis-induced hemorrhage also are valid operative indications. Because pancreatectomy carries a high mortality and does not reduce the incidence of complications, it has been abandoned as a therapy for acute pancreatitis.

COMPLICATIONS OF ACUTE PANCREATITIS

INFECTIOUS

Infectious complications are the most common cause of death in acute pancreatitis, accounting for 25% of all fatalities. Common infections include pancreatic or diaphragmatic abscess, cholangitis, urinary tract infection, and peritonitis. When necrotic areas or fluid collections are visualized in the region of the pancreas, CT-guided fine-needle aspiration has proven to be a safe and effective diagnostic method. Whenever possible, antibiotic therapy should be guided by Gram's stain and culture of appropriate body fluids. When uncertainty exists regarding the site of origin or infecting organism, however, antibiotic coverage should include drugs directed against gram-negative aerobes, anaerobes, and *Staphylococci*. The most common bacteria recovered from pancreatic tissue are listed in Table 38.7.

PULMONARY

Hypoxemia occurs in as many as two-thirds of all patients with pancreatitis; one in three patients develops infiltrates, atelectasis, or pleural effusions. Hydrostatic pulmonary edema frequently complicates unmonitored fluid replacement. Although pleural effusions usually are exudative in character and left-sided, bilateral or right-sided effusions are possible. Most effusions should be tapped to exclude the possibility of empyema, particularly if fluid appears suddenly or late in the clinical course. Pneumonia and fat embolism are not uncommon. ARDS, the most dreaded complication, occurs in 10 to 20% of all cases of pancreatitis, most commonly in patients with severe disease. The etiology of ARDS is unknown but possibly relates to the circulatory release of activated enzymes.

COAGULATION

Pancreatic inflammation commonly activates the coagulation cascade, but clinical evidence of coagulopathy is unusual. Although bleeding disorders are more common than inappropriate clotting, splenic or portal vein thrombosis may complicate acute pancreatitis.

ELECTROLYTES

A variety of fluid and electrolyte disorders are common in acute pancreatitis (see Chapter 13, Fluid and Electrolyte Disorders). Hypocalcemia may persist for weeks after the onset of acute pancreatitis. Total and ionized calcium levels usually reach a nadir of 7 to 8 mg/dL approximately 5 days after pain begins. Even though biochemical hypocalcemia is frequent, symptoms are rare. Mechanisms include the formation of intra-abdominal calcium complexes, hypoalbuminemia, and increased release of glucagon or thyrocalcitonin. Treatment parallels that of any case of symptomatic hypocalcemia. In a minority of patients with hypotension refractory to volume replacement and vasopressor therapy, administration of calcium chloride may rapidly elevate blood pressure.

Serum magnesium may be reduced by vomiting, diarrhea, poor oral intake, or deposition in necrotic fat. Hypomagnesemia, especially common in alcohol-induced acute pancreatitis, may precipitate refractory hypokalemia and hypocalcemia.

HEMORRHAGE

Pancreatic inflammation and pseudocysts can erode into major vessels, resulting in massive hemorrhage into the GI tract, peritoneal cavity, or retroperitonium. Vascular erosion presumably is due to the effects of proteolytic enzymes and direct pressure necrosis in the case of pseudocysts. Patients developing pancreatitis are prone to develop other hemorrhagic problems, including gastric stress ulceration, peptic ulcer disease, variceal bleeding, and splenic vein thrombosis.

Although only 10% of patients bleed directly into the pancreatic parenchyma, this condition (hemorrhagic pancreatitis) carries a very high mortality, related largely to subsequent infection in the devitalized tissue. Hemorrhagic pancreatitis has no distinctive clinical features. Although the diagnosis is suggested by methemoglobin in peritoneal fluid, virtually any source of intraperitoneal blood can produce this finding. Coagulation disorders that accompany acute pancreatitis worsen the hemorrhagic tendency, regardless of bleeding source. Attempts at specific treatment of hemorrhagic acute pancreatitis, including pancreatectomy and peritoneal lavage, have limited effectiveness.

RENAL

Oliguric acute renal failure occurs in approximately 25% of all patients with acute pancreatitis and carries an associated mortality of nearly 80%. Hypovolemia, hypotension, sepsis, and drug-induced renal damage are the most frequent causes.

ASCITES

Acute pancreatitis can produce ascites when transudative fluid crosses the retroperitoneal boundary or when ductal disruption causes spillage into the peritoneum. When pancreatic secretions leak into the peritoneal cavity, intense inflammation of the lining membrane causes massive exudation ("pancreatic ascites"). Overt disruption of the pancreatic duct commonly accompanies traumatic or hemorrhagic acute pancreatitis. When ductal disruption occurs, amylase levels in ascitic fluid typically exceed the corresponding serum levels, often rising to higher than 1000 IU/L. Three to 6 weeks of bed rest and nutritional support may be required for spontaneous healing of the pancreatic leak and resolution of the ascites. Surgical repair is indicated in refractory cases and should be guided by preoperative ERCP.

LOCAL COMPLICATIONS

Five local complications occur in acute pancreatitis. Pseudocysts, collections of fluid, form in about one-half of all cases of acute pancreatitis, and usually develop within the first 3 weeks of illness. Pseudocysts are most commonly associated with severe cases of acute pancreatitis. Initial detection is by abdominal examination in approximately 40% of cases and by ultrasound or CT scan in the remainder. Luckily, one-half of all pseudocysts resolve promptly. In the remainder, 6 months or longer may be required for spontaneous resolution. Although pseudocyst drainage or excision often proves difficult, operative intervention should be considered for those with acute complications or persistent, incapacitating symptoms. A drop in hematocrit with signs of shock and abdominal distention are reasons for immediate operation.

Phlegmons are solid masses of indurated pancreas that may be detected as abdominal masses on examination or by CT scanning. Phlegmons should be suspected in patients with persistent fever, abdominal pain, and tenderness, especially if leukocytosis persists. Most phlegmons resolve spontaneously within 10 to 14 days.

Pancreatic abscess is a poorly defined term applied to a variety of necrotic pancreatic tissue collections. The current, more descriptive terminology for this problem currently is "infected necrotic pancreatitis." Infected necrosis is uncommon, occurring in only 1 to 10% of all cases, but is much more frequent in clinically severe cases, especially those resulting from biliary tract obstruction. Infection forms in the pancreatic bed late in the course (usually after 3 to 4 weeks of illness), often after a period of apparent improvement. Abscess formation is suggested radiographically by air–fluid levels in the lesser sac or gas bubbles in the pancreatic bed. Slightly more than one-half of infected peripancreatic collections are polymicrobial, with a predominance of enteric gram-negative rods. Surgical or catheter drainage and culture-directed antibiotics are indicated in such cases (catheter drainage is less successful than surgery). External drainage often is sufficient for early suppuration, but later complications usually require internal drainage. By locally invasive autodigestion, acute pancreatitis can lead to the formation of fistulas. Fistulas connect the pancreas to the colon, stomach, duodenum, bile duct, small bowel, or skin surface.

Repeated bouts of acute pancreatitis may incite chronic pancreatitis, a disease characterized by pain and deficiency of endocrine and exocrine pancreatic function (diabetes and malabsorption).

KEY POINTS

1. Ethanol and gallstones account for most cases of acute pancreatitis. Of these two entities, gallstone-induced pancreatitis is the more important diagnosis to make because biliary obstruction usually requires surgical intervention for survival, and prompt surgical or endoscopic decompression of the biliary tract can abort some episodes of acute pancreatitis.

2. The diagnosis of pancreatitis usually can be made on clinical grounds, with confirmation by amylase or lipase determinations. Both measurements are nonspecific, however, and often are altered by renal insufficiency.

3. Ultrasound can detect pancreatitis-associated gallstones and bile duct obstruction with high reliability but is much more limited in visualizing peripancreatic edema of non–gallstone-induced pancreatitis. CT scanning is the optimal imaging procedure to detect and stage pancreatitis, and CT-scan-based scoring systems can provide prognostic information.

4. The therapy of pancreatitis is largely supportive: fluid and electrolyte replacement and antimicrobial therapy of infection are keystones of support. In cases caused by biliary obstruction, relief of the blockage is essential for optimal outcome.

5. Surgical therapy for pancreatitis is of limited value, being most helpful for patients requiring biliary tract decompression or drainage of necrotic pancreatic material.

SUGGESTED READINGS

1. Agarwal N, Pitchumoni CS. Assessment of severity in acute pancreatitis. Am J Gastroenterol 1991;86:1385–1391.
2. Agarwal N, Pitchumoni CS, Sivaprasad AV. Evaluating tests for acute pancreatitis. Am J Gastroenterol 1990;85:356–366.
3. Balthazar EJ, Freeny PC, vanSonnenberg E. Imaging and intervention in acute pancreatitis. Radiology 1994;193:297–306.
4. Bradley EL. Antibiotics in acute pancreatitis—current status and future directions. Am J Surg 1989;158:472–477.
5. Calleja GA, Barkin JS. Acute pancreatitis. Med Clin North Am 1993;77:1037–1056.
6. Epstein BM, Herttzanu Y. Clinical presentations of acute pancreatitis. The value of computed tomography. Am J Gastroenterol 1984;79:55–58.
7. del-Castillo FC, Rattner DW, Warshaw AL. Acute pancreatitis. Lancet 1993;342:475–479.
8. Finch WT, Sawyers JL, Schenker S. A prospective study to determine the efficacy of antibiotics in acute pancreatitis. Ann Surg 1976;183:667–671.
9. Frey CF. Hemorrhagic pancreatitis. Am J Surg 1979;137:616–623.
10. Gumaste V, Singh V, Dave P. Significance of pleural effusion in patients with acute pancreatitis. Am J Gastroenterol 1992;87:871–874.
11. Larvin M, McMahon MJ. APACHE II score for assessment and monitoring of acute pancreatitis. Lancet 1989;2:201–205.
12. Levant JA, Secrist DM, Resin H, et al. Nasogastric suction in the treatment of alcoholic pancreatitis. A controlled study. JAMA 1974;229(1):51–52.
13. Marshall JB. Acute pancreatitis: a review with emphasis on new developments. Arch Intern Med 1993;153:1185–1198.
14. Martin JK, van Heerden JA, Bess MA. Surgical management of acute pancreatitis. Mayo Clin Proc 1984;59:259–267.
15. Mayer AD, McMahon MJ, Corfield AP, et al. Controlled clinical trial of peritoneal lavage for the treatment of severe acute pancreatitis. N Engl J Med 1985;312(7):399–404.
16. Moossa AR. Diagnostic tests and procedures in acute pancreatitis. N Engl J Med 1984;311(10):639–643.
17. Neoptolemos JP, Hall AW, Finlay DF, et al. The urgent diagnosis of gallstones in acute pancreatitis: a prospective study of three methods. Br J Surg 1984;71:230–233.
18. Nordestgarrd AG, Wilson SE, William HA. Early computed tomography as a predictor of outcome in acute pancreatitis. Am J Surg 1986;152:127–132.
19. Pederzoli P, Bassi C, Vesentini S, et al. A randomized multicenter trial of antibiotic prophylaxis of septic complications in acute necrotizing pancreatitis with imipenem. Surg Gynecol Obstet 1993;176:480–483.
20. Potts JR. Acute pancreatitis. Surg Clin North Am 1988;68:281–289.
21. Ranson JHC. Etiological and prognostic factions in human acute pancreatitis: a review. Am J Gastroenterol 1982;77:633–638.
22. Ranson JHC, Balthazar E, Caccavale R, et al. Computed tomography in the prediction of pancreatic abscesses in acute pancreatitis. Ann Surg 1982;201:656–665.
23. Ranson JHC, Turner JW, Rose DH, et al. Respiratory complications in acute pancreatitis. Ann Surg 1974;179:557–566.
24. Schwartz MS, Brandt LJ. The spectrum of pancreatic disorders in patients with the acquired immune deficiency syndrome. Am J Gastroenterol 1989;84:459–462.

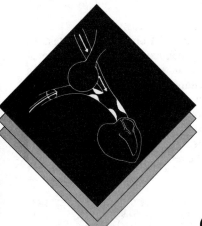

Gastrointestinal Bleeding

INTRODUCTION

Bleeding from the gastrointestinal (GI) tract is a common problem that usually manifests in one of three ways: (*a*) overt, severe upper GI bleeding in a young, otherwise healthy patient prompting admission; (*b*) less brisk, lower GI bleeding in an older but healthy patient; or (*c*) the onset of upper GI bleeding in a patient in the ICU who has multiple failing organ systems. The latter presentation has become much less common with the widespread use of pharmacologic prophylaxis, early enteral nutrition, and greater attention to reestablishing and maintaining systemic oxygenation and perfusion. Significant upper GI bleeding that precipitates admission to the ICU is the most frequent and straightforward of these presentations and, will be the primary focus of this discussion. The most difficult clinical situation occurs when GI bleeding (upper or lower) develops in a critically ill patient but its source remains obscure despite extensive evaluation.

Regardless of source, several factors predicting a poor prognosis have been identified for patients with GI bleeding: large volume hemorrhage, bleeding from an obscure site, advanced age, or presence of multiple organ failures. Specifically, the combination of renal failure and hepatic parenchymal failure carries a dismal prognosis.

INITIAL EVALUATION AND THERAPY

In patients with conspicuous upper or lower GI bleeding, attention should first be turned to ob-taining a brief history and noting vital signs, ensuring a stable airway and ventilation, and establishing intravenous access. Next, an attempt to differentiate upper from lower GI bleeding should be made to optimally direct diagnostic and therapeutic interventions. In this regard, the history can be very revealing. The duration and volume of bleeding, history of peptic ulcer disease, nonsteroidal anti-inflammatory drug use, and alcohol consumption are key points. The site of blood loss from the body (oral or rectal) also provides a valuable guide. Simply stated, a history of vomiting blood rarely is the result of lower GI bleeding. In contrast, red blood from the rectum can result from upper or lower GI bleeding.

On examination, pallor is of little help in judging the severity of bleeding. Bruises may be a clue to an underlying coagulopathy. Cutaneous or mucous membrane arteriovenous malformations may signal the presence of Rendu-Osler-Weber syndrome or von Willebrand's disease. Fever is rare in patients with GI bleeding unless infection coexists. Tachypnea can be an appropriate compensatory response to profound hemorrhage and resultant metabolic acidosis, the result of aspirating vomited blood, or a manifestation of anxiety alone. Likewise, tachycardia suggests volume depletion but may be present in patients with minimal volume loss. Assessment of intravascular volume status is best quickly gauged by examining the pulse and blood pressure response to postural change. A 20-mm Hg decrease in blood pressure when a patient is shifted from the supine to erect position indicates a 20% or greater loss of intravascular volume. Shock observed in the supine position suggests a 40% circulating volume loss. Stupor or coma can result from hypotension alone but often signals the presence of hepatic encephalopathy. In patients with altered mental status due to hepatic encephalopathy, the physical stigmata of cirrhosis (e.g., jaundice, palmar erythema, gynecomastia, ascites, ecchymoses, spider angiomata, caput medusa) are commonly present.

Regardless of bleeding source, at least two large-bore (16- to 14-gauge) peripheral intravenous catheters should be inserted to allow rapid fluid and blood administration. A central venous catheter is not always necessary. At the time of catheter insertion, blood should be obtained for analysis of hematocrit, electrolytes, creatinine, liver function tests, prothrombin time, and platelet count. Samples also should be sent for typing and cross-matching. The basic principles of support of the circulation and transfusion are presented in Chapters 3 and 14, respectively; however, a few points deserve emphasis. First, the major pathophysiologic defect in severe GI bleeding is intravascular volume depletion. Therefore, the best initial therapy is not vasopressor infusion but rather isotonic crystalloid replacement until blood is available. Colloid therapy offers no demonstrated advantage over crystalloid resuscitation, despite the fact that a smaller volume of the former is required to produce a similar degree of volume expansion. Colloids risk allergic reaction, are not always immediately available, and are substantially (10–100 times) more expensive than crystalloid for an equivalent degree of volume expansion. Blood replacement is best accomplished using specific component therapy with serial assessments of hematocrit, platelet count, and prothrombin time. Whole blood is unnecessary. Thrombocytopenia or soluble clotting factor deficiencies should be corrected rapidly to assist in achieving hemostasis. Reasonable targets for transfusion are a platelet count higher than 100,000/mm^3, a normal prothrombin time, and a hematocrit level of 30%. Higher standards for hematocrit may be appropriate in patients with ongoing critical oxygen supply problems, such as myocardial ischemia or stroke.

For most patients with upper GI bleeding, gentle placement of a nasogastric (NG) or orogastric (OG) tube is safe and useful to monitor the rate of bleeding. Although controversial, possible exceptions include patients with known or suspected esophageal varices or Mallory-Weiss tears in whom tube placement theoretically could aggravate bleeding. Patients with impaired liver function may benefit from purging intestinal blood that may precipitate hepatic encephalopathy, but blood is an excellent laxative, making other cathartics unnecessary. Gastric lavage does not decrease the rate of upper GI bleeding, even when the solution is cooled or fortified with norepinephrine. Furthermore, gastric lavage with water may induce hyponatremia, whereas saline may cause fluid overload.

LOCALIZING THE BLEEDING SITE

Examination of vomitus or gastric contents and the appearance of the stool greatly helps to localize the site of bleeding. If present, hematemesis is a reliable sign of upper GI bleeding. For patients without hematemesis, a nasogastric aspirate helps diagnose an upper GI site and assess activity of bleeding. An upper GI bleed is unlikely if the aspirate does not reveal fresh blood or at least "coffee ground" material, although as many as 15% of patients with upper GI bleeding have negative gastric aspirates. These "false–negative" aspirates usually occur when a competent pylorus prevents the gastric reflux of blood originating in the distal duodenum. Testing gastric contents for occult blood rarely is helpful or necessary and may produce false–positive results in patients who have recently eaten meat or who have an alkaline stomach pH.

Even though massive upper GI hemorrhage can produce bright red rectal bleeding, hematochezia originates from a lower site in more than 90% of cases. As little as 15 mL of blood in the upper GI tract may produce guaiac-positive stools, but melena (black, tarry stools formed by the digestion of blood by acid and bacteria) requires a loss of more than 100 mL of blood over a relatively brief period. Because blood in the gut speeds transit time, melena seldom results from lower GI bleeding unless it originates in the proximal (right) colon and is delayed in passage. More commonly, significant bleeding from the right colon produces maroon-colored stools, whereas bleeding from the left colon results in bright red blood emanating from the rectum. A mixture of formed stool with bright red blood is highly suggestive of a distal colonic (sigmoid colon or rectal) source. Once the general area of bleeding has been determined, specific diagnostic tests are indicated to isolate the exact site.

UPPER GI BLEEDING

A relatively small number of conditions are responsible for most cases of upper GI bleeding (Table 39.1). Peptic ulcer disease (gastric and duodenal ulcer) leads the list, followed closely by gastric and esophageal erosive disease and variceal bleeding. When an upper GI bleeding source is suspected on the basis of history and physical examination, making a definitive diagnosis usually is fairly straightforward. The typical evaluation is outlined in Figure 39.1. Fortunately, regardless of cause, upper GI bleeding stops spontaneously in most (70–80%) in most patients.

Esophagogastroduodenoscopy (EGD) is the initial procedure of choice to obtain a precise diagnosis, gain prognostic information, and possibly control bleeding. Early endoscopy (performed during or within 24 hours of bleeding cessation) has a high diagnostic yield. When a discrete amenable lesion is identified, endoscopic intervention can improve rebleeding and mortality rates. EGD is useful to: (*a*) definitively demonstrate a bleeding site; (*b*) identify esophageal varices; (*c*) predict the likelihood for rebleeding and, hence, the need for surgery; (*d*) permit endoscopic control of some bleeding lesions; (*e*) reduce operating room time by guiding a planned approach to a bleeding lesion preoperatively. EGD has several limitations, however: (*a*) an optimal examination requires patients to take nothing by mouth (NPO) for 6 hours; (*b*) rapid bleeding can obscure the view; (*c*) sedation may compromise ventilation in patients with borderline respiratory status; (*d*) the procedure proves dangerous as well as unre-

TABLE 39–1

SOURCES OF UPPER GI BLEEDING

Source	Approximate Frequency
Peptic ulcer disease	50%
Erosive gastritis–esophagitis	25%
Variceal bleeding	15%
Mallory-Weiss tears	5%
Others*	5–10%

* Carcinomas, vascular malformations, etc.

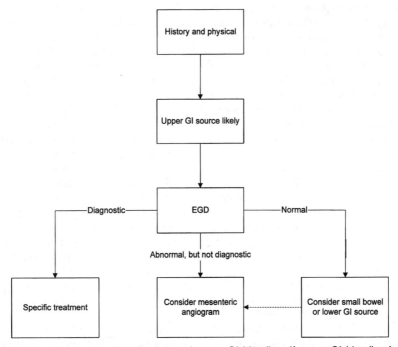

FIG. 39–1. Typical diagnostic evaluation of suspected upper GI bleeding. If upper GI bleeding is believed to be likely after obtaining a history and performing a physical examination, esophagogastroduodenoscopy (EGD) is usually performed. If EGD is diagnostic, therapy directed at the specific lesion should be instituted. For example, histamine blockers for ulcer disease. If the EGD is normal, the small bowel or lower GI tract should be considered as a bleeding source. When the EGD is abnormal but non-diagnostic, consideration should be given to mesenteric angiography which is sometimes diagnostic.

warding when a viscus perforates or the patient fails to cooperate.

Bipolar/multipolar electrocoagulation, heater probe coagulation, YAG laser therapy, and injection therapy using ethanol, epinephrine, or other sclerosants are four methods that can be used during EGD to terminate upper GI bleeding. Few comparative trials have been conducted using these techniques, but most data indicate that there is not one technique superior in efficacy or safety. Therefore, the technique used to halt bleeding is determined largely by the personal preference of the endoscopist.

If a technically satisfactory EGD fails to reveal a bleeding source, two possibilities exist: the bleeding lesion is beyond the reach of the endoscope (i.e., in the small bowel or colon) or bleeding from an upper GI site has stopped spontaneously. If no upper GI source for blood loss exists, evaluation of the lower GI tract is indicated; however, it is not prudent to hastily dismiss the possibility of an upper GI source even after "negative" EGD. More often than expected, bleeding from an esophageal varix goes unrecognized as volume depletion collapses the normally distended veins and spontaneously arrests hemorrhage. Often not until circulating volume is restored do patients again begin to bleed visibly.

When EGD fails to reveal a bleeding site but an upper GI source is still considered likely or when EGD is unable to define a specific lesion because of brisk bleeding, angiography probably is the next most useful procedure. Furthermore, angiography probably is the procedure of first choice to diagnose hemorrhage from the small bowel. During angiography, bleeding may be arrested by infusing vasoconstrictors or by placing embolizing material in the bleeding vessel.

In the evaluation of upper or lower GI bleeding, plain abdominal radiographs rarely help unless they demonstrate free air (indicating perforation of a viscus) or "thumbprinting" of the large bowel (suggesting ischemic colitis). Contrast upper GI series are no longer indicated for evaluation of acute upper GI bleeding because they are seldom diagnostic, revealing only gross anatomic features, but failing to show more subtle lesions (varices, gastritis, and Mallory-Weiss tears). Furthermore, even if the upper GI series detects an abnormality, it never directly confirms it as the bleeding site. Finally, swallowed barium compromises subsequent tests, including CT scanning, angiography, and colonoscopy, and makes surgery technically more difficult. Barium studies also require transport of potentially unstable patients to the radiography suite.

PREVENTION OF UPPER GASTROINTESTINAL BLEEDING

Over the last decade, the incidence of upper GI bleeding in the ICU has declined dramatically. Although this is partly the result of the widespread use of histamine blockers and other gastroprotective agents, many other practices that could contribute to the reduction in bleeding rates have also changed. For example, it is now recognized that enteral feeding helps maintain or restore enteric mucosal integrity and may decrease the risk of GI bleeding when compared to starvation or parenteral nutrition (TPN). It also has become clear that some medications have ulcerogenic potential for the stomach and small bowel and should be avoided in high-risk patients whenever possible. Examples include corticosteroids, slow-release potassium tablets, and aspirin or other nonsteroidal anti-inflammatory agents. Because hypotension also has been shown to be a potent reversible risk factor for mucosal ulceration and mesenteric ischemia, it is possible that more aggressive resuscitation practices are partly responsible for the reduced risk of bleeding.

Not all patients in the ICU require pharmacologic "ulcer prophylaxis;" however, routine prophylaxis probably is indicated for patients undergoing prolonged (>48 hours) mechanical ventilation, and for patients with coagulation disorders (e.g., thrombocytopenia, consumptive, hereditary, or pharmacologic coagulation disorders). For patients who are eating normally or receiving near-target rates of enteral tube feeding, gastric acid suppression probably adds risk and cost without potential benefit, especially for nonventilated patients. If mucosal protection or pharmacologic gastric acid buffering is indicated, histamine blockers, proton pump inhibitors, sucralfate, and antacids are available to accomplish the task. Histamine blockers and antacids have comparable effectiveness as long as the gastric pH is maintained greater than 4.0. Potential side effects of antacid therapy include diarrhea, phosphate binding, and (in patients with renal insufficiency) magnesium toxicity. Because sucralfate requires acid for dissolution and tissue binding, it is ineffective if administered concurrently with antacids or histamine blockers. There are no clinically significant differences in effectiveness of the currently available H_2-blocking drugs. When using histamine blockers, drug selection, route of administration, and dosing frequency can have a dramatic effect on cost. Because efficacy is equal, the least expensive histamine blocker should be chosen. Continuous intravenous infusions are expensive and not necessary to achieve protection—intermittent H_2 blocker injection is equally effective. In fact, most patients can have an H_2 blocker given intermittently via the nasogastric or orogastric tube, with equal efficacy to intravenous dosing. In general, the side effects of H_2 blockers include altered drug metabolism, thrombocytopenia, and central nervous system disturbances. The latter have been reported most commonly with cimetidine in elderly patients.

Although somewhat controversial, gastric acid suppression is associated with a modestly increased risk of nosocomial pneumonia as a result of gastric overgrowth of bacteria and subsequent aspiration. It seems that not only is gastric pH important, so are stomach volume and patient position. This is evidenced by the finding that the risk of nosocomial pneumonia is comparable when using histamine blockers or sucralfate but modestly higher when using large volumes of antacids. Clearly, the simplest and most effective measure to lower the risk of nosocomial pneumonia is to elevate the head of the bed to 30° for all patients who can tolerate such positioning. Doing so reduces the reflux of gastric contents and the potential for aspiration.

SPECIFIC CONDITIONS CAUSING UPPER GI BLEEDING

Peptic Ulcer Disease

One-half of all cases of upper GI bleeding in the ICU are due to peptic ulceration, even though bleeding is an uncommon initial manifestation. Most ambulatory patients with peptic ulcers relate a history of epigastric pain (particularly nocturnal) relieved by food, histamine blockers, or antacids. A similar history rarely is provided by patients in the ICU. As noted above, EGD is the diagnostic procedure of choice because it is safe, rapidly performed, and may facilitate control of bleeding with electrocoagulation or laser therapy. Even in situations in which bleeding cannot be controlled, information gained from the endoscopy permits precise planning of a definitive surgical procedure.

The overall risk of recurrent bleeding from peptic ulcer disease approaches 20 to 30%, but certain

TABLE 39–2

RISK OF RECURRENT UPPER GI BLEEDING BASED ON ENDOSCOPIC FINDINGS

Endoscopic Finding	Approximate Risk of Rebleeding
Visible spurting vessel	~100%
Active oozing	30–80%
Nonbleeding vessel	50%
Esophageal varices	50%
Red or black "spot"	5–10%
Clean ulcer base	1%

specific endoscopic findings portend a higher risk, suggesting that more aggressive or earlier intervention is indicated. Visualization of persistent active bleeding from a visible vessel mandates endoscopic, angiographic, or surgical intervention because of the almost certain risk of continued or recurrent hemorrhage. When a nonbleeding vessel is seen in an ulcer crater, the risk of rebleeding may be as high as 80%, suggesting that surgical intervention probably is indicated. Visualization of an adherent clot overlying an ulcer crater predicts rebleeding in as many as one in three patients, whereas a lesion oozing blood without a visible vessel has only about a 10% risk of bleeding. Flat pigmented spots or smooth ulcer bases carry a low (1–10%) risk of rebleeding and therefore usually are not treated. The risks of rebleeding associated with various endoscopic findings are summarized in Table 39.2. Location of the ulcer may also provide an indication of the likelihood of rebleeding. Ulcers high on the lesser gastric curvature (over the left gastric artery) and on the posterior–inferior wall of the duodenum (overlying the gastroduodenal artery) are the most ominous.

Fortunately, most gastric and duodenal peptic ulcers stop bleeding spontaneously with supportive care and control of gastric pH and do not require endoscopic or surgical therapy. Persistent severe hemorrhage should prompt consideration of endoscopic intervention, surgery, or angiographic occlusion.

Stress Ulceration

Erosive gastritis–esophagitis or gastric stress ulceration—is the second most common cause of GI bleeding in the ICU and is particularly common in critically ill patients with respiratory failure, sepsis, hypotension, or burns. Although "superficial,'' stress ulceration may result in severe bleeding, particularly in patients with underlying coagulopathy. These erosions result from the combined actions of acid, ulcerogenic drugs, and ischemia on mucosal surfaces, typically developing 5 to 7 days after admission to the ICU. Histamine blockers, omeprazole, antacids, and sucralfate all can reduce the incidence of stress ulceration, but the best preventative measures are avoidance of hypotension and hypoxia and early provision of enteral nutrition. For unclear reasons, the incidence of gastric stress ulceration seems to be decreasing.

Mallory-Weiss Tears

Forceful retching may disrupt the mucosa of the gastroesophageal (GE) junction, resulting in a Mallory-Weiss tear. These lacerations of the mucosa account for at least 5 to 10% of all upper GI bleeding and are much more common in men than in women. Precipitating or contributing factors include (*a*) alcohol usage, (*b*) intractable vomiting, and (*c*) food impaction within the esophagus. Rarely, coughing, seizures, heavy lifting, pregnancy, and upper GI endoscopy have been associated with such lesions. Interestingly, no precipitating cause is determined in approximately 20% of cases. Even though these lesions commonly lead to massive hemorrhage, bleeding almost always stops spontaneously. The diagnosis is suggested by a history of forceful, painless hematemesis and is confirmed by EGD demonstrating linear tears on the gastric side of the GE junction. (Because of the small size of the tears, an upper GI series usually is unrevealing.) Supportive treatment includes antiemetics, control of gastric pH, and expectant observation. EGD is an important diagnostic test because balloon tamponade (directed at presumed variceal bleeding) may splay the mucosa, extending the laceration and aggravating the bleeding. In the rare instance in which bleeding does not abate spontaneously, EGD with

electrocoagulation, therapeutic injection, or laser coagulation can halt bleeding. Surgery to control hemorrhage rarely is necessary unless the tear involves preexisting esophageal varices.

Portal Hypertension and Variceal Bleeding

Varices are fragile, bulbous venous channels that shunt portal blood to the systemic circuit in an attempt to circumvent portal hypertension. These native shunts usually are the result of cirrhosis induced by ethanol or viral hepatitis, but portal hypertension has many potential causes, spanning the anatomic spectrum from the portal to hepatic vein (Table 39.3). The largest of these collateral channels tend to form at the gastroesophageal junction; however, hemorrhoidal and retroperitoneal veins also may dilate and bleed. As many as 40% of all patients with cirrhosis eventually develop variceal hemorrhage characterized by abrupt, painless, massive upper GI bleeding. The history of such patients often is remarkably similar to that of patients with Mallory-Weiss tears.

The risk of bleeding roughly correlates with the size of the varices, the severity of the underlying liver disease, and the magnitude of the hepatic venous pressure gradient. (Bleeding is uncommon when the pressure gradient is less than 12 mm Hg.) The hemorrhage of variceal bleeding often is difficult to treat because of accompanying coagulation abnormalities. In this patient group, soluble clotting factor disorders are common as a result of malnutrition or impaired hepatic synthetic function. Furthermore, the direct toxic effects of ethanol on the bone marrow and portal-hypertension-induced hypersplenism often result in thrombocytopenia. The acute mortality of variceal bleeding approaches 50%. Even when the initial hemorrhage ceases, variceal bleeding recurs in at least 50% of patients, many times within just a few weeks of the initial hemorrhage. Because patients with varices tend to be chronically ill with impaired clotting, immune, and renal function, it is not surprising that

TABLE 39–3

CAUSES OF PORTAL HYPERTENSION

Extrahepatic	Intrahepatic	Sinusoidal	Hepatic Vein
Portal vein thrombosis	Schistosomiasis	Cirrhosis	Budd-Chiari syndrome
Congenital			Veno-occlusive disease
Septic			
Traumatic			
Malignancy			

nearly two-thirds of patients die within 12 months of the first bleeding episode.

Treatment

Because 30 to 40% of all bleeding episodes in patients with known esophageal varices originate in nonvariceal sources (e.g., ulcers, Mallory-Weiss tears, etc.), it is important to determine the bleeding site before instituting definitive therapy. Obviously, hemodynamic stabilization and stomach evacuation must be achieved before diagnostic procedures are attempted. As with all massive GI bleeding, fluid resuscitation, hemoglobin maintenance, and correction of coagulation abnormalities are key components of therapy. For patients with variceal bleeding, some clinicians preferentially use vasopressors over fluid replacement to restore mean arterial pressure, theorizing that the hepatic vein/portal pressure gradient will be reduced and thus the risk of hemorrhage will be lowered. Unfortunately, no human data exist to support this contention and volume depletion can result in hypoperfusion of other vital organ systems. Similarly, there is no evidence that gentle NG tube insertion aggravates variceal bleeding; however, such tubes may induce esophagitis and gastric erosion if left in place for prolonged periods. The accumulation of massive ascites can contribute to an increased hepatic vein/portal vein pressure gradient. Therefore, for some patients, large-volume paracentesis can be a useful adjunct to reduce the driving pressure for hemorrhage. Aspiration pneumonitis also is extremely common in patients with variceal bleeding because of depressed mental status, massive vomiting, and esophageal instrumentation with scopes and tubes. Avoiding oral feeding in stuporous patients and elevating the head of the bed are sensible. For many patients, early ''prophylactic'' intubation is reasonable to avoid massive aspiration.

When airway and circulatory stability have been achieved and variceal bleeding is confirmed, six methods are available to control the bleeding: pharmacotherapy, variceal tamponade, variceal obliteration, decompressive shunting, devascularization, and liver transplantation. One commonly used plan to gain control of variceal hemorrhage is outlined in Figure 39.2.

Pharmacotherapy

Vasopressin, a splanchnic vasoconstrictor, often initially gains control of variceal bleeding by decreasing portal blood flow through hepatic and collateral vascular channels, but it is not known whether vasopressin lowers the incidence of rebleeding. (Initial bleeding control can be obtained in more than 50% of cases using vasopressin, but as many as 10% of patients will have potentially lethal side effects from the therapy.) Vasopressin usually is administered as a continuous intravenous infusion of 0.2 to 0.8 units per minute, given in a peripheral vein and continued 24 hours after clinical bleeding has stopped. Direct administration into a bleeding visceral artery may be useful for patients with diverticular or peptic ulcer hemorrhage but offers no advantage for variceal bleeding. Vasopressin-associated complications include arrhythmias (especially bradycardia), myocardial and mesenteric ischemia, congestive heart failure, stroke, and renal insufficiency. Randomized trials suggest that the addition of nitroglycerin to vasopressin not only improves the success rate of bleeding control but also reduces the risk of vasopressin-induced complications. In this setting, nitroglycerin is best administered by constant intravenous infusion at a starting dose of 40 μg/minute, which is then titrated upward to achieve a target systolic blood pressure of 90 to 100 mm Hg. Unfortunately, neither vasopressin alone nor in combination with nitroglycerin has been demonstrated to reduce the mortality rate of this highly lethal condition.

Somatostatin and octreotide, its synthetic analog, are promising splanchnic vasoconstrictors that inhibit release of gastrointestinal hormones. Initial trials have shown a superior rate of bleeding control using these agents compared to vasopressin, but decreased renal perfusion, reduced systemic vascular resistance, and decreased gut motility suggest that further study is necessary before they should be accepted widely. Like vasopressin, somatostatin has not been proven to reduce mortality.

Propranolol has been used chronically to decrease portal blood flow and portal pressure, reducing the risk of variceal rebleeding in cirrhosis by as much as 50% during the first year of therapy. Although propranolol may decrease rebleeding episodes in patients with varices, β-blockade blunts compensatory cardiovascular responses and therefore should not be used to treat active variceal bleeding.

Variceal Tamponade

Balloon tamponade controls esophageal bleeding in 70 to 90% of patients, many of whom are

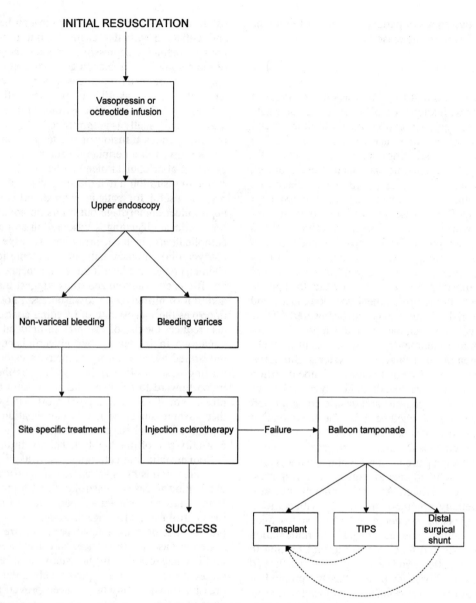

INITIAL RESUSCITATION

Vasopressin or
octreotide infusion

Upper endoscopy

Non-variceal bleeding

Bleeding varices

Site specific treatment

Injection sclerotherapy ──Failure──▶ Balloon tamponade

SUCCESS

Transplant

TIPS

Distal
surgical
shunt

FIG. 39–2. One plan for managing variceal bleeding. After initial stabilization, an infusion of the vasoconstrictors vasopressin or octreotide may reduce or control variceal hemorrhage. In most cases upper endoscopy is then performed to confirm a variceal bleeding source. If varices are bleeding, injection sclerotherapy is utilized to prevent recurrent hemorrhage. If the combination of a vasoconstrictor infusion and endoscopic injection fails to control hemorrhage, balloon tamponade followed by a procedure (transplant or shunt) to directly lower portal pressures may be considered.

refractory to other modalities. Unfortunately, because balloon tamponade can only be used for 72 hours, all patients treated with balloon tamponade need immediate consideration of definitive therapy at the time the tube is inserted. Unfortunately, one-half of all patients treated with tamponade re-

bleed on decompression. Currently, a four-lumen device with gastric and esophageal balloons (e.g., the Minnesota tube) is preferred over the three-lumen Sengstaken-Blakemore tube because it enables the evacuation of the proximal esophagus, possibly reducing the risk of aspiration.

The Minnesota tube is inserted through the mouth into the stomach. Appropriate positioning of the gastric balloon is then checked by radiograph before inflation to prevent fatal esophageal rupture. In emergent situations, the tube may be passed a minimum of 50 cm before the gastric balloon is inflated to 100 mL. Any evidence of patient discomfort indicates potential esophageal positioning. If the 100-mL gastric balloon inflation is well tolerated, the balloon should be inflated to 400 to 450 mL and then placed on gentle traction against the gastroesophageal junction. (Tension usually is maintained by taping the tube to a football helmet placed on the patient.) The esophageal balloon should be inflated only if bleeding continues with the gastric balloon inflated, and then only to a maximum pressure of 40 mm Hg. Upon completion of this inflation sequence, it is crucial to confirm the proper configuration by radiograph. The tube should be kept in place for at least 24 hours after cessation of bleeding but no longer than 72 hours. Without meticulous technique and monitoring, complications occur in a high percentage of patients who undergo balloon tamponade. Aspiration remains the most frequent complication despite recent modifications of tube design. It is so frequent that many physicians advocate "prophylactic" endotracheal intubation before insertion of a Minnesota or Blakemore tube. Cephalad migration may produce upper airway obstruction, a catastrophic event for the patient whose airway is unsecured. (Scissors should be kept at the bedside for immediate tube transection if airway obstruction occurs.) Esophagogastric rupture, another devastating complication, usually results from improper tube placement and inflation of the gastric balloon in the esophagus. Pressure necrosis of the nose, mouth, and gastroesophageal mucosa also are common.

Variceal Obliteration

Endoscopy with variceal injection of a sclerosing agent (injection sclerotherapy) has become the procedure of choice for variceal bleeding because it at least temporarily controls the hemorrhage in more than 90% of cases. During the procedure, the varices or surrounding tissue are injected with a small volume of chemical sclerosant. Injection sclerotherapy has a lowered rate of early rebleeding (20–30%) versus 50 to 60% for balloon tamponade and offers a better short-term survival rate. Sclerotherapy also reduces transfusion require-

ments and is less dangerous than emergent surgical shunting. (Overall, long-term survival is similar in groups treated by injection sclerotherapy or shunting, however.) After the control of acute bleeding, repeated sclerotherapy may obliterate the dilated vessels and reduce the incidence of late rebleeding. There is no significant difference in efficacy or complication rates among the various sclerosing agents currently available, although a 1 to 3% solution of sodium tetradecyl sulfate is used most commonly. Minor complications (fever, chest pain, and tachycardia) occur in almost one-half of all patients. Major complications of sclerotherapy occur in 15 to 40% of patients and include (a) aspiration; (b) pulmonary dysfunction (acute respiratory distress syndrome [ARDS]) secondary to aspiration, sepsis, or sclerosants; and (c) local esophageal problems, including ulceration, perforation, stricture, dysmotility, and abscess formation. A rare complication, perforation of the esophagus, may produce empyema, mediastinitis, or mediastinal hematoma. Occasionally, sclerotherapy incites bacteremia.

Unfortunately, sclerotherapy is not uniformly successful for esophageal varices and generally is not effective for gastric varices. After controlling the acute bleeding episode, more than 90% of patients undergoing sclerotherapy eventually will rebleed unless repeated sclerotherapy is performed until the varices are obliterated. Repetitive sclerotherapy may reduce long-term mortality from variceal bleeding by approximately 25%, an effect that is comparable to long-term administration of propranolol. An alternative that seems to be equally effective to injection sclerotherapy is endoscopic variceal ligation, in which tight constrictive bands are placed around the bases of the varices, causing them to thrombose and slough off.

Decompressive Shunting

Both surgical and nonsurgical options are now available to control variceal bleeding by lowering the hepatic–portal vein pressure gradient. These decompressive shunts target GI bleeding and are best performed in patients with good hepatic parenchymal function and those patients considered to be future candidates for liver transplantation. No shunting procedure results in an improvement in hepatic function; therefore, all variants represent poor choices for patients with severely impaired liver function.

Most widely employed of the "nonsurgical"

options is the transjugular, intrahepatic, portosystemic shunt (TIPS). In this procedure, a needle is forced from the hepatic vein to the portal vein, through which a guide wire is placed. Expandable stents are then passed over the guidewire and dilated until the portohepatic pressure gradient is lowered to an acceptable level. This form of "intrahepatic" shunt at least temporarily lowers the distending pressure for the gastroesophageal varices. The long-term patency and risk:benefit ratio of TIPS is not yet known. Therefore, although TIPS cannot yet be widely advocated, it may stem bleeding in high-risk patients who are not amenable or responsive to injection sclerotherapy. The TIPS procedure probably is best viewed as a "bridge" to liver transplant, not a permanent solution to the problem of portal hypertension. Therefore, nontransplant candidates do not represent good TIPS candidates.

Surgical shunts may be classified as total or "selective," based on the degree of blood flow diverted around the liver. Total shunts, such as portocaval and mesocaval shunts, provide a decompressive anastomosis of a portion of the portal vein to the inferior vena cava. The size and position of the anastomosed vessels determines the vascular pressure and blood flow through the liver. When large, such shunts divert nearly all portal blood flow from the liver, resulting in a high risk of hepatic encephalopathy and liver failure. Smaller shunts reduce this risk but may fail to lower the portohepatic gradient sufficiently to avert bleeding.

More selective procedures, such as the distal splenorenal or Warren shunt, decompress portal circulation by joining the splenic and left renal vein. Selective shunts better preserve hepatic perfusion while decreasing portal pressure and varix diameter, thereby reducing bleeding risk. In experienced centers, selective shunts are the preferred operations for elective decompression but are time consuming and therefore not feasible in unstable patients. Unfortunately, selective shunts do not improve long-term survival; however, they do change the cause of death from GI hemorrhage to encephalopathy and liver failure. Surgical shunting procedures do not preclude consideration of liver transplant at a later time.

Devascularization

Variceal bleeding also can be arrested by techniques that devascularize the varices. This extensive operation usually involves splenectomy, gastric and esophageal devascularization, and esophageal transection. Even though interruption of the esophagus or stomach is transiently effective at controlling variceal bleeding, portal pressure remains elevated and bleeding elsewhere often becomes a problem. Furthermore, esophageal transection represents a radical lifestyle change that is unacceptable for many patients.

Liver Transplant

Although liver transplantation corrects portal hypertension, the primary indication for transplantation is hepatic failure, not variceal bleeding. Therefore, hepatic transplant should be reserved for stable patients with parenchymal liver failure. Patients with good hepatic reserve (Childs A) should first be considered for a selective shunt procedure before liver transplant. Patients with the more severe Childs C disease who lack other contra-indications may be considered for liver transplant. Liver transplantation is a complex and expensive procedure that carries a significant risk of rejection and opportunistic infection secondary to the required immunosuppression.

Aortoenteric Fistulas

On rare occasion, prosthetic aortic grafts may erode into the GI tract, causing massive hemorrhage. Exsanguination often follows a moderate to large "herald" bleed that stops spontaneously. Aortoenteric fistulas usually occur in the distal duodenum and occasionally cause pulsatile bleeding from the mouth or nasogastric tube. Endoscopy and aortography are the only methods currently available to establish this diagnosis but rarely can be accomplished before death. Immediate laparotomy should be undertaken in patients with a confirmed diagnosis or intractable bleeding otherwise unexplained in a predisposed patient.

Vascular Malformations

Angiodysplasia is the most common form of enteric vascular abnormality, a category that also includes arteriovenous malformations (AVMs) and vascular telangiectasia. Although angiodysplasia occurs most commonly in the large bowel, it is a common cause of upper GI bleeding in patients with renal failure, aortic stenosis, and von Willebrand's disease. Angiodysplasia is second only to erosive gastritis as a cause of bleeding in patients with renal failure. Most microvascular malformations involving the upper GI tract are located in the duodenum. The diagnosis must be made by angiography or by EGD. (EGD diagnosis can be difficult because of the small size of most of these lesions, but when located, they can be ablated by laser, heat, or electrocoagulation.)

Miscellaneous Causes of Upper GI Bleeding

Hemobilia, a rare cause of upper GI bleeding, occurs when hepatic blood drains via the bile ducts into the duodenum. Hemobilia may be due to tumor involvement of the bile ducts or liver but most commonly follows blunt chest or abdominal trauma. Hemobilia should also be suspected in patients with pancreatitis and those having recently undergone ERCP. The triad of abdominal pain, jaundice, and upper GI bleeding should prompt consideration of this condition. Hemobilia is seldom massive and spontaneously resolves in most cases.

Although pancreatic disease is an unusual primary cause of upper GI bleeding, hemorrhage may occur when pseudocysts or pancreatic tumors erode the posterior duodenal wall. Patients with acute pancreatitis frequently bleed from gastritis, ulcers, Mallory-Weiss tears, or esophageal varices unrelated to their pancreatitis. Coagulation disorders that accompany pancreatitis worsen the bleeding tendency.

THE ROLE OF SURGERY

Unfortunately, those most in need of surgery often are the worst operative candidates because of their limited tolerance of anemia and hypotension. For patients with ulcer-related upper GI bleeding who are not good surgical candidates, consideration should be given to endoscopic injection of epinephrine and to laser or thermal coagulation. Angiography with embolization or selective vasopressin infusion also may be helpful if general anesthesia must be avoided. Several indications prompt surgical intervention in upper GI bleeding: (a) a visible or spurting vessel in the base of an ulcer crater, even if initially controlled by nonsurgical means; (b) brisk hemorrhage from a lesion that perforates a GI viscus; (c) massive ongoing blood losses from any source (more than 1500 mL or 6–10 units of blood in the first 24 hours).

TABLE 39–4

CAUSES OF SIGNIFICANT LOWER GASTROINTESTINAL BLEEDING

Condition	Approximate Frequency
Angiomas	35%
Polyps — carcinoma	15%
Upper GI source	15%
Other — miscellaneous	15%
Diverticular disease	10%
Unknown	10%
Ischemic and inflammatory colitis	5%

LOWER GI BLEEDING

If history and examination suggest lower GI hemorrhage, the diagnostic approach should vary with the severity of bleeding and whether or not bleeding is ongoing. Hemorrhage from a lower GI source tends to be less profuse and intermittent and can arise from sources over a much larger anatomic area than that of upper GI bleeding. Therefore, the site of lower GI bleeding often is more difficult to diagnose with certainty. The most common causes of significant lower GI bleeding and their frequency are shown in Table 39.4. Several points deserve emphasis: a significant proportion (perhaps 10–15%) of ''lower GI'' bleeding actually is the result of blood flowing downstream from an upper GI source. This is in distinct contrast to upper GI bleeding, which rarely arises from the lower GI tract. Angiomatous disease leads the list of bleeding sources, being almost twice as likely as the next most common etiologies, polyps and neoplasms. Finally, in contrast to upper GI hemorrhage, which is almost always accurately and rapidly diagnosed, lower tract bleeding remains undiagnosed in 10 to 15% of patients. Fortunately, most lower GI bleeding episodes (nearly 80%) spontaneously cease. Unfortunately, rebleeding occurs in as many as 25% of patients.

THE DIAGNOSTIC APPROACH

The diagnostic evaluation of lower GI bleeding is significantly more difficult than that for upper GI hemorrhage. One suggested schema for the evaluation of lower GI bleeding is presented in the Figure 39.3, and specific diagnostic tests are discussed below.

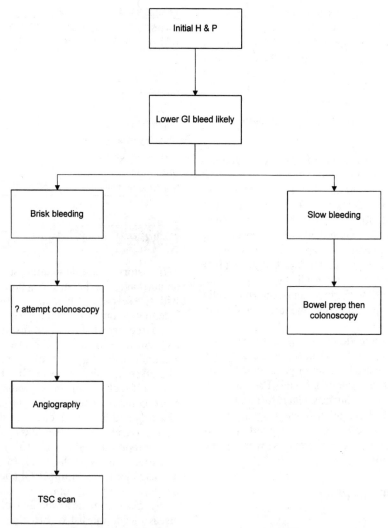

FIG. 39–3. Typical evaluation of suspected lower GI bleeding. When history and physical examination reveal lower GI bleeding to be likely, the diagnostic sequence is often dictated by the rate of bleeding. When bleeding is slow, a thorough bowel preparation followed by colonoscopy is most likely to yield a diagnosis. When bleeding is brisk, angiography or technetium sulfur colloid scan (TSC) are often diagnostic where colonoscopy fails.

Colonoscopy

Colonoscopy following thorough bowel preparation (oral purging) probably is the diagnostic procedure with the highest yield for lower GI bleeding. A bedside procedure, colonoscopy, reveals a bleeding site in one-half to three-fourths of all cases of lower GI bleeding, and if not diagnostic, does not preclude subsequent diagnostic procedures. Unfortunately, the volume of colonic blood and lack of purging before emergent colonoscopy often precludes an adequate examination.

Because visualization often is impaired severely, perforation of the colon is more likely in this setting. If no diagnosis is reached after colonoscopy and bleeding continues briskly or recurs, a nuclear medicine scan or angiogram should be considered. A tagged red blood cell (RBC) scan or angiogram are at least as likely to yield a diagnosis as colonoscopy when bleeding is active.

Angiography

A diagnostic angiogram requires a skilled radiologist, a cooperative patient, and a relatively rapidly bleeding lesion. To demonstrate extravasation of contrast, patients must be bleeding at a rate 0.5 mL/minute or more. Success rates for detection of bleeding sites vary widely, depending on patient characteristics, the angiographer's experience, and the source of bleeding. Advantages of angiography include localization of bleeding when positive, the ability to be performed on the unprepared bowel, and the option of injecting emboli or vasoconstrictors to halt hemorrhage. The combined incidence of allergic dye reactions, contrast-induced renal failure, vascular perforation, and cholesterol embolization from this procedure is approximately 10%, even in experienced centers.

GI Bleeding Scans

Nuclear scans are more helpful than endoscopy or arteriography in detecting intermittent lower bleeding. Three tests used to detect GI bleeding include the technetium-sulphur colloid (TSC) scan, the technetium-labeled RBC scan, and the Meckel's scan.

Meckel's diverticuli may be localized using a radioactive tracer secreted by ectopic gastric mucosa lining the diverticulum. Although highly sensitive and specific, false-positive Meckel's scans are seen in non-fasting patients and in those with large arteriovenous malformations.

TSC studies are accomplished by rapidly scanning the abdomen after injection of a radioactive tracer that has a very short (3 minute) circulating life. The abdomen is then examined to look for "puddling" of tracer at the site of bleeding. TSC scanning requires active bleeding to occur at the time the radioactive material is injected. Although the technique can localize as little as 0.5 ml/minute bleeding, it is diagnostic in only about 10% of cases. With a longer half-life than technetium, tagged red cell scans allow repeated scanning for up to 24 hours, a feature that may be particularly useful in patients with intermittent bleeding. Because of its superior sensitivity, RBC labeled scans are usually preferred to TSC scans.

Imprecision is the major problem with all radionuclide scanning. Therefore, although the general region of GI bleeding may be confirmed, precise localization usually requires endoscopy or arteriography. In addition, some tracers concentrate in the liver and spleen, while others are secreted into the gut lumen, obscuring underlying bleeding sites or resulting in "false positive" studies. False positive scans may be minimized by using continuous nasogastric (NG) suction to rid the stomach of secreted radionuclide. About half of all positive studies are diagnostic within minutes. Nonetheless, these tests may be time consuming, occasionally requiring 6–18 hours for definitive results. Delayed scanning (at 24 hours) improves sensitivity but decreases specificity because of the gastric secretion of isotopes. A second major disadvantage of nuclear scans is the frequent need for repeated trips from the ICU to the nuclear medicine department with the associated risks and costs. An obvious major advantage of nuclear scans is that no bowel preparation is necessary.

Barium Enema

The barium enema is not a useful test in active lower GI bleeding because it only grossly defines colonic structure. Therefore, while contrast may demonstrate inflammatory bowel disease, diverticulosis, or colon carcinoma it does not prove any of these to be the source of bleeding, and these studies lack the resolution necessary to define angiodysplasia or rectal ulceration.

SPECIFIC CONDITIONS CAUSING LOWER GI BLEEDING

Angiodysplasia

Most angiodysplastic lesions never bleed and are incidental findings in the elderly at the time of colonoscopy. There are no unique historical features that distinguish angiodysplastic from diverticular bleeding. However, the venous bleeding of angiodysplasia is usually less severe than the arterial bleeding of diverticulosis. The previously reported association of aortic stenosis murmurs with angiodysplasia is probably not significant. Like diverticular bleeding, angiodysplastic bleeding almost always spontaneously stops, but recurs even more commonly (25–50%) than diverticular bleeding. Like diverticular bleeding, angiodysplastic hemorrhage most frequently originates in the right colon and terminal ileum. Colonoscopy can detect bleeding angiodysplastic lesions in 70–80% of cases when the colon is optimally prepared. Angiography less reliably displays vascular malformations (35–70%) and, unfortunately, confirms hemorrhage much less often. Because of the high incidence of rebleeding, endoscopic electrocoagulation, laser ablation or surgical removal of the involved portion of colon should be considered if hemorrhaging angiodysplastic vessels are demonstrated.

Polyps and Colon Carcinoma

Colon carcinoma more commonly produces slow, continuous blood loss than massive GI hemorrhage. It is left colonic and rectal neoplasms that are most likely to cause gross bleeding. Premonitory symptoms include a change in bowel habits, melena, and crampy abdominal pain, with or without weight loss. Sequential rectal examination, and colonoscopy are likely to reveal the cancerous site of blood loss.

Diverticulosis

Diverticulosis is generally a disease of patients over the age of 40 years. Although diverticular disease accounts for a substantial percentage of guaiac positive stools, only 10–15% of significant lower GI bleeding episodes can be attributed to diverticuli. Diverticular bleeding is sudden in onset, painless in nature, and usually self limited, but it recurs in 10–25% of patients. Although most diverticuli arise in the left colon, usually diverticular bleeding originates from the right side (50–70%). Interestingly, diverticular bleeding does not usually occur in patients with acute diverticulitis (characterized by fever and lower abdominal pain). Angiography demonstrates the site of active bleeding in $\frac{1}{2}$–$\frac{3}{4}$ of cases and offers the therapeutic option of intra-arterial vasopressin infusion. The barium enema is rarely helpful, and the value of colonoscopy is usually compromised by large amounts of colonic blood and stool in the unprepared patient. The value of tagged RBC studies varies with the severity of bleeding, and even when localized to the colon, such studies do not distinguish between diverticular disease, angiodysplasia and carcinoma.

Other Causes of Lower GI Bleeding

Ischemic colitis and bowel infarction due to mesenteric thrombosis or embolism may produce mucosal sloughing, bowel necrosis, and lower GI bleeding (see Chapter 37, The Acute Abdomen). Significant blood loss in ischemic colitis is unusual, and most episodes stop spontaneously. The splenic flexure and descending colon are the most common sites. Inflammatory bowel disease may cause massive lower GI bleeding in the young. In such patients bloody diarrhea is commonly super-imposed upon chronic, crampy abdominal pain. The diagnosis is by colonoscopy and therapy is medical unless massive persistent hemorrhage necessitates colectomy. Rectal ulcers are another rare but potentially fatal cause of massive lower GI bleeding occurring most frequently in patients with chronic renal failure. Rectal varices can produce massive hematochezia in patients with portal hypertension.

LOWER GI BLEEDING THERAPY

In lower GI bleeding only a small minority (~20%) of patients need any sort of intervention to stop bleeding. Colonoscopy using laser or heated probe coagulation can almost always stop bleeding following polypectomy; often stops the bleeding of angiodysplasia; and occasionally controls the bleeding of diverticulosis. Complications include perforation and exacerbation of the bleeding.

Angiographic techniques to stop lower GI bleeding include intra-arterial vasopressin infusion and embolization. Vasopressin is effective in approximately 90% of episodes of angiodysplasia or diverticulosis. Such therapy leads to a 5–15% complication rate and a ~50% incidence of rebleeding. In non-surgical candidates who fail vasopressin, intraarterial embolization using small distal gel-foam plugs may terminate the bleeding. Embolization via angiographic catheter or selective infusion of vasopressin may be temporarily helpful in patients with diverticular or angiodysplastic lesions. Because of the high incidence of rebleeding in angiodysplasia, however, resection is usually recommended.

In patients with massive lower GI bleeding of undetermined origin, exploratory laparotomy will identify the bleeding site in only $\frac{1}{3}$ of cases. If the bleeding site cannot be found at the time of laparotomy, a right hemicolectomy is usually favored because both bleeding diverticuli and angiodysplastic lesions are more common there. Emergent blind segmental resection of the colon is associated with a mortality rate of 30–40%, with a similar chance of rebleeding. Localization of the bleeding site by angiography or colonoscopy reduces mortality to < 10% and minimizes the risk of rebleeding. Because of the operative risks of emergent colectomy, resection should be considered only for patients with massive bleeding who fail angiography and embolization, patients with numerous angiodysplastic lesions, and patients with angiodysplasia who fail electrocoagulation therapy.

KEY POINTS

1. Prophylactic treatments can reduce the incidence of upper gastrointestinal bleeding in patients at high risk (e.g., chronic mechanical ventilation, coagulation disorders). Prophylactic methods include acid suppression or neutralization, or gastric mucosal coating. The best prophylaxis, however seems to be maintenance of good splanchnic perfusion and provision of enteral feeding as early as tolerated.

2. Upper GI bleeds are usually readily distinguished from lower tract bleeds by simple history and physical examination. Vomiting blood is a highly reliable sign of upper Gi bleeding, whereas hematochezia may result from an upper or lower source.

3. EGD provides a rapid, safe, and precise method to diagnose the source of upper GI bleeding, offers several therapeutic options (injection therapy, heater probe or multi-polar coagulation), and provides useful prognostic information regarding the risk of rebleeding.

4. With the possible exception of varices and ulcers containing visible vessels, most GI bleeding ceases spontaneously; hence, therapy is supportive.

5. Significant lower GI bleeding is less common than bleeding from an upper source. If the bowel can be evacuated, colonoscopy provides an etiologic diagnosis in a majority of cases. With briskly bleeding lower GI lesions, angiography or tagged red blood cell scans offer other good diagnostic options.

SUGGESTED READINGS

1. Aboujaoude MM, Grant DR, Ghent CN, et al. Effect of porta systemic shunts on subsequent transplantation of the liver. Surg Gynecol Obstet 1991;172:215–219.
2. Agusti A, Roca J, Bosch J, et al. The lung in patients with cirrhosis. J Hepatol 1988;10:251–257.
3. Alexandrino PT, Alves MM, Pinto Correia J. Propranolol or endoscopic sclerotherapy in the prevention of recurrence of variceal bleeding. A prospective, randomized controlled trial. J Hepatol 1988;7:175–185.
4. ASGE Publication. The role of endoscopy in the patient with lower gastrointestinal bleeding: guidelines for clinical application. Gastrointest Endosc 1988;34:23S.
5. Athanasoulis CA, Baum SAR, Rosch J, et al. Mesenteric arterial infusions of vasopressin for hemorrhage from colonic diverticulosis. Am J Surg 1975;129:212.
6. Bismuth H, Adam R, Mathur S, et al. Options for elective treatment of portal hypertension in cirrhotic patients in the transplantation era. Am J Surg 1990;160:105–110.
7. Bornman PC, Theodorou NA, Suttleworth RD, et al. Importance of hypovolemic shock and endoscopic signs in predicting recurrent hemorrhage for peptic ulceration: a prospective evaluation. Br Med J 1985;291:245.
8. Bosch J, Groszmann RJ, Groszmann RJ, et al. Association of transdermal nitroglycerin to vasopressin infusion in the treatment of variceal hemorrhage: a placebo-controlled trial. Hepatology 1989;10:962–968.
9. Brandt LJ, Boley SJ. The role of colonoscopy in the diagnosis and management of lower intestinal bleeding. Scand J Gastroenterol 1984;19(Suppl 102):61.
10. Browder W, Cerise EJ, Litwin MS. Impact of emergency angiography in massive lower gastrointestinal bleeding. Ann Surg 1986;204:530.
11. Bubrick MP, Lundeen JW, Onstad GR, et al. Mallory-Weiss syndrome: analysis of fifty-nine cases. Surgery 1980;88:400.
12. Buchman TG, Bulkley GB. Current management of patients with liver gastrointestinal bleeding. Surg Clin North Am 1987;67:651.
13. Bunker SR, Lull RJ, Tanaseco DE, et al. Scintigraphy of gastrointestinal hemorrhage. Am J Radiol 1984;143:543.
14. Carson J, Strom B, Soper L, et al. The association of nonsteroidal anti-inflammatory drugs with upper gastrointestinal tract bleeding. Arch Intern Med 1987;147:85–90.
15. Chung SCS, Leung JWC, Lo KK, et al. Natural history of the sentinel clot. An endoscopic study. Gastroenterology 1990;98:A31.
16. DeFelice C. Endoscopic injection treatments in patients with shock and gastrointestinal bleeding or stigma of recent hemorrhage. Endoscopy 1987;18:1985.
17. Gomes AS, Lois JF, McCoy RD. Angiographic treatment of gastrointestinal hemorrhage: comparison of vasopressin infusion and embolization. Am J Roentgenol 1986;146:1031.
18. Gupta PK, Fleisher DE. Nonvariceal upper gastrointestinal bleeding. Med Clin North Am 1993;77:973–992.
19. Helmich GA, Stallworth JR, Brown JJ. Angiodysplasia: characterization, diagnosis, and advances in treatment. South Med J 1990;83:1450.
20. Hui WM, Ng MMT, Lok ASF, et al. A randomized comparative study of laser photocoagulation, heater probe, and bipolar electrocoagulation in the treatment of actively bleeding ulcers. Gastrointest Endosc 1981;37:299.
21. Hunter JM, Pezim ME. Limited value of technetium 99m-labeled red cell scintigraphy in localization of lower gastrointestinal bleeding. Am J Surg 1990;159:504.
22. Jensen DM, Machicado GA. Diagnosis and treatment of severe hematochezia: the role of urgent colonoscopy after purge. Gastroenterology 1988;95:1569.
23. Leitman MI, Paull DE, Shires GT. Evaluation and man-

agement of massive lower gastrointestinal hemorrhage. Ann Surg 1989;209:175.

24. Matthewson D, Swain CP, Bland M, et al. Randomized comparison of Nd:YAG laser heater probe and no endoscopic therapy for bleeding peptic ulcers. Gastroenterology 1990;98:1239.

25. Moulton S, Adams M, Johanson K. Aortoenteric fistula: a seven year urban experience. Am J Surg 1986;151:607.

26. Nicholson ML, Neoptolemos JP, Sharp JF, et al. Localization of lower gastrointestinal bleeding using in vivo technetium 99m labeled red blood cell scintigraphy. Br J Surg 1989;76:358.

27. O'Connor KW, Lehman G, Yune H, et al. Comparison of three nonsurgical treatments for bleeding esophageal varices. Gastroenterology 1989;96:899–906.

28. Oxner RB, Simmonds NJ, Gertner DJ, et al. Endoscopic injection for bleeding peptic ulcers. Lancet 1992;339:966.

29. Pottter GD, Sellin JH. Lower gastrointestinal bleeding. Gastrointestinal Clin North Am 1988;17:341.

30. Proceedings of the Consensus Conference on Therapeutic Endoscopy in Bleeding Ulcers. Gastrointest Clin North Am 1990;36:S1–S65.

31. Rege RV, Nahrwold DL. Diverticular disease. Curr Probl Surg 1989;26:133.

32. Richter JM, Christensen MR, Colditz GA, et al. Angiodysplasia: natural history and efficacy of therapeutic interventions. Dig Dis Sci 1989;34:1542.

33. Ring EJ, Lake JR, Roberts JP, et al. Using transjugular intrahepatic portosystemic shunts to control variceal bleeding before liver transplantation. Ann Intern Med 1992;116:304–309.

34. Rosen AM, Leischer DE. Lower GI bleeding: updated diagnosis and management. Geriatrics 1989;44:49.

35. Rossini FP, Ferrari A, Spandre M, et al. Emergent colonoscopy. World J Surg 1989;13:190.

36. Schrock TR. Colonoscopic diagnosis and treatment of lower gastrointestinal bleeding. Surg Clin North Am 1989;69:1309.

37. Spencer J. Lower gastrointestinal bleeding. Br J Surg 1989;76:3.

38. Sutton FM. Upper gastrointestinal bleeding in patients with esophageal varices. Am J Med 1987;83:273–275.

39. Swain CP, Storey DW, Bown SG, et al. Nature of the bleeding vessel in recurrently bleeding ulcers. Gastroenterology 1986;90:595.

40. Terblanche J, Bornman PJC. Endoscopic sclerotherapy. Surg Clin North Am 1990;70:341–359.

41. Teres J, Bordas JM, Bravo D, et al. Sclerotherapy vs. distal splenorenal shunt in the elective treatments of variceal hemorrhage: a randomized controlled trial. Hepatology 1987;7:430–436.

42. Tsai YT, Lay CS, Lai KH, et al. Controlled trial of vasopressin plus nitroglycerin vs. vasopressin alone in the treatment of bleeding esophageal varices. Hepatology 1986;6:406–409.

43. Valenzuela JE, Schubert T, Fogel MR, et al. A multicenter, randomized, double-blind trial of somatostatin in the management of acute hemorrhage from esophageal varices. Hepatology 1989;10:958–961.

44. Van Stiegmann G, Yamamaoto M. Endoscopic techniques for the management of active variceal bleeding. Gastrointest Clin N Am 1992;2:59–75.

45. Wara P, Stodkilde H. Bleeding pattern before admission as guideline for emergency endoscopy. Scand J Gastroenterol 1985;20:76–78.

46. Warren WD, Henderson JM, Millikan W, et al. Distal splenorenal shunt versus endoscopic sclerotherapy for long-term management of variceal bleeding. Preliminary report of a prospective randomized trial. Ann Surg 1986;203:454–462.

47. Westaby D, Polson RJ, Gimson AE, et al. A controlled trial of injection sclerotherapy for active variceal bleeding. Hepatology 1989;9:274–277.

48. Westaby D, Polson RJ, Gimson AE, et al. A controlled trial of oral propranolol compared with injection sclerotherapy for the long-term management of variceal bleeding. Hepatology 1990;11:353–359.

49. Wood RP, Shaw BW Jr, Rikkers LF. Liver transplantation for variceal hemorrhage. Surg Clin North Am 1990;70:449–461.

50. Zemel G, Katzen BT, Becfker GJ, et al. Percutaneous transjugular portosystemic shunt. JAMA 1991;266:390–393.

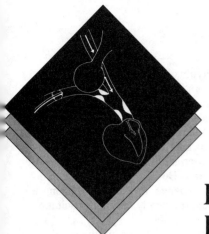

CHAPTER 40

Burns and Inhalational Injury

BURN EVALUATION

Mortality rates for burn victims vary widely, depending on the depth and size of the burn, the patient's underlying health and age, and the occurrence of associated inhalational injury. Most deaths from fires result from smoke inhalation, which usually proves fatal before patients reach the hospital. Upon reaching the hospital, hypovolemic shock and smoke-induced airflow obstruction are predominant early complications; sepsis is the most common late fatal complication. Inhalational injury is a major determinant of outcome; its occurrence may double the mortality rate of any given burn. Age also is a powerful predictor of mortality. For example, a 20-year-old individual sustaining a 50% full-thickness burn has nearly a 75% chance of survival, whereas the same burn is nearly always fatal for a 70-year-old individual. After the airway has been secured and hemodynamics have stabilized, the patient should be examined carefully to determine the depth and extent of thermal injury, and the burns should be gently washed and dressed.

SEVERITY

Burns are classified by their depth (partial or full thickness) or by severity of injury (first to third degree) (Table 40.1).

ESTIMATION OF BURN SIZE

In adults, the percentage of body surface affected by burn injury can be estimated by the "rule of nines." This rule assigns percentages of the total body surface area (BSA) to the anterior and posterior surfaces of the head, limbs, and trunk (see Fig. 40.1). As another useful measure, the palm of the patient's hand is approximately 1% of total BSA. Estimation of the total area involved by second- and third-degree burns is useful in determining fluid requirements and expected mortality. Adults with extensive or severe burns and most burned children require admission. Criteria for hospital admission are given in Table 40.2.

INITIAL MANAGEMENT

Initial management of the patient with severe burns should include careful assessment of the airway and vital signs to ensure adequate ventilation and perfusion. Inadequate ventilation or perfusion demand immediate attention. If carbon monoxide poisoning is known or even highly suspected, 100% oxygen should be administered to accelerate the clearance of carbon monoxide. After securing the airway and ensuring oxygenation, repletion of circulating volume should be undertaken. Hypovolemic shock is the most common cause of death in the first 24 hours after admission. Most adult patients with burns that require vigorous volume repletion should have urinary and central venous or pulmonary artery catheters inserted for assessment of volume status. Although invasive monitoring increases the risk of line-related infection, as many as one-half of all patients will have suboptimal resuscitation when

TABLE 40–1

CLASSIFICATION OF BURNS BY SEVERITY

Severity	Skin Examination	Sensation
First*	Erythema	Painful
Second**	Erythema/blisters/edema	Painful
Third**	White or charred Firmly indurated	Anesthetic

* Partial thickness
** Full thickness

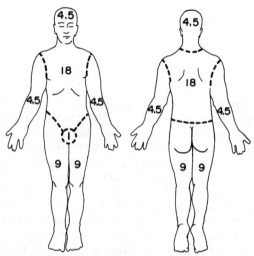

FIG. 40–1. Burn wound diagram illustrating the surface area of selected body regions. Numbers correspond to percentages of total BSA.

TABLE 40–2

CRITERIA FOR HOSPITAL ADMISSION: ADULTS

Second-degree burn >20% BSA

Third-degree burn >5% BSA

Any second-degree or third-degree burn in a patient ≥60 years

Inhalation injury

Circumferential burns of trunk or extremities

Burns of hand, face, feet, or perineum

fluid replacement is guided by vital signs, mental status, and urine output alone (see Chapter 3, Support of Failing Circulation). Difficulties in achieving resuscitation of burn patients often can be traced to transient myocardial dysfunction, presumably the result of humoral myocardial depressant factors, such as tumor necrosis factor α.

FLUID THERAPY

Burns cause hypovolemia as a result of massive shifts of fluid from intravascular to extravascular compartments and by exudation through injured skin. Hemoconcentration (due to intravascular fluid losses) or anemia (due to hemolysis induced by thermal effects and vascular damage) also may occur. With appropriate fluid resuscitation, hemoconcentration is rare. Because the packed cell volume (PCV) can change in either direction, it should be checked frequently during resuscitation with a target of 30 to 40%.

Numerous strategies have been advocated for replacing circulating volume. A central feature of all plans is to administer large volumes of salt-containing fluid during the initial 24 hours. The Parkland Formula is one good fluid replacement strategy in which 3 to 4 mL of normal saline per kilogram per percentage of BSA burn are given in the first day (Table 40.3). Customarily, one-half of the fluid deficit is replaced in the first 8 hours, with the remainder administered over the next 16 hours. (For purposes of fluid replacement, burn areas calculated to be more than 50% are considered to be exactly 50% BSA). Patients with concomitant inhalational injury may require up to 50% more fluid for successful resuscitation (up to 6 mL/kg/percent BSA burn). All fluid replacement strategies are associated with the development of tissue edema; however, the use of hypertonic (250 mmol/L) saline solution may achieve hemodynamic resuscitation with less tissue edema. Although it usually is difficult to administer too much fluid to a burn victim, one clinical clue to excessive fluid replacement is a urine out-

TABLE 40–3

FLUID REPLACEMENT STRATEGY

First 24 hours:	3–4 mL/kg/% BSA burn of Ringer's solution or normal saline
	Replace one-half of the deficit in first 8 hours
	Replace second half of the deficit in next 16 hours

After first 24 hours:
  Continue tailored crystalloid support. Colloid optional after first day
  Supplemental free water (D5W) and potassium usually required
  Goals: Adequate central vascular pressure
      Adequate blood pressure
      Urinary output of 0.5–1.0 mL/kg/hour

TABLE 40–4

CLUES TO INHALATION INJURY

Enclosed space exposure
Loss of consciousness
Nasal, oral, or facial burns
Carbonaceous sputum
Hoarseness or stridor
Upper airway changes by bronchoscopy
Chest radiograph showing pulmonary edema

put consistently exceeding 2 mL/kg/hour. After fluid replacement, dopamine may be required to maintain adequate cardiac output, blood pressure, and urine flow. High doses of α-adrenergic agonists (e.g., norepinephrine) should be avoided, if possible, because of their tendency to decrease nutritive blood flow to already injured skin.

After 24 hours, sodium requirements decline and permeability of leaky vessels decreases. Free water and colloid are then administered in larger quantities to maintain circulating volume and electrolyte balance. After the first 24 hours, evaporative water losses may be estimated by the following formula: hourly water loss (in mL) = (25 + % area of burn) × (total BSA in m²). This formula predicts that a patient with a 25% burn and a 2-m² BSA will lose approximately 100 mL of water per hour. Within the first 24 hours of the burn event, colloids offer little advantage over crystalloid because the newly injured vasculature fails to retain even the larger colloid molecules.

RESPIRATORY MANAGEMENT

Airway complications are a common cause of early death in burn patients. The history and physical examination provide valuable clues to the extent of inhalational injury (see Table 40.4). Burns and inhalation injuries cause respiratory complications through five basic mechanisms: (a) airway obstruction; (b) toxin inhalation; (c) increased metabolism and ventilation requirement; (d) impairment of host defenses; (e) production of late obstructive and restrictive lung disease.

Airway Obstruction

Hot gases, particularly steam (because of its high specific heat) can rapidly cause upper airway obstruction and bronchospasm; however, heat-related tissue edema can progress for 24 to 48 hours after the injury. Patients with burns of the face or neck that appear inconsequential at the time of admission may quickly experience swelling that leads to life-threatening airway obstruction. Therefore, as a rule, patients with second- or third-degree burns of the face or neck should be intubated in the first hours of hospitalization to avoid airway obstruction. Failure to follow this principle will lead to situations in which massive tissue swelling precludes intubation. If intubation is required, a large-diameter orotracheal tube should be placed to facilitate clearance of voluminous secretions and performance of bronchoscopy should the need arise. Prophylactic intubation generally should continue for at least 72 hours. When the need for intubation is uncertain, laryngoscopy or bronchoscopy can evaluate the severity of airway edema and need for endotracheal intubation. Intubation should be performed if there is any clinical evidence of airway obstruction or if laryngoscopy demonstrates supraglottic edema. Bedside tests of pulmonary function, especially flow–volume loops, can be helpful in questionable cases. Hypoxemia or diffuse radiographic infiltrates noted at the time of admission are also poor prognostic signs which indicate the need for early intubation and mechanical ventilation. A normal chest radiograph or PaO_2, however, by no means excludes inhalational injury.

For patients not requiring immediate intubation for airway obstruction or hypoxemia, aggressive respiratory therapy with bronchodilators and humidified oxygen may avert the need for mechanical ventilation. Inhalation of a low-viscosity mixture of helium and oxygen can be a useful temporizing measure for patients with mild airway edema, as can nebulization of racemic epinephrine. Neither therapy, however, should delay intubation for patients with facial burns or symptomatic airway obstruction. Bronchospasm and bronchorrhea commonly develop after inhalational injury to the lower airway. Although effective early on, bronchodilators are of less value late in the course of post-burn airway obstruction. Corticosteroids do not reduce airway edema and substantially increase mortality by predisposing patients to infection. Simple measures such as elevating the head of the bed to 30° during initial resuscitation may help to decrease the degree of airway edema. Clearly, the rate of fluid administration should not be decreased in burns involving the airway; inadequate fluids may allow underperfusion and worsening of airway damage.

TABLE 40–5

TOXIC COMPONENTS OF SMOKE

Material Burned	Toxic Product	Physiologic Effect
Wood, paper, cotton	Acrolein, acetaldehyde Formaldehyde, acetic acid	Airway irritation, bronchospasm Mucosal sloughing
Plastics	Phosgene, chlorine Hydrogen chloride	Airway irritation Acute lung injury
Synthetic (nylon, rayon)	Hydrogen cyanide Oxides of nitrogen	Cyanide poisoning, tissue hypoxia Pulmonary edema
All of the above	Carbon monoxide	Tissue hypoxia

Increased Ventilatory Requirements

Minute ventilation may be extraordinarily high after large burns because of increased metabolism; a 50 to 60% burn may double caloric requirements and CO_2 production. Although hyperpnea usually is due to the burn-induced hypermetabolic state, alternative explanations (e.g., hyperthyroidism, drug or alcohol withdrawal, pneumonia, acute respiratory distress syndrome [ARDS], pulmonary embolism, or uncontrolled pain) should be considered in every case. The increased ventilatory requirements may be sufficient to overwhelm the capacity of patients with underlying lung disease, resulting in respiratory failure.

Toxic Gas Inhalation

Depending on the fuel consumed, fires may produce dozens to hundreds of toxic compounds that can cause respiratory inflammation and systemic toxicity (Table 40.5). Inhaled gases produce injury in three ways: (*a*) by acting as asphyxiants, (*b*) by causing airway irritation, or (*c*) by functioning as systemic toxins. Any gas (e.g., nitrogen, helium, carbon dioxide) may be a lethal asphyxiant when it displaces oxygen from the atmosphere, resulting in a hypoxic gas mixture. Water-soluble gases usually act as airway irritants because they are deposited rapidly in high concentrations on the mucous membranes of the moist upper airway. Airway edema and bronchospasm usually result from the high-solubility gases such as chlorine, ammonia, and sulfur dioxide. In contrast, low-solubility toxins are more likely to gain access to the lower respiratory tract, as are potent acids or aldehydes carried there by inhaled particulates. Phosgene and nitrogen dioxide are good examples of such poorly soluble toxins. Obviously, when victims are trapped in a closed space, even highly soluble gases may reach the lower respiratory tract. The injury resulting from lower airway gas exposure is very similar to acid aspiration, presenting as diffuse bronchoconstriction, reduced lung compliance, and ventilation–perfusion mismatching. Chemical injury is suggested by erythema below the level of the vocal cords or by scintigraphic demonstration of ventilation–perfusion mismatching. The mucosal edema of chemical injury builds for 24 to 48 hours after exposure and severely impairs mucociliary transport. In addition, the inflammatory mediators and white cells released into the airways promote secretion formation, atelectasis development, and ventilation–perfusion mismatching. Copious secretions, bronchospasm, airway obstruction, and ciliary damage warrant aggressive respiratory therapy. In cases of severe inhalational injury, the airway mucosa sloughs at about 72 hours and requires 7 to 14 days to regenerate. Bacterial superinfection and pneumonitis are common during this time.

Carbon Monoxide and Cyanide

Carbon monoxide (CO) is the primary cause of death in 75% of fire fatalities. CO competes directly with oxygen for hemoglobin binding and displaces the oxyhemoglobin dissociation curve leftward, resulting in impaired release of O_2 to the tissues. Because the affinity of CO for hemoglobin is roughly 250 times greater than that of oxygen, concentrations of inspired CO as low as 0.1% can rapidly produce fatally high levels of nonfunctional carboxyhemoglobin (CO-Hgb). The sensitivity of a patient to CO poisoning is influenced strongly by underlying health; patients with diseases of the central nervous system or heart are unusually susceptible. The clinical symptoms of acute CO poisoning are those of tissue hypoxia and correlate well with the CO-Hgb

TABLE 40–6

CORRELATION OF CARBOXYHEMOGLOBIN LEVELS AND SYMPTOMS IN CARBON MONOXIDE POISONING*

Carboxyhemoglobin Level	Symptoms
<15%	Usually none
15–20%	Headache, confusion
20–40%	Disorientation, visual impairment, nausea
40–60%	Hallucinations, coma, shock
>60%	Death

* Absence of detectible carboxyhemoglobin does not rule out carbon monoxide exposure.

level (Table 40.6). However, because of delays in extrication and transport of victims to the hospital and prehospital use of oxygen, low or undetectable initial levels of CO-Hgb should not be used as evidence of an absence of CO effect. Unfortunately, the correlation between acute CO-Hgb levels and late neuropsychiatric effects is poor.

Two principles underpin treatment of CO poisoning: maximization of tissue O_2 delivery and use of high concentrations of O_2 to promote CO excretion. While breathing air, the elimination half-life ($t\frac{1}{2}$) of CO is 2 to 3 hours. When breathing pure O_2 at ambient pressure, the $t\frac{1}{2}$ declines to 20 to 30 minutes. Because O_2 profoundly affects CO clearance, the most important therapy in patients with suspected CO poisoning is to immediately administer 100% oxygen. CO-Hgb levels exceeding 25% in normal subjects or 15% in patients with ischemic heart disease should be treated aggressively. High fractions of inspired O_2 should be used until the CO-Hgb concentration falls below 10%.

The use of hyperbaric oxygen (HBO) therapy remains controversial. Although HBO can further speed removal of CO from the body, hyperbaric chambers complicate patient management and are not widely available. Furthermore, after the first hour, HBO offers little demonstrated advantage over 100% oxygen at ambient pressure in reducing CO-Hgb levels. It is possible that HBO has unproven beneficial effects unrelated to its ability to accelerate CO clearance from the body. Randomized studies do not suggest that the late complications (especially behavioral disturbances) after CO exposure are reduced by HBO. A reasonable compromise position is to use HBO, if locally available, for symptomatic (i.e., unconscious at

the fire scene or on arrival, altered neurologic status, hemodynamically unstable) CO exposure victims and for patients with documented high CO-Hgb levels, even if asymptomatic. Presently, it does not seem that the benefits of HBO exceed the risks of transporting acutely ill, unstable patients long distances to receive the therapy. Although the beneficial effects of hyperbaric therapy diminish if administered more than 6 hours after exposure, anecdotal evidence suggests that some manifestations of CO exposure may be reversed by HBO days or even weeks after CO exposure.

Closed-space fires also generate cyanide (CN) through the combustion of wood, silk, nylon, and polyurethane. Because a diagnostic test is not available, CN exposure often goes unrecognized. CN binds to tissue cytochrome enzymes, impairing normal O_2 use and causing lactic acidosis. Hyperbaric O_2 therapy is not useful in CN toxicity because the pathophysiologic defect is in O_2 usage at the cellular level, not one of O_2 delivery. Tissue hypoxia from CO or CN usually is evident immediately after exposure and should be suspected in burn patients with apparently normal clinical indices of perfusion but an unexplained metabolic (lactic) acidosis.

In CO poisoning arterial blood gases may demonstrate a nearly normal PaO_2 but decreased measured O_2 content and hemoglobin saturation. In contrast, PO_2, O_2 saturation and O_2 content may all be normal in CN intoxication. Unlike CO poisoning, mixed venous O_2 saturations are inappropriately high in cyanide intoxication due to underuse of delivered O_2. The treatment of CN poisoning includes use of inhaled amyl nitrate, intravenous sodium nitrite, and intravenous sodium thiosulfate.

OTHER IMPORTANT CONSIDERATIONS

Major burns impair the ability to conserve heat and maintain normal body temperature. Therefore, after burn cleansing, wounds should be covered with clean warm coverings and body temperature monitored closely. Ileus commonly follows major burns, and gastric distention or markedly diminished bowel sounds should prompt insertion of an oral or nasogastric tube connected to suction. After wound cleansing, a topical antibiotic should be applied to limit skin colonization by bacteria. Systemic antibiotics offer no demonstrated advantage in prophylaxis. Without confirmation of recent immunization, tetanus toxoid should be administered. Pain and anxiety relief, particularly in partial thickness burns, is critical to allow debridement, cleansing, and other patient manipulations (see Chapter 17, Analgesia, Sedation, and Paralysis). Full-thickness burns are frequently anesthetic so that patients often require little or no pain medication.

LATE COMPLICATIONS OF BURNS

The late complications of burns include: (*a*) infection/sepsis/multiple organ failure; (*b*) gastrointestinal bleeding; (*c*) hypermetabolism; and (*d*) local wound problems.

INFECTION AND SEPSIS

Infection presents the greatest threat to life of burn patients after the first 36 hours; pneumonia and burn wound sepsis represent the most common and lethal conditions. Immunocompetence of burned patients, including T-cell, monocyte, and macrophage function, are significantly depressed. Clearly, nosocomial pneumonitis is an ever-present risk for the intubated patient, particularly when inhalation injury has compromised host defenses (see Chapters 26 and 27).

Devastating infection also can result from skin disruption. Massive numbers of bacteria may invade the burn wound and adjacent tissue. In the first 3 to 5 days after a burn, *Staphylococci* are the most common invading organisms, but after 5 days, gram-negative rods (especially *Pseudomonas*) predominate. In addition to standard methods of infection control, meticulous wound care, including the use of topical antibiotics, early wound debridement and closure, and use of gowns, masks, and gloves decrease the infection risk. Prophylactic systemic antibiotics are not of benefit. When antibiotics are used, it should be kept in mind that burned patients have accelerated clearance of some drugs, most notably aminoglycosides. Increased basal temperature renders the detection of wound infection difficult. Because the normal body temperature of burn patients may rise as high as 38.5°C as a result of hypermetabolism, fever to this degree does not necessarily warrant the institution of parenteral antibiotics. When burn wound sepsis is suspected, quantitative cultures of burned skin, subcutaneous tissue, and adjacent normal skin should be performed. Growth of more than 10^5 organisms per gram of tissue or histologic evidence of invasion of adjacent unburned skin are highly suggestive of severe complicating infection, even though substantial sampling error may occur in quantitative culturing methods. Long before the results of these tests are available, however, antibiotics must be instituted on clinical grounds if high spiking fever, leukocytosis and neutrophilia, or other signs of sepsis are present.

Burns can produce sepsis syndrome and multiple organ failure (see Chapter 27, Sepsis Syndrome). It is not clear whether the burn wound itself, an undetectable infection, or the release of toxins across the gut wall (e.g., endotoxin) causes this clinical syndrome. The occurrence of sepsis syndrome can be minimized by early wound excision and grafting, aggressive nutritional support, avoidance of corticosteroids, and prompt diagnosis and treatment of infections.

GASTROINTESTINAL BLEEDING

Gastrointestinal (GI) bleeding due to stress (curling) ulceration occurs commonly in burn patients. Burn victims are one of the few groups to clearly benefit from empiric stress ulceration prophylaxis. Effective prophylaxis uses histamine blockers or sucralfate. Antacids are more expensive and more labor intensive but less effective at maintaining gastric pH above 4.0 than are histamine blockers. Furthermore, antacids are associated with higher rates of nosocomial pneumonia; therefore, they represent third-line therapy.

HYPERMETABOLIC STATE

Metabolic rate may double in patients with second- and third-degree burns that exceed 50% BSA. Indeed, extensive burns represent the single greatest sustained metabolic stress experienced by humans. Full expression of hypermetabolism may require 5 to 7 days. Patients with major burns raise resting body temperature and dedicate a large fraction of energy consumption to the heat production that maintains the gradient with ambient temperature; therefore, establishing higher environmental temperature reduces caloric expenditure. Aggressive nutritional support is required and usually is given parenterally to circumvent the high incidence of gastrointestinal malfunction. However, parenteral nutrition usually is withheld during the first 24 to 36 hours of hospitalization because of the complexities of fluid management in the period of initial resuscitation. In the initial phase of treatment, the daily calorie requirement may be roughly estimated as 25 times the weight

TABLE 40–7

TOPICAL ANTIMICROBIAL THERAPY

	Silver Sulfadiazine	Sodium Nitrate	Mafenide (Sulfamylon)
Advantages:	Painless Easily applied Wide spectrum	Painless Wide spectrum	Easily applied Good eschar penetration
Disadvantages:	Poor eschar penetration Leukopenia Thrombocytopenia	Poor eschar penetration Skin staining Leaches NaCl from tissue	Metabolic acidosis (carbonic anyhydrase inhibitor) Narrow bacterial spectrum (GNR) Rare aplastic crisis

GNR, gram-negative rods.

in kilograms plus 40 times the percentage of BSA burned. Giving 50 to 60% of the estimated caloric requirement as glucose minimizes catabolic losses of nitrogen. Administration of glucose at rates above 5 to 7 mL/kg/minute, however, may lead to glucose intolerance and increased CO_2 associated with overfeeding. Lipid may be used as the source for the remaining 40% of nonprotein calories. Increased lipid clearance observed in burn victims supports the argument for raising the percentage of calories given as fat. Two grams of protein usually are given per kilogram of body weight. High-protein enteral diets with a calorie:nitrogen ratio of 100:1 may increase survival. Because enteral feeding preserves mucosal integrity, buffers gastric acid, and increases resistance of patients to infection, the transition from parenteral to enteral feeding should be made at the earliest possible time. (For a complete discussion of nutrition therapy, see Chapter 16 [Nutritional Assessment and Support].)

BURN WOUND CARE

The goals of burn wound care are to (*a*) prevent infection, (*b*) limit discomfort, (*c*) accelerate healing, and (*d*) maximize ultimate function. In general, these goals are best accomplished by the use of early debridement, topical antibiotics, and skin grafting. Topical antibiotics are applied to the skin once or twice daily to limit wound colonization. Wounds should be cleaned and debrided before application of new antibiotic, a process often requiring narcotic analgesia. Several topical antibiotics are available, each with unique advantages, antibacterial spectra, and complications (Table 40.7). If long-term topical antibiotics are needed, changing the agent used at 7- to 10-day intervals may prevent the overgrowth of resistant organisms. When burn wound sepsis is suspected,

empirical antibiotic regimens should cover *Pseudomonas aeruginosa* and *Staphylococci*. The recent development of *in vitro* cultured skin is a promising development in the therapy for patients previously requiring extensive grafting procedures.

Many of the same principles that apply to chemical, electrical, and thermal burns are useful for patients with extensive skin damage as the result of toxic epidermal necrolysis or Stevens-Johnson syndrome. Fortunately, such patients rarely require debridement or grafting.

Mechanical Problems of the Burn Wound

Patients with circumferential burns of the trunk or an extremity and those with burns of the face, hands, feet, or perineum unequivocally require hospital admission and immediate consultation by a burn specialist. Eschar frequently encases the trunk or extremities. These limiting shells may prevent the tissue expansion required to accommodate the massive edema that follows burn injury. Edema occurring in both burned and unburned tissues reaches maximal severity 12 to 48 hours after injury. Ischemia and/or necrosis may result from the consequent rise in tissue pressure if unrelieved. Furthermore, eschar-related limitation of chest expansion may lead to respiratory failure. In the extremities, edema can be minimized by elevating the burned limb. Decreased capillary refill, cyanosis, paresthesia, and deep pain in tissues distal to the burn site dictate the need for escharotomy. Doppler ultrasound examination demonstrating a diminished pulse amplitude distal to the eschar confirms high tissue pressures and potential vascular compromise. In circumferential burns of the trunk, reduced thoracic compliance (noted during mechanical ventilation), severe tachypnea, or ventilatory distress suggests the need for escharotomy. Escharotomy is performed by incising devitalized wound tissue along the entire lateral and medial aspects of the trunk or affected limb. After the healing process has begun, hydrotherapy debridement may become an important adjunct to the process.

NONTHERMAL BURN INJURIES

CHEMICAL INJURY

Copious irrigation with clear water comprises the primary initial treatment of chemical burns of all types. Care must be taken to avoid extending the chemical injury by allowing the patient to lie in contaminated flush solution. Removal of contaminated clothing and irrigation in a shower is preferable. After flushing, chemical burns should be treated like thermal burns. Although alkaline and acidic chemicals injure tissue by altering its pH, strong neutralizing solutions should not be used because they may precipitate exothermic reactions, risking additional thermal damage. The adequacy of irrigation in pH-related chemical injury may be assessed by testing the area with litmus paper to ensure neutral pH.

ELECTRICAL BURNS

Electrical burns inflicted by lightning or another high-voltage source may produce extensive tissue damage with little external evidence of injury. Bone and muscle damage are frequent. Electrical injury may cause severe exit wounds at the hands, knees, or feet—sites frequently overlooked in the initial evaluation. (Such wounds are analogous to projectile injuries, which produce small entrance but large exit wounds.) For all patients with electrical injury, an electrocardiogram should be performed to look for evidence of arrhythmias, myocardial injury, or conduction disturbance. Even in the absence of overt cardiac injury, short-term observation in a monitored bed setting probably is prudent. Because of the high incidence of associated rhabdomyolysis, volume loading in conjunction with osmotic and loop diuretics and sodium bicarbonate may be indicated to avert renal failure.

KEY POINTS

1. For burn victims, the keystones of initial therapy are large-volume crystalloid resuscitation and maintenance of the airway. Commonly, isotonic crystalloid (3 to 4 mL/kg/percentage BSA burn) is required for volume resuscitation during the first 24 hours after a burn injury.

2. Inhalational damage is a very common early injury that is usually best managed initially by intubation and administration of 100% oxygen. The role of hyperbaric oxygen therapy remains controversial but perhaps is best limited to comatose patients with high carboxyhemoglobin levels who can be treated promptly.

3. Burn wounds are metabolically taxing, requiring huge amounts of energy and patient work to maintain an often dramatically elevated minute ventilation and cardiac output. Patients with marginal ventilatory status can develop respiratory failure from excessive ventilatory demands.

4. The hypermetabolic state and intercompartmental fluid shifts often dramatically alter drug therapy in the patient with burns. In many cases, drug doses must be significantly increased to achieve therapeutic effect.

5. Sepsis is the most common late fatal complication of burns, usually related to gram-negative rod infection of the burn wound.

SUGGESTED READINGS

1. Alexander JW, MacMillian BG, Stinnett JD, et al. Beneficial effects of aggressive protein feeding in severely burned children. Ann Surg 1980;192:505–517.
2. Baxter CR. Fluid volume and electrolyte changes in the early postburn period. Clin Plast Surg 1974;1:693–703.
3. Boswick JA, ed. Burns. Surg Clin North Am 1987;67(1).
4. Cahalane M, Demling RH. Early respiratory abnormalities from smoke inhalation. JAMA 1984;251(6):771–773.
5. Choi IS. Delayed neuropsychiatric sequelae in carbon monoxide intoxication. Arch Neurol 1983;40:433–435.
6. Deitch EA. The management of burns. N Engl J Med 1990;323:1249–1253.
7. Deitch EA. A policy of early excision and grafting in elderly burn patients shortens hospital stay and improves survival. Burns 1985;12:109–114.
8. Demling RH, Frye E, Read T. Effect of sequential early

burn wound excision and closure on postburn oxygen consumption. Crit Care Med 1991;19:861–866.

9. Demling RH. Burns. N Engl J Med 1985;313(22): 1389–1398.
10. Demling RH. Fluid resuscitation after major burns. JAMA 1983;250(11):1438–1440.
11. Dries DJ, Waxman K. Adequate resuscitation of burn patients may not be measured by urine output and vital signs. Crit Care Med 1991;19:327–329.
12. Gorman DF, Clayton D, Gillegan JE, Webb RK. A longitudinal study of 100 consecutive admissions for carbon monoxide poisoning to the Royal Adelaide Hospital. Anaesth Intensive Care 1992;20:311–316.
13. Herndon DN, Curreri PW, Abston S, et al. Treatment of burns. Curr Probl Surg 1987;24:341–397.
14. Herndon DN, Traber DL, Traber LD. The effect of resuscitation on inhalation injury. Surgery 1986;100:248–251.
15. Ilano Al, Raffin TA. Management of carbon monoxide poisoning. Chest 1990;97:165–169.
16. Luterman A, Dacso CC, Curreri PW. Infections in burn patients. Am J Med 1986;81(Suppl 1A):45–52.
17. Mathieu D, Nolf M, Durocher A, et al. Acute carbon monoxide poisoning: risk of late sequelae and treatment by hyperbaric oxygen. Clin Toxicol 1985;23:315–324.

18. Myers RAM, Snyder SK, Emhoff TA. Subacute sequelae of carbon monoxide poisoning. Ann Emerg Med 1985; 14:1163–1167.
19. Navar PD, Saffle JR, Warden GD. Effect of inhalation injury on fluid resuscitation requirements after thermal injury. Am J Surg 1985;150:716–720.
20. Norkool DN, Kirkpatrick JN. Treatment of acute carbon monoxide poisoning with hyperbaric oxygen: a review of 115 cases. Ann Emerg Med 1985;14:1168–1171.
21. Shirani KZ, Pruitt BA, Mason AD. The influence of inhalation injury and pneumonia on burn mortality. Ann Surg 1987;205:82–87.
22. Sloan EP, Murphy DG, Hart R, et al. Complications and protocol considerations in carbon monoxide-poisoned patients who require hyperbaric oxygen therapy: report from a ten-year experience. Ann Emerg Med 1989;18:629–634.
23. Sykes RA, Mani MM, Hiebert JM. Chemical burns: retrospective review. J Burn Care Rehabil 1986;7(4):343–347.
24. Venus B, Matsuda T, Copiozo JB, et al. Prophylactic intubation and continuous positive airway pressure in the management of inhalation injury in burn victims. Crit Care Med 1981;9:519–523.
25. Winter PM, Miller JN. Carbon monoxide poisoning. JAMA 1976;236(13):1502–1504.

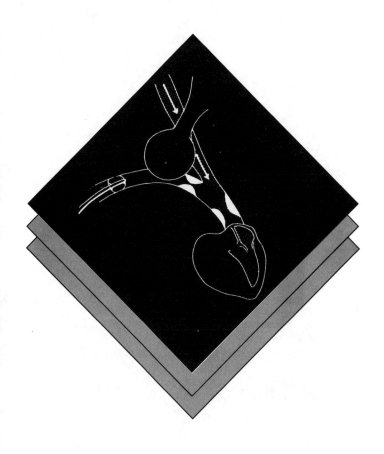

Appendix

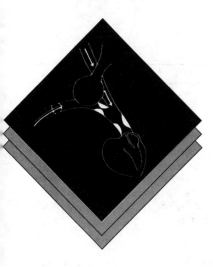

Definitions and Normal Values

CONVERSION FACTORS

Temperature
  Fahrenheit to centigrade: $°C = (°F - 32) \times 5/9$.
  Centigrade to fahrenheit: $°F = (°C \times 9/5) + 32$.

Pressure
  1 mmHg = 1.36 cmH$_2$O (A pressure of 10 mmHg = 13.6 cmH$_2$O.)
  1 cm H$_2$O = 0.73 mmHg

Length
  1 inch (in) = 2.54 cm
  1 cm = 0.394 in

Weight
  1 pound (lb) = 0.454 kg
  1 kilogram (kg) = 2.2 lb
  1 grain (g) = 60 mg

Work
  1 joule = 1 watt·second
  1 joule = 0.1 kg·m
  1 joule = (10 cmH$_2$O)/(1 liter)

Resistance
  1 hybrid (Wood) unit = 80 dyne·cm·sec^{-5}

USEFUL RENAL FORMULAS AND NORMAL VALUES[a]

Quantity	Formula	Normal
Estimated creatinine clearance (Cl_{Cr})	$\dfrac{(140\text{-age})(\text{wt in kg})}{72 \times \text{serum } [Cr]}$	>100 ml/min
Renal failure index (RFI)	$\dfrac{\text{Urine } [Na^+] \times \text{serum } [Cr]}{\text{Urine } [Cr]}$	<1 Pre-renal >1 Intra-renal
Fractional excretion of sodium (FENa)	$\dfrac{(\text{Urine } [Na^+] \times \text{serum } [Cr])}{(\text{Serum } [Na^+] \times \text{urine } [Cr])}$	<1 Pre-renal >1 Intra-renal
Anion gap (AG)	$[Na^+] - ([Cl^-] + [HCO_3^-])$	8–12 mEq/l
Calculated osmolality (Osm)	$2 \times [Na^+] + [\text{glucose}]/18 + [\text{BUN}]/2.8$	285–295 mOsm/l
Calculated H_2O deficit (liters)	$0.6 \,(\text{wt in kg}) \times ([Na^+] - 140)/140$	
Corrected $[Ca^{2+}]$	If albumin ↓ by 1 gm/dl $[Ca^{2+}]$ ↓ by 0.8 mg/dl	
Colloid osmotic pressure (COP)	$1.4 \,[\text{globulin}]^* + 5.5 \,[\text{albumin}]^*$	24 ± 3 mmHg

[a] wt, weight; ↑, increased; ↓, decreased; *, (gm/dl).

USEFUL CIRCULATORY FORMULAS AND NORMAL VALUES[a]

Quantity	Formula	Normal
Mean arterial pressure (MAP)	$(P_{sys} + 2\,P_{dia})/3$	>70 mmHg
Heart rate max (HR_{max})	$220 - \text{age}$	
Central venous pressure (CVP)		5–12 cmH$_2$O
Mean pulmonary artery pressure (P_{PA})		10–17 mmHg
Mean pulmonary capillary wedge (P_W)		5–12 mmHg
Cardiac output (CO)	$HR \times SV$	>5 l/min
Body surface area (BSA)	$0.202 \times \text{wt}_{kg}^{0.425} \times \text{ht}_{m}^{0.725}$	1.5–2.0 m^2
Stroke volume (SV)	CO/HR	>60 ml
Cardiac index (CI)	CO/BSA	>2.5 l/min/m^2
Systemic vascular resistance (SVR)	$(MAP - CVP) \times 80/CO$	900–1200 dyne·sec·cm^{-5} 11–15 Wood units
Pulmonary vascular resistance (PVR)	$(P_{\overline{PA}} - P_w) \times 80/CO$	150–250 dyne·sec·cm^{-5} 2–3.1 Wood units
Ejection fraction (EF)	$SV/\text{end-diastolic volume}$	LV >65%, RV >50%
Circulating blood volume	≈ 70 ml/kg	≈ 5000 ml
Oxygen delivery	$CO \times CaO_2$	≈ 700 ml O$_2$/min/m^2

[a] LV, left ventricle; RV, right ventricle; wt, weight; ht, height; P_{sys}, systolic pressure; P_{dia}, diastolic pressure.

USEFUL RESPIRATORY FORMULAS AND NORMAL VALUES[a]

Quantity	Formula	Normal
Tidal volume (V_T)	6–7 ml/kg	≈500 ml
Vital capacity (VC)		65–70 ml/kg
Maximal inspiratory pressure (MIP)		>75–100 cmH$_2$O
Deadspace (V_D)	≈⅓ V_T	1 ml/pound or 0.45 ml/kg
Deadspace ratio (V_D/V_T)	(PaCO$_2$ − P$_E$ECO$_2$)/PaCO$_2$	0.25–0.40
Minute ventilation (V_E)		5–10 l/min
Maximal ventilatory volume (MVV)	≈35 × FEV$_1$	
Peak flow	(height, age, sex dependent)	>7 l/sec or > 425 l/min
Dynamic characteristic	V_T/(P$_{aw}$ − PEEP)	Flow dependent
Static compliance (C$_{stat}$)	V_T/(P$_{plat}$ − PEEP)	80 ml/cmH$_2$O
Resistance to airflow (R$_L$)	(P$_{dyn}$ − P$_{plat}$)/flow	<4 cmH$_2$O/l/sec
Alveolar partial pressure of O$_2$ (P$_A$O$_2$)	(P$_b$ − P$_{H_2}$O) × FiO$_2$ − (PaCO$_2$)/0.8	>100 mmHg
Arterial-alveolar difference (A-aDO$_2$)	P$_A$O$_2$ − PaO$_2$	<10 mmHg @ FiO$_2$ = 0.21
Arterial PaO$_2$/FiO$_2$ ratio (P/F)	PaO$_2$/FiO$_2$	>400
Arterial/alveolar ratio (a/A)	PaO$_2$/P$_A$O$_2$	>0.9
Arterial O$_2$ tension (PaO$_2$)	100 − (age/3)	80–95 mmHg
Arterial O$_2$ saturation (SaO$_2$)		SaO$_2$ > 90%
Arterial CO$_2$ tension (PaCO$_2$)		37–43 mmHg
Mixed venous O$_2$ tension (Pv̄O$_2$)		≈35–40 mmHg
Mixed venous O$_2$ saturation (Sv̄O$_2$)		>70%
Mixed venous CO$_2$ tension (Pv̄CO$_2$)		≈45 mmHg
Arterial O$_2$ content (CaO$_2$)	(Hgb × 1.34)SaO$_2$ + (PaO$_2$ × .003)	≈20 ml/dl
Venous O$_2$ content (Cv̄O$_2$)	(Hgb × 1.34) Sv̄O$_2$ + (Pv̄O$_2$ × .003)	≈15 ml/dl
Oxygen consumption (V̇O$_2$)	CO$_l$ × C(a-v)O$_2$ml/dl × 10	≈250 ml/min
Extraction ratio	C (a-v̄)O$_2$/CaO$_2$	≈0.25
Pulmonary capillary O$_2$ content (CcO$_2$)	(Hgb × 1.34) + (P$_A$O$_2$ × .003)	≈20 ml/dl
Shunt fraction (venous admixture) % (Q̇$_s$/Q̇$_T$)	(CcO$_2$ − CaO$_2$)/(CcO$_2$ − Cv̄O$_2$) × 100	<5%
Arterio-venous O$_2$ content difference C(a-v̄)O$_2$	CaO$_2$ − Cv̄O$_2$	≈5 ml/dl

CONTENT OF COMMON INTRAVENOUS FLUIDS

	Electrolytes (mEq/l)						Calories and Osmolality	
Type	Na$^+$	Cl$^-$	K$^+$	Ca^{2+}	Lactate	HCO$_3^-$	mOsm/l	kcal/l
D5W	0	0	0	0	0	0	252	170
D50W	0	0	0	0	0	0	2530	1700
½ NS	77	77	0	0	0	0	154	0
NS	154	154	0	0	0	0	308	0
Ringer's lactate	130	109	4	3	28	0	273	0
3% NaCl	513	513	0	0	0	0	1026	0
D5½NS	77	77	0	0	0	0	406	170
NaHCO$_3$	1000					1000	2000	0
20% Mannitol	0	0	0	0	0	0	1098	

TEMPERATURE CORRECTION FACTORS FOR BLOOD pH AND GAS MEASUREMENTS (ADD TO OBSERVED VALUE)

Patient's Temperature				
°F	°C	pH	PCO_2 (%)	PO_2 (%)
110	43	−.09	+22	+35
107	41.5	−.07	+17	+27
106	41	−.06	+16	+25
105	40.5	−.05	+14	+22
104	40	−.04	+12	+19
103	39.5	−.04	+10	+16
102	39	−.03	+8	+13
101	38.5	−.02	+6	+10
100	38	−.01	+4	+7
98–99	**37**	**None**	**None**	**None**
97	36	+.01	−4	−7
96	35.5	+.02	−6	−10
95	35	+.03	−8	−13
94	34.5	+.04	−10	−16
93	34	+.04	−12	−19
92	33.5	+.05	−14	−22
91	33	+.06	−16	−25
90	32	+.07	−19	−30
88	31	+.09	−22	−35
86	30	+.10	−26	−39
84	29	+.12	−29	−43
82	28	+.13	−32	−47
80	26	+.15	−36	−53
75	24	+.19	−43	−60

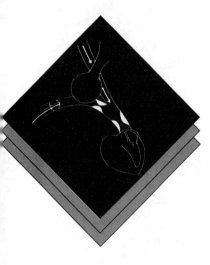

Index

Page numbers in *italics* represent figures; page numbers with *t* indicate tables.

See Chapter 22, *Hypertensive Emergencies*. (Close monitoring of hemody-namic response critical for safe use.)   *Usual concentration.

LABETALOL

Bolus Technique: 10–20 mg. i.v., then 40–80 mg i.v. q 10–20 minutes (maximum 300 mg).

Infusion Technique: Mix: 200 mg in 200 mL D5W, final (1 mg/mL). Begin 2 at mg/minute. Titrate upward at 5- to 15-minute intervals. Effect usually seen within 200 mg total dose.

Notes: Predominantly β blocker with mild α blocking effects. Use cautiously in asthma, COPD, CHF, liver failure, and in patients with cardiac conduction defects.

NICARDIPINE

Mix: 25 mg/250 mL, final (0.1 mg/mL)

Infuse: Begin 5 mg/hr, increase by 5 mg/hr every 15 minutes (maximum, 15 mg/hr). Reduce dose to 3–5 mg/hr when BP begins to decline. (Usual maintenance dose: 3–5 mg/hr.)

Notes: Potent calcium antagonist vasodilator, "stepped infusion dosing." Hypo-tension or tachycardia rare. Renal clearance. Oral form available.

NITROGLYCERIN

Mix: 200 mg in 500 mL saline, final (400 µg/mL)*

Infuse: Begin 5 µg/minute, double dose q 5–15 minutes for effect. (Usual dose, 5–400 µg/minute.)

Notes: Higher range doses needed for HTN crisis, lower doses for angina. Predominant effects on venous side. Side effects: "Antabuse effect," methemoglobinemia, headache, tachyphylaxis.

NITROPRUSSIDE

Mix: 100 mg/500 mL saline, final (200 µg/mL)

Infuse: Begin 0.5 µg/kg/minute. Double dose q 5–15 minutes to effect. (Usual dose, 0.5–5.0 µg/kg/minute.)

Notes: Potent vasodilator. Lower doses often sufficient for CHF. High-range doses needed for hypertensive crisis. Protect from light. Use cautiously in renal and hepatic failure (cyanide/thiocyanate toxicity possible). Avoid use alone in aortic dissection (reflex tachycardia).

PHENTOLAMINE

Bolus Technique: 0.5 mg i.v. test dose, then 1–5 mg i.v. q 5–15 minutes as needed.

Notes: Nonselective α blocker. Overshoot hypotension common.

TRIMETHAPHAN

Mix: 500 mg in 500 mL D5W, final (1 mg/mL)

Infuse: Begin at 1 mg/min. Titrate upward at 1- to 5-minute intervals. (Usual dose, 1–15 mg/minute.)

Notes: Ganglionic blocker, most useful for aortic dissection. Side effects common: ileus, vomiting, urinary retention, cycloplegia, orthostasis, respiratory arrest.

See Chapter 3, *Support of the Circulation*. (Close monitoring of hemodynamic response critical for safe use.)   *Usual concentration.

DOBUTAMINE

Mix: 500 mg in 500 mL, final (1000µg/mL)*

Dose: Begin at 2–5 µg/kg/minute. Titrate to desired effect. (Usual dose, 5–15 µg/kg/minute.)

Notes: Minimal alpha effects. Inotrope and systemic vasodilator. May precipitate hypotension in patients with profound hypovolemia or peripheral vasocon-striction.

DOPAMINE:

Mix: 400 mg/500 mL, final (800 µg/mL)*

Dose: Begin at 2 µg/kg/minute. Double dose q 5–15 minutes to desired effect or toxicity. (Usual range, 2–20 µg/kg/minute)

Notes: Lower doses: β (chronotropic) and dopaminergic (renal vasodilating) effects predominate. High doses: vasoconstriction more prominent. Consider adding epinephrine or norepinephrine if >10–20 µg/kg/minute needed for hypotension. Arrhythmogenic.

EPINEPHRINE

Mix: 2 mg/500 mL, final (4 µg/mL)*

Dose: Begin at 2 µg/minute. Double dose q 5–15 minutes to desired effect. (Usual range, 2–20 µg/minute.)

Notes: Chronotrope, inotrope, and vasoconstrictor. (Less vasoconstrictive than norepinephrine.) May have profound hypertensive effect in patients on β blockers.

ISOPROTERENOL

Mix: 2 mg/250 mL, final (8 µg/mL)*

Dose: Begin 2 µg/minute. Rapidly titrate to achieve desired heart rate. (Usual range, 2–10 µg/minute.)

Notes: β agonist (chronotrope, inotrope, bronchodilator and vasodilator). Useful in refractory bradycardia and in *Torsades* to shorten QT interval.

PHENYLEPHRINE

Mix: 30 mg/250 mL, final (120 µg/mL)*

Dose: Begin at 2 µcg/kg/minute. Double dose q 5–15 minutes to desired effect. (Usual dose, 2–20 µg/minute.)

Notes: Essentially pure α agonist.

NOREPINEPHRINE

Mix: 8 mg/500 mL, final (16 µg/mL)

Dose: Begin 1–2 µg/minute. Double dose q 5–15 minutes to desired effect. (Usual range, 5–20 µg/minute.)

Notes: Most potent α agonist (vasoconstrictor). Modestly less β (chronotropic) action than epinephrine. β effects predominate at doses <10 µg/minute. High doses risk tissue ischemia. Often combined with low-dose dopamine.

ANTIARRHYTHMICS

See Chapter 4, *Arrhythmias, Pacing, and Cardioversion.* (Accurate diagnosis of arrhythmia critical for optimal drug selection. Therapy usually should be administered under ECG guidance.)

ADENOSINE
- Bolus: 6–12 mg i.v. by rapid bolus. Infusion not indicated.
- Notes: Often produces brief periods of "asystole." Rapid administration essential.

BRETYLIUM
- Mix: 500 mg/500 mL D5W, final (1 mg/mL)
- Infuse: Initial bolus dose 5 mg/kg i.v. over 30 minutes then infuse 1–2 mg/minute. Reserve more rapid administration for hypotensive patients with refractory ventricular arrhythmias.
- Notes: Infusion may induce hypotension. Renal insufficiency requires reduced dose. Nausea and vomiting common.

DILTIAZEM
- Mix: 100 mg/250 mL, final (0.4 mg/mL)
- Infuse: Bolus with 0.25 mg/kg. Begin infusion at 5–10 mg/hr. Titrate to achieve rhythm control or maximum of 15–20 mg/hr.
- Notes: High-grade AV block possible. May facilitate conduction via bypass tracts in patients with Wolff-Parkinson-White and its variants.

ESMOLOL
- Bolus: 500 µg/kg
- Mix: 2500 mg/250 mL, final (10 mg/mL)
- Infuse: Begin at 50 µg/kg/min. Titrate upward at 5- to 15-minute intervals to desired effect. (Usual dose, 50–200 µg/kg/minute.)
- Notes: Ultra-short-acting β blocker.

LIDOCAINE
- Bolus: 1–1.5 mg/kg
- Mix: 4 gm in 500 mL saline, final (8 mg/mL)
- Infuse: 1–4 mg/minute
- Notes: Neurotoxicity seen with overdose. Clearance reduced in older patients and those with liver disease or congestive heart failure.

PROCAINAMIDE
- Bolus: 10 mg/kg at a rate ≤50 mg/minute
- Mix: 4 gm in 500 mL, final (8 mg/mL)
- Infuse: 1–4 mg/minute
- Notes: Immunologic reactions common with long-term use. Hepatic metabolism, renal clearance.

ANTICOAGULANT & THROMBOLYTIC DRUGS

See Chapter 21, *Angina and Myocardial Infarction,* and Chapter 23, *DVT and Pulmonary Embolism.* (Hemorrhagic complications possible, close monitoring essential.)

STREPTOKINASE
- MI dose: 1.5 million units i.v. over 1 hour
- DVT-PE dose: 250,000 U i.v. load, then 100 U/hr infusion for 24–72 hours.
- Notes: Allergic reactions possible, especially in patients with recent *Streptococcal* infections. Least expensive thrombolytic.

UROKINASE
- DVT-PE dose: 4,400 U load, then 4,400 U/kg/hr infusion for 12–48 hours.
- Notes: Allergic reactions less common than with streptokinase. Intermediate in cost.

TISSUE PLASMINOGEN ACTIVATOR (TPA)
- MI dose: 15 mg i.v. bolus, then–0.75 mg/kg (not to exceed 50 mg) i.v. over 30 minutes, then–
  0.5 mg/kg (not to exceed 35 mg) i.v. over 60 minutes.
- DVT-PE dose: 100 mg i.v. over 2 hours.
- Notes: Allergic reactions rare. Most costly thrombolytic.

ANISOYLATED PLASMINOGEN STREPTOKINASE ACTIVATOR COMPLEX (APSAC)
- MI dose: 30 U i.v. over 5 minutes.
- Notes: Expensive. Alternative to streptokinase.

HEPARIN (Full-dose anticoagulation: target PTT > 1.5 x control)
- Bolus: 70–150 U/kg
- Infusion: 15–40 U/kg/hr (usual maintenance, 20 U/kg/hr)
  Check PTT in 6 hours:
  If <1.5 x control: rebolus with 70–150 U/kg and increase infusion rate by 20%.
  If PTT 1.5–3 x control: recheck PTT in 6–12 hours. After consecutive PTTs in therapeutic range, switch to once daily monitoring.
  If PTT > 3 x control but no clinical evidence of bleeding: reduce infusion rate by 20% and recheck PTT in 6 hours.
  If patient has clinical hemorrhage, interrupt heparin and reconsider antithrombotic options.